CANCER CHEMOPREVENTION

CANCER DRUG DISCOVERY AND DEVELOPMENT

BEVERLY A. TEICHER, SERIES EDITOR

CANCER CHEMOPREVENTION

VOLUME 1: PROMISING CANCER CHEMOPREVENTIVE AGENTS

Edited by

GARY J. KELLOFF, MD
ERNEST T. HAWK, MD, MPH

National Institutes of Health
Rockville, MD

CAROLINE C. SIGMAN, PhD

CCS Associates
Mountain View, CA

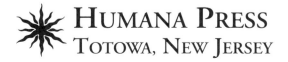

HUMANA PRESS
TOTOWA, NEW JERSEY

© 2004 Humana Press Inc.
999 Riverview Drive, Suite 208
Totowa, New Jersey 07512
www.humanapress.com

Production Editor: Mark J. Breaugh

Cover design by Patricia F. Cleary.

This publication is printed on acid-free paper. ∞
ANSI Z39.48-1984 (American National Standards Institute)
Permanence of Paper for Printed Library Materials

For additional copies, pricing for bulk purchases, and/or information about other Humana titles, contact Humana at the above address or at any of the following numbers: Tel.:973-256-1699; Fax: 973-256-8341; Email: humanapr.com; or visit our Website: http://humanapress.com

Photocopy Authorization Policy:
Authorization to photocopy items for internal or personal use, or the internal or personal use of specific clients, is granted by Humana Press Inc., provided that the base fee of US $25.00 per copy is paid directly to the Copyright Clearance Center at 222 Rosewood Drive, Danvers, MA 01923. For those organizations that have been granted a photocopy license from the CCC, a separate system of payment has been arranged and is acceptable to Humana Press Inc. The fee code for users of the Transactional Reporting Service is: [1-58829-076-X/04 $25.00].

Printed in the United States of America. 10 9 8 7 6 5 4 3 2 1

Library of Congress Cataloging-in-Publication Data

E-ISBN:1-59259-767-X

Cancer chemoprevention / edited by Gary J. Kelloff, Ernest T. Hawk, Caroline C. Sigman.
      p. ; cm. -- (Cancer drug discovery and development)
  Includes bibliographical references and index.
  ISBN 1-58829-076-X (v. 1 : alk. paper)
  1. Cancer--Chemoprevention.
  [DNLM: 1. Anticarcinogenic Agents--therapeutic use. 2. Neoplasms--prevention & control. 3. Chemoprevention--methods. QZ 267 C2144 2004] I. Kelloff, Gary. II. Hawk, Ernest T. III. Sigman, Caroline C. IV. Series.
  RC268.15.C3612 2004
  616.99'4061--dc22
                        2004000342

PREFACE

The past three decades have seen significant advances in cancer treatment and early detection. Particularly noteworthy are decreased mortality from childhood leukemia, and increased screening for breast, colon, and prostate cancer, resulting in the detection of smaller, less advanced lesions with concomitant improved treatment and, in some cases, improved outcomes. Nonetheless, during this same period overall cancer incidence has increased; morbidity associated with surgery, radiation, and chemotherapy is still considerable; and disappointingly, overall cancer survival has remained relatively flat *(1,2)*. However, there has been an enormous gain in our understanding of carcinogenesis and cancer progression, owing in large part to the technology allowing exploration of signal transduction pathways, identification of cancer-associated genes, imaging of tissue architecture, and molecular and cellular function.

This knowledge has focused cancer therapeutics on drugs that take advantage of cellular control mechanisms to selectively eradicate cancer cells. Several of these new drugs are now on the market—notably, the monoclonal antibody trazumutab (Herceptin®) and imatinib mesylate (Gleevec®). Trazumutab blocks ligand binding to human epidermal growth factor receptor-2 (HER2; also called ErbB2, Neu) *(3)*. HER2/Neu has tyrosine kinase (TK) activity that activates signal transduction involved in cell growth and development, and is associated with cancer progression and resistance to chemotherapy. Trazumutab is approved for use in treatment of metastatic breast cancer that overexpresses HER-2/Neu. Imatinib mesylate is an oral small molecule inhibitor that targets the *bcr-abl* TK that results from the Philadelphia (Ph) chromosome, which is found in 95% of chronic myeloid leukemias (CML) *(4)*. The drug is approved for treatment of CML. Imatinib mesylate also inhibits platelet-derived growth factor receptor and c-Kit TKs, and has been approved to treat unresectable or metastatic c-kit-positive gastrointestinal stromal tumors *(5)*.

Most importantly, knowledge of carcinogenesis has provided new and promising opportunities to prevent cancer—that is, to treat precancer or inhibit carcinogenesis (a process often involving 20–30 years in human epithelial cancers) rather than waiting to treat the cancer. Sporn *(6)* coined the term chemoprevention to describe this discipline in oncology: use of drugs, biologics, or nutrients that can be applied at any time in the process before invasive disease to inhibit, delay, or reverse carcinogenesis. Since that time, remarkable progress has been made in developing chemoprevention strategies, started by Sporn's (e.g., *6*) and Wattenberg's (e.g., *7,8*) research on mechanisms of chemopreventive drugs and assays for evaluating these drugs in animal models, and Hong's early clinical studies on prevention of head and neck carcinogenesis *(9,10)*. In the early 1980s, the US National Cancer Institute (NCI), recognizing the promise of chemoprevention, established a chemoprevention drug development program that has grown to incorporate and support mechanistic research on potential chemopreventive agents, in vitro and animal efficacy screening, efficacy modeling of human cancers, development of cancer biomarkers as potential surrogate endpoints, preclinical toxicology and pharmacology, clinical safety and pharmacology, and clinical efficacy studies. In the mid-1990s, NCI and FDA scientists worked together to develop guidance for developing and obtaining marketing approval for chemoprevention drugs *(11)*. The chemopreventive agent development program has been complemented by worldwide research efforts in screening and early diagnosis, epidemiology of cancer prevention, mechanisms of carcinogenesis, and agent discovery. The 1990s saw the first fruits of chemopreventive agent development—FDA approvals for tamoxifen in prevention of breast cancer *(12)* and celecoxib in treatment of colorectal precancers *(13)*.

The general strategy for developing chemopreventive agents, as described in the NCI/FDA guidance *(11, see also 14–18)*, is to first characterize the efficacy of candidate drugs using in vitro transformation modulation, chemoprevention-related mechanistic assays, and animal tumor models of carcinogenesis. As for most other drug indications, the most promising efficacious agents then undergo preclinical toxicity, pharmacokinetics, and pharmacodynamics evaluation. Clinical development is planned and implemented for those agents that meet criteria for acceptable toxicity as well as efficacy. Often, additional efficacy and toxicity testing is done to test alternative routes of agent delivery, dosage regimens, new target tissues, and combinations of agents for increased efficacy and decreased toxicity, and to evaluate toxicities seen in early clinical studies.

Clinical development of chemopreventive agents, as for other pharmaceuticals, is carried out primarily in Phase I, II, and III trials. Phase I clinical trials are safety, pharmacokinetics, and pharmacodynamics studies. These trials include single-dose studies in both fasting and nonfasting normal subjects to characterize single dose pharmacokinetics and acute toxicity. Also, repeated daily-dose studies assess multiple-dose pharmacokinetics and chronic toxicity using multiple-dose levels for a period of 1–3 months in normal subjects or up to 12 months in subjects at increased risk of cancer(s) for which the drug demonstrates efficacy in preclinical evaluation. Participation of normal subjects for more than one month is considered based on available information (toxicity, clinical experience, etc.) for each drug on a case-by-case basis. In most cases, the Phase I studies evaluate drug effects as well as serum (and sometimes agent tissue) levels of the agent. Agent effects believed to be potentially associated with chemopreventive activity are measured. For example, in studies of nonsteroidal antiinflammatories (NSAIDs), serum and tissue levels of prostaglandins (e.g., PGE_2) would be measured. In studies with the irreversible ornithine decarboxylase (ODC) inhibitor eflornithine, tissue levels of polyamines are measured.

Phase II trials are initial efficacy studies. These randomized, double-blind, placebo-controlled trials emphasize the evaluation of phenotyic and genotypic (molecular) biomarkers that are highly correlated to cancer incidence and may serve as surrogate endpoints for cancer incidence reduction. Phase III studies are randomized, blinded, placebo-controlled clinical efficacy trials. These studies are typically large and have the objectives of demonstrating a significant reduction in incidence or delay in occurrence of cancer, validating surrogate endpoints, further assessing drug toxicity, and further characterizing the relationship of dose and/or pharmacokinetics to efficacy and toxicity.

Cancer Chemoprevention Volume 1 is a comprehensive survey of promising cancer chemopreventive agents, grouped by pharmacological and/or mechanistic classes. The agent classes presented vary widely in terms of stage of development as chemopreventives, ranging from such extensively studied groups as NSAIDs and antiestrogens to drugs with recently identified potential based on mechanistic activity (e.g., protein kinase inhibitors, histone deacetylase inhibitors, and anti-angiogenesis agents), as well as agents yet to be evaluated in chemoprevention settings (e.g., proteasome and chaperone protein inhibitors). Attention is devoted to food-derived agents (such as tea, curcumin, soy isoflavones), vitamins, and minerals because of their high promise for prevention in healthy populations. For each agent class, the discussion addresses considerations for chemopreventive drug discovery and development outlined above as they apply to the class in general and to specific agents within the class. Methods for evaluating chemopreventive activity and strategies for chemoprevention in major cancers are described in detail in the second volume of *Cancer Chemoprevention*.

Antimutagens (Chapters 1–4) block the activity of carcinogens by preventing carcinogen activation (e.g., modifiers of cytochrome P450s described in Chapters 2 and 4) and promoting carcinogen detoxification (e.g., phase 2 enzyme enhancers described in Chapters 1 and 3). The interest in developing phase 2 enzyme enhancers, particularly glutathione-S-transferase (GST) inducers, is considerable because they are found in foods (e.g., cruciferous vegetables, garlic), may be effective in restoring effects of genes masked by hypermethylation (e.g., GST genes), and have demonstrated preclinical chemopreventive activity in multiple cancer targets (e.g., oltipraz).

Antiinflammatories and their derivatives (Chapters 5–11), particularly NSAIDs (Chapters 5 and 6), may be the best substantiated chemopreventive agents. A wealth of mechanistic, epidemiologic, animal efficacy, and clinical intervention (e.g., celecoxib, sulindac, and aspirin) data support the chemopreventive potential of antiinflammatories, as well as their activities against other diseases of aging. Toxicity presents some problems for antiinflammatories. Gastrointestinal bleeding and ulceration are associated with chronic NSAID use, caused by this interference with cyclooxygenase (COX) products (the primary mechanism of action of NSAIDs is COX inhibition). As described in Chapters 5 and 6, several strategies have been explored to limit this toxicity, including use of agents specific for inhibition of COX-2, the inducible, inflammation-associated form of COX, thus sparing normal cell function mediated by COX-1. Other strategies include topical instead of systemic delivery of drug as described for corticosteroids in Chapter 9.

Steroid hormones and their nuclear receptors are targets for chemoprevention because they exert tissue-specific proliferative effects on cells by modulating transcription. Although some of these effects are associated with carcinogenesis and other toxicities, many can be beneficial (e.g., bone-protecting effects of estrogens). Two strategies have been explored for chemoprevention in hormone-responsive tissues—reducing levels of hormones (by inhibiting steroid aromatase and 5α-reductase) and selectively blocking hormone receptors (Chapters 12–16). Antiestrogens have shown high promise as chemopreventive agents (e.g., tamoxifen), and mechanistic studies have suggested that tissue and receptor-specific activities can be exploited to develop third and fourth generation selective estrogen receptor modulators (SERMs) that maximize beneficial activities (Chapters 12 and 16). Although current androgen receptor antagonists have side effects that limit their use in treating asymptomatic men, selective androgen receptor antagonists (SARA) may have activities in androgen-sensitive tissues similar to SERM activities in estrogen-sensitive tissues (the theoretical basis for SARA is described in Chapter 14). Other members of the steroid superfamily—vitamin D, retinoids, and dehydroepiandrostenedione (DHEA)—have shown potent chemopreventive activity, but also have some dose-related safety issues. As for the steroid hormones and receptors, much research has been devoted to strategies that avert toxic side effects. For example, Chapters 17 and 19 describe the design of vitamin D and DHEA analogs with reduced toxicity that retain chemopreventive activity. Many side effects of retinoids (e.g., night blindness and dermatitis) result from vitamin A depletion. Chapter 18 describes the design of retinoids that interact selectively with retinoid receptor isoforms associated with carcinogenesis and its inhibition (and may have less effect on vitamin A activities), as well as study designs that lessen toxicity (e.g., retinoid drug holidays and combinations with other chemopreventive agents).

As noted earlier, cellular control mechanisms are of great interest for cancer therapy, and molecules on signal transduction pathways that mediate these mechanisms are potentially good targets for cancer drugs. Because many of these molecular targets are overexpressed, amplified, or mutated in precancers, signal transduction pathways are also of interest as mechanisms for chemoprevention. Chapters 20–28 outline the rationale and potential strategies for chemoprevention at some of these targets: EGFR, ODC, *ras*, *raf*, cyclic GMP phosphodiesterase, Hsp90, and molecules involved in cell cycle control. Because signal transduction pathways are also critical to normal cell function, chemoprevention strategies involving these pathways are designed to minimize effects on normal cells. For example, potential chemopreventive agents inhibit targets expressed or depleted only in rapidly proliferating cells or focus on targets at points on the pathways that allow normal cells to function via alternative routes. A few drugs have shown chemopreventive efficacy at these targets (e.g., EGFR and *ras* inhibitors); however, side effects resulting from their primary mechanisms of action and correlating with their potency raise concerns about safety and tolerability for long-term use in asymptomatic people. For that reason, food-derived agents that demonstrate pleiotropic inhibitory effects on signal transduction are interesting potential chemopreventives because of their expected relatively low toxicity. Soy isoflavones, which are also antiestrogens (Chapter 24) and monoterpenes (Chapter 25), are examples of food-derived agents that have demonstrated chemopreventive efficacy.

Dietary antioxidants (e.g., tea polyphenols, flavonoids) and modulators of fat metabolism (e.g., 4-3 fatty acids, conjugated linoleic acid), vitamins and their analogs (e.g., carotenoids, vitamin C, folic acid), vitamin antioxidants (e.g., lycopene, vitamin E) and minerals (e.g., calcium and selenium) have demonstrated chemopreventive efficacy in animal and, in some cases, clinical and epidemiological cancer settings (Chapters 29–39). However, the development of chemopreventive agents from these sources is complicated. In some cases, identification and use of a key component in the complex dietary mixture (e.g., epigallocatechin gallate in tea) has proven to be a useful sentinel. In most cases, it has only been possible to demonstrate chemopreventive activity of vitamins in deficiency states, making it difficult to evaluate vitamin agents in a clinical setting. These issues are discussed in Chapters 31–37. Activity with tea (Chapter 30) and other dietary polyphenols presents the issues and strategies for identifying chemopreventive activity of complex dietary mixtures.

Recently, interest has increased in evaluating potential chemopreventive agents that may not work directly on precancer cells, but modify the activity of cellular and tissue machinery (Chapters 40–43). Angiogenesis, which requires stimulation of endothelial tissue and is required for growth of neoplastic tissue, has been a target of chemoprevention in particular (Chapter 40). Also, proteasomes can be involved in cell proliferation by promoting activation of transcription factors (e.g., NfB) and their inhibition may have a role in chemoprevention (Chapter 41). Epigenetic modulation of DNA is another new and potentially very productive mechanism for chemoprevention—e.g., by modulation of DNA methylation (Chapter 42) and inhibition of histone deacetylases (Chapter 43). Proof of principle studies have shown chemopreventive efficacy of the DNA methylating agent, azacytidine, and the histone deacetylase inhibitor SAHA in animal studies.

As this volume demonstrates, much progress has been made in discovering and developing of agents that have shown or have promise to become chemopreventive drugs. The pace of this progress is increasing because of advances in many scientific disciplines that contribute to our understanding, not least of which is delineation of genetic progression models that define the carcinogenesis process from precancer to invasive disease in both humans and preclinical models. These models provide the information and opportunity to discover and develop agents targeted to the specific molecular abnormalities that define carcinogenesis. Data derived from diverse disciplines continue to prove that disruption of carcinogenesis is always more successful when the intervention is early in the neoplastic process, that is, when genetic lesions are less numerous and dysregulation of key pathways is minimal. Therefore, the promise that chemopreventive drug intervention can reduce the human cancer burden is very great. Limited success in achieving this goal thus far relates more to the difficulty and need of obtaining data that candidate drugs are safe on chronic administration than questions of relative efficacy. The dose relationship of antioxidants becoming prooxidants depending on tissue microenvironments, of antihormones becoming agonists based on tissue-specific context, and of signal transduction inhibitors disturbing normal cell function while successfully inhibiting carcinogenesis, are but a few examples of this phenomenon. The field of chemoprevention drug discovery and development will move forward by access to and recruitment of numerous scientific disciplines that allow incremental developments documenting efficacy/safety and net therapeutic benefit at each stage. Important components of this process include definition of molecular targets, creation of in vitro and in vivo models to evaluate inhibition of the targets, establishing assays for measuring drug effect biomarkers, establishing therapeutic dose and incremental safety, stratifying human subjects for cancer risk and presence of relevant molecular targets, and developing biomarkers that can serve as surrogates of clinical response and clinical benefit—all so that human trials of short duration and limited size can be conducted to establish clear clinical benefit or provide data compelling enough to justify large trials.

This volume describes the relevant drug classes, drugs, mechanisms of action, and relevant drug effect markers. Volume 2, *Strategies in Chemoprevention*, describes exciting methodologies that will help accelerate progress in this field, and includes a comprehensive review of the state of clinical development of chemoprevention in the various human cancer target organs.

Gary J. Kelloff, MD
Ernest T. Hawk, MD, MPH
Caroline C. Sigman, PhD

REFERENCES

1. Sporn MB. The war on cancer. Lancet 1996;347:1377–1381.
2. Jemal A, Murray T, Samuels A, et al. Cancer Statistics, 2003. CA Cancer J Clin 2003;53:5–26.
3. Yarden Y, Sliwkowski MX. Untangling the ErbB signalling network. Nat Rev Mol Cell Biol 2001;2:127–137.
4. Druker BJ, Talpaz M, Resta D, et al. Efficacy and safety of a specific inhibitor of the Bcr-Abl tyrosine kinase in chronic myeloid leukemia. N Engl J Med 2001;344:1031–1037.
5. DeMatteo RP. The GIST of targeted cancer therapy: a tumor (gastrointestinal stromal tumor), a mutated gene (c-kit), and a molecular inhibitor (STI571). Ann Surg Oncol 2002;9:831–839.
6. Sporn MB. Approaches to prevention of epithelial cancer during the preneoplastic period. Cancer Res 1076;36:2699–2702.
7. Wattenberg LW. Inhibition of chemical carcinogenesis. J Natl Cancer Inst 1978;60:11–18.
8. Wattenberg LW. Chemoprevention of cancer. Cancer Res 1985;45:1–8.
9. Hong WK, Endicott J, Itri LM, et al. 13-cis-Retinoic acid in the treatment of oral leukoplakia. N Engl J Med 1986;315:1501–1505.
10. Hong WK, Lippman SM, Itri LM, et al. Prevention of second primary tumors with isotretinoin in squamous-cell carcinoma of the head and neck. N Engl J Med 1990;323:795–801.
11. Kelloff GJ, Johnson JJ, Crowell JA, et al. Approaches to the development and marketing approval of drugs that prevent cancer. Cancer Epidemiol Biomarkers Prev 1995;4:1–10.
12. Fisher B, Costantino JP, Wickerham DL, et al. Tamoxifen for prevention of breast cancer: report of the National Surgical Adjuvant Breast and Bowel Project P-1 Study. J Natl Cancer Inst 1998;90(18):1371–1388.
13. Steinbach G, Lynch PM, Phillips RK, et al. The effect of celecoxib, a cyclooxygenase-2 inhibitor, in familial adenomatous polyposis. N Engl J Med 2000;342:1946–1952.
14. Kelloff GJ, Boone CW, Steele VE, et al. Progress in cancer chemoprevention: perspectives on agent selection and short-term clinical intervention trials. Cancer Res 1994;54:2015s–2024s.
15. Kelloff GJ, Hawk ET, Crowell JA, et al. (1996) Strategies for identification and clinical evaluation of promising chemopreventive agents. Oncology 1996;10:1471–1484.
16. Kelloff GJ, Hawk ET, Karp JE, et al. Progress in clinical chemoprevention. Semin Oncol 1997;24:241–252.
17. Kelloff GJ, Sigman CC, Johnson KM, et al. Perspectives on surrogate endpoints in the development of drugs that reduce the risk of cancer. Cancer Epidemiol Biomarkers Prev 2000;9:127–134.
18. O'Shaughnessy JA, Kelloff GJ, Gordon GB, et al. Treatment and prevention of intraepithelial neoplasia: an important target for accelerated new agent development: recommendations of the American Association for Cancer Research Task Force on the Treatment and Prevention of Intraepithelial Neoplasia. Clin Cancer Res 2002;8:314–346.

CONTENTS

CONTRIBUTORS

JULIAN ADAMS, PhD • *Millennium Pharmaceuticals, Inc., Cambridge, MA*

VAQAR M. ADHAMI, PhD • *Division of Dermatology, Department of Medicine, University of Wisconsin Medical School, Madison, WI*

FARRUKH AFAQ, PhD • *Division of Dermatology, Department of Medicine, University of Wisconsin Medical School, Madison, WI*

NIHAL AHMAD, PhD • *Division of Dermatology, Department of Medicine, University of Wisconsin Medical School, Madison, WI*

ADRIANA ALBINI, PhD • *Molecular Biology Laboratory, National Cancer Research Institute (IST), Genoa, Italy*

STEVEN D. AVERBUCH, MD • *AstraZeneca Pharmaceuticals, Wilmington, DE*

MARIA BAGNASCO • *Department of Health Sciences, Section of Hygiene and Preventive Medicine, University of Genoa, Italy*

ROUMEN BALANSKY • *Department of Health Sciences, Section of Hygiene and Preventive Medicine, University of Genoa, Italy*

STEPHEN BARNES, PhD • *Departments of Pharmacology and Toxicology, Biochemistry and Molecular Genetics, Comprehensive Cancer Center, University of Alabama at Birmingham; Purdue-UAB Botanicals Center for Age-Related Disease, Birmingham, AL*

JOHN A. BARON, MD, MS, MSC • *Departments of Medicine and Community and Family Medicine, Dartmouth Medical School, Lebanon, NH*

SONJA BERNDT, PharmD • *Department of Epidemiology, Johns Hopkins Bloomberg School of Public Health, Baltimore, MD*

PAUL A. BUNN JR., MD • *University of Colorado Cancer Center, Denver, CO*

BRENDA CARTMEL, PhD • *Department of Epidemiology and Public Health, Yale University School of Medicine, New Haven, CT*

BRUCE C. CASTO, SCD • *Division of Environmental Health Sciences, School of Public Health, The Ohio State University, Columbus, OH*

WILLIAM Y. CHANG, DVM, PhD • *Department of Pharmacology, Ligand Pharmaceuticals Inc., San Diego, CA*

ROBERT S. CHAPKIN, PhD • *Faculty of Nutrition, Texas A&M University, College Station, TX*

MARK S. CHAPMAN, PhD • *Department of Molecular and Cell Biology, Ligand Pharmaceuticals, Inc., San Diego, CA*

EUN JOO CHUNG, PhD • *Medical Oncology Clinical Research Unit, Center for Cancer Research, National Cancer Institute, National Institutes of Health, Bethesda, MD*

ANDREAS I. CONSTANTINOU, PhD • *Department of Surgical Oncology, College of Medicine, University of Illinois, Chicago, IL*

PAMELA L. CROWELL, PhD • *Department of Biology, Indiana University-Purdue University, Indianapolis, Indianapolis, IN*

FRANCESCO D'AGOSTINI • *Department of Health Sciences, Section of Hygiene and Preventive Medicine, University of Genoa, Genoa, Italy*

SILVIO DE FLORA, MD • *Department of Health Sciences, Section of Hygiene and Preventive Medicine, University of Genoa, Genoa, Italy*

KAPIL DHINGRA, MBBS • *Hoffman-La Roche Inc., Nutley, NJ*

JOHN DIGIOVANNI, PhD • *Science Park Research Division, University of Texas MD Anderson Cancer Center, Smithville, TX*

ETHAN DMITROVSKY, MD • *Department of Pharmacology and Toxicology, Department of Medicine, Dartmouth Medical School; Norris Cotton Cancer Center, Lebanon, NH*

MITCHELL DOWSETT, PhD • *Academic Department of Biochemistry, Royal Marsden Hospital, London, UK*

JENNIFER E. DRISKO, DVM, PhD • *Merck Research Laboratories, Rahway, NJ*

RAYMOND N. DuBOIS, MD, PhD • *Departments of Medicine and Cancer Biology, Vanderbilt University Medical Center and Vanderbilt-Ingram Cancer Center, Nashville, TN*

KARAM EL-BAYOUMY, PhD • *Institute for Cancer Prevention, American Health Foundation Cancer Center, Valhalla, NY*

SUSAN M. FISCHER, PhD • *Department of Carcinogenesis, University of Texas MD Anderson Cancer Center, Smithville, TX*

SARAH J. FREEMANTLE, PhD • *Department of Pharmacology and Toxicology, Dartmouth Medical School, Lebanon, NH*

BALZ FREI, PhD • *Linus Pauling Institute, Oregon State University, Corvallis, OR*

JUDY E. GARBER, MD • *Division of Cancer Epidemiology and Control, Dana-Farber Cancer Institute, Boston, MA*

MARK W. GERACI, MD • *University of Colorado Comprehensive Cancer Center, University of Colorado Health Sciences Center, Denver, CO*

EUGENE W. GERNER, PhD • *Arizona Cancer Center, University of Arizona, Tucson, AZ*

GARY B. GORDON, MD, PhD • *Abbott Laboratories, Abbott Park, IL*

MICHAEL N. GOULD, PhD • *McArdle Laboratory for Cancer Research, Department of Oncology, University of Wisconsin-Madison, Madison, WI*

KATHRYN Z. GUYTON, PhD, DABT • *CCS Associates, Mountain View, CA*

YUKIHIKO HARA, PhD • *Tokyo Food Techno Co., Tokyo, Japan*

CURTIS C. HARRIS, MD • *Laboratory of Human Carcinogenesis, National Cancer Institute, National Institutes of Health, Bethesda, MD*

STEPHEN S. HECHT, PhD • *University of Minnesota Cancer Center, Minneapolis, MN*

KATHY J. HELZLSOUER, MD, MHS• *Department of Epidemiology, Johns Hopkins Bloomberg School of Public Health, Baltimore, MD*

JANE HIGDON, PhD • *Linus Pauling Institute, Oregon State University, Corvallis, OR*

KIRK HOFFMAN, PhD • *Cell Pathways, Inc., Horsham, PA*

LORNE J. HOFSETH, PhD • *Laboratory of Human Carcinogenesis, National Cancer Institute, National Institutes of Health, Bethesda, MD*

HAN-YAO HUANG, MPH, PhD • *Department of Epidemiology, Johns Hopkins Bloomberg School of Public Health, Baltimore, MD*

S. PERWEZ HUSSAIN, PhD • *Laboratory of Human Carcinogenesis, National Cancer Institute, National Institutes of Health, Bethesda, MD*

ALBERTO IZZOTTI • *Department of Health Sciences, Section of Hygiene and Preventive Medicine, University of Genoa, Italy*

ROBERT L. KEITH, MD • *Denver VA Medical Center, University of Colorado Health Sciences Center; University of Colorado Comprehensive Cancer Center, Denver, CO*

GARY J. KELLOFF, MD • *Biomedical Imaging Program, Division of Cancer Treatment and Diagnosis, National Cancer Institute, National Institutes of Health, Bethesda, MD*

THOMAS W. KENSLER, PhD, DABT • *Department of Environmental Health Sciences, Johns Hopkins Bloomberg School of Public Health, Baltimore, MD*

FADLO R. KHURI, MD • *Winship Cancer Institute, Emory University School of Medicine, Atlanta, GA*

SUTISAK KITAREEWAN, PhD • *Department of Pharmacology and Toxicology, Dartmouth Medical School, Hanover, NH*

RUSSELL D. KLEIN, PhD • *Department of Carcinogenesis, University of Texas MD Anderson Cancer Center, Smithville, TX*

HEATHER E. KLEINER, PhD • *Department of Carcinogenesis, Science Park Research Division, University of Texas MD Anderson Cancer Center, Smithville, TX*

NANCY E. KOHL, PhD • *Cancer Research Department, Merck Research Laboratories, West Point, PA*

DEBORA L. KRAMER, PhD • *Department of Pharmacology and Therapeutics, Roswell Park Cancer Institute, Buffalo, NY*

DAVID KRITCHEVSKY, PhD • *The Wistar Institute, University of Pennsylvania, Philadelphia, PA*

CORAL A. LAMARTINIERE, PhD • *Department of Pharmacology and Toxicology, Comprehensive Cancer Center, University of Alabama at Birmingham, Birmingham, AL*

JULIA A. LAWRENCE, DO • *Louisiana State University Health Sciences Center, New Orleans, LA*

SUNMIN LEE, MS • *Medical Oncology Clinical Research Unit, Center for Cancer Research, National Cancer Institute, National Institutes of Health, Bethesda, MD*

WILLIAM W. LI, MD • *The Angiogenesis Foundation, Cambridge, MA*

ANDREA LOAIZA-PEREZ, PhD • *Medical Oncology Clinical Research Unit, Center for Cancer Research, National Cancer Institute, National Institutes of Health, Bethesda, MD*

JOANNE R. LUPTON, PhD • *Faculty of Nutrition, Texas A&M University, College Station, TX*

YAN MA, BM • *Department of Pharmacology and Toxicology, Dartmouth Medical School, Lebanon, NH*

SUSAN T. MAYNE, PhD • *Department of Epidemiology and Public Health, Yale University School of Medicine, New Haven, CT*

FRANK MCCORMICK, PhD, FRS • *Comprehensive Cancer Center and Cancer Research Institute, University of California, San Francisco, CA*

YORK E. MILLER, MD • *Denver VA Medical Center; University of Colorado Health Sciences Center; University of Colorado Comprehensive Cancer Center, Denver, CO*

JEFFREY N. MINER, PhD • *Department of Molecular and Cell Biology, Ligand Pharmaceuticals Inc., San Diego, CA*

HASAN MUKHTAR, PhD • *Division of Dermatology, Department of Medicine, University of Wisconsin Medical School, Madison, WI*

PATRICK NANA-SINKAM, MD • *University of Colorado Health Sciences Center, Denver, CO*

ANDRÉS NEGRO-VILAR, MD, PhD • *Department of Molecular and Cell Biology, Ligand Pharmaceuticals, Inc., San Diego, CA*

RAPHAEL A. NEMENOFF, PhD • *University of Colorado Comprehensive Cancer Center, University of Colorado Health Sciences Center, Denver, CO*

HO JUNG OH, PhD • *Medical Oncology Clinical Research Unit, Center for Cancer Research, National Cancer Institute, National Institutes of Health, Bethesda, MD*

RIFAT PAMAKCU, MD, PhD • *Cell Pathways Inc., Horsham, PA*

MICHAEL W. PARIZA, PhD • *Food Research Institute, University of Wisconsin, Madison, WI*

LAURA L. PASHKO, PhD • *Fels Institute for Cancer Research and Molecular Biology, Temple University School of Medicine, Philadelphia, PA*

IAN PITHA-ROWE, BA • *Department of Pharmacology and Toxicology, Dartmouth Medical School, Lebanon, NH*

GARY H. POSNER, PhD • *Department of Chemistry, Johns Hopkins University, Baltimore, MD*

CHINTHALAPALLY V. RAO, PhD • *American Health Foundation, Valhalla, NY*

BANDARU S. REDDY, DVM, PhD • *Institute for Cancer Prevention, American Health Foundation Cancer Center, Valhalla, NY*

MELISSA K. REEDER, PhD • *Cell Pathways Inc., Horsham, PA*

EDWARD A. SAUSVILLE, MD, PhD • *Medical Oncology Clinical Research Unit, Center for Cancer Research, National Cancer Institute, National Institutes of Health, Bethesda, MD*

TOMOHIRO SAWA, PhD • *Laboratory of Human Carcinogenesis, National Cancer Institute, National Institutes of Health, Bethesda, MD*

DAVID S. SCHRUMP, MD • *Thoracic Oncology Section, Surgery Branch, Center for Cancer Research, National Cancer Institute, National Institutes of Health, Bethesda, MD*

ARTHUR G. SCHWARTZ, PhD • *Department of Microbiology, Fels Institute for Cancer Research and Molecular Biology, Temple University School of Medicine, Philadelphia, PA*

ALESSANDRO SGAMBATO, MD, PhD • *Institute of General Pathology, Catholic University, Rome, Italy*

CAROLINE C. SIGMAN, PhD • *CCS Associates, Mountain View, CA*

CAROLYN L. SMITH, PhD • *Molecular & Cellular Biology, Baylor College of Medicine, Houston, TX*

GARY D. STONER, PhD • *Division of Environmental Health Sciences, School of Public Health, The Ohio State University, Columbus, OH*

PAUL TALALAY, MD • *Department of Pharmacology and Molecular Sciences, Johns Hopkins University, Baltimore, MD*

W. JOSEPH THOMPSON, PhD • *Cell Pathways Inc., Horsham, PA*

JANE B. TREPEL, MD • *Medical Oncology Clinical Research Unit, Center for Cancer Research, National Cancer Institute, National Institutes of Health, Bethesda, MD*

RICHARD B. VAN BREEMEN, PhD • *Department of Medicinal Chemistry and Pharmacognosy, College of Pharmacy, University of Illinois, Chicago, IL*

LEE W. WATTENBERG, MD • *Department of Laboratory Medicine and Pathology, University of Minnesota, Minneapolis, MN*

I. BERNARD WEINSTEIN, MD • *Herbert Irving Comprehensive Cancer Center, College of Physicians and Surgeons, Columbia University, New York, NY*

TIMOTHY S. WIEDMANN, PhD • *Department of Pharmaceutics, University of Minnesota, Minneapolis, MN*

WALTER C. WILLETT, MD, DRPH • *Harvard School of Public Health, Brigham and Women's Hospital, Harvard Medical School, Boston, MA*

PAUL WORKMAN, PhD • *Cancer Research UK Centre for Cancer Therapeutics, The Institute of Cancer Research, Belmont, Sutton, Surrey, England*

SIU-LONG YAO, MD • *Merck Research Laboratories, Rahway, NJ*

SHUMIN M. ZHANG, MD, SCD • *Harvard School of Public Health, Brigham and Women's Hospital, Harvard Medical School, Boston, MA*

I ANTIMUTAGENS

1

Inducers of Enzymes That Protect Against Carcinogens and Oxidants

Drug- and Food-Based Approaches with Dithiolethiones and Sulforaphane

Thomas W. Kensler, PhD, DABT and Paul Talalay, MD

CONTENTS

INTRODUCTION
MECHANISMS OF PHASE 2 ENZYME INDUCTION
OLTIPRAZ AND OTHER DITHIOLETHIONES
SULPHORAFANE
REFERENCES

1. INTRODUCTION

The multiple stages of carcinogenesis offer many potential strategies for protection. However, in the majority of tests conducted in animal models, protection has been achieved by administering the chemopreventive agent prior to and/or concurrently with the exposure to the carcinogen. Considering this temporal relationship between the administration of anticarcinogen and carcinogen, it seems likely that these agents act—at least in part—to alter the metabolism and disposition of carcinogens, thereby altering events that are critical to the initial interactions of chemical carcinogens with biomolecules.

Many chemical carcinogens require metabolic activation to reactive intermediates to exert carcinogenic activity. Two types of reactive intermediates are principally responsible for carcinogenic damage to DNA: electrophiles, largely of exogenous origin, and reactive oxygen species (ROS) originating in part from exogenous sources, but arising in substantial quantities as byproducts of normal cellular oxidations. ROS production can be augmented by inflammation and oxidative stress. As highlighted in Fig.1, the conversion of generally innocuous procarcinogens to highly reactive "ultimate" carcinogens can be catalyzed by a number of enzymes, particularly those that comprise the cytochrome P450 superfamily. A second metabolic

step involves the transfer or conjugation of an endogenous, water-soluble substrate to the functional group introduced during phase 1 biotransformation, thereby facilitating elimination of the carcinogen. These phase 2 reactions—which include sulfation, acetylation, glucuronidation, and conjugation with glutathione—typically lead to carcinogen detoxification. Thus, the amount of ultimate carcinogen available for interaction with its target represents, in part, a balance between competing activating and detoxifying reactions. Although this balance is under genetic control, both phase 1 and phase 2 enzymes are inducible by a wide variety of agents: their activities are readily modulated by a variety of factors including nutritional status, age, hormones, phytochemicals, and exposure to drugs or other xenobiotics. In this setting, chemopreventive agents can profoundly modulate the constitutive metabolic balance between activation and inactivation of carcinogens through their actions on both phase 1 and phase 2 enzymes.

It has been known for several decades that antioxidants such as butylated hydroxyanisole, butylated hydroxytoluene (BHT), and ethoxyquin can exert a chemopreventive effect when administered simultaneously with a carcinogen (1). Perhaps the earliest study to indicate a role for the induction of phase 2 enzymes in

From: Cancer Chemoprevention, Volume 1: Promising Cancer Chemoprevention Agents
Edited by: G. J. Kelloff, E. T. Hawk, and C. C. Sigman © Humana Press Inc., Totowa, NJ

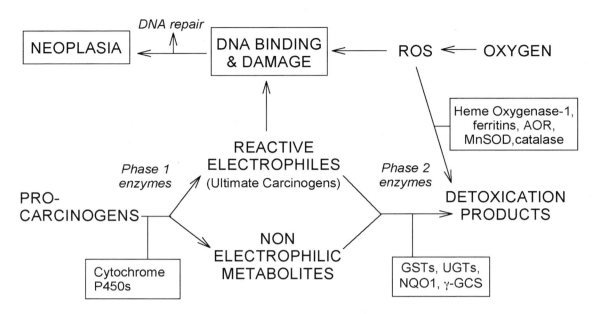

Fig. 1. Role of metabolism in chemical carcinogenesis. Susceptibility to carcinogen damage is partly controlled by the balance between phase 1 activation and phase 2 detoxication. ROS, reactive oxygen species; NQO1, quinone reductase, GSTs, glutathione *S*-transferases; UGTs, UDP-glucuronosyl transferases; γ-GCS, γ-glutamylcysteine synthase; MnSOD, manganese superoxide dismutase; AOR, NAD(P)H:alkenal/one oxidoreductase.

the protective actions of these antioxidants was that of Talalay and colleagues *(2)*. They showed that liver and extra-hepatic cytosols from butylated hydroxyanisole- or ethoxyquin-fed rats or mice exhibited much higher activities of phase 2 enzymes than controls. Moreover, cytosols prepared from the livers of the treated rodents eliminated the mutagenic activity in urine collected from mice treated with benzo*[a]*pyrene (B*[a]*P). More recently, substantial experimental evidence has been gathered to support the view that induction of phase 2 enzymes is a critical mechanism sufficient to engender protection against the toxic and carcinogenic actions of reactive intermediates. As indicated in recent reviews (3–5), the major elements of the supportive findings are:

- Enzyme induction and chemoprotection in animals are produced by the same compounds (of many chemical classes), occur at similar doses, and have similar tissue specificities.
- Natural sensitivity or resistance to carcinogens correlates with expression of phase 2 enzymes (e.g., aflatoxin B_1-induced hepatocarcinogenesis and glutathione *S*-transferases (GST) expression in rats vs mice).
- Overexpression of inducible phase 2 enzymes (e.g., GSTs and aflatoxin aldehyde reductase) by cDNA transfection protects cells against carcinogen-induced DNA damage and/or cytotoxicity.

- Loss of expression of GST-P activity, in vitro and in vivo, leads to enhanced DNA adduct formation and enhanced sensitivity to carcinogenesis, respectively.
- Deficiencies in expression of phase 2 enzymes may be important determinants for susceptibility to cancer in humans (e.g., polymorphisms in GSTs, quinone reductase (NQO1), *N*-acetyltransferases).
- Monitoring of enzyme induction has led to the isolation from natural sources, recognition, and synthesis of novel, potent chemoprotective agents (e.g., sulforaphane, dithiolethiones, dimethyl fumarate, terpenoids).

2. MECHANISMS OF PHASE 2 ENZYME INDUCTION

Initial molecular studies in rats and subsequent studies in humans indicated that increases in mRNA and protein levels of several phase 2 genes in response to a number of chemoprotective agents were mediated through the transcriptional activation of these genes *(6,7)*. Two families of phase 2 enzyme inducers exist, based upon their ability to also elevate phase 1 enzymatic profiles. Prochaska and Talalay *(8)* have coined the terms *bifunctional* and *monofunctional* inducers to describe these families. Bifunctional inducers (e.g., polycyclic hydrocarbons, dioxins, azo dyes, flavones) can all be characterized as large planar polycyclic aromatics, and elevate phase 2 as well as selected phase 1 enzymatic activities such as aryl hydrocarbon hydroxylase. These compounds are potent ligands for the aryl hydrocarbon *(Ah)* receptor, and the direct participation of the *Ah* receptor in the activation of aryl hydrocarbon hydroxylase gene transcription has been demonstrated *(9)*. Moreover, since phase 2 enzyme inducibility by bifunctional inducers segregates in mice that possess functional *Ah* receptors, it is believed that these enzymes are under the direct control of the *Ah* receptor. Monofunctional inducers (phenols, lactones, isothiocyanates, dithiocarbamates, and 1,2-dithiole-3-thiones) elevate phase 2 enzymatic activities without significantly elevating the phase 1 activities described here, and do not possess obvious defining structural characteristics. Several—but not all—phase 2 enzyme inducers have also been shown to inhibit the activities of some cytochrome P450 enzymes, but the contribution of this component to their chemoprotective actions in vivo is unclear *(10)*.

There is no evidence at this time to suggest that monofunctional inducers function through a receptor-mediated pathway. However, Talalay et al. *(11)* have identified a chemical signal present in some monofunctional inducers: the presence or acquisition of an electrophilic center. Isothiocyanates are highly electrophilic. Many monofunctional inducers are Michael reaction acceptors (e.g., olefins or acetylenes conjugated to an electron-withdrawing group such as a carbonyl function), and potency is generally paralleled by their efficiency as Michael reaction acceptors. These generalizations can explain the inducer activity of many types of chemopreventive agents, and have led to the identification of other novel classes of inducers, including acrylates, fumarates, maleates, vinyl ketones, and vinyl sulfones. Other classes of monofunctional inducers—notably peroxides, vicinal dimercaptans, heavy metals, arsenicals, and the 1,2-dithiole-3-thiones—exhibit a common capacity for reaction with sulfhydryls by either oxidoreduction or alkylation *(12)*.

Several regulatory elements that control the expression and inducibility of the Ya subunit of rodent GSTs by bifunctional and monofunctional inducers have been characterized *(13,14)*. A 41-basepair element in the 5'-flanking region of the rat GST Ya gene, termed the Antioxidant Response Element (ARE), has been identified using a series of 5' deletion mutants fused to the chloramphenicol acetyl transferase gene and then transfected into hepatoma cells. To date,

AREs have been detected in the promoters of nearly a score of genes. All share a common RTGACnnnGC motif *(15)*. Prestera et al. *(12)* observed that members of eight distinct chemical classes of monofunctional inducers stimulate expression of a reporter gene, growth hormone, through the ARE when an ARE-growth hormone construct is transfected into murine hepatoma cells. Comparisons of potency for induction of reporter-gene expression and quinone reductase NQO1 activity in the same cells indicated a striking concordance over a 4-log range for the two endpoints. Furthermore, when 25 dithiolethiones and related analogs were evaluated for their activities as inducers of NQO1 and as activators of the transfected ARE construct in this model system, a strong correlation was seen in the potencies of 21 active 1,2-dithiole-3-thiones to elicit the two responses *(16)*. Moreover, no dithiolethiones were inactive in only one system. As a whole, these results suggest that the ARE mediates most—if not all—of the phase 2 enzyme-inducer activity of these compounds.

The transcription factors that bind to the ARE consensus sequence have not been fully identified, and are likely to vary between cell types and species. Nrf1 and Nrf2, members of the basic-leucine zipper NF-E2 family of transcription factors that regulate the expression of globin genes during erythroid development *(17,18)* are known to bind and activate the ARE. Overexpression of either Nrf1 or Nrf2 in human hepatoma cells enhances the basal and inducible transcriptional activity of an ARE reporter gene *(19)*. Because other basic-leucine zipper transcription factors typically form heterodimers, Nrf1/Nrf2 may also dimerize with other factors in order to activate the ARE. The tissue-specific expression profiles of a number of transcription factors suggest that an Nrf2/small Maf heterodimer most closely mirrors the pattern for induction of phase 2 genes in vivo. Using recombinant Nrf2 and mafK proteins in an electromobility shift assay with the promoter sequence of the murine GST Ya gene, Yamamoto and colleagues *(20)* demonstrated binding of the heterodimer complex to this promoter. Oligonucleotides that contained the ARE effectively competed for the binding of this heterodimeric complex to the GST Ya promoter. This group has also directly examined this issue by exploring the effects of disruption of the *nrf2* gene in vivo on induction of phase 2 enzymes. The phenolic antioxidant butylated hydroxyanisole vigorously induced GST and other phase 2 activities and mRNA expression in several tissues of wild-type and heterozygous mutant mice, but not

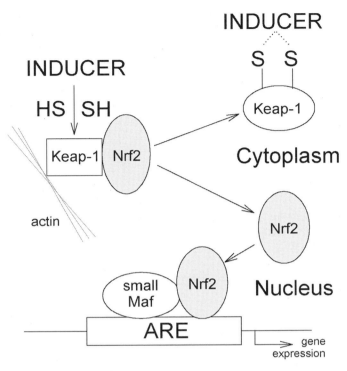

Fig. 2. General scheme for the roles of Keap1 and Nrf2 in the induction of phase 2 enzymes through the Antioxidant Response Element (ARE).

in the homozygous *nrf2*-mutant mice *(20)*. Comparable effects have been observed with 3*H*-1,2-dithiole-3-thione *(21)* and sulforaphane *(22)*. Collectively, these results suggest that Nrf2/small Maf heterodimers may be one of the key regulators of phase 2 gene expression. The relative balance between levels of Nrf2 and small maf proteins may be important determinants for expression or repression of phase 2 genes.

As depicted in Fig.2, under basal conditions Nrf2 is largely bound in the cytoplasm to Keap1, which is anchored to the actin cytoskeleton. When inducers disrupt the Keap1-Nrf2 complex, Nrf2 migrates to the nucleus and enhances gene transcription through binding to the ARE *(23)*. Inducers appear to disrupt the interaction of Keap1 and Nrf2 through specific interactions with cysteine residues in the intervening region (IVR) of Keap1 *(24)*. An understanding of the molecular signaling pathways for enzyme induction and a knowledge of the factors that control the specificity of action of enzyme inducers will be extremely helpful in the design and isolation of more efficient and selective inducers. The importance of the Keap1/Nrf2 system in chemoprevention is highlighted by studies in which mice that were deficient in Nrf2 were shown to be much more susceptible to the hepatic toxicity of

acetaminophen *(25)*, the pulmonary toxicities of butylated hydroxytoluene (BHT) *(26)*, and hyperoxia *(27)*, and to gastric carcinogenesis by B*[a]*P *(28)*. Unlike wild-type controls, these animals are not protected against tumor formation by the phase 2 inducers oltipraz and sulforaphane *(28,29)*.

Since the early studies of Wattenberg, Talalay, and Bueding on the induction of GSTs by phenolic antioxidants, and then dithiolethiones, the list of genes that are coordinately regulated by these chemopreventive agents has been expanding. The classic enzymatic analyses of these investigators has been followed by approaches targeted at measuring changes in gene-transcript levels, initially by subtractive hybridization and differential display *(30)*, and subsequently using microarray techniques *(31,32)* on samples prepared from tissues of rodents treated with enzyme inducers. Collectively, these analyses have led to the recognition that the actions of "phase 2 inducers" far exceed the original formulation of the concept of two phases of xenobiotic metabolism *(33)* that defined phase 2 enzymes. Phase 2 enzymes also play major roles in protecting against oxidative stresses *(34–36)*. Thus, the genes that are coordinately regulated by Nrf2 exert actions against electrophiles and oxidants.

Phase 2 enzymes exert highly versatile and important protective functions through a variety of mechanisms, including: direct inactivation of toxic electrophiles by conjugation with endogenous ligands such as glutathione (GSH) by GSTs and glucuronides by uridine 5' diphosphate (UDP)-glucuronosyltransferases; disarming of reactive centers of molecules, such as the reduction of electrophilic quinines to hydroquinones by NQO1, and hydrolysis of epoxides to diols by epoxide hydrolase; reduction of toxic alkyl hydroperoxides and DNA base hydroperoxides by the peroxidase activities of GSTs; reductions by GSTs of hydroxyalkenals, which are free radical-initiated lipid peroxidation products and excellent GST substrates; salvage by GSTs of adenine and thymine propenals that are produced by radiation and hydroxyl radicals; efficient GST-catalyzed conjugations of the o-quinone metabolites of catecholamines with GSH, thereby suppressing the generation of ROS by redox cycling of these quinones; elevation of cellular GSH, the principal cellular antioxidant, by upregulation of γ-glutamylcysteine synthetase; antioxidant function of NQO1 that prevents the redox cycling of quinones and the depletion of cellular GSH, maintains other cellular antioxidants (ubiquinone and α-tocopherylquinone) in their active and reduced forms, thereby protecting membranes against oxidative damage; generation of the powerful antioxidant bilirubin by heme oxygenase-1; and finally, elevation of ferritin levels, thereby scavenging intracellular iron that may otherwise contribute to oxidative stress. In light of the profound importance of ROS in the genesis of malignancy (37), it is noteworthy that these antioxidative activities of phase 2 enzymes are "indirect" because the enzymes are not consumed in exerting their antioxidant functions (unlike direct antioxidants such as vitamin C), and that these enzymes have far longer half-lives and presumably more prolonged actions than direct antioxidants (38). The protracted pharmacodynamic action of these inducers is a very appealing component of their mode of action (39).

3. OLTIPRAZ AND OTHER DITHIOLETHIONES

1,2-dithiole-3-thiones (Fig. 3) are five-membered cyclic sulfur-containing compounds used commercially as antioxidants in rubber, greases, and oils. Two substituted 1,2-dithiole-3-thiones with chemotherapeutic, radioprotective, and chemoprotective properties are

used medicinally. The drug oltipraz (5-methyl-4-[2-pyrazinyl]-1,2-dithiole-3-thione) has shown significant antischistosomal activity in experimental animals and humans. Cure rates of up to 90% have been achieved with single doses of oltipraz in field trials. The other 1,2-dithiole-3-thione in clinical use is anethole dithiolethione (5-[p-methoxyphenyl]-1,2-dithiole-3-thione, ADT), an approved drug used in Canada, Europe, and other countries to counteract dry mouth caused by psychotropic drugs and radiation. It is also marketed as a choleretic and hepatoprotective agent.

During the course of studies on the mechanism of antischistosomal activity of oltipraz, Bueding et al. (40) initially noted that administration of the drug to mice infected with *Schistosoma mansoni* caused a reduction in the GSH stores of the worms. Subsequent investigations have suggested that inactivation of GSH reductase with its subsequent effects on GSH pools in the parasite was an important component of the antischistosomal activity of oltipraz (41). Inhibition of schistosome oxidant defense systems in turn renders the parasites susceptible to killing by the ROS produced during the inflammatory response of the host (42). In contrast to the effects on the worms, Ansher et al. (43) observed that the administration of oltipraz, ADT, and several other substituted 1,2-dithiole-3-thiones to mice resulted in substantial increases in the levels of GSH in the liver, lung, kidney, forestomach, and upper jejunal mucosa. In addition to raising GSH levels, these dithiolethiones were found to enhance the activities of phase 2 enzymes. Similar, although less potent, effects were previously noted with the antioxidants butylated hydroxyanisole and ethoxyquin, compounds also known to be anticarcinogens. Collectively, these findings led Budeing to predict that oltipraz, ADT, and related 1,2-dithiole-3-thiones may be excellent candidate compounds for cancer chemoprevention studies. Remarkably, 1,2-dithiole-3-thiones represent the first of a very limited set of classes of compounds for which anticarcinogenic activity in vivo was solely predicted from biochemical measurements.

3.1. Efficacy in Animal Models

The initial confirmation that 1,2-dithiole-3-thiones may exert chemoprotective effects in vivo came from the demonstration by Ansher et al. (44) that oltipraz and ADT each protected against the hepatotoxicity of carbon tetrachloride and acetaminophen in mice. Subsequent studies have demonstrated protection by oltipraz against the acute hepatotoxicities of allyl

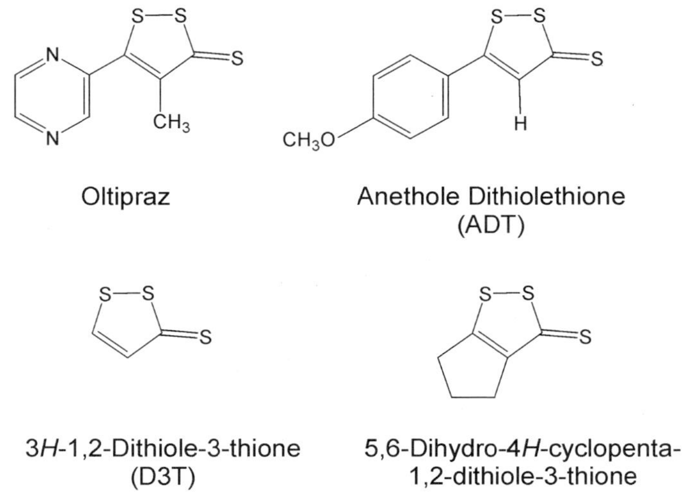

Fig. 3. Structures of oltipraz (4-methyl-5-[2-pyrazinyl-1,2-dithiole-3-thione, anethole] dithiolethione [5-(*p*-methoxyphenyl]-1,2-dithiole-3-thione), 3*H*-1,2-dithiole-3-thione and 5,6-dihydro-4*H*-cyclopenta-1,2-dithiole-3-thione; especially promising members of the dithiolethione class of enzyme-inducing chemopreventive agents.

alcohol and acetaminophen in the hamster *(45)* and aflatoxin B$_1$ (AFB$_1$) in the rat *(46)*. Toxin-induced elevations in liver-function tests were blunted in all cases. Substantial reductions in aflatoxin-induced fibrosis have been observed with oltipraz *(47)*. Pretreatment with oltipraz also substantially reduced the mortality produced by either single or chronic exposure to AFB$_1$ *(46)*. Kim and colleagues recently demonstrated that oltipraz inhibits dimethlynitrosamine-induced liver fibrosis in the rat liver, apparently through suppression of expression of transforming growth factor(TGF)-β1 and tumor necrosis factor(TNF)-α *(48)*. A more dramatic observation by this group is that oltipraz reverses cirrhosis in dimethylnitrosamine-treated rats *(49)*. Hepatic fibrosis and cirrhosis are well-known consequences of severe hepatic injury, and are related to hepatocarcinogenesis *(50)*.

To directly test the cancer chemoprotective activity of oltipraz, Wattenberg and Bueding examined the capacity of oltipraz to inhibit carcinogen-induced neoplasia in mice *(51)*. Oltipraz was administered either 24 or 48 h before treatment with each of three chemically diverse carcinogens: diethylnitrosamine, uracil mustard, and B*[a]*P. This sequence of oltipraz and carcinogen administration was repeated once a week for 4–5 wk. Oltipraz reduced the number of both pulmonary adenomas and tumors of the forestomach induced by B*[a]*P by nearly 70%. Pulmonary adenoma formation induced by uracil mustard or diethylnitrosamine was also significantly reduced by oltipraz

pretreatment, but to a lesser extent. Oltipraz has now shown chemopreventive activity against different classes of carcinogens that target the small intestine *(52)*, colon *(53)*, pancreas *(54)*, urinary bladder *(55)*, blood cells *(56)*, trachea *(57)*, liver *(58)*, mammary gland *(59)*, and skin *(60)*. The most dramatic actions of oltipraz occur in the colon and liver, where dietary administration results in significant reductions in both tumor incidence and multiplicity. Pharmacokinetic studies in rodents indicate that these two organs are among those with the highest tissue concentrations following oral administration of the drug *(61)*. Complete protection against AFB$_1$-induced hepatocarcinogenesis is achieved when oltipraz is fed before and during administration; however, such an exposure-intervention paradigm is not directly relevant to most human populations. Bolton et al. *(47)* observed that a delayed and transient intervention with oltipraz relative to the period of aflatoxin administration offers significant protection against the formation of presumptive preneoplastic lesions in the liver. These results are consistent with observations that oltipraz protects against the genotoxic and cytotoxic actions of AFB$_1$. However, administration of oltipraz solely after exposure to AFB$_1$ has no protective effect *(62)*. By contrast, Reddy et al. *(53)* observed that the protective effects of oltipraz against azoxymethane-induced colon carcinogenesis in rats was nearly equi-effective, regardless of whether oltipraz was administered during or after carcinogen administration.

ADT has undergone more limited evaluation as a cancer chemopreventive agent. Although it is equipotent with oltipraz in the induction of phase 2 enzymes in murine liver cells in culture (16), it is less effective than oltipraz at inhibiting hepatic preneoplastic lesion formation in aflatoxin-treated rats (63). ADT inhibits the formation of azoxymethane-induced colon tumors (64). ADT also affects mammary carcinogenesis (65). 7,12-dimethylbenz[a]anthracene (DMBA)-treated female rats fed 200 ppm ADT had a 40% lower multiplicity of mammary tumors. Tumor latency was also significantly increased; however, no effect on final tumor incidence was observed.

3.2. Clinical Trials

3.2.1. PHARMACOKINETICS AND SAFETY

During the course of evaluation of oltipraz for anti-schistosomal activities, nearly a score of clinical trials were conducted. In these trials, 1.0–4.5 g of oltipraz was administered during a period of 1–3 d and greater than 90% cure rates were reported (reviewed in 66). The most frequent side effects among the 1284 patients exposed to oltipraz were related to the digestive system—namely, nausea, abdominal pain/distress, vomiting, and diarrhea. Headaches, dizziness, and paresthesia and fingertip pain were also frequently reported (67). The later two effects appeared to increase after exposure to sunlight. Most of these effects were reported to be mild, subsided within 1–2 days, and did not require discontinuation of the drug. No significant changes were noted in blood chemistry and hematology. Because of concerns about photosensitivity, oltipraz is no longer used to treat schistosomiasis.

Unlike trials for the chemotherapy of schistosomiasis, chemoprevention trials require evaluation of lower but sustained dosing. Several Phase I chemoprevention clinical trials have been conducted to characterize the pharmacokinetics and side effects of oltipraz in this setting. As reviewed by Benson (68), a 6-mo Phase I trial was completed in which participants were given oral daily doses of oltipraz at 125 or 250 mg. The maximum tolerated dose of oltipraz was determined to be 125 mg daily. Grade I/II toxicities of photosensitivity/heat intolerance, as well as gastrointestinal disturbances and neurotoxicities, were reported. Peak plasma concentrations exhibited wide variability. In another Phase I study, a single oral dose of oltipraz was given to normal volunteers at dose levels of 125, 250, 375, and 500 mg. There was no significant difference

in half-life between the four dose levels (6–9 h). Peak plasma levels of ≥1.0 µg/mL were achievable, with marked inter-individual variability. A series of small trials evaluating single oral doses of oltipraz for up to 28 d (dosing range 1–3 mg/kg) also showed short half-lives, a sustained steady state without variation after a loading dose, and increased serum and urine concentrations of oltipraz or metabolites with consumption of a high-fat diet (69).

A more recent study (70) evaluated single doses varying from 125–1000 mg/m². Concentration-time profiles were highly variable among individuals, and the occurrence of secondary concentration peaks suggested substantial enterohepatic cycling. Absorption was rapid, with an observed t_{max} of 2 h. Maximum plasma concentration values were proportional to the dose. The elimination half-lives of oltipraz ranged from a mean of 9–22 h, and the latter value was obtained at the lowest dose level. The half-life values at the three higher dose levels were similar, and are in agreement with those obtained during the high-dose schistosomiasis studies.

A small trial examined the combination of oltipraz with N-acetyl-l-cysteine (NAC) in healthy volunteer smokers who received daily NAC (1200 mg/d) and were randomized to weekly placebo, 200 mg oltipraz, or 400 mg oltipraz (71). The combination was selected on the basis of non-overlapping toxicities for the two drugs and an untested expectation that the combination would exert augmented biochemical action on enzyme induction. The study was closed early because of toxicities. Both NAC alone (placebo group) and the combination with the high dose of oltipraz contributed to the high incidence of side effects.

Several Phase II clinical trials of oltipraz have evaluated the side effects of oltipraz with the benefit of blinding through the use of a placebo arm. In a randomized, double-blind placebo-controlled trial conducted in Qidong, China and described here (72), participants received either placebo daily, 125 mg oltipraz daily, or 500 mg oltipraz weekly for 2 mo. Overall, 11.3% of the placebo group reported an adverse event; this proportion was significantly lower than the clinical events occurring among the 125-mg arm (29.0%) or the 500-mg arm (25.6%). The majority of adverse events (AEs) occurred within the first week of treatment. Numbness, tingling, and occasional pain in the extremities were the most frequently reported symptoms, and were the only AEs significantly more reported in the oltipraz arms compared to the placebo arm. In a follow-up Phase IIb chemoprevention trial conducted in the same region of China, participants were administered either placebo (250 mg), or 500 mg oltipraz once a week for 48 wk. One month into the intervention, following a dramatic seasonal shift in weather patterns, symptoms of numbness and tingling in the extremities, as well as a propensity to develop sunburn, were reported in nearly 10% of the participants who received active drug. A halving of the dose and distribution of sunscreen to participants eliminated the further manifestation of these symptoms over the duration of the study. All symptoms resolved within 1 wk.

3.2.2. PHARMACODYNAMICS

Several studies have demonstrated that oltipraz can modulate the expression and activities of both phase 1 and 2 enzymes in humans. Many enzyme inducers, including oltipraz, also inhibit certain isoforms of phase 1 enzymes—notably, cytochrome P450s. Kinetic studies with heterologously expressed human P450s 1A2 and 3A4 indicate competitive inhibition with apparent K_is of pharmacologically achievable, low-micromolar concentrations (73). Consistent with this in vitro finding, Sofowora et al. (74) reported that a single 125-mg dose of oltipraz reduced CYP1A2 activity by 75% in healthy individuals phenotyped by monitoring drug effect on caffeine metabolism.

Oltipraz induces the expression of several isoforms of GSTs in primary cultures of human hepatocytes (73,75). Gupta et al. (76) reported a doubling in the specific activity of GST in peripheral lymphocytes obtained from Phase I study participants 10 h after administration of 125 mg oltipraz. Elevations in levels of GSH were also observed. In a dose-finding study with 125, 250, 500, or 1000 mg/m^2 oltipraz as a single oral dose, increases in GST activities were seen in peripheral mononuclear cells and colon mucosa biopsies at the lower, but not higher, doses (77). Four- to fivefold increases in mRNA transcripts for γ-glutamylcysteine synthetase and NQO1 were seen in colon mucosa at 250 mg/m^2. Higher doses were not more effective. mRNA content increased after dosing to reach a peak on d 2 and declined to baseline levels during the subsequent week. In another study by Benson and colleagues (78), a persistent elevation of lymphocyte GSH content was noted over a 6-mo dosing period with 100 mg oltipraz daily (but not with either 20 or 50 mg q.d.); however, no inductive effect was seen at any dose on lymphocyte GST activities. Collectively, these results demonstrate that oltipraz triggers the expression of

phase 2 enzymes in humans, although relationships between dose, duration, magnitude of induction, and gene sets have not been well-characterized.

To more directly test the hypothesis that oltipraz can modulate the metabolism of carcinogens in humans, a Phase IIa intervention trial with oltipraz was conducted. Study participants were recruited from residents of Daxin Township, Qidong, China, where dietary exposures to aflatoxins and the risk for hepatocellular carcinoma are high. This trial with oltipraz was a randomized, placebo-controlled, double-blind study,in which 240 adults in general good health with no history of major chronic illnesses and with detectable serum aflatoxin-albumin adduct levels at baseline were randomized into one of three intervention arms: placebo; 125 mg oltipraz administered daily; or 500 mg oltipraz administered weekly. The methods, participant characteristics, compliance, and adverse events, as well as initial results on modulation of biomarkers from this trial, have been reported (72,79,80).

Urine samples were collected at 2-wk intervals throughout the active 8-wk intervention period as well as during the 8-wk follow-up period. Aflatoxin metabolites were assayed in urine samples from one cross-section in time, and after the first month on the active intervention (71). Sequential immunoaffinity and liquid chromatography coupled to mass spectrometry and fluorescence detection was used to identify and quantify the phase 1 metabolite, aflatoxin M_1 and the phase 2 metabolite, aflatoxin-mercapturic acid, in these urine samples. One month of weekly administration of 500 mg oltipraz led to a significant decrease (51%) in median levels of M_1 excreted in urine compared to placebo, but had no effects on levels of aflatoxin-mercapturic acid. By contrast, daily intervention with 125 mg of oltipraz led to a significant, 2.6-fold increase in the median levels of aflatoxin-mercapturic acid excretion, but had only a modest effect on excreted M_1 levels. Thus, sustained low-dose oltipraz increased phase 2 conjugation of aflatoxin, yielding higher levels of mercapturic acid, but did not appreciably affect formation of aflatoxin M_1. Intermittent high-dose oltipraz inhibited the phase 1 activation of aflatoxin, as reflected by lowered excretion of aflatoxin M_1. Potential effects of induction of phase 2 enzymes (e.g., GSTs) in this arm appears to be masked by the inhibition of aflatoxin-8,9-epoxide formation. Indeed, Langouët et al. (81) have reported two- to fourfold increases in the protein levels of alpha and mu classes of GSTs in primary human hepatocytes treated with 50 μM oltipraz, but found that this inductive effect was not associated with an increased formation of aflatoxin-GSH conjugates because it was overcome by the inhibitory effect of oltipraz on aflatoxin B_1 activation. Studies with experimental models indicate that both mechanisms are likely to contribute to reduced genotoxicity and other chemopreventive actions of this drug (82).

In addition to the cross-sectional measurements of effects of oltipraz on urinary aflatoxin metabolites, longitudinal analyses of the effects of slopes of aflatoxin-in-albumin adducts have been conducted (79). Aflatoxin albumin adducts are formed via the epoxide pathway in a reaction of aflatoxin-diol with lysine residues in albumin. These adducts are useful biomarkers because they share a common activation pathway with the DNA adducts, but, also reflect cumulative exposures because of the relatively long (~21 d) half-life of circulating albumin. There were no consistent changes in albumin-adduct levels in the placebo arm, or in the 125-mg oltipraz daily arm during the 16-wk observation period. However, individuals who received 500 mg oltipraz once a wk for 8 wk showed a triphasic response to oltipraz. No effect was observed during the first month of the intervention, whereas a significant diminution in adduct levels was observed during the second month of active intervention and during the first month of follow-up. A partial rebound in adduct levels toward baseline values was observed during the second month of follow-up. Linear regression models up to wk 13 confirmed a significant weekly decline in biomarker levels in this group. Because modulation of aflatoxin-albumin adducts and diminution of aflatoxin M_1 levels were both observed in the 500-mg weekly arm, comparisons of the albumin adduct slopes with levels of aflatoxin M_1 were made. Individuals ranked in the lowest tertile of aflatoxin M_1 levels showed the greatest decline in aflatoxin-albumin adduct levels. This moderate correlation suggests that inhibition of cytochrome P450 activity could contribute to the observed decline in albumin adducts.

The only chemoprevention trial with ADT was a very recent Phase IIb study examining the protective effects of ADT in smokers with bronchial dysplasia (83). One hundred twelve current and former smokers with a smoking history of at least 30 pack-yr and at least one site of bronchial dysplasia identified by an autofluorescence bronchoscopy-directed biopsy were randomly assigned to receive placebo or ADT at 25 mg 3× daily for 6 mo. Changes in histopathologic grade and nuclear morphometry index were used as primary

and secondary end point biomarkers, respectively. One hundred one participants had a follow-up bronchoscopy-directed biopsy. In a lesion-specific analysis, the progression rate of preexisting dysplastic lesions by two or more grades and/or appearance of new lesions was significantly lower in the ADT group (8%) than in the placebo group (17%). In a person-specific analysis, the disease progression rate was significantly lower in the ADT group (32%) than in the placebo group (59%). Bronchial dysplasia is a useful surrogate intermediate end point to evaluate the efficacy of chemopreventive agents because the morphological criteria for these pre-invasive lesions are defined, and grading appears to be consistent among pulmonary pathologists. Thus, this study suggests that ADT is a promising chemopreventive agent for lung cancer. Notably, although nearly half the participants on the active arm of the trial underwent dose reduction because of abdominal bloating or flatulence, no severe toxicities were noted. Nonetheless, a more sustainable dosing regimen that preserves efficacy must be defined. In addition, both ADT and oltipraz exert effects on gene expression that are independent of the Nrf2 pathway (49,84,85), and which may therefore be independent of phase 2 induction. It has not been determined whether enzyme induction contributed to the protective actions observed against bronchial dysplasia in these smokers.

3.3. Prospects for 1,2-Dithiole-3-Thiones

The larger question of whether modulation of carcinogen metabolism—by enzyme inhibition, enzyme induction, or other mechanisms—can substantively reduce the risk of cancer in individuals at high risk for exposure to environmental carcinogens remains open. A Phase IIb intervention trial with oltipraz in Qidong was conducted recently to evaluate the efficacy of 250 mg or 500 mg oltipraz given weekly to modulate levels of aflatoxin biomarkers over a 1-yr period in comparison to a placebo group. Biomarkers exploring the multiple mechanisms of action of oltipraz are currently being measured. The Phase IIb study could serve as a foundation for selecting a safe and effective dose for subsequent studies. However, issues of availability and the cost of oltipraz coupled with the consistent manifestation of annoying but not life-threatening side effects suggest that oltipraz may have a very limited future in clinical chemoprevention. Oltipraz has been a drug of expedience for establishing a "proof of principle" regarding the utility of enzyme inducers in cancer chemoprevention. Although oltipraz may have the broadest range of chemopreventive efficacy of any agent tested to date in animal models, it is not a particularly potent enzyme inducer, even among the dithiolethione class of molecules. Its development as a clinical chemopreventive agent, although dependent upon its efficacy in animal studies, is a direct result of the pre-existing clinical investment and development during its phase as a chemotherapeutic drug for schistosomiasis. Chemopreventive 1,2-dithiole-3-thiones that are at least one order of magnitude more potent than oltipraz in vivo have been developed subsequently *(16,86)*. Many of these compounds are considerably less expensive in their synthesis and purification than oltipraz. Although efficacy for several lead compounds has been established, the rate-limiting step in their development is safety evaluation. Two of these lead compounds—the unsubstituted parent molecule, 1,2-dithiole-3-thione, and 5,6-dihydro-4H-cyclopenta-1,2-dithiole-3-thione—are currently undergoing further preclinical development under the auspices of the National Cancer Institute. Although no formal understanding of the structural or molecular basis for the toxicity of oltipraz has been developed, it can be hoped that a chemical dissociation of the protective and toxic actions may arise in some of these analog molecules, much as dissociations between the antischistosomal and chemopreventive properties have been reported *(40)*. ADT also provides a useful perspective because it is equipotent to oltipraz as an enzyme inducer in vitro, and a less potent inhibitor of hepatic tumorigenesis in vivo, but is devoid of major side effects at its recommended dosing levels (25 mg, 3× daily). Thus, the ideal inducer molecules will not rely on potency alone, but rather a desirable prophylactic index that maximally separates efficacy and toxicity. Because enzyme inducers are likely to be primarily targeted at individuals in the general population with low to moderate risk of cancer, the importance of tolerability (safety) cannot be underestimated.

Agents that are structurally unrelated to dithiolethiones with 100 or more-fold greater potency as phase 2 inducers have been identified with cell-culture screening assays (87–89). Although some, such as arsenicals and mercurials, are *de facto* unsuitable for human use, some of these potent inducers are found in foods, making them potentially more accessible and acceptable for the general population. Natural products are not intrinsically safer than synthetic agents, although patterns of long-term ingestion of certain food types provide guidelines for identifying promising compounds or foods themselves *(90)*. The following section describes the identification and development of one phytochemical, sulforaphane, as a promising inducer agent that now has established anticarcinogenic efficacy in animals and is undergoing clinical evaluation.

4. SULFORAPHANE

4.1. History

Numerous epidemiological studies from many regions of the world report strikingly lower cancer risks among individuals who consume large quantities of fruit and vegetables (reviewed in refs. *91–94*). Individuals who eat high levels of yellow and green vegetables, particularly those of the family Cruciferae (mustards) and the genus *Brassica* (cauliflower, Brussels sprouts, broccoli, and cabbage), reduce their susceptibility to cancer at a variety of organ sites *(95,96)*. The mechanisms responsible for these protective effects are multiple, probably involve complex interactions, and are not fully understood *(97)*. However, it is striking that a number of epidemiological studies strongly suggest that the specific consumption of crucifers (in comparison to total fruit and vegetable intake) is especially effective in reducing cancer risk *(96)*. Thus, the risks of prostate cancer *(97–99)*, breast cancer *(100)*, and non-Hodgkin's lymphoma in women *(101)* are all lower in high crucifer consumers. Interestingly, no relationship was observed between bladder cancer risk and high fruit and vegetable intake, but the multivariate risk reduction ratio for cruciferous vegetables alone was highly significant *(102)*. The phytochemistry of crucifers is unusual because they contain high concentrations of glucosinolates that are hydrolyzed enzymatically by plant myrosinase and by mammalian gastrointestinal flora to isothiocyanates *(103)*. Since many isothiocyanates are potent inducers of phase 2 genes and also block chemical carcinogenesis *(104–106)*, induction of enzymes that detoxify electrophiles and ROS are very likely to be of importance in the protective action of vegetables against cancer. Several clinical trials have also supported this notion: Boogards et al. *(107)* found that consumption of Brussels sprouts raises the levels of α-class GSTs in human serum, similar to its effects on α- and π-class GST in rectal mucosa *(108)*. Surrogate biomarkers for phase 2 enzymes have been used with varying success to detect inducer activity in humans given a lyophilized broccoli preparation *(109)*. Finally, a number of studies have demonstrated that the "whole body" metabolism of test compounds was accelerated by the ingestion of vegetables and other foods (110–112).

A simple system to rapidly detect and measure potencies of phase 2 enzyme inducers, based on the direct assay of the specific activity of NQO1 in murine hepatoma cells grown in microtiter-plate wells, was developed in our laboratory *(113–115)*. A survey of extracts of a variety of commonly consumed, organically and conventionally grown vegetables for NQO1-inducer potency identified crucifers (and particularly those of the genus *Brassica*) as singularly rich sources *(114)*. The assay system also measures toxicity, which was unrelated to inducer potency among the vegetable extracts examined. By monitoring NQO_1 induction in a subsequent study *(116)*, Zhang and colleagues *(103)* isolated and identified (−)-1–isothio-cyanato-(4*R*)-(methylsulfinyl)butane [CH_3–SO–(CH_2)$_4$–NCS] (sulforaphane) as the major and very potent phase 2 enzyme inducer in mature, market-stage broccoli *(Brassica oleracea italica cv. Saga)*. Sulforaphane is a monofunctional inducer of phase 2 genes *(8)* that is active at submicromolar concentrations in cells in culture. Sulforaphane is the most potent naturally occurring monofunctional inducer thus far characterized.

4.2. Efficacy in Animal Models

The anticarcinogenic properties of isothiocyanates were recognized more than 30 years ago, and have attracted considerable attention in several laboratories (reviewed in refs. *104–106*). A variety of isothiocyanates inhibit the formation of tumors elicited by many different types of carcinogens at several target organ sites. However, the anticarcinogenicity of sulforaphane has not been widely evaluated. Following the isolation of sulforaphane from broccoli, Zhang et al. *(117)* observed that administration of 75 or 150 µmol of sulforaphane per d for 5 d around the time of exposure to the carcinogen DMBA significantly reduced the incidence and multiplicity of mammary tumors in rats. Comparable efficacy was observed with a synthetic norbornane analog (*exo*-2-acetyl-*exo*-6-isothio-cyanatonorbornane) originally designed as a potent enzyme inducer. Two other analogs, *endo*-2-acetyl-*exo*-6-isothiocyanatonorbornane and *exo*-2-acetyl-*exo*-5-isothiocyanatonorbornane, were less effective anticarcinogens. Sulforaphane and another synthetic analog (sulforamate: ±4-methylsulfinyl-1-(*S*-methyldithiocarbamyl)-butane) were potent inhibitors of preneoplastic lesion formation in mouse mammary glands treated

with a polycyclic aromatic hydrocarbon (PAH) in organ culture (84% and 78% inhibition at 1 µM, respectively) *(118)*. Sulforaphane also inhibits B*[a]*P- and 1,6-dinitropyrene-DNA adduct formation in human mammary epithelial cells *(119)*. Chung et al. *(120)* have reported that sulforaphane significantly blocked the formation of aberrant crypt foci (ACF) in the colons of rats treated with azoxymethane, regardless of whether sulforaphane was administered concurrently with or after the carcinogen. Sulforaphane also inhibits B*[a]*P-induced gastric tumorigenesis. However, this protective effect is lost in *nrf2*-deficient mice in which phase 2 enzymes are low and not inducible, highlighting the importance of phase 2 induction in the protective actions of sulforaphane *(29)*.

4.3. Actions of Sulforaphane in Cell Culture

Studies of the inducer properties of a series of isothiocyanates have revealed that the isothiocyanates that induced phase 2 enzymes accumulated to remarkably high concentrations (e.g., 100-fold in 30 min at 37°C) compared to extracellular concentrations in cells in culture; those that did not accumulate were not inducers. Millimolar intracellular concentrations of sulforaphane can be obtained, so that the potency of sulforaphane as an inducer may directly relate to its ability to accumulate in cells *(121)*. Several key characteristics of the accumulation process have been established (121–123): initial accumulation rates are linearly related to time and concentration, and cannot be saturated; peak levels and time-course of intracellular accumulation are dependent on the structure of the isothiocyanate; areas under the accumulation-time curves correlate closely with inducer potencies of isothiocyanates; isothiocyanates accumulate principally as GSH conjugates (dithiocarbamates), and GSH levels are depleted by the accumulations; accumulation of isothiocyanates can be controlled by regulating intracellular GSH levels; and the accumulation process occurs in a wide variety of cell types. Sulforaphane is also rapidly exported from cells as a GSH conjugate through membrane pumps *(124)*. Thus, cellular exposure to sulforaphane in vivo may be very pulsatile, a kinetic feature that is nonetheless sufficient to trigger phase 2 enzyme induction. Moreover, the thio-conjugates of sulforaphane and other isothiocyanates may contribute to their pharmacodynamic action *(125,126)*. Both sulforaphane and its mercapturic acid (NAC conjugate) mediated growth arrest and apoptosis in human prostate cancer cells *(126)*. Expression of cyclin D1 and

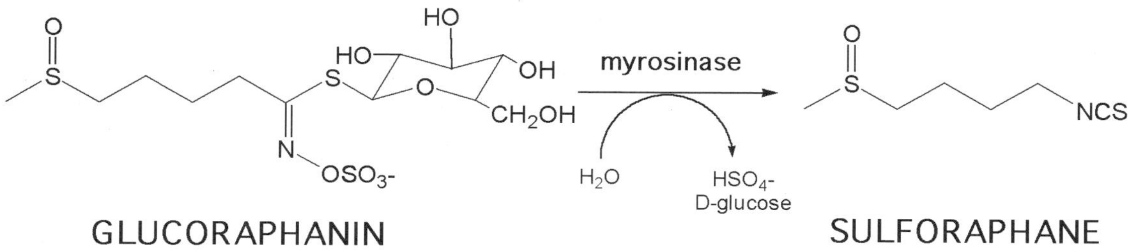

Fig. 4. Myrosinase reaction yielding sulforaphane from glucoraphanin.

DNA synthesis were inhibited along with G_1 cell-cycle block. Caspase activation and DNA-strand breaks accompany apoptosis in these cells. Increased apoptotic-cell fraction has also been observed in human T-cell leukemia cells (127) and HT29 human colon cancer cells (128) following treatment with sulforaphane. Dramatic protection against the toxicity of oxidants by sulforaphane has also been reported. The cytotoxicities of four oxidant stressors (menadione, t-butyl hydroperoxide, 4-hydroxynonenal, and peroxynitrite) in human adult retinal pigment epithelial cells were blunted by treatment with low micromolar concentrations of sulforaphane in a time- and concentration-dependent manner (38). The protection was prolonged, and persisted for several days after removal of sulforaphane before returning to control levels. The degree and time-course of antioxidant protection was closely correlated with the elevations of NQO1 activities and of GSH levels.

One action of sulforaphane that may not be directly related to its inducer properties is the recent finding that this isothiocyanate is a potent bacteriostatic/bacterioci-dal agent against the growth of many clinical isolates of *Helicobacter pylori*, including strains that are resistant to conventional antibiotics (29). Moreover, sulforaphane eliminated intracellular reservoirs of *H. pylori* that are notoriously difficult to eradicate. Infections with *H. pylori* are known to cause gastritis and peptic ulcers, and dramatically enhance the risk of gastric cancer. Since high concentrations of sulforaphane can probably be delivered by the dietary route to the gastric mucosa, the dual antitumor and antibacterial actions of sulforaphane are worthy of consideration as strategies to reduce the previously mentioned gastric pathologies.

4.4. Broccoli Sprouts as a Rich Source of Sulforaphane

The biosynthetic precursors of isothiocyanates in plants are glucosinolates. Glucosinolates are β-thioglucoside N-hydroxysulfates, and some 120 glu-cosinolates with different R groups (e.g., alkyl, alkenyl, alkylthioalkyl, aryl, and indolyl) have been identified in plants (103). The conversion of glucosinolates to isothiocyanates is catalyzed by myrosinase (a thioglucosidase), which invariably accompanies glucosinolates in plant cells. Myrosinase is normally com-partmentalized in the intact plant, and is released upon plant injury. The glucosinolate precursor of sulforaphane is glucoraphanin (Fig. 4).

A method for the simultaneous and complete extraction from plant tissues of both isothiocyanates and glucosinolates, although blocking their interconversion by myrosinase (115), revealed for the first time that these compounds exist in the fresh plant almost entirely as glucosinolates. Isothiocyanates are active phase 2 gene inducers in cell cultures, whereas glucosinolates require hydrolysis by myrosinase in order to display inducer activity. A survey of solvent extract of marketed broccoli heads for inducer activity (after myrosinase treatment) revealed that this activity was highly variable and unrelated to the physical appearance of the vegetable. A surprising finding was that broccoli seeds contain much higher concentrations of inducer glucosinolates, and that 3-day-old sprouts, grown from selected seeds (by exposure to water and light), contain 20–50× higher concentrations of inducers than market-stage broccoli. Extracts of 3-d-old sprouts grown from seeds of 55 random commercial cultivars of broccoli produced inducer potencies (measured as NQO1 induction in Hepa 1c1c7 cells) ranging from 92,500–769,000 U/g fresh weight. Repetitive Kg-scale harvests of 3-d-old broccoli (cultivar SAGA) sprouts yielded an average of 511,000 U / g fr. wt. Moreover, analysis of 3-d-old broccoli sprouts by a paired-ion chromatography method (129,130) showed quite clearly that more than 90% of the inducer activity was attributable to glucoraphanin. The ability to grow sprouts under highly controlled conditions, and to produce 3-d-old plants that contain

250,000–750,000 U of inducer activity per g (as compared to 35,000 U/g in market-stage broccoli) have been an enormous advantage for studies in animal models as well as clinical studies.

Aqueous extracts of 3-d-old broccoli sprouts (containing either glucoraphanin or sulforaphane as the principal enzyme inducer) were evaluated as inhibitors of mammary carcinogenesis in DMBA-treated female Sprague-Dawley rats. Treatment with either glucosinolate or isothiocyanate at the time of carcinogen administration was highly effective in reducing the incidence, multiplicity, size, and rate of development of mammary tumors in these animals. Importantly, the tumor-inhibitory potencies of these broccoli-sprout extracts were comparable to equivalent doses of pure sulforaphane when tested in the same animal model, suggesting that the presence of unrecognized tumor inhibitors in the broccoli sprout extracts was unlikely *(115,117)*. These results established that small quantities of crucifer sprouts may protect against the risk of cancer as effectively as much larger quantities of mature vegetables of the same variety *(115)*.

4.5. Clinical Trials

Clinical studies with pure sulforaphane have not yet begun; however, a number of Phase I studies have been completed using broccoli sprouts or other foods containing sulforaphane and its precursor glucosinolate, glucoraphanin. Isothiocyanates such as sulforaphane readily conjugate with GSH, yielding a series of dithiocarbamate products—principally NAC conjugates (mercapturic acids) *(131–133)*. The first step in the formation in vivo of such NAC derivatives is conjugation with GSH catalyzed by GSTs, producing the corresponding dithiocarbamates. The resulting conjugates are successively hydrolyzed to the cysteinylglycine and the cysteinyl derivatives by γ-glutamyltranspeptidase and cysteinylglycinase, respectively, and the cysteine derivatives are finally acetylated by *N*-acetyltransferase action *(134)*. Both isothiocyanates and dithiocarbamates, but not glucosinolates, can be measured in biological fluids with high sensitivity and specificity by cyclocondensation with 1,2-benzenedithiol *(135–139)*.

Use of the cyclocondensation assay in pharmacokinetic studies has indicated that although absolute levels varied, there was remarkably little inter-subject variation in the extent of dithiocarbamate excretion after dosing volunteers with different cruciferous vegetables *(137–139)*. In intact broccoli sprouts, inducer activity is present largely in the form of glucosinolates. To

determine the extent to which glucosinolates are converted to isothiocyanates in the absence of plant myrosinase, a small crossover study was conducted to compare urinary dithiocarbamate excretion after equimolar doses of glucosinolate or the cognate isothiocyanate preparation *(138)*. Broccoli sprouts were plunged into boiling water to destroy myrosinase activity, and were homogenized (the glucosinolate preparation). A portion of this glucosinolate preparation was then treated with a daikon sprout extract rich in myrosinase to create the isothiocyanate preparation. Urinary dithiocarbamate levels fell below the limit of detection during an initial 3-d washout period, then peaked within 8 h after each dosing. Although the glucosinolate and isothiocyanate doses were equal (100 µmol), the isothiocyanate preparation yielded nearly 7× more urinary dithiocarbamates (88.9 ± 5.5 µmol) than the glucosinolate preparation (13.1 ± 1.9 µmol). Also, dicarbamate excretion was higher when intact sprouts were chewed thoroughly rather than swallowed. This study indicates that even in the absence of plant myrosinase activity, glucosinolates are converted to isothiocyanates in humans, and that isothiocyanates are much more bioavailable than glucosinolates. Thorough chewing of fresh sprouts also exposes the glucosinolates to plant myrosinase and significantly increases dithiocarbamate excretion. To determine whether enteric microflora contribute to glucosinolate metabolism in humans, the effect of a standard preoperative bowel preparation on dithiocarbamate excretion after ingestion of glucosinolates from mature broccoli was evaluated *(137)*. The bowel preparation consisted of mechanical cleansing followed by antibiotic treatment, a regimen that reduces enteric bacteria by five logs. After an initial 3-d washout period, glucosinolates were administered on d 4 and 7 (before the bowel prep) and on d 12 and 15 (after the bowel prep). There was a dramatic reduction in dithiocarbamate excretion after the bowel preparation (from 11.3 ± 3.1% before, to 1.3 ± 1.3% of dose after). This result provides compelling evidence that in the absence of plant myrosinase, most or all glucosinolate-to-isothiocyanate conversion in humans is mediated by enteric microflora. Pharmacokinetic measurements have been made in four human volunteers who received single doses of approx 200 µmol of broccoli-sprout isothiocyanates (largely sulforaphane). Isothiocyanates were absorbed rapidly, reached peak concentration of 0.9 to 2.3 µmol/ml in plasma, serum, and erythrocytes at 1 h after feeding, and declined with first-order kinetics (half-life

1.8 h). The cumulative excretion at 8 h was 58% of the administered dose.

Studies evaluating the pharmacodynamic action of broccoli-sprout preparations through induction of phase 2 enzymes and modulation of carcinogen disposition in humans are currently underway. The conduct of clinical trials with discrete foods rather than formulated drugs presents additional challenges in study design, conduct, and evaluation. In the case of studies with broccoli sprouts, the ability to grow plants with well-defined levels of an anticarcinogen, the availability of a highly sensitive and precise cyclocondensation assay for monitoring isothiocyanate kinetics and study compliance, and the use of well-established biomarkers for evaluating efficacy have set the stage for high-quality, informative studies.

REFERENCES

1. Wattenberg LW. Inhibition of carcinogenic and toxic effects of polycyclic hydrocarbons by phenolic antioxidants and ethoxyquin. *J Natl Cancer* Inst 1972;48:1425–1430.
2. Benson AM, Batzinger RP, Ou S-Y L, et al. Elevation of hepatic GST activities and protection against mutagenic metabolites of B[a]P by dietary antioxidants. *Cancer Res* 1978;38:4486–4495.
3. Kensler TW. Chemoprevention by inducers of carcinogen detoxication enzymes. *Environ Health Perspect* 1997;105S4:965–970.
4. Fahey JW, Talalay P. Antioxidant functions of sulforaphane: a potent inducer of phase II detoxication enzymes. *Food Chem Toxicol* 1999;37:973–979.
5. Hayes JD, McLellan LI. Glutathione and glutathione-dependent enzymes represent a coordinately regulated defense against oxidative stress. *Free Radic Res* 1999;31:273–300.
6. Rushmore TH, King RG, Paulson KE, Pickett CB. Regulation of glutathione S-transferase Ya subunit gene expression: Identification of a unique xenobiotic-responsive element controlling inducible expression by planar aromatic compounds. *Proc Natl Acad Sci USA* 1990;87:3826–3830.
7. Pearson WB, Windle JJ, Morrow JF, et al. Increased synthesis of glutathione S-transferase in response to anticarcinogenic antioxidants. Cloning and measurement of messenger RNA. *J Biol Chem* 1983;258:2052–2062.
8. Prochaska HJ, Talalay P. Regulatory mechanisms of monofunctional and bifunctional anticarcinogenic enzyme inducers in murine liver. *Cancer Res* 1988;48:4776–4782.
9. Fisher JM, Wu L, Denison MS, Whitlock JP, Jr. Organization and function of a dioxin-responsive enhancer. *J Biol Chem* 1990;265:9676–9681.
10. Langouët S, Coles B, Morel F, et al. Inhibition of CYP1A2 and CYP3A4 by oltipraz results in reduction of aflatoxin B_1 metabolism in human hepatocytes in primary culture. *Cancer Res* 1995;55:5574–5579.
11. Talalay P, DeLong MJ, Prochaska HJ. Identification of a common chemical signal regulating the induction of enzymes that protect against chemical carcinogenesis. *Proc Natl Acad Sci USA* 1988;85:8261–8265.
12. Prestera T, Holtzclaw WD, Zhang Y, Talalay P. Chemical and molecular regulation of enzymes that detoxify carcinogens. *Proc Natl Acad Sci USA* 1993;90:2965–2969.
13. Friling RS, Bensimon A, Tichauer Y, Daniel V. Xenobiotic-inducible expression of murine glutathione S-transferase Ya subunit gene is controlled by an electrophile-responsive element. *Proc Natl Acad Sci USA* 1990;87:6258–6262.
14. Jaiswal AK. Antioxidant response element. *Biochem Pharmacol* 1994;48:439–444.
15. Wasserman WW, Fahl WE. Functional antioxidant responsive elements. *Proc Natl Acad Sci USA* 1997;94:5361–5366.
16. Egner PA, Kensler TW, Prestera T et al. Regulation of phase 2 enzyme induction by oltipraz and other dithiolethiones. *Carcinogenesis* 1994;15:177–181.
17. Chan JY, Han X, Kan YW. Cloning of Nrf1, an NF-E2-related transcription factor, by genetic selection in yeast. *Proc Natl Acad Sci USA* 1993;90:11,366–11,370.
18. Moi P, Chan K, Asunis I, et al. Isolation of NF-E2-related factor 2 (Nrf2), a NF-E2-like basic leucine zipper transcriptional activator that binds to the tandem NF-E2/AP1 repeat of the β-globin locus control region. *Proc Natl Acad Sci USA* 1993;91:9926–9930.
19. Venugopal R, Jaiswal AK. Nrf1 and Nrf2 positively and c-Fos and Fra1 negatively regulate the human antioxidant response element-mediated expression of NAD(P)H:quinone oxidoreductase$_1$ gene. *Proc Natl Acad Sci USA* 1996;93:14,960–14,965.
20. Itoh K, Chiba T, Takahashi S, et al. An Nrf2/small Maf heterodimer mediates the induction of phase II detoxifying enzyme genes through antioxidant response elements. *Biochem Biophys Res Comm* 1997;236:313–322.
21. Kwak M-K, Itoh K, Yamamoto M, et al. Role of transcription factor Nrf2 in the induction of hepatic phase 2 and antioxidative enzymes in vivo by the chemoprotective agent 3H-1,2-dithiole-3-thione. *Mol Med* 2001;7:135–145.
22. McMahon M, Itoh K, Yamamoto M, et al. The Cap'n'Collar basic leucine zipper transcription factor Nrf2 (NF-E2 p45-related factor 2) controls both constitutive and inducible expression of intestinal detoxification and glutathione biosynthetic enzymes. *Cancer Res* 2001;61:3299–3307.
23. Itoh K, Wakabayashi N, Katoh Y, et al. Keap1 represses nuclear activation of antioxidant responsive elements by Nrf2 through binding to the amino-terminal Neh2 domain. *Genes Dev* 1999;13:76–86.
24. Dinkova-Kostova AT, Holtzclaw WD, Cole RN, et al. Direct evidence that sulfhydryl groups of Keap1 are the sensors regulating induction of phase 2 enzymes that protect against carcinogens and oxidants. *Proc Natl Acad Sci USA* 2002;99:11,908–11,913.
25. Enomoto A, Itoh K, Nagayoshi E, et al. High sensitivity of Nrf2 knockout mice to acetaminophen hepatotoxicity associated with decreased expression of ARE-regulated drug metabolizing enzymes and antioxidant genes. *Toxicol Sci* 2001;59:169–177.
26. Chan K, Kan YW. Nrf2 is essential for protection against acute pulmonary injury in mice. *Proc Natl Acad Sci USA* 1999;96:12,731–12,736.
27. Cho HY, Jedlicka AE, Reddy SPM, et al. Role of nrf2 in protection against hyperoxic lung injury in mice. *Am J Respir Cell Mol Biol* 2002;26:175–182.

28. Ramos-Gomez M, Kwak MK, Dolan PM, et al. Sensitivity to carcinogenesis is increased and chemoprotective efficacy of enzyme inducers is lost in *nrf2* transcription factor deficient mice. *Proc Natl Acad Sci USA* 2001;98:3410–3415.

29. Fahey JW, Haristoy X, Dolan PM, et al. Sulforaphane inhibits extracellular, intracellular and antibiotic-resistant strains of *Helicobacter pylori* and prevents benz[*a*]pyrene-induced stomach cancers. *Proc Natl Acad Sci USA* 2002;99:7610–7615.

30. Primiano T, Gastel JA, Kensler TW, Sutter TR. Isolation of cDNAs representing dithiolethione-responsive genes. *Carcinogenesis* 1996;17:2297–2303.

31. Li J, Lee JM, Johnson JA. Microarray analysis reveals an antioxidant responsive element-driven gene set involved in conferring protection from an oxidative stress-induced apoptosis in IMR-32 cells. *J Biol Chem* 2002;277:388–394.

32. Thimmulappa RK, Mai KH, Srisuma S, et al. Identification of Nrf2 regulated genes by oligonucleotide microarray: potential role in cancer chemoprevention. *Cancer Res* 2002;62:5196–5203.

33. Williams RT. Comparative patterns of drug metabolism. *Fed Proc* 1967;26:1029–1039.

34. Primiano T, Sutter TR, Kensler TW. Redox regulation of genes that protect against carcinogens. *Comp Biochem Physiol* 1997;118B:487–497.

35. Fahey JW, Talalay PT. Antioxidant functions of sulforaphane: a potent inducer of phase 2 detoxication enzymes. *Food Chem Toxicol* 1999;37:973–979.

36. Hayes JD, McLellan LI. Glutathione and glutathione-dependent enzymes represent a coordinately regulated defense against oxidative stress. *Free Radic Res* 1999;31:273–300.

37. Guyton KZ, Kensler TW. Oxidative mechanisms in carcinogenesis. *Br Med Bull* 1993;49:523–544.

38. Gao X, Dinkova-Kostova AT, Talalay P. Powerful and prolonged protection of human retinal pigment epithelial cells, keratinocytes, and mouse leukemia cells against oxidative damage: the indirect antioxidant effects of sulforaphane. *Proc Natl Acad Sci USA* 2001;98:15,221–15,226.

39. Primiano T, Egner PA, Sutter TR, et al. Intermittent dosing with oltipraz: relationship between chemoprevention of aflatoxin-induced tumorigenesis and induction of glutathione S-transferases. *Cancer Res* 1995;55:4319–4324.

40. Bueding E, Dolan P, Leroy JP. The antischistosomal activity of oltipraz. *Res Commun Chem Pathol Pharmacol* 1982;37:293–303.

41. Moreau N, Martens T, Fleury MB, Leroy JP. Metabolism of oltipraz and glutathione reductase inhibition. *Biochem Pharmacol* 1990;40:1299–1305.

42. Mkoji GM, Smith JM, Pritchard RK. Effect of oltipraz on the susceptibility of adult *Schistosoma mansoni* to killing by mouse peritoneal exudates cells. *Parisitol Res* 1990;76:435–439.

43. Ansher SS, Dolan P, Bueding E. Biochemical effects of dithiolthiones. *Food Chem Toxicol* 1986;24:405–415.

44. Ansher SS, Dolan P, Bueding E. Chemoprotective effects of two dithiolethiones and of butylhydroxyanisole against carbon tetrachloride and acetaminophen toxicity. *Hepatology* 1983;3:932–935.

45. Davies MH, Schamber GJ, Schnell RC. Oltipraz-induced amelioration of acetaminophen hepatotoxicity in hamsters. *Toxicol Appl Pharmacol* 1991;109:17–28.

46. Liu LY, Roebuck BD, Yager JD, et al. Protection by 5-(2-pyrazinyl)-4-methyl-1,2-dithiole-3-thione (oltipraz) against the hepatotoxicity of aflatoxin B$_1$ in the rat. *Toxicol Appl Pharmacol* 1988;93:442–451.

47. Bolton MG, Muñoz A, Jacobson LP, et al. Transient intervention with oltipraz protects against aflatoxin-induced hepatic tumorigenesis. *Cancer Res* 1993;53:3499–3504.

48. Kang KW, Choi SH, Ha JR, et al. Inhibition of dimethylnitrosamine-induced liver fibrosis by [5-(2-pyrazinyl)-4-methyl-1,2-dithiol-3-thione] (oltipraz) in rats: suppression of transforming growth factor-β1 and tumor necrosis factor-α expression. *Chem Biol Interactions* 2002;139:61–77.

49. Kang KW, Kim YG, Cho MK, et al. Oltipraz regenerates cirrhotic liver through CCAAT/enhancer binding protein-mediated stellate cell inactivation. *FASEB J* 2002;16:1988–1990.

50. Newberne PM, Harrington DH, Wogan GN. Effects of cirrhosis and other liver insults on induction of liver tumors by aflatoxin in rats. *Lab Investig* 1966;15:962–969.

51. Wattenberg LW, Bueding E. Inhibitory effects of 5-(2-pyrazinyl)-4-methyl-1,2-dithiol-3-thione (oltipraz) on carcinogenesis induced by B[*a*]P, diethylnitrosamine and uracil mustard. *Carcinogenesis* 1986;7:1379–1381.

52. Rao CV, Tokomo K, Kelloff G, Reddy BS. Inhibition by dietary oltipraz of experimental intestinal carcinogenesis induced by azoxymethane in male F344 rats. *Carcinogenesis* 1991;12:1051–1055.

53. Rao CV, Rivenson A, Katiwalla M, et al. Chemopreventive effect of oltipraz during different stages of experimental colon carcinogenesis induced by azoxymethane in male F344 rats. *Cancer Res* 1993;53:2505–2506.

54. Clapper ML, Wood M, Leahy K, et al. Chemopreventive activity of oltipraz against *N*-nitrosobis(2-oxopropyl)amine (BOP)-induced ductal pancreatic carcinoma development and effects on survival of Syrian golden hamsters. *Carcinogenesis* 1995;16:2159–2165.

55. Moon RC, Kelloff GJ, Detrisac CJ, et al. Chemoprevention of OH-BBN induced bladder cancer in mice by oltipraz, alone or in combination with 4-HPR and DFMO. *Anticancer Res* 1994;14:5–11.

56. Rao CV, Rivenson A, Zang E, et al. Inhibition of 2-amino-1-methyl-6-phenylimidazo[4,5]pyridine-induced lymphoma formation by oltipraz. *Cancer Res* 1996;56:3395–3398.

57. Moon RC, Rao KVN, Detrisac CJ, et al. Chemoprevention of respiratory tract neoplasia in the hamster by oltipraz, alone and in combination. *Int J Oncol* 1994;4:661–667.

58. Roebuck BD, Liu YL, Rogers AR, et al. Protection against aflatoxin B$_1$-induced hepatocarcinogenesis in F344 rats by 5-(2-pyrazinyl)-4-methyl-1,2-dithiole-3-thione (oltipraz): predictive role for short-term molecular dosimetry. *Cancer Res* 1991;51:5501–5506.

59. Moon RC. Evaluation of chemopreventive agents by in vivo screening assays. Prepared for National Cancer Institute by IIT Research Institute under Contract No. N01-CN-55448-04. Final Report, 1988.

60. Helmes CT, Becker RA, Seidenberg JM, et al. Chemoprevention of mouse skin tumorigenesis by dietary oltipraz. Proc Am Assoc *Cancer Res* 1989;30:177.

61. Heusse D, Marland M, Bredenbac J, et al. Disposition of 14C-oltipraz in animals. Pharmacokinetics in mice, rats and monkeys. Comparison of the biotransformation in the infect-

ed mouse and in schistosomes. *Arzneimittelforschung* 1985;35:1431–1436.

62. Maxuitenko YY, MacMillan DL, Kensler TW, Roebuck BD. Evaluation of the post-initiation effects of oltipraz on afla-toxin B_1-induced preneoplastic foci in a rat model of hepatic tumorigenesis. *Carcinogenesis* 1993;14:2423–2425.

63. Kensler TW, Primiano T, Sutter TR, et al. Mechanisms of chemoprotection by 1,2-dithiole-3-thiones$_8$. In Proceedings of the International Symposium on Natural Antioxidants: Molecular Mechanisms and Health Effects. Packer L, Traber MG, Xin W, eds. AOCS Press Champaign IL, 1996:243–250.

64. Reddy BS, Rao CV, Rivenson A,Kelloff GJ. Chemopreven-tion of colon carcinogenesis by organosulfur compounds. *Cancer Res* 1993;53:3493–3498.

65. Lubet RA, Steele VC, Eto I, et al. Chemopreventive efficacy of anethole trithione, *N*-acetyl-L-cysteine, miconazole and phenethylisothiocyanate in the DMBA-induced rat mammary cancer model. *Int J Cancer* 1997;72:95–101.

66. Archer S. The chemotherapy of schistosomiasis. *Annu Rev Pharmacol* 1985;25:485–508.

67. Oltipraz—Investigational Drug Brochure, Chemoprevention Branch, National Cancer Institute, 1994.

68. Benson AB III. Oltipraz: a laboratory and clinical review. *J Cell Biochem* 1993;17F Suppl:278–291.

69. Dimitrov NV, Bennett JL, McMillan J, et al. Clinical phar-macology studies of oltipraz – a potential chemopreventive agent. *Invest New Drugs* 1992;10: 89–298.

70. O'Dwyer PJ, Szarka C, Brennan JM, et al. Pharmacokinetics of the chemopreventive agent oltipraz and of its metabolite M3 in human subjects after a single oral dose. *Clin Cancer Res* 2000;6:4692–4696.

71. Pendyala L, Schwartz G, Bolanowska-Higdon W, et al. Phase I/pharmacodynamic study of *N*-acetylcysteine/ oltipraz in smokers: early termination due to excessive toxi-city. *Cancer Epidemiol Biomarkers Prev* 2001;10:269–272.

72. Jacobson LP, Zhang BC, Zhu YR, et al. Oltipraz Chemoprevention Trial in Qidong, People's Republic of China: Study Design and Clinical Outcomes. *Cancer Epidemiol Biomarkers Prev* 1997;6,257–265.

73. Langouët S, Furge LL, Kerriguy N, et al. Inhibition of human cytochrome P450 enzymes by 1,2-dithiole-3-thione, oltipraz, and its derivatives, and sulforaphane. *Chem Res Toxicol* 2000;13:245–251.

74. Sofowora GG, Choo EF, Mayo YS, Wilkinson GR. In vivo inhibition of human CYP1A2 activity by oltipraz. *Cancer Chemother Pharmacol* 2001;47:505–510.

75. Morel F, Fardel O, Meyer DJ, et al. Preferential increase of glutathione *S*-transferase class alpha transcripts in cultured human hepatocytes by phenobarbital, 3-methylcholanthrene and dithiolethiones. *Cancer Res* 1993;53:231–234.

76. Gupta E, Olopade OI, Ratain MJ, et al. Pharmacokinetics and pharmacodynamics of oltipraz as a chemopreventive agent. *Clin Cancer Res* 1995;1:1133–1138.

77. O'Dwyer PJ, Szarka CE, Yao KS, et al. Modulation of gene expression in subjects at risk for colorectal cancer by the chemopreventive dithiolethione oltipraz. *J Clin Investig* 1996;98:1210–1217.

78. Benson AB III, Olopade OI, Ratain MJ, et al. Chronic low dose of 4-methyl-5-(2-pyrazinyl)-1,2-dithiole-3-thione (oltipraz) in patients with previously resected colon polyps

79. Kensler TW, He X, Otieno M, et al. Oltipraz chemoprevention trial in Qidong, People's Republic of China: modulation of serum aflatoxin albumin adduct biomarkers. *Cancer Epidemiol Biomarkers Prev* 1998;7:127–134.

80. Wang JS, Shen X, He X, Zhu YR, et al. Protective alterations in phase 1 and 2 metabolism of aflatoxin B_1 by oltipraz in residents of Qidong, People's Republic of China. *J Natl Cancer Inst* 1998;91:347–354.

81. Langouët S, Coles B, Morel F, et al. Inhibition of CYP1A2 and CYP3A4 by oltipraz results in reduction of aflatoxin B_1 metabolism in human hepatocytes in primary culture. *Cancer Res* 1995;55:5574–5579.

82. Kensler TW, Groopman JD, Sutter TR, et al. Development of cancer chemopreventive agents: oltipraz as a paradigm. *Chem Res Toxicol* 1999;12:113–126.

83. Lam S, MacAulay C, le Riche JC, et al. A randomized phase IIb trial of anethole dithiolethione in smokers with bronchial dysplasia. *J Natl Cancer Inst* 2002;94:1001–1009.

84. Ben-Mahdi MH, Gozin A, Driss F, et al. Anethole dithio-lethione regulates oxidant-induced tyrosine kinase activation in endothelial cells. *Antioxid Redox Signal* 2000;2:789–799.

85. Le Ferrec E, Lagadic-Grossmann D, Rauch C, et al. Transcriptional induction of CYP1A1 by oltipraz in human Caco-2 cells is aryl hydrocarbon receptor- and calcium-dependent. *J Biol Chem* 2002;277:24,780–24,787.

86. Maxiutenko YY, Curphey TJ, Libby AH, et al. Identification of dithiolethiones with better chemopreventive properties than oltipraz. Carcinogenesis 1998;19:1609–1615.

87. Prochaska HJ, Santamaria AB, Talalay P. Rapid detection of inducers of enzymes that protect against carcinogens. *Proc Natl Acad Sci USA* 1992;89:2394–2398.

88. Zhang Y, Talalay P, Cho C-G, Posner GH. A major inducer of anticarcinogenic protective enzymes from broccoli: isola-tion and elucidation of structure. *Proc Natl Acad Sci USA* 1992;89:2399–2403.

89. Pezzutto JM. Plant-derived anticancer agents. *Biochem Pharmacol* 1997;53:121–133.

90. Talalay P, Talalay P. The importance of using scientific prin-ciples in the development of medicinal agents from plants. *Acad Med* 2001;76:238–247.

91. Block G, Patterson B, Subar A. Fruit, vegetables and cancer prevention: a review of the epidemiological evidence. *Nutr Cancer* 1992;18:1–29.

92. Steinmetz KA, Potter JD. Vegetables, fruit, and cancer. I. Epidemiology. *Cancer Causes Control* 1991;2:325–357.

93. Steinmetz KA, Potter JD. Vegetables, fruit, and cancer pre-vention: a review. *J Am Diet Assoc* 1996;96:1027–1039.

94. World Cancer Research Fund. *Food, Nutrition and the Prevention of Cancer: A Global Perspective.* American Institute for Cancer Research, Washington, DC, 1997

95. Beecher CWW. Cancer preventive properties of varieties of *Brassica oleracea*: a review. *Am J Clin Nutr* 1994;59 Suppl:1165–1170.

96. Talalay P, Fahey JW. Phytochemicals from cruciferous plants protect against cancer by modulating carcinogen metabolism. *J Nutr* 2001;131:3027S–3033S.

97. Steinmetz KA, Potter, JD. Vegetables, fruit, and cancer. II. Mechanisms. *Cancer Causes Control* 1991;2:427–442.

98. Kolonel LN, Hankin JH, Whittemore AS, et al. Vegetables, fruits, legumes and prostate cancer: a multi-

center case-control study. *Cancer Epidemiol Biomarkers Prev* 2000;9:795–804.

99. Cohen JH, Kristal AR, Stanford JL. Fruit and vegetable intake and prostate cancer risk. *J Natl Cancer Inst* 2000;92: 61–68.

100. Terry P, Wolk A, Persson, I. Magnusson C. Brassica vegetables and breast cancer risk. *J Am Med Assoc* 2001;286:2975–2977.

101. Zhang SM, Hunter DJ, Rosner BA, et al. Intake of fruits, vegetables, and related nutrients and the risk of non-Hodgkin's lymphoma among women. *Cancer Epidemiol Biomarkers Prev* 2000;9:477–485.

102. Michaud DS, Spiegelman D, Clinton SK, et al. Fruit and vegetable intake and incidence of bladder cancer in a male prospective cohort. *J Natl Cancer Inst* 1999;91:605–613.

103. Fahey JW, Zalcmann A, Talalay P. The chemical diversity and distribution of glucosinolates and isothiocyanates among plants. *Phytochemistry* 2001;56:5–51.

104. Zhang Y, Talalay P. Anticarcinogenic activities of organic isothiocyanates: chemistry and mechanisms. *Cancer Res* (Suppl) 1994;54:1976s–1981s.

105. Hecht SS. Chemoprevention by isothiocyanates. *J Cell Biochem* (Suppl) 1995;22:195–209.

106. Hecht SS. Chemoprevention by modifiers of carcinogen metabolism, In *Phytochemicals as Bioactive Agents*. Bidlack WR, Omaye ST, Meskin MS, Topham DKW, eds. Technomic Publishing Co., Lancaster, PA, 2000; pp. 43–74.

107. Boogards JJP, Verhagen H, Willems MI, et al. Consumption of Brussels sprouts results in elevated alpha-class glutathione *S*-transferase levels in human blood plasma. *Carcinogenesis* 1994;15:1073–1075.

108. Nijhoff WA, Grubben MJAL, Nagengast FM, et al. Effects of consumption of Brussels sprouts on intestinal and lymphocytic glutathione *S*-transferases in humans. *Carcinogenesis* 1995;16:2125–2128.

109. Clapper ML, Szarka CE, Pfeiffer GR, et al. Preclinical and clinical evaluation of broccoli supplements as inducers of glutathione *S*-transferase activity. *Clin Cancer Res* 1997;3:25–30.

110. Conney AH, Pantuck EJ, Hsiao K-C, et al. Enhanced phenacetin metabolism in human subjects fed charcoal-broiled beef. *Clin Pharmacol Ther* 1976;20:633–643.

111. Conney AH, Pantuck EJ, Hsiao KC, et al. Regulation of drug metabolism in man by environmental chemicals and diet. *Fed Proc* 1977;36:1647–1652.

112. Conney AH, Buening NM, Pantuck EJ, et al. Regulation of human drug metabolism by dietary factors. CIBA *Found Symp* 1980;76:147–167.

113. Prochaska HJ, Santamaria AB. Direct measurement of NAD(P)H: quinone reductase from cells in cultured microtiter wells: a screening assay for anticarcinogenic enzyme inducers. *Anal Biochem* 1988;169:328–336.

114. Prochaska HJ, Santamaria AB, Talalay P. Rapid detection of inducers of enzymes that protect against cancer. *Proc Natl Acad Sci USA* 1992;89:2394–2398.

115. Fahey JW, Zhang Y, Talalay P. Broccoli sprouts: an exceptionally rich source of inducers of enzymes that protect against chemical carcinogens. *Proc Natl Acad Sci USA* 1997;94:10,367–10,372.

116. Zhang Y, Talalay P, Cho CG, Posner GH. A major inducer of anticarcinogenic protective enzymes from broccoli: isolation and elucidation of structure. *Proc Natl Acad Sci USA* 1992;89:2399–2403.

117. Zhang Y, Kensler TW, Cho CG, et al. Anticarcinogenic activities of sulforaphane and structurally related synthetic norbornyl isothiocyanates. *Proc Natl Acad Sci USA* 1994;91:3147–3150.

118. Gerhauser C, You M, Liu J, et al. Cancer chemopreventive potential of sulforamate, a novel analog of sulforaphane that induces phase 2 drug-metabolizing enzymes. *Cancer Res* 1997;57:272–278.

119. Singletary K, MacDonald C. Inhibition of benzo[*a*]pyrene- and 1,6-dinitropyrene-DNA adduct formation in human mammary epithelial cells by dibenzoylmethane and sulforaphane. *Cancer Lett* 2000;155: 47–54.

120. Chung FL, Conaway CC, Rao CV, Reddy BS. Chemoprevention of colonic aberrant crypt foci in Fischer rats by sulforaphane and phenethyl isothiocyanate. *Carcinogenesis* 2000;21:2287–2291.

121. Zhang Y, Talalay P. Mechanisms of differential potencies of isothiocyanates as inducers of anticarcinogenic phase 2 enzymes. *Cancer Res* 1998;58:4632–4639.

122. Zhang Y, Talalay P. Role of glutathione in the accumulation of anticarcinogenic isothiocyanates and their glutathione conjugates in murine hepatoma cells. *Carcinogenesis* 2000;21:1175–1182.

123. Zhang Y. Molecular mechanism of rapid cellular accumulation of anticarcinogenic isothiocyanates. *Carcinogenesis* 2001;22:425–431.

124. Zhang Y, Callaway EC. High cellular accumulation of sulforaphane, a dietary anticarcinogen, is followed by rapid transporter-mediated export as a glutathione conjugate. *Biochem J* 2002;365:301–307.

125. Conaway CC, Krzeminsik J, Amin S, Chung FL. Decomposition rates of isothiocyanate conjugates determine their activity as inhibitors of cytochrome P450 enzymes. *Chem Res Toxicol* 2002;14:1170–1176.

126. Chiao JW, Chung FL, Kancheria R, et al. Sulforaphane and its metabolite mediate growth arrest and apoptosis in human prostate cancer cells. *Int J Oncol* 2002;20:631–636.

127. Fimognari C, Nusse M, Cesari R, et al. Growth inhibition, cell-cycle arrest and apoptosis in human T-cell leukemia by the isothiocyanate sulforaphane. *Carcinogenesis* 2002;23:581–586.

128. Gamet-Payrastre L, Li P, Lumeau S, et al. Sulforaphane, a naturally occurring isothiocyanate, induces cell cycle arrest and apoptosis in HT29 human colon cancer cells. *Cancer Res* 2000;60:1426–1433.

129. Prestera T, Fahey JW, Holtzclaw WD, et al. Comprehensive chromatographic and spectroscopic methods for the separation and identification of intact glucosinolates. *Anal Biochem* 1996;239:168–179.

130. Troyer JK, Stephenson KK, Fahey JW. Analysis of glucosinolates from broccoli and other cruciferous vegetables by hydrophilic interaction liquid chromatography. *J Clin Chromatography* 2001;919:299–304.

131. Chung F-L, Morse MA, Elklind KI, Lewis J. Quantitation of human uptake of the anticarcinogen phenethyl isothiocyanate after a watercress meal. *Cancer Epidemiol Biomark Prev* 1992;1:383–388.

132. Jiao D, Ho CT, Foiles P, Chung FL. Identification and quantitation of the N-acetylcysteine conjugate of allyl isothiocyanate in human urine after ingestion of mustard. *Cancer Epidemiol Biomark Prev* 1994;3:487–492.

133. Mennicke WH, Görler K, Krumbiegel G, et al. Studies on the metabolism and excretion of benzyl isothiocyanate in man. *Xenobiotica* 1988;4:441–447.

134. Brüsewitz G, Cameron BD, Chasseaud LF, et al. The metabolism of benzyl isothiocyanate and its cysteine conjugate. *Biochem J* 1977;162:99–107.

135. Zhang Y, Cho C-G, Posner GH, Talalay P. Spectroscopic quantitation of organic isothiocyanates by cyclocondensation with vicinal dithiols. *Anal Biochem* 1992;205:100–107.

136. Zhang Y, Wade KL, Prestera T, Talalay P. Quantitative determination of isothiocyanates, dithiocarbamates, carbon disulfide, and related thiocarbonyl compounds by cyclocondensation with 1,2-benzenedithiol. *Anal Biochem* 1996;239:160–167.

137. Shapiro TA, Fahey JW, Wade KL, et al. Human metabolism and excretion of cancer chemoprotective glucosinolates and isothiocyanates of cruciferous vegetables. *Cancer Epidemiol Biomark Prev* 1998;7:1091–1100.

138. Shapiro TA, Fahey JW, Wade KL, et al. Chemoprotective glucosinolates and isothiocyanates of broccoli sprouts: metabolism and excretion in humans. *Cancer Epidemiol Biomark Prev* 2001;10:501–508.

139. Ye L, Dinkova-Kostova AT, Wade KL, et al. Quantitative determination of dithiolecarbamates in human plasma, serum, erythrocytes and urine: pharmacokinetics of broccoli sprout isothiocyanates in humans. *Clin Chim Acta* 2002;316:43–53.

2 Chemoprevention by Isothiocyanates

Stephen S. Hecht, PhD

CONTENTS

1. INTRODUCTION

Isothiocyanates are among the most effective known chemopreventive agents *(1)*. Examples of complete inhibition of carcinogenicity in laboratory animals through relatively low doses of isothiocyanates are not unusual. Many isothiocyanates occur naturally as glucosinolate conjugates in frequently consumed cruciferous vegetables *(2)*. Consistent with the animal carcinogenicity data, three recent epidemiologic studies have demonstrated that human consumption of isothiocyanates in vegetables decreases lung cancer risk *(3–5)*. Other studies have shown that consumption of genus *Brassica* vegetables is protective against lung cancer *(6)*. Collectively, these data indicate that isothiocyanates have substantial potential for chemoprevention of human cancers.

More than 100 structurally distinct glucosinolates that are precursors of isothiocyanates have been isolated from plants, and these studies have been extensively reviewed *(2,7,8)*. Significant amounts of glucosinolates are found in commonly consumed cruciferous vegetables such as broccoli, cabbage, cauliflower, turnip, horseradish, watercress, and Brussels sprouts. When the raw vegetables are chewed or otherwise macerated, cells are broken and myrosinase—an enzyme that is normally separated cellularly from the glucosinolates—comes into contact with them and catalyzes hydrolysis, as illustrated in Fig.1. Isothiocyanates are common products of this reaction, although other products such as indole-3-carbinol, in the case of glucobrassican

(R=3-indolyl-), are also formed. Normal portions of these raw vegetables will release multi-milligram amounts of isothiocyanates, but cooking, which inactivates myrosinase, sharply decreases the isothiocyanate dose. The daily dose of isothiocyanates from raw vegetables greatly exceeds the dose of strong carcinogens from cigarettes *(1)*. Isothiocyanates are plant defense compounds, and are responsible for the sharp taste often associated with these vegetables. Some of these naturally occurring isothiocyanates have received considerable attention as chemopreventive agents. Prominent among these are 2-phenylethyl isothiocyanate (PEITC), which is found in watercress and Chinese cabbage as its conjugate gluconasturtiin (R = $PhCH_2CH_2$-), and sulforaphane, which is found in broccoli as its conjugate glucoraphanin (R = $CH_3S(O)CH_2CH_2CH_2CH_2$-). PEITC has entered human clinical trials. Broccoli sprouts, which are rich in glucoraphanin, are now sold as dietary supplements and can be found on the shelves of upscale grocery stores.

Synthetic isothiocyanates—in many cases structural analogs of naturally occurring isothiocyanates with chemopreventive activity—have also been investigated. Several of these compounds have chemopreventive properties that are many orders of magnitude greater than those of the naturally occurring compounds. However, problems with toxicity—and in some cases, enhancement of carcinogenicity—have hindered the development of these compounds as chemopreventive agents.

This chapter reviews efficacy data for isothiocyanates as inhibitors of carcinogenesis and discusses recent

From: Cancer Chemoprevention, Volume 1: Promising Cancer Chemoprevention Agents
Edited by: G. J. Kelloff, E. T. Hawk, and C. C. Sigman © Humana Press Inc., Totowa, NJ

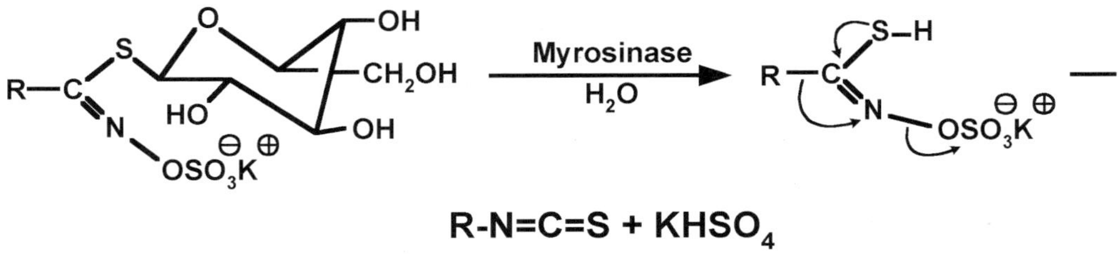

Fig. 1. Conversion of glucosinolates to isothiocyanates, catalyzed by myrosinase.

developments related to our understanding of mechanisms of chemoprevention by isothiocyanates.

2. CHEMOPREVENTIVE EFFICACY OF ISOTHIOCYANATES

Table 1 summarizes the literature on inhibition of carcinogenesis by isothiocyanates. A significant number of isothiocyanates, both naturally occurring and synthetic, have been tested. Naturally occurring isothiocyanates with chemopreventive activity include benzyl isothiocyanate (R = PhCH$_2$, BITC), PEITC, 3-phenylpropyl isothiocyanate (R = PhCH$_2$CH$_2$CH$_2$, PPITC), and sulforaphane. Among these, BITC and PEITC are the most extensively studied.

BITC is an effective inhibitor of rat mammary and mouse lung tumorigenesis by the polycyclic aromatic hydrocarbons (PAH) 7,12-dimethylbenz[a]anthracene (DMBA) and benzo[a]pyrene (B[a]P) (9–12). In mouse lung tumorigenesis experiments, gavage of BITC 15 min prior to treatment with B[a]P inhibits lung-tumor multiplicity by as much as 80%, greater than achieved under the same conditions with equimolar doses of either sulforaphane or the well-known antioxidant chemopreventive agent butylated hydroxyanisole (13). Gavaged BITC is also a strikingly potent inhibitor of lung-tumor induction by two other PAH: 5-methylchrysene (5-MeC) and dibenz[a,h]anthracene (DB[a,h]A) (13). This may be significant because PAH are acknowledged to be important carcinogens in tobacco smoke and certain occupational environments (14,15). BITC appears to be less effective when given in the diet, perhaps because palatability limits the dose. Mixed results have been obtained in studies of BITC as an inhibitor of nitrosamine carcinogenesis. It has no effect on mouse lung tumor induction by the tobacco-specific carcinogen 4-(methylnitrosamino)-1-(3-pyridyl)-1-butanone (NNK) or by N-nitrosodiethylamine (DEN), and it has no effect on esophageal tumor

induction in rats by N-nitrosobenzylmethylamine (NBMA) (12,16–18). It inhibited rat liver tumor induction by DEN, but enhanced rat bladder tumor induction by a mixture of DEN and N-butyl-N-(4-hydroxybutyl)nitrosamine (OH-BBN) (19,20).

In contrast to BITC, PEITC has broad inhibitory activity against tumors induced by N-nitrosamines. This includes inhibition of lung tumorigenesis in mice and rats by NNK, inhibition of liver tumor induction by DEN in the mouse, inhibition of esophageal-tumor induction by NBMA in the rat, and inhibition of lung and pancreatic tumorigenesis by N-nitrosobis(2-oxopyropyl)amine (BOP) in the hamster.

Inhibition of NNK-induced pulmonary carcinogenesis by PEITC has been demonstrated in multiple studies in mice and rats (16,21–26). Dietary PEITC is particularly effective. In one study, complete inhibition of lung-tumor induction was achieved in F344 rats treated with NNK in the drinking water and PEITC in the diet (3 μmol/g diet) (23). Dietary PEITC is also an effective inhibitor of lung-tumor induction by NNK in mice (21). PEITC (3 or 6 μmol/g diet) completely inhibited esophageal tumor induction by NBMA in rats (27). When PEITC (100 or 10 μmol) was given by gavage 2 h prior to treatment of hamsters with BOP, virtually complete inhibition of lung tumor induction was observed (28). Pancreatic tumorigenesis was also inhibited at the higher dose of PEITC. These striking results clearly demonstrate the efficacy of PEITC in these models. However, PEITC has limited efficacy against PAH. Both gavaged and dietary PEITC failed to inhibit B[a]P-induced lung tumorigenesis in mice (11,21,29). Mixed results have been obtained in the DMBA rat mammary tumor model. Initial studies by Wattenberg, in which PEITC was given by gavage, showed inhibition of mammary tumorigenesis (9). A study by Lubet et al. in which PEITC was given in the diet showed no effect or somewhat enhanced mammary tumorigenesis by DMBA (30). However, another dietary study demonstrated that carcinoma volume, but

Table 1

Inhihition of Carcinogenesis by Isothiocyanates

Isothiocyanate R-N = C = S; R=	Naturally Occurring?[a]	Carcinogen[b]	Species and Target Organ	Effect	Reference
α-Naphthyl–	No	3'-Me-DAB	Rat liver	inhibition	112
		Ethionine	Rat liver	inhibition	113
		AAF	Rat liver	inhibition	113
		DAB	Rat liver	inhibition	114
		m-toluylenediamine	Rat liver	inhibition	115
		DEN	Rat liver	no effect	116
		OH-BBN	Rat bladder	inhibition	117
β-Naphthyl–	No	DAB	Rat liver	inhibition	114
Ph–	No	DMBA	Rat mammary	inhibition	9
		NNK	Mouse lung	no effect	16
PhCH₂–	Yes	DMBA	Rat mammary	inhibition	9,10
			Mouse forestomach	inhibition	9
			Mouse lung	inhibition	9
		B[a]P	Mouse lung	inhibition	11–13
			Mouse forestomach	inhibition or no effect	11,12
		5-MeC	Mouse lung	inhibition	13
		DB[a,h]A	Mouse lung	inhibition	13
		NNK	Mouse lung	no effect	16,17
		DEN	Mouse forestomach	inhibition	12
			Mouse lung	no effect	12
			Rat liver	inhibition	19
		MAM	Rat small intestine/colon	inhibition	118
		NBMA	Rat esophagus	no effect	18
		DEN + OH-BBN	Rat bladder	enhancement	20
		B[a]P + NNK	Mouse lung	no effect	21
Ph(CH₂)₂–	Yes	DMBA	Rat mammary	inhibition or no effect	9,30,31
			Mouse forestomach	inhibition	9
			Mouse lung	inhibition	9
		NNK	Rat lung	inhibition	22–24
			Rat nasal cavity, liver	no effect	24
			Mouse lung	inhibition	16,25,26,32,46,119,120

(continued)

23

Table 1 (*continued*)

Isothiocyanate R-N=C=S; R=	Naturally Occurring?[a]	Carcinogen[b]	Species and Target Organ	Effect	Reference
		DEN	Mouse lung	no effect	17
			Mouse liver	inhibition	120
		NBMA	Rat esophagus	inhibition or no effect	18,27,122
		BOP	Hamster pancreas and lung	inhibition or no effect	28,123
			Hamster liver	no effect	
		B[a]P	Mouse lung	no effect	11,21,29
			Mouse skin	no effect	11
		DEN + OH-BBN	Rat bladder	enhancement	20
		B[a]P + NNK	Mouse lung	inhibition or no effect	21
		Environmental tobacco smoke, gas phase	Mouse lung	no effect	124
PhCH₂- + Ph(CH₂)₂-	Yes	B[a]P + NNK	Mouse lung	inhibition or no effect	21
		Environmental tobacco smoke, gas phase	Mouse lung	no effect	34
Ph(CH₂)₃-	Yes	NNK	Mouse lung	inhibition	25,26
		NBMA	Rat esophagus	inhibition	18
		BOP	Hamster lung	inhibition	38
			Hamster pancreas, liver, kidney	no effect	38
		NNN	Rat esophagus	inhibition	36
		B[a]P + NNK	Mouse lung	inhibition	37
Ph(CH₂)₄-	Yes	NNK	Mouse lung	inhibition	25,26
		NBMA	Rat esophagus	inhibition	18
		BOP	Hamster pancreas and lung	inhibition	43
			Hamster liver	enhancement	43
Ph(CH₂)₅-	No	NNK	Mouse lung	inhibition	26
Ph(CH₂)₆-	No	NNK	Mouse lung	inhibition	26,46,119
		B[a]P	Rat lung	inhibition	22,125
			Mouse skin	no effect	11
		NBMA	Rat esophagus	enhancement or no effect	50,52
		AOM	Rat colon	enhancement	51

24

Ph(CH$_2$)$_8$–	No	NNK	Mouse lung	inhibition	42
Ph(CH$_2$)$_{10}$–	No	NNK	Mouse lung	inhibition	42
PhCH(Ph)CH$_2$–	No	NNK	Mouse lung	inhibition	42
PhCH$_2$CH(Ph)–	No	NNK	Mouse lung	inhibition	42
CH$_2$=CHCH$_2$–	Yes	NNK	Mouse lung	no effect	42
CH$_3$(CH$_2$)$_5$–	Yes	NNK	Mouse lung	inhibition	42
CH$_3$(CH$_2$)$_3$CH(CH$_3$)–	?	NNK	Mouse lung	inhibition	42
CH$_3$(CH$_2$)$_{11}$–	No	NNK	Mouse lung	inhibition	42,44
3-PyrC(CH$_2$)$_3$– (||O)	No	NNK	Mouse lung	no effect	25
9-Phenanthryl–	No	B[a]P	Mouse skin	no effect	11
9-Methylenephenanthryl–	No	B[a]P	Mouse skin	no effect	11
6-Chrysenyl–	No	B[a]P	Mouse skin	no effect	11
6-Benzo[a]pyrenyl–	No	B[a]P	Mouse skin	no effect	11
CH$_3$S(CH$_2$)$_4$– (||O)	Yes	DMBA	Rat mammary	inhibition	39
		B[a]P	Mouse lung	no effect	13
CH$_3$S(CH$_2$)$_6$-	Yes	NNK	Mouse lung	inhibition	126
(bicyclic structure, O=C, H$_3$C)	No	DMBA	Rat mammary	inhibition	39
(bicyclic structure, H$_3$C–C=O)	No	DMBA	Rat mammary	inhibition	39
(bicyclic structure, O=C, H$_3$C)	No	DMBA	Rat mammary	inhibition	39

[a]Based on Fenwick et al. (8)

[b]Abbreviations: AAF, 2-acetylaminofluorene; AOM, azoxymethane; B[a]P, benzo[a]pyrene; BOP, N-nitrosobis(2-oxopropyl)amine; 3'-Me-DAB, 3'-methyl-4-dimethylaminoazobenzene; DAB, 4-dimethylaminoazobenzene; DB[a,h]A, dibenz[a,h]anthracene; DEN, N-nitrosodiethylamine; DMBA, 7,12-dimethylbenz[a]anthracene; MAM, methylazoxymethanol acetate; 5-MeC, 5-methylchrysene; NBMA, N-nitrosobenzylmethylamine; NNK, 4-(methylnitrosamino)-1-(3-pyridyl)-1-butanone; OH-BBN, N-butyl-N-(4-hydroxybutyl)nitrosamine

25

not multiplicity or incidence, was decreased by PEITC (31). The effects of PEITC on carcinogenesis by PAH require further investigation.

The contrasting effects of BITC and PEITC on tumorigenesis by PAH and N-nitrosamines are interesting and require further study. Gavaged, but not dietary, BITC is a very effective inhibitor of PAH-induced mouse-lung tumorigenesis yet has little effect on tumorigenesis by nitrosamines. Dietary PEITC is a strong inhibitor of tumorigenesis in several N-nitrosamine models. In mice, dietary PEITC appears to be more effective than gavaged PEITC as an inhibitor of NNK-induced lung tumorigenesis (21,32). PEITC has little impact on tumorigenesis by PAH in mice. With these results in mind, mixtures of BITC and PEITC have been tested as inhibitors of lung tumor induction in mice by mixtures of NNK and B[a]P (21). Dietary BITC plus PEITC inhibited lung tumor induction by a mixture of NNK and B[a]P. Dietary BITC alone had no effect against NNK and B[a]P, and dietary PEITC did not inhibit lung tumorigenesis by B[a]P. Therefore, it was concluded that inhibition of NNK plus B[a]P-induced lung tumorigenesis by dietary BITC plus PEITC was mainly caused by inhibition of NNK-induced lung tumors by PEITC. Mechanistic studies support this conclusion (33). Gavaged PEITC plus BITC had modest or no effect on lung tumor induction by a mixture of NNK and B[a]P (21).

Recently, a model has been developed in which "environmental tobacco smoke," consisting of 89% sidestream and 11% mainstream cigarette smoke, induces a small but reproducible and significant increase in lung tumor multiplicity in A/J mice (34). Studies have shown that this increase in tumor multiplicity is the result of a component of the gas phase of tobacco smoke, and not B[a]P, NNK, or other well-known carcinogens in the particulate phase. These results appear to conflict with much of the available data on tumor induction by tobacco smoke and its constituents (35). A potential problem with the model is the significant weight loss among the mice treated with smoke. Dietary PEITC and a mixture of dietary BITC and PEITC were tested in this model, but neither had any effect on lung tumor multiplicity (34).

PPITC is a very effective inhibitor of carcinogenesis by N-nitrosamines. PPITC (0.4, 1.0, or 2.5 μmol/g diet) inhibited NBMA-induced esophageal tumorigenesis in rats by 90–100% (18). It also virtually completely inhibited esophageal tumorigenesis in rats induced by the tobacco-specific N-nitrosamine N'-nitrosonornico-

tine (NNN) (36). PPITC was more effective than PEITC in the rat NBMA esophageal tumor model, and was also more effective than PEITC as an inhibitor of lung tumorigenesis induced by NNK in mice (18,26). It was also a strong inhibitor of lung tumor igenesis induced by a mixture of B[a]P and NNK in mice (37). PPITC was a very effective inhibitor of lung tumorigenesis induced in hamsters by BOP, but less effective than PEITC in this model (38). It had no effect on pancreatic tumors induced by BOP, in contrast to the inhibitory effects of PEITC.

Limited data are available on chemoprevention by sulforaphane, perhaps because it is expensive and difficult to synthesize in large quantities. It inhibited rat mammary tumor induction by DMBA but was ineffective as an inhibitor of mouse lung tumor induction by B[a]P (13,39). Sulforaphane also had no effect on lung tumor induction by NNK in mice (40). Sulforaphane and PEITC both significantly reduced the formation of colonic aberrant crypt foci (ACF) in F344 rats treated with azoxymethane (41). Reduction was observed in both the initiation and promotion stages of the experiment. The N-acetyl-cysteine (NAC) conjugates of sulforaphane and PEITC were also effective in the post-initiation phase.

Structure-activity studies demonstrate that increased isothiocyanate lipophilicity increases inhibitory potency against NNK-induced lung tumorigenesis in the A/J mouse (42). Thus, single doses of 10-phenyldecyl isothiocyanate or 1-dodecyl isothiocyanate as low as 0.04–1 μmol are sufficient to inhibit mouse-lung tumorigenesis induced by a single dose of 10 μmol NNK. However, different relationships were found in other tumor models. In the rat esophagus, PPITC was a better inhibitor than PEITC, but extension of the chain length to 4-phenylbutyl (PBITC) decreased activity (18). In the hamster lung, PBITC was less effective than either PPITC or PEITC (43). Other studies have shown that the isothiocyanate group, but not the phenyl ring, is necessary for inhibition, and that lower reactivity with glutathione (GSH) leads to better inhibitory potency in the NNK mouse lung-tumor model (42,44). Several isothiocyanates containing a PAH moiety were tested as potential inhibitors of B[a]P-induced mouse-skin tumorigenesis, but no inhibition of tumorigenicity was observed (11). Synthetic rigid analogs of sulforaphane were effective as inhibitors of rat mammary tumorigenesis in the DMBA model (39).

Isothiocyanates are metabolized by conjugation with GSH, and are ultimately excreted as their NAC conjugates (45). GSH and NAC conjugates of PEITC inhibit lung tumorigenesis induced in A/J mice by NNK when given before the carcinogen (46). NAC conjugates of PEITC and PPITC administered in the diet during the period of carcinogen treatment decreased lung tumorigenesis induced in A/J mice by a mixture of B[a]P and NNK, but the NAC conjugate of BITC was ineffective (37). Higher doses of dietary NAC conjugates of BITC and PEITC inhibited B[a]P-induced lung tumorigenesis in A/J mice when given after the carcinogen, suggesting that isothiocyanates and their conjugates may possess a general ability to inhibit carcinogenesis above and beyond modification of carcinogen metabolism (47). The NAC conjugate of PEITC also inhibits the growth rate of prostate-cancer cells and human leukemia cells in culture (48,49)

Enhancement of tumorigenesis has been observed in some studies of isothiocyanates. Both BITC and PEITC promote urinary-bladder carcinogenesis in rats treated with DEN and OH-BBN, although the dose used was higher than that used for chemoprevention (20). 6-Phenylhexyl isothiocyanate (R = Ph(CH$_2$)$_6$, PHITC), which is not known to be naturally occurring, enhances colon and esophageal carcinogenesis in rat-tumor models (50,51). PHITC administered to rats after the esophageal carcinogen NMBA had modest but insignificant promoting activity, and did not have a significant effect on esophageal cell proliferation (52).

3. MECHANISMS OF CHEMOPREVENTION BY ISOTHIOCYANATES

Most isothiocyanates are active as chemopreventive agents when administered before, or concurrently with, the carcinogen. There are relatively few examples of chemoprevention by isothiocyanates given after carcinogen treatment. This indicates that the major effect of isothiocyanates is favorable modulation of carcinogen metabolism—e.g., inhibition of phase 1 enzymes involved in carcinogen activation and induction of phase 2 enzymes involved in carcinogen detoxification. There is now a large body of evidence in support of this concept. The literature on isothiocyanates and related compounds as inhibitors of phase 1 enzymes and inducers of phase 2 enzymes has been extensively reviewed (1,53–56). More recently, it has become apparent that isothiocyanates and their NAC conjugates have a variety of other cellular

effects that may be pertinent to chemoprevention. Important among these is the induction of apoptosis. This chapter examines the conclusions of the pertinent reviews, and discusses studies that are relevant to mechanisms of isothiocyanate chemoprevention, focusing on those published since 2000.

3.1. Effects on Cytochrome P450 Enzymes

Cytochrome P450 enzymes (P450s) play a critical role in the activation of carcinogens to electrophiles that bind to DNA, producing DNA adducts. The formation of DNA adducts is a necessary step for cancer induction by many carcinogens. Inhibition of P450s involved in carcinogen activation to DNA adducts frequently results in inhibition of tumor formation. Isothiocyanates can selectively inhibit P450s by binding to the apoprotein or heme moiety, or by serving as competitive inhibitors. Inhibition depends both on the structure of the isothiocyanate and the particular cytochrome P450. P450s 1A2, 2B1, and 2E1 are among those that are inhibited by isothiocyanates.

Nakajima et al. studied the inhibition and inactivation of human P450s by PEITC using microsomes from baculovirus-infected insect cells expressing specific human P450s (57). PEITC competitively inhibited P450 1A2 and, to a lesser extent, P450 2A6. PEITC was found to be a very strong noncompetitive inhibitor of P450 2B6. PEITC was also a noncompetitive inhibitor of P450 2C9, and was a mechanism-based inactivator of P450 2E1.

Nakajima's results are generally consistent with other studies. Smith et al. demonstrated that PEITC inhibited P450 1A2-catalyzed metabolism of NNK (58). We found that consumption of watercress, an abundant source of PEITC, altered NNK metabolism in smokers, consistent with inhibition of P450 1A2 (59,60). However, our results do not support an effect of watercress consumption on P450 2A6 activity in humans. Watercress consumption failed to alter metabolism of nicotine to cotinine, and did not significantly affect 7-hydroxylation of coumarin (61,62). Both of these reactions are catalyzed by P450 2A6. Others have observed the inhibitory effects of watercress consumption on P450 2E1-catalyzed reactions in humans (63,64).

The strong inhibitory effect of PEITC on P450 2B6 observed by Nakajima et al. is potentially interesting because this enzyme is a good catalyst of NNK activation (Murphy SE, unpublished data). Conaway et al. also observed that PEITC inhibited P450 2B1-related activities in rat liver microsomes (65).

The effects of BITC on rat and human P450s were studied by Hollenberg's group. BITC is a potent mechanism-based inactivator of rat P450 2B1; inactivation occurs primarily through protein modification (66). BITC is also a mechanism-based inactivator of rat P450s 1A1, 1A2, and 2E1 and human P450s 2B6 and 2D6. It was most effective in inactivating P450s 2B1, 2B6, 1A1, and 2E1. Analysis of BITC metabolites in the P450 2B1 reactions indicated that benzylamine was the major metabolite, suggesting conversion of BITC to benzyl isocyanate, which modified the P450 apoprotein or was hydrolyzed to benzylamine (67). In related work, the inactivation of P450 2E1 by *t*-butyl isothiocyanate was explored (68). The results suggested that *t*-butyl isothiocyanate inactivated P450 2E1 by binding to a critical active-site amino acid residue, which may have acted as the sixth ligand to heme, thus interfering with oxygen and substrate binding. PEITC inactivated P450 2E1, as well as a mutant in which the conserved threonine at position 303 was replaced by alanine (69). BITC did not inactivate the mutant, but inhibited it in a competitive manner. These results indicate differences in the mechanisms by which PEITC and BITC interact with P450 2E1.

Conaway et al. investigated the inhibition of P450-mediated reactions by thiol conjugates of isothiocyanates, which have chemopreventive properties that are analogous to those of the parent isothiocyanates (70). Inhibition of pentoxyresorufin O-dealkylation, for P450 2B1, and ethoxyresorufin O-dealkylation, for P450 1A1, roughly paralleled the extent of decomposition of the conjugates to their parent isothiocyanates, suggesting that the parent compounds were responsible for the observed inhibition.

3.2. Effects on Phase 2 Enzymes

Isothiocyanates accumulate in high concentrations in cultured cells, and the resulting levels are related to their abilities to induce phase 2 enzymes such as NAD(P)H:quinone reductase (QR) (71). The intracellular forms of sulforaphane and BITC were found to be dithiocarbamates resulting from GSH conjugation, suggesting that conjugation with GSH is responsible for accumulation of isothiocyanates in murine hepatoma cells (71). Initial uptake rates of four isothiocyanates in MCF-7 human breast cancer cells correlated with GSH conjugation, but not lipophilicity. It was concluded that GSH conjugation is the dominant mechanism affecting isothiocyanate uptake in cells (72). Intracellular accumulation of BITC, PEITC, sulforaphane and allyl isothiocyanate in mouse-skin papilloma cells correlated with elevations in GSH content, QR activity, and glutathione-*S*-transferase (GST) activity. The elevations were mediated by the DNA regulatory antioxidant/electrophile-response element (ARE/EpRE) (73).

Isothiocyanates are good inducers of QR. The 5'-promoter region of the human QR gene contains the *cis*-acting AP-1 and NFκB transcription factor-binding sites. Exposure of HT29 human colon cells to BITC caused an increase in AP-1 and NFκB binding, and activation of c-Jun N-terminal kinase (JNK), which phosphorylates c-Jun, a component of AP-1. These results suggest that JNK is involved in QR induction as an initial event that precedes an increase in transcription-factor binding (74). 6-(Methylsulfinyl)hexyl isothiocyanate, an active principal of wasabi, induced QR in Hepa 1c1c7 cells. Induction of QR transcription involved activation of ARE/EpRE (75). The related compounds 7-(methylsulfinyl)heptyl and 8-(methylsulfinyl)octyl isothiocyanates were also shown to be potent inducers of QR. These isothiocyanates are found in watercress at far lower concentrations than PEITC, but are stronger inducers of QR (76). Several other methyl(sulfinylalkyl) isothiocyanates were also shown to be inducers of QR (77). Sulforaphane was found to be a potent inducer of QR activity in human prostate-cancer-cell lines (78).

BITC is an inducer of GST activity. Nakamura et al. examined the induction of GST by BITC in rat liver epithelial RL34 cells (79). BITC specifically enhanced GSTP1. Addition of BITC to cells resulted in an immediate increase in reactive oxygen intermediates. With different isothiocyanates, the induction of *GSTP1* closely correlated with production of reactive oxygen intermediates. The *GSTP1* enhancer I-containing region was essential for induction of the *GSTP1* gene. These data suggest that production of reactive oxygen intermediates is involved in the induction of *GSTP1* by BITC. Expression of multidrug resistance-associated protein 2 (MRP2), which is an efflux pump that contributes to biliary secretion of xenobiotics, was increased in primary rat and human hepatocytes treated with sulforaphane. Sulforaphane-related formation of reactive oxygen intermediates may have contributed to the MRP2 induction (80).

Kong et al. and Kwak et al. have reviewed the activation of the ARE/EpRE present in many phase 2 genes (54,55). Basic leucine-zipper transcription factors, including nuclear factor-erythroid 2 (NF-E2)-related factor-1 (Nrf1), Nrf2, and small Maf, have been implicated in the binding and transcriptional activation of ARE/EpRE sequences. Activation of the mitogen-activated protein kinase (MAPK) pathway by various isothiocyanates—including PEITC, BITC, and sulforaphane—has been observed, ultimately leading to phase 2 enzyme induction via ARE/EpRE.

The favorable effects of isothiocyanates on phase 1 and phase 2 enzymes should be reflected in decreased DNA binding of carcinogens that are metabolized by these enzymes. Previous studies of isothiocyanate effects on NNK and NBMA provide support for this hypothesis (reviewed in ref. *1*). Decreased DNA binding of NNK in the mouse and rat lung is consistent with decreased lung tumorigenesis in animals treated with PEITC. This has been attributed to inhibition by PEITC of specific pulmonary P450s involved in the metabolic activation of NNK *(1)*. In a recent study, we investigated the effects of dietary BITC and PEITC on DNA adduct formation in A/J mice treated with a mixture of B[*a*]P and NNK *(33)*. Dietary PEITC, or dietary BITC plus PEITC, inhibited the formation of pyridyloxobutyl-DNA adducts of NNK. There were no effects of dietary isothiocyanates on levels of O^6-methylguanine (from NNK) or N^2-(7,8,9-trihydroxy-7,8,9,10-tetrahydrobenzo[*a*]pyrene-10-yl)deoxyguanosine (from B[*a*]P). These results were consistent with our previous studies of the effects of PEITC on NNK-DNA binding in rats, supporting a role for inhibition of pyridyloxobutyl-DNA adducts as a mechanism of inhibition of tumorigenesis by dietary PEITC or BITC plus PEITC. However, the observed inhibition was modest, suggesting that other effects of isothiocyanates were involved.

We also investigated the role of DNA adduct modification in the contrasting effects of BITC and PEITC on lung tumorigenesis in A/J mice treated with B[*a*]P *(81)*. As discussed previously, BITC but not PEITC inhibits B[*a*]P-induced tumorigenesis. DNA adducts were measured under conditions closely similar to those used in the tumor studies. Both BITC and PEITC inhibited B[*a*]P -DNA adduct formation in the lung. Inhibition was modest, and there was no difference between adduct levels in the mice treated with BITC and B[*a*]P vs PEITC and B[*a*]P. These results suggest that other effects of BITC may be involved in inhibition of B[*a*]P-induced lung tumorigenesis in the A/J mouse.

3.3. Other Cellular Effects

These results suggest that isothiocyanates have effects other than modification of DNA adduct formation that are important in chemoprevention. Prominent

among these is induction of apoptosis. A considerable body of evidence now indicates that isothiocyanates induce apoptosis in various systems. BITC and PEITC both induce sustained activation of JNK, and this is associated with induction of apoptosis in various cell types *(82)*. Treatment with isothiocyanates under conditions of apoptosis induction causes rapid and transient induction of caspase-3/CPP32-like activity *(83)*. PEITC induces apoptosis in mouse epidermal JB6 cells through a *p53*-dependent pathway *(84)*. PEITC induces apoptosis in human leukemia cells and inhibits cell growth in this system *(48,85)*. Further studies have shown that the formation of GSH conjugates of PEITC is important during the induction of apoptosis, and that this may lead to depletion of cellular GSH *(86)*. The caspase pathway plays an essential role, and the JNK pathway a supporting role in the induction of apoptosis in HL60 cells by PEITC and allyl isothiocyanate *(87)*. A recent study demonstrates that PEITC further increases apoptosis induced in the respiratory tract of rats by cigarette smoke *(88)*. BITC and sulforaphane induce apoptosis in human colon cancer cells (89–91).

Yang et al. investigated the effects of the NAC conjugates of BITC and PEITC on molecular events associated with apoptosis in the A/J mouse lung *(47)*. Both compounds inhibited B[*a*]P-induced lung tumorigenesis when administered after the carcinogen. There was a significant increase in apoptosis in the lung. The MAPK pathway was activated in animals treated with the NAC conjugates. The phosphorylation of *p38* and extracellular signal-regulated kinases (ErKs) 1 and 2 was also induced, and AP-1 activity was increased. Phosphorylation of *p53* was also higher in the groups treated with the NAC conjugates of BITC and PEITC.

Sulforaphane has antiinflammatory properties. It decreased lipopolysaccharide-induced secretion of pro-inflammatory and pro-carcinogenic signaling factors in cultured Raw 264.7 macrophages. It caused reduction of inducible nitric oxide synthase (iNOS) and cyclooxygenase (COX-2) protein expression. NFκB was identified as the key mediator of these responses *(92)*.

It is apparent that isothiocyanates affect a number of signal-transduction pathways. Kong et al. hypothesize that at low concentrations, isothiocyanates and other chemopreventive agents may activate the MAPK pathway, leading to induction of gene expression such as phase 2 enzymes resulting in protection or survival mechanisms *(93)*. At higher concentrations, they will activate the MAPK pathway and the caspase pathway will also be activated, leading to apoptotic cell death. This intriguing hypothesis merits further investigation.

3.4. Isothiocyanate Metabolism and its Relationship to Epidemiologic Results

Conjugation of isothiocyanates with GSH and excretion in the urine as NAC conjugates is a well-established metabolic pathway for BITC, PEITC, and allyl isothiocyanate in rats and humans (45,94–99). The disposition and pharmacokinetics of PEITC and PHITC were compared in rats with the goal of gaining insight into the higher efficacy of PHITC as a chemopreventive agent against lung cancer (100). In contrast to PEITC, a relatively small proportion of PHITC metabolites was excreted in urine, and higher effective doses of PHITC were found in the lung and other tissues, which may in part explain its higher activity.

Chung and colleagues have developed a urinary biomarker for total isothiocyanates in human urine (101). Results of analyses of human urine for this biomarker correlated well with levels of NAC conjugates of PEITC or allyl isothiocyanate that were independently analyzed. Application of this assay to urine samples from Singapore residents demonstrated a highly significant positive association between dietary intake and urinary excretion levels of total isothiocyanates (102). Levels of total isothiocyanates in the urine of individuals who consumed fresh or cooked watercress, or fresh or steamed broccoli, were compared. The results demonstrate that, because of the inactivation of myrosinase during cooking or steaming, the total isothiocyanate dose is considerably less upon consumption of cooked or steamed vegetables compared to raw vegetables (103,104). Broccoli sprouts were shown to be a good source of glucosinolates and isothiocyanates, based on analysis of their urinary NAC conjugates (105).

GSH conjugation is important in isothiocyanate metabolism. GSTM1, GSTP1, GSTA1, and GSTA2 are involved to varying extents in the catalysis of isothiocyanate conjugation with GSH (106). These genes are polymorphic in the human population (107–109). It is proposed that individuals with low or null activity would have higher levels of free circulating isothiocyanates, and could potentially be protected against cancer more effectively than those in whom the isothiocyanates were conjugated (110). Lin et al. demonstrated that individuals exposed to dietary broccoli and who have the GSTM1-null phenotype are less at risk for colon cancer than those who are GSTM1-positive (111). This is consistent with a lower conjugation of isothiocyanates in the GSTM1-null individuals. These results demonstrate the potential confounding effects of GST genotype, since GSTM1-null individuals would also be expected to detoxify carcinogens less readily, and therefore would be at higher risk. There is a balance between GST catalysis of isothiocyanate conjugation vs carcinogen detoxification.

Three recent epidemiologic studies have examined the relationship between isothiocyanate intake, GST genotype, and lung cancer. London et al. examined the relationship between total isothiocyanate concentrations in urine, collected before diagnosis, and the subsequent risk of lung cancer among 232 incident cases of lung cancer and 710 matched controls from a cohort of 18,244 men in Shanghai, China (3). Individuals with detectable isothiocyanates in urine were at decreased risk of lung cancer, and the protective effect was seen primarily among individuals with homozygous deletion of GSTM1, and particularly with deletion of both GSTM1 and GSTT1. Spitz et al. examined the relationship of isothiocyanate consumption and GST status to lung cancer in 503 newly diagnosed lung cancer cases and 465 controls (4). Cases reported significantly lower isothiocyanate intake per day than controls. Low isothiocyanate intake and GSTM1- and GSTT1-null genotypes were associated with increased lung cancer risk in current smokers. Zhao et al. evaluated the link between dietary isothiocyanate intake, GSTM1 and GSTT1 polymorphisms, and lung cancer risk in 420 Chinese women (5). Higher weekly intake of isothiocyanates reduced the risk of lung cancer to a greater extent in smokers than in nonsmokers. The inverse association was stronger among subjects with homozygous deletion of GSTM1 and/or GSTT1. These results illustrate the complexity of gene-carcinogen and gene-chemopreventive agent interactions in molecular epidemiology. However, there generally was a consistent relationship between isothiocyanate intake and decreased cancer risk.

4. CONCLUSIONS

Isothiocyanates are now firmly established as effective chemopreventive agents in a wide range of animal models. Inhibition is observed in many different tissues and in animals treated with a variety of carcinogens. Complete inhibition of tumor formation is not an unusual occurrence in these studies. Although some isothiocyanates can enhance carcinogenesis in certain models, the overwhelming proportion of evidence is toward protection. A large body of evidence clearly demonstrates that isothiocyanates can inhibit specific cytochrome P450 enzymes responsible for carcinogen activation, and can induce a variety of phase 2 enzymes responsible for carcinogen detoxification. The mechanisms of inhibition and induction are now very well understood. These combined properties can explain much of the observed tumor-inhibitory effects of isothiocyanates. However, a rapidly increasing number of studies now indicate that isothiocyanates as well as their NAC conjugates have cellular effects above and beyond the alteration of carcinogen metabolism. Isothiocyanates induce a cascade of signal-transduction events that lead to apoptosis. Other potentially beneficial effects have also been observed. Humans receive large doses of isothiocyanates upon consumption of normal amounts of cruciferous vegetables. Robust biomarkers for quantifying these doses are now available. The application of these biomarkers in epidemiologic studies and consideration of gene-isothiocyanate interactions have produced encouraging results indicating that isothiocyanates protect against cancer in humans.

ACKNOWLEDGMENT

Research in the author's laboratory on isothiocyanates is supported by NCI grant CA-46535 from the National Cancer Institute.

REFERENCES

1. Hecht SS. Inhibition of carcinogenesis by isothiocyanates. *Drug Metabol Rev 2000*; 32:395–411.
2. Fahey JW, Zalcmann AT, Talalay P. The chemical diversity and distribution of glucosinolates and isothiocyanates among plants. *Phytochemistry* 2001;56:5–51.
3. London SJ, Yuan JM, Chung FL, et al. Isothiocyanates, glutathione *S*-transferase M1 and T1 polymorphisms, and lung-cancer risk: a prospective study of men in Shanghai, China. *Lancet* 2000;356:724–729.
4. Spitz MR, Duphorne CM, Detry MA, et al. Dietary intake of isothiocyanates: evidence of a joint effect with glutathione *S*-transferase polymorphisms in lung cancer risk. *Cancer Epidemiol Biomarkers Prev* 2000;9:1017–1020.
5. Zhao B, Seow A, Lee EJ, et al. Dietary isothiocyanates, glutathione *S*-transferase -M1, -T1 polymorphisms and lung cancer risk among Chinese women in Singapore. *Cancer Epidemiol Biomark Prev* 2001;10:1063–1067.
6. Verhoeven DTH, Goldbohm RA, van Poppel G, et al. Epidemiological studies on *Brassica* vegetables and cancer risk. *Cancer Epidemiol Biomark Prev* 1996;5:733–748.
7. Tookey HL, VanEtten CH, Daxenbichler ME. Glucosinolates, in *Toxic Constituents of Plant Stuffs.* Liener IE, ed. Academic Press, New York, 1980, pp.103–142.
8. Fenwick GR, Heaney RK, Mawson R. Glucosinolates, in *Toxicants of Plant Origin, vol. II: Glycosides.* Cheeke PR, ed. CRC Press, Inc., Boca Raton, FL 1989,pp. 2–41.
9. Wattenberg LW. Inhibition of carcinogenic effects of polycyclic hydrocarbons by benzyl isothiocyanate and related compounds. *J Natl Cancer Inst* 1977;58:395–398.
10. Wattenberg LW. Inhibition of carcinogen-induced neoplasia by sodium cyanate, tert-butyl isocyanate, and benzyl isothiocyanate administered subsequent to carcinogen exposure. *Cancer Res* 1981;41:2991–2994.
11. Lin JM, Amin S, Trushin N, Hecht SS. Effects of isothiocyanates on tumorigenesis by benzo[a]pyrene in murine tumor models. *Cancer Lett* 1993;74:151–159.
12. Wattenberg LW. Inhibitory effects of benzyl isothiocyanate administered shortly before diethylnitrosamine or benzo[a]pyrene on pulmonary and forestomach neoplasia in A/J mice. *Carcinogenesis* 1987;8:1971–1973.
13. Hecht SS, Kenney PMJ, Wang M, Upadhyaya P. Benzyl isothiocyanate: an effective inhibitor of polycyclic aromatic hydrocarbon tumorigenesis in A/J mouse lung. *Cancer Lett* 2002;187:87–94.
14. Hecht SS. Tobacco smoke carcinogens and lung cancer. *J Natl Cancer Inst* 1999;91:1194–1210.
15. International Agency for Research on Cancer. Polynuclear Aromatic Compounds, Part 1, Chemical, Environmental, and Experimental Data. IARC Monographs on the Evaluation of the Carcinogenic Risk of Chemicals to Humans. Lyon, France, IARC, 1983, pp. 62–66.
16. Morse MA, Amin SG, Hecht SS, Chung FL. Effects of aromatic isothiocyanates on tumorigenicity, O^6-methylguanine formation, and metabolism of the tobacco-specific nitrosamine 4-(methylnitrosamino)-1-(3-pyridyl)-1-butanone in A/J mouse lung. *Cancer Res* 1989;49:2894–2897.
17. Morse MA, Reinhardt JC, Amin SG, et al. Effect of dietary aromatic isothiocyanates fed subsequent to the administration of 4-(methylnitrosamino)-1-(3-pyridyl)-1-butanone on lung tumorigenicity in mice. *Cancer Lett* 1990;49:225–230.
18. Wilkinson JT, Morse MA, Kresty LA, Stoner GD. Effect of alkyl chain length on inhibition of *N*-nitrosomethylbenzylamine-induced esophageal tumorigenesis and DNA methylation by isothiocyanates. *Carcinogenesis* 1995;16:1011–1015.
19. Sugie S, Okumura A, Tanaka T, Mori H. Inhibitory effects of benzyl isothiocyanate and benzyl thiocyanate on diethylnitrosamine-induced hepatocarcinogenesis in rats. *Jpn J Cancer* Res 1993;84:865–870.
20. Hirose M, Yamaguchi T, Kimoto N, et al. Strong promoting activity of phenylethyl isothiocyanate and benzyl isothiocyanate on urinary bladder carcinogenesis in F344 male rats. *Int J Cancer* 1998;77:773–777.
21. Hecht SS, Kenney PMJ, Wang W, et al. Effects of phenethyl isothiocyanate and benzyl isothiocyanate, individually and in combination, on lung tumorigenesis induced in A/J mice by benzo[a]pyrene and 4-(methylnitrosamino)-1-(3-pyridyl)-1-butanone. *Cancer Lett* 1999;150:49–56.
22. Chung FL, Kelloff G, Steele V, et al. Chemopreventive efficacy of arylalkyl isothiocyanates and N-acetylcysteine for lung tumorigenesis in Fischer rats. *Cancer Res* 1996;56:772–778.
23. Hecht SS, Trushin N, Rigotty J, et al. Complete inhibition of 4-(methylnitrosamino)-1-(3-pyridyl)-1-butanone induced rat

lung tumorigenesis and favorable modification of biomarkers by phenethyl isothiocyanate. *Cancer Epidemiol Biomarkers Prev* 1996;5:645–652.

24. Morse MA, Wang CX, Stoner GD, et al. Inhibition of 4-(methylnitrosamino)-1-(3-pyridyl)-1-butanone-induced DNA adduct formation and tumorigenicity in lung of F344 rats by dietary phenethyl isothiocyanate. *Cancer Res* 1989;49:549–553.

25. Morse MA, Eklind KI, Amin SG, et al. Effects of alkyl chain length on the inhibition of NNK-induced lung neoplasia in A/J mice by arylalkyl isothiocyanates. *Carcinogenesis* 1989;10:1757–1759.

26. Morse MA, Eklind KI, Hecht SS, et al. Structure-activity relationships for inhibition of 4-(methylnitrosamino)-1-(3-pyridyl)-1-butanone lung tumorigenesis by arylalkyl isothiocyanates in A/J mice. *Cancer Res* 1991;51:1846–1850.

27. Stoner GD, Morrissey D, Heur YH, et al. Inhibitory effects of phenethyl isothiocyanate on N-nitrosobenzylmethylamine carcinogenesis in the rat esophagus. *Cancer Res* 1991;51:2063–2068.

28. Nishikawa A, Furukawa F, Uneyama C, et al. Chemopreventive effects of phenethyl isothiocyanate on lung and pancreatic tumorigenesis in N-nitrosobis(2-oxopropyl)amine-treated hamsters. *Carcinogenesis* 1996;17:1381–1384.

29. Adam-Rodwell G, Morse MA, Stoner GD. The effects of phenethyl isothiocyanate on benzo[a]pyrene-induced tumors and DNA adducts in A/J mouse lung. *Cancer Lett* 1993;71:35–42.

30. Lubet RA, Steele VE, Eto I, et al. Chemopreventive efficacy of anethole trithione, N-acetyl-L-cysteine, miconazole and phenethylisothiocyanate in the DMBA-induced rat mammary cancer model. *Int J Cancer* 1997;72:95–101.

31. Futakuchi M, Hirose M, Miki T, et al. Inhibition of DMBA-initiated rat mammary tumour development by 1-O-hexyl-2,3,5-trimethylhydroquinone, phenylethyl isothiocyanate, and novel synthetic ascorbic acid derivatives. *Eur J Cancer Prev* 1998;7:153–159.

32. El Bayoumy K, Upadhyaya P, Desai DH, et al. Effects of 1,4-phenylenebis(methylene)selenocyanate, phenethyl isothiocyanate, indole-3-carbinol, and d-limonene individually and in combination on the tumorigenicity of the tobacco-specific nitrosamine 4-(methylnitrosamino)-1-(3-pyridyl)-1-butanone in A/J mouse lung. *Anticancer Res* 1996;16:2709–2712.

33. Sticha KRK, Kenney PMJ, Boysen G, et al. Effects of benzyl isothiocyanate and phenethyl isothiocyanate on DNA adduct formation by a mixture of benzo[a]pyrene and 4-(methylnitrosamino)-1-(3-pyridyl)-1-butanone in A/J mouse lung. *Carcinogenesis* 2002;23:1433–1439.

34. Witschi H. Successful and not so successful chemoprevention of tobacco smoke-induced lung tumors. *Exp Lung Res* 2000;26:743–755.

35. International Agency for Research on Cancer. Tobacco Smoking. IARC Monographs on the Evaluation of the Carcinogenic Risk of Chemicals to Humans. Lyon, FR: IARC, 1986;37–375.

36. Stoner GD, Adams C, Kresty LA, et al. Inhibition of N'-nitrosonornicotine-induced esophageal tumorigenesis by 3-phenylpropyl isothiocyanate. *Carcinogenesis* 1998;19:2139–2143.

37. Hecht SS, Upadhyaya P, Wang M, et al. Inhibition of lung tumorigenesis in A/J mice by N-acetyl-S-(N-2-phenethylthiocarbamoyl)-L-cysteine and *myo*-inositol, individually and in combination. *Carcinogenesis* 2002;23:1455–1461.

38. Nishikawa A, Furukawa F, Ikezaki S, et al. Chemopreventive effects of 3-phenylpropyl isothiocyanate on hamster lung tumorigenesis initiated with N-nitrosobis(2-oxopropyl)amine. *Jpn J Cancer Res* 1996;87:122–126.

39. Zhang Y, Kensler TW, Cho CG, et al. Anticarcinogenic activities of sulforaphane and structurally related synthetic norbornyl isothiocyanates. *Proc Natl Acad Sci USA* 1994;91:3147–3150.

40. Chung FL, Jiao D, Conaway CC, et al. Chemopreventive potential of thiol conjugates of isothiocyanates for lung cancer and a urinary biomarker of dietary isothiocyanates. *J Cell Biochem* [suppl] 1997;27:76–85.

41. Chung FL, Conaway CC, Rao CV, Reddy BS. Chemoprevention of colonic aberrant crypt foci in Fischer rats by sulforaphane and phenethyl isothiocyanate. *Carcinogenesis* 2000;21:2287–2291.

42. Jiao D, Eklind KI, Choi CI, et al. Structure-activity relationships of isothiocyanates as mechanism-based inhibitors of 4-(methylnitrosamino)-1-(3-pyridyl)-1-butanone-induced lung tumorigenesis in A/J mice. *Cancer Res* 1994;54:4327–4333.

43. Son HY, Nishikawa A, Furukawa F, et al. Modifying effects of 4-phenylbutyl isothiocyanate on N-nitrosobis(2-oxopropyl)amine-induced tumorigenesis in hamsters. *Cancer Lett* 2000;160:141–147.

44. Jiao D, Smith TJ, Kim S, et al. The essential role of the functional group in alkyl isothiocyanates for inhibition of tobacco-nitrosamine-induced lung tumorigenesis. *Carcinogenesis* 1996;17:755–759.

45. Brüsewitz G, Cameron BD, Chasseaud LF, et al. The metabolism of benzyl isothiocyanate and its cysteine conjugate. *Biochem J* 1977;162:99–107.

46. Jiao D, Smith TJ, Yang CS, et al. Chemopreventive activity of thiol conjugates of isothiocyanates for lung tumorigenesis. *Carcinogenesis* 1997;18:2143–2147.

47. Yang Y-M, Conaway CC, Chiao JW, et al. Inhibition of benzo(a)pyrene-induced lung tumorigenesis in A/J mice by dietary N-acetylcysteine conjugates of benzyl and phenethyl isothiocyanates during the post-initiation phase is associated with activation of MAP kinases and p53 activity and induction of apoptosis. *Cancer Res* 2002;62:2–7.

48. Chiao JW, Chung FL, Krzeminski J, et al. Modulation of growth of human prostate cancer cells by the N-acetylcysteine conjugate of phenethyl isothiocyanate. *Int J Oncol* 2000;16:1215–1219.

49. Xu K, Thornalley PJ. Studies on the mechanism of the inhibition of human leukaemia cell growth by dietary isothiocyanates and their cysteine adducts in vitro. *Biochem Pharmacol* 2000;60:221–231.

50. Stoner GD, Siglin JC, Morse MA, et al. Enhancement of esophageal carcinogenesis in male F344 rats by dietary phenylhexyl isothiocyanate. *Carcinogenesis* 1995;16:2473–2476.

51. Rao CV, Rivenson A, Simi B, et al. Enhancement of experimental colon carcinogenesis by dietary 6-phenylhexyl isothiocyanate. *Cancer Res* 1995;55:4311–4318.

52. Hudson TS, Carlton PS, Gupta A, et al. Investigation of the enhancement of N-nitrosomethylbenzylamine-induced esophageal tumorigenesis by 6-phenylhexyl isothiocyanate. *Cancer Lett* 2001;162:19–26.

53. Smith TJ, Yang CS. Effect of organosulfur compounds from garlic and cruciferous vegetables on drug metabolism enzymes. *Drug Metabol Drug Interact* 2000;17:23–49.

54. Kwak MK, Egner PA, Dolan PM, et al. Role of phase 2 enzyme induction in chemoprotection by dithiolethiones. *Mutat Res* 2001;480-481:305–315.

55. Zhang Y, Talalay P. Anticarcinogenic activities of organic isothiocyanates: chemistry and mechanism. *Cancer Res* [suppl] 1994;54:1976s–1981s.

56. Kong AN, Owuor E, Yu R, et al. Induction of xenobiotic enzymes by the map kinase pathway and the antioxidant or electrophile response element (ARE/EpRE). *Drug Metab Rev* 2001;33:255–271.

57. Nakajima M, Yoshida R, Shimada N, et al. Inhibition and inactivation of human cytochrome P450 isoforms by phenethyl isothiocyanate. *Drug Metab Dispos* 2001;29:1110–1113.

58. Smith TJ, Guo Z, Guengerich FP, Yang CS. Metabolism of 4-(methylnitrosamino)-1-(3-pyridyl)-1-butanone (NNK) by human cytochrome P450 1A2 and its inhibition by phenethyl isothiocyanate. *Carcinogenesis* 1996;17:809–813.

59. Hecht SS, Chung FL, Richie JP Jr, et al. Effects of watercress consumption on metabolism of a tobacco-specific lung carcinogen in smokers. *Cancer Epidemiol Biomarkers Prev* 1995;4:877–884.

60. Carmella SG, Borukhova A, Akerkar SA, Hecht SS. Analysis of human urine for pyridine-*N*-oxide metabolites of 4-(methylnitrosamino)-1-(3-pyridyl)-1-butanone, a tobacco-specific lung carcinogen. *Cancer Epidemiol Biomark Prev* 1997;6:113–120.

61. Hecht SS, Carmella SG, Murphy SE. Effects of watercress consumption on urinary metabolites of nicotine in smokers. *Cancer Epidemiol Biomark Prev* 1999;8:907–913.

62. Murphy SE, Johnson LM, Losey LM, et al. Effects of watercress consumption on coumarin metabolism in humans. *Drug Metab Dispos* 2001;29:786–788.

63. Chen L, Mohr SN, Yang CS. Decrease of plasma and urinary oxidative metabolites of acetaminophen after consumption of watercress by human volunteers. *Clin Pharmacol Ther* 1996;60:651–660.

64. Leclercq I, Desager JP, Horsmans Y. Inhibition of chlorzoxazone metabolism, a clinical probe for CYP2E1, by a single ingestion of watercress. *Clin Pharmacol Ther* 1998;64:144–149.

65. Conaway CC, Jiao D, Chung FL. Inhibition of rat liver cytochrome P450 isozymes by isothiocyanates and their conjugates: a structure-activity relationship study. *Carcinogenesis* 1996;17:2423–2427.

66. Goosen TC, Kent UM, Brand L, Hollenberg PF. Inactivation of cytochrome P450 2B1 by benzyl isothiocyanate, a chemopreventative agent from cruciferous vegetables. *Chem Res Toxicol* 2000;13:1349–1359.

67. Goosen TC, Mills DE, Hollenberg PF. Effects of benzyl isothiocyanate on rat and human cytochromes P450: identification of metabolites formed by P450 2B1. *J Pharmacol Exp Ther* 2001;296:198–206.

68. Kent UM, Roberts-Kirchhoff ES, et al. Spectral studies of tert-butyl isothiocyanate-inactivated P450 2E1. *Biochemistry* 2001;40:7253–7261.

69. Moreno RL, Goosen T, Kent UM, et al. Differential effects of naturally occurring isothiocyanates on the activities of

cytochrome P450 2E1 and the mutant P450 2E1 T303A. *Arch Biochem Biophys* 2001;391:99–110.

70. Conaway CC, Krzeminski J, Amin S, Chung FL. Decomposition rates of isothiocyanate conjugates determine their activity as inhibitors of cytochrome P450 enzymes. *Chem Res Toxicol* 2001;14:1170–1176.

71. Zhang Y. Role of glutathione in the accumulation of anticarcinogenic isothiocyanates and their glutathione conjugates by murine hepatoma cells. *Carcinogenesis* 2000;21:1175–118.

72. Zhang Y. Molecular mechanism of rapid cellular accumulation of anticarcinogenic isothiocyanates. *Carcinogenesis* 2001;22:425–431.

73. Ye L, Zhang Y. Total intracellular accumulation levels of dietary isothiocyanates determine their activity in elevation of cellular glutathione and induction of Phase 2 detoxification enzymes. *Carcinogenesis* 2001;22:1987–1992.

74. Patten EJ, DeLong MJ. Temporal effects of the detoxification enzyme inducer, benzyl isothiocyanate: activation of c-Jun *N*-terminal kinase prior to the transcription factors AP-1 and NF kappa B. *Biochem Biophys Res Commun* 1999;257:149–155.

75. Hou DX, Fukuda M, Fujii M, Fuke Y. Transcriptional regulation of nicotinamide adenine dinucleotide phosphate: quinone oxidoreductase in murine hepatoma cells by 6-(methylsufinyl)hexyl isothiocyanate, an active principle of wasabi (Eutrema wasabi Maxim). *Cancer Lett* 2000;161:195–200.

76. Rose P, Faulkner K, Williamson G, Mithen R. 7-Methylsulfinylheptyl and 8-methylsulfinyloctyl isothiocyanates from watercress are potent inducers of phase II enzymes. *Carcinogenesis* 2000;21:1983–1988.

77. Hou DX, Fukuda M, Fujii M, Fuke Y. Induction of NADPH:quinone oxidoreductase in murine hepatoma cells by methylsulfinyl isothiocyanates: methyl chain length-activity study. *Int J Mol Med* 2000;6:441–444.

78. Brooks JD, Paton VG, Vidanes G. Potent induction of phase 2 enzymes in human prostate cells by sulforaphane. *Cancer Epidemiol Biomark Prev* 2001;10:949–954.

79. Nakamura Y, Ohigashi H, Masuda S, et al. Redox regulation of glutathione S-transferase induction by benzyl isothiocyanate: correlation of enzyme induction with the formation of reactive oxygen intermediates. *Cancer Res* 2001;60:219–225.

80. Payen L, Courtois A, Loewert M, et al. Reactive oxygen species-related induction of multidrug resistance-associated protein 2 expression in primary hepatocytes exposed to sulforaphane. *Biochem Biophys Res Commun* 2001;282:257–263.

81. Sticha KR, Staretz ME, Liang H, et al. Effects of benzyl isothiocyanate and phenethyl isothiocyanate on benzyl[*a*]pyrene metabolism and DNA adduct formation in the A/J mouse. *Carcinogenesis* 2000;21:1719–1711.

82. Chen YR, Wang W, Kong ANT, Tan TH. Molecular mechanisms of c-Jun *N*-terminal kinase-mediated apoptosis induced by anticarcinogenic isothiocyanates. *J Biol Chem* 1998;273:1769–1775.

83. Yu R, Mandlekar S, Harvey KJ, et al. Chemopreventive isothiocyanates induce apoptosis and caspase-3-like protease activity. *Cancer Res* 1998;58:402–408.

84. Huang C, Ma W, Li J, et al. Essential role of p53 in phenethyl isothiocyanate (PEITC)-induced apoptosis. *Cancer Res* 1998;58:4102–4106.

85. Xu K, Thornalley PJ. Inhibition of leukaemia growth and apoptosis induced by phenethyl isothiocyanate and cysteine conjugate. *Br J Cancer* 1999;81:574–575.

86. Xu K, Thornalley PJ. Involvement of glutathione metabolism in the cytotoxicity of the phenethyl isothiocyanate and its cysteine conjugate to human leukaemia cells in vitro. *Biochem Pharmacol* 2001;61:165–177.

87. Xu K, Thornalley PJ. Signal transduction activated by the cancer chemopreventive isothiocyanates: cleavage of BID protein, tyrosine phosphorylation and activation of JNK. *Br J Cancer* 2001;84:670–673.

88. D'Agostini F, Balansky RM, Izzotti A, et al. Modulation of apoptosis by cigarette smoke and cancer chemopreventive agents in the respiratory tract of rats. *Carcinogenesis* 2001;22:375–380.

89. Kirlin WG, Cai J, DeLong M, et al. Dietary compounds that induce cancer preventive phase 2 enzymes activate apoptosis at comparable doses in HT29 colon carcinoma cells. *J Nutr* 1999;129:1827–1835.

90. Bonnesen C, Eggleston IM, Hayes JD. Dietary indoles and isothiocyanates that are generated from cruciferous vegetables can both stimulate apoptosis and confer protection against DNA damage in human colon cell lines. *Cancer Res* 2001;61:6120–6130.

91. Gamet-Payrastre L, Li P, Lumeau S, et al. Sulforaphane, a naturally occurring isothiocyanate, induces cell cycle arrest and apoptosis in HT29 human colon cancer cells. *Cancer Res* 2000; 60:1426–1433.

92. Heiss E, Herhaus C, Klimo K, et al. Nuclear factor kappa B is a molecular target for sulforaphane-mediated anti-inflammatory mechanisms. *J Biol Chem* 2001;276:32,008–32,015.

93. Kong AN, Yu R, Hebbar V, et al. Signal transduction events elicited by cancer prevention compounds. *Mutat Res* 2001;480–481:231–241.

94. Gorler K, Krumbiegel G, Mennicke WH. The metabolism of benzyl isothiocyanate and its cysteine conjugate in guinea-pigs and rabbits. *Xenobiotica* 1982;12:535–542.

95. Mennicke WH, Gorler K, Krumbiegel G. Metabolism of some naturally occurring isothiocyanates in the rat. *Xenobiotica* 1983;13:203–207.

96. Mennicke WH, Görler K, Krumbiegel G, et al. Studies on the metabolism and excretion of benzyl isothiocyanate in man. *Xenobiotica* 1988;18:441–447.

97. Ioannou YM, Burka LT, Matthews HB. Allyl isothiocyanate: comparative disposition in rats and mice. *Toxicol Appl Pharmacol* 1984;75:173–181.

98. Eklind KI, Morse MA, Chung FL. Distribution and metabolism of the natural anticarcinogen phenethyl isothiocyanate in A/J mice. *Carcinogenesis* 1990;11:2033–2036.

99. Chung FL, Morse MA, Eklind KI, Lewis J. Quantitation of human uptake of the anticarcinogen phenethyl isothiocyanate after a watercress meal. *Cancer Epidemiol Biomark Prev* 1992;1:383–388.

100. Conaway CC, Jiao D, Kohri T, et al. Disposition and pharmacokinetics of phenethyl isothiocyanate and 6-phenylhexyl isothiocyanate in F344 rats. *Drug Metabol Dispos* 1999;27:13–20.

101. Chung FL, Jiao D, Getahun SM, Yu MC. A urinary biomarker for uptake of dietary isothiocyanates in humans. *Cancer Epidemiol Biomark Prev* 1998;7:103–108.

102. Seow A, Shi CY, Chung FL, et al. Urinary total isothiocyanate (ITC) in a population-based sample of middle-aged and older Chinese in Singapore: relationship with dietary total ITC and glutathione *S*-transferase M1/T1/P1 genotypes. *Cancer Epidemiol Biomark Prev* 1998;7:775–781.

103. Getahun SM, Chung FL. Conversion of glucosinolates to isothiocyanates in humans after ingestion of cooked watercress. *Cancer Epidemiol Biomark Prev* 1999;8:447–451.

104. Conaway CC, Getahun SM, Liebes LL, et al. Disposition of glucosinolates and sulforaphane in humans after ingestion of steamed and fresh broccoli. *Nutr Cancer* 2000;38:168–178.

105. Shapiro TA, Fahey JW, Wade KL, et al. Chemoprotective glucosinolates and isothiocyanates of broccoli sprouts: metabolism and excretion in humans. *Cancer Epidemiol Biomark Prev* 2001;10:501–508.

106. Meyer DJ, Crease DJ, Ketterer B. Forward and reverse catalysis and product sequestration by human glutathione *S*-transferases in the reaction of GSH with dietary aralkyl isothiocyanates. *Biochem J* 1995;306:565–569.

107. Spivack SD, Fasco MJ, Walker VE, Kaminsky LS. The molecular epidemiology of lung cancer. *Crit Rev Toxicol* 1997;27:319–365.

108. Watson MA, Stewart RK, Smith GBJ, et al. Human glutathione *S*-transferase P1 polymorphisms: relationship to lung tissue enzyme activity and population frequency distribution. *Carcinogenesis* 1998;19:275–280.

109. Coles BF, Morel F, Rauch C, et al. Effect of polymorphism in the human glutathione *S*-transferase A1 promoter on hepatic GSTA1 and GSTA2 expression. *Pharmacogenetics* 2001;11:663–669.

110. Ketterer B. Dietary isothiocyanates as confounding factors in the molecular epidemiology of colon cancer. *Cancer Epidemiol Biomark Prev* 1998;7:645–646.

111. Lin HJ, Probst-Hensch NM, Louie AD et al. Glutathione transferase null genotype, broccoli, and lower prevalence of colorectal adenomas. *Cancer Epidemiol Biomark Prev* 1998;7:647–652.

112. Sasaki S. Inhibitory effects by α-naphthyl-isothiocyanate on liver tumorigenesis in rats treated with 3'-methyl-4-dimethylaminoazobenzene. *J Nara Med Assoc* 1963;14:101–2115.

113. Sidransky H, Ito N, Verney E. Influence of α-naphthyl-isothiocyanate on liver tumorigenesis in rats ingesting ethionine and *N*-2-fluorenylacetamide. *J Natl Cancer Inst* 1966;37:677–686.

114. Lacassagne A, Hurst L, Xuong MD. Inhibition, par deux naphthylisothiocyanates, de l'hepatocancérogenèse produit, chez le rat, par le p-diméthylaminoazobenzène (DAB). *C R Séances Society Biol Fil* 1970;164:230–233.

115. Ito N, Hiasa Y, Konishi Y, Marugami M. The development of carcinoma in liver of rats treated with m-toluylenediamine and the synergistic and antagonistic effects with other chemicals. *Cancer Res* 1969;29:1137–1145.

116. Makiura S, Kamamoto Y, Sugihara S, et al. Effect of 1-naphthyl isothiocyanate and 3-methylcholanthrene on hepatocarcinogenesis in rats treated with diethylnitrosoamine. *Jpn J Cancer Res* 1973;64:101–104.

117. Ito N, Matayoshi K, Matsumura K, et al. Effect of various carcinogenic and non-carcinogenic substances on development of bladder tumors in rats induced by *N*-butyl-*N*-(4-

hydroxybutyl)nitrosoamine. *Jpn J Cancer Res* 1974; 65:123–130.

118. Sugie S, Okamoto K, Okumura A, et al. Inhibitory effects of benzyl thiocyanate and benzyl isothiocyanate on methylazoxymethanol acetate-induced intestinal carcinogenesis in rats. *Carcinogenesis* 1994;15:1555–1560.

119. Morse MA, Eklind KI, Amin SG, Chung FL. Effect of frequency of isothiocyanate administration on inhibition of 4-(methylnitrosamino)-1-(3-pyridyl)-1-butanone-induced pulmonary adenoma formation in A/J mice. *Cancer Lett* 1992;62:77–81.

120. Matzinger SA, Crist KA, Stoner GD, et al. K-ras mutations in lung tumors from A/J and A/JxTSG-*p53* F$_1$ mice treated with 4-(methylnitrosamino)-1-(3-pyridyl)-1-butanone and phenethyl isothiocyanate. *Carcinogenesis* 1995;16:2487–2492.

121. Pereira MA. Chemoprevention of diethylnitrosamine-induced liver foci and hepatocellular adenomas in C3H mice. *Anticancer Res* 1995;15:1953–1956.

122. Siglin JC, Barch DH, Stoner GD. Effects of dietary phenethyl isothiocyanate, ellagic acid, sulindac and calcium on the induction and progression of *N*-nitrosomethylbenzylamine-induced esophageal carcinogenesis in rats. *Carcinogenesis* 1995;16:1101–1106.

123. Nishikawa A, Furukawa F, Kasahara K, et al. Failure of phenethyl isothiocyanate to inhibit hamster tumorigenesis induced by *N*-nitroso*bis*(2-oxopropyl)amine when given during the post-initiation phase. *Cancer Lett* 1999;141:109–115.

124. Witschi H, Espiritu I, Yu M, Willits NH. The effects of phenethyl isothiocyanate, *N*-acetylcysteine and green tea on tobacco smoke-induced lung tumors in strain A/J mice. *Carcinogenesis* 1998;19:1789–1794.

125. Hecht SS, Trushin N, Rigotty J, et al. Inhibitory effects of 6-phenylhexyl isothiocyanate on 4-(metshylnitrosamino)-1-(3-pyridyl)-1-butanone metabolic activation and lung tumorigenesis in rats. *Carcinogenesis* 1996;17:2061–2067.

126. Yano T, Yajima S, Virgona N, et al. The effect of 6-methylthiohexyl isothiocyanate isolated from *Wasabia japonica* (wasabi) on 4-(methylnitrosamino)-1-(3-pyridyl)-1-buatnone-induced lung tumorigenesis in mice. *Cancer Lett* 2000;155:115–120

3

Antigenotoxic and Cancer Preventive Mechanisms of *N*-Acetyl-*l*-Cysteine

Silvio De Flora, MD, Alberto Izzotti, Adriana Albini, PhD, Francesco D'Agostini, Maria Bagnasco, and Roumen Balansky

CONTENTS

INTRODUCTION
BIOCHEMICAL AND PHARMACOLOGICAL ISSUES
EFFICACY OF NAC AS A MODULATOR OF MUTAGENESIS AND CARCINOGENESIS
PROTECTIVE MECHANISMS OF NAC IN MUTAGENESIS AND CARCINOGENESIS
CONCLUSIONS
ACKNOWLEDGMENTS
REFERENCES

1. INTRODUCTION

The aminothiol *N*-acetyl-*l*-cysteine (NAC) is an analog and precursor of reduced glutathione (GSH). During the last four decades, it has been extensively used as a mucolytic agent. In addition, because of its multiple protective mechanisms, NAC has been proposed for a broad array of applications, both preventive and therapeutic. The scientific community has a continuously growing interest in this molecule, which is being used with increasing frequency in both clinical investigations and experimental studies. As of February 1, 2002, a total of 5153 scientific papers were available in MEDLINE under the query term "acetyl-cysteine," with an impressive growth during the last 10 years. In one month alone (January 2002), 134 new papers were added to this database.

Several review articles that examine the cancer chemopreventive properties of NAC are available in the literature *(1–9)*. The objective of this chapter is to update the state of the art on this subject. First, we delineate some biochemical and pharmacological features of this drug, also including original data regarding the safety of NAC as evaluated by multigene expression technology (Subheading 2). We then review studies related to the efficacy of NAC as a modulator of mutagenesis and carcinogenesis, as evaluated in in vitro test systems, in animal models that evaluate intermediate biomarkers and tumors at various sites, and in chemoprevention clinical trials (Subheading 3). Finally, we follow a mechanistic approach by discussing the multiple points at which NAC intervenes in the mutagenesis and carcinogenesis processes (Subheading 4).

2. BIOCHEMICAL AND PHARMACOLOGICAL ISSUES

2.1. NAC and the Glutathione System

GSH (γ-glutamyl-*l*-cysteinyl glycine) is known to play a central physiological role in maintaining body homeostasis and in protecting cells against oxidants, toxicants, DNA-damaging agents, and carcinogens of either exogenous or endogenous source *(10,11)*. The intracellular ratio of GSH to oxidized glutathione (GSSG) is approx 100:1. This ratio is maintained by the GSH redox cycle, which involves the activities of GSH peroxidase and NADPH-dependant GSSG reductase. The main supply of NADPH is provided by glucose 6-phosphate dehydrogenase (G6PD) and 6-phosphogluconate dehydrogenase (6PGD) in erythrocytes, and additionally by isocitric dehydrogenase and malic dehydrogenase in other tissues *(12)*. Most of the biological functions of GSH depend on the reactivity of

From: Cancer Chemoprevention, Volume 1: Promising Cancer Chemoprevention Agents
Edited by: G. J. Kelloff, E. T. Hawk, and C. C. Sigman © Humana Press Inc., Totowa, NJ

the thiol group of its cysteinyl residue *(13)*. The reaction rate of GSH with electrophiles is greatly enhanced by GSH *S*-transferases (GST), which catalyze conjugation processes resulting in detoxification and excretion of water-soluble conjugates *(13–15)*. Genetic polymorphisms have been detected within this broad family of phase 2 isoenzymes. Two of the GST-encoding genes, identified as *GSTM1* (μ) and *GSTT1* (θ), have a null genotype in humans caused by deletion of both paternal and maternal alleles, resulting in a lack of active proteins *(16)*. The absence of these genes has been associated with cancer in various organs *(17)* as well as with disease occurrence and oxidative DNA damage in glaucoma *(18)*, and with DNA adduct levels in atherosclerotic lesions *(19)*. In addition, we hypothesised that *GSTM1* and *N*-acetyltransferase *(NAT2)* polymorphisms may affect responsiveness to treatment with NAC, as a first tentative approach to the pharmacogenomics of chemopreventive agents (*see* Subheading 3.3.2.).

Unfortunately, the large GSH molecule is not transported efficiently into cells, and *l*-cysteine, which is the rate-limiting amino acid in the intracellular synthesis of this tripeptide, is toxic to humans *(11)*. The nontoxic molecule of NAC is readily deacetylated in cells to yield *l*-cysteine, thereby promoting intracellular synthesis of GSH, which is catalyzed by γ-glutamylcysteine synthetase *(8)*. Moreover, NAC can increase GSH intracellular stores by inducing GSSG reductase activity, as shown both in vitro *(20)* and in humans *(21)*. In addition to acting as a GSH precursor, NAC is *per se* responsible for protective effects in the extracellular environment, mainly because of its nucleophilic and antioxidant properties *(8,9)*.

Administration of NAC can be particularly useful in the case of GSH depletion, which is known to occur under conditions of oxidative stress and exposure to toxic and carcinogenic agents *(10,11)*. Moreover, GSH stores appear to be depleted in chronic infections caused by at least three viruses (e.g., hepatitis B virus [HBV], hepatitis C virus [HCV;], and human immunodeficiency virus [HIV]) typically associated with cancer. In fact, both humans infected with HBV and woodchucks infected with woodchuck hepatitis virus display enhanced metabolic activation of chemical hepatocarcinogens, accompanied in woodchucks by GSH depletion related to the amounts of virus in hepatocytes *(22–24)*. GSH levels decreased in both plasma and peripheral-blood lymphocytes of patients chronically infected with HCV *(25)*. In HIV-infected healthy carriers or AIDS patients, GSH levels were decreased in plasma *(26,27)*, epithelial lining-fluid *(27)*, and peripheral-blood monocellular cells *(26)*. It is noteworthy that low thiol levels are associated with impaired survival *(28,29)*.

GSH depletion has also been shown to occur during physical exercise, which may induce oxidative stress. Blood GSH oxidation is a marker of exercise-induced oxidative stress in humans. Studies in GSH-deficient animals clearly indicate the central importance of having adequate tissue GSH to protect exercise-induced oxidative stress. Among the various thiol supplements studied, NAC and α-lipoic acid hold the most promise *(30)*.

2.2. Pharmacokinetics and Safety of NAC

The apparent uptake of GSH occurs largely, if not entirely, through pathways involving prior breakdown to dipeptides and amino acids, transport of these, and intracellular synthesis of the tripeptide *(11)*. NAC easily penetrates cell membranes, and in humans, the intestinal absorption of NAC occurs rapidly. Although bioavailability is less than 10% *(31)*, this is much higher than absorption of GSH, which is not taken up intact to a significant extent into the portal blood from the gastrointestinal tract *(11)*. In the organism, NAC can be present in different forms, such as *N,N'*-diacetylcysteine or *N*-acetylcysteine-cysteine, and metabolism gives rise to a number of products, such as cysteine, cystine, methionine, GSH, and mixed disulphides, which are the predominant form in the plasma *(32)*. Therefore, the pharmacokinetics of NAC are difficult to evaluate, and contradictory results are reported in the literature. For instance, in one study oral NAC increased the levels of plasma cysteine and GSH in both plasma and bronchoalveolar lavage (BAL) fluid *(33)*, and another study found an increase of free cysteine but no change in total cysteine or GSH *(32)*. Still another one found no change of free or total cysteine or GSH in plasma *(21)*. These patterns hamper the evaluation of compliance in clinical trials using NAC, but also show that NAC has little influence on normal homeostasis.

NAC has very low toxicity in both experimental animals and treated humans. In fact, LD_{50} by the oral route is greater than 10 g/kg body wt in both mice and rats, and LD_{50} following intravenous administration is 4.6 g/kg in mice and 2.8 g/kg in rats *(34)*. A daily dose of 1 g/kg body wt given *per os* to rats for 18 consecutive mo had

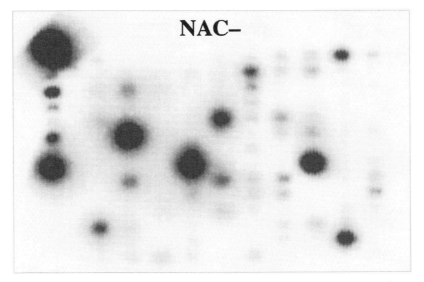

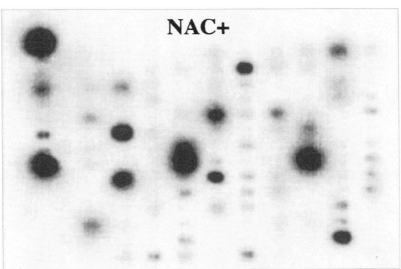

Fig. 1. Appearance of electronic autoradiographs of cDNA arrays (Atlas™ Mouse Stress Array) hybridized with ^{32}P-labeled probes–obtained by reverse transcription of mRNA from the lung of A/J mice, either untreated (NAC) or receiving NAC in the drinking water, at the dose of 1 g/kg body wt, for five consecutive days (NAC+). None of the 36 expressed genes, from a total of 149 examined genes, varied more than twofold in the lungs of NAC-treated mice. The expressed genes could be classified into four main functional categories: (A) metabolism of xenobiotics, including a series of cytochrome P450 isoenzymes (CYP1A1, CYP2B29, CYP2E1, CYP2F2, CYP4B1, and CYP21A1), dimethylaniline oxidase 1, soluble epoxide hydrolase, DT-diaphorase, and nucleophosmin; (B) response to stress, including extracellular superoxide dismutase precursor, heme oxygenase 1, endoplasmic reticulum protein (ERP) 99, ER-60 precursor, ERP72, cyclophilin-40, vimentin, FK-506-binding protein and its precursor FKBP13; (C) protein removal and DNA repair, including T-complex protein 1 theta, eta and zeta sub-units, endonuclease III homolog 1, ATP-dependent DNA helicase II 70-kDa subunit rad52, DNA mismatch repair protein MSH3, mdm2 p53-associated protein, and BRCA2; (D) housekeeping genes, including ubiquitin, phospholipase A2, hypoxantine-guanine phosphoribosyl transferase, glyceraldehyde-3-phosphate dehydrogenase, myosin I alpha, cytoplasmic beta-actin, 45kDa calcium-binding protein precursor, and 40S ribosomal protein. The list of 113 genes whose electronic signal was less than twofold higher than background levels can be inferred, by exclusion, from the Atlas™ Mouse Stress Array gene list (available on the website http://atlas/info.clontech.com)

no detrimental effects *(34)*. In humans, doses of 0.5 g/kg body wt *per os (35)* or 0.3 g/kg body wt intravenously *(36)* were given when NAC was used as an antidote to acute intoxications. Other details regarding NAC safety in clinical trials are reported in Subheading 3.3.

All modulating effects of NAC described in the following sections were detected in a variety of situations leading to toxicity, imbalances of the redox state, or changes in homeostasis. At the molecular level, the safety of a chemopreventive agent can be evaluated by evaluating the lack of influence on gene expression under physiological conditions, especially regarding those genes involved in damage to macromolecules and stress response. For this purpose, we used cDNA array technology to investigate expression of multiple genes in the lung of A/J mice, either untreated or receiving NAC in the drinking water, at a dose of 1g/kg body wt, for five consecutive days. Regardless of treatment with NAC, 36 of the 149 genes included in the Atlas™ Mouse Stress Array (Clontech Laboratories, Inc., Palo Alto, CA) exhibited an electronic signal more than twofold higher than background levels. As shown in Fig. 1 and confirmed by software analysis (Atlas™ Image and Atlas™ Navigator 1.5, Clontech), none of the genes expressed varied more than twofold between the NAC-treated mice and untreated mice. Thus, even at the very high doses used in animal models to modulate intermediate biomarkers, prevent preneoplastic lesions and tumors, exert anti-angiogenic effects, and attenuate invasion and metastasis of cancer cells (as described in this chapter), oral NAC did not alter the background expression of a number of genes in the mouse lung. We plan to undertake similar studies in tissues of humans before and after treatment with NAC.

2.3. Pharmacological Applications of NAC

NAC was introduced as a mucolytic agent in the early 1960s. Its capacity to reduce mucus viscosity depends on breakage of disulphide bridges and depolymerization of mucin molecules. This drug has found extensive clinical application in the therapy and prophylaxis of respiratory diseases. Aside from acute bronchitis, NAC was proposed for the treatment of chronic obstructive broncopulmonary disease *(37)* and its re-exacerbations, as documented by the meta-analysis of 15 clinical trials *(38)*, acute respiratory distress syndrome (ARDS), influenza-like syndromes *(39)*, and idiopathic pulmonary fibrosis *(40)*. Moreover, NAC has been proposed to treat a variety of conditions that share alterations of the redox status and GSH depletion

as common pathogenetic determinants *(41)*. For instance, clinical trials have shown the ability of NAC to improve the renal function in hepatorenal syndrome *(42)*, prevent reduction in renal function induced by radiographic contrast agents *(43)*, decrease the risk of graft-vs-host disease (GVHD) in transplanted patients *(44)*, lower plasma homocysteine levels *(45)*, and limit the size of heart infarct *(46)*.

NAC has also been used as an antidote for acute intoxications. The prototype of this application is to treat overdosage of the analgesic drug acetaminophen (paracetamol) *(36)*, whose cytotoxicity is mediated by the reactive metabolite *N*-acetyl-*p*-benzoquinoneimine, a strongly electrophilic and oxidizing agent formed in the liver via cytochrome P450 monooxygenase, and in the kidney via prostaglandin synthetase system *(32)*. Other possible applications of NAC in clinical toxicology include protection against hepatorenal damage induced by the potent GSH-depleting toxins chloroform, carbon tetrachloride, 1,2-dichloropropane, and α-amanitine (contained in *Amanita phalloides*), bone-marrow toxicity of chloramphenicol, cardiorespiratory arrest caused by acrylonitrile, liver necrosis induced by bromobenzene, multiple lesions produced by mustard gas (dichlorodiethyl sulfide), and methemoglobinemia, hemolysis, and cataract induced by naphthalene *(32)*. Furthermore, NAC has been used to attenuate the side effects of cytostatic drugs—e.g., cardiomyopathy caused by doxorubicin (adriamycin) and the hemorrhagic cystitis caused by cyclophosphamide and iphosphamide *(32)*.

As described in this chapter, NAC has been extensively investigated for possible applications in the prevention of genotoxic damage and oxidative stress in cancer and other chronic degenerative diseases.

3. EFFICACY OF NAC AS A MODULATOR OF MUTAGENESIS AND CARCINOGENESIS

3.1. In Vitro Test Systems

3.1.1. ACELLULAR SYSTEMS

NAC inhibited single-strand breakage in plasmid DNA exposed to aqueous extracts of cigarette smoke and a nitric oxide-releasing compound, which forms potent reactive species such as peroxynitrite *(47)*. NAC prevented oxidative damage to calf thymus DNA produced in Fenton-type reactions, which generate hydroxyl radicals (·OH). In particular, NAC inhibited DNA fragmentation and formation of ^{32}P postlabeled nucleotide modifications and 8-hydroxy-2'-deoxyguanosine

(8-OH-dG) in DNA exposed to either H_2O_2 or a mixture of H_2O_2 and $CuSO_4$ *(48)* as well as formation of the 8-OH-dG tautomer 8-oxo-2'-deoxyguanosine (8-oxo-dG) in DNA exposed to a mixture of H_2O_2, $CuSO_4$, nitrilotriacetic acid, and ascorbic acid *(49)*. NAC also inhibited formation of adducts to calf thymus DNA metabolically activated *N*-nitrosopyrrolidine *(50)*. Conversely, NAC did not inhibit the formation of ^{32}P postlabeled DNA adducts by metabolically activated benzo*[a]*pyrene (B*[a]*P) *(51)* and dibenzo*(a,l)*pyrene *(52)*. As discussed in Subheading 3.1.2., these findings are consistent with results of bacterial mutagenicity test systems using liver preparations from rats treated with enzyme inducers.

3.1.2. BACTERIA

Several studies evaluated the ability of NAC to modulate genotoxicity of either direct-acting mutagens or promutagens in *Salmonella typhimurium his*⁻ strains and, in some cases, in *Escherichia coli* strains with differential DNA repair capacities. Activity profiles for a variety of mutagens are available *(53)*.

Fifteen years ago we demonstrated that, like other thiols, NAC dose-dependently decreases "spontaneous" mutagenicity in strain TA104 *(54–56)*. This effect was confirmed by another laboratory *(57)*. Since inhibition of "spontaneous" revertants did not occur in TA102, which has different DNA repair capacities than TA104, we hypothesized that inhibition of "spontaneous" mutations by thiols depends not only on their antioxidant properties but also by possible effects on DNA repair mechanisms *(56)*.

NAC is known to act as a radioprotector *(58)*. However, NAC did not affect the mutagenicity, in strain TA102 and TA104, of ultraviolet (UV) radiation emitted either by monochromatic sources at 254 nm *(1)* or 365 nm *(8)* or by fluorescent *(8)* or halogen lamps *(59)*.

NAC attenuated the direct mutagenicity of peroxides, including cumene hydroperoxide *(1)* and hydrogen peroxide *(20)*, in TA102 and TA104 as well as DNA-damaging activity of hydrogen peroxide in *E. coli (60)*. Crocidolite, chrysotile fibers, and man-made vitreous fibre-21 increased 8-OH-dG levels in calf-thymus DNA and were mutagenic to TA100, and more potently, to its GSH-deficient derivatives TA100/NG-54 and TA100/NG-57. Pretreatment with NAC reduced the number of revertants to less than that of the parent strains *(61)*. Moreover, as reported in Subheading 4.2., NAC inhibited the bacterial genotox-icity of reactive oxygen species (ROS) generated in vitro by electron-transfer reactions *(55,62)* or produced by human phagocytic leukocytes *(63)*. With the exception of nitrofurantoin *(1)* and of sodium azide *(1,64)*, tested in strain TA100 and TA100NR, NAC was found to inhibit mutagenicity to *S. typhimurium his* strains of many direct mutagens that belong to a variety of chemical families and functional categories. The list includes the pesticides captan and folpet in TA100 *(8)*; the antitumor drugs 2-methoxy-6-chloro-9-[3-(2-chloroethyl)aminopropylamino]-acridine (ICR 191) in TA1537 *(8)*, and doxorubicin (adri-amycin) in TA98 *(65)*; glutaraldehyde and formaldehyde, also in the form of vapors, in TA102 and TA104 *(54)*; β-propiolactone in TA100 *(8)*; hydralazine in TA98 *(8)*, quercetin in TA98 *(8)*; 4-nitroquinoline 1-oxide in TA100 *(20,66)*; *N*-methyl-*N'*-nitro-*N*-nitrosoguanidine (MNNG) in TA1530 *(64)* and TA100 *(67)*, as well as in the differential DNA repair assay in *E. coli (67)*; 2-nitrofluorene in TA1538 and TA98 *(64)*; 1-nitropyrene, 1,8-dinitropyrene, and diesel extracts in TA98, TA100 and TA104 *(57)*; vinyl carbamate epoxide in TA1535 *(68)*; epichlorohydrin in TA1535 *(20)*; and sodium dichromate in TA102 *(20)*.

The effect of NAC on promutagens and S9-requiring complex mixtures is more difficult to interpret. Some data suggest a protective role of NAC—for instance, in the case of promutagens such as benzidine activated by hamster liver S9 *(69)*, aflatoxin B_1 activated by wood-chuck liver regardless of infection with hepatitis virus *(23)*, and doxorubicin, whose mutagenicity was inhibited by NAC in the absence of—and even more efficiently, in the presence of—rat liver S9 *(65)*. In other cases, modulation by NAC was more uncertain, ranging from lack of inhibition to inhibition at high doses only to enhancement of mutagenicity. The tested compound included the aromatic amines 2-aminoanthracene, 2-acetylaminofluorene (2AAF) and 2-aminofluorene in TA1538 and TA98 *(20,64,70)*; aflatoxin B_1 in TA98 and TA100 *(20,70–72)*; cyclophosphamide in TA1535 *(20,70)*; 3-amino-1-methyl-5*H*-pyrido[4,3-*b*]indole (Trp-P-2) in TA98 *(20)*; B*[a]*P in TA1538, TA98 and TA100 *(20,64)*; and complex mixtures, including cigarette smoke *(66)* and cigarette smoke condensate (CSC) *(20)*. All uncertain or inconsistent results were observed when the promutagens were tested in the presence of rat liver S9, and the outcome depended on pretreatment of rats with enzyme inducers. As previously discussed in more detail *(8)*, these patterns occur because NAC does not inhibit and may even stimulate metabolic activation. The resulting reactive metabolites are detoxified by coordinated blocking because of the nucleophilicity of this molecule and, to some extent, by stimulation of phase 2 enzymes (see Subheading 4.4.). In fact, the same promutagens were efficiently counteracted by NAC in animal models (see Subheading 3.2.1.) while, both in mutagenicity test systems (this Subheading) and acellular systems (see Subheading 3.1.1.), S9 mix cannot fully mimic the complexity of the in vivo situation. For instance, S9 mix lacks co-factors for phase II enzymes (73).

3.1.3. CULTURED MAMMALIAN CELLS

NAC exerted protective effects in genotoxicity and cell-transformation assays in cultured mammalian cells. As evaluated by single-cell electrophoresis (COMET assay), NAC inhibited the genotoxicity of both acrolein and water-soluble cigarette smoke in human lymphoid cells containing Epstein-Barr episomes (74). Using the micronucleus test, NAC attenuated the genotoxicities of arsenite in cultured human fibroblasts (75) and of the oxidizing agent paraquat in human endothelial cells (76). Moreover, NAC inhibited induction of sister chromatid exchanges in Chinese hamster ovary cells co-cultivated with phagocytic leukocytes, which generate ROS (77).

In particular cases, however, GSH contributes to metabolic activation of certain genotoxic agents. Accordingly, depending on the situation, NAC may exert adverse effects. This has been shown to be the case for MNNG, as assessed by evaluating either 6TG-resistant mutations in V79 Chinese hamster cells (78) or his^+ reversions in strain TA100 of S. typhimurium (67). In both prokaryotic and eukaryotic cells, NAC enhanced mutagenicity when reacting intracellularly, although mutagenicity was enhanced when MNNG reacted intracellularly with NAC derivatives. NAC also enhanced DNA-strand breakage induced by potassium bromate in cultured human lymphocytes (79). NAC did not affect formation of DNA adducts by dibenzo(a,l)pyrene in the human breast-cell line MCF-7 (80). Tumor-promoting activity of H_2O_2 in rat liver-epithelial oval cells was decreased by NAC, which inhibited phosphorylation of connexin 43 and disruption of gap-junctional intercellular communications (81). NAC attenuated the ability of B[a]P to induce transformation of cultured rat tracheal-epithelial cells. This system appears to identify chemopreventive compounds that act at early stages of the carcinogenesis process (82).

In addition, a number of studies provided evidence that NAC displays anticytotoxic (Subheading 4.9.) and antiproliferative effects (Subheading 4.14.), and modulates apoptosis (Subheading 4.10.) in cultured mammalian cells.

3.2. Animal Models

3.2.1. BIOMARKERS AND PRENEOPLASTIC LESIONS

Many studies have provided evidence that, almost invariably, NAC exerts protective effects toward alterations of biomarkers induced in rodents by individual carcinogens and carcinogenic complex mixtures. The biomarkers that have been studied include adducts to hemoglobin and mitochondrial DNA, and adducts to nuclear DNA in various tissues; oxidative alterations of nucleotides; DNA fragmentation; DNA-protein crosslinks (DPXL); apoptosis; alterations of nuclear enzymes; cytogenetic damage; and preneoplastic lesions, such as altered foci in the liver, aberrant crypt foci (ACF) in the colon, and morphological and functional alterations in the respiratory tract.

3.2.1.1. The Respiratory Tract NAC was found to modulate a variety of biomarkers and/or preneoplastic lesions in isolated cells of the respiratory tract such as BAL cells, particularly pulmonary alveolar macrophages (PAM); and in tissues such as nasal, tracheal, bronchial, and bronchiolar epithelia, as well as in the mixed-cell population of the lung. Changes in the respiratory tract were induced in rodents exposed whole-body to cigarette smoke, either mainstream, sidestream or environmental, or receiving intratracheal instillations either of lung carcinogens, such as B[a]P or chromium(VI), or of complex mixtures, such as air-particulate extracts.

NAC decreased the levels of DNA adducts, detected by ^{32}P postlabeling analysis in the dissected nasal epithelium of Sprague-Dawley rats exposed to mainstream cigarette smoke for 40 d (Izzotti A, Balansky R, unpublished data).

PAM, which are the predominant cells in BAL, are sentinel cells that phagocytize foreign particles and can both activate and detoxify carcinogens. Therefore, they are ideal for evaluating the modulation of biomarkers in both humans and experimental animals (83). NAC given by gavage inhibited formation of DNA adducts detected by synchronous fluorescence spectrophotometry (SFS) in the lung of Sprague-Dawley rats exposed whole-body to mainstream cigarette smoke (84). A similar effect detected by ^{32}P postlabeling was observed in BAL cells of Sprague-Dawley rats that were exposed whole-body to environmental cigarette smoke and received NAC in drinking water *(85)*. Formation of micronucleated and polynucleated PAM was significantly attenuated by oral NAC in BDF_1 mice that were exposed whole-body to mainstream cigarette smoke *(86)*, and in Sprague-Dawley rats that received intra-tracheal instillations of B*[a]*P *(87)* or air-particulate extracts *(88)* or exposed whole-body to mainstream cigarette smoke *(89)* or to environmental cigarette smoke *(85)*. In the last study, the effect of NAC, given in drinking water was enhanced by co-administration of oltipraz in the diet *(85)*. Moreover, NAC was capable of normalizing BAL cellularity, which in BDF_1 mice was still altered 11 wk after discontinuation of exposure to mainstream cigarette smoke because of an almost 10-fold increase of polymorphonucleates and a parallel decrease of PAM *(86)*.

A variety of biomarkers were evaluated in the lung mixed-cell population of Sprague-Dawley rats. Oral NAC suppressed formation of adducts to mitochondrial DNA in the lungs of rats exposed whole-body to mainstream cigarette smoke *(90)*, which may be a factor in the pathogenesis of several chronic degenerative diseases. NAC inhibited formation of SFS-positive adducts to nuclear DNA in the lungs of rats that received intra-tracheal instillations of B*[a]*P *(87,91)* or exposed whole-body to mainstream cigarette smoke *(84)*. NAC significantly decreased levels of ^{32}P postlabeled DNA adducts in the lungs of rats exposed to environmental cigarette smoke (85), yet in another study it had no effect on sidestream cigarette smoke *(92)*[a]. Interestingly, NAC interacted synergistically with oltipraz to decrease environmental cigarette smoke-induced DNA adducts in the lung *(85)*. NAC also decreased oxidative DNA damage (8-OH-dG) in the rat lung following exposure to environmental cigarette smoke *(85)*.

In the lungs of rats that received intra-tracheal instillations of air-particulate extracts, both SFS and ^{32}P postlabeling analyses demonstrated the ability of NAC to decrease the levels of DNA adducts. Moreover, NAC counteracted the induction of micronuclei in PAM and epithelial cells of the respiratory tract, and the induction of polynucleated PAM. In the same animals' lungs, NAC attenuated stimulation of the nuclear enzyme poly(ADP ribose) polymerase (PARP), produced by the lung by exposure to air-particulate extracts *(88)*. NAC also affected genotoxic effects produced in vivo by chromium(VI), which is a lung carcinogen when inhaled at high doses *(94)*. In fact, NAC significantly decreased pre-genotoxic and genotoxic alterations produced by intra-tracheal instillations of sodium dichromate to rats, as shown by inhibition of ^{32}P-postlabeled nucleotide modifications, DNA fragmentation, and DPXL *(95)*.

The histological structure of the rat trachea resembles that of the human bronchus, the major site of smoking-related cancer in humans *(96)*, and inhaled cigarette smoke induces preneoplastic changes in rat tracheal-epithelial cells *(97)*. In two separate experiments in Sprague-Dawley rats exposed to mainstream cigarette smoke, oral NAC inhibited formation of DNA adducts in the dissected tracheal epithelium *(98)*. Similarly, NAC diminished DNA adduct levels in the dissected tracheal epithelium of the same rat strain following exposure to environmental cigarette smoke *(85)*. However, in another laboratory, dietary NAC did not significantly influence the levels of most major and minor lipophilic DNA adducts formed in the whole trachea of rats exposed to sidestream cigarette smoke *(92)*[a]. Exposure to cigarette smoke, either mainstream or environmental, is a strong inducer of apoptosis in the respiratory tract, as evaluated both by morphological analysis and the TdT-mediated nick-end labeling (TUNEL) method *(99)*. Administration of NAC in drinking water significantly attenuated induction of apoptosis both in bronchial/bronchiolar epithelium of mainstream cigarette smoke-exposed rats and in PAM of environmental cigarette smoke-exposed rats. This effect was ascribed to the ability of NAC to inhibit the genotoxic effects and other events that trigger the apoptotic process *(99)*. Recently we demonstrated that the oral administration of NAC during pregency prevents birth-related genomic and transcriptional attentions in mouse lung *(100)*.

NAC was also shown to protect rat respiratory airways from morphological and functional alterations

---

[a]Comparative experiments have provided evidence that the contrasting conclusions generated in these studies are methodological in nature, depending on the chromatographic conditions used to separate DNA adducts. In fact, the chromatographic system used in ref. *92*, employing isopropanol/ammonium hydroxide as developing buffer, yields much lower amounts of DNA adducts and fails to detect the massive diagonal radioactive zone (DRZ). The DRZ, which can be detected by using urea-containing developing buffer, expresses a multitude of DNA-binding agents that are present in cigarette smoke *(85,93)*.

produced by cigarette smoke. For instance, administration of NAC in drinking water significantly prevented epithelial secretory-cell hyperplasia, especially in the smallest bronchioli, as well as hypersecretion of mucus in the larynx and trachea of Wistar rats exposed whole-body to mainstream cigarette smoke *(101)*. In addition, treatment of Sprague-Dawley rats with NAC by gavage inhibited mainstream cigarette smoke-induced severe histopathological changes in terminal airways, including an intense inflammation of bronchial and bronchiolar mucosae accompanied by multiple hyperplastic and metaplastic foci of micropapillomatous growth, and a severe emphysema accompanied by extensive disruption of alveolar walls *(89)*. Oral NAC also prevented alterations in morphometry, consisting of airway-wall thickening of small, medium, and large bronchi, and alterations in ventilation distribution after exposure of rats to cigarette smoke for 10 wk *(102)*.

3.2.1.2. The Digestive System

Oral NAC produced a significant shift from severe to mild preneoplastic lesions in the esophagus of BD_6 rats treated with *N,N*-diethylnitrosamine (DEN) and diethyldithiocarbamate (DEDTC) (*see* Subheading 3.2.2.2).

NAC was evaluated for the ability to inhibit the formation of ACF, putative precancerous lesions, in the colon of rats receiving subcutaneous(SC) injections of azoxymethane (AOM). In F344 rats, NAC (2 g/kg diet) significantly reduced the number of AOM-induced lesions from 228 to 151 ACF/animal *(103)*. However, this result was not confirmed in a further study carried out in the same laboratory under similar experimental conditions *(104)*. In F344 rats, the conjugate of NAC with phenylethyl isothiocyanate (PEITC), given by gavage, reduced the formation of total foci and multicrypt foci when administered during the post-initiation stage, but was ineffective as an anti-initiator *(105)*.

Administration of NAC in drinking water significantly decreased levels of adducts to mtDNA in the liver of Sprague-Dawley rats treated with 2AAF by gavage *(90)*. In Wistar rats that received the same carcinogen, co-administration of NAC in diet protected the nuclear enzyme PARP from the damage produced by 2AAF, either according to the Teebor and Becker protocol *(106)* or the Solt and Farber model *(8)*. Oral NAC significantly decreased the levels both of SFS-positive DNA adducts in the livers of Sprague-Dawley rats receiving intra-tracheal instillations of B*[a]*P *(87)*, and of ^{32}P-postlabeled DNA adducts in the liver of Sprague-Dawley rats that received 7,12-

dimethylbenz*(a)*anthracene (DMBA) by gavage (Izzotti A et al., unpublished data). NAC had a strong antagonistic effect on formation of hepatic lipid hydroperoxides in Sprague-Dawley rats treated with an intraperitoneal (ip) injection of the hepatocarcinogen safrole *(107)*. In a study on the protective role of thiols on induction of DNA damage in the liver of Sprague-Dawley rats, as determined by the alkaline elution technique, an ip injection of NAC greatly reduced the genotoxicity of MNNG, yet it did not affect the genotoxicity of *N*-methyl-*N*-nitrosourea (MNU) *(108)*.

The transplacental exposure of Swiss albino mice to environmental cigarette smoke resulted in the enhancement of bulky DNA adduct and 8-OH-dG levels, along with overexpression of a large number of genes in the fetus liver. Administration of NAC in drinking water to environmental cigarette smoke-exposed pregnant mice significantly attenuated these alterations *(109)*.

In two separated studies, NAC inhibited and delayed the formation of γ-glutamyltranspeptidase (GGT)-positive foci in the liver of Wistar rats fed a 2AAF-supplemented diet for four consecutive cycles, according to the Teebor and Becker protocol *(110)*.

3.2.1.3. Hair Follicle Cells

Oral NAC prevented the alopecia induced in C57BL/6 mice by doxorubicin, which typically causes oxidative DNA damage *(111)*. In the same mouse strain, whole-body exposure to environmental cigarette smoke induced grey hair and alopecia, accompanied by apoptosis of hair follicle cells. Administration of NAC in drinking water totally prevented these effects *(112)*.

3.2.1.4. Mammary Glands

In a study using blind coded samples, administration of dietary NAC (10 g/kg diet) significantly decreased DNA adducts levels in mammary epithelial cells of Sprague-Dawley rats that received a single DMBA dose (12 mg/rat) by gavage (our unpublished data, in collaboration with the University of Alabama at Birmingham and the U.S. National Cancer Institute, Chemoprevention Branch).

3.2.1.5. The Cardiovascular System

Oral NAC inhibited the formation of SFS-positive DNA adducts in the hearts of Sprague-Dawley rats that received intra-tracheal instillations of B*[a]*P *(87)* or exposed whole-body to mainstream cigarette smoke *(84)*. Similarly, NAC significantly decreased levels of DNA adducts in the heart of the same rat strain following exposure to environmental cigarette smoke, as assessed by ^{32}P postlabeling *(85)*, but had no effect in another study using rats exposed to sidestream cigarette smoke *(92)*.

In the aorta of Sprague-Dawley rats, NAC significantly reduced the level of DNA adducts, as detected by SFS in mainstream cigarette smoke-exposed rats *(91)* or by ^{32}P-postlabeling in environmental cigarette smoke-exposed rats *(113)*.

3.2.1.6. The Urogenital Tract Administration of NAC by gavage significantly decreased the levels of DNA adducts in Sprague-Dawley rats exposed to mainstream cigarette smoke, as detected by SFS in kidney or by ^{32}P postlabeling in the testis *(8)*.

NAC significantly reduced dominant lethal mutations in Sprague-Dawley rats treated with ethyl methanesulfonate *(114)*.

3.2.1.7. Bone Marrow and Peripheral Blood In Sprague-Dawley rats exposed whole-body to environmental cigarette smoke, treatment with NAC in drinking water strongly reduced levels of adducts to hemoglobin of 4-aminobiphenyl and B*(a)*P-7,8-diol-9,10-epoxide, typical constituents of cigarette smoke. This effect was further potentiated by combining NAC with oltipraz in diet *(85)*.

Several studies have investigated the ability of NAC to modulate systemic genotoxic effects in rodents, either untreated or treated with cigarette smoke, polycyclic aromatic hydrocarbons (PAH), aromatic amines, or urethane. These effects were usually determined by evaluating the frequency of micronucleated (MN) polychromatic erythrocytes (PCE), either in fetal liver or adult bone marrow, and of MN normochromatic erythrocytes (NCE) in the peripheral blood.

Lifetime administration of NAC in the drinking water, at 0.1 or 0.5 g/kg body wt, did not affect "spontaneous" levels of MN PCE in the peripheral blood of both male and female BDF$_1$ mice (Balansky R et al., unpublished data).

In BDF$_1$ mice exposed whole-body to mainstream cigarette smoke, NAC often decreased smoke-induced formation of MN PCE in bone marrow, but not to a significant extent, and significantly attenuated the formation of MN NCE in peripheral blood *(86)*. Following exposure of Sprague-Dawley rats to mainstream cigarette smoke, NAC decreased toxicity in bone marrow, as shown by normalization of the PCE:NCE ratio, but failed to attenuate the frequency of MN PCE *(89)*. Administration of NAC in drinking water and its combination with dietary oltipraz significantly decreased the frequency of MN PCE in

bone marrow of Sprague-Dawley rats exposed to environmental cigarette smoke *(85)*. NAC, given in drinking water during pregnancy, significantly decreased frequency of MN PCE in the liver of fetuses of Swiss albino mice whose mothers had been exposed to environmental cigarette smoke during pregnancy *(109)*.

NAC failed to inhibit the induction of MN PCE in the bone marrow of C57BL/6 mice treated with DMBA by gavage *(115)*. Conversely, the frequency of MN PCE was significantly attenuated by NAC in BDF$_1$ mice that received a single ip injection either of the aromatic amine 2AAF or of the chromium(VI) salt sodium dichromate, and in Balb/c mice that received a single ip injection of urethane (Balansky R et al., unpublished data). Moreover, the frequency of MN PCE, periodically monitored in Balb/c mice treated with ip injections of urethane, was significantly decreased by NAC in a dose-related fashion, which predicted the subsequent inhibition of urethane-induced lung tumors *(116)*.

3.2.2. Tumors

3.2.2.1. The Respiratory Tract In Fischer rats that received sc injections of the tobacco-specific nitrosamine 4-(methylnitrosamino)-1-(3-pyridyl)-1-butanone (NNK),1.5 mg/kg body wt 3×/wk for 21 wk, the incidence of nasal cavity tumors was decreased from 78% of controls to 61% and 47% when the diet was supplemented with NAC at 6.5 and 13.1 g/kg diet, respectively *(117)*.

Dietary NAC (6.8 g/kg diet) significantly inhibited the formation of squamous carcinomas in the tracheas of Syrian golden hamsters that received a local application of 5% MNU once per wk for 15 wk *(118)*.

The effect of oral NAC on lung adenomas induced by urethane was evaluated in three mouse strains. Administration of NAC (2 g/kg diet) in the diet significantly decreased both tumor incidence and multiplicity in Swiss albino mice treated with a single ip administration of urethane at the dose of 1 g/kg body wt *(119)*. A significant and dose-dependent decrease of lung-tumor multiplicity was produced by NAC (0.1 or 0.5 g/kg body wt) in the drinking water of Balb/c mice treated with 10 daily ip injections (0.4 g/kg body wt each) of urethane *(116)*. A significant decrease of tumor multiplicity was observed when NAC was given (2 g/kg diet) to A/J mice treated with a single ip injection of urethane at 0.25 g/kg body wt, but no protective effect occurred when the carcinogen was dosed at either 1 or 0.1 g/kg body wt *(120)*. In a further study of A/J mice treated with a single ip injection of urethane (1 g/kg body wt), administration of NAC in the drinking water (1 g/kg body wt) significantly decreased tumor multiplicity; this effect was further enhanced by combining NAC with ascorbic acid at the same dose *(121)*.

NAC failed to affect the lung tumor yield in A/J mice exposed whole-body to environmental cigarette smoke for 5 mo, followed by 4 mo of recovery in filtered air *(120)*. As confirmed by our laboratory *(122)*, this treatment results in a weak but significant increase of lung tumors. Notably, with the exception of combined treatment with *myo*-inositol and dexamethasone *(123,124)*, all tested chemopreventive agents, including PEITC *(120)* and its combination with benzyl isothiocyanate (BITC) *(123)*, decaffeinated green tea *(120)*, acetylsalicylic acid *(123)*, D-limonene, and 1,4-phenylenbis(methylene)selenoisocyanate *(124)*, were unsuccessful in attenuating the increase in lung tumors produced by environmental cigarette smoke in this experimental model.

Dietary administration of NAC, at either 6.5 or 13.1 g/kg diet, did not affect lung-tumor incidence in Fischer rats that received sc injections of NNK (1.5 mg/kg body wt) 3×/wk for 21 wk. Determination of lung-tumor multiplicity was not possible in this study *(117)*. Similarly, administration of NAC at either 13.1 or 26.2 g/kg diet did not affect the lung tumor yield 16 wk after a single (10 µmol) ip injection of NNK in A/J mice. However, incidence of NNK-induced lung adenocarcinomas significantly decreased by 26.2 g NAC/kg diet 52 wk after carcinogen administration, indicating that NAC retards malignant progression in the lungs of NNK-treated A/J mice *(125)*.

The fact that isothiocyanates are excreted as NAC conjugates via the mercapturic acid pathway has prompted studies intended to evaluate the ability of conjugates of NAC with either PEITC, 3-phenylhexyl isothiocyanate, or BITC to modulate the lung-tumor yield in NNK-treated A/J mice. Although the protective effects of isothiocyanate in this model were not potentiated following conjugation with NAC, it was concluded that use of NAC conjugates may be convenient because of their reduced toxicity compared to isothiocyanate alone and their higher lipophilicity, which facilitates absorption and gradual dissociation of NAC and isothiocyanates in the body *(126)*. These conjugates also significantly inhibited lung tumors in A/J mice when given after an injection of NNK *(127)*.

Moreover, administration of the NAC conjugates of BITC and PEITC with the diet, after a single dose of B*[a]*P by gavage, significantly reduced the lung-tumor multiplicity *(128)*.

3.2.2.2. The Digestive System NAC given in drinking water (0.4 g/kg body wt) produced a significant shift from severe to mild preneoplastic lesions (hyperplasia and keratosis/acanthosis) and an inhibition of tumor multiplicity (papillomas and squamocellular carcinomas) in the esophagus in BD$_6$ rats treated with 8 weekly ip injections of DEN (50 mg/kg body wt) followed in 4 h with ip injections of DEDTC (50 mg/kg body wt) *(129)*.

The ability of NAC to attenuate chemically induced colon tumors was demonstrated in two rat models. The administration of NAC with drinking water (1 g/L) in Wistar rats treated with 15 weekly sc injections of 1,2-dimethylhydrazine (DMH) significantly decreased both the incidence and multiplicity of intestinal tumors *(130)*. In F344 rats treated with two weekly sc injections of AOM, the administration of NAC with the diet, at either 0.6 or 1.2 g/kg diet, significantly decreased the multiplicity of colon adenocarcinomas *(131)*. In C57BL/6J mice treated for 12 weeks with dextran sulfate sodium in the drinking water and iron-enriched diet, followed by a 10 day recovery period, administration of NAC with the diet (2 g/kg in the diet) significantly decreased both incidence and multiplicity of colorectal adenocarcinomas as well as chronic ulcerative colitis *(132)*.

Conversely, NAC failed to inhibit liver tumor formation in rodents treated with DEN. This lack of protective effects was observed in C3H mice that received ip injections of NAC (30 mg/kg body wt) on d 13, 14, and 15, followed by administration of this agent in the diet (2 g/kg) starting at 21 d of age; DEN was administered ip, at 4 mg/kg body wt, on d 15 of age *(133)*. Moreover, under the same conditions reported for the esophagus, NAC did not affect the yield of benign and malignant liver tumors in BD$_6$ rats treated with DEN and DEDTC *(129)*.

3.2.2.3. Skin NAC inhibited the formation of skin papillomas in mice treated with DMBA and 12-*O*-tetradecanoyl-13-phorbol acetate (TPA) *(134)*. Unlike GSH, topical application of NAC to skin papillomas did not significantly inhibit progression to squamous cell carcinomas *(135)*. Benign and malignant skin tumors were produced by the topical application of B*[a]*P (64 µg/mouse), twice /wk for 7 wk, in *p53* haploinsufficient Tg.AC (v-Ha-*ras*) mice, which contain activated, carcinogen-inducible *ras* oncogene and an inactivated *p53* tumor-suppressor gene. NAC, given at a dosage of 30 g/kg diet, significantly delayed the appearance of skin lesions, reduced tumor multiplicity by 43%, and improved survival by 5 wk. However, malignant spindle-cell tumors were only observed in 25% of NAC-fed mice, and not in controls *(136)*.

3.2.2.4. Mammary Glands NAC, given with the diet (8 g/kg diet) inhibited the formation of mammary adenocarcinomas in rats treated with methylnitrosourea (MNU) *(118)*. NAC (1 μM) inhibited the formation of DMBA-induced hyperplastic alveolar nodules in mouse mammary-organ culture *(6)* and inhibited the formation of DNA adducts in both liver and mammary epithelial cells of DMBA-treated rats (A. Izzotti et al., unpublished data). However, given with the diet (4 or 8 g/kg diet), NAC failed to inhibit the formation of mammary adenocarcinomas in Sprague-Dawley rats treated with a single dose of DMBA (12 mg/rat) by gavage *(137)*.

3.2.2.5. The Bladder Dietary NAC (0.2 g/kg diet) significantly inhibited the formation of transitional-cell bladder carcinomas in mice treated with *N*-butyl-*N*-(hydroxybutyl)nitrosamine (OH-BBN) *(138)*.

3.2.2.6. The Brain Intravenous injection of ethylnitrosourea to pregnant rats on d 18 of gestation resulted in formation of gliomas in the offspring, which had a shortened life expectancy. Diet supplementation with NAC produced no effect on the formation of brain tumors, but life expectancy was significantly improved *(139)*. Interestingly, a pharmacokinetic study had shown that radiolabeled NAC was taken up by most of the investigated mouse tissues, except the brain and spinal cord *(140)*.

3.2.2.7. Other Sites In Wistar rats that received 2AAF with the diet (0.5 g/kg diet), according to the Teebor and Becker model, co-administration of NAC (1 g/kg diet) inhibited the formation of Zymbal gland squamous-cell carcinomas *(110)*.

In F344 rats receiving sc injections of NNK (1.5 mg/kg body wt) 3×/wk a wk for 21 wk, administration of NAC with the diet, at 13.1 g/kg, reduced the incidence of Leydig-cell tumors of the testis from 27/36 (75%) to 11/36 (30.5%) *(117)*.

In the same study, in the absence of NNK administration, no tumor was detected in the pancreas of NAC-treated rats, vs a 25% incidence recorded in untreated controls *(117)*.

Administration of NAC with drinking water at 0.055 g/kg body wt did not inhibit the formation of tumors (fibrosarcomas, osteosarcomas, and carcinomas) in the hind legs of Wistar rats treated with local X-irradiation (16 Gy) and hyperthemia (60 min at 43°C), either individually or in combination *(141)*.

3.3. Chemoprevention Studies in Humans

3.3.1. PHASE I CLINICAL TRIALS

In addition to extensive clinical experience demonstrating the safety of NAC, even at very high doses (*see* Subheading 2.2.), a Phase I trial specifically evaluated the pharmacokinetics and pharmacodynamics of NAC as a potential cancer chemopreventive agent. This trial involved the escalation of both the NAC dose and the number of the treated subjects. The highest nontoxic dose was 800 mg/m²/d (0.12 mmol/kg body wt) in most of the subjects. Minimal side effects were seen at daily doses of 1600 mg/m² for 4 wk; the maximum tolerated dose was 6400 mg/m²/d (1 mmol/kg body wt), which caused bad taste and gastrointestinal disturbance in 40% of subjects *(21)*. The Euroscan trial randomized 2592 patients to NAC (600 mg/d), retinyl palmitate, a combination of both agents, or no treatment (*see* Subheading 3.3.3.). NAC was the least toxic, and 17.9% of patients failed to complete 2 y of treatment, vs 25.8% in the retinyl palmitate and 25.2% in the combined treatment arm *(142)*. In a Phase II trial, 21 smoking volunteers received 600 mg NAC in two daily doses for 6 mo (*see* Subheading 3.3.2.); all subjects tolerated the treatment and completed the study, although one participant experienced minor side effects *(143)*. Another Phase I/pharmacodynamic study evaluated the association of NAC (six smokers, 1,200 mg/d) with oltipraz at either 200 mg/d (four smokers) or 400 mg/d (nine smokers). The study was closed as a result of the side effects of treatments *(144)*.

3.3.2. PHASE II CLINICAL TRIALS

The urinary excretion of cigarette smoke genotoxic metabolites was evaluated in the *his⁻* strain YG1024 of *S. typhimurium* and in *E. coli* strains with distinctive DNA repair capacities. After treatment with oral NAC (600–800 mg/d), 7 out of 10 smokers significantly decreased excretion of genotoxic metabolites. This effect was already evident after 1 d of NAC administration, and was reversible upon withdrawal of treatment *(145)*.

Oral NAC, given for up to 142 d in three daily doses of 600 mg to 11 nonsmoking patients suffering from alveolar pulmonary fibrosis, significantly lowered levels of 4-aminobiphenyl-hemoglobin adducts *(146)*. Mechanistically, it is noteworthy that NAC is a good precursor of GSH in red blood cells *(70)*, and that GSH and hemoglobin compete for reaction with nitrosobiphenyl, a reactive metabolite of 4-aminobiphenyl *(147)*.

Agents such as NAC, which have antimutagenic activity, may protect against the numerous mutagenic events that occur throughout colon carcinogenesis *(148)*. Preliminary data suggested that NAC can decrease the recurrence rate of adenomatous polyps *(149)*. Moreover, a significant decrease in the proliferation index of colonic crypts occurred in 34 patients with previous adenomatous colonic polyps, after treatment with oral NAC (800 mg/d) for 12 mo. No variation of the same index was observed in 30 subjects who received a placebo *(150)*.

A battery of biomarkers was evaluated in healthy smoking volunteers in a double-blind Phase II chemoprevention trial in which 21 subjects were given a placebo and 20 subjects were treated with NAC (600 mg oral tablets/d), for a period of 6 mo. Although the placebo group had no significant variation in any of the investigated biomarkers, the NAC group showed a significant decrease in levels of both 8-OH-dG and lipophilic DNA adducts in BAL cells as well as in the frequency of micronuclei in the mouth floor and soft palate cells *(143)*.

Thus, several studies showed that oral NAC is capable of modulating certain biomarkers involved in carcinogenesis. Certainly, there is a broad interindividual variability in the response to treatment. As a first pharmacogenomic approach in chemoprevention research, we stratified the subjects involved in the previously mentioned Phase II trial *(143)* according to their metabolic genotypes. The decrease in micronucleus frequency in buccal cells of smokers after 6 mo of treatment with NAC became even more evident in subjects who were either *NAT2* slow acetylators or had a null *GSTM1* genotype, although there was no significant decrease either in *NAT2* fast acetylators or *GSTM1*-positive subjects (our unpublished data, in collaboration with van Schooten FJ et al.). These preliminary data suggest that metabolic genetic polymorphisms can influence responsiveness to NAC treatment in terms of reducing a genotoxicity biomarker. In particular, subjects who are slow acetylators or lack the *GSTM1* genotype thus have lower detoxifying capacities, and appear to derive greater benefit from NAC administration.

The "mutagen sensitivity" assay, which measures chromosomal damage induced by bleomycin in cultures of peripheral blood lymphocytes, has been proposed as a method to evaluate the efficacy of chemopreventive

agents *(151,152)*. However, it has also been shown that sensitivity to bleomycin is constitutional *(153)*. NAC, in doses ranging from 0.1–10 mmol/L, decreased by 23–73% the number of bleomycin-induced chromosomal breaks in freshly cultured lymphocytes from head and neck cancer patients *(151,152)*. However, sensitivity to bleomycin was not changed in lymphocytes from head and neck cancer patients who received oral NAC (600 mg/d for 3–9 mo), as compared to lymphocytes from untreated patients *(153)*.

3.3.3. Phase III Clinical Trials

A multicentric clinical trial (Euroscan) evaluated 2592 patients previously treated for head and neck cancer or lung cancer. The patients were mostly previous or current smokers, and were randomly assigned to four groups that received either no treatment, retinyl palmitate, NAC (600 mg/d), or both drugs for a period of 2 yr. After a median followup of 49 mo, 916 patients had experienced local/regional recurrences, second primary tumors, distant metastasis, and/or death. There was no significant difference among the four intervention arms *(142)*. Clearly, the target of this Phase III trial was different from that of the previously reported Phase II trial in smokers *(143)*, which evaluated the effects of NAC in healthy subjects, thereby reproducing a primary prevention setting.

4. PROTECTIVE MECHANISMS OF NAC IN MUTAGENESIS AND CARCINOGENESIS

In addition to evaluating the efficacy of putative chemopreventive agents, it is essential to understand their mechanisms of action. Inhibition of mutagenesis and carcinogenesis can be achieved by a variety of mechanisms, which are often interconnected and reiterated in various stages of carcinogenesis. During the last 15 years, we proposed several classifications of mechanisms of inhibitors and carcinogenesis, and provided examples of protective agents within each category (for instance, *see* refs. 154–157). Some chemopreventive agents have pleiotropic properties and have multiple points of intervention, which renders them effective in different stages of the pathogenetic process and efficacious toward a broader spectrum of mutagens and carcinogens. As discussed here, NAC is a typical example of an agent that acts via many different mechanisms, ranging from inhibition of mutation and cancer initiation to prevention of angiogenesis, invasion, and metastasis of cancer cells. In reviewing the protective mechanisms of NAC it should be considered that as for any other chemopreventive agent, it is often difficult to distinguish whether modulation of a given end point is a genuine mechanism or rather a secondary effect—e.g., the epiphenomenon of other mechanisms acting upstream in the chain of events that ultimately regulate the observed end point. Another preliminary consideration is that many mechanisms of NAC depend on its ability to act as a precursor of intracellular *l*-cysteine and GSH. However, other mechanisms, especially in the extracellular environment, can be ascribed to NAC itself.

4.1. Nucleophilicity

As discussed in the following subsection, the SH group of NAC and other aminothiols renders them highly reactive toward electrophilic compounds and metabolites, thereby preventing their binding to nucleophilic sites of DNA and other molecules that are critical targets in carcinogenesis. This property of NAC is broadly supported by results obtained in in vitro test systems with direct-acting mutagens (*see* Subheading 3.1.). The blocking of proximal or ultimate metabolites of carcinogens by NAC has also been demonstrated by analytical methods, as with aflatoxin B$_1$, whose difuran region is bound by NAC *(71)*, and of formic acid 2-[4-(5-nitro-furyl)-2-thiazolyl]-hydrazide (FNT), a renal carcinogen with a reactive intermediate produced by peroxidation via prostglandin H synthetase capable of forming 5-*(S)*-substituted thioether conjugates with GSH and NAC *(158)*.

4.2. Antioxidant Activity

Together with nucleophilicity, antioxidant activity represents a crucial mechanism of NAC, to such an extent that this molecule is more and more extensively used as a prototype agent to evaluate the role of oxidative mechanisms in a wide range of physiological and pathological processess.

The main mechanism of NAC as an antioxidant is scavenging ROS. ROS are endogenously generated by all aerobic cells, and are known to participate in a wide variety of deleterious reactions *(159)* and to be closely associated with alterations in gene expression *(160)*. NAC has been reported to react rapidly with hydroxyl radical (•OH) and hypochlorous ion ($^-$OCl), and more slowly with superoxide anion radical (O$^-_2$) and hydrogen peroxide (H$_2$O$_2$) *(161,162)*. The reaction of NAC with H$_2$O$_2$ involves a non-enzymic reduction of the peroxide with concomitant formation of NAC disulfide *(163)*. NAC and other thiols react with singlet oxygen

('O$_2$), presumably by formation of corresponding disulfides *(164)*. In bacterial test systems, NAC attenuated the genotoxicity of peroxides, such as H$_2$O$_2$ *(20,60)* and cumene hydroperoxide *(1)*. NAC also inhibited the mutagenicity of •OH released by human phagocytic leukocytes *(63)*. NAC exerted protective effects when ROS were generated by monoelectronic reduction of O$_2$ in the reaction of xanthine oxidase with hypoxanthine, which forms H$_2$O$_2$. Mutagenicity at this stage was ascribed to O$^-_2$, since catalase had no significant effect. A further enhancement of mutagenicity was observed by accelerating O$^-_2$ dismutation upon addition of superoxide dismutase (SOD), leading to the formation of H$_2$O$_2$. In any case, NAC efficiently decreased the mutagenicity of ROS *(55)*. Moreover, NAC attenuated the genotoxic effects produced by volatile ROS generated by illuminating the chromophore rose bengal, which results both in electron transfer reactions (O$^-_2$, H$_2$O$_2$, and •OH) and energy transfer reactions ('O^2) *(62)*. By using ^{32}P postlabeling methods, NAC was found to inhibit the formation of 8-OH-dG *(48)* and 8-oxo-dG *(49)* in DNA exposed to •OH-generating Fenton-type reactions. In addition, NAC protected DNA from reactive nitrogen species (RNS), such as peroxynitrite resulting from the reaction between cigarette smoke and a nitric oxide-releasing compound *(47)*.

Lipid peroxidation is an important mechanism involved in the pathogenesis of diverse diseases. NAC inhibited the lipid peroxidation induced by inflammatory reactions of malondialdehyde in vivo *(165)*, and counteracted the effects of 4-hydroxy-2-nonenal *(166)*.

Recently, NAC has also been shown to inhibit cyclooxygenases (COX). For instance, it inhibited the expression of COX-2 in colorectal cancer (CRC) cells *(167)* and in vascular muscle cells *(168)*. NAC was found to be a strong inhibitor of NNK-induced prostaglandin E$_2$ (PGE$_2$) synthesis by decreasing COX-1 expression in cultured human macrophages. It was suggested that ROS, generated during pulmonary metabolism of NNK, could act as signal-transduction messengers and activate NFκB, which induces COX activity and increases PGE$_2$ synthesis *(169)*.

Although many studies have documented the antioxidant properties of NAC, a few studies show that, under certain conditions, this thiol may behave as a pro-oxidant. For instance, in the presence of Cu(II), NAC induced DNA damage by generating H$_2$O$_2$ *(170)*. A similar situation also occurs with other typical antioxidants, and has frequently been reported with ascorbic acid (AsA) (121). In this respect, it is noteworthy that GSH has been shown, both in vitro and in vivo, to maintain a reducing intracellular milieu that can reduce dehydroascorbic acid (171,172). A similar effect was produced by combining AsA with NAC (121).

4.3. Inhibition of the Nitrosation Reaction and Blocking of the Nitrosation Products

The nitrosation reaction mainly occurs in the acidic stomach environment, and represents an important source of endogenously formed carcinogens. We comparatively evaluated the ability of NAC, GSH, and ascorbic acid to affect the nitrosation reaction and to block the nitrosation products of famotidine and ranitidine in a simulated acidic environment. Compared to ascorbic acid, a prototype inhibitor of nitrosation, the two thiols were much slower in reacting with sodium nitrite. However, they were much more efficient in blocking the mutagenicity of nitrosoderivatives of both famotidine and ranitidine (173).

4.4. Modulation of Xenobiotic Metabolism

NAC appears to behave as a weak bifunctional inducer of xenobiotic metabolism. In fact, it poorly influences phase 1 enzymes that are involved in the metabolic activation of procarcinogens, and stimulates phase 2 enzymes to some extent (8).

In particular, NAC did not affect the levels of total cytochromes P450 when assayed either in vitro in chicken embryo hepatocytes (174) or in vivo in the rat liver and lung (70). Dietary NAC slightly—but significantly—induced aryl hydrocarbon hydroxylase (AHH) activity in the liver of Wistar rats (2), yet did not affect the increase of AHH in the lung and of 7-ethoxyresorufin O-deethylase (EROD) and epoxide hydrolase induced by the exposure of Sprague-Dawley rats to mainstream cigarette smoke (175).

Several studies have provided evidence that NAC is capable of modulating cytosolic enzyme activities that are directly or indirectly related to the GSH cycle (see Subheading 2.1.). In fact, dietary NAC stimulated G6PD, 6PGD, GSSG reductase, and NAD(P)H-dependent diaphorases in the hepatic and pulmonary S105 fractions of Sprague-Dawley rats (70). It also stimulated G6PD, 6PGD, NAD(P)H-dependent diaphorases, chromium(VI) reduction, and GST in PAM S12 fractions from the same animals (176). Stimulation of GSSG reductase was also found to occur in peripheral-blood lymphocytes of human volunteers who took oral NAC (21).

GST, a crucial phase 2 enzyme, has been proposed as a marker for potential inhibitors of chemical carcinogenesis (177). GST was slightly but significantly induced in the liver of Swiss albino mice (119) and F344 rats (132) that received NAC with the diet. NAC is an inducer of GSTP1 gene, an effect largely mediated by the activator protein-1 (AP-1) site (178). Interestingly, from a total of 688 tested genes by cDNA array technology, GSTM2 and GSTP1 were the only genes overexpressed in the liver of Swiss albino fetuses whose mothers had received NAC in drinking water (Izzotti A et al., manuscript in preparation).

4.5. Effects in Mitochondria

NAC has shown protective effects in mitochondria. As discussed in Subheading 3.2.1.1., its oral administration inhibited the formation of adducts to mtDNA in the lungs of rats exposed to mainstream cigarette smoke (90). In mice, NAC protected against the age-related increase in oxidized proteins in synaptic mitochondria (179) and the decline of oxidative phosphorylation in liver mitochondria, whereas NAC significantly increased the specific activity of complex I, IV, and V (180). In vitro, NAC enhanced adenosine 5'triphosphate (ATP) levels in bovine retinal pigment epithelium cells subjected to oxidative stress (181) and prevented the tobacco-smoke-induced disruption of deltapsim (mitochondrial membrane potential) that resulted in apoptotic death of human monocytes (182).

4.6. Decrease of Biologically Effective Carcinogen Dose

Adducts to macromolecules are crucial steps in carcinogenesis. Accordingly, in principle, inhibition of their formation in treated animals or exposed humans would be expected to predict a decreased risk of developing the disease (183). As reported in greater detail in Subheading 3.2.1. and in the references cited therein, oral NAC significantly decreased the levels of adducts to hemoglobin and adducts to nuclear DNA in isolated cells (BAL cells, mammary epithelial cells), tissues (tracheal epithelium), and organs (lung, liver, heart, kidney, testis) of rodents exposed to carcinogens, such as B[a]P and DMBA, and complex mixtures, such as air-particulate extracts, mainstream cigarette smoke, and environmental cigarette smoke. In humans, oral NAC significantly decreased hemoglobin adduct levels in non-smokers and DNA adduct levels in BAL cells of smokers (see Subheading 3.3.2.).

4.7. Effects on DNA Repair

The differential ability of NAC and other thiols to decrease the "spontaneous" mutagenicity in strain TA104 of *S. typhimurium* but not in TA102, which has a deletion of the *uvrB* gene encoding for an error-free DNA excision-repair system, suggests that NAC may influence DNA-repair processes *(56)*. Using three different hepatocarcinogenesis models (Teebor and Becker, Solt and Faber, and Druckey) in Wistar rats, dietary NAC prevented the 2AAF-induced depletion of PARP, a nuclear enzyme that modulates changes in chromatin architecture during DNA replication or DNA excision repair *(106)*. Depletion of GSH is known to lead to methionine deficiency thereby impairing the methylation process *(184)*.

4.8. Modulation of Gene Expression and Signal-Transduction Pathways

As discussed in Subheading 2.2., even high doses of NAC have little effect on the expression of a number of genes in the mouse lung under physiological conditions. However, in recent years, an impressive number of studies have documented that NAC is capable of modulating a variety of signal-transduction pathways altered by toxic agents, carcinogens, cytokines, and changes of the redox potential. For example, the following effects were produced by NAC: the post-transcriptional increase of *p53* expression *(185)*; decrease of retinoblastoma (RB) protein phosphorylation which leads to reversal of RB-mediated growth inhibition *(186)*; decrease of c-*fos* and c-*jun* induction *(187)*; inhibition of activation *(188)* and binding activity *(189)* of the transcription factor activator protein-1 (AP-1); inhibition of activation *(188,190)*; and nuclear translocation *(191)* of the transcription factor NFκB; inhibition of activity of the transcription factor-signal-transducer and activator of transcription (STAT1) *(192)*; inhibition of overexpression of NFκB-inducing kinase (NIK) and IκB kinases (IKK-α and IKKβ) *(190)*; inactivation of proteine kinase C (PKC) *(193)*; blocking the expression of *GADD153* gene *(194)*; uncoupling signal transduction from *ras* to mitogen-activated protein kinase (MAPK) *(185)*; activation of phosphorylation of extracellular signal-regulated kinase (ERK)-MAPK *(195)*; induction of *p16 (INK4a)* and *p21 (WAF/CIP1)* expression and prolongation of cell-cycle transition through the G_1 phase *(196)*; inhibition of tumor necrosis factor-α (TNFα) release *(191)* and TNFα induced sphingomyelin hydrolysis and ceramide generation *(197)*; decrease of the biological activity of transforming growth factor-β (TGFβ) as a result of a direct effect on the TGFβ molecule *(198)*; suppression of epidermal growth factor (EGF) dimerization, activation of the EGF cellular receptor and EGF-induced activation of c-*ras (199)*; inhibition of c-Ha-*ras* expression *(200)*.

4.9. Anticytotoxic Activity

In addition to the studies which specifically deal with modulation of apoptosis (*see* Subheading 4.10.), many reports have examined the anticytotoxic activity of NAC, to such an extent that this molecule has been defined as a pluripotent protector against cell death *(201)*. To give a few examples, NAC prevented the GSH-depleting effects of cigarette smoke in the isolated perfused rat lung *(202)* and counteracted the toxicity of cigarette smoke in cultured rat hepatocytes and lung cells *(203)*, human bronchial cells *(203)*, alveolar macrophages *(204)*, and monocytes *(205)*. NAC was by far the most effective of the agents studied in protecting rat cardiomyocytes from the toxicities of the *N*-hydroxyl amino metabolites of the heterocyclic amines 2-amino-3-methylimidazo[4,5-*f*]quinoline (IQ) and 2-amino-2-methyl-6-phenylimidazo[4,5-*b*]pyridine (PHiP) *(206)*. NAC inhibited the toxicity to endothelial cells of cigarette smoke extracts *(205)*, hyperoxia *(207)*, and ROS generated in the hypoxanthine-xanthine oxidase system *(208)*. NAC resulted in a significant inhibition of chromium(VI)-induced cell death in NFκB-inhibited cells, which suggested that NFκB is essential for inhibiting ROS-dependent cytotoxicity *(209)*.

4.10. Modulation of Apoptosis

More than 100 data dealing with modulation of apoptosis by NAC were selected from MEDLINE in a survey carried out in November 2000. Test cells included both normal cells from different systems (respiratory, cardiovascular, haematopoietic, digestive, nervous, and endocrine) and tumor cells (carcinomas, sarcomas, and tumors of the hematopoietic system) from a variety of species, including humans, bovines, felines, and rodents. Many different inducers were used in order to elicit apoptosis via ROS-mediated mechanisms. They included peroxides, such as H_2O_2 *(210–215)* and *tert*-butylhydroperoxide *(216)*; ROS donors *(215,217–221)*; NO *(222,223)* and NO_x donors *(220,222,224)*; GSH depletors *(225–227)*; modulators of metabolism, such as reducing sugars *(228–230)*, glutamate *(231,232)*, methylglyoxal, and 3-deoxyglucosone *(233,234)*; L-DOPA *(235)*; dopamine *(236–240)*; 7-ketocholesterol *(241)*; neopterin, biopterin, and folate *(242)*, complex I (NADH dehydrogenase) inhibitors *(243)*, glucose deprivation *(244)*, and trophic factor deprivation *(209)*; signal-trasduction modulators, such as NGF deprivation *(245,246)*, TNF-α(247–250), TNFα plus HIV-1 Tat *(251)*, TGF-α1 *(214)*, HGF *(252)*, antagonist G *(253)*, overexpression of *c-myc (254)*, antibodies toward *fas (221,255,256)* or CD3 *(246)*, and the lipid-signalling molecule ceramide *(257–259)*; a variety of chemical agents such as bleomycin *(260)*, actinomycin D *(261)*, daunorubicin *(262,263)*, doxorubicin *(264)*, nitrogen mustard *(265)*, pyrrolo-1,5-benzoxazepines *(266)*, retinoids (267–269), etoposide *(241,270,271)*, cycloheximide *(241)*, butyl hydroxytoluene *(272)*, and vanilloid compounds *(273)*; caffeic acid derivatives *(274)*; nordihydroguaiaretic acid *(275)*, selenite *(276)*, arsenite *(277,278)*, copper *(279)*, manganese *(280)*, and cadmium *(281)*; complex mixtures, such as cigarette smoke *(99)* and diesel exhaust particles *(282,283)*; mitogenic stimuli *(284)*; toxins, such as ricin *(285)*, endotoxin *(286)*, and 1-methyl-4-(2'-ethylphenyl)-1,2,3,6-tetrahydropyridine *(280)*; hormones and analogs or modulators, such as tamoxifen and derivatives *(287)*, glucocorticoid hormones *(288)*, methylprednisolone *(289)*, and dexamethasone *(271)*; viral infections caused by HIV *(290,291)*, feline immunodeficiency virus *(292)*, Sindbis virus *(293)*, and bovine viral diarrhea virus *(294)*; physical agents, such as asbestos *(295)*; and suboptimal growth temperature *(296)*. Actually, all cited agents work via a variety of mechanisms, which are often interconnected and share the common property of causing an imbalance of redox potential that leads to apoptosis. In several cases, the authors of the studies mentioned here have specified that certain effects of NAC were independent of its antioxidant properties and ability to replenish GSH stores.

On the whole, 91 of the 104 data (89.5%) reported with in vitro studies showed that NAC inhibits apoptosis. Ten data (9.6%) were consistent with lack of effect of NAC on apoptosis, and three data only (2.9%) showed an enhancement of apoptosis by NAC. Interestingly, in one of these three studies, NAC induced apoptosis in several transformed cell lines and transformed primary cultures, but not in normal cells *(297)*. It is important to consider that modulation of apoptosis has multiple meanings. Thus, stimulation of apoptosis is a mechanism shared by certain chemopreventive agents and a number of chemothera-

peutical drugs *(298)*. In the case of chemopreventive agents, however, one should discriminate between the induction of apoptosis as an anticarcinogenic mechanism and inhibition of apoptosis as an epiphenomenon of protective mechanisms that modulate apoptosis signalling *(156)*. In other degenerative diseases, especially those that affect post-mitotic tissues, the inhibition of apoptosis is clearly a protective mechanism *(299)*.

In the in vivo studies, oral NAC protected the respiratory tract of Sprague-Dawley rats from cigarette smoke-induced apoptosis, as shown by inhibition of apoptosis in the bronchial and bronchiolar epithelia of mainstream cigarette smoke-exposed rats and in the PAM of environmental cigarette smoke-exposed rats *(99)*. Moreover, oral NAC prevented hair follicle-cell apoptosis and alopecia in C57BL/6 mice exposed to environmental cigarette smoke *(112)*. The protective effect of NAC toward smoke-induced apoptosis in the respiratory tract may be relevant in lung carcinogenesis as well as in other pulmonary diseases *(300–302)*. Further studies demonstrated the ability of NAC to inhibit ROS-mediated apoptosis in situations which may play a role in other pathological conditions, such as experimental diabetes in pancreatic β cells of mice *(303)*, balloon-catheter injury in the rabbit carotid artery *(304)*, and tectal-cell lesions in the eye retinal ganglion of chicken embryos *(305)*.

4.11. Antiinflammatory Activity

It is well-known that NAC has antiinflammatory properties which act through mechanisms which are also involved in carcinogenesis. For instance, oral NAC normalized BAL cellularity after cessation of exposure of mice to mainstream cigarette smoke *(86)*. Its administration to rats decreased lung NFκB activation, cytokine-induced neutrophil chemoattractant mRNA expression in lung tissue, and endotoxin-induced neutrophilic alveolitis *(306)*. In another rat model of lung injury, NAC decreased all tested parameters of lung injury, such as lipid peroxidation, production of nitrite/nitrate, TNFα, and interleukin (IL) 1β *(307)*. Interestingly, the infusion of NAC at high doses reduced respiratory burst, but augmented neutrophil phagocytosis in intensive care unit patients *(308)*. NAC was consistently found to inhibit either gene expression, production, or secretion of variously induced pro-inflammatory cytokines, such as TNFα *(309)* and IL-8 *(310–312)*, and intracellular adhesion molecule-1 (ICAM-1) *(309)*. Another antiinflammatory mechanism of NAC involves the previously discussed inhibition of COX-2 *(167,168)*.

4.12. Protective Effects in Tumor-Associated Viral Diseases

As discussed in Subheading 2.1., GSH depletion occurs in viral diseases associated with tumors in humans. NAC has been shown to exert protective effects in infections caused by HBV and HCV, which are associated with primary hepatocellular carcinoma; in HIV infection, which is associated with Kaposi's sarcoma (KS) and other tumors; and in Epstein-Barr virus (EBV) infection, which is associated with Burkitt's lymphoma, sinonasal angiocentric T-cell lymphoma, immunosuppression-related lymphoma, Hodgkin's disease, and nasopharyngeal carcinoma.

NAC was found to inhibit HBV replication by disturbing the virus assembly *(313)*. It counteracted the induction of the transcription factors STAT-3 and NFκB by the HBV X (HBx) protein, which plays vital roles in viral replication and in the generation of hepatocellular carcinoma *(314)*. NAC potently suppressed the induction of κB-controlled reporter genes by the HBV middle surface (MHBs) antigen *(315)*. Moreover, NAC inhibited activation of aflatoxin B$_1$ to mutagenic metabolites in the presence of liver preparations from woodchucks, either uninfected or infected with woodchuck hepatisis virus or also bearing primary hepatocellular carcinoma *(23)*.

Oral NAC increased the levels of GSH in plasma and peripheral blood lymphocytes of patients who were chronically infected with HCV *(25)*. NAC eliminated the activation of STAT-3 and NFκB by the HCV nonstructural protein 5A (NS5A) *(316)*. However, NAC did not enhance the benefit of conventional therapy with interferon-α in chronic HCV patients *(317)*.

NAC displayed several beneficial effects in HIV infection, which correlates with the clinical finding that its oral administration combined with antiretroviral therapy significantly reduced mortality in AIDS patients *(28,29)*. NAC replenished GSH levels in plasma and T lymphocytes of HIV carriers *(318)*, and inhibited HIV reverse transcriptase in chronically infected T lymphocytes *(319)*, monocellular cells *(320,321)*, and macrophages *(322)*, which resulted in the suppression of HIV replication in the absence of cytotoxic or cytostatic effects. HIV production was also inhibited by NAC thrugh the inhibition of cytokines *(323)*. It is noteworthy that, as reported in Subheading 4.18., oral NAC strongly inhibited the growth of KS in nude mice *(324)*.

NAC has been proposed as a good candidate for controlling EBV infection, based on its ability to suppress CD21, a receptor for EBV *(325)*.

4.13. Protection of Gap-Intercellular Communications

Gap-junctional intercellular communications (GJIC) play a role in carcinogenesis, especially in tumor promotion. NAC was found to inhibit disruption of GJIC and hyperphosphorylation of connexin 43 in cultures of rat-liver epithelial cells initiated with MNNG and further treated with H$_2$O$_2$ as a tumor promoter *(81)*.

4.14. Inhibition of Proliferation

A number of studies have pointed out the possible antiproliferative effects of NAC in cultured mammalian cells via a variety of mechanisms. For instance, NAC inhibited the TPA-mediated induction of cyclin D$_1$ and DNA synthesis *(326)*, and inhibited the abnormal cell-cycle progression mediated by the *p38* MAPK cascade *(327)*. NAC reduced the elevation of *c-fos* and decreased the proliferation of rat tracheal smooth-muscle cells *(328)*. It induced *p16* (INK4a) and *p21* (WAF/CIP1) gene expression, and prolonged cell-cycle transition through G$_1$ phase in various types of mammalian cells. This finding suggested a potentially novel molecular basis for chemoprevention by NAC, as increased intracellular GSH was not required for G$_1$ arrest, and other antioxidants whose action is limited to scavenging radicals did not induce G$_1$ arrest *(195)*. Both L-NAC (GSH precursor) and D-NAC (non-precursor of GSH) slowed cell-cycle progression by inhibiting topoisomerase-IIα activity *(329)*. The remarkable decrease of cyclin D$_1$ expression and increase of pancreatic carcinoma cells in G$_1$ phase suggest the possible utility of NAC as an antitumor agent *(330)*.

There are also indications that NAC can exert antiproliferative effects in humans. For instance, oral NAC attenuated the proliferative index in the colon in patients with previous adenomatous colonic polyps *(149)*, and its topical application was successfully used for the treatment for lamellar hycthyosis, based on the observed inhibition of proliferation in cultured human keratinocytes *(331)*.

4.15. Stimulation of Differentiation

The prolonged culture of mesangial cells, derived from isolated rat glomeruli, produced multifocal nodule structures, known as "hillocks," which consist of cells and the extracellular matrix. Exposure of mesangial cells to NAC dramatically facilitated hillock formation. These results indicated that, through a redox-sensitive mechanism, NAC induces mesangial cells to create a three-dimensional cytoarchitecture that underlies cellular differentiation (332).

4.16. Modulation of Tumor Progression

In addition to its effects on cell proliferation (Subheading 4.14.) and angiogenesis (Subheading 4.18), as previously reported (Subheading 3.2.2.1.), NAC retarded malignant progression in the lungs of NNK-treated A/J mice (125).

4.17. Modulation of Immune Functions

A number of studies have evaluated the immunological effects of NAC. To give a few examples, NAC enhanced natural killer (NK) function in cells of aging mice, which is a favorable response because aging mice have decrease NK function and a higher incidence of neoplasia (333,334).Administration of NAC to mice enhanced the immunogenic potential of tumor cells (335). The topical application of NAC prevented suppression of contact hypersensitivity in UVB-exposed mice at a site distant from the site of application, which demonstrated the ability of NAC to prevent systemic immunosuppression (336). In randomized clinical trials, NAC was found to improve immune functions in asymptomatic HIV-infected subjects (337).

4.18. Inhibition of Angiogenesis

The "angiogenic switch" refers to acquisition of an angiogenic phenotype by tumor cells, generally triggered by the release of angiogenic factors such as vascular endothelial growth factor (VEGF), interleukin 8 (IL-8),TGFβ),and basic-fibroblast-like growth factor (bFGF). Tumor angiogenesis is known to play a critical role in tumor progression, but is also an early event in tumorigenesis that favors the expansion of hyperplastic foci and subsequent tumor development (338). Diverse cancer chemopreventive agents appear to interfere with common pathways in the angiogenic cascade by blocking the angiogenic switch and maintaining tumor dormancy. Several chemopreventive agents share this mechanism, suggesting that it may be a key factor; we thus propose the novel concept of "angioprevention" (338).

Several in vitro and in vivo studies have provided evidence that NAC is a potent antiangiogenic agent (338). NAC strongly inhibits expression or production of VEGF, either secreted under basal conditions by human cancer cells, such as melanoma (339) and KS (324), or induced by a variety of agents such as H_2O_2 (340), IL-1 (341), arsenite (342), hypoxia-inducible factor 1α (HIF-1) (342), epithelial growth factor, and TPA (343). NAC also inhibited adverse effects of VEGF, such as the induction of expression of monocyte chemoattractant protein-1 (MCP-1), a chemochine that has been proposed to recruit leukocytes to sites of inflammation, neovascularization, and vascular injury (344). NAC also inhibited invasion, chemotaxis, and gelatinolytic activity of human endothelial cell lines EAhy926 and HUVE cells (345) and highly vascularized KS-Imm cells (324). At the same time, NAC inhibited TGFβ-induced apoptosis and genotoxic damage produced by the oxidizing agent paraquat in EAhy926 cells (76).

Antiangiogenic activity of NAC was further supported by two in vivo studies in mice. In the first, sponges of Matrigel (a reconstituted basement membrane matrix) containing heparin and highly angiogenic KS-cell supernatants were implanted subcutaneously in C57BL/6 mice. After 72 h, these sponges became highly vascularized and hemorragic. Administration of NAC in drinking water (2 g/kg body wt) significantly reduced the formation of new blood vessels, by an average of 70%, and reduced hemoglobin content in the Matrigel implants (345). In another study, KS-Imm cells were injected subcutaneously in the flank region of (CD-1)BR nude mice. After established tumor masses were detectable in all mice, NAC was given in the drinking water (2 g/kg body wt). Consistent with the higher KS frequency in males as compared to females, the tumor volume in control mice at the end of the experiment was significantly higher in males (3.2 ± 0.5 cm^3) than in females (1.0 ± 0.3 cm^3). NAC-treated mice had significantly reduced growth in both genders, and the tumor volume was 1.1 ± 1.0 cm^3 in males and 0.3 ± 0.2 cm^3 in females. Most NAC-treated females and one-half of the male animals showed an evident trend of tumor mass regression (324). In a survival experiment, NAC again significantly reduced tumor volume (9.8 ± 6.2 cm^3 in control mice as opposed to 1.3 ± 1.1 cm^3 in NAC-treated mice when all mice were still alive) and increased median survival time (45 d in controls vs 108 d in treated animals). Two-thirds of treated mice showed regression of the neoplastic mass after 15–55 d, which in one-half of the responders appeared to be complete. These mice showed a high and significant correlation between tumor volume and either VEGF or proliferation markers PCNA and Ki-67, which accordingly were significantly lower in NAC-treated mice than in controls. This correlated with reduced VEGF production in NAC-treated cultures *(324)*.

4.19. Inhibition of Invasion and Metastasis of Cancer Cells

Inhibition of angiogenesis by NAC, as discussed in Subheading 4.18., interferes with growth of the neoplastic mass and prevents possible contact between cancer cells and vessels, a prerequisite for invasion of blood and lymphatic streams by cancer cells and their subsequent colonization in distant tissues to form metastases. Several additional lines of evidence from both in vitro and in vivo experiments provide evidence for NAC's ability to prevent invasion and metastasis.

A crucial role in invasion is played by degradation of type IV collagen in vessel basement membranes. This process is accomplished by enzymes that are produced by cancer cells, particularly matrix metalloproteases (MMP) known as type IV collagenases, such as MMP-2 (gelatinase A) and MMP-9 (gelatinase B) *(346)*. These enzymes are thus key targets for inhibitors of invasion and metastasis. In agreement with preliminary data reported by another laboratory *(347)*, we showed that NAC completely inhibits both MMP-2 and MMP-9 produced by murine melanoma cells (K1735 and B16-BL6) and Lewis lung carcinoma cells (C87) *(348)*. Furthermore, it has been shown that NAC inhibited the invasion of T24 human bladder cancer cells by decreasing MMP-9 production *(349)*. Inhibition of type IV collagenases by NAC can be ascribed to the fact that sulfhydryl groups chelate a zinc ion that is essential for the activity of these enzymes *(350)*. In addition, as reported in Subheading 4.8., NAC inhibits activation *(188)* and binding activity *(189)* of AP-1, a heterodimeric complex encoded by proto-oncogenes c-*jun* and c-*fos* that is involved in collagenase gene transcription *(189)*.

Additional protective effects of NAC may result from its ability to attenuate oxidative mechanisms (Subheading 4.2.) and inflammation (Subheading 4.11.), which have been shown to play a role in invasion and metastasis. For instance, H_2O_2 may contribute to retention or extravasion of circulating tumor cells, and O_2^- released by tumor cells may be involved in basement membrane degradation *(351)*. Similar observations have also been made in studies on noncancerous cells. NAC inhibited intrinsic O_2^- generation as a byproduct of macrophages and neutrophils in human fetal membranes, and dramatically suppressed MMP-9 activity *(352)*. During acute endotoxemia, NAC blocked MMP-2 and MMP-9 activation in rat lung *(353)*. In normal human bronchial cells, NAC inhibited expression of MMP-9 induced by TNFα via the NFκB-mediated pathway *(354)*. Moreover, NAC inhibited MMP production in macrophage-derived foam cells *(355)* and alveolar macrophages *(356)* via oxidant-sensitive pathways.

Using the Boyden chamber assay, which evaluates in vitro the ability of cancer cells to invade a reconstituted basement membrane (Matrigel), provides information on three properties of malignant cells— e.g., adhesion to basement membranes, degradation, and invasion. At nontoxic concentrations, NAC inhibited chemotactic and invasive activities of five cancer cell lines of either human or murine origin in a dose-dependent manner *(348)*.

A number of experiments have provided evidence for the in vivo modulation of tumor- and malignant-cell metastasis by NAC. Particularly in experimental metastasis assays, in which formation of a primary tumor is bypassed by intravenous (iv) injection of B16-F10 melanoma cells in (CD-1)BR nude mice resulting in development of lung metastases, NAC reduced the metastatic burden. In spontaneous metastasis assays, B16-BL6 melanoma cells were injected subcutaneously into the footpad of C57BL/6 mice, resulting in local primary tumors and the subsequent spread of lung metastases. Oral administration of NAC (0.5, 1, and 2 g/kg body wt) resulted in a sharp decrease of experimental metastases, in a dose-related decrease of the weight of locally formed primary tumors, and in the reduction of spontaneous metastases *(348)*. Using the same murine models, six separate experiments showed that NAC given with drinking water and doxorubicin given parenterally behaved synergistically in reducing the weight and frequency of primary tumors and local recurrences, and the number of both experimental and spontaneous metastases *(357)*. This conclusion was further supported by an additional study in which administration of NAC alone and in combination with doxorubicin was found to significantly improve survival rates of mice treated with cancer cells *(111)*. These experiments found that oral NAC prevents alopecia induced by doxorubicin in C57BL/6 mice *(111)*. Therefore, NAC appears to exert several protective effects toward important side effects of doxorubicin, including ROS-dependent congestive cardiomyopathy *(358)*, genotoxicity in vitro *(65)*, and alopecia in mice (111). At the same time, NAC and doxorubicin appear to work synergistically to prevent metastases in mice (111,357).

Several independent studies have confirmed the antitumoral and antimetastatic properties of NAC. For instance, oral NAC inhibited tumor appearance in more than one-third (18 of 50) of B6D2F1 mice injected with L1210 lymphoma cells. The same animals were resistant to a second inoculation of L1210 cells with no further treatment with NAC (359). The iv administration of NAC, coupled with high hydrostatic pressure, provoked an anti-tumor response capable of eradicating metastatic nodules formed by Lewis lung carcinoma cells in C57BL/6 and Balb/c mice (335). In spontaneous hypertensive (SHR) rats, ER-1 cells treated for 1 mo with EGF produced tumor nodules in the peritoneum after intraperitoneal (ip) injection, and formed lung metastases after iv injection. Both peritoneal tumors and lung metastases were significantly reduced when ER-1 cells were co-treated with EGF and 5 or 10 mM NAC (360).

4.20. Inhibition of Multidrug Resistance Genes

Overexpression of multidrug resistance (mdr) genes and their encoded P-glycoproteins mediates the adenosine 5' triphosphate (ATP)-efflux of lipophilic xenobiotics and anticancer drugs, and is a major mechanism for the development of resistance of cancer cells to chemotherapy. The addition of H_2O_2 to the culture medium of primary rat hepatocytes resulted in mdrb-1 mRNA and P-glycoprotein overexpression, which was markedly suppressed by NAC (361). Similarly, NAC was found to inhibit the NFκB-mediated activation of mdrb-1 by the hepatocarcinogen 2AAF (362).

4.21. Extension of Lifespan in Experimental Test Systems

Because of mechanisms such as antioxidant activity (Subheading 4.2.), effects in mitochondria (Subheading 4.5.), and stimulation of immune functions during aging (Subheading 4.17.), NAC would be expected to have anti-aging properties. In fact, under in vitro conditions, NAC markedly extended the lifespan of human diploid fibroblasts. Since the GSH depletor L-buthionine-(R,S)-sulfoximine (BSO) had an opposite effect, it was concluded that cellular GSH level is a determinant of the lifespan of these cells (363). A study in Drosophila melanogaster showed that dietary NAC resulted in a significant and dose-dependent increase of the lifespan. The largest effect was obtained at a

NAC concentration of 10 mg/mL food and corresponded to a 27% extension of the lifespan. At this dose, NAC treatment did not influence the feeding behavior or the physical activity of the flies (364). These results corroborate the finding that aging in the mosquito is correlated with a GSH loss that may be caused by cysteine deficiency (365).

4.22. Improvement of Quality of Life for Cancer Patients

Studies in humans have led to the conclusion that NAC may improve the quality of life of cancer patients. In fact, NAC increased the body-cell mass both in healthy subjects with high plasma cysteine/thiol ratios and in cancer patients. The body-cell mass is the sum of the oxygen-consuming, potassium-rich, and glucose-oxidizing cells and—in practical terms—is the total body mass minus body fat and extracellular mass. In addition, NAC increased albumin level and functional capacity in cancer patients, in the absence of detectable changes in the GSH status. These studies showed a substantial change in the plasma thiol/disulfide redox state in human senescence and wasting, and suggested that this change may be a causative factor and a potential target for clinical intervention. The effect of NAC treatment on the albumin level was considered particularly important because of earlier unsuccessful attempts to improve this parameter by nutritional therapy, and because the albumin level is a strong predictor of hospital survival and the cost of hospitalization (366).

5. CONCLUSIONS

Cancer chemopreventive agents should have certain essential requirements, including low cost, practicality of use, lack of side effects, and efficacy (183). There is no doubt that NAC meets the first three requirements. As to efficacy, NAC showed an impressive variety of protective effects and mechanisms in vitro, in animal models, and also in humans at the level of intermediate biomarkers. As for most drugs assayed in intervention trials, its efficacy as a cancer chemopreventive agent has not yet been established in humans. Studies designed to evaluate whether regular NAC intake in healthy individuals can actually lower the risk of developing cancer are particularly imortant. Moreover, the anti-angiogenic and anti-invasive properties of NAC, which have a solid mechanistic foundation, warrant studies aimed at evaluating whether this molecule—possibly at high doses and in combination with cytostatic drugs—could help to inhibit the progression of cancer in humans.

ACKNOWLEDGMENTS

The studies reported in this article were supported by grants from the US National Cancer Institute, the Italian Association for Cancer Research (AIRC), and the Italian Ministry of University and Research (MIUR).

We thank Dr. Sofia Ceravolo for her skillful assistance in editing the manuscript.

REFERENCES

1. De Flora S, Bennicelli C, Serra D, et al. Role of glutathione and *N*-acetylcysteine as inhibitors of mutagenesis and carcinogenesis, in *Absorption and Utilization of Amino Acids, Vol. III*. Friedman M, ed. CRC Press, Boca Raton, FL, 1989, pp.19–53.
2. De Flora S, Camoirano A, Izzotti A, et al. Antimutagenic and anticarcinogenic mechanisms of aminothiols, in *Anticarcinogenesis and Radiation Protection III*. Nygaard F, Upton AC, eds. Plenum Press, New York, 1991, pp.275–285.
3. De Flora S, Izzotti A, D'Agostini F, Cesarone CF. Antioxidant activity and other mechanisms of thiols in chemoprevention of mutation and cancer. *Am J Med* 1991;91 suppl 3C:122–130.
4. De Flora S, Izzotti A, D'Agostini F, et al. Chemopreventive properties of *N*-acetylcysteine and other thiols, in *Cancer Chemoprevention*. Wattenberg L, Lipkin M, Boone CW, Kelloff GJ, eds. CRC Press, Boca Raton, FL, 1992, pp.183–194.
5. De Vries N, De Flora S. *N*-Acetyl-L-cysteine. *J Cell Biochem* 1993; 17F suppl:270–278.
6. Kelloff GJ, Crowell JA, Boone CW, et al. Clinical development plans for cancer chemopreventive agents: *N*-acetylcysteine. *J Cell Biochem* 1994;20:63–73.
7. De Flora S, Cesarone CF, Balansky RM, et al. Chemopreventive properties and mechanisms of *N*-acetylcysteine. The experimental background. *J Cell Biochem* 1995;58 suppl. 22:33–41.
8. De Flora S, Balansky R, Bennicelli C, et al. Mechanisms of anticarcinogenesis: The example of *N*-acetylcysteine, in *Drugs, Diet and Disease, Vol. 1. Mechanistic Approaches to Cancer*. Ioannides C, Lewis DFV, eds. Ellis Horwood, Hemel Hempstead, 1995, pp.151–203.
9. De Flora S, Izzotti A, D'Agostini F, Balansky RM. Mechanisms of *N*-acetylcysteine in the prevention of DNA damage and cancer, with special reference to smoking-related endpoints. *Carcinogenesis* 2001;22:999–1013.
10. Harington JS. The sulfhydryl group and carcinogenesis. *Adv Cancer Res* 1967;10:247–309.
11. Meister A. Metabolism and function of glutathione, in *Glutathione: Chemical, Biochemical and Medical Aspects*. Dolphin D, Poulson R, Avramovis O, eds. John Wiley, New York, 1989, pp.367–374.
12. Cohen G, Hochstein P. Glutathione peroxidase: the primary agent for the elimination of hydrogen peroxide in erythrocytes. *Biochemistry* 1963;2:1420–1428.
13. Chasseaud LF. The role of glutathione and glutathione *S*-transferases in the metabolism of chemical carcinogens and other electrophilic agents. *Adv Cancer Res* 1979;29:175–274.
14. Ketterer B, Harris JM, Talaska G, et al. The human glutathione *S*-transferase supergene family, its polymorphism, and its effect on susceptibility to lung cancer. *Environ Hlth Perspect* 1992;98:87–94.
15. Hayes JD, Pulford DJ. The glutathione-*S*-transferase supergene family: regulation of GST and the contribution of isoenzyme to cancer chemoprotection and drug resistance. *Crit Rev Biochem Mol Biol* 1995;30:445–600.
16. Seidegård J, Vorachek WR, Pero RW, Pearson WR. Hereditary differences in the expression of the human glutathione transferase active on *trans*-stilbene oxide are due to a gene deletion. *Proc Natl Acad Sci USA* 1988;85:7293–7297.
17. Tanningher M, Malacarne D, Izzotti A, et al. Drug metabolism polymorphisms as modulators of cancer susceptibility. *Mutat Res* 1999;436:227–261.
18. Izzotti.A, Saccà SC, Cartiglia C, De Flora S. Oxidative DNA damage in the eye of glaucoma patients. *Am J Med*, 2003;114:638–646.
19. Izzotti A, Cartiglia C, Lewtas J, De Flora S. Increased DNA alterations in atherosclerotic lesions of individuals lacking the *GSTM1* genotype. *FASEB J* 2001;15:752–757.
20. De Flora S, Bennicelli C, Zanacchi P, et al. In vitro effects of *N*-acetylcysteine on the mutagenicity of direct-acting compounds and procarcinogens. *Carcinogenesis* 1984;5:505–510.
21. Pendyala L, Creaven PJ. Pharmacokinetic and pharmacodynamic studies of *N*-acetylcysteine, a potential chemopreventive agent during a phase I trial. *Cancer Epidemiol Biomark Prev* 1995;4:245–251.
22. De Flora S, Hietanen E, Bartsch H, et al. Enhanced metabolic activation of chemical hepatocarcinogens in woodchucks infected with hepatitis B virus. *Carcinogenesis* 1989;10:1099–1106.
23. De Flora S, Bennicelli C, Camoirano A, et al. Metabolic activation of food hepatocarcinogens in hepatitis B virus-infected humans and animals, in *Mutagens and Carcinogens in the Diet*. Pariza MW, Aeschbacher H-U, Felton JS, Sato S, eds. New York, Wiley-Liss, 1990, pp.167–172.
24. Izzotti A, Scatolini L, Lewtas J, et al. Enhanced levels of DNA adducts in the liver of woodchucks infected with hepatitis virus. *Chem-Biol Inter* 1995;97:273–285.
25. Suàrez M, Beloqui O, Prieto J. GSH and chronic hepatitis C virus (Abstract), in *Preventive and Therapeutic Strategies for Lung Protection: The Role of Glutathione System*. ESI Stampa Medica, San Donato Milanese, 1992, p.20.
26. Eck HP, Gmünder H, Hartmann M, et al. Low concentrations of acid-soluble thiol (cysteine) in the blood plasma of HIV-1-infected patients. *Biol Chem Hoppe-Seyler* 1989;370:101–108.
27. Buhl R, Holroyd KJ, Mastrangeli A, et al. Systemic glutathione deficiency in symptom-free HIV-seropositive individuals. *Lancet* 1989; ii:1294–1298.
28. Herzenberg LA, De Rosa SC, Dubs JG, et al. Glutathione deficiency is associated with impaired survival in HIV disease. *Proc Natl Acad Sci USA* 1997;94:1967–1972.
29. Marmor M, Alcabes P, Titus S, et al. Low serum thiol levels predict shorter times-to-death among HIV-infected injecting drug users. *AIDS* 1997;11:1389–1393.
30. Sen CK, Packer L. Thiol homeostasis and supplements in physical exercise. *Am J Clin Nutr* 2000;72 Suppl 2:653S–669S.

31. Burgunder JM, Varriale A, Lauterberg BH. Effect of *N*-acetylcysteine and glutathione following paracetamol administration. *Eur J Clin Pharmacol* 1989;36:127–131.

32. Flanagan RJ, Meredith TJ. Use of *N*-acetylcysteine in clinical toxicology. *Am J Med* 1991;91:131–139.

33. Bridgeman MME, Marsden M, MacNee W, et al. Cysteine and glutathione concentrations in plasma and bronchoalveolar lavage fluid after treatment with *N*-acetylcysteine. *Thorax* 1991;46:39–42.

34. Johnston RE, Hawkins HC, Weikel JH Jr. The toxicity of *N*-acetylcysteine in laboratory animals. *Semin Oncol* 1983;10 suppl. 1:17–24.

35. Mulvaney W, Quilter T, Mortera A. Experiences with acetylcysteine in cystinuric patients. *J. Urol* 1975;114:107–108.

36. Prescott LF, Illingworth RN, Critchley JAJH, et al. Intravenous *N*-acetylcysteine: the treatment of choice for paracetamol poisoning. *Br Med J* 1979;2:1097–1100.

37. Repine JE, Bast A, Lankhorst I, The Oxidative Stress Study Group. Oxidative stress in chronic obstructive pulmonary disease. *Am J Respir Crit Care Med* 1997;56:341–357.

38. Stey C, Steurer J, Bachmann S, et al. The effect of oral *N*-acetylcysteine in chronic bronchitis: a quantitative systematic review. *Eur Respir J* 2000;16:253–262.

39. De Flora S, Grassi C, Carati L. Attenuation of influenza-like symptomatology and improvement of cell-mediated immunity with long-term *N*-acetylcysteine treatment. *Eur Respir J* 1997;10:1535–1541.

40. Meyer A, Buhl R, Kampf S, Magnussen H. Intravenous *N*-acetylcysteine and lung glutathione of patients with pulmonary fibrosis and normals. *Am J Crit Care Med* 1995;152:1055–1060.

41. Crystal RG, Bast A (eds). Oxidants and antioxidants: pathophysiologic determinants and therapeutic agents. *Am J Med* 1991;91:1–145.

42. Holt S, Goodier D, Marley R, et al. Improvement in renal function in hepatorenal syndrome with *N*-acetylcysteine. *Lancet* 1999;353:294–295.

43. Tepel M, van der Giet M, Schwarzfeld C, et al. Prevention of radiographic-contrast-agent-induced reductions in renal function by acetylcysteine. *N Engl J Med* 2000;343:180–184.

44. Colombo AA, Alessandrino EP, Bernasconi P, et al. *N*-acetylcysteine in the treatment of steroid-resistant acute graft-versus-host-disease: preliminary results. Gruppo Italiano Trapianto di Midollo Osseo (GITMO). *Transplantation* 1999;68:1414–1416.

45. Wiklund O, Fager G, Anderson A, et al. *N*-acetylcysteine treatment lowers plasma homocysteine but not serum lipoprotein(a) levels. *Atherosclerosis* 1996;119:99–106.

46. Sochman J, Vrbska J, Musilova B, Rocek M. Infarct size limitation: acute *N*-acetylcysteine defense (ISLAND trial): preliminary analysis and report after the first 30 patients. *Clin Cardiol* 1996;19:94–100.

47. Yoshie Y, Ohshima H. Synergistic induction of DNA strand breakage by cigarette tar and nitric oxide. *Carcinogenesis* 1997;18:1359–1363.

48. Izzotti A, Orlando M, Gasparini L, et al. In vitro inhibition by *N*-acetylcysteine of oxidative DNA modifications detected by ^{32}P postlabeling. *Free Radic Res* 1998;28:165–178.

49. Srinivasan P, Vadhanan MV, Arif JM, Gupta RC. Evaluation of antioxidant potential of natural and synthetic agents *in vitro* (Abstract). *Proc Am Ass Cancer Res* 2000;41:663–664.

50. Wang M, Nishikawa A, Chung FL. Differential effects of thiols on DNA modifications via alkylation and Michael addition by alpha-acetoxy-*N*-nitrosopyrrolidine. *Chem Res Toxicol* 1992;5:528–531.

51. Smith WA, Gupta RC. Use of a microsome-mediated test system to assess efficacy and mechanisms of cancer chemopreventive agents. *Carcinogenesis* 1996;17:1285–1290.

52. Smith WA, Arif JM, Gupta RC. Effect of cancer chemopreventive agents on microsome-mediated DNA adduction of the breast carcinogen dibenzo*[a,l]*pyrene. *Mutat Res* 1998;412:307–314.

53. Waters MD, Stack HF, Jackson MA, et al. Activity profiles of antimutagens. In vitro and in vivo data. *Mutat Res* 1996;350:109–129.

54. De Flora S, Bennicelli C, Camoirano A, et al. Inhibition of mutagenesis and carcinogenesis by *N*-acetylcysteine, in *Anticarcinogenesis and Radiation Protection*. Cerutti PA, Nygaard O, Simic MG, eds. Plenum Press, New York and London, 1987, pp.373–379.

55. De Flora S, Bennicelli C, Zanacchi P, et al. Mutagenicity of active oxygen species in bacteria and its enzymatic or chemical inhibition. *Mutat Res* 1989;214:153–158.

56. De Flora S, Bennicelli C, Rovida A, et al. Inhibition of the "spontaneous" mutagenicity in *Salmonella typhimurium* TA102 and TA104. *Mutat Res* 1994;307:157–167.

57. Barale R, Micheletti R, Sbrana C, et al. *N*-acetylcysteine inhibits diesel extract mutagenicity in the Ames test and SCE induction in human lymphocytes in *Antimutagenesis and Anticarcinogenesis Mechanisms III*. Bronzetti G, Hayatsu H, De Flora S, et al., eds. Plenum Press, New York, 1993, pp.149–160.

58. Selig C, Nothdurft W, Fliedner TM. Radioprotective effect of *N*-acetylcysteine on granulocyte/macrophage colony-forming cells of human bone marrow. *J Cancer Res Clin Oncol* 1993; 115:346–349.

59. De Flora S, Camoirano A, Izzotti A, Bennicelli C. Potent genotoxicity of halogen lamps, compared to fluorescent light and sunlight. *Carcinogenesis* 1990;11:2171–2177.

60. De Flora S. Detoxification of genotoxic compounds as a threshold mechanism limiting their carcinogenicity. *Toxicol Pathol* 1984;12:337–343.

61. Howden PJ, Faux SP. Glutathione modulates the formation of 8-hydroxydeoxy-guanosine in isolated DNA and mutagenicity in *Salmonella typhimurium* TA100 induced by mineral fibres. *Carcinogenesis* 1996;17:2275–2277.

62. Camoirano A, De Flora S, Dahl T. Genotoxicity of volatile and secondary reactive oxygen species generated by photosensitization. *Env Mol Mutag* 1993;21:219–228.

63. Weitzman SA, Stossel TP. Effects of oxygen radical scavengers and antioxidants on phagocyte-induced mutagenesis. *J Immunol* 1982;128:2770–2772.

64. Wilpart M, Mainguet P, Geeroms D, Roberfroid M. Desmutagenic effects of *N*-acetylcysteine on direct and indirect mutagens. *Mutat Res* 1985;142:169–177.

65. De Flora S, Camoirano A, Izzotti A, et al. Antimutagenic and anticarcinogenic mechanisms of aminothiols, in *Anticarcinogenesis and Radiation Protection III*. Nygaard F, Upton AC eds. Plenum Press, New York, 1991, pp.275–285.

66. Camoirano A, Balansky RM, Bennicelli C, et al. Experimental databases on inhibition of the bacterial mutagenicity of 4-nitroquinoline 1-oxide and cigarette smoke. *Mutat Res* 1994;317: 89–109.

67. Camoirano A, Badolati GS, Zanacchi P, et al. Dual role of thiols in N-methyl-N-nitro-N-nitrosoguanidine genotoxicity. *Life Science Adv-Exp Oncol* 1988;7:21–25.

68. Park K, Liem A, Stewart BC, Miller JA. Vinyl carbamate epoxide, a major strong elecrophilic, mutagenic and carcinogenic metabolite of vinyl carbamate and ethyl carbamate (urethane). *Carcinogenesis* 1993;14:441–450.

69. Josephy PD, Carter MH, Goldberg MT. Inhibition of benzidine mutagenesis by nucleophiles: a study using the Ames test with hamster hepatic activation. *Mutat Res* 1985;143:5–10.

70. De Flora S, Bennicelli C, Camoirano A, et al. In vivo effects of N-acetylcysteine on glutathione metabolism and on the biotransformation of carcinogenic and/or mutagenic compounds. *Carcinogenesis* 1985;6:1735–1745.

71. Friedman M, Wehr CM, Schade JE, MacGregor JT. Inactivation of aflatoxin B_1 mutagenicity by thiols. *Food Chem Toxicol* 1982;20:887–892.

72. Shetty TK, Francis AR, Bhattacharya RK. Modifying role of dietary factors on the mutagenicity of aflatoxin B_1: in vitro effect of sulphur-containing amino acids. *Mutat Res* 1989;222:403–407.

73. Ioannides C, Ayrton AD, Lewis DFW, Walker R. Extrapolation of in vitro antimutagenicity to the in vivo situation: the case for anthraflavic acid. *Basic Life Sci* 1993;61:103–110

74. Yang Q, Hergenhahn M, Weninger A, Bartsch H. Cigarette smoke induces direct DNA damage in the human B-lymphoid cell line Raji. *Carcinogenesis* 1999;20:1769–1775.

75. Yih LH, Lee TC. Effects of exposure protocols on induction of kinetochore-plus and -minus micronuclei by arsenite in diploid human fibroblasts. *Mutat Res* 1999;440:75–82.

76. Aluigi MG, De Flora S, D'Agostini F,et al. Antiapoptotic and antigenotoxic effects of N-acetylcysteine in human cells of endothelial origin. *Anticancer Res* 2000;20:3183–3187.

77. Weitberg AB, Weitzman SA, Clark EP, Stossel TP. Effects of antioxidants on oxidant-induced sister chromatid exchange formation. *J Clin Investig* 1985;75:1835–1841.

78. Romert L, Jenssen D. Mechanism of N-acetylcysteine (NAC) and other thiols as both positive and negative modifiers of MNNG-induced mutagenicity in V79 Chinese hamster cells. *Carcinogenesis* 1987;8:1531–1535.

79. Parsons JL, Chipman JK. The role of glutathione in DNA damage by potassium bromate in vitro. *Mutagenesis* 2000;15:311–316.

80. Smith WA, Freeman JW, Gupta RC. Effect of chemopreventive agents on DNA adduction induced by the potent mammary carcinogen dibenzo[a,l]pyrene in the human breast cells MCF-7. *Mutat Res* 2001;480-481:97–108.

81. Huang R-P, Peng A, Hossain MZ, et al. Tumor promotion by hydrogen peroxide in rat liver epithelial cells. *Carcinogenesis* 1999;20:485–492.

82. Steele VE, Kelloff GJ, Wilkinson BP, Arnold JT. Inhibition of transformation in cultured rat tracheal epithelial cells by potential chemopreventive agents. *Cancer Res* 1990;50:2068–2074.

83. De Flora S, Izzotti A, D'Agostini F, et al. Pulmonary alveolar macrophages in molecular epidemiology and chemoprevention of cancer. *Environ Health Perspect* 1993;99:249–252.

84. Izzotti A, Balansky R, Coscia N, et al. Chemoprevention of smoke-related DNA adduct formation in rat lung and heart. *Carcinogenesis* 1992;13:2187–2190.

85. Izzotti A, Balansky RM, D'Agostini F, et al. Modulation of biomarkers by chemopreventive agents in smoke-exposed rats. *Cancer Res* 2001;61:2472–2479.

86. Balansky R, D'Agostini F, De Flora S. Induction, persistence and modulation of cytogenetic alterations in cells of smoke-exposed mice. *Carcinogenesis* 1999;20:1491–1497.

87. De Flora S, D'Agostini F, Izzotti A, Balansky R. Prevention by N-acetylcysteine of benzo(a)pyrene clastogenicity and DNA adducts in rats. *Mutat Res* 1991;250:87–93.

88. Izzotti A, Camoirano A, D'Agostini F, et al. Biomarker alterations produced in rat lung by intratracheal instillations of air particulate extracts, and chemoprevention with oral N-acetylcysteine. *Cancer Res* 1996;56:1533–1538.

89. Balansky R, D'Agostini F, De Flora S. Protection by N-acetylcysteine of the histopathological and cytogenetical damage produced by exposure of rats to cigarette smoke. *Cancer Lett* 1992;64:123–131.

90. Balansky R, Izzotti A, Scatolini L, et al. Induction by carcinogens and chemoprevention by N-acetylcysteine of adducts to mitochondrial DNA in rat organs. *Cancer Res* 1996;56:1642–1647.

91. Izzotti A, D'Agostini F, Bagnasco M, et al. Chemoprevention of carcinogen-DNA adducts and chronic degenerative diseases. *Cancer Res* 1994;54 suppl:1994s–1998s.

92. Arif JM, Gairola CG, Glauert HP, et al. Effects of dietary supplementation of N-acetylcysteine on cigarette smoke-related DNA adducts in rat tissues. *Int J Oncol* 1997;11:1227–1233.

93. Izzotti A, Bagnasco M, D'Agostini F, et al. Formation and persistence of nucleotide alterations in rats exposed whole-body to environmental cigarette smoke. *Carcinogenesis* 1999;20:1499–1505.

94. De Flora S. Threshold mechanisms and site specificity in chromium(VI) carcinogenesis. *Carcinogenesis* 2000;21:533–541.

95. Izzotti A, Orlando M, Bagnasco M, Camoirano A, De Flora S. DNA fragmentation, DNA-protein crosslinks, ^{32}P postlabeled modifications and formation of 8-hydroxy-2'-deoxyguanosine in the lung but not in the liver of rats receiving intratracheal instillations of chromium(VI). Chemoprevention by N-acetylcysteine. *Mutat Res* 1998;400:233–244.

96. Kendrick J, Nettesheim P, Hammos AS. Tumor induction in tracheal grafts. A new experimental model for respiratory carcinogenesis studies. *J Natl Cancer Inst* 1974;52:1317–1325.

97. Thomassen DG, Chen BT, Mauderly JL, et al. Inhaled cigarette smoke induces preneoplastic changes in rat tracheal epithelial cells. *Carcinogenesis* 1989;10:2359–2361.

98. Izzotti A, Balansky RM, Scatolini L, et al. Inhibition by N-acetylcysteine of carcinogen-DNA adducts in the tracheal epithelium of rats exposed to cigarette smoke. *Carcinogenesis* 1995;16:669–672.

99. D'Agostini F, Balansky RM, Izzotti A, et al. Modulation of apoptosis by cigarette smoke and cancer chemopreventive agents in the respiratory tract of rats. *Carcinogenesis* 2001;22:375–380.

100. Izzotti A, Balansky RM, Camoirano A, et al. Birth-related genomic and transcripional changes in mouse lung. Modulation by transplacental N-acetylcysteine. *Mutat. res (rev Mutat Res)* 2003;544:441–449.

101. Rogers DF, Turner NC, Marriot C, Jeffery PK. Oral N-acetylcysteine or S-carboxymethylcysteine inhibit cigarette smoke-induced hypersecretion of mucus in rat larynx and trachea in situ. *Eur Respir J* 1989;2:955–960.

102. Rubio ML, Sanchez-Cifuentes MV, Ortega M, et al. *N*-acetylcysteine prevents cigarette smoke induced small airways alterations in rats. *Eur Resp J* 2000;15:505–511.

103. Pereira MA, Khoury MD. Prevention by chemopreventive agents of azoxymethane-induced foci of aberrant crypts in rat colon. *Cancer Lett* 1991;61:27–33.

104. Pereira MA, Barnes LH, Rassman VL, et al. Use of azoxymethane-induced foci of aberrant crypts in rat colon to identify potential cancer chemopreventive agents. *Carcinogenesis* 1994;15:1049–1054.

105. Chung FL, Conaway CC, Rao CV Reddy BS. Chemoprevention of colonic aberrant crypt foci in Fisher rats by sulforaphane and phenethyl isothiocyanate. *Carcinogenesis* 2000;21:2287–2291.

106. Cesarone CF, Menegazzi M, Scarabelli L, et al. Protection of molecular enzymes by aminothiols, in *Anticarcinogenesis and Radiation Protection, Vol. 2*. Nygaard F, Upton AC, eds. Plenum Press, New York, 1991, pp.261–268.

107. Liu TY, Chen CC, Chi CW. Safrole-induced oxidative damage in the liver of Sprague-Dawley rats. *Food Chem Toxicol* 1999;37:697–702.

108. Chan JYH, Stout DL, Becker FK. Protective role of thiols in carcinogen-induced DNA damage in rat. *Carcinogenesis* 1986;7:1621–1624.

109. Izzotti A, Balansky RM, Cartiglia C, et al. Genomic and transcriptional alterations in mouse fetus liver after transplacental exposure to cigarette smoke. *FASEB J* 2003;17:1127–1129.

110. Cesarone C F, Scarabelli L, Orunesu M, et al. Effects of aminothiols in 2-acetylaminofluorene-treated rats. I. Damage and repair of liver DNA, hyperplastic foci, and Zymbal gland tumors. *In Vivo* 1987;1:85–91.

111. D'Agostini F, Bagnasco M, Giunciuglio D, et al. Oral *N*-acetylcysteine inhibition of doxorubicin-induced clastogenicity and alopecia: Interaction between the two drugs in preventing primary tumors and lung micrometastases in mice. *Int J Oncol* 1998;13:217–224.

112. D'Agostini F, Balansky R, Pesce CM, et al. Alopecia and hair follicle cell apoptosis in mice exposed to environmental cigarette smoke. *Toxicol Lett* 2000;114:117–123.

113. Izzotti A, Camoirano A, Cartiglia C, et al. Formation of DNA adducts in the aorta of smoke-exposed rats. Modulation by five chemopreventive agents. *Mutat Res* 2001;494:97–106.

114. Gandy J, Bates HK, Conder LA, Harbison RD. Effects of reproductive tract glutathione enhancement and depletion on ethyl methanesulfonate-induced dominant lethal mutations in Sprague-Dawley rats. *Teratog Carcinog Mutagen* 1992;12:61–70.

115. Doyle CE, Mackay JM, Ashby J. Failure of *N*-acetylcysteine to protect the mouse bone marrow against the clastogenicity of 7,12-dimethylbenzanthracene. *Mutagenesis* 1993;8:583–584.

116. Balansky R, De Flora S. Chemoprevention by *N*-acetylcysteine of urethane-induced lung tumors in mice, as related to the time-course monitoring of micronuclei in peripheral blood erythrocytes. *Int J Cancer* 1998;77:302–305.

117. Chung FL, Kelloff GJ, Steele VE, et al. Chemopreventive efficacy of arylalkylisothiocyanates and *N*-acetylcysteine for lung tumorigenesis in Fischer rats. *Cancer Res* 1996;56:772–778.

118. Boone CW, Steele VE, Kelloff GJ. Screening for chemopreventive (anticarcinogenic) compounds in rodents. *Mutat Res* 1992;267:251–255.

119. De Flora S, Astengo M, Serra D, Bennicelli C. Inhibition of urethan-induced lung tumors in mice by dietary *N*-acetylcysteine. *Cancer Lett* 1986;32:235–241.

120. Witschi H, Espiritu I, Yu M, Willits NH. The effects of phenethyl isothiocyanate, *N*-acetylcysteine and green tea on tobacco smoke-induced lung tumors in strain A/J mice. *Carcinogenesis* 1998,19:1789–1794.

121. D'Agostini F, Balansky R, Camoirano A, De Flora S. Interactions between *N*-acetylcysteine and ascorbic acid in modulating mutagenesis and carcinogenesis. *Int J Cancer* 2000;88:702–707

122. D'Agostini F, Balansky RM, Bennicelli C, et al. Pilot studies evaluating the lung tumor yield in cigarette smoke-exposed mice. *Int J Oncol* 2001,18:607–615.

123. Witschi H, Espiritu I, Uyeminami D. Chemoprevention of tobacco smoke-induced lung tumors in A/J strain mice with dietary *myo*-inositol and dexamethasone. *Carcinogenesis* 1999;20:1375–1378.

124. Witschi H, Uyeminami D, Moram D, Espiritu I. Chemoprevention of tobacco smoke lung carcinogenesis in mice after cessation of smoke exposure. *Carcinogenesis* 2000;21:977–982.

125. Conaway CC, Jiao D, Kelloff GJ, et al. Chemopreventive potential of fumaric acid, *N*-acetylcysteine, *N*-(4-hydroxyphenyl) retinamide and beta-carotene for tobacconitrosamine-induced lung tumors in A/J mice. *Cancer Lett* 1998;124:85–93.

126. Jiao D, Smith TJ, Yang C-S, et al. Chemopreventive activity of thiol conjugates of isothiocyanates for lung tumorigenesis. *Carcinogenesis* 1997;18:2143–2147.

127. Conaway CC, Krzeminski J, Amin S, et al. *N*-acetylcysteine conjugates of isothiocyanates inhibit lung tumors induced by a tobacco carcinogen at post-initiation stages (Abstract). *Proc Am Assoc Cancer Res* 2000;41:660.

128. Yang Y-M, Conaway CC, Chiao JW, et al. Inhibition of benzo(*a*)pyrene-induced lung tumorigenesis in A/J mice by dietary *N*-acetylcysteine conjugates of benzyl and phenethyl isothiocyanates during the postinitiation phase is associated with activation of mitogen-activated protein kinases and p53 activity and induction of apoptosis. *Cancer Res* 2002;62:2–7.

129. Balansky RM, Ganchev G, D'Agostini F, De Flora S. Effects of *N*-acetylcysteine in an oesophageal carcinogenesis model in rats treated with diethylnitrosamine and diethyldithiocarbamate. *Int J Cancer* 2002;98:493–497.

130. Wilpart M, Speder A, Roberfroid M. Anti-initiation activity of *N*-acetylcysteine in experimental colonic carcinogenesis. *Cancer Lett* 1986;31:319,324.

131. Reddy BS, Rao CV, Rivenson A, Kelloff GJ. Chemoprevention of colon carcinogenesis by organosulfur compounds. *Cancer Res* 1993;53:3493–3498.

132. Seril DN, Liao J, Ho KLK et al. Inhibition of chronic ulcerative colitis-associated colorectal adenocarcinoma development in a murine model by *N*-acetylcysteine. *Carcinogenesis* 2002;23:993–1001.

133. Pereira MA. Chemoprevention of diethylnitrosamine-induced liver foci and hepatocellular adenomas in C3H mice. *Anticancer Res* 1995;15:1953–1956.

134. Rotstein JB, Slaga TJ. Anticarcinogenic mechanisms, as evaluated in the multistage mouse skin model. *Mutat Res* 1988;202:421–427.

135. Rotstein JB, Slaga TJ. Effect of exogenous glutathione on tumor progression in the murine skin multistage carcinogenesis model. *Carcinogenesis* 1988;9:1547–1551.

136. Martin KR, Trempus C, Saulnier M, et al. Dietary *N*-acetyl-L-cysteine modulates benzo(*a*)pyrene-induced skin tumors in cancer-prone p53 haploinsufficient Tg.AC (*v-Ha-ras*) mice. *Carcinogenesis* 2001;22:1373–1378.

137. Lubet RA, Steele VE, Eto I, et al. Chemopreventive efficacy of anethole trithione, *N*-acetyl-L-cysteine, miconazole and phenethyl isothiocyanate in the DMBA-induced rat mammary cancer model. *Int J Cancer* 1997;72:95–101.

138. Kelloff GJ, Boone CW, Malone WF, et al. Development of chemopreventive agents for bladder cancer *J Cell Biochem* 1992;161:1–12.

139. Ross DA, Kish P, Muraszko KM, et al. Effect of dietary vitamin A or *N*-acetylcysteine in ethylnitrosourea-induced rat gliomas. *J Neurooncol* 1998;40:29–38.

140. McLellan LI, Lewis AD, Holl DJ, et al. Uptake and distribution of *N*-acetylcysteine in mice: tissue-specific effects on glutathione concentrations. *Carcinogenesis* 1995; 16:2099–2106.

141. Sminia P, van der Kracht AHW, Frederiks WM, Jansen W. Hyperthermia, radiation carcinogenesis and the protective potential of vitamin A and *N*-acetylcysteine. *J Cancer Res Clin Oncol* 1996;122:343–350.

142. van Zandwijk N, Dalesio O, Pastorino U, et al. EUROSCAN, a randomized trial of vitamin A and *N*-acetylcysteine in patients with head and neck cancer or lung cancer. *J Natl Cancer Inst* 2000;92:977–986.

143. Van Schooten FJ, Nia AB, De Flora S, et al. Effects of oral *N*-acetylcysteine: a multi-biomarker study in smokers. *Cancer Epidemiol Biomark Prev* 2002;11:176–175.

144. Pendyala L, Schwartz G, Bolanowska-Higdon W, et al. Phase I/pharmacodynamic study of *N*-acetylcysteine/oltipraz in smokers. Early termination due to excessive toxicity. *Cancer Epidemiol Biomark Prev* 2001;10:269–272.

145. De Flora S, Camoirano A, Bagnasco M, et al. Smokers and urinary genotoxins. Implications for selection of cohorts and modulation of endpoints in chemoprevention trials. *J Cell Biochem* 1996;25 suppl:92–98.

146. Rösler S, Behr J, Richter E. *N*-acetylcysteine treatment lowers 4-aminobiphenyl haemoglobin adduct levels in non-smokers. *Eur J Cancer Prev* 1999;8:469–472.

147. Bryant MS, Skipper PL, Tannenbaum SR, Maclure M. Haemoglobin adducts of 4-aminobiphenyl in smokers and nonsmokers. *Cancer Res* 1987;47:602–608.

148. Greenwald P, Kelloff GJ, Boone CW, McDonald SS. Genetic and cellular changes in colorectal cancer: proposed targets of chemopreventive agents. *Cancer Epidemiol Biomark Prev* 1995;4:691–702.

149. Ponz de Leon M, Roncucci L. Chemoprevention of colorectal tumors: role of lactulose and of other agents. *Scand J Gastroenterol* 1997;222:72–75.

150. Estensen RD, Levy M, Klopp SJ, et al. *N*-acetylcysteine suppression of the proliferative index in the colon of patients with previous adenomatous colonic polyps. *Cancer Lett* 1999;147:109–114.

151. Trizna Z, Schants SP, Hsu TC. Effects of *N*-acetyl-L-cysteine and ascorbic acid on mutagen-induced chromosomal sensitivity in patients with head and neck cancers. *Am J Surg* 1991;162:294–298.

152. Trizna Z, Schants SP, Lee JJ, et al. In vitro protective effects of chemopreventive agents against bleomycin-induced genotoxicity in lymphoblastoid cell lines and peripheral blood lymphocytes of head and neck cancer patients. *Cancer Detect Prev* 1993;17:575–583.

153. Cloos J, Bongers V, Lubsen H, et al. Lack of effect of daily *N*-acetylcysteine supplementation on mutagen sensitivity. *Cancer Epidemiol Biomark Prev* 1996;5:941–944.

154. De Flora S, Ramel C. Mechanisms of inhibitors of mutagenesis and carcinogenesis. Classification and overview. *Mutat Res* 1988;202:285–306.

155. De Flora S, Izzotti A, Bennicelli C. Mechanisms of antimutagenesis and anticarcinogenesis. Role in primary prevention, in *Antimutagenesis and Anticarcinogenesis Mechanisms III*. Bronzetti G, Hayatsu H, De Flora S, et al., eds. Plenum Press, New York, 1993, pp.1–16.

156. De Flora S. Mechanisms of inhibitors of mutagenesis and carcinogenesis. *Mutat Res* 1998;402:151–158.

157. De Flora S, Izzotti A, D'Agostini F, et al. Multiple points of intervention in the prevention of cancer and other mutation related diseases. *Mutat Res* 2001;480–481:9–22.

158. Walters FP, Wise RW, Lakshmi VM, et al. Metabolism of the renal carcinogen FNT by peroxidases. *Carcinogenesis* 1986;7:1411–1414.

159. Allen RG. Oxidative stress and superoxide dismutase in development, aging and gene regulation. *Age* 1998;21:47–76.

160. Allen RG, Tresini M. Oxidative stress and gene regulation. *Free Radic Biol Med* 2000;28:463–499.

161. Aruoma OI, Halliwell B, Hoey B M, Butler J. The antioxidant action of *N*-acetylcysteine: its reaction with hydrogen peroxide, hydroxyl radical, superoxide, and hypochlorous acid. *Free Radic Biol Med* 1989,6, 593–597.

162. Doelman CJ, Bast A. Oxygen radicals in lung pathology. *Free Radic Biol Med.* 1990;9:381–400.

163. Moldéus P, Cotgreave IA, Berggren M. Lung protection by a thiol-containing antioxidant: *N*-acetylcysteine. *Respiration* 1986;50 Suppl 1: 31–42.

164. Rougée M, Bensasson RV, Land EJ, Pariente R. Deactivation of singlet molecular oxygen by thiols and related compounds, possible protectors against skin photosensitivity. *Photochem Photobiol* 1988;47:485–489.

165. Christen S, Schaper M, Lykkesfeldt J, et al. Oxidative stress in brain during experimental bacterial meningitis: differential effects of α-phenyl-*tert*-butyl nitrone and *N*-acetylcysteine treatment. *Free Radic Biol Med* 2001;31:754–762.

166. Watanabe T, Pakala R, Katagiri T, Benedict CR. Lipid peroxidation product 4-hydroxy-2-nonenal acts synergistically with serotonin in inducing vascular smooth muscle cell proliferation. *Atherosclerosis* 2001;155:37–44.

167. Chinery R, Beauchamp RD, Shyr Y, et al. Antioxidants reduce cyclooxygenase-2 expression, prostaglandin production, and proliferation in colorectal cancer cells. *Cancer Res* 1998;58:2323–2327.

168. Yan Z, Subbaramaiah K, Camilli T, et al. Benzo(*a*)pyrene induces the transcription of cyclooxygenase-2 in vascular smooth muscle cells. Evidence for the involvement of extracellular signal-regulated kinase and NF-κB. *J Biol Chem* 2000;18:4949–4955.

169. Rioux N, Castonguay A. The induction of cyclooxygenase-1 by a tobacco carcinogen in U937 human macrophages is

correlated to the activation of NF-κB. *Carcinogenesis* 2000;21:1745–1751.

170. Oikawa S, Yamada K, Yamashita N, et al. *N*-acetylcysteine, a cancer chemopreventive agent, causes oxidative damage to cellular and isolated DNA. *Carcinogenesis* 1999;20:1485–1490.

171. Meister A. Glutathione, ascorbate, and cellular protection. *Cancer Res* 1994;54 Suppl:1969s–1975s.

172. Winkler BS, Orselli SM, Rex TS. The redox couple between glutathione and ascorbic acid: a chemical and physiological perspective. *Free Radic Biol Med* 1994;17:339–349.

173. De Flora S, Cesarone CF, Bennicelli C, et al. Antigenotoxic and anticarcinogenic effects of thiols. In vitro inhibition of the mutagenicity of drug nitrosation products and protection of rat liver ADP-ribosyl transferase activity, in *Chemical Carcinogenesis: Models and Mechanisms.* Feo F, Pani P, Columbano A, Garcea R, eds. Plenum Press, New York, 1988, pp.75–86.

174. Cupo DJ, Wetterhahn KE. Modification of chromium(VI)-induced DNA damage by glutathione and cytochromes P-450 in chicken embryo hepatocytes. *Proc Natl Acad Sci USA* 1985;82:6755–6759.

175. Bagnasco M, Bennicelli C, Camoirano A, et al. Metabolic alterations produced by cigarette smoke in rat lung and liver, and their modulation by oral *N*-acetylcysteine. *Mutagenesis* 1992;7:295–301.

176. De Flora S, Romano M, Basso C, et al. Detoxifying activities in alveolar macrophages of rats treated with acetylcysteine, diethyl maleate and/or Aroclor. *Anticancer Res* 1986;6:1009–1012.

177. Wattenberg LW. Inhibition of neoplasia by minor dietary constituents. *Cancer Res* 1983;43:2448s–2453s.

178. Xia C, Hu J, Ketterer B, Taylor JB. The organization of the human *GSTP1-1* gene promoter and its response to retinoic acid and cellular redox status. *Biochem J* 1996;313:155–161.

179. Banaclocha MM, Hernandez AI, Martinez N, Ferrandiz ML. *N*-acetylcysteine protects against age-related increase in oxidized proteins in mouse synaptic mitochondria. *Brain Res* 1997;762:256–258.

180. Miquel J, Ferrandiz ML, De Juan E, et al. *N*-acetylcysteine protects against age-related decline of oxidative phosphorylation in liver mitochondria. *Eur J Pharmacol* 1995;292:333–335.

181. Palmero M, Bellot JL, Castillo M, et al. An in vitro model of ischemic-like stress in retinal pigmented epithelium cells: protective effects of antioxidants. *Mech Ageing Dev* 2000;114:185–190.

182. Banzet N, Franáois D, Polla BS. Tobacco smoke induces mitochondrial depolarization along with cell death: effects of antioxidants. *Redox Rep* 1999;4:229–236.

183. De Flora S, Balansky R, Scatolini L, et al. Adducts to nuclear DNA and mitochondrial DNA as biomarkers in chemoprevention, in *Principles of Chemoprevention.* Stewart BW, McGregor D, Kleihues P, eds. IARC Sci. Publ. No. 139. International Agency for Research on Cancer, Lyon, France, 1996, pp.291–301.

184. Lertratanangkoon K, Orkiszewski RS, Scimeca JM. Methyl-donors deficiency due to chemically induced glutathione depletion. *Cancer Res* 1996;56:995–1005.

185. Liu M, Pelling JC, Ju J, et al. Antioxidant action *via p53*-mediated apoptosis. *Cancer Res* 1998;58:1723–1729.

186. Nargi JL, Ratan RR, Griffin DE. p53-independent inhibition of proliferation and p21(WAF1/Cip1)-modulated induction of cell death by the antioxidants *N*-acetylcysteine and vitamin E. *Neoplasia* 1999;1:544–556.

187. Janssen YM, Heintz NH, Mosman BT. Induction of c-*fos* and c-*jun* proto-oncogene expression by asbestos is ameliorated by *N*-acetyl-L-cysteine in mesothelial cells. *Cancer Res* 1995;55:2085–2089.

188. Kamata H, Tanaka C, Yagisawa H, et al. Suppression of nerve growth factor-induced neuronal differentiation of PC12 cells. *J Biol Chem* 1996;271:33,018–33,025.

189. Bergelson S, Pinkus R, Daniel V. Intracellular glutathione levels regulate *Fos/Jun* induction and activation of glutathione *S*-transferase gene expression. *Cancer Res* 1994;54:36–40.

190. Ho E, Chen G, Bray TM. Supplementation of *N*-acetylcysteine inhibits NFκB activation and protects against alloxan-induced diabetes in CD-1 mice. *FASEB J* 1999;13:1845–1854.

191. Oka S, Kamata H, Kamata K, et al. *N*-acetylcysteine suppresses TNF-induced NF-κB activation through inhibition of IκB kinases. *FEBS Lett* 2000;472:196–202.

192. Maziere C, Dantin F, Dubois F, et al. Biphasic effects of UVA radiation on STAT1 activity and tyrosine phosphorylation in cultured human keratinocytes. *Free Radic Biol Med* 2000;28:1430–1437.

193. Ward NE, Pierce DS, Chung SE, et al. Irreversible inactivation of protein kinase C by glutathione. *J Biol Chem* 1998;273:12,558–12,566.

194. Luethy JD, Holbrook NJ. The pathway regulating *GADD153* induction in response to DNA damage is independent of protein kinase C and tyrosine kinases. *Cancer Res* 1994;54 Suppl:1902s–1906s.

195. Li WQ, Dehnade F, Zafarullah M. Thiol antioxidant, *N*-acetylcysteine, activates extracellular signal-regulated kinase signaling pathway in articular chondrocytes. *Biochem Biophys Res Commun* 2000;275:789–794.

196. Liu M, Wikonkal NM, Brash D. Induction of cyclin-dependent kinase inhibitors and G$_1$ prolongation by the chemoprevenive agent *N*-acetylcysteine. *Carcinogenesis* 1999;20:1869–1872.

197. Liu B, Andrieu-Abadie N, Levade T, et al. Glutathione regulation of neutral sphingomyelinase in tumor necrosis factor-alpha-induced cell death. *J Biol Chem* 1998;273:11,313–11,320.

198. White AC, Maloney EK, Lee SL, et al. Reduction of endothelial cell related TGF-α activity by thiols. *Endothelium* 1999;6:231–239.

199. Kamata H, Shibukawa Y, Oka SI, Hirata H. Epidermal growth factor receptor is modulated by redox through multiple mechanisms. Effects of reduction and H$_2$O$_2$. *Eur J Biochem* 2000;267:1933–1944.

200. Kerzee JK, Ramos KS. Activation of c-Ha-*ras* by benzo(*a*)pyrene in vascular smooth muscle cells involves redox stress and aryl hydrocarbon receptor. *Mol Pharmacol* 2000;58:152–158.

201. Mayer M, Noble M. *N*-acetyl-L-cysteine is a pluripotent protector against cell death and enhancer of trophic factor-mediated cell survival *in vitro*. *Proc Natl Acad Sci USA* 1994;91:7496–7500.

202. Moldéus P, Cotgreave IA, Berggren M. Lung protection by a thiol-containing antioxidant: *N*-acetylcysteine. *Respiration* 1986;50 suppl:31–42.

203. Moldéus P, Berggren M, Grafstrom R. *N*-acetylcysteine protection against the toxicity of cigarette smoke and cigarette smoke condensates in various tissues and cells *in vitro*. *Eur J Respir Dis* 1985;139 suppl:123–129.

204. Voisin C, Aerts C, Wallaert B. Prevention of in vitro oxidant-mediated alveolar macrophage injury by cellular glutathione and precursors. *Bull Eur Physiopath Respir* 1987;23:309–313.

205. Pinot F, el Yaagoubi A, Christie P, et al. Induction of stress proteins by tobacco smoke in human monocytes: modulation by antixodants. *Cell Stress Chaperones* 1997;2:156–161.

206. Davis CD, Snyderwine EG. Protective effect of *N*-acetylcysteine against heterocyclic amine-induced cardiotoxicity in cultured myocyets and in rats. *Food Chem Toxicol* 1995;33:641–651.

207. Ota Y, Kugiyama K, Sugiyama S, et al. Impairment of endothelium-dependent relaxation of rabbit aortas by cigarette smoke extract. Role of free radicals and attenuation by captopril. *Atherosclerosis* 1997;131:195–202.

208. Junod AF, Jornot L, Grichting G. Comparative study on the selenium- and *N*-acetylcysteine-related effects on the toxic action of hyperoxia, paraquat and the enzyme reaction hypoxanthine-xanthine oxidase in cultured endothelial cells. *Agents Actions* 1987;22:176–183.

209. Chen F, Bower J, Leonard SS, et al. Protective roles of NF-κB for chromium(VI)-induced cytotoxicity is revealed by expression of IκB kinase-b mutant. *J Biol Chem* 2001;277:3342–3349.

210. Kurata S. Selective activation of p38 MAPK cascade and mitotic arrest caused by low level oxidative stress. *J Biol Chem* 2000;275:23413–23416.

211. Kanno S, Ishikawa M, Takayanagi M, et al. Exposure to hydrogen peroxide induces cell death via apoptosis in primary cultured mouse hepatocytes. *Biol Pharm Bull* 1999;22:1296–1300.

212. Kanno S, Ishikawa M, Takayanagi M, et al. Characterization of hydrogen peroxide-induced apoptosis in mouse primary cultured hepatocytes. *Biol Pharm Bull* 2000;23:37–42.

213. Rimpler MM, Rauen U, Schmidt T, et al. Protection against hydrogen peroxide cytotoxicity in rat-1 fibroblasts provided by the oncoprotein *Bcl-2*: maintenance of calcium homoeostasis is secondary to the effect of *Bcl-2* on cellular glutathione. *Biochem J* 1999;340:291–297.

214. Lafon C., Mathieu C, Guerrin M, et al. Transforming growth factor beta 1-induced apoptosis in human ovarian carcinoma cells: protection by the antioxidant *N*-acetylcysteine and *bcl-2*. *Cell Growth Differ* 1996;7:1095–1104.

215. Suhr SM, Kim DS. Comparison of the apoptotic pathways induced by L-amino acid oxidase and hydrogen peroxide. *J Biochem Tokyo* 1999;125:305–309.

216. Jiang S, Wu MW, Sternberg P, Jones DP. *Fas* mediates apoptosis and oxidant-induced cell death in cultured hRPE cells. *Investig Ophthalmol Vis Sci* 2000;41:645–655.

217. Chen SH, Liu SH,, Liang YC, et al. Death signaling pathway induced by pyrrolidine dithiocarbamate-Cu(2+) complex in the cultured rat cortical astrocytes. *Glia* 2000;31:249–261.

218. Galle J, Heermeier, Wanner C. Atherogenic lipoproteins, oxidative stress, and cell death. *Kidney Int* 1999;56 Suppl 71:S62–S65.

219. Ma Y, Ogino T, Kawabata T, et al. Cupric nitrilotriacetate-induced apoptosis in HL-60 cells association with lipid peroxidation, release of cytochrome c from mitochondria, and activation of caspase-3. *Free Radic Biol Med* 1999;27:227–233.

220. Foresti R, Sarathchandra P, Clark JE, et al. Peroxynitrite induces haem oxygenase-1 in vascular endothelial cells: a link to apoptosis. *Biochem J* 1999;339:729–736.

221. Lepri E, Gambelunghe C, Fioravanti A, et al. *N*-acetylcysteine increases apoptosis induced by H_2O_2 and mo-antiFas triggering in a 3DO hybridoma cell line. *Cell Biochem Funct* 2000;18:201–208.

222. Khan S, Kayahara M, Joashi U, et al. Differential induction of apoptosis in Swiss 3T3 cells by nitric oxide and the nitrosonium cation. *J Cell Sci* 1997;110:2315–2322.

223. Umansky V, Rocha, M. Breitkreuz R, et al. Glutathione is a factor of resistance of Jurkat leukemia cells to nitrite oxide-mediated apoptosis. *J Cell Biochem* 2000;78:578–587.

224. Lee JW, Beckham C, Michel BR, et al. HLA-DR-mediated signals for hematopoiesis and induction of apoptosis involve but are not limited to a nitric oxide pathway. *Blood* 1997;90:217–225.

225. Dvorakova K, Payne CM, Tome ME, et al. Induction of oxidative stress and apoptosis in myeloma cells by the aziridine-containing agent imexon. *Biochem Pharmacol* 2000;60:749–758.

226. Haddad JJ, Land SC. The differential expression of apoptosis factors in the alveolar epithelium is redox sensitive and requires NF-kB (RelA)-selective targeting. *Biochem Biophys Res Commun* 2000;271:257–267.

227. Watson RW, Rotstein OD, Nathens AB, et al. Thiol-mediated redox regulation of neutrophil apoptosis. *Surgery* 1996;120:150–158.

228. Kletsas D, Barbieri D, Stathakos D, et al. The highly reducing sugar 2-deoxy-D-ribose induces apoptosis in human fibroblasts by reduced glutathione depletion and cytoskeletal disruption. *Biochem Biophys Res Commun* 1998;243: 416–425.

229. Kaneto H, Fujii, J, Myint T, et al. Reducing sugars trigger oxidative modification and apoptosis in pancreatic beta-cells by provoking oxidative stress through the glycation reaction. *Biochem J* 1996;320:855–863.

230. Barbieri D, Grassilli E, Monti D, et al. D-Ribose and deoxy-D-ribose induce apoptosis in human quiescent peripheral blood mononuclear cells. *Biochem Biophys Res Commun* 1994;201:1109–1116.

231. Higuchi Y, Matsukawa S. Active oxygen-mediated chromosomal 1-2 Mbp giant DNA fragmentation into internucleosomal DNA fragmentation in apoptosis of glioma cells induced by glutamate. *Free Radic Biol Med* 1998;24:418–426.

232. Froissard P, Monrocq H, Duval D. Role of glutathione metabolism in the glutamate-induced programmed cell death of neuronal-like PC12 cells. *Eur J Pharmacol* 326:93–99.

233. Kikuchi S, Shinpo K, Moriwaka F, et al. Neurotoxicity of methylglyoxal and 3-deoxyglucosone on cultured cortical neurons: synergism between glycation and oxidative stress, possibly involved in neurodegenerative diseases. *J Neurosci Res* 1999;57:280–289.

234. Okado A, Kawasaki Y, Hasuike Y, et al. Induction of apoptotic cell death by methylglyoxal and 3-deoxyglucosone in

macrophage-derived cell lines. *Biochem Biophys Res Commun* 1996;225:219–224.

235. Migheli R, Godani C, Sciola L, et al. Enhancing effect of manganese on L-DOPA-induced apoptosis in PC12 cells: role of oxidative stress. *J Neurochem* 1999;73:1155–1163.

236. Dhalla NS, Elmoselhi AB, Hata T, Makino N. Status of myocardial antioxidants in ischemia-reperfusion injury. *Cardiovasc Res* 2000;47:446–456.

237. Luo Y. Umegaki H, Wang X, et al. Dopamine induces apoptosis through an oxidation-involved SAPK/JNK activation pathway. *J Biol Chem* 1998;273:3756–3764.

238. Hoyt KR, Reynolds IJ, Hastings TG. Mechanisms of dopamine-induced cell death in cultured rat forebrain neurons: interactions with and differences from glutamate-induced cell death. *Exp Neurol* 1997;143:269–281.

239. Masserano JM, Gong L, Kulaga H, et al. Dopamine induces apoptotic cell death of a catecholaminergic cell line derived from the central nervous system. *Mol Pharmacol* 1996;50:1309–1315.

240. Offen D, Ziv I, Sternin H, et al. Prevention of dopamine-induced cell death by thiol antioxidants: possible implications for treatment of Parkinson's disease. *Exp Neurol* 1996;141:32–39.

241. Lizard G, Gueldry S, Sordet O, et al. Glutathione is implied in the control of 7-ketocholesterol-induced apoptosis, which is associated with radical oxygen species production. *FASEB J* 1998;12:1651–1663.

242. Spottl N, Wirleitner B, Bock G, et al. Reduced pteridine derivatives induce apoptosis in human neuronal NT2/HNT cells. *Immunobiology* 2000;201: 478–491.

243. Seaton TA, Cooper JM, Schapira AH. Free radical scavengers protect dopaminergic cell lines from apoptosis induced by complex 1 inhibitors. *Brain Res* 1997;777:110–118.

244. Song SH, Lee KH, Kang MS, Lee,Y.J. Role of paxillin in metabolic oxidative *stress-induced cy*toskeletal reorganization involvement of SAPK signal transduction pathway and PTP-PEST gene expression. *Free Radic Biol Med* 2000;29:61–70.

245. *Fer*rari G, Yan CY, Greene LA. *N*-acetylcysteine (D- and L-stereoisomers) prevents apoptotic death of neuronal cells. *J Neurosci 1995*;15:2857–2866.

246. Schultz JB, Bremen D, Reed JC, et al. Cooperative interaction of neuronal apoptosis by *BCL-2* and *BAG-1* expression: prevention of caspase activation and reduced production of reactive oxygen species. *J Neurochem* 1997; 69:2075–2086.

247. Singh I, Pahan K, Khan M, Singh AK Cytokine-mediated induction of ceramide production is redox-sensitive. Implication to proinflammatory cytokine-mediated apoptosis in demyelinating diseases. *J Biol Chem* 1998;23:20,354–20,362.

248. Liu B, Andrieu-Abadie N, Levade T, et al. Glutathione regulation of neutral sphingomyelinase in tumor necrosis factor-alpha-indu*c*ed cell death. *J Biol Chem* 1998;273:11,313–11,320.

249. Cossarizza A, Franceshi C, Monti D, et al. Prote*ctive effect* of *N*-acetylcysteine in tumor necrosis factor-alpha-induced apoptosis in U937 cells: the role of mitochondria. *Exp Cell Res* 1996;220:232–240.

250. Giardina C, Boulares H, Inan MS. NSAIDs and butyrate sensitize a human colorectal cancer cell line to TNF-alpha

and *Fas* ligation: the role of reactive oxygen species. *Biochim Biophys Acta* 1999;1448:425–438.

251. Shi B, Raina J, Lorenzo A, et al. Neuronal apoptosis induced by HIV-1 *Tat protein* and TNF-alpha: potentiation of neurotoxicity mediated by oxidative stress and implcations for HIV-1 dementia. *J Neurovirol* 1998;4:281–290.

252. Arakaki N, Kajihara T, Arakaki R, et al. Involvement of oxidative stress in tumor cytotoxic activity of hepatocyte growth factor/scatter factor. *J Biol Chem* 1999;274:13,541–13,546.

253. MacKinnon AC, Waters C, Rahman I, et al. [Arg(6),D-Trp(7,9),*N*(me)Phe(8)]-substance P (6–11) (antagonist G) induces AP-1 transcription and sensitizes cells to chemotherapy. *Br J Cancer* 2000;83: 941–948.

254. Yildiz D, Ercal N, Frank RL, Matthews RH Effect of 4-hydroxynonenal and *N*-acetyl-L-cysteine on *Myc*-induced apoptosis. *Toxicol Lett* 1996;89:215–221.

255. Furuke K, Bloom ET. Redox-sensi*tive* events in *Fas*-induced apoptosis in human NK cells include ceramide generation and protein tyrosine dephosphorylation. *Int Immunol* 1998;10:1261–1272.

256. Um HD, Orenstein JM, Wahl SM. *Fas* mediates apoptosis in human monocytes by a reactive oxygen intermediate dependent pathway. *J Immunol* 1996;156:3469–3477.

257. Cao LC, Honeyman T, Jonassen J, Scheid C. Oxalate-induced ceramide accumulation in Madin-Darby canine kidney and LLC-PK1 cells. *Kidney Int* 2000;57: 2403–2411.

258. Davis MA, Flaws JA, Young M, et al. Effect of ceramide on intracellular glutathione determines apoptotic or necrotic cell death of JB6 tumor cells. *Toxicol Sci* 2000;53:48–55.

259. Quillet-Mary A, Jaffrezou JP, Mansat V, et al. Implication of mitochondrial hydrogen peroxide generation in ceramide-induced apoptosis. *J Biol Chem* 1997;272:21,388–21,395.

260. Hug H, Strand S, et al. Reactive oxygen intermediates are involved in the induction of CD95 ligand mRNA expression by cytostatic drugs in hepatoma cells. *J Biol Chem* 1997;272:28,191–28,193.

261. Ando K, Hagiwara T, Beppu M, Kikugawa K. Naturally ocurring anti-band 3 antibody binds to apoptotic human T-lymphoid cell line Jurkat through sialylated poly-*N*-acetyl-lactosaminyl saccharide chains on the cell surface. *Biochem Biophys Res Commun* 2000;275:412–417.

262. Sawyer DB, Fukazawa R, Arstall MA, Kelly RA. Daunorubicin-induced apoptosis in rat cardiac myocytes is inhibited by dexrazoxane. *Circ Res* 1999;84:257–265.

263. Quillet-Mary A, Mansat V, Duchayne E, et al. Daunorubicin-induced internucleosomal DNA fragmentation in acute myeloid cell lines. *Leukemia* 1996;10:417–425.

264. Friesen C, Fulda S, Debatin KM Induction of CD95 ligand and apoptosis by doxorubicin is modulated by the redox state in chemosensitive- and drug-resistant tumor cells. *Cell Death Differ* 1999;6:471–480.

265. Weltin D, Aupeix K, Iltis C, et al. *N*-acetylcysteine protects lymphocytes from nitrogen mustard-induced apoptosis. *Biochem Pharmacol* 1996;51:1123–1129.

266. Zisterer DM, Campiani G, Nacci V, Williams DC. Pyrrolo-1,5-benzoxazepines induce apoptosis in HL-60, Jurkat, and Hut-78 cells: a new class of apoptotic agents. *J Pharmacol Exp Ther* 2000;293:48–59.

267. Shen JC, Wang TT, Chang S, Hursting SD. Mechanistic studies of the effects of the retinoid *N*-(4-hydroxyphenyl)reti-

namide on prostate cancer cell growth and apoptosis. *Mol Carcinog* 1999;24:160–168.

268. Furuke K, Sasada T, Ueda-Taniguchi Y, et al. Role of intracellular redox status in apoptosis induction of human T-cell leukemia virus type I-infected lymphocytes by 13-*cis*-retinoic acid. *Cancer Res* 1997;57:4916–4923.

269. Delia D, Aiello A, Meroni L, et al. Role of antioxidants and intracellular free radicals in retinamide-induced cell death. *Carcinogenesis* 1997;18:943–948.

270. Eymin B, Dubrez L, Allouche M, Solary E. Increased *gadd153* messenger RNA level is associated with apoptosis in human leukemic cells treated with etoposide. *Cancer Res* 1997;57:686–695.

271. Fésüs L, Szondy Z, Uray I. Probing the molecular program of apoptosis by cancer chemopreventive agents. *J Cell Biochem* 1995;22 Suppl:151–161.

272. Palomba L., Sestili P, Cantoni O. The antioxidant butylated hydroxytoluene induces apoptosis in human U937 cells: the role of hydrogen peroxide and altered redox state. *Free Radic Res* 1999;31:93–101.

273. Macho A, Blazquez MV, Navas P, Munoz E. Induction of apoptosis by vanilloid compounds does not require *de novo* gene transcription and activator potein 1 activiy. *Cell Growth Differ* 1998;9:277–286.

274. Chiao C., Carothers AM, Grunberger D, et al. Apoptosis and altered redox state induced by caffeic acid phenethyl ester (CAPE) in transformed rat fibroblast cells. *Cancer Res* 1995;55:3576–3583.

275. Biswal SS, Datta K, Shaw SD, et al. Glutathione oxidation and mitochondrial depolarization as mechanisms of nordihydroguaiaretic acid-induced apoptosis in lipoxygenase-deficient FL5.12 cells. *Toxicol Sci* 2000; 53:77–83.

276. Shen H, Yang, C, Liu J, Ong C. Dual role of glutathione in selenite-induced oxidative stress and apoptosis in human hepatoma cells. *Free Radical Biol Med* 2000;28:1115–1124.

277. Wedi B, Straede J, Wieland B, Kapp A. Eosinophil apoptosis is mediated by stimulators of cellular oxidative metabolism and inhibited by antioxidants: involvement of a thiol-sensitive redox regulation in eosinophil cell death. *Blood* 1999;94:2365–2373.

278. Watson RW, Redmond HP, Wang JH, et al. Mechanisms involved in sodium arsenite-induced apoptosis of human neutrophils. *J Leukoc Biol* 1996;60:625–632.

279. Pang JH., Chau LY. Copper-induced apoptosis and immediate early gene expression in macrophages. *Atherosclerosis* 1999;146:45–52.

280. Desole MS, Sciola L, Delogu MR, et al. Role of oxidative stress in the manganese and 1-methyl-4-(2'-ethylphenyl)-1,2,3,6-tetrahydropyridine-induced apoptosis in PC12 cells. *Neurochem Int* 1997;31:169–176.

281. Thevenod F, Friedmann JM, Katsen AD, Hauser IA. Up-regulation of multidrug resistance P-glycoprotein via nuclear factor-κB activation protects kidney proximal tubule cells from cadmium- and reactive oxygen species-induced apoptosis. *J Biol Chem* 2000;275:1887–1896.

282. Hiura TS, Li N, Kaplan R, et al. The role of a mitochondrial pathway in the induction of apoptosis by chemicals extracted from diesel exhaust particles. *J Immunol* 2000;165:2703–2711.

283. Hiura TS, Kaszubowski MP, Li N, Nel AE. Chemicals in diesel exhaust particles generate reactive oxygen radicals and

induce apoptosis in macrophages. *J Immunol* 1999;163:5582–5591.

284. Sandstrom PA, Mannie MD, Buttke TM. Inhibition of activation-induced death in T cell hydridomas by thiol antioxidants: oxidative stress as a mediator of apoptosis. *J Leukoc Biol* 1994;55:221–226.

285. Oda T, Iwaoka J, Komatsu N, Muramatsu T. Involvement of *N*-acetylcysteine-sensitive pathways in ricin-induced apoptotic cell death in U937 cells. *Biosci Biotechnol Biochem* 1999;63:341–348.

286. Abello PA, Fidler SA, Buchman TG. Thiol reducing agents modulate induced apoptosis in porcine endothelial cells. *Shock* 1994;2:79–83.

287. Hayon T, Dvilansky A, Oriev L, Nathan I. Non-steroidal antiestrogens induce apoptosis in HL-60 and MOLT3 leukemic cells: involvement of reactive oxygen radicals and protein kinase C. *Anticancer Res* 1999;19:2089–2093.

288. Fernandez A, Kiefer J, Fosdick L, McConkey DJ. Oxygen radical production and thiol depletion are required for Ca(2+)-mediated endogenous endonuclease activation in apoptotic thymocytes. *J Immunol* 1995;155:5133–5139

289. Jones DP, Maellaro E, Jiang S, et al. Effects of *N*-acetyl-L-cysteine on T-cell apoptosis are not mediated by increased cellular glutathione. *Immunol Lett* 1995;45:205–209.

290. Sandstrom PA, Roberts B, Folks TM, Buttke TM. HIV gene expression enhances T cell susceptibility to hydrogen peroxide-induced apoptosis. *AIDS Res Hum Retroviruses* 1993;9:1107–1113.

291. Malorni W, Rivabene R, Santini MT Donelli G. *N*-acetylcysteine inhibits apoptosis and decreases viral particles in HIV-chronically infected U937 cells. *FEBS Lett* 1993;327:75–78.

292. Mortola E, Okuda M, Ohno K, et al. Inhibition of apoptosis and virus replication in feline immunodeficiency virus-infected cells by *N*-acetylcysteine and ascorbic acid. *J Vet Med Sci* 1998;60:1187–1193.

293. Lin KI, Lee SH, Narayanan R, et al. Thiol agents and *Bcl-2* identify an alphavirus-induced apoptotic pathway that requires activation of the transcription factor NF-kB. *J Cell Biol* 1995;131:1149–1161.

294. Schweizer M, Peterhans E. Oxidative stress in cells infected with bovine viral diarrhoea virus: a critical step in the induction of apoptosis. *J Gen Virol* 1999;80:1147–1155.

295. Jimenez LA, Zanella C, Fung H, et al. Role of extracellular signal-regulated protein kinases in apoptosis by asbestos and H_2O_2. *Am J Physiol* 1997;273:L1029–L1035.

296. Shimura M, Osawa Y, Yuo A, et al. Oxidative stress as a necessary factor in room temperature-induced apoptosis in HL-60 cells. *J Leukoc Biol* 2000;68:87–96.

297. Liu M, Pelling JC, Ju J, et al. Antioxidant action via *p53*-mediated apoptosis. *Cancer Res* 1998;58:1723–1729.

298. Thompson CB Apoptosis in the pathogenesis and treatment of disease. *Science* 1995;267:1456–1462.

299. Kinscherf R, Deigner HP, Haberkorn,U. Apoptosis modulators in the therapy of neurodegenerative diseases. *Expert Opin Investig Drugs* 2000;9:747–764.

300. Ortiz LA, Moroz K, Liu J-Y, et al. Alveolar macrophage apoptosis and TNF-alpha, but not p53, expression correlate with murine response to bleomycin. *Am J Physiol* 1998;275:L1208–L1218.

301. Kuwano K, Miyazaki H, Hagimoto N, et al. The involvement of Fas-Fas ligand pathway in fibrosis lung diseases. *Am J Resp Cell Mol Biol* 1999;20: 53–60.

302. Guinee D Jr, Brambilla E, Fleming M, et al. The potential role of BAX and BCL-2 expression in diffuse alveolar damage. *Am J Pathol* 1997;151:999–1007.

303. Kaneto H, Kajimoto Y, Miyagawa J, et al. Beneficial effects of antioxidants in diabetes: possible potection of pancreatic beta-cells against glucose toxicity. *Diabetes* 1999;48:2398–2406.

304. Pollman MJ, Hall JL, Gibbons GH. Determinants of vascular smooth muscle cell apoptosis after balloon angioplasty injury. Influence of redox state and cell phenotype. *Circ Res* 1999;84:113–121.

305. Castagne V, Clarke PG. Axotomy-induced retinal ganglion cell death in development: its time-course and its diminution by antioxidants. *Proc R Soc Lond B Biol Sci* 1996;263:1193–1197.

306. Blackwell TS, Blackwell TR, Holden EP, et al. In vivo antioxidant treatment suppresses nuclear factor-κB activation and neutrophilic lung inflammation. *J Immunol* 1996;157:1630–1637.

307. Cuzzocrea S, Mazzon E, Dugo L, et al. Protective effects of *N*-acetylcysteine on lung injury and red blood cell modification induced by carrageenan in the rat. *FASEB J* 2001;15:1187–1200.

308. Heller AR, Groth G, Heller SC, et al. *N*-acetylcysteine reduces respiratory burst but augments neutrophil phagocytosis in intensive care unit patients. *Crit Care Med* 2001;29:272–276.

309. Sakurada S, Kato T, Okamoto T. Induction of cytokines and ICAM-1 by proinflammatory cytokines in primary rheumatoid synovial fibroblasts and inhibition by *N*-acetyl-L-cysteine and aspirin. *Int Immunol* 1996; 8:1483–1493.

310. Matsumoto K, Hashimoto S, Gon Y, et al. *N*-acetylcysteine inhibits IL-1 alpha-induced IL-8 secretion by bronchial epithelial cells. *Respir Med* 1998;92:512–515.

311. Sato M, Miyazaki T, Nagaya T, et al. Antioxidants inhibit tumor necrosis factor-alpha mediated stimulation of interleukin-8, monocyte chemoattractant protein-1, and collagenase expression in cultured human synovial cells. *J Rheumatol* 1996;23:432–438.

312. Kawasaki S, Takizawa H, Takami K, et al. Benzene-extracted components are important for the major activity of diesel exhaust particles: effect of interleukin-8 gene expression in human bronchial epithelial cells. *Am J Respir Cell Mol Biol* 2001;24:419–426.

313. Weiss L, Hildt E, Hofschneider PH. Anti-hepatitis B virus activity of *N*-acetyl-L-cysteine (NAC): new aspects of a well-established drug. *Antiviral Res* 1996;32:43–53.

314. Waris G, Huh KW, Siddiqui A. Mitochondrially associated hepatitis B virus X protein constitutively activates transcription factors STAT-3 and NF-κB via oxidative stress. *Mol Cell Biol* 2001;21:7721–7730.

315. Meyer M, Caselmann WH, Schluter V, et al. Hepatitis B virus transactivator MHBst: activation of NF-κB, selective inhibition by antioxidants and integral membrane localization. *EMBO J* 1992;11:2991–3001.

316. Gong G, Waris G, Tanveer R, Siddiqui A. Human hepatitis C virus NS5A protein alters intracellular calcium levels, induces oxidative stress, and activates STAT-3 and NF-κB. *Proc Natl Acad Sci USA* 2001;98:9599–9604.

317. Grant PR, Black A, Garcia N, et al. Combination therapy with interferon-alpha plus *N*-acetylcysteine for chronic hepatitis C: a placebo controlled double-blind multicentre study. *J Med Virol* 2000;61:439–442.

318. De Rosa SC, Zaretsky MD, Dubs JG, et al. *N*-acetylcysteine replenishes glutathione in HIV infection. *Eur J Clin Invest* 2000;30:915–929.

319. Harakeh S, Jariwalla R.J. Comparative study of the anti-HIV activities of ascorbate and thiol-containing reducing agents in chronically HIV-infected cells. *Am J Clin Nutr* 1991;54 Suppl 6:1231S–1235S.

320. Ho WZ, Douglas SD. Glutathione and *N*-acetylcysteine suppression of human immunodeficiency virus replication in human monocyte/macrophages in vitro. *AIDS Res Hum Retroviruses* 1992;8:1249–1253.

321. Lioy J, Ho WZ, Cutilli JR, et al. Thiol suppression of human immunodeficiency virus type 1 replication in primary cord blood monocyte-derived macrophages in vitro. *J Clin Investig* 1993;91:495–498.

322. Kalebic T, Kinter A, Poli G, et al. Suppression of human immunodeficiency virus expression in chronically infected monocytic cells by glutathione, glutathione ester, and *N*-acetylcysteine. *Proc Natl Acad Sci USA* 1991; 88:986–990.

323. Roederer M, Staal FJ, Raju PA, et al. Cytokine-stimulated human immunodeficiency virus replication is inhibited by *N*-acetyl-L-cysteine. *Proc Natl Acad Sci USA* 1990;87:4884–4888.

324. Albini A, Morini MD, D'Agostini F, et al. Inhibition of angiogenesis-driven Kaposi's sarcoma tumor growth in nude mice by oral *N*-acetylcysteine. *Cancer Res* 2001;61:8171–8178.

325. Nishinaka Y, Nakamura H, Okada N, et al. Redox control of EBV infection: prevention by thiol-dependent modulation of functional CD21/EBV receptor expression. *Antiox Redox Signal* 2001;3:1075–1087.

326. Huang TS, Duyster J, Wang JY. Biological response to phorbol ester determined by alternative G1 pathways. *Proc Natl Acad Sci USA* 1995;92:4793–4797.

327. Kurata S. Selective activation of p38 MAPK cascade and mitotic arrest caused by low level oxidative stress. *J Biol Chem* 2000;275:23,413–23,416.

328. Brar SS, Kennedy TP, Whorton AR, et al. Requirement for reactive oxygen species in serum-derived growth factor-induced growth of airway smooth muscle. *J Biol Chem* 1999;274:20,017–20,026.

329. Grdina DJ, Murley JS, Roberts JC. Effects of thiols on topoisomerase-II α activity and cell cycle progression. *Cell Prolif* 1998;31:217–229.

330. Kusano C, Takao S, Noma H, et al. *N*-acetylcysteine inhibits cell cycle progression in pancreatic carcinoma cells. *Hum Cell* 2000;13:213–220.

331. Redondo P, Bauza A. Topical *N*-acetylcysteine for lamellar ichthyosis [Letter]. *Lancet* 1999;354:1880.

332. Kitamura M. The antioxidant *N*-acetylcysteine induces mesangial cells to create three-dimensional cytoarchitecture that underlies cellular differentiation. *J Am Soc Nephrol* 1999;10:746–751.

333. Breithaupt TB, Vazquez A, Baez I, Eylar EH. The suppression of T cell function and NF-κB expression by serine protease inhibitors is blocked by *N*-acetylcysteine. *Cell Immunol* 1996;173:124–130.

334. Ferrandez MD, Correa R, Del Rio M, De la Fuente M. Effects in vitro of several antioxidants on the natural killer function of aging mice. *Exp Gerontol* 1999;34:675–685.

335. Goldman Y, Peled A, Shinitzky M. Effective elimination of lung metastases induced by tumor cells treated with hydrostatic pressure and *N*-acetyl-L-cysteine. *Cancer Res* 2000;60:350–358.

336. Van den Broeke LT, Beijersbergen Van Henegouwen GMJ. Topically applied N-acetylcysteine as a protector against UVB-induced systemic immune suppression. *J Photochem Photobiol B*: 1995;27:61–65.

337. Breitkreutz R, Pittack N, Nebe CT, et al. Improvement of immune functions in HIV infection by sulfur supplementation: two randomized trials. *J Mol Med* 2000;78:55–62.

338. Tosetti F, Ferrari N, De Flora S, Albini A. "Angioprevention:" Angiogenesis is a common and key target for cancer chemopreventive agents. *FASEB J* 2002;16:2–14.

339. Redondo P, Bandres E, Solano T, et al. Vascular endothelial growth factor (VEGF) and melanoma. *N*-acetylcysteine downregulates VEGF production in vitro. *Cytokine* 2000;12:374–378.

340. Chua CC, Hamdy RC, Chua BH. Upregulation of vascular endothelial growth factor by H_2O_2 in rat heart endothelial cells. *Free Radic Biol Med* 1998;15:891–897.

341. Tsuji F, Matsuoka H, Aono H, et al. Effects of sulfhydryl compounds on interleukin-1-induced vascular endothelial growth factor production in human synovial stromal cells. *Biol Pharm Bull* 2000;23:663–665.

342. Duyndam MC, Hulscher TM, Fontijn D, et al. Induction of vascular endothelial growth factor expression and hypoxia-inducible factor 1 alpha protein by the oxidative stressor arsenite. *J Biol Chem* 2001;276:48,066–48,076.

343. Redondo P, Jimenez E, Perez A, Garcia-Foncillas J. *N*-acetylcysteine downregulates vascular endothelial growth factor production by human keratinocytes in vitro. *Arch Dermatol Res* 2000; 292:621–628.

344. Marumo T, Schini-Kert VB, Busse R. Vascular endothelial growth factor activates nuclear factor-κB and induces monocyte chemoattractant protein-1 in bovine retinal endothelial cells. *Diabetes* 1999;48:1131–1137.

345. Cai T, Fassina GF, Giunciuglio D, et al. *N*-Acetylcysteine inhibits endothelial cell invasion and angiogenesis while protecting from apoptosis. *Lab Investig* 1999;79:1151–1159.

346. Morini M, Cai T, Aluigi MG, et al. The role of the thiol *N*-acetylcysteine in the prevention of tumor invasion and angiogenesis. *Int J Biol Markers* 1999;14:268–271.

347. Masiero L, Mazzieri R; Kalebic T, et al. Modulation of expression and activity of MMP-2 by reducing agents and uPA plasmin (Abstract). *Eur J Histochem* 1993; 37 Suppl:60–61.

348. Albini A, D'Agostini F, Giunciuglio D, et al. Inhibition of invasion, gelatinase activity, tumor take and metastasis of malignant cells by *N*-acetylcysteine. *Int J Cancer* 1995;61:121–129.

349. Kawakami S, Kageyama Y, Fujii Y, et al. Inhibitory effect of *N*-acetylcysteine on invasion and MMP-9 production of T24 human bladder cancer cells. *Anticancer Res* 2001;21:213–219.

350. Stetler-Stevenson GW, Talano J, Gallagher M, et al. Inhibition of human type IV collagenase by a highly conserved peptide sequence derived from its prosegment. *Am J Med Sci* 1991;302:163–170.

351. Nonaka Y, Iwagaki H, Kimura T, et al. Effect of reactive oxygen intermediates on the *in vitro* invasive capacity of tumor cells and liver metastasis in mice. *Int J Cancer* 1993;54:983–986.

352. Buhimschi IA, Kramer WB, Buhimschi CS, et al. Reduction-oxidation (redox) state regulation of matrix metalloproteinase activity in human fetal membranes. *Am J Obstet Gynecol* 2000;182:458–464.

353. Lois M, Brown LA, Moss IM, et al. Ethanol ingestion increases activation of matrix metalloproteinases in rat lungs during acute endotoxemia. *Am J Respir Crit Care Med* 1999;160:1354–1360.

354. Hozumi A, Nishimura Y, Nishiuma T, et al. Induction of MMP-9 in normal human bronchial epithelial cells by TNF-alpha via NF-κB-mediated pathway. *Am J Physiol Lung Cell Mol Physiol* 2001;281:L1444–L1452.

355. Galis ZS, Asanuma K, Godin D, Meng X. *N*-acetylcysteine decreases the matrix-degrading capacity of macrophage-derived foam cells; new target for antioxidant theraphy? *Circulation* 1998;97:2445–2453.

356. Yoshida M, Korfhagen TR, Whitsett JA. Surfactant protein D regulates NF-κB and matrix metalloproteinase production in alveolar macrophages via oxidant-sensitive pathways. J Immunol 2001;166:7514–7519.

357. De Flora S, D'Agostini F, Masiello L, et al. Synergism between *N*-acetylcysteine and doxorubicin in the prevention of tumorigenicity and metastasis in murine models. *Int J Cancer* 1996;62:842–848.

358. Doroshow JH, Locker JY, Ifrim I, Myers CE. Prevention of doxorubicin cardiac toxicity in the mouse by *N*-acetylcysteine. *J Clin Investig* 1981;68:1053–1064.

359. Delneste Y, Jeannin P, Potier L, et al. *N*-acetyl-L-cysteine exhibits antitumoral activity by increasing tumor necrosis factor alpha-dependent T-cell cytotoxicity. *Blood* 1997;90:1124–1132.

360. Hamada J-i, Nakata D, Nakae D, et al. Increased oxidative DNA damage in mammary tumor cells by continuous epidermal growth factor stimulation. *J Natl Cancer Inst* 2001;93:214–219.

361. Ziemann C, Bürkle A, Kahl GF, Hirsch-Ernst KI. Reactive oxygen species participate in mdr1b mRNA and P-glycoprotein overexpression in primary rat hepatocytes cultures. *Carcinogenesis* 1999;20:407–414.

362. Deng L, Lin-Lee YC, Claret FX, Kuo MT. 2-Acetylaminofluorene up-regulates rat mdr1b expression through generating reactive oxygen species that activate NF-κB pathway. *J Biol Chem* 2001;276:413–420.

363. Honda S, Matsuo M. Relationships between the cellular glutathione level and *in vitro* life span of human diploid fibroblasts. *Exp Gerontol* 1988;23:81–86.

364. Brack C, Bechter-Thuring E, Labuhn M. *N*-acetylcysteine slows down ageing and increases the life span of *Drosophila melanogaster*. *Cell Mol Life Sci* 1997;53:960–966.

365. Richie JPJ, Lang CA. A decrease in cysteine levels causes the glutathione deficiency of aging in the mosquito. *Proc Soc Exp Biol Med* 1988;187:235–240.

366. Hack V, Breitkreutz R, Kinscherf R, et al. The redox state as a correlate of senescence and wasting and as a target for therapeutic intervention. *Blood* 1998;92:59–67.

Modifiers of Cytochrome(s) P450

John DiGiovanni, PhD
and Heather E. Kleiner, PhD

CONTENTS

1. INTRODUCTION

1.1. Overview of P450 Superfamily

Cytochromes P450 (CYPs) belong to a superfamily of enzymes that have different, but overlapping, substrate specificities and tissue distribution. The highest concentration of CYPs is in the liver endoplasmic reticulum, but P450 is found in most other tissues of the body. CYPs are heme-containing enzymes that can either detoxify or bioactivate xenobiotics (foreign chemicals). The following seven types of reactions are catalyzed by CYPs: i) hydroxylation of an aliphatic or aromatic carbon; ii) epoxidation of a double bond; iii) heteroatom (*S*-, *N*-, and *I*-) oxygenation and *N*-hydroxylation; iv) heteroatom (*O*-, *S*-, and *N*-) dealkylation; v) oxidative group transfer; vi) cleavage of esters; and vii) dehydrogenation (*1*). In humans, the predominant isoform of P450 in the liver is CYP1A2. Other human liver P450s include CYP 2A6, 2B6, 2C8, 2C9, 2C19, 2D6, 2E1, and 3A4 (reviewed in ref. *1*). CYP1A1 is expressed in extrahepatic sites including human lung, the intestines, the skin, lymphocytes, and the placenta. Human CYP1B1 catalyzes the activation of a number of diverse pro-carcinogens (*2*), and is expressed in a variety of extra-hepatic sites, including steroid-responsive and steroidogenic tissues (*3–5*).

CYPs are involved in the bioactivation of many pro-carcinogens (Table 1). CYP1A2 catalyzes the *N*-hydroxylation of aromatic amines such as 4-aminobiphenyl and 2-aminonaphthalene, which is the first step in the bioactivation of these compounds. CYP1A2

is also involved in the activation of aflatoxin B_1 (AFB_1), heterocyclic amines, and certain nitroaromatic compounds. CYP1A1 is induced by cigarette smoke, charcoal-broiled meat (polycyclic aromatic hydrocarbons or PAH), cruciferous vegetables (indoles), and omeprazole (*6,7*). Studies with human microsomal CYPs and mutagenesis assays have implicated CYPs 1A1 and 1B1 in the first oxidation step of PAHs, but the second bioactivation step leading to the diol epoxides may be catalyzed by the CYPs 1A1, 1B1, 3A4, 1A2, 2B6, and 2C9 (reviewed in ref. *8*). Studies also suggest that AFB_1 may be bioactivated by CYPs 3A4 and 1A2. CYPs 1A1, 1A2, 1B1, 3A4, and 2B5 have been implicated in the *N*-hydroxylation of arylamines. Furthermore, the tobacco-specific *N*-nitrosamines may be bioactivated by CYPs 2E1, 3A4, and 2A6. Dietary carcinogens such as heterocyclic aromatic amines are *N*-hydroxylated by the CYP1 family, mainly 1A2. CYPs can also mediate the activation of estrogenic compounds into putative carcinogenic metabolites. CYPs 3A4 and 3A5 have been reported to catalyze the 16α-hydroxylation of estrone, and CYP1B1 catalyzes the 4-hydroxylation of estrogen (reviewed in ref. *8*).

2. MODIFIERS OF P450

2.1. Organosulfur Compounds

Oltipraz (5-(2-pyrazinyl)-4-methyl-1,2-dithiole-3-thione) is a synthetic derivative of the plant product 1,2-dithione-3-thione. Oltipraz has been shown to inhibit carcinogenesis in a number of animal models,

From: Cancer Chemoprevention, Volume 1: Promising Cancer Chemoprevention Agents
Edited by: G. J. Kelloff, E. T. Hawk, and C. C. Sigman © Humana Press Inc., Totowa, NJ

Table 1

P450 Isoforms Involved in Carcinogen Activation

P450 Isoform	Reaction	Pro-Carcinogen	Examples
1A2	N-hydroxylation	Aromatic amines PhIP	4-aminobiphenyl, 2-aminonaphthalene, 2-aminofluorene, NNK, 2-acetylamino fluorene
1A1	Hydroxylation, epoxidation	PAH	Benzo[a]pyrene, Dibenzo[a,l]pyrene
1B1	Hydroxylation, epoxidation	PAH	Benzo[a]pyrene, Dibenzo[a,l]pyrene
3A4		PAH, AFB$_1$, Nitrosamines	
2E1		Nitrosamines, AOM	

including AFB$_1$ hepatocarcinogenesis in rats *(9–11)* and 2-amino-1-methyl-6-phenylimidazo[4,5-b]pyridine (PhIP)-induced lymphoma *(12)*. It was previously recognized that the chemopreventive effects of oltipraz against AFB$_1$ hepatocarcinogenesis might be the result of its ability to induce alpha-class glutathione *S*-transferase (GST) *(13,14)*. However, other investigators have demonstrated that oltipraz can also modulate CYP1A1/1A2 and 2B1/2B2 *(15)*. In this regard, oltipraz was found to be a reversible inhibitor of rat-liver microsomal ethoxyresorufin (EROD) and pentoxyresorufin *O*-dealkylase (PROD) activities *(15)*. However, oltipraz was also found to also induce CYP1A1/1A2 and 2B1/2B2 protein and mRNA levels in rat-liver primary cultures. oltipraz inhibited AFB$_1$ metabolism to AFM$_1$ and AFB-glutathione conjugate in primary cultures. oltipraz inhibited caffeine metabolism when co-administered or when administered 4 h prior to caffeine, but increased caffeine metabolism when administered 24 h or more before caffeine treatment. In rats, oltipraz increased EROD and PROD activities, and elevated CYP1A and 2B mRNAs but not 2C11. AFB$_1$ can be metabolized to the *exo*-epoxides—primarily by CYP3A4, but also CYP1A2 (reviewed in ref. *16*). Oltipraz is currently under clinical investigation in Qidong, P.R. China *(17)*. Oltipraz (125 mg p.o. daily) significantly increased the excretion of aflatoxin mercapturic acid. At 500 mg once a week, it reduced levels of AFM$_1$, an oxidative metabolite of AFB$_1$. These observations suggest that the mechanism of anti-carcinogenesis may be the result of GST induction as well as, CYP modulation.

2.1.1. GARLIC AND ONION COMPOUNDS

Garlic *(Allium sativa)* and onions *(Allium cepa)* contain numerous organosulfur compounds (OSCs)

that have been studied for their anticarcinogenic properties. Epidemiological studies have indicated that consumption of garlic or onions is associated with a reduced risk of cancers, particularly stomach and colon cancer (reviewed in ref. *18*). Studies in animal models have supported these observations. Pretreatment with diallyl sulfide (DAS) prior to carcinogens inhibits esophageal carcinogenesis by *N*-nitrosomethylbenzylamine (NBMA) *(19)*, and benzo[a]pyrene (B[a]P)-induced pulmonary and forestomach tumorigenesis in rodents *(20)*. In addition, female Sprague-Dawley rats co-treated with diallyl disulfide (DAD) (200 ppm in the diet) and PhIP (85 mg/kg p.o.) fed a high-fat diet had a lesser incidence and multiplicity of mammary tumors *(21)*.

Although it has been stated that the antimutagenic activities of OSCs against several ultimate carcinogens are closely related to their abilities to induce phase 2 enzymes *(22,23)*, OSCs can also modulate CYPs. For example, rats fed a diet supplemented with 20% onion powder daily for 9 d showed a significant increase in hepatic EROD (CYP1A1) activity, and a significant decrease (by 35%) in *p*-nitrophenol hydroxylase (CYP2E1) activity *(24)*. Onion powder contains a variety of different compounds, including flavonols (quercetin and its glucosides; isorhamnetin glucosides); alk(en)yl polysulfides (di-, tri-, and tetrasulfides); dimethyl thiophenes; polysulfides; dipropyl disulfide; and lacrimatory factors *(24)*. Thus, other compounds in addition to the OSCs in onion powder may also participate in its CYP-modulating activity. The reduction of CYP2E1 activity by OSCs suggests the possibility of blocking the activation of nitrosamines, which are bioactivated by CYP2E1. DAS, a competitive inhibitor of rat liver microsomal CYP2E1 *p*-nitrophenol hydroxylase activity *(25)*, is metabolized by rat liver microsomes to diallyl sulfone, which is both a competitive and mechanism-based inhibitor of CYP2E1 *(25)*. It has been shown that CYP2A6 may contribute to the mutagenic bioactivation of *N*-nitrosamines *(26,27)*, including tobacco-related *N*-nitrosamines *(28,29)*. DAS inhibited mouse CYP2A5 activity toward acetaminophen (APAP) metabolism *(30)*. DAD protected against *N*-nitrosodiethylamine carcinogenesis in mice and rats *(31,32)*. Structure-activity relationship studies of various OSCs showed that 4,4'-dipyridyl disulfide and 4,4'-dipyridyl sulfide were the most effective inhibitors of CYP2A6 coumarin 7-hydroxylase activity in *Escherichia coli* cells that expressed human CYP and OR *(33)*. These two compounds exhibited competitive inhibition, and were relatively selective for CYP2A6. They possess two pyridine rings, similar to metyrapone, another CYP inhibitor *(34)*. Furthermore, dialkyl disulfides were more potent inhibitors of CYP2A6 activity than dialkyl sulfide, suggesting that the sulfur atom may be important in the inhibitory activity *(33)*. Whereas DAS and other OSCs did not inhibit constitutive pulmonary or hepatic CYP1A1 activity in A/J mice (25 µmol, p.o.) *(23)*, another study found that DAS (200 mg/kg) and garlic extract (50 mg/kg) significantly blocked 2,3,7,8-tetrachlorodibenzo-*p*-dioxin (TCDD) induction of pulmonary CYP1A1 activity, mRNA, and protein levels *(35)*, and had moderate effects on CYP1A1 in the liver.

2.2. Curcuminoids

Curcumin [1,7-*bis*(4-hydroxy-3-methoxyphenyl)-1,6-heptadiene-3,5-dione; diferuloyol methane] is the major yellow pigment extracted from turmeric, a spice from the rhizome of *Curcuma longa* Linn used in seasonings such as curry powder. As a potential modifier of CYPs, curcumin's anti-carcinogenic activities have been demonstrated in a variety of models—for example, topical pretreatment of mice with curcumin inhibited epidermal B*[a]*P-DNA adduct formation in female CD-1 mice *(36)*. Topical pretreatment of mice with curcumin also inhibited skin-tumor initiation by B*[a]*P and 7,12-dimethylbenz[a]anthracene (DMBA) in a two-stage protocol *(36)*. Furthermore, curcumin (0.2% in the diet) administered 4 d prior to initiation with diethyl nitrosamine and continued until the end of the study inhibited hepatocellular carcinoma incidence by 62% and tumor multiplicity by 80% *(37)*. Curcumin (0.5% and 2% in the diet) also blocked B*[a]*P forestomach tumorigenesis in A/J mice when administered during either the initiation period or

the post-initiation period *(38)*. Curcumin (2% in the diet) also blocked azoxymethane (AOM)-induced colon adenoma and adenocarcinoma formation in female CF-1 mice when administered during the initiation period, the post-initiation period, or both *(38)*. AOM is metabolized by CYP2E1 *(39)*.

Dibenzoylmethane (DBM) is a chemical analog of curcumin. Both compounds contain a central β-diketone group in conjugation with unsaturated carbon groups that are subject to enolization of the β-diketone group. DBM differs from curcumin because it lacks the hydroxyl and methoxy side chains. Administration of DBM during carcinogen treatment at a dose of 0.2–1% in the diet significantly blocked DMBA DNA adduct formation in the mammary glands of female SENCAR mice *(40)*. Moreover, a significant reduction in DMBA mammary tumorigenesis was observed in female SENCAR mice treated with 1% DBM in the diet for 2 wk before DMBA treatment until the end of the study *(41)*. In addition, both 1% DBM and 2% curcumin in the diet significantly reduced the formation of lymphomas, leukemias, and ovarian tumors in the mice, but DBM was more effective than curcumin *(41)*. It has been suggested that curcumin is less active because it is not as well-absorbed in the gut as DBM *(41)*.

Although the anti-promoting and antioxidant effects of curcumin play a role in its anticarcinogenic effects *(42)*, mechanistic studies have demonstrated that it also modulates CYPs. In Sprague-Dawley rat liver microsomes, curcumin, demethoxycurcumin, and *bis*-demethoxycurcumin inhibited EROD (CYP1A1), methoxyresorufin-*O*-dealkylase (MROD) (CYP1A2), and PROD (CYP2B1) activities with IC_{50} values ranging from 2.5–20 µ*M (43)*. However, curcumin also triggered a 2.5-fold induction of CYP1A1 in 101L cells, which are derived from human hepatoma HepG2 cells that are stably transfected with a human CYP1A1 promoter and a 5'-flanking sequence linked to a luciferase reporter gene *(44)*. Another study describes curcumin as a bifunctional inducer, because it induces both GST activity and the expression of *Cyp1a1* and *1b1* mRNA in oral human squamous cell carcinoma cell lines *(45)*. It was shown that curcumin stimulates the translocation and formation of aryl hydrocarbon receptor (Ahr)-ARNT complex. Despite the activation of Ahr, curcumin inhibited the formation of tetraols from B*[a]*P-7,8-diol in both the squamous cell carcinoma cells and in human oral tissue samples *(45)*. Studies with DBM have also shown an activating effect on Ahr. Repeated oral administration of DBM at 100 or 200 mg/kg body wt caused a four- to sixfold induction of rat liver microsomal EROD activity *(46)*. However, administration of DBM prior to DMBA treatment blocked DMBA induction of EROD activity in rat-liver microsomes *(46)*. It was shown that DBM competitively inhibited EROD activity in DMBA-induced rat liver microsomes incubated with DBM (up to 10 µM), with an IC_{50} of 1.1 µM *(46)*. DBM also inhibited DMBA induction of hepatic *Cyp1a1, 1a2*, and *1b1* mRNA expression, but DBM alone actually increased expression of these Cyp genes *(46)*. Similarly, in HepG2 cells, DBM inhibited the induction of EROD activity induced by TCDD or DMBA, but by itself induced EROD activity. DBM blocked Ahr activation by TCDD in HepG2 cells, but by itself caused the activation of Ahr. Ligand-binding assays showed that DBM blocked [^{3}H]TCDD ligand binding to the Ahr at a 2500-molar excess*(46)*. Thus, although DBM is a ligand for Ahr, it has relatively weak affinity compared to TCDD or DMBA. Whether the effects of DBM on Ahr activation play a role in its anticarcinogenic effects has not yet been determined.

2.3. Flavonoids

Flavonoids are polyphenolic antioxidants that occur ubiquitously in plants. Their structures include flavones, isoflavones (e.g., genistein, daidzein), flavonols (e.g., quercetin), flavonones, flavanols (e.g., catechins), and anthocyanidins, and more than 4000 have been identified as naturally occurring (reviewed in ref. *47*). Flavonoids are abundant in the human diet in citrus, apples, tea (catechins), legumes and soybeans (isoflavones), cruciferous vegetables, cherries, grapes, berries, red wine (catechins), and herbs. The estimated intake of all flavonoids in the U.S. diet has ranged from a few hundred mg per d to up to 650 mg per d as the aglycones (reviewed in refs. *47,48*). Flavonoids possess multiple mechanisms of action for their anticarcinogenic effects, including antioxidant activity, but they have also been shown to block the initiation stages of carcinogenesis. For example, when administered in the diet during either initiation or postinitiation, diosmin (a flavone) and hesperidin (a flavanone), found in the peel of citrus fruits, blocked mouse-bladder carcinogenesis induced by *N*-butyl-*N*-(4-hydroxybutyl)nitrosamine (OH-BBN)*(49)*. Furthermore, mutagenicity assays in hamster-embryo V79 cells have shown apigenin, acacetin, chrysin, and kaempferide to be effective against B*[a]*P. Quercetin

blocked mutagenicity by the heterocyclic amine 2-amino-3-methylimidazo[4,5-f]quinoline (IQ) *(50,51)*, and was also shown to significantly inhibit lung-tumor incidence by *N*-nitrosodiethylamine in mice *(52)*.

Mechanistic studies have shown that flavones (e.g., acacetin, diosmetin) were more potent inhibitors of human cDNA lymphoblastoid-expressed CYPs 1A1, 1B1, and 1A2 than flavanones (e.g., eriodictyol, hesperetin, homoeriodictyol, naringenin); this may be because of the double bond on the 2,3 position of the C ring *(53)*. Lineweaver-Burke plots showed that hesperetin is a competitive inhibitor of CYP1B1 *(53)*. All were more effective at blocking CYP1B1 than 1A1 or 1A2. In fact, homoeriodictyol was a rather selective inhibitor of CYP1B1 with an IC50 of 0.24 µM. Also, many inhibitors of CYPs are actually substrates for the enzyme. It was also shown that ^{3}H-hesperetin is *O*-demethylated by CYP1A1 and 1B1, but not CYP1A2, 3A4, or human-liver microsomes *(53)*. Some other flavones shown to have inhibitory activities against CYPs in vitro include 3-, 5-, or 7-hydroxyflavones, 3,7-dihydroxyflavone, and 3,5,7-trihydroxyflavone (also known as galangin, which is found in honey). These flavones inhibited human cDNA-expressed MROD activities of CYPs 1A1 and 1A2, with IC50s ranging from 0.2–0.02 µM *(54)*. Differential effects on mechanisms and selectivity were observed among the various substituted flavones. Galangin was the most potent inhibitor of CYP1A2 (mixed inhibition), and 7-hydroxyflavone was the most effective inhibitor of CYP1A1 (competitive inhibition) *(54)*. A water extract of the root of *Scutellaria baicalensis* (which contains flavonoids) and wogonin, one of the components of this product, inhibited liver microsomal CYP1A1/1A2 production of AFM_1 from AFB_1 *(55)*. In addition, prenylated flavonoids isolated from hops, *Humulus lupulus*, inhibited cDNA-expressed human CYP 1A1, 1B1, and 1A2 EROD activities. In addition, these compounds (e.g., 8-prenylnaringenin and isoxanthohumol) inhibited CYP1A2 metabolic activation and covalent binding (to DNA or protein) of AFB_1 *(56,57)*.

The effects of flavonoids on CYP activities in vivo have also been investigated. Baicalein and wogonin are two flavonoids isolated from the root of *Scutellaria baicalensis*. When fed to C57BL/6 mice in a liquid diet for 1 wk, both compounds inhibited B*[a]*P hydroxylase (AHH) activities in the mouse liver by ~50% at 5 *mM (58)*. Unlike the inhibitory effects observed in the liver, wogonin increased AHH activities in the kidney, and both compounds increased EROD and AHH activities in the lung *(58)*. Wogonin also inhibited the expression of CYP1A1/1A3, 2E1, and 3A in the mouse liver, but both baicalein and wogonin increased CYP1A protein expression in lung *(58)*. However, these compounds did not change the liver, kidney, or lung weight in the mice *(58)*.

Although they are not naturally occurring, 7,8-benzoflavone (7,8-BF) (also called *alpha*-naphthoflavone) and 5,6-benzoflavone (5,6-BF) (also called *beta*-naphthoflavone) have been extensively studied, and warrant discussion here. 5,6-BF is an Ah receptor agonist, and induces CYP 1A enzyme activities *(59–61)*. Administration of 5,6-BF during the initiation phase blocked DMBA mammary carcinogenesis in female Sprague-Dawley rats, but was ineffective when administered during the post-initiation stage *(62,63)*, so it was suggested that its action occurs via modulation of phase 1 enzymes. It was later shown that 5,6-BF administered in the diet blocked DMBA-DNA adduct formation in liver and mammary tissues of female Sprague-Dawley rats *(64)*. Furthermore, prior administration of 5,6-BF to rabbits inhibited the formation of AFB_1-DNA adducts in isolated rabbit lung cells incubated with AFB_1 *(65)*. It also increased the formation of AFM_1, a detoxification product, because of selective induction of CYPs *(65)*. Feeding 5,6-BF in the diet while administering AFB_1 to rats also inhibited AFB_1 hepatocarcinogenesis, presumably by increased detoxification of AFB_1 to AFM_1 *(66)*. However, in rainbow trout, low doses of 5,6-BF inhibited AFB_1 DNA adduct formation in the absence of EROD induction *(67)*. Instead, 5,6-BF inhibited the 8,9-epoxidation of AFB_1 *(67)*, which is metabolized by CYP2K1 in rainbow trout *(68)*. Thus, the effects of 5,6-BF may not be caused solely by its induction of CYP enzymes.

Unlike 5,6-BF, which primarily induces CYPs, 7,8-BF is a potent and selective inhibitor of the CYP 1 family. When administered in the diet, both 5,6-BF and 7,8-BF suppressed 2-amino-1-methyl-6-phenylimidazo-(4,5-*b*)pyridine (PhIP)-induced mammary carcinogenesis in female Sprague-Dawley rats *(69)*. As PhIP is bioactivated by CYP1A2, the proposed mechanism of suppression of PhIP mammary carcinogenesis by 7,8-BF is by inhibition of CYP1A2 *(69)*. However, since 5,6-BF induces CYPs 1A1/1A2, these authors suggested that its ability to induce phase 2 enzymes may play a role in its inhibitory effects on PhIP mammary carcinogenesis *(69)*. Previous studies from several

laboratories have shown 7,8-BF to be an effective inhibitor of DMBA skin tumor initiation, but not B*[a]*P skin tumor initiation *(70,71)*. Later, it was shown that 7,8-BF may be a highly selective inhibitor of mouse CYP1B1 *(72)*. However, species differences have been observed, because it was shown that 7,8-BF may be a more effective inhibitor of CYP1A1 in human cells compared to mouse cells *(73)*. Consistent with this observation, it has previously been reported that 7,8-BF inhibits human CYP1A1, although at higher concentrations than for CYP1B1 *(74,75)*. Notably, 7,8-BF can also act as a partial agonist of Ahr *(76)*.

Evidence suggests that certain naturally occurring flavonoids may be agonists/antagonists of Ahr. It has been shown by gel-shift analysis that quercetin and keampferol are Ahr ligands *(77)*. Furthermore, galangin, which inhibited DMBA metabolism and DNA adduct formation in MCF-7 cells, blocked the induction of CYP1A1 mRNA by TCDD or DMBA *(78)*. However, in the absence of these inducers, galangin induced CYP1A1 expression by itself *(78)*. Thus, the effects of flavonoids on carcinogen bioactivation may be a result of inhibition of CYP activity in addition to their effects on Ahr.

2.4. Green Tea Polyphenols

Epicatechin derivatives make up ~74% of the total green tea polyphenols (GTP), or ~6% (w/w) of total green tea leaves *(79)*. Of these, (–)–epigallocatechin-3-gallate (EGCG), (–)–epigallocatechin (EGC), (–)–epicatechin (EC), and (–)–epicatechin-3-gallate (ECG) represent ~55%, 14%, 2.2%, and 2.5% of the total GTP, respectively *(79)*. Both GTP and EGCG blocked mutagenicity of B*[a]*P, 2-aminofluorene, and AFB_1 in *Salmonella typhimurim* TA98 supplemented with a hepatic S9 system *(80)*. GTP blocked rat-liver microsomal activities of AHH, EROD, and 7-ethoxycoumarin *O*-deethylase (ECD) *(81)*. Of the (–)–EC derivatives, the most effective inhibitors of AHH activities in rat liver microsomes were EGCG>ECG>EGC>EC, at concentrations ranging from 0.1–1.0 m*M* *(81)*. It has been suggested that the mechanism of inhibition of CYP monooxygenase activities by these compounds may be the result of impairment of electron flow *(81)*. Indeed, (–)EC derivatives do not appear to be selective for specific isoforms of CYP, since they block AHH, ECD, and EROD activities at relatively high concentrations compared to other CYP inhibitors.

Topical administration of EGCG to SENCAR mice inhibited formation of B*[a]*P and DMBA epidermal

DNA adducts *(79)*. When administered prior to DMBA dosing, EGCG also inhibited tumorigenesis in a DMBA-12-*O*-tetradecanoylphorbol-13-acetate (TPA) two-stage skin tumorigenesis model *(79)*. Furthermore, topical administration of GTP prior to DMBA dosing also blocked mouse skin tumorigenesis in a DMBA-TPA two-stage model *(82)*. In a rat mammary tumorigenesis model, when green tea was administered in the drinking water for the entire study (including during carcinogen dosing period), it decreased the number of tumors, tumor weight, and latency time *(83)*. However, since green tea was administered during the entire study, it is difficult to determine whether CYP modulation played a role in its anti-tumorigenic effects.

2.5. Indoles

Indole glucosinolates are found as decomposition products in members of the *Brassica* family (e.g., watercress, cauliflower, brussels sprouts). Incubation of indole-3-carbinol (I3C) at pH 5.0 produces condensation products [likely 3,3'-diindolylmethane, or DIM, and 2,3-*bis*(indole-3-ylmethyl)indole], which induce CYP1A1 and 2B1/2-mediated EROD and PROD activities, respectively, in the liver, kidneys, and colon of rats treated with the condensate *(84)*. Also, it has been reported that I3C induces Ahr *(85)*. The active agent may be 5,11-dihyroindolo[3,2-b]carbazole, as it has high affinity for Ahr, and I3C is only effective in inducing Ahr when administered orally *(86,87)*. It has been suggested that acid condensation products are responsible for the effects of orally administered I3C, rather than I3C itself. Another acid condensation product, DIM, is a potent, noncompetitive inhibitor of trout CYP1A1-mediated EROD activity. It also inhibits rat liver microsomal EROD (CYP1A1) and PROD (CYP2B1/20 activities, human CYP1A1 and 1A2 EROD activities, and microsomal metabolism of AFB_1 *(88)*. As with many inhibitors of CYPs, DIM was found to be a substrate for rat hepatic microsomal mono-oxygenase activity, resulting in the formation of a monohydroxylated product *(88)*. In addition to I3C, *N*-methoxyindole-3-carbinol was also found to induce CYP1A1 in rat liver and Hepa1c1c7 (Hepa-1) rat hepatoma cells, and was more potent than I3C *(89)*. Furthermore, this compound inhibited EROD activity of hepatic microsomes *(89)*. This bifunctional effect has been reported with I3C acid condensation products elsewhere *(90)*. The induction of CYP1A1 by *N*-methoxyindole-3-carbinol was shown to occur via Ahr because it induced the Ahr DNA response

element (DRE) complex, did not induce EROD in Arnt-deficient Hepa-1 mutant cells line B13, and induced CAT activity in cells that were stably transfected with DRE-CAT reporter *(89)*.

The effects of I3C in the diet have shown some promise for chemoprevention. When I3C was administered to rats in the diet (0.02%, 0.1%, w/w), it inhibited PhIP DNA adduct formation in several organs, including the spleen, pancreas, lung, colon, cecum, liver, stomach, and small intestines, but not mammary epithelial cells *(91)*. When administered either by gavage or in the diet, I3C induced CYP1A1/1A2 RNA expression in the liver and 1A1 expression in the colon *(91)*. It also induced EROD (CYP1A1) and MROD (CYP1A2) activities in the liver *(91)*. I3C administered in the diet also reduced the amount of unmetabolized PhIP excreted in the urine, indicating that it accelerated the metabolism of PhIP *(91)*. This has also been shown to occur using acid condensation products of I3C in rats, in which I3C increased the overall metabolism of PhIP by 2.5 times *(84)*. Interestingly, the metabolism of PhIP was shifted from a ratio of 4'-hydroxy-PhIP (catalyzed by CYP1A1)/*N*-hydroxy-PhIP (catalyzed by CYP1A2) of 3.8 in control rats to 0.8 in rats treated with the acid condensation products of I3C *(84)*. Grubbs and colleagues showed that administration of I3C to female rats either during the initiation stage or during the entire study effectively blocked mammary tumorigenesis by *N*-methyl-*N*-nitrosourea (MNU) (a direct-acting carcinogen) and DMBA (an indirect-acting carcinogen) *(92)*. I3C induced MROD (CYP1A2), EROD (CYP1A1), and benzyloxyresorufin-*O*-dealkylase (CYP2B1/2) activities and induced mRNA expression in the liver, in addition to induction of phase 2 enzymes *(92)*. Therefore, it was concluded that the anticarcinogenic activity of I3C in rats was the result of an acid condensation product generated in the stomach, and that induction of CYPs and phase 2 enzymes contributed to its anticarcinogenic effects. However, other mechanisms (such as changes in estrogen metabolism) may be involved, since I3C also inhibited tumorigenesis by a direct-acting carcinogen *(92)*. Indeed, it was suggested that since I3C induced CYP1A1 activity, it may shift the carcinogen-induced metabolism of estrogen from the 16α-hydroxylation toward C2-hydroxylation *(93)*.

Despite I3C's anticarcinogenic effects, it may not be appropriate as a chemopreventive agent in humans *(94)*, because it can be converted to mutagenic nitrosamines in the stomach in the presence of acid and nitrite *(95,96)*. Also, in the mouse epidermis, I3C enhanced ornithine decarboxylase induction by TPA *(97)*. Conversely, when given with TPA, I3C inhibited skin tumorigenesis in a DMBA-TPA two-stage model *(98)*. Although I3C is considered an antiestrogen, it is a promoter in the liver and colon. In a multi-organ tumor study, I3C delayed mammary-tumor latency induced by DMBA; in the colon, it inhibited the formation of aberrant crypt foci (ACF) by AOM by 40% *(94)*. In the liver, I3C induced GST-P foci in AFB$_1$-treated and vehicle control rats *(94)*.

2.6. Isothiocyanates

The isothiocyanates are found in cruciferous vegetables. Many studies have been done to evaluate their chemopreventive potential. Since this class of compounds is discussed in another part of this book, we will discuss isothiocyanates only briefly. It has been shown that phenethyl isothiocyanate (PEITC) is an effective inhibitor of tumorigenesis in A/J mouse lung by 4-(methylnitrosamino)-1-(3-pyridyl)-1-butanone (NNK), but not by B[*a*]P (*(99,100)*. In contrast, benzyl isothiocyanate (BITC) effectively inhibits A/J mouse lung tumorigenesis by B[*a*]P, DMBA, 5-methylchrysene, and dibenzo[*a,h*]anthracene *(101,102)*, but not by NNK *(103,104)*. PEITC only inhibited NNK lung tumorigenesis when given prior to carcinogen treatment *(105)*, indicating that its mechanism of action may be partly caused by inhibition of carcinogen metabolism. It also appeared that the differences in PEITC and BITC to block tumorigenesis may be the result of differences in specificity of CYP modulation. PEITC did not block B[*a*]P DNA adduct formation in the lungs of A/J mice *(100)* as expected, based on its inability to block lung tumorigenesis by B[*a*]P. Interestingly, despite the role of O^6-methyl guanine in tobacco carcinogenesis, PEITC did not block formation of O^6-methyl guanine, although it did significantly block formation of 4-hydroxy-1-(3-pyridyl)-1-butanone-releasing adducts *(106)*. On the other hand, BITC pretreatment inhibited the formation of anti-B[*a*]P 7,8-diol-9,10-epoxide (BPDE) DNA adducts in mice treated with B[*a*]P *(106)*. It was also demonstrated that BITC can inactivate CYP1A1, 1A2, 2B1, and 2E1 activities *(107,108)*. In lung microsomes of mice treated with BITC or PEITC, NNK metabolism to the keto aldehyde, keto alcohol, and NNK-*N*-oxide were inhibited by PEITC, but not BITC *(109)*. In contrast, BITC inhibited EROD and PROD activity, but PEITC did not *(110)*. These results explain the effectiveness of BITC

for PAH, which are known to be bioactivated primarily by the CYP1 family. Furthermore, PEITC blocked the in vitro metabolic activation of NNK by reconstituted CYP1A2. PEITC competitively inhibited CYP1A2-mediated metabolism of NNK to the keto alcohol at a K$_i$ of 0.18 μ*M* *(111)*.

As with other CYP modulators, many are capable of inhibiting CYPs as well as inducing them. It was shown that oral administration of PEITC in rats caused an initial reduction in hepatic EROD (CYP1A), erythromycin *N*-demethylase (CYP3A), and *N*-nitrosodimethylamine demethylase (CYP2E1) activities, but that CYP1A and 3A activities recovered by 24 h. The inhibition of CYP2E1 activities was even more profound, and recovery back to control levels was slow. In contrast, PROD (CYP2B1/2) activities increased significantly over a period of 24 h *(112)*. The role of hepatic PROD induction in PEITC inhibition of NNK lung tumorigenesis is unclear.

2.7. Coumarins

Coumarins are widely distributed in nature, and are found in all parts of plants *(113)*. These compounds are especially common in grasses, orchids, citrus fruits, and legumes *(113,114)*. Because they are so abundant in nature, coumarins make up an important part of the human diet. Based on chemical structure, they can be broadly classified as simple coumarins (e.g., coumarin); furanocoumarins of the linear (e.g. imperatorin), or angular (e.g., angelicin) type; and pyranocoumarins of the linear (e.g., xanthyletin) or angular (e.g., seselin) type. Simple coumarins are very widely distributed in the plant kingdom *(113)*. Citrus oils, in particular, contain abundant amounts of both simple coumarins and furanocoumarins *(115)*. Furthermore, umbelliferous plants used in Chinese herbal medicine contain furanocoumarins. For example, isoimperatorin, imperatorin, and oxypeucedanin have been isolated from the active fraction of the crude drug "Tang-Bai'Zhi" *(116)*.

Earlier studies demonstrated that, as a general class, coumarins can modulate the metabolism of PAH and possibly other carcinogens. For example, the inhibitory effects of several 8-acyl-7-hydroxycoumarins on 3-methylcholanthrene (3-MCA)-induced rat hepatic AHH activities were reported *(117)*. Imperatorin and several derivatives were reported to inhibit various drug-metabolizing enzymes *(118)*. Notably, imperatorin was an effective antimutagen for 2-aminoanthracene and B[*a*]P in *S. typhimurium* in the presence of a hepatic 9000g supernatant (S_9) activating system (*119*). Several other coumarins also displayed antimutagenic activity to varying degrees in this system, including coumarin, umbelliferone, psoralen, and osthol. Bergapten and xanthotoxin, when added in vitro, inhibited hepatic microsomal 7-ethoxycoumarin-*O*-deethylase (ECD), B[*a*]P-hydroxylase, aminopyrene-*N*-demethylase, and hexobarbital hydroxylase (*120,121*). Xanthotoxin was reportedly a potent inhibitor of the in vivo phase 1 metabolism of phenytoin, hexobarbital, caffeine, and theophylline (*122,123*). This furanocoumarin was also found to be an inducer of hepatic ECD, AHH, and ethylmorphine-deethylase, when administered orally to rats at relatively low doses over a period of several days (*124,125*). Xanthotoxin was also found to be metabolically activated to intermediates that bind covalently to liver microsomal protein, leading to the inactivation of CYPs through covalent modification of the apoprotein (*120,126,127*). Coriandrin was reported to be metabolized very rapidly by rat-liver microsomal preparations (*128*). Bergamottin was reported to be a mechanism-based inactivator of CYP3A4 in human liver microsomes (*129*). It was also shown that 8-MOP is a mechanism-based inactivator of purified reconstituted human CYP2A6 and 2B1 (*130,131*). $H_2^{18}O$ incorporation studies support the idea that 8-MOP is initially oxidized to an epoxide intermediate, which either binds covalently to the apoprotein or undergoes hydrolytic ring opening (*130,131*). Finally, Maenpaa and colleagues (*132*) reported that several coumarins, especially the linear furanocoumarins, inhibited mouse CYP2A5-mediated coumarin 7-hydroxylase activity.

The potential inhibitory effects of coumarins against chemically induced cancer in rodents have been examined in several studies. Orally administered coumarin and 4-methyl-coumarin were moderately effective inhibitors of DMBA-induced mammary tumors in the rat, and showed inhibitory activity for B[*a*]P-induced neoplasia of the mouse forestomach. Limettin was a less effective inhibitor of DMBA-induced mammary tumors, and was inactive for B[*a*]P-induced neoplasia of the mouse forestomach (*133,134*). In general, simple coumarins with polar substituents were found to be relatively poor inhibitors of tumorigenesis in these model systems. A strong correlation between ability to elevate GST and inhibit B[*a*]P-induced forestomach tumors was noted for a series of compounds (*135*). Dietary treatment with coumarin was also found to

inhibit AFB_1 hepatocarcinogenesis in rats (*136*), which correlated with its ability to induce phase 2 enzymes in the liver, especially GSTs. We have shown that bergamottin, coriandrin, ostruthin, and imperatorin inhibited tumor initiation by B[*a*]P in a two-stage carcinogenesis protocol (*137*). In contrast, bergamottin slightly enhanced tumor initiation by DMBA. However, imperatorin was an effective inhibitor of skin tumorigenesis induced by DMBA, using both a two-stage and a complete carcinogenesis protocol. The effects of bergamottin on B[*a*]P skin-tumor initiation was hypothesized to be the result of selective inhibition of CYP1A1-mediated metabolism to B[*a*]P-7,8-dihydrodiol (*138*). These studies also supported the hypothesis that B[*a*]P and DMBA are bioactivated by different isoforms of CYP in mouse skin, and that bergamottin and imperatorin selectively inhibit different isoforms of mouse CYPs. To further understand the selective nature of CYP inhibition by different coumarins, we used mouse-cell lines that primarily express either CYP1B1 or CYP1A1 (*72*). Mouse embryo fibroblast C3H/10T1/2 (10T1/2) cells, and mouse hepatoma-derived 1c1c7 (Hepa-1) cells, which preferentially express CYP1B1 and CYP1A1 (*3,139*) respectively, were co-incubated with 2 μM bergamottin, imperatorin, and isopimpinellin, along with DMBA (2 μM). Bergamottin inhibited DMBA metabolism to DMBA-3,4-diol, and blocked DNA adduct formation in Hepa-1 cells, but had little effect in 10T1/2 cells. In contrast, imperatorin and isopimpinellin inhibited DMBA bioactivation in both cell lines. These results indicated that bergamottin is a more selective inhibitor of CYP1A1, and overall a less effective inhibitor of the metabolic activation of DMBA in the mouse epidermis. In contrast, imperatorin and isopimpinellin, which block metabolic activation of DMBA in the mouse epidermis, appear to inhibit both CYP1B1 and 1A1.

Oral and topical administration of isopimpinellin inhibited mouse-skin tumorigenesis by DMBA in the two-stage model (*140*). Isopimpinellin and imperatorin also reduced PAH DNA adducts in several tissues when given orally together with B[*a*]P or DMBA (*140*). In many of these tissues, EROD and PROD activities were reduced following multiple oral doses of imperatorin and isopimpinellin. Our results demonstrate that certain coumarins have the ability to block skin tumor initiation and complete carcinogenesis by PAHs such as B[*a*]P and DMBA through inhibition of the CYPs that are involved in the metabolic activation of these hydrocarbons. Our data also support the hypothesis that coumarins with inhibitory activity against both CYP1A1 and 1B1 are the most effective inhibitors of PAH skin carcinogenesis.

Interestingly, oral administration of imperatorin and isopimpinellin to mice resulted in an initial decrease in EROD activities in the liver, followed by an increase in EROD and PROD activities in liver at 24 h (140). In vivo toxicity studies showed no overt signs of systemic toxicity by orally administered isopimpinellin or imperatorin (141). However, there was an increase in liver weight, which is common with hepatic enzyme inducers. We are currently investigating the mechanism(s) of CYP induction in the livers of mice following oral administration of coumarins.

2.8. Miscellaneous

The coffee-specific diterpenes cafestol and kahweol (C + K) have also been studied for their chemopreventive properties. In a hamster cheek-pouch model, it was shown that C + K administered in the diet prevented DMBA tumorigenesis by 35%, mainly by decreasing the tumor number (142). It was later shown that C + K in the diet could block in vitro genotoxicity of AFB_1 in rat liver microsomes or S9 fractions (143). Two potential mechanisms were observed in the rat liver following dietary treatment of C + K: induction of GST, and reduction in protein and mRNA expression of CYP2C11 and 3A2 (143). Similarly, C + K treatment in vitro blocked protein expression of CYP3A2 and 2C11 and induced GSTs in primary rat hepatocytes (144). Pretreatment of cells with C + K prior to AFB_1 treatment blocked the formation of AFB_1 DNA adducts in primary rat hepatocytes (144). However, co-treatment of C+K and AFB_1 for 3 h was not effective at blocking AFB_1 DNA adduct formation, ruling out the possibility of a direct inhibitory effect in primary rat hepatocytes (144). In a human cell line of hepatocyte origin (THLE cells) stably transfected with AFB_1 activating CYPs, pretreatment of C+K blocked AFB_1 DNA adduct formation in cells transfected with CYP1A2 or 2B6, but was cytotoxic in cells transfected with CYP3A4 (144). In contrast to the results observed in rat hepatocytes, co-incubation of C + K and AFB_1 in human THLE cells transfected with CYP2B6 also inhibited the formation of AFB_1 DNA adducts (144). Thus, the inhibitory effects of C + K may be the result of a dual mechanism, inhibition of CYP expression, and induction of GST. However, hypercholesterolemia has been observed both in humans (145,146) and in rats and gerbils (147) as a side effect

of treatment with C + K. Hypercholesterolemic effects may be a result of the dose; it may be possible to find doses that have chemopreventive properties without negative side effects.

Rosemary extract, from the plant *Rosmarinus officinalis* L., has also been studied for its chemopreventive properties. Topical administration of rosemary to mice prior to B[a]P or DMBA initiation blocked skin tumor incidence and multiplicity in mice (148). Rosemary also blocked epidermal B[a]P DNA adduct formation (148). In addition to its effects on blocking tumor initiation, it was also shown that rosemary could block the tumor-promoting effects of TPA in the mouse epidermis (148). Later, it was found that rosemary extract and carnosol, but not ursolic acid, when administered intraperitoneal for 5 d prior to DMBA treatment, inhibited palpable mammary-tumor incidence and multiplicity in rats (149). Furthermore, carnosol and rosemary extract inhibited DMBA DNA adduct formation in rat mammary glands (149). Rosemary and carnosol, but not ursolic acid, increased liver GST and NQO1 in female rats, but this is unlikely to be the mechanism for inhibition of PAH skin tumor initiation. It was also demonstrated that in human bronchial epithelial cells, rosemary extract and carnosol induced GST pi and NQO1, decreased EROD activity, and blocked formation of B[a]P DNA adducts (150). Rosemary contains numerous compounds, including flavonoids (e.g., rosmarinic acid, caffeic acid, hydroxy-apigenin), phenolic diterpenes (e.g., carnosic acid, carnosol, rosmanol), and volatile terpenes (151). Administration of different extracts of rosemary to rats for 2 wk resulted in induction of several drug-metabolizing enzymes. Both the water-soluble extract and the essential oils caused an increase in EROD, PROD, and MROD activity, but no change in p-nitrophenol hydroxylase activity (CYP2E1).

Although many of the compounds described in this chapter have multiple actions, including induction and inhibition of CYPs and induction of phase 2 enzymes, the aryl acetylenes have been studied mainly as CYP inhibitors. These synthetic compounds are mechanism-based inactivators of CYPs, and have very selective actions. 1-ethynylpyrene (1-EP), 1-vinylpyrene (VP), and 2-ethynylnaphthalene (EN) inhibited B[a]P and DMBA DNA adduct formation in mouse epidermis (152). Of the three compounds, 1-EP was the most potent, and was more selective for DMBA than B[a]P (152). In a two-stage skin carcinogenesis study, 1-EP

Table 2
Inhibitors of P450

P450 Isoform	Inhibitor	Examples
1A2	Curcumin, flavonoids, isothiocyanates	Galangin, 7,8-BF, BITC, PEITC
1A1	Curcumin, flavonoids, diindolylmethane, isothiocyanates, coumarins	7-hydroxyflavone, 7,8-BF, BITC, bergamottin
1B1	Flavonoids, coumarins	Hesperetin, 7,8-BF, imperatorin, isopimpinellin
2A5	Coumarins	Linear furanocoumarins
2B6	Curcumin, diindolylmethane, isothiocyanates	BITC
3A4	Coumarins, coffee-specific diterpenes	Bergamottin, cafestol + kahweol
2E1	Organosulfur compound isothiocyanates	Olitpraz, diallyl sulfide, BITC

effectively blocked the number of papillomas per mouse induced by DMBA by up to 95% at 44 nmol, and VP and EN were also effective, but required higher doses to achieve similar levels of inhibition (up to 4400–132,000 nmol) (152). 1-EP and VP also blocked B[a]P skin-tumor initiation, but required higher doses than for DMBA (152). None of the three aryl acetylenes were very effective against MNNG tumor initiation (152).

3. SUMMARY AND CONCLUSIONS

From this review, it can be seen that many natural and synthetic compounds have been shown to modulate CYPs, and possess anticarcinogenic activities against a variety of chemical carcinogens in a number of tissues (summarized in Table 2). In summary, organosulfur compounds such as those present in garlic and onions have been shown to inhibit activities of CYPs 2E1, 2A6, and 1A1, and to block the metabolic bioactivation of nitrosamines. Curcuminoids inhibit CYPs 1A and 2B, and possess anticarcinogenic activities toward PAHs and AOM. Flavonoids inhibit the CYP1 family, and block the activation of nitrosamines, aflatoxins, and PAH. The green tea polyphenols also block CYP1 family activities, and inhibit bioactivation of PAH and AFB_1. Indoles, such as those from the *Brassica* family, can both induce and inhibit members of the CYP1 family, and have demonstrated anticarcinogenic activity against the food-borne carcinogens PhIP and AFB_1. Isothiocyanates, which have varying specificities against members of the CYP1 family, can inhibit bioactivation of tobacco-specific NNK and PAHs. Naturally occurring coumarins, which inhibit CYP1 family members and CYP3A4, block PAH and AFB_1 bioactivation and tumorigenesis. Finally, aryl acetylenes are potent synthetic inhibitors of CYPs and block PAH activation.

Inhibition of CYPs as a strategy for the chemoprevention of cancer has been studied for many years. Numerous compounds have been shown to inhibit specific CYPs, and block metabolism and metabolic activation of specific carcinogens, as summarized in this and other reviews (153–156). Many of these compounds also inhibit chemical carcinogenesis in experimental animals. A knowledge of the CYPs involved in metabolic activation of specific classes of carcinogens is essential for determining the usefulness and effectiveness of specific CYP inhibitors. Based on availability, we believe that the most practical CYP inhibitors are those that have a broad spectrum of inhibitory activities against multiple members of a specific CYP family. In addition, those compounds that possess inhibitory activities across several CYP families involved in the metabolic activation of carcinogens are also of considerable interest and practicality. Although there are occupational settings and some environmental settings in which humans may be exposed to predominantly one or very few carcinogenic compounds, humans are generally most often exposed to chemical mixtures containing more than one carcinogenic agent. CYP inhibitors with broader activities are more likely to block the effects of such mixtures. In addition, since multiple CYPs can metabolize a single compound—some leading to detoxification and others leading to activation—CYP inhibitors with broader activities are likely to be more effective, even against single carcinogenic agents. These points can be easily illustrated with our own studies using certain flavonoids and naturally occurring linear furanocoumarins (72,73).

Finally, human carcinogenesis is likely to involve both complete carcinogenesis and initiation-promotion-type processes. With regard to the former process, humans are constantly exposed to low levels of carcinogens through the air, water, and food (e.g., PAH). Except for very unusual situations, humans are usually not exposed to sufficient quantities of carcinogens in single doses to lead to carcinogenesis, or even initiation. Any modifying factor that reduces the effective dose of a carcinogen (e.g., DNA adducts) in a specific target tissue may have a dramatic effect on overall cancer incidence, especially if the initiation process requires cumulative exposure to reach a threshold. Therefore, an understanding of specific dietary constituents that may reduce or block metabolic activation of carcinogens is an important goal. Such information could lead to the development of specific chemopreventive agents, to specific dietary recommendations regarding foods containing substantial quantities of certain types of chemicals, or to approaches using mixtures of agents (e.g., a broad-spectrum P450 inhibitor plus an antioxidant and/or an electrophile trapping agent). Although it may seem difficult to time inhibitor exposure directly with carcinogen exposure in humans, chemicals that are ingested virtually every day would not necessitate such stringent timing requirements. Therefore, additional research intended to identify CYP inhibitors with the most appropriate properties, as noted here, seems most critical.

REFERENCES

1. Parkinson A. Biotransformation of xenobiotics, in *Casarett and Doull's Toxicology: The Basic Science of Poisons*, 5th ed. Klaasen C, ed. McGraw-Hill, New York, 1996, pp.113–186.

2. Shimada T, Hayes CL, Yamazaki H, et al. Activation of chemically diverse procarcinogens by human cytochrome P-450 1B1. *Cancer Res* 1996;56:2979–2984.

3. Alexander DL, Eltom SE, Jefcoate CR. Ah receptor regulation of CYP1B1 expression in primary mouse embryo-derived cells. *Cancer Res* 1997;57:4498–4506.

4. Brake PB, Jefcoate CR. Regulation of cytochrome P4501B1 in cultured rat adrenocortical cells by cyclic adenosine 3',5'-monophosphate and 2,3,7,8-tetrachlorodibenzo-p-dioxin. *Endocrinology* 1995;136:5034–5041.

5. Savas U, Bhattacharyya KK, Christou M, et al. Mouse cytochrome P-450EF, representative of a new 1B subfamily of cytochrome P-450s. Cloning, sequence determination, and tissue expression. *J Biol Chem* 1994;269:14,905–14,911.

6. McLemore TL, Adelberg S, Liu MC, et al. Expression of CYP1A1 gene in patients with lung cancer: evidence for cigarette smoke-induced gene expression in normal lung tissue and for altered gene regulation in primary pulmonary carcinomas. *J Natl Cancer Inst* 1990;82:1333–1339.

7. Song BJ, Gelboin HV, Park SS, et al. Monoclonal antibody-directed radioimmunoassay detects cytochrome P-450 in human placenta and lymphocytes. *Science* 1985;228:490–492.

8. Hasler JA, Estabrook R, Murray M, et al. Human cytochromes P450. *Mol Aspects Med* 1999;20:1–137.

9. Kensler TW, Egner PA, Trush MA, et al. Modification of aflatoxin B1 binding to DNA in vivo in rats fed phenolic antioxidants, ethoxyquin and a dithiothione. *Carcinogenesis* 1985;6:759–763.

10. Kensler TW, Egner PA, Dolan PM, et al. Mechanism of protection against aflatoxin tumorigenicity in rats fed 5-(2-pyrazinyl)-4-methyl-1,2-dithiol-3-thione (oltipraz) and related 1,2-dithiol-3-thiones and 1,2-dithiol-3-ones. *Cancer Res* 1987;47:4271–4277.

11. Kensler TW, Groopman JD, Eaton DL, et al. Potent inhibition of aflatoxin-induced hepatic tumorigenesis by the monofunctional enzyme inducer 1,2-dithiole-3-thione. *Carcinogenesis* 1992;13:95–100.

12. Rao CV, Rivenson A, Zang E, et al. Inhibition of 2-amino-1-methyl-6-phenylimidazo[4,5]pyridine-induced lymphoma formation by oltipraz. *Cancer Res* 1996;56:3395–3398.

13. Meyer DJ, Harris JM, Gilmore KS, et al. Quantitation of tissue- and sex-specific induction of rat GSH transferase subunits by dietary 1,2-dithiole-3-thiones. *Carcinogenesis* 1993;14:567–572.

14. Raney KD, Meyer DJ, Ketterer B, et al. Glutathione conjugation of aflatoxin B1 exo- and endo-epoxides by rat and human glutathione S-transferases. *Chem Res Toxicol* 1992;5:470–478.

15. Langouet S, Maheo K, Berthou F, et al. Effects of administration of the chemoprotective agent oltipraz on CYP1A and CYP2B in rat liver and rat hepatocytes in culture. *Carcinogenesis* 1997;18:1343–1349.

16. Guengerich FP, Johnson WW, Shimada T, et al. Activation and detoxication of aflatoxin B1. *Mutat Res* 1998;402:121–128.

17. Kensler TW, Curphey TJ, Maxiutenko Y, Roebuck BD. Chemoprotection by organosulfur inducers of phase 2 enzymes: dithiolethiones and dithiins. *Drug Metabol Drug Interact* 2000;17:3–22.

18. Le Bon AM, Siess MH. Organosulfur compounds from Allium and the chemoprevention of cancer. *Drug Metabol Drug Interact* 2000;17:51–79.

19. Wargovich MJ, Woods C, Eng VW, et al. Chemoprevention of N-nitrosomethylbenzylamine-induced esophageal cancer in rats by the naturally occurring thioether, diallyl sulfide. *Cancer Res* 1988;48:6872–6875.

20. Sparnins VL, Barany G, Wattenberg LW. Effects of organosulfur compounds from garlic and onions on benzo[*a*]pyrene-induced neoplasia and glutathione S-transferase activity in the mouse. *Carcinogenesis* 1988;9:131–134.

21. Suzui N, Sugie S, Rahman KM, et al. Inhibitory effects of diallyl disulfide or aspirin on 2-amino-1-methyl-6-phenylimidazo[4,5-b]pyridine-induced mammary carcinogenesis in rats. *Jpn J Cancer Res* 1997;88:705–711.

22. Guyonnet D, Belloir C, Suschetet M, et al. Antimutagenic activity of organosulfur compounds from Allium is associated with phase 2 enzyme induction. *Mutat Res* 2001;495:135–145.

23. Srivastava SK, Hu X, Xia H, et al. Mechanism of differential efficacy of garlic organosulfides in preventing

benzo(*a*)pyrene-induced cancer in mice. *Cancer Lett* 1997;118:61–67.

24. Teyssier C, Amiot MJ, Mondy N, et al. Effect of onion consumption by rats on hepatic drug-metabolizing enzymes. *Food Chem Toxicol* 2001;39:981–987.

25. Brady JF, Ishizaki H, Fukuto JM, et al. Inhibition of cytochrome P-450 2E1 by diallyl sulfide and its metabolites. *Chem Res Toxicol* 1991;4:642–647.

26. Yamazaki H, Inui Y, Yun CH, et al. Cytochrome P450 2E1 and 2A6 enzymes as major catalysts for metabolic activation of *N*-nitrosodialkylamines and tobacco-related nitrosamines in human liver microsomes. *Carcinogenesis* 1992;13:1789–1794.

27. Patten CJ, Smith TJ, Friesen MJ, et al. Evidence for cytochrome P450 2A6 and 3A4 as major catalysts for *N'*-nitrosonornicotine alpha-hydroxylation by human liver microsomes. *Carcinogenesis* 1997;18:1623–1630.

28. Kushida, H., Fujita, K., Suzuki, A., et al. Development of a Salmonella tester strain sensitive to promutagenic *N*-nitrosamines: expression of recombinant CYP2A6 and human NADPH-cytochrome P450 reductase in *S. typhimurium* YG7108. *Mutat Res* 2000;471:135–143.

29. Kushida, H., Fujita, K., Suzuki, A., et al. Metabolic activation of *N*-alkylnitrosamines in genetically engineered *Salmonella typhimurium* expressing CYP2E1 or CYP2A6 together with human NADPH-cytochrome P450 reductase. *Carcinogenesis* 2000;21:1227–1232.

30. Genter MB, Liang HC, Gu J, et al. Role of CYP2A5 and 2G1 in acetaminophen metabolism and toxicity in the olfactory mucosa of the Cyp1a2(–/–) mouse. *Biochem Pharmacol* 1998;55:1819–1826.

31. Wattenberg LW, Sparnins VL, Barany G. Inhibition of *N*-nitrosodiethylamine carcinogenesis in mice by naturally occurring organosulfur compounds and monoterpenes. *Cancer Res* 1989;49:2689–2692.

32. Takahashi S, Hakoi K, Yada H, et al. Enhancing effects of diallyl sulfide on hepatocarcinogenesis and inhibitory actions of the related diallyl disulfide on colon and renal carcinogenesis in rats. *Carcinogenesis*1992;13:1513–1518.

33. Fujita K, Kamataki T. Screening of organosulfur compounds as inhibitors of human CYP2A6. *Drug Metab Dispos* 2001;29:983–989.

34. Testa B, Jenner P. Inhibitors of cytochrome P-450s and their mechanism of action. *Drug Metab Rev* 1981;12:1–117.

35. Hong JY, Wang ZY, Smith TJ, et al. Inhibitory effects of diallyl sulfide on the metabolism and tumorigenicity of the tobacco-specific carcinogen 4-(methylnitrosamino)-1-(3-pyridyl)-1-butanone (NNK) in A/J mouse lung. *Carcinogenesis* 1992;13:901–904.

36. Huang MT, Wang ZY, Georgiadis CA, et al. Inhibitory effects of curcumin on tumor initiation by benzo[*a*]pyrene and 7,12-dimethylbenz[*a*]anthracene. *Carcinogenesis* 1992;13:2183–2186.

37. Chuang SE, Kuo ML, Hsu CH, et al. Curcumin-containing diet inhibits diethylnitrosamine-induced murine hepatocarcinogenesis. *Carcinogenesis* 2000;21:331–335.

38. Huang MT, Lou YR, Ma W. et al. Inhibitory effects of dietary curcumin on forestomach, duodenal, and colon carcinogenesis in mice. *Cancer Res* 1994;54:5841–5847.

39. Sohn OS, Ishizaki H, Yang CS, Fiala ES. Metabolism of azoxymethane, methylazoxymethanol and *N*-nitrosodi-

methylamine by cytochrome P450IIE1. *Carcinogenesis* 1991;12:127–131.

40. Lin CC, Lu YP, Lou YR, et al. Inhibition by dietary dibenzoylmethane of mammary gland proliferation, formation of DMBA-DNA adducts in mammary glands, and mammary tumorigenesis in Sencar mice. *Cancer Lett* 2001;168:125–132.

41. Huang MT, Lou YR, Xie JG, et al. Effect of dietary curcumin and dibenzoylmethane on formation of 7,12-dimethylbenz[*a*]anthracene-induced mammary tumors and lymphomas/leukemias in Sencar mice. *Carcinogenesis* 1998;19:1697–1700.

42. Kawamori T, Lubet R, Steele VE, et al. Chemopreventive effect of curcumin, a naturally occurring anti-inflammatory agent, during the promotion/progression stages of colon cancer. *Cancer Res* 1999;59: 597–601.

43. Thapliyal R, Maru GB. Inhibition of cytochrome P450 isozymes by curcumins in vitro and in vivo. *Food Chem Toxicol* 2001;39:541–547.

44. Allen SW, Mueller L, Williams SN, et al. The use of a high-volume screening procedure to assess the effects of dietary flavonoids on human cyp1a1 expression. *Drug Metab Dispos* 2001;29:1074–1079.

45. Rinaldi AL, Morse MA, Fields HW, et al. Curcumin activates the aryl hydrocarbon receptor yet significantly inhibits (–)-benzo(*a*)pyrene-7R-trans-7,8-dihydrodiol bioactivation in oral squamous cell carcinoma cells and oral mucosa. *Cancer Res* 2002;62:5451–5456.

46. MacDonald CJ, Ciolino HP, Yeh GC. Dibenzoylmethane modulates aryl hydrocarbon receptor function and expression of cytochromes P50 1A1, 1A2, and 1B1. *Cancer Res* 2001;61:3919–3924.

47. Hollman PC, Katan MB. Dietary flavonoids: intake, health effects and bioavailability. *Food Chem Toxicol* 1999;37:937–942.

48. Yang CS, Landau JM, Huang MT, Newmark HL. Inhibition of carcinogenesis by dietary polyphenolic compounds. *Annu Rev Nutr* 2001;21:381–406.

49. Yang M, Tanaka T, Hirose Y, et al. Chemopreventive effects of diosmin and hesperidin on *N*-butyl-*N*-(4- hydroxybutyl)nitrosamine-induced urinary-bladder carcinogenesis in male ICR mice. *Int J Cancer* 1997;73:719–724.

50. Lautraite S, Musonda AC, Doehmer J, et al. Flavonoids inhibit genetic toxicity produced by carcinogens in cells expressing CYP1A2 and CYP1A1. *Mutagenesis* 2001;17:45–53.

51. Chae YH, Ho DK, Cassady JM, et al. Effects of synthetic and naturally occurring flavonoids on metabolic activation of benzo[*a*]pyrene in hamster embryo cell cultures. *Chem Biol Interact* 1992;82:181–193.

52. Khanduja KL, Gandhi RK, Pathania V, Syal N. Prevention of N-nitrosodiethylamine-induced lung tumorigenesis by ellagic acid and quercetin in mice. *Food Chem Toxicol* 1999;37:313–318.

53. Doostdar H, Burke MD, Mayer RT. Bioflavonoids: selective substrates and inhibitors for cytochrome P450 CYP1A and CYP1B1. *Toxicology* 2000;144:31–38.

54. Zhai S, Dai R, Wei X, et al. Inhibition of methoxyresorufin demethylase activity by flavonoids in human liver microsomes. *Life Sci* 1998;63:L119–L123.

55. Kim BR, Kim DH, Park R, et al. Effect of an extract of the root of *Scutellaria baicalensis* and its flavonoids on aflatoxin

B1 oxidizing cytochrome P450 enzymes. *Planta Med* 2001;67:396–399.

56. Miranda CL, Yang YH, Henderson MC, et al. Prenylflavonoids from hops inhibit the metabolic activation of the carcinogenic heterocyclic amine 2-amino-3-methylimidazo[4, 5-f]quinoline, mediated by cDNA-expressed human CYP1A2. *Drug Metab Dispos* 2000;28:1297–1302.

57. Henderson MC, Miranda CL, Stevens JF, et al. In vitro inhibition of human P450 enzymes by prenylated flavonoids from hops, *Humulus lupulus. Xenobiotica* 2000;30:235–251.

58. Ueng YF, Shyu CC, Lin YL, et al. Effects of baicalein and wogonin on drug-metabolizing enzymes in C57BL/6J mice. *Life Sci* 2000;67:2189–2200.

59. Boobis AR, Nebert DW, Felton JS. Comparison of beta-naphthoflavone and 3-methylcholanthrene as inducers of hepatic cytochrome(s) P-448 and aryl hydrocarbon (benzo[a]pyrene) hydroxylase activity. *Mol Pharmacol* 1977;13:259–268.

60. Nebert DW, Jensen NM, Shinozuka H, et al. The Ah phenotype. Survey of forty-eight rat strains and twenty inbred mouse strains. *Genetics* 1982;100:79–87.

61. Blank JA, Tucker AN, Sweatlock J, et al. alpha-Naphthoflavone antagonism of 2,3,7,8-tetrachlorodibenzo-p-dioxin-induced murine lymphocyte ethoxyresorufin-O-deethylase activity and immunosuppression. *Mol Pharmacol* 1987;32:169–172.

62. Wattenberg L, Leong JL. Inhibition of the carcinogenic action of 7,12-dimethylbenz[a]anthracene by beta-naphthoflavone. *Proc Soc Exp Biol Med* 1968;128:940–943.

63. Malejka-Giganti D, Niehans GA, Reichert MA, Bliss RL. Post-initiation treatment of rats with indole-3-carbinol or beta-naphthoflavone does not suppress 7, 12-dimethylbenz[a]anthracene-induced mammary gland carcinogenesis. *Cancer Lett* 2000;160:209–218.

64. Izzotti A, Camoirano A, Cartiglia C, et al. Patterns of DNA adduct formation in liver and mammary epithelial cells of rats treated with 7,12-dimethylbenz*(a)*anthracene, and selective effects of chemopreventive agents. *Cancer Res* 1999;59:4285–4290.

65. Im SH, Bolt MW, Stewart RK, Massey TE. Modulation of aflatoxin B1 biotransformation by beta-naphthoflavone in isolated rabbit lung cells. *Arch Toxicol* 1996;71:72–79.

66. Gurtoo HL, Koser PL, Bansal SK, et al. Inhibition of aflatoxin B1-hepatocarcinogenesis in rats by beta-naphthoflavone. *Carcinogenesis* 1985;6:675–678.

67. Takahashi N, Harttig U, Williams DE, Bailey GS. The model Ah-receptor agonist beta-naphthoflavone inhibits aflatoxin B1-DNA binding in vivo in rainbow trout at dietary levels that do not induce CYP1A enzymes. *Carcinogenesis* 1996;17:79–87.

68. Takahashi N, Miranda CL, Henderson MC, et al. Inhibition of in vitro aflatoxin B1-DNA binding in rainbow trout by CYP1A inhibitors: alpha-naphthoflavone, beta-naphthoflavone and trout CYP1A1 peptide antibody. *Comp Biochem Physiol C Pharmacol Toxicol Endocrinol* 1995;110:273–280.

69. Mori H, Sugie S, Rahman W, Suzui N. Chemoprevention of 2-amino-1-methyl-6-phenylimidazo [4,5-b]pyridine-induced mammary carcinogenesis in rats. *Cancer Lett* 1999;143:195–198.

70. DiGiovanni J, Slaga TJ, Viaje A, et al. The effects of 7,8-benzoflavone on skin-tumor initiating activities of various

71. Slaga TJ, Thompson S, Berry DL, et al. The effects of benzoflavones on polycyclic hydrocarbon metabolism and skin tumor initiation. *Chem Biol Interact* 1977;17:297–312.

72. Kleiner HE, Vulimiri SV, Reed MJ, et al. Role of cytochrome P450 1a1 and 1b1 in the metabolic activation of 7,12-dimethylbenz[a]anthracene and the effects of naturally occurring furanocoumarins on skin tumor initiation. *Chem Res Toxicol* 2002;15: 226–235.

73. Kleiner HE, Reed MJ, DiGiovanni J. Naturally occurring coumarins inhibit human cytochromes P450 and block benzo[a]pyrene and 7,12-dimethylbenz[a]anthracene DNA adduct formation in MCF-7 cells. *Chem Res Toxicol* 2003 (in press).

74. Shimada T, Yamazaki H, Foroozesh M, et al. Selectivity of polycyclic inhibitors for human cytochrome P450s 1A1, 1A2, and 1B1. *Chem Res Toxicol* 1998;11:1048–1056.

75. Shimada T, Gillam EM, Sutter TR, et al. Oxidation of xenobiotics by recombinant human cytochrome P450 1B1. *Drug Metab Dispos* 1997;25:617–622.

76. Merchant M, Arellano L, Safe S. The mechanisms of action of a-naphthoflavone as an inhibitor of 2,3,7,8-tetrachlorodibenzo-p-dioxin-induced CYP1A1 gene expression. *Arch Biochem Biophys* 1990;281:84–89.

77. Ciolino HP, Daschner PJ, Yeh GC. Dietary flavonols quercetin and kaempferol are ligands of the aryl hydrocarbon receptor that affect CYP1A1 transcription differentially. *Biochem J* 1999;340:715–722.

78. Ciolino HP, Yeh GC. The flavonoid galangin is an inhibitor of CYP1A1 activity and an agonist/antagonist of the aryl hydrocarbon receptor. *Br J Cancer* 1999;79:1340–1346.

79. Katiyar SK, Agarwal R, Wang ZY, et al. (−)-Epigallocatechin-3-gallate in *Camellia sinensis* leaves from Himalayan region of Sikkim: inhibitory effects against biochemical events and tumor initiation in Sencar mouse skin. *Nutr Cancer* 1992;18:73–83.

80. Wang ZY, Cheng SJ, Zhou ZC, et al. Antimutagenic activity of green tea polyphenols. *Mutat Res* 1989;223:273–285.

81. Wang ZY, Das M, Bickers DR, Mukhtar H. Interaction of epicatechins derived from green tea with rat hepatic cytochrome P-450. *Drug Metab Dispos* 1988;16:98–103.

82. Huang MT, Ho CT, Wang ZY, et al. Inhibitory effect of topical application of a green tea polyphenol fraction on tumor initiation and promotion in mouse skin. *Carcinogenesis* 1992;13:947–954.

83. Kavanagh KT, Hafer LJ, Kim DW, et al. Green tea extracts decrease carcinogen-induced mammary tumor burden in rats and rate of breast cancer cell proliferation in culture. *J Cell Biochem* 2001;82:387–398.

84. Vang O, Frandsen H, Hansen KT, et al. Modulation of drug-metabolising enzyme expression by condensation products of indole-3-ylcarbinol, an inducer in cruciferous vegetables. *Pharmacol Toxicol* 1999;84:59–65.

85. Loub WD, Wattenberg LW, Davis DW. Aryl hydrocarbon hydroxylase induction in rat tissues by naturally occurring indoles of cruciferous plants. *J Natl Cancer Inst* 1975;54:985–988.

86. Bjeldanes LF, Kim JY, Grose KR, et al. Aromatic hydrocarbon responsiveness-receptor agonists generated from indole-3-carbinol in vitro and in vivo: comparisons with

7- and 12-substituted derivatives of 7,12-dimethyl-benz[a]anthracene. *J Natl Cancer Inst* 1978;61:135–140.

2,3,7,8- tetrachlorodibenzo-p-dioxin. *Proc Natl Acad Sci USA* 1991;88:9543–9547.

87. Kleman MI, Poellinger L, Gustafsson JA. Regulation of human dioxin receptor function by indolocarbazoles, receptor ligands of dietary origin. *J Biol Chem* 1994;269:5137–5144.

88. Stresser DM, Bjeldanes LF, Bailey GS, Williams DE. The anticarcinogen 3,3'-diindolylmethane is an inhibitor of cytochrome P-450. *J Biochem Toxicol* 1995;10:191–201.

89. Stephensen PU, Bonnesen C, Schaldach C, et al. N-methoxyindole-3-carbinol is a more efficient inducer of cytochrome P- 450 1A1 in cultured cells than indol-3-carbinol. *Nutr Cancer* 2000;36:112–121.

90. Chen YH, Riby J, Srivastava P, et al. Regulation of CYP1A1 by indolo[3,2-b]carbazole in murine hepatoma cells. *J Biol Chem* 1995;270:22,548–22,555.

91. He YH, Friesen MD, Ruch RJ, Schut HA. Indole-3-carbinol as a chemopreventive agent in 2-amino-1-methyl-6-phenylimidazo[4,5-b]pyridine (PhIP) carcinogenesis: inhibition of PhIP- DNA adduct formation, acceleration of PhIP metabolism, and induction of cytochrome P450 in female F344 rats. *Food Chem Toxicol* 2000;38:15–23.

92. Grubbs CJ, Steele VE, Casebolt T, et al. Chemoprevention of chemically-induced mammary carcinogenesis by indole-3-carbinol. *Anticancer Res* 1995;15:709–716.

93. Tiwari RK, Guo L, Bradlow HL, et al. Selective responsiveness of human breast cancer cells to indole-3-carbinol, a chemopreventive agent. *J Natl Cancer Inst* 1994;86: 126–131.

94. Stoner G, Casto B, Ralston S, et al. Development of a multi-organ rat model for evaluating chemopreventive agents: efficacy of indole-3carbinol. *Carcinogenesis* 2002;23:265–272.

95. Tiedink HG, Davies JA, Visser NA, et al. The stability of the nitrosated products of indole, indole-3-acetonitrile, indole-3-carbinol and 4-chloroindole. *Food Chem Toxicol* 1989;27:723–730.

96. Sasagawa C, Matsushima T. Mutagen formation on nitrite treatment of indole compounds derived from indole-glucosinolate. *Mutat Res* 1991;250:169–174.

97. Birt DF, Walker B, Tibbels MG, Bresnick E. Anti-mutagenesis and anti-promotion by apigenin, robinetin and indole-3-carbinol. *Carcinogenesis* 1986;7:959–963.

98. Srivastava B, Shukla Y. Antitumour promoting activity of indole-3-carbinol in mouse skin carcinogenesis. *Cancer Lett* 1998;134:91–95.

99. Lin JM, Amin S, Trushin N, Hecht SS. Effects of isothiocyanates on tumorigenesis by benzo[a]pyrene in murine tumor models. *Cancer Lett* 1993;74:151–159.

100. Adam-Rodwell G, Morse MA, Stoner GD. The effects of phenethyl isothiocyanate on benzo[a]pyrene-induced tumors and DNA adducts in A/J mouse lung. *Cancer Lett* 1993;71: 35–42.

101. Hecht SS. Inhibition of carcinogenesis by isothiocyanates. *Drug Metab Rev* 2000;32:395–411.

102. Hecht S, Kenney P, Wang M, Upadhyaya P. Benzyl isothiocyanate: an effective inhibitor of polycyclic aromatic hydrocarbon tumorigenesis in A/J mouse lung. *Cancer Lett* 2002;187:87–94.

103. Hecht SS, Kenney PM, Wang M, et al. Effects of phenethyl isothiocyanate and benzyl isothiocyanate, individually and in combination, on lung tumorigenesis induced in A/J mice by benzo[a]pyrene and 4-(methylnitrosamino)-1-(3-pyridyl)-1-butanone. *Cancer Lett* 200;150:49–56.

104. Morse MA, Amin SG, Hecht SS, Chung FL. Effects of aromatic isothiocyanates on tumorigenicity, O6-methyl-guanine formation, and metabolism of the tobacco-specific nitrosamine 4-(methylnitrosamino)-1-(3-pyridyl)-1-butanone in A/J mouse lung. *Cancer Res* 1989;49:2894–2897.

105. Morse MA, Reinhardt JC, Amin SG, et al. Effect of dietary aromatic isothiocyanates fed subsequent to the administration of 4-(methylnitrosamino)-1-(3-pyridyl)-1-butanone on lung tumorigenicity in mice. *Cancer Lett* 1990;49:225–230.

106. Sticha KR, Kenney PM, Boysen G, et al. Effects of benzyl isothiocyanate and phenethyl isothiocyanate on DNA adduct formation by a mixture of benzo[a]pyrene and 4-(methylnitrosamino)-1-(3-pyridyl)-1-butanone in A/J mouse lung. *Carcinogenesis* 2002;23:1433–1439.

107. Goosen TC, Kent UM, Brand L, Hollenberg PF. Inactivation of cytochrome P450 2B1 by benzyl isothiocyanate, a chemopreventative agent from cruciferous vegetables. *Chem Res Toxicol* 2000;13:1349–1359.

108. Kent UM, Juschyshyn MI, Hollenberg PF. Mechanism-based inactivators as probes of cytochrome P450 structure and function. *Curr Drug Metab* 2001;2:215–243.

109. Guo Z, Smith TJ, Wang E, et al. Structure-activity relationships of arylalkyl isothiocyanates for the inhibition of 4-(methylnitrosamino)-1-(3-pyridyl)-1-butanone metabolism and the modulation of xenobiotic-metabolizing enzymes in rats and mice. *Carcinogenesis* 1993;14: 1167–1173.

110. Smith TJ, Guo Z, Li C, et al. Mechanisms of inhibition of 4-(methylnitrosamino)-1-(3-pyridyl)-1-butanone bioactivation in mouse by dietary phenethyl isothiocyanate. *Cancer Res* 1993;53:3276–3282.

111. Smith TJ, Guo Z, Guengerich FP, Yang CS. Metabolism of 4-(methylnitrosamino)-1-(3-pyridyl)-1-butanone (NNK) by human cytochrome P450 1A2 and its inhibition by phenethyl isothiocyanate. *Carcinogenesis* 1996;17:809–813.

112. Guo Z, Smith TJ, Wang E, et al. Effects of phenethyl isothiocyanate, a carcinogenesis inhibitor, on xenobiotic-metabolizing enzymes and nitrosamine metabolism in rats. *Carcinogenesis* 1992;13:2205–2210.

113. Murray RDH, Mendez J, Brown SA, eds. *The Natural Coumarins: Occurrence, Chemistry and Biochemistry.* John Wiley & Sons, Ltd., New York, 1982, pp.97–111.

114. Robinson T. Aromatic compound, in *The Organic Constituents of Higher Plants: Their Chemistry and Interrelationships.* Robinson T, ed. Burgess Publishing Co., Minneapolis, MN, 1967, pp.47–76.

115. Stanley W, Jurd L. Citrus coumarins. *J Agr Food Chem* 1971;19:1106–1110.

116. Okuyama T, Takata M, Nishino H, et al. Studies on the anti-tumor-promoting activity of naturally occurring substances. II. Inhibition of tumor-promoter-enhanced phospholipid metabolism by umbelliferous materials. *Chem Pharm Bull* (Tokyo) 1990;38:1084–1086.

117. Stupans I, Ryan A. In vitro inhibition of 3-methylcholan-threne-induced rat hepatic acyl hydrocarbon hydroxylase by 8-acyl-7-hydroxycoumarins. *Biochem Pharmacol* 1984;33:131–139.

118. Woo W, Shin K, Lee C. Effect of naturally occurring coumarins on the activity of drug metabolizing enzyme. *Biochem Pharmacol* 1983;32:1800–1803.

119. Wall ME, Wani MC, Hughes TJ, Taylor H. Plant antimutagens, in *Antimutagenesis and Anticarcinogenesis Mechanism II.* Karuda Y, Shankel DM, Walters MD, eds. Plenum Press, New York, 1990, pp. 61–78.

120. Fouin-Fortunet H, Tinel M, Descatoire V, et al. Inactivation of cytochrome P450 by the drug methoxsalen. *J Pharmacol Exp Ther* 1986:236:237–247.

121. Letteron P, Descatoire V, Larrey D, et al. Inactivation and induction of cytochrome P450 by various psoralen derivatives in rats. *J Pharmacol Exp Ther* 1986;238:685–692.

122. Mays D, Nawoot S, Hilliard J, et al. Inhibition and induction of drug biotransformation in vivo by 8-methoxypsoralen: studies of caffeine, phenytoin and hexobarbital metabolism in the rat. *J Pharmacol Exp Ther* 1987;243:227–233.

123. Apseloff G, Sheppard D, Chambers M, et al. Inhibition and induction of theophylline metabolism by 8-methoxypsoralen: in vivo study in rats and humans. *Drug Metabol Dispos* 1990;18:298–303.

124. Tsamboas D, Vizethum W, Goerz G. Effect of oral 8-methoxypsoralen on rat liver microsomal cytochrome P-450. *Arch Dermatol Res* 1978;263:339–342.

125. Bickers D, Mukhtar H, Molica S, Pathak M. The effect of psoralens on hepatic and cutaneous drug metabolizing enzymes and cytochrome P450. *J Investig Dermatol* 1982;79:201–205.

126. Mays D, Hilliard J, Wong D, Gerber N. Activation of 8-methoxypsoralen by cytochromes P-450 enzyme kinetics of covalent binding and influence of inhibitors and inducers of drug metabolism. *Biochem Pharmacol* 1989;38:1647–1655.

127. Mays D, Hilliard J, Wong D, et al. Bioactivation of 8-methoxypsoralen and irreversible inactivation of cytochrome P450 in mouse liver microsomes: modification by monoclonal antibodies, inhibition of drug metabolism and distribution of covalent adducts. *J Pharmacol Exp Ther* 1990;254:720–731.

128. Ashwood-Smith MJ, Warrington PJ, Jenins M, et al. Photobiological properties of a novel, naturally occurring furoisocoumarin, coriandrin. *Photochem Photobiol* 1989;50: 745–751.

129. He K, Iyer KR, Hayes RN, et al. Inactivation of cytochrome P450 3A4 by bergamottin, a component of grapefruit juice. *Chem Res Toxicol* 1998;11:252–259.

130. Koenigs LL, Trager WF. Mechanism-based inactivation of P450 2A6 by furanocoumarins. *Biochemistry* 1998;37: 10,047–10,061.

131. Koenigs LL, Trager WF. Mechanism-based inactivation of cytochrome P450 2B1 by 8-methoxypsoralen and several other furanocoumarins. *Biochemistry* 1998;37:13,184–13,193.

132. Maenpaa J, Sigusch H, Raunio H, et al. Differential inhibition of coumarin 7-hydroxylase activity in mouse and human liver microsomes. *Biochem Pharm* 1993;45:1035–1042.

133. Feuer G, Kellen J. Inhibition and enhancement of mammary tumorigenesis by 7,12-dimethylbenz (a)anthracene in the female Sprague-Dawley rat. *Int J Clin Pharmacol* 1974;9:62–69.

134. Feuer G, Kellen JA, Kovacs K. Suppression of 7,12-dimethylbenzo(a)anthracene-induced breast carcinoma by coumarin in the rat. *Oncology* (Basel) 1976;33:35–39.

135. Sparnins V, Wattenberg L. Enhancement of glutathione-*S*-transferase activity of the mouse forestomach by inhibitors of benzo(a)pyrene-induced neoplasia of the forestomach. *J Natl Cancer Inst* 1981;66: 769–771.

136. Kelly VP, Ellis EM, Manson MM, et al. Chemoprevention of aflatoxin B1 hepatocarcinogenesis by coumarin, a natural benzopyrone that is a potent inducer of aflatoxin B1-aldehyde reductase, the glutathione *S*-transferase A5 and P1 subunits, and NAD(P)H:quinone oxidoreductase in rat liver. *Cancer Res* 2000;60:957–969.

137. Cai Y, Kleiner H, Johnston D, et al. Effect of naturally occurring coumarins on the formation of epidermal DNA adducts and skin tumors induced by benzo[a]pyrene and 7,12-dimethylbenz[a]anthracene in SENCAR mice. *Carcinogenesis* 1997;18:1521–1527.

138. Cai Y-N, Baer-Dubowska W, Ashwood-Smith M, DiGiovanni J. Inhibitory effects of naturally occurring coumarins on the metabolic activation of benzo[a]pyrene and 7,12-dimethylbenz[a]anthracene in cultured mouse keratinocytes. *Carcinogenesis* 1997;18:215–222.

139. Pottenger L, Jefcoate C. Characterization of a novel cytochrome P450 from the transformable cell line, C3H/10T1/2. Carcinogenesis 1990;11:321–327.

140. Kleiner HE, Vulimiri SV, Miller L, et al. Oral administration of naturally occurring coumarins leads to altered phase I and II enzyme activities and reduced DNA adduct formation by polycyclic aromatic hydrocarbons in various tissues of SENCAR mice. *Carcinogenesis* 2001;22:73–82.

141. Kleiner HE, Vulimiri SV, Starost MF, et al. Oral administration of the citrus coumarin, isopimpinellin, blocks DNA adduct formation and skin tumor initiation by 7,12-dimethylbenz[a]anthracene in SENCAR mice. *Carcinogenesis* 2002;23:1667–1675.

142. Miller EG, McWhorter K, Rivera-Hidalgo F, et al. Kahweol and cafestol: inhibitors of hamster buccal pouch carcinogenesis. *Nutr Cancer* 1991;15:41–46.

143. Cavin C, Holzhauser D, Constable A, et al. The coffee-specific diterpenes cafestol and kahweol protect against aflatoxin B1-induced genotoxicity through a dual mechanism. *Carcinogenesis* 1998;19:1369–1375.

144. Cavin C, Mace K, Offord EA, Schilter B. Protective effects of coffee diterpenes against aflatoxin B1-induced genotoxicity: mechanisms in rat and human cells. *Food Chem Toxicol* 2001;39:549–556.

145. Urgert R, Katan MB. The cholesterol-raising factor from coffee beans. *J R Soc Med* 1996;89:618–623.

146. de Roos B, Katan MB. Possible mechanisms underlying the cholesterol-raising effect of the coffee diterpene cafestol. *Curr Opin Lipidol* 1999;10:41–45.

147. Terpstra AHM, Katan MB, Weusten-van der Wouw B, et al. The hypercholesterolemic effect of cafestol in coffee oil in gerbils and rats. *J Nutr Biochem* 2000;11:311–317.

148. Huang MT, Ho CT, Wang ZY, et al. Inhibition of skin tumorigenesis by rosemary and its constituents carnosol and ursolic acid. *Cancer Res* 1994;54:701–708.

149. Singletary K, MacDonald C, Wallig M. Inhibition by rosemary and carnosol of 7,12-dimethylbenz[a]anthracene (DMBA)-induced rat mammary tumorigenesis and in vivo DMBA-DNA adduct formation. *Cancer Lett* 1996;104:43–48.

150. Offord EA, Mace K, Ruffieux C, et al. Rosemary components inhibit benzo[a]pyrene-induced genotoxicity in human bronchial cells. *Carcinogenesis* 1995;16:2057–2062.

151. Debersac P, Heydel JM, Amiot MJ, et al. Induction of cytochrome P450 and/or detoxication enzymes by various extracts of rosemary: description of specific patterns. *Food Chem Toxicol* 2001;39:907–918.

152. Viaje A, Jui-yun L, Hopkins NE, et al. Inhibition of the binding of 7,12-dimethylbenz[a]anthracene and benzo[a]pyrene to DNA in mouse epidermis by aryl acetylates. *Carcinogenesis* 1990;11:1139–1143.

153. DiGiovanni J, Slaga TJ, Juchau MR. Inhibitory effects of environmental chemicals on polycyclic aromatic hydrocarbon in carcinogenesis, in *Carcinogenesis, Modifiers of Chemical Carcinogenesis, Vol. 5.* Raven Press, New York, 1980, pp.145–168.

154. DiGiovanni J, Slaga TJ. Modification of polycyclic aromatic hydrocarbon carcinogenesis, in *Polycyclic Hydrocarbons and Cancer, Vol. 3.* Gelboin HV, Tso POP, eds. Academic Press, New York, 1981, pp.259–292.

155. Slaga TJ, DiGiovanni J. Inhibition of carcinogenesis, in *Chemical Carcinogens, Vol. II.* Searle CE, ed. ACS Monograph, 1984, pp.1279–1321.

156. DiGiovanni J. Inhibition of chemical carcinogenesis, in *Handbook of Experimental Pharmacology, Part II: Carcinogenesis and Mutagenesis.* Grover PL, Cooper CS, eds. Springer Verlag, Heidelberg, Germany, 1990, pp.159–332.

II ANTIINFLAMMATORIES

5 Antiinflammatories and Chemoprevention

NSAIDs and Other Inhibitors of Arachidonic Acid Metabolism

Gary B. Gordon, MD, PhD, Gary J. Kelloff, MD and Caroline C. Sigman, PhD

CONTENTS

1. INTRODUCTION

As demonstrated in this and the following chapters of this volume, there has been a virtual explosion of interest in the prostanoids—their formation, metabolism and catabolism, physiologic roles, and pathophysiologic involvement in the related disease processes of inflammation and carcinogenesis. With the understanding that there are two major forms of cyclooxygenase (COX-1 and COX-2), an enzyme that is critical to prostanoid synthesis, and the development of pharmacologic and genetic tools to selectively inhibit each form and examine the consequences of their activity, it is possible to conduct meaningful animal experiments and human trials to establish or repudiate their clinical importance. This opportunity has opened many challenging and valuable discussions within and among the academic, regulatory, patient, and pharmaceutical communities.

The information presented in these chapters supports the theory that carcinogenesis is a disease process that leads first to premalignant states of hyperplasia and dysplasia and then to frank cancer, just as inflammation can first cause clinical symptoms of pain and redness that ultimately lead to joint destruction and damage in other organs. Perhaps earlier intervention will prove to be valuable to patients in both of these disease settings. In the following sections, selected aspects of prostanoid metabolism are reviewed.

1.1. Prostanoid Metabolism

As the understanding of the physiologic effects of prostanoids grows, so does the understanding of their metabolism, catabolism, and mechanism(s) of action. The enzymatic release of arachidonic acid (AA) from cellular stores by phospholipase A_2 (PLA_2) is the initiating step in this process. AA can then be metabolized either through a series of enzymatic steps to prostaglandins (PGs) and thromboxanes via the COX pathway, or to hydroxyeicosatetraenoic acids (HETEs) and leukotrienes (LTs) via the lipoxygenase (LOX) pathway. These products then act directly, or through receptors on signaling pathways that are not fully understood. It is clear that some components of these pathways, such as COX-1, are constitutive or housekeeping, and are thus important for normal physiologic

From: Cancer Chemoprevention, Volume 1: Promising Cancer Chemoprevention Agents
Edited by: G. J. Kelloff, E. T. Hawk, and C. C. Sigman © Humana Press Inc., Totowa, NJ

function. Others, such as COX-2, are inducible and may be associated with one or more pathophysiologic states or reactions. In addition, as with many enzymatic systems, there appear to be situations in which alternative exogenous substrates may be used by some of these enzymes, resulting in other forms of insult to the organism. Furthermore, some of the metabolic steps in this pathway can generate reactive oxygen species (ROS), which also may cause insults. Despite this relatively complex and evolving situation, as the relationships of various arms of the metabolic and functional pathways are revealed, new and more specific means of targeting the pathways are being developed. Such agents may be more or less specific inhibitors of the COXs or the LOXs, they may be agents that block the actions of specific pathway products, or they may be agents that prevent the induction of various elements of the metabolic pathways. Understanding the value of such approaches and potentially how to block these pathways at multiple steps should enhance the therapeutic risk-benefit ratio that can be determined. As discussed here and in Chapter 6 of this volume, perhaps the best example of this evolution is the development of COX-2-specific inhibitors. Such compounds were developed in response to the understanding that although the COX-1 isoenzyme is primarily of housekeeping importance, COX-2 is inducible, and associated with inflammation and its cellular pathophysiology. The structural differences between these forms have provided the opportunity to develop COX-2-specific agents that are effective antiinflammatory drugs, demonstrate cancer-preventive activity, and have a better gastrointestinal safety profile than agents that inhibit both forms of COX.

2. AA METABOLIC PATHWAYS PROVIDE MOLECULAR TARGETS FOR CANCER CHEMOPREVENTION BY ANTIINFLAMMATORIES

The role of AA metabolism in carcinogenesis has been extensively reviewed (See refs.1–6) as have cancer prevention strategies based on modulation of the AA metabolic pathways (7–13). As described here, AA metabolism begins with intracellular release of AA catalyzed by phospholipases (14). Cytokines (e.g., interleukins [ILs] and tumor necrosis factor [TNF]) can activate PLA_2 (15). AA is then metabolized to PGs, thromboxanes, LTs, and HETEs via oxidative enzymes (6). The nature of the products are partly regulated by the AA content of the membrane

(modulated by the composition of the diet) as well as tissue-specific expression and activity of the various components of the pathway. Activated oxygen species and alkylperoxy species are formed throughout this process. PG and LT synthesis are associated strongly with carcinogenesis; both are inhibited by antioxidants and antiinflammatory agents.

2.1. Prostaglandin Synthesis and Carcinogenesis

The first step in the PG synthetic pathway is mediated by the enzyme prostaglandin H synthase (PHS). It is this enzyme that is traditionally considered the target of antiinflammatories such as the nonsteroidal antiinflammatory drugs (NSAIDs). PHS has two activities—COX, which catalyzes the formation of prostaglandin G_2 (PGG_2) from AA, and hydroperoxidase, which catalyzes the reduction of PGG_2 to PGH_2 (5,16). In order to return to its native state, hydroperoxidase requires a reducing cosubstrate. Under some circumstances this role can be played by exogenous procarcinogens—for example, arylamino and arylnitro compounds, which are then activated via oxidation to fre radical and electrophilic carcinogens that can form adducts with DNA and thereby initiate carcinogenesis. The expected product of the reaction, PGH_2, is further metabolized to form other PGs (PGE_2, $PGF_{2\alpha}$, PGD_2), thromboxanes, and prostacyclin (PGI_2). As mentioned, the specific products formed are tissue- and cell type-dependent, and these products in turn are autocrine and paracrine signal-transduction mediators through a family of cell- and ligand-specific G-protein-coupled receptors. For example, PGE_2, which appears to play an important role in carcinogenesis, acts through receptor subtypes EP_1–EP_4 (6,17). PGs may also interact with other cellular receptors to modulate signal transduction—for example, PGE_2 transactivates epidermal growth-factor receptor (EGFR) (18). As shown in Fig. 1, the PG pathway can be inhibited by antiinflammatories in at least six ways: inhibition of COX activity (e.g., preventing the formation of PGG_2); inhibition of peroxidase activity; blocking formation of reactive intermediates; scavenging reactive intermediates (e.g., by glutathione [GSH] conjugation); blocking PG receptors; and inhibition of COX gene expression. Of these, the inhibition of COX activity has been investigated most extensively, particularly through NSAIDs which derive their pharmacological activity specifically from inhibition of COX activity. More recently, inhibition of COX gene expression has been of great interest as a potential

Table 1

Cell Signaling and COX-2 Gene Expression

Cell Signal Factor[1]	Reference(s)
Associated with COX-2 Upregulation	
Growth factors (EGF, PDGF, TGFβ$_1$, VEGF, bFGF)	4,22,55,143,144
p53 (mutated)	4,145,146
Interleukins	4,22
TNFα	4,22
LPS	4,22
Hormones	4,22
NFκB	4,8
Ha-ras	4
v-src	4
EGFR	18,146,147
HER-2/neu	33,148,149
Bcl-2	39,146
PI3K/akt	150
MAPK	4,31–33
uPA	18
Jun	4
AP-1	151–154
CREB/p300	30,153,154
wnt-1	146,155
MMP	63,146
n-6-PUFA	30
Modulation of COX-2 Translation	24
HuR (RNA-binding protein)	25,156
CUGBP2 (RNA-binding protein)	157
Activated on COX-2 Expression	
PPARγ, α, δ	12,158–160
EP1–EP4 (PG Receptors)	6,12,17

[1]CREB, cyclic AMP response element-binding protein; EGF, epidermal growth factor; EGFR, epidermal growth factor receptor; FGF, fibroblast growth factor; LPS, lipopolysaccharide; MAPK, mitogen-activated protein kinase; MMP, matrix metalloproteinase; NFκB, nuclear factor kappa B; PDGF, platelet-derived growth factor; PG, prostaglandin; PI3K, phosphatidylinositol-3-kinase; PPAR, peroxisome proliferator-activated receptor; PUFA, polyunsaturated fatty acid; TGF, transforming growth factor; TNF, tumor necrosis factor; uPA, urinary plasminogen activator; VEGF, vascular endothelial growth factor.

strategy for chemoprevention. To add more complexity, PGH$_2$ itself breaks down to form a direct-acting mutagen known as malondialdehyde (19).

As described here, PGs and other PHS products are essentially hormones with multiple tissue- and cell-specific activities required, in part, for normal physiological activity. The need to provide cells with sufficient COX products to function normally has challenged the development of COX inhibitors as drugs for chronic use (20, 21). For example, PGE$_2$ in the gut promotes protective mucosal secretions, and lowered gut PG levels resulting from NSAID administration are associated with one of the major side effects of long-term NSAID treatment, gastrointestinal (GI) ulceration and bleeding

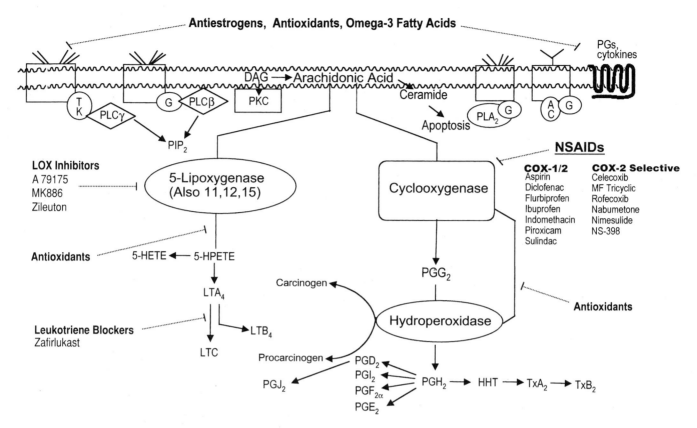

Fig. 1. Inhibitors of arachidonic acid (AA) metabolism with potential chemopreventive activity. A schematic of AA metabolism highlighting the cyclooxygenase (COX) and 5-lipoxygenase (5-LOX) is shown with sites of inhibition (————|) by NSAIDs and other agents that have demonstrated chemopreventive activity in animal models of carcinogenesis. Abbreviations are as follows: AC, adenyl cyclase; DAG, diacylglycerol; G, G-coupled protein; HETE, hydroxyeicosatetraenoic acid; HHT, 12-hydroxyheptadeca-trienoic acid; HPETE, hydroperoxyeicosatetraenoic acid; LT, leukotriene; PG, prostaglandin; PIP$_2$, phosphatidylinositol diphosphate; PKC, protein kinase C; PL, phospholipase; TK, tyrosine kinase; TX, ythromboxane.

(5). Likewise, PGs in the kidney and thromboxanes in platelets are important to normal physiological function. Their loss is associated with renal tubule toxicity and excessive bleeding, respectively *(5).* The discovery of an inducible form of COX (COX-2), which predominates in sites of inflammation in macrophages and in synovio-cytes, and is strongly associated with carcinogenesis, has provided a feasible approach to minimizing the toxicity of COX inhibition. The constitutive COX-1 isoform predominates in the sites of potential toxicity—stomach, the GI tract, platelets, and kidneys. Drugs that selectively inhibit COX-2 activity at pharmacological doses (e.g., celecoxib, rofecoxib) have shown potentially lower rates of GI toxicity than traditional NSAIDs (e.g., ibuprofen, sulindac, piroxicam), which inhibit both COX isoforms *(21).*

As an alternative to inhibiting COX activity, leaving constitutive COX activity and expression intact through selective interference with inducible COX-2 gene expression may be an effective way to avoid toxicities caused by PG depletion. COX-2 is located in both endoplasmic reticulum and nuclear membranes; gene expression is upregulated via signal-transduction pathways in response to growth factors, tumor promoters, cytokines, and oncogenes (reviewed in *4,5,22*), and COX-2 message stability may also be modulated *(23–26)* (Table 1).

2.2. Leukotriene Synthesis and Carcinogenesis

The burst of lipoxygenase (LOX) activity that is observed during inflammation is the first step in the formation of LTs from AA. Available evidence suggests that the immediate products of LOX activity, HETEs and their hydroperoxy precursors (HPETEs), mediate cell-proliferative aspects of carcinogenesis *(27).* For example, antioxidant and antiinflammatory

Table 2

COX-2 and 5-LOX Expression in Human Neoplasia[1]

Target Organ	COX-2 Precancer	COX-2 Cancer	5-LOX Cancer
Colon	√[2]	√	√
Bladder	√	√	ND
Esophagus	√	√	ND
Skin	√	√	√
Melanoma	ND	√?	√
Head and neck	√	√	√
Leukemia/lymphoma	ND	√?	√
Multiple myeloma	ND	√	ND
Lung	√	√	√
Breast	√	√	√
Prostate	√[3]	√?	ND
Pancreas	√	√	√
CNS	ND	√	√
Cervix	√	√	ND
Endometrium	ND	√	ND
Ovary	ND	√?	ND
Liver	ND	√	ND
Stomach	ND	√	ND

[1]Based on (*9,11*). *See also* (*26,30,45,54,56,161–168*).

[2]√, Expression observed; √?, Expression reported but not clear that data are significant; ND, no significant data showing increased expression found; most studies were in human cancer or precancer cell lines.

[3]PIA, prostatic inflammatory atrophy.

compounds that suppress formation of these free radicals and electrophiles (e.g., vitamin E, flavonoids, curcuminoids, and tea polyphenols) inhibit tumor progression in mouse skin.

The LOXs are a family of non-heme iron-containing dioxygenases that catalyze stereospecific oxygenation of the 5-, 12-, or 15-carbon atoms of AA to form corresponding HETEs, which are metabolized to LTs or lipoxins through additional sequential cell-specific reactions (*6,15,27,28*). For example, in the presence of 5-LOX activating protein (FLAP), 5-LOX catalyzes oxygenation of AA to 5-HPETE, which is then dehydrated to form the epoxide LTA_4. LTA_4 is further metabolized to either LTB_4 via stereoselective hydration by LTA_4 hydrolase, or to LTC_4 through GSH conjugation catalyzed by LTC_4 synthase. Sequential metabolic reactions, catalyzed by γ-glutamyl transferase and a specific membrane-bound dipeptidase, convert LTC_4 into LTD_4 and LTE_4, respectively (the slow-reacting substances of anaphylaxis). In the lung, sulfidopeptide LTs are known to act on a single high-affinity, smooth-muscle receptor, the *cys*-LT_1 receptor, resulting in bronchoconstriction and changes in vascular permeability and mucous secretion in this tissue. LTs are produced primarily in eosinophils, mast cells, and basophils.

Similar to PG interaction with cellular receptors, LTs act through tissue- and cell-specific receptors to modulate the growth of several normal human cell types (T-lymphocytes, skin fibroblasts, epidermal keratinocytes, and glomerular epithelial cells). Both LTB_4 and LTC_4 increase growth of arterial smooth-muscle cells, airway-epithelial cells, and mitogen-stimulated lymphocytes in vitro. LTs also play a role in the regulation of hematopoiesis. LOX inhibition and blockade of LT receptors are the predominant methods of interference with carcinogenesis-associated activities on this pathway (Fig. 1). Inhibition of LOX has been proposed as a potentially more effective chemoprevention strategy because of the associated reduced production of oxygen radical intermediates *(27)*.

The remainder of this chapter focuses primarily on two molecular targets on the AA metabolic pathways that, as indicated previously, have thus far shown the greatest promise as targets for chemopreventive intervention—COX-2 on the PG pathway and 5-LOX on the LT pathway. Subheading 2 summarizes research findings that qualify COX-2, and to a lesser extent 5-LOX, as targets for cancer-preventive intervention and progress in developing cancer prevention strategies involving specific modulation of these targets. Chapters 6 (COX-2) and 7 (LOX) of this volume describe in detail the research evidence supporting the chemopreventive potential of agents directed at these targets. Subheading 3 considers antiinflammatory and antioxidant agents that affect LOX and COX less specifically—by interactions at the cellular membrane, with nuclear receptors, and as free-radical scavengers. Many of these activities are also described in Chapters 9, 10, 29–31, and 39 of this volume. Subheading 4 addresses possible lines of future research on chemoprevention strategies based on blocking COX and LOX.

3. COX-2 AND 5-LOX AS IDEAL MOLECULAR TARGETS FOR CANCER PREVENTION

Criteria that characterize an effective molecular target for chemoprevention are as follows: the target is mutated or overexpressed in precancers and possibly cancers; a mechanistic rationale(s) exists for the target's participation in carcinogenesis; chemopreventive modulation of the target is associated with low toxicity; and target modulation provides clinical benefit, directly or indirectly related to chemopreventive potential. Ideally, the modulation of the target can be quantified directly or via a closely related activity. COX-2 and 5-LOX meet these criteria, as summarized in the following paragraphs.

3.1. COX-2 as a Target for Cancer Prevention

The hypothesis that COX-2 inhibition can prevent cancer is supported by several lines of evidence that are reviewed here (*see also* refs. *7–13*). Briefly, there is extensive epidemiologic evidence that chronic NSAID use is associated with a reduced risk of developing various cancers and premalignant conditions. COX-2 itself is overexpressed in most solid tumors and their associated premalignant lesions. In animals, inhibition

of COX-2 by either knockout of the gene or the use of selective agents reduces the incidence of pre-cancers and cancers in genetically predisposed and chemically induced animal models. Furthermore, the use of selective COX-2 inhibitors decreases proliferation and increases apoptosis in such models. Perhaps related to these observations are the effects that COX-2 inhibitors have on reducing angiogenesis and cell migration and invasion. Most importantly, traditional NSAIDs—and to a lesser extent selective COX-2 inhibitors—reduce the incidence of or actually treat premalignant lesions in people (diclofenac for actinic keratoses and sulindac and celecoxib for polyps), as reported in randomized trials. Selected aspects of these observations are described more extensively here.

3.1.1. COX-2 EXPRESSION IN CARCINOGENESIS

COX-2 is expressed nearly ubiquitously in cancer and precancerous tissues (*see* Table 2). It has been found in epithelial cancer cells, but the body of evidence suggests that its activity in the stroma (fibroblasts, immune cells, endothelial cells) may also be critical to carcinogenesis (*8,21,26,29*). It is induced by cellular stress, such as during inflammation, and is thus expected to be present at very low or undetectable levels in unaffected cells. As described here, mechanisms that control transcription, mRNA stability, and translation appear to contribute to elevated COX-2 expression (*see also* Table 1). Furthermore, cellular and tissue functions in carcinogenesis are associated with COX-2 expression, including increased proliferation, reduced apoptosis, angiogenesis, and cell migration and invasiveness (e.g., *see 4,8,26,30*).

3.1.1.1. Proliferation COX-2-derived PGs can increase cell proliferation by modulating growth-factor receptor (e.g., EGFR)-mediated signaling or by affecting downstream molecular targets in signal-transduction pathways such as mitogen-activated protein kinase (MAPK) *(31–33)*. Chronic inflammation and suppressed immune response are associated with elevated COX-2 expression, and are known risk factors for epithelial carcinogenesis *(7,34)*; COX-2 overexpression may lead to stimulation of the signal-transduction pathways involved in cell proliferation, as stated here. For example, in colorectal cancer, production of PGs is associated with immune suppression and loss of HLA antigens *(35,36)*. PGE_2 produced by monocytes and macrophages suppresses factors required for immune surveillance, including lymphokines, T- and B-cell proliferation, and natural killer (NK) cell cyto-

Table 3

COX and LOX Inhibitors with Chemopreventive Activity in Animal Carcinogenesis Models (Published Studies)[1]

| | *NSAIDs* | | *LOX* |
Target Organ	*Non-Selective*	*COX-2 Selective*	*Inhibitors*
Colon	Flurbiprofen	Celecoxib	—
	Piroxicam	MF Tricyclic	
	Sulindac	Tilmacoxib	
		Nimesulide	
		NS-398	
		Rofecoxib	
Bladder	Aspirin	Celecoxib	—
	Ibuprofen	Nimesulide	
	Indomethacin		
	Ketoprofen		
	Piroxicam		
	Sulindac		
Skin	Diclofenac	Celecoxib	—
	Indomethacin	SC-58125	
	Piroxicam		
	Sulindac		
Head and neck	—	Nimesulide	—
Lung	Aspirin	NS-398	A 79175
	Sulindac		MK-886
			Zafirlukast
			Zileuton
Breast	Aspirin	Celecoxib	NDGA
	Ibuprofen	Nabumetone	Esculetin
	Indomethacin	Nimesulide	
Pancreas	—	Nimesulide	Zileuton

[1]Data adapted from (*13*). *See also* (*10,11,169–171*).

toxic activity. COX-2 inhibitors suppress inflammatory response and stimulate immune response. In ultraviolet-exposed-skin, topical application of the COX-2-selective inhibitor celecoxib was shown to effectively decrease edema, dermal neutrophil infiltration and activation, PGE_2 levels, and production of sunburn cells (*37*).

3.1.1.2. COX-2 and Apoptosis Reduced apoptosis is prevalent in carcinogenesis and is associated with COX-2 expression (*38,39*)—for example, through COX-2-dependent upregulation of *bcl-2* (*39*). Induction of apoptosis is a potentially important cancer preventive mechanism of COX inhibitors, which have been found to induce apoptosis in the colon (*40,41*), bladder (*42*), stomach (*43*), prostate (*44*), pancreas (*45*), esophagus (*46,47*), lung (*48,49*), and head and neck (*50*) cancer cells.

3.1.1.3. COX-2 and Angiogenesis PGs stimulate tumor cell growth through neovascularization (*51–53*), and COX-2 is expressed in the angiogenic vasculature within tumors and pre-existing vasculature adjacent to tumors in the human breast, lung, pancreas, prostate, bladder, and colon cancers (reviewed in refs. *54–56*). COX inhibitors also decrease tumor blood vessel and capillary formation, inhibit expression of angiogenic growth factors such as vascular endothelial growth factor

Table 4

Representative Clinical Cancer Chemoprevention Studies of the COX-2 Selective Inhibitor Celecoxib[1]

Target Organ/Agent	Study Cohort	Objective(s)
Colon		
Celecoxib	FAP[2] patients ≥18 yr old	Regression /prevention of colorectal adenomas;of duodenal dysplasia; modulation of biomarkers *(76,77)*
Celecoxib ± Eflornithine	FAP patients ≥18 yr old	Regression/prevention of colorectal adenomas; modulation of duodenal dysplasia; modulation of biomarkers
Celecoxib	FAP genotype ≥10 yr old without FAP phenotype	Delay time to expression of FAP phenotype
Celecoxib	HNPCC	Modulation of biomarkers
Celecoxib	Previous colorectal adenoma	Prevention of colorectal adenomas; modulation of ACF and other biomarkers
Celecoxib	Previous colorectal adenoma	Prevention of colorectal adenomas
Celecoxib	Previous colorectal adenoma and ≥5 rectal ACF	Modulation of ACF and other biomarkers
Bladder		
Celecoxib	Superficial TCC (Ta, T1/TIS) post- BCG	Increased time to recurrence of superficial TCC; modulation of biomarkers
Breast		
Celecoxib	Premenopausal women ages 18–55 at high risk for ER– breast cancer (based on age-related Gail risk, BRCA1/2 mutation,family history, previous ADH,LCIS, DCIS or early stage ER-invasive breast cancer	COX-2 expression; ductal-cell proliferation; serum proteomics compared with mammographic density
Esophagus		
Celecoxib	Barrett's esophagus	Regression of Barrett's dysplasia
Celecoxib ±SeMet	Esophageal squamous dysplasia	Regression of dysplasia
Head and Neck		
Celecoxib	OPL	Regression of OPL; modulation of bio markers; PGE_2 levels
Lung		
Celecoxib	Chronic smokers (mild COPD)	Modulation of biomarkers
Celecoxib	Previous stage I NSCLC	Prevention of lung cancers cancers; modulation of precancerous changes
Prostate		
Celecoxib	Prostate cancer (scheduled for radical prostatectomy)	Modulation of biomarkers; pharmacodynamics

Skin

Celecoxib	Fitzpatrick Skin Type I–IV photosensitivity	Decreased UV damage; modulation of bio markers
Celecoxib	BCNS with previous BCC	Prevention of BCC
Celecoxib	AK (10–40 on upper extremities neck and head)	Prevention and regression of AK; modulationof carcinogenesis biomarkers

[1]*See* cancertrials.nih.gov for more information on these studies.

[2]Abbreviations: ACF, aberrant crypt foci; ADH, atypical ductal hyperplasia; AK, actinic keratosis; BCC, basal cell carcinoma; BCG, *Bacillus Calmette-Guerin*; BCNS, basal cell nevus syndrome; COPD, chronic obstructive pulmonary disease; DCIS, ductal carcinoma *in situ*; ER, estrogen receptor; FAP, familial adenomatous polyposis; HNPCC, hereditary nonpolyposis colorectal cancer; LCIS, lobular carcinoma *in situ*; NSCLC, non-small cell lung cancer; OPL, oral premalignant lesions; PG, prostaglandin; SeMet, *l*-selenomethionine; TCC, transitional cell carcinoma; TIS, transitional cell carcinoma *in situ*.

(VEGF) and basic fibroblast growth factor (bFGF), inhibit αVβ3 integrin, and are agonists of the anti-angiogenic PPARγ *(29,57)*.

3.1.1.4. COX-2 and Invasiveness and Cell Migration COX -2 expression has been directly associated with increased tumor cell adhesion, growth of endothelial cells, and invasiveness *(30,55,58–62)*. For example, human colon cancer cells with upregulated COX-2 expression showed increased invasiveness, activation of matrix metalloproteinase-2 (MMP-2), and increased MMP expression; the COX inhibitor sulindac reversed invasiveness and MMP activation *(63)*.

3.1.2. Epidemiological Evidence Associates the Use of COX Inhibitors with Cancer Prevention

Chronic use of COX inhibitors has been associated with reduced cancer risk in many cancer target organs—colorectum, bladder, breast, esophagus (and the precancerous Barrett's esophagus), lung (specifically, smokers' lung), pancreas, prostate, skin (melanoma and non-melanoma), and stomach *(9,30,64,65)*. The association of leukemias and lymphomas with chronic inflammation suggests that NSAIDs may also reduce the risk of these cancers *(30)*. The evidence that NSAIDs reduce cancer risk is most striking for colorectal cancer (CRC). More than 20 studies have found a reduced incidence of CRCs or precancerous adenomas associated with chronic use of aspirin or other NSAIDs (reviewed in ref. 9). Since use of COX-2 selective inhibitors is just beginning to be evaluated in epidemiological studies, these observations are based on the use of aspirin and other nonselective COX inhibitors. However, it is very probable that the cancer preventive activity observed is at least partly the result of COX-2 inhibition. A preliminary report of

a recent study comparing the recurrence of superficial bladder cancer in users of celecoxib, other NSAIDs, acetaminophen, and none of these antiinflammatories suggests that COX-2 is involved in risk reduction. Patients using celecoxib or NSAIDs had a significantly lower risk of recurrence (≈30%) than those using acetaminophen or none of these drugs (≈60%) *(66)*.

3.1.3. COX-2 Inhibitors Show Chemopreventive Efficacy in Animal Models of Carcinogenesis

NSAIDs have shown chemopreventive efficacy in many animal carcinogenesis models *(11)*. This activity has been observed most consistently in studies of colon carcinogenesis, and activity has also been observed in the bladder, skin, head and neck, lung, mammary gland, and pancreatic cancer models. COX-2 involvement is suggested by the observation that the chemopreventive effects of COX-2-selective inhibitors are equal to or more profound than those of traditional NSAIDs (Table 3 summarizes published studies on COX-2-selective inhibitors). One interesting observation drawn from these studies is that the COX-2-selective inhibitors may be more effective in reducing cancer progression than cancer incidence. This effect has been found in the colon, skin, and bladder. For example, in the rat bladder, the COX-2-selective inhibitor celecoxib reduced cancer incidence and multiplicity, but was most effective in preventing the progression of dysplasia to cancers *(67)*. Similarly, papilloma incidence was reduced in UV-induced mouse skin, but the most dramatic effects of 500 ppm celecoxib in the diet were reductions in papilloma multiplicity (2/mouse in the celecoxib treatment group vs 18/mouse in the UV control group) and size (1.3% >2 mm diameter in the celecoxib group vs 12.5% > 2 mm in the UV control group) *(68,69)*.

3.1.4. COX-2 INHIBITORS IN CLINICAL INTERVENTION STUDIES: A PRIMARY TARGET IS REGRESSION AND PREVENTION OF INTRA-EPITHELIAL NEOPLASIA (IEN)

Strong scientific rationales, evidence, and strategies support the use of IEN end points for clinical cancer prevention studies (7,70–72). Particularly convincing evidence supports the use of colorectal adenomas. Several chemoprevention trials with colorectal adenoma recurrence and regression as end points have been undertaken with COX inhibitors in familial adenomatous polyposis (FAP) patients. The traditional NSAID sulindac has shown dramatic effects in causing total or almost total regression of colorectal adenomatous polyps and preventing the recurrence of high-grade adenomas in patients with FAP (73,74), although it did not prevent new adenomas in subjects with the FAP genotype in whom the FAP adenoma phenotype had not yet been seen (75). A study completed in 1999 examined the effect of the COX-2-selective inhibitor celecoxib at two doses against colorectal polyps in subjects with FAP (76). In the randomized, double-blind, placebo-controlled study of 77 FAP patients, a 6-mo intervention with 800 mg/d celecoxib significantly reduced polyps the number of 28%, and 53% of treated subjects showed a ≥25% reduction. A blinded physicians' assessment indicated a qualitative improvement in the colon and rectum, and to a lesser extent in the duodenum, of treated subjects (77). This trial led to accelerated FDA marketing approval of celecoxib as an adjunct to standard care for regression and reduction of adenomatous polyps in FAP patients. Follow-up studies of celecoxib in patients with FAP as well as in subjects with sporadic adenomas are in progress to evaluate the relative effect of celecoxib on polyp regression and prevention, and to determine whether greater efficacy will result from combination therapy of celecoxib with other agents (such as eflornithine). Rofecoxib is also being evaluated for preventing sporadic colorectal adenomas (78).

As noted here, abundant epidemiological evidence associates the use of aspirin and other nonselective NSAIDs with a reduced risk of colorectal adenomas and cancers. Despite the potential toxicity of these drugs, low-dose aspirin is interesting because it provides the possibility of simultaneously reducing cardiovascular risk, although careful risk:benefit analyses may be needed to define appropriate populations for intervention. Two randomized, controlled studies have shown that aspirin may have potential as a cancer chemopreventive. The first study of aspirin (325 mg qd) in patients with previously resected CRC (Duke's stage A, B1, B2, or C) was terminated early when the difference between treatment groups reached statistical significance (79). Compared with the placebo group, fewer aspirin patients had adenomas (17% vs 27%, p = 0.004), and the adjusted relative risk for adenoma recurrence was 0.65 (95% CI, 0.46–0.91). Adenoma number (0.2 vs 0.49, p = 0.003) and time to adenoma recurrence were lower with aspirin treatment. In the second study in patients with previous adenomas, 81 mg qd (but not 325 mgqd) aspirin reduced adenoma incidence by 19% (80). Compared with placebo, relative risks for any adenoma were 0.81 (95% CI, 0.69–0.96) and 0.96 (95% CI, 0.81–1.13) for 81 or 325 mg qd aspirin, respectively; respective relative risks for adenomas ≥1 cm were 0.59 (95% CI, 0.38–0.92) and 0.83 (95% CI, 0.55–1.23).

Celecoxib is the COX-2-selective NSAID that has been evaluated most extensively in clinical chemoprevention studies. Representative cancer prevention studies with this agent using IEN along with earlier carcinogenesis-associated markers as end points are summarized in Table 4. In addition to the studies in the colon described here, celecoxib is being evaluated in the prevention of superficial bladder cancers, regression and prevention of actinic keratosis, modulation of progression to basal cell carcinomas in patients with basal cell nevus syndrome, regression of Barrett's esophagus (a precursor of esophageal adenocarcinoma) and esophageal dysplasia (a precursor of squamous cell carcinoma of the esophagus), and modulation of bronchial metaplasia/dysplasia and oral premalignant lesions (OPL), as well as modulation of biomarkers of prostate and breast carcinogenesis.

3.1.5. COX-2-SELECTIVE INHIBITORS SHOW LOW TOXICITY AND HAVE THE POTENTIAL TO PROVIDE CLINICAL BENEFIT IN SEVERAL CHRONIC DISEASES

COX inhibitors are already widely used to treat chronic inflammatory conditions, particularly osteo- and rheumatoid arthritis. It is speculated—although it is far from clear—that these compounds may have additional indications in cardiovascular disease, and potentially in neurodegenerative (Alzheimer's) disease (21). As described here, significant toxicity is associated with use of nonselective COX inhibitors that inhibit formation of tissue-protective PGs catalyzed by constitutive COX-1. For example, an estimated 16,000 deaths in the United States were associated with NSAID use in 1997 (20). Incidence of the most prevalent of these toxicities, GI ulceration, and bleeding, were reduced in patients using COX-2-selective drugs in comparative studies of chronically administered COX-2-selective inhibitors with nonselective COX inhibitors (reviewed in ref. *5*). Although the evidence indicates that COX-2-selective inhibitors are safe for chronic use, a very limited study suggests that use of COX-2-selective NSAIDs may increase the risk of heart attack *(81)*. Cardiotoxicity associated with inhibition of the vasodilator COX product PGI$_2$ without concomitant inhibition of vasoconstricting thromboxanes has been raised as a possible concern in high-risk patients *(12,82)*. Also, because little COX-2 is found in platelets, a primary site for thromboxane formation, selective COX-2 inhibitors— unlike NSAIDs, which inhibit COX-1—are not effective as cardioprotective thromboxane inhibitors. It is also possible that the inhibition of COX-2 may affect kidney and reproductive function *(20,21)*.

3.2. LOX as a Target for Cancer Prevention
3.2.1. LOX Expression in Carcinogenesis

Although the body of evidence is less than for COX and PGs, LOX products, LTs and HETEs, also contribute to carcinogenesis because of their oxidant activity and through modulation of signal-transduction pathways. LOX expression (particularly, 12-LOX) has been well-documented in many types of cancers, including the prostate, breast, lung, head and neck, colon, and skin *(27,83,84)*. The presence of the 12-LOX product 12(S)-HETE has been correlated to the metastatic potential of some cancer cells, including prostate cancer cells *(83)*. 12(S)-HETE also participates in signal transduction; it stimulates protein kinase C (PKC) and mediates the effects of growth factors such as EGF, bFGF, and platelet-derived growth factor (PDGF), and cytokines (e.g., TNF, granulocyte-macrophage colony-stimulating factor [GM-CSF], and ILs) on signal transduction *(27,85–90)*. PKC activation by 12(S)-HETE leads to the release and secretion of cathepsin B, a cysteine protease involved in tumor metastasis and invasion *(84)*. 12(S)-HETE also stimulates adhesion by upregulating integrin receptors *(91,92)*. 5-LOX metabolites, particularly 5-HETEs, have been shown to stimulate prostate cancer cell growth *(93, 94)*.

As inflammatory mediators, LTs elicit vessel-wall adhesion, smooth-muscle contraction, granulocyte degranulation, chemotaxis, and increased mucous secretion and vascular permeability *(28)*. A number of drugs that specifically inhibit the LOX metabolic pathway have been developed to treat inflammatory diseases such as asthma, ulcerative colitis, arthritis, and psoriasis, and it has been proposed that these drugs may have potential as chemopreventive agents *(27)*, particularly drugs that affect the 5-LOX pathway—5-LOX inhibitors such as zileuton, FLAP inhibitors, and LTB$_4$-receptor antagonists such as zafirlukast, montelukast, and pranlukast.

3.2.2. Cancer Preventive Potential of LOX Pathway Inhibition

The most compelling data for 5-LOX inhibitors as chemopreventive agents are in the lung *(95)*. 5-LOX inhibitors have been shown to reduce lung adenomas induced by *N*-nitrosonornicotine (NNK) in Strain A/J mice *(96)*. In human lung-cancer cells, LOX inhibitors reduced 5-HETE-stimulated proliferation *(97)*. Although no cancer-preventive efficacy studies on LOX inhibitors in the prostate have been reported, several studies have shown that LOX products (particularly 5-HETE) stimulate prostate cancer cell growth and LOX-specific inhibitors reduce this growth *(93, 94)*. 5-HETE stimulates growth of human breast cancer cells, and this growth is inhibited (apoptosis is increased) by 5-LOX and FLAP inhibitors *(98)*. Available data suggest that fatty acid metabolites—including products of the LOX pathways—enhance tumorigenesis, and compounds that are nonspecific inhibitors of the LOX pathways, nordihydroguaiaretic acid (NDGA) and esculetin, prevent development of *N*-methyl-*N*-nitrosourea (MNU)- and 7,12-dimethylbenz(a)anthracene (DMBA)-induced rat mammary gland tumors *(99,100)*. The relevant studies in these three targets, as well as data suggesting roles for LOX inhibition in cancer prevention of head and neck carcinogenesis, melanoma, and leukemia, are described briefly in the following paragraphs.

3.2.2.1. The Lung In the lung-cancer prevention study cited here, the FLAP inhibitor MK 886 and the 5-LOX inhibitor A 79175 reduced the multiplicity of NNK-induced tumors in strain A/J mice; A 79175 also reduced tumor incidence *(96)*. Interestingly, in the same study, the COX-inhibitor aspirin reduced tumor multiplicity and the combination of aspirin and A 79175 (e.g., inhibiting both COX and LOX pathways) had synergistic activity in lowering tumor incidence and multiplicity. LOX metabolites have also been found to stimulate lung cancer cell growth. 5-LOX is stimulated by two autocrine growth factors, gastrin-releasing peptide

(GRP) and insulin-like growth factor (IGF), to increase production of 5-HETE (*101*). 5-HETE stimulated the growth of lung cancer cells, and 5-LOX inhibitors NDGA, AA-861, and MK 886 decreased proliferation; aspirin had little effect. Expression of 5-LOX and FLAP mRNA by lung cancer cell lines was confirmed using reverse transcriptase-polymerase chain reaction (RT-PCR), and the presence of 5-LOX mRNA was identified in samples of primary lung-cancer tissue, including both small-cell and non-small-cell lung carcinomas (NSCLC). Also relevant to the lung are studies demonstrating that LOXs mediate oxidation of potent carcinogens such as benzidine,*o*-dianisidine and benzo[*a*]pyrene (B[*a*]P); this activation can be blocked by LOX inhibitors NDGA and esculetin (*102*).

3.2.2.2. The Prostate Reduced levels of AA have been observed in prostate cancer, and 10-fold greater turnover of AA in malignant vs benign prostatic tissue suggested a possible increase in AA metabolism (*103,104*). In human prostate-cancer cells, linoleic acid stimulated cell growth, and COX inhibitors and a LOX inhibitor blocked it, substantiating the involvement of AA metabolism in prostate-cancer-cell proliferation (*105*). COX-specific inhibitors alone did not reduce human prostate PC3 cell DNA synthesis, and the AA antagonist eicosatetraynoic acid (ETYA) did reduce synthesis, suggesting the involvement of LOX products in prostate cancer cell proliferation. A 5-LOX-specific inhibitor (A 63162) also reduced DNA synthesis and growth in prostate cancer cells (*106*). Also, 5-HETE— and particularly the 5-oxo-eicosatetraenoic form (5-oxo-ETE)—stimulated PC3 cell growth similarly to AA; LTs had no effect. 5-HETEs also effectively reversed growth inhibition produced by the FLAP inhibitor MK 886. Both MK 886 and AA 861 effectively blocked prostate-tumor proliferation induced by AA; in the same study, the COX inhibitor ibuprofen and the nonspecific 12-LOX inhibitors baicalein and *N*-benzyl-*N*-hydroxy-5-phenylpentanamide were ineffective (*93*).

3.2.2.3. The Breast 5-LOX and FLAP inhibitors reduce growth and increase apoptosis and G_1 phase arrest in human breast-cancer cells; PPARγ and PPARα are upregulated and may help to mediate these effects (*98*). Nonspecific and 12-LOX inhibition reduce growth and invasiveness of MDA-MB-435 breast-cancer cells. For example, esculetin blocked linoleic acid-enhanced invasion of these cells, and COX-specific inhibitor piroxicam had no effect (*107*). The nonspecific LOX inhibitor NDGA inhibited adhesion to collagen IV induced by either A 23187 or AA.

In BT-20 breast-cancer cells, NDGA inhibited LOX-mediated metabolism of linoleic acid to 13-hydroxyoctadecadienoic acid (13-HODE) and blocked EGF-induced DNA synthesis, suggesting a role for LOX in the EGFR signaling pathway (*108*). NDGA administered post-initiation reduced mammary gland tumor multiplicity in rats induced with MNU (*99*). Esculetin significantly reduced DMBA-induced mammary gland tumor incidence and volume in rats fed high- and low-fat diets; piroxicam had no effect (*100*). Both the COX-specific inhibitors nabumetone and esculetin reduced MNU-induced mammary gland tumor incidence in rats fed a standard diet (*109*).

3.2.2.4. Other Cancers—Colon, Head and Neck, Melanoma, and Leukemia SC 41930, a competitive LTB_4 antagonist, inhibited LTB_4-induced growth stimulation in HT-29 colon cancer cells; a similar inhibition was reported in mouse colon adenocarcinoma cell lines MAC16, MAC13, and MAC26 treated with other 5-LOX inhibitors, including BWA4C, BWB70C, and zileuton (*110,111*). BWA4C was the most effective inhibitor in male NMRI mice transplanted with fragments of MAC26 or MAC16 colon tumors, decreasing both tumor volume and tumor growth rate after 8–13 d of treatment.

12- and 15-HETE are major AA metabolites in squamous epithelial carcinomas of the head and neck. Also, 12(S)-HETE is the predominant metabolic product of metastatic B16 melanoma cells (*112*). Additionally, excess LT production, specifically LTC_4, has been documented in cells from patients with both acute and chronic leukemias (*113,114*). The addition of the 5-LOX-specific inhibitors SC 41661A and A 63162 to these cells reduced DNA labeling and decreased cell numbers within 72 h (*113*). Other LOX inhibitors, including piriprost, NDGA, and BW755C, also inhibited growth of human hematopoietic cancer cell lines (*115,116*).

3.2.3. OTHER CONSIDERATIONS IN USING LOX INHIBITORS FOR CANCER PREVENTION

In contrast to the extensive clinical development activity for COX-2-selective inhibitors in cancer prevention, there have been relatively few studies on LOX inhibitors. Since oral 5-LOX pathway-blocking agents are efficacious as anti-asthmatics, the lung has a high priority for future cancer prevention studies and applications of LOX inhibitors and LTA-receptor antagonists. Cancer prevention testing of approved pharmaceuticals in this class, such as zileuton, pranlukast, and zafirlukast, has been considered with oral formulations. In fact, a Phase II clinical trial has been initiated to evaluate the effects of zileuton on lung dysplasia.

As suggested here, LOX inhibition may be more effective for cancer prevention than LT-receptor antagonism. However, current 5-LOX inhibitors available as anti-asthmatics have shown evidence of potentially significant liver toxicity. A manufacturer-sponsored long-term safety study of zileuton evaluated liver function in 2,458 patients who recieved zileuton plus normal asthma medications (117). After 12 mo of treatment, liver transaminase levels increased by 4.6% (3× the upper limit of normal) in the zileuton-treated group, compared with a 1.1% increase in patients who recieved only the other asthma medications. Sixty-one percent of liver enzyme elevations occurred within the first 2 mo of zileuton treatment. Such toxicity could limit the use of these drugs for cancer prevention in asymptomatic populations.

Future studies may include the development of inhalant formulations, which may potentially reduce toxicity and allow for higher dose levels. Whether inhalant formulations of these agents would remain efficacious and exert cancer-preventive activity has not yet been determined. The prostate is also a cancer target of great interest, based on the high rate of AA metabolism and antiproliferative activity of LOX inhibitors in prostate cancer cells. In this regard, inhibitors of the 12-LOX pathway may prove to be better candidates for cancer preventive intervention; however, this research will depend on production and availability of such agents.

4. RECEPTOR INHIBITION AND FREE-RADICAL TRAPPING: OTHER CHEMOPREVENTIVE MECHANISMS THAT AFFECT COX AND LOX METABOLIC PATHWAYS

Antioxidants that are potent inhibitors of AA metabolism perform perhaps the most prominent oxygen free-radical scavenging activity associated with inhibition of carcinogenesis. Numerous chemicals with this activity, as here, are proving to be effective chemopreventive agents. Compounds such as vitamin E, which scavenges lipoxygenase products, and GSH-S-transferase inhibitors, which enhance detoxifying conjugation of electrophiles with GSH, inhibit tumor promotion in mouse skin (118). Likewise, lipoxygenase inhibitors such as curcumin, flavonoids, and tea

polyphenols, stable one-electron donors that competitively inhibit production of unstable free radicals and electrophiles by PHS, also inhibit tumor promotion in mouse skin (118).

The control of AA release by diacerylglycerol kinase and phospholipases may be mediated through signal-transduction pathways. Compounds that block signal transduction at the membrane level, including antiestrogens, flavonoids, curcuminoids, vitamin E, and triterpenoids, may be chemopreventive through inhibition of AA metabolism (118). PGE_2 is known to suppress immune response in certain tumor cells (1,22). Inhibitors of PHS may relieve this suppression.

Antiinflammatory corticosteroids (e.g., dexamethasone, budesonide) have a wide range of biological activities that may impact on AA metabolism, including the inhibition of phospholipase A_2 and interaction with nuclear transcription factors via the glucucorticoid receptor (119,120). Wattenberg has demonstrated the chemopreventive activity of oral and aerosolized corticosteroids (budesonide) in B[a]P-induced mouse lung, and budesonide is now being studied for prevention and regression of bronchial dysplasia in chronic smokers (121–123) (see also Chapter 9).

NSAIDs may also block carcinogen activation by cytochrome P450s. For example, PGE_2 induces steroid aromatase, that can lead to increased proliferation of estrogen-sensitive tissues such as the breast (124).

5. PROMISING FUTURE RESEARCH ON AA METABOLIC PATHWAYS IN CANCER CHEMOPREVENTION

Overwhelming evidence shows that AA metabolic pathways provide good targets for cancer preventive strategies, particularly COX- and potentially LOX-mediated arms. Future strategies will focus on optimizing the cancer-preventive therapeutic index (TI) based on modulation of lead targets, particularly COX-2, as well as identifying and developing strategies for other targets on these pathways.

One method to optimize TIs is by combination therapy—pairing agents with complementary mechanisms of activity to enhance efficacy and/or reduce toxicity. Enhanced cancer preventive activity over either agent alone has been observed in combining a COX inhibitor with an inducible nitric oxide synthase (iNOS) inhibitor SC-51 (125), EGFR inhibitor EKI-569 (126), and a potent antiproliferative eflornithine (an irreversible inhibitor of ornithine decarboxylase)

(67,127,128). In these examples, efficacy was seen at doses low enough to avoid or reduce associated toxicities. Single agents combining two potential chemopreventive mechanisms involving AA and other antiinflammatory pathways are also very intriguing. One example is dual COX/LOX inhibitors such as ML3000 *(129)*. Although these drugs have not been evaluated for cancer preventive activity, they exhibit potent antiinflammatory activity in the colon, with no GI toxicity. A second example, nitric oxide (NO)-releasing NSAIDs (e.g., NO conjugated with aspirin, sulindac, or ibuprofen), inhibit iNOS and are more potent inhibitors of colon cancer cell (HT-29) growth than corresponding NSAIDs *(130,131)*. NO-aspirin has also been shown to prevent aberrant crypt foci (ACF) development in the rat colon *(132)*.

Other molecular targets for cancer prevention have been associated with COX and LOX pathways. For example, R-flurbiprofen, an antiinflammatory that inhibits COX-2 expression but not COX-2 activity, has shown cancer preventive activity in the Min mouse colon and TRAMP mouse prostate carcinogenesis models *(133,134)*. Evidence suggests that the agent blocks COX-2 expression by inhibiting NFκB-mediated activation. Also, PPARγ agonists such as PGJ_2 and GW1929 inhibit COX-2 expression in a human neuroblastoma cell line, at least partly through blocking AP-1 transcription factor binding to the response site in the COX-2 gene promoter *(135)*.

Other enzymes may also contribute to increased levels of PGE_2 in many precancers and cancers, including colorectal adenomas and adenocarcinomas. Yoshimatsu et al. *(136)* have reported that an inducible microsomal PGE synthase (mPGES-1) is overexpressed in colorectal lesions and may provide a target for chemopreventive agents. Interestingly, various molecular factors associated with carcinogenesis showed some differential effects on mPGES-1 and COX-2 induction.

PGI_2, formed from PGH_2 via PGI synthase (PGIS), is one of the main products of AA in vascular tissue; it is a potent vasodilator and it inhibits proliferation and DNA synthesis in smooth muscle. Reduced levels of PGIS have been seen in non-small cell lung cancer (NSCLC) compared with paired normal lung tissue, suggesting that upregulation of PGIS or PGI_2 may have potential as a chemopreventive strategy in lung (*see* Chapter 11).

Like inhibitors of COX activity and expression, inhibitors of PG receptors have potential as cancer-preventive agents. ONO-8711, a selective PGE receptor EP_1 antagonist, inhibited the formation of ACF and adenomas in Min mice *(137)*. This agent has also shown activity against rat mammary-gland tumors induced by 2-amino-1-methyl-6-phenylimidazo(4,5-β)pyridine (PhIP) *(138)*. Elevated levels of COX-2 and PGE_2 in breast cancers compared with surrounding tissue, coupled with evidence that PGE_2 stimulates transcription of the steroid aromatase gene (CYP19) via binding to EP receptors *(124)*, suggested EP-receptor antagonism as a potential target for decreasing estrogen biosynthesis and associated proliferative activity in breast carcinogenesis. Similarly, ONO-AE2-227 is an EP_4 antagonist that has been shown to inhibit azoxymethane (AOM)-induced ACF in C57BL/6Cr mice and polyp formation in Min mice *(43)*.

In the LOX pathway, 15-LOX-1 and its product 13-S-HODE have been implicated as potential effectors of cancer preventive activity, and 15-LOX-1 has been suggested as a non-COX target for NSAID cancer-preventive activity *(139,140)*. NSAIDs were found to induce apoptosis in colorectal cancer and esophageal cancer cells while upregulating 15-LOX-1.

Finally, PLA_2 activity effectors show both the promise and complexity of modulating AA metabolism in cancer prevention *(141,142)*. As stated in Subheading 1, PLA_2 catalyzes release of AA from membrane phospholipids, and thus is a potential target for cancer preventive intervention. Group IV cytosolic PLA_2-deficient Min mice showed reduced polyp burdens. However, not all PLA_2 isoforms promote carcinogenesis. Min mice with Group IIA secretory PLA_2 isoform deficiency exhibited an increased tumor burden *(142)*. As also been observed in the LOX and COX pathways, these contradictory findings may be a result of tissue- and cell type-specific control of PLA_2.

ACKNOWLEDGMENT

The authors wish to gratefully acknowledge Dr. Andrew J. Dannenberg, Cornell University Weill Medical College and Strang Cancer Prevention Center, for his review of the material presented in this chapter.

REFERENCES

1. Zenser TV, Davis BB. Arachidonic acid metabolism, in *Cellular and Molecular Targets for Chemoprevention*. Steele VE, Stoner GD, Boone CW, Kelloff GJ, eds. CRC Press, Boca Raton, FL 1992, pp. 225–243.
2. Taketo MM. Cyclooxygenase-2 inhibitors in tumorigenesis (part II). *J Natl Cancer Inst* 1998;90:1609–1620.
3. Taketo MM. Cyclooxygenase-2 inhibitors in tumorigenesis (part I). *J Natl Cancer Inst* 1998;90:1529–1536.

4. Herschman HR. Function and regulation of prostaglandin synthase 2. *Adv Exp Med Biol* 1999;469:3–8.

5. FitzGerald GA, Patrono C. The coxibs, selective inhibitors of cyclooxygenase-2. *N Engl J Med* 2001;345:433–442.

6. Funk CD. Prostaglandins and leukotrienes: advances in eicosanoid biology. *Science* 2001;294:1871–1875.

7. Kelloff GJ. Perspectives on cancer chemoprevention research and drug development. *Adv Cancer Res* 2000;78:199–334.

8. Gupta RA, DuBois RN. Colorectal cancer prevention and treatment by inhibition of cyclooxygenase-2. *Nat Rev Cancer* 2001;1:11–21.

9. Anderson WF, Umar A, Viner JL, Hawk ET. The role of cyclooxygenase inhibitors in cancer prevention. *Curr Pharm Des* 2002;8:1035–1062.

10. Howe LR, Dannenberg AJ. A role for cyclooxygenase-2 inhibitors in the prevention and treatment of cancer. *Semin Oncol* 2002;29:111–119.

11. Kelloff GJ, Steele VE, Sigman CC. Chemoprevention of cancer by NSAIDs and selective COX-2 blockade, in *COX-2 Blockade in Cancer Prevention and Therapy*. Harris RE, ed. Humana Press, Totowa, NJ, 2002, pp.279–300.

12. Marnett LJ, DuBois RN. COX-2: A Target for Colon Cancer Prevention. *Annu Rev Pharmacol Toxicol* 2002;42:55–80.

13. Kelloff GJ, Sigman CC. Arachidonic acid pathway in cancer prevention, in *Mechanisms in Carcinogenesis and Cancer Prevention*. Vainio HU, Hietanen E, eds. H Springer-Verlag, Heidelberg, Germany, 2003, pp.187–210.

14. Samuelsson B. An elucidation of the arachidonic acid cascade. Discovery of prostaglandins, thromboxane and leukotrienes. *Drugs* 1987;33 Suppl 1:2–9.

15. Needleman P, Turk J, Jakschik BA, et al. Arachidonic acid metabolism. *Annu Rev Biochem* 1986;55:69–102.

16. Smith WL, Marnett LJ, DeWitt DL. Prostaglandin and thromboxane biosynthesis. *Pharmacol Ther* 1991;49:153–179.

17. Watanabe K, Kawamori T, Nakatsugi S, et al. Role of the prostaglandin E receptor subtype EP1 in colon carcinogenesis. *Cancer Res* 1999;59:5093–5096.

18. Adam L, Mazumdar A, Sharma T, et al. A three-dimensional and temporo-spatial model to study invasiveness of cancer cells by heregulin and prostaglandin E2. *Cancer Res* 2001;61:81–87.

19. Marnett LJ. Aspirin and the potential role of prostaglandins in colon cancer. *Cancer Res* 1992;52:5575–5589.

20. Wolfe MM, Lichtenstein DR, Singh G. Gastrointestinal toxicity of nonsteroidal antiinflammatory drugs. *N Engl J Med* 1999;340:1888–1899.

21. Kulkarni SK, Jain NK, Singh A. Cyclooxygenase isoenzymes and newer therapeutic potential for selective COX-2 inhibitors. *Methods Find Exp Clin Pharmacol* 2000;22:291–298.

22. Smith WL, DeWitt DL, Garavito RM. Cyclooxygenases: structural, cellular, and molecular biology. *Annu Rev Biochem* 2000;69:145–182.

23. Sheng H, Shao J, DuBois RN. K-Ras-mediated increase in cyclooxygenase 2 mRNA stability involves activation of the protein kinase B1. *Cancer Res* 2001;61:2670–2675.

24. Cok SJ, Morrison AR. The 3'-untranslated region of murine cyclooxygenase-2 contains multiple regulatory elements that alter message stability and translational efficiency. *J Biol Chem* 2001;276:23,179–23,185.

25. Dixon DA, Tolley ND, King PH, et al. Altered expression of the mRNA stability factor HuR promotes cyclooxygenase-2 expression in colon cancer cells. *J Clin Investig* 2001;108:1657–1665.

26. Subbaramaiah K, Dannenberg AJ. Cyclooxygenase 2: a molecular target for cancer prevention and treatment. *Trends Pharmacol Sci* 2003;24:96–102.

27. Steele VE, Holmes CA, Hawk ET, et al. Lipoxygenase inhibitors as potential cancer chemopreventives. *Cancer Epidemiol Biomark Prev* 1999;8:467–483.

28. Samuelsson B, Dahlen SE, Lindgren JA, et al. Leukotrienes and lipoxins: structures, biosynthesis, and biological effects. *Science* 1987;237:1171–1176.

29. Masferrer J. Approach to angiogenesis inhibition based on cyclooxygenase-2. *Cancer J* 2001;7 Suppl 3:S144–S150.

30. Harris RE. Cyclooxygenase-2 blockade in cancer prevention and therapy: widening the scope of impact, in *COX-2 Blockade in Cancer Prevention and Therapy*. Harris RE, ed. Humana Press Totowa, NJ, 2002,pp.341–365.

31. Xie W, Herschman HR. Transcriptional regulation of prostaglandin synthase 2 gene expression by platelet-derived growth factor and serum. *J Biol Chem* 1996;271:31,742–31,748.

32. Herschman HR, Reddy ST, Xie W. Function and regulation of prostaglandin synthase-2. *Adv Exp Med Biol* 1997;407:61–66.

33. Subbaramaiah K, Norton L, Gerald W, Dannenberg AJ. Cyclooxygenase-2 is overexpressed in HER-2/neu-positive breast cancer: evidence for involvement of AP-1 and PEA3. *J Biol Chem* 2002;277:18,649–18,657.

34. Weitzman SA, Gordon LI. Inflammation and cancer: role of phagocyte-generated oxidants in carcinogenesis. *Blood* 1990;76:655–663.

35. Balch CM, Dougherty PA, Cloud GA, Tilden AB. Prostaglandin E2-mediated suppression of cellular immunity in colon cancer patients. *Surgery* 1984;95:71–77.

36. McDougall CJ, Ngoi SS, Goldman IS, et al. Reduced expression of HLA class I and II antigens in colon cancer. *Cancer Res* 1990;50:8023–8027.

37. Wilgus TA, Ross MS, Parrett ML, Oberyszyn TM. Topical application of a selective cyclooxygenase inhibitor suppresses UVB mediated cutaneous inflammation. *Prostaglandins Other Lipid Mediat* 2000;62:367–384.

38. Bedi A, Pasricha PJ, Akhtar AJ, et al. Inhibition of apoptosis during development of colorectal cancer. *Cancer Res* 1995;55:1811–1816.

39. Tsujii M, DuBois RN. Alterations in cellular adhesion and apoptosis in epithelial cells overexpressing prostaglandin endoperoxide synthase 2. *Cell* 1995;83:493–501.

40. Hara A, Yoshimi N, Niwa M, et al. Apoptosis induced by NS-398, a selective cyclooxygenase-2 inhibitor, in human colorectal cancer cell lines. *Jpn J Cancer Res* 1997;88:600–604.

41. Sheng H, Williams CS, Shao J, et al. Induction of cyclooxygenase-2 by activated Ha-ras oncogene in Rat-1 fibroblasts and the role of mitogen-activated protein kinase pathway. *J Biol Chem* 1998;273:22,120–22,127.

42. Mohammed SI, Knapp DW, Bostwick DG, et al. Expression of cyclooxygenase-2 (COX-2) in human invasive transitional cell carcinoma (TCC) of the urinary bladder. *Cancer Res* 1999;59:5647–5650.

43. Sawaoka H, Tsuji S, Tsujii M, et al. Expression of the cyclooxygenase-2 gene in gastric epithelium. *J Clin Gastroenterol* 1997;25 Suppl 1:S105–S110.

44. Liu XH, Yao S, Kirschenbaum A, Levine AC. NS398, a selective cyclooxygenase-2 inhibitor, induces apoptosis and down-regulates bcl-2 expression in LNCaP cells. *Cancer Res* 1998;58:4245–4249.

45. Ding XZ, Tong WG, Adrian TE. Blockade of cyclooxygenase-2 inhibits proliferation and induces apoptosis in human pancreatic cancer cells. *Anticancer Res* 2000;20:2625–2631.

46. Zimmermann KC, Sarbia M, Weber AA, et al. Cyclooxygenase-2 expression in human esophageal carcinoma. *Cancer Res* 1999;59:198–204.

47. Hida T, Kozaki K, Muramatsu H, et al. Cyclooxygenase-2 inhibitor induces apoptosis and enhances cytotoxicity of various anticancer agents in non-small cell lung cancer cell lines. *Clin Cancer Res* 2000;6:2006–2011.

48. Yao R, Rioux N, Castonguay A, You M. Inhibition of COX-2 and induction of apoptosis: two determinants of nonsteroidal anti-inflammatory drugs' chemopreventive efficacies in mouse lung tumorigenesis. *Exp Lung Res* 2000;26:731–742.

49. Li M, Lotan R, Levin B, et al. Aspirin induction of apoptosis in esophageal cancer: a potential for chemoprevention. *Cancer Epidemiol Biomark Prev* 2000;9:545–549.

50. Nishimura G, Yanoma S, Mizuno H, et al. A selective cyclooxygenase-2 inhibitor suppresses tumor growth in nude mouse xenografted with human head and neck squamous carcinoma cells. *Jpn J Cancer Res* 1999;90:1152–1162.

51. Tsujii M, Kawano S, Tsuji S, et al. Cyclooxygenase regulates angiogenesis induced by colon cancer cells. *Cell* 1998;93:705–716.

52. Tomozawa S, Tsuno NH, Sunami E, et al. Cyclooxygenase-2 overexpression correlates with tumour recurrence, especially haematogenous metastasis, of colorectal cancer. *Br J Cancer* 2000;83:324–328.

53. Uefuji K, Ichikura T, Mochizuki H. Cyclooxygenase-2 expression is related to prostaglandin biosynthesis and angiogenesis in human gastric cancer. *Clin Cancer Res* 2000;6:135–138.

54. Koki AT, Leahy KM, Masferrer JL. Potential utility of COX-2 inhibitors in chemoprevention and chemotherapy. *Expert Opin Investig Drugs* 1999;8:1623–1638.

55. Masferrer JL, Koki A, Seibert K. COX-2 inhibitors. A new class of antiangiogenic agents. *Ann NY Acad Sci* 1999;889:84–86.

56. Koki A, Khan NK, Woerner BM, et al. Cyclooxygenase-2 in human pathological disease. *Adv Exp Med Biol* 2002;507:177–184.

57. Dormond O, Foletti A, Paroz C, Ruegg C. NSAIDs inhibit alpha V beta 3 integrin-mediated and Cdc42/Rac-dependent endothelial-cell spreading, migration and angiogenesis. *Nat Med* 2001;7:1041–1047.

58. Jones MK, Wang H, Peskar BM, et al. Inhibition of angiogenesis by nonsteroidal anti-inflammatory drugs: insight into mechanisms and implications for cancer growth and ulcer healing. *Nat Med* 1999;5:1418–1423.

59. Sawaoka H, Tsuji S, Tsujii M, Gunawan ES, Sasaki Y, Kawano S, et al. Cyclooxygenase inhibitors suppress angiogenesis and reduce tumor growth in vivo. *Lab Invest* 1999;79:1469–1477.

60. Suh N, Wang Y, Williams CR, et al. A new ligand for the peroxisome proliferator-activated receptor-gamma (PPAR-gamma), GW7845, inhibits rat mammary carcinogenesis. *Cancer Res* 1999;59:5671–5673.

61. Majima M, Hayashi I, Muramatsu M, et al. Cyclo-oxygenase-2 enhances basic fibroblast growth factor-induced angiogenesis through induction of vascular endothelial growth factor in rat sponge implants. *Br J Pharmacol* 2000;130:641–649.

62. Mehta RG, Williamson E, Patel MK, Koeffler HP. A ligand of peroxisome proliferator-activated receptor gamma, retinoids, and prevention of preneoplastic mammary lesions. *J Natl Cancer Inst* 2000;92:418–423.

63. Tsujii M, Kawano S, DuBois RN. Cyclooxygenase-2 expression in human colon cancer cells increases metastatic potential. *Proc Natl Acad Sci USA* 1997;94:3336–3340.

64. Thun MJ, Henley SJ, Patrono C. Nonsteroidal anti-inflammatory drugs as anticancer agents: mechanistic, pharmacologic, and clinical issues. *J Natl Cancer Inst* 2002;94:252–266.

65. Sorensen HT, Friis S, Norgard B, et al. Risk of cancer in a large cohort of nonaspirin NSAID users: a population-based study. *Br J Cancer* 2003;88:1687–1692.

66. Sheey OE, Zhao SZ, Raymoundo AL, et al. Celecoxib associated with reduced risk of superficial bladder cancer (SBC) recurrence. *Proc Amer Soc Clin Oncol Abstract* 2003;1539.

67. Grubbs CJ, Lubet RA, Koki AT, et al. Celecoxib inhibits N-butyl-N-(4-hydroxybutyl)-nitrosamine-induced urinary bladder cancers in male B6D2F1 mice and female Fischer-344 rats. *Cancer Res* 2000;60:5599–5602.

68. Fischer SM, Lo HH, Gordon GB, et al. Chemopreventive activity of celecoxib, a specific cyclooxygenase-2 inhibitor, and indomethacin against ultraviolet light-induced skin carcinogenesis. *Mol Carcinog* 1999;25:231–240.

69. Fischer SM, Conti CJ, Viner J, et al. Celecoxib and difluoromethylornithine in combination have strong therapeutic activity against UV-induced skin tumors in mice. *Carcinogenesis* 2003;24:945–952.

70. Kelloff GJ, Sigman CC, Johnson KM, et al. Perspectives on surrogate end points in the development of drugs that reduce the risk of cancer. *Cancer Epidemiol Biomark Prev* 2000;9:127–137.

71. O'Shaughnessy JA, Kelloff GJ, Gordon GB, et al. Treatment and prevention of intraepithelial neoplasia: an important target for accelerated new agent development. *Clin Cancer Res* 2002;8:314–346.

72. Metz DC, Alberts DS. Gastrointestinal cancer prevention in the United States: the road ahead. *Cancer Epidemiol Biomark Prev* 2003;12:81–83.

73. Giardiello FM, Hamilton SR, Krush AJ, et al. Treatment of colonic and rectal adenomas with sulindac in familial adenomatous polyposis. *N Engl J Med* 1993;328:1313–1316.

74. Cruz-Correa M, Hylind LM, Romans KE, Booker SV, Giardiello FM. Long-term treatment with sulindac in familial adenomatous polyposis: a prospective cohort study. *Gastroenterology* 2002;122:641–645.

75. Giardiello FM, Yang VW, Hylind LM, et al. Primary chemoprevention of familial adenomatous polyposis with sulindac. *N Engl J Med* 2002;346:1054–1059.

76. Steinbach G, Lynch PM, Phillips RK, et al. The effect of celecoxib, a cyclooxygenase-2 inhibitor, in familial adenomatous polyposis. *N Engl J Med* 2000;342:1946–1952.

77. Phillips RK, Wallace MH, Lynch PM, et al. A randomised, double blind, placebo controlled study of celecoxib, a selec-

tive cyclooxygenase 2 inhibitor, on duodenal polyposis in familial adenomatous polyposis. *Gut* 2002;50:857–860.

78. Oshima M, Murai N, Kargman S, et al. Chemoprevention of intestinal polyposis in the Apcdelta716 mouse by rofecoxib, a specific cyclooxygenase-2 inhibitor. *Cancer Res* 2001;61:1733–1740.

79. Sandler RS, Halabi S, Baron JA, et al. A randomized trial of aspirin to prevent colorectal adenomas in patients with previous colorectal cancer. *N Engl J Med* 2003;348:883–890.

80. Baron JA, Cole BF, Sandler RS, Haile RW, Ahnen D, Bresalier R, et al. A randomized trial of aspirin to prevent colorectal adenomas. *N Engl J Med* 2003;348:891–899.

81. Mukherjee D, Nissen SE, Topol EJ. Risk of cardiovascular events associated with selective COX-2 inhibitors. *JAMA* 2001;286:954–959.

82. McAdam BF, Catella-Lawson F, Mardini IA, et al. Systemic biosynthesis of prostacyclin by cyclooxygenase (COX)-2: the human pharmacology of a selective inhibitor of COX-2. *Proc Natl Acad Sci USA* 1999;96:272–277.

83. Honn KV, Tang DG, Gao X, et al. 12-lipoxygenases and 12(S)-HETE: role in cancer metastasis. *Cancer Metastasis Rev* 1994;13:365–396.

84. Honn KV, Timar J, Rozhin J, et al. A lipoxygenase metabolite, 12-(S)-HETE, stimulates protein kinase C-mediated release of cathepsin B from malignant cells. *Exp Cell Res* 1994;214:120–130.

85. Schade UF, Ernst M, Reinke M, Wolter DT. Lipoxygenase inhibitors suppress formation of tumor necrosis factor in vitro and in vivo. *Biochem Biophys Res Commun* 1989;159:748–754.

86. Masferrer JL, Rimarachin JA, Gerritsen ME, et al. 12(R)-hydroxyeicosatrienoic acid, a potent chemotactic and angiogenic factor produced by the cornea. *Exp Eye Res* 1991;52:417–424.

87. Liu B, Maher RJ, Hannun YA, et al. 12(S)-HETE enhancement of prostate tumor cell invasion: selective role of PKC alpha. *J Natl Cancer Inst* 1994;86:1145–1151.

88. Liu YW, Chen BK, Chen CJ, et al. Epidermal growth factor enhances transcription of human arachidonate 12-lipoxygenase in A431 cells. *Biochim Biophys Acta* 1997;1344:38–46.

89. Liu B, Maher RJ, De Jonckheere JP, et al. 12(S)-HETE increases the motility of prostate tumor cells through selective activation of PKC alpha. *Adv Exp Med Biol* 1997;400B:707–718.

90. Dethlefsen SM, Shepro D, D'Amore PA. Arachidonic acid metabolites in bFGF-, PDGF-, and serum-stimulated vascular cell growth. *Exp Cell Res* 1994;212:262–273.

91. Chopra H, Timar J, Chen YQ, et al. The lipoxygenase metabolite 12(S)-HETE induces a cytoskeleton-dependent increase in surface expression of integrin alpha IIb beta 3 on melanoma cells. *Int J Cancer* 1991;49:774–786.

92. Tang DG, Honn KV. 12-Lipoxygenase, 12(S)-HETE, and cancer metastasis. *Ann NY Acad Sci* 1994;744:199–215.

93. Ghosh J, Myers CE. Central role of arachidonate 5-lipoxygenase in the regulation of cell growth and apoptosis in human prostate cancer cells. *Adv Exp Med Biol* 1999;469:577–582.

94. Myers CE, Ghosh J. Lipoxygenase inhibition in prostate cancer. *Eur Urol* 1999;35:395–398.

95. Moody TW, Leyton J, Martinez A, et al. Lipoxygenase inhibitors prevent lung carcinogenesis and inhibit non-small cell lung cancer growth. *Exp Lung Res* 1998;24:617–628.

96. Rioux N, Castonguay A. Prevention of NNK-induced lung tumorigenesis in A/J mice by acetylsalicylic acid and NS-398. *Cancer Res* 1998;58:5354–5360.

97. Rioux N, Castonguay A. Inhibitors of lipoxygenase: a new class of cancer chemopreventive agents. *Carcinogenesis* 1998;19:1393–1400.

98. Avis I, Hong SH, Martinez A, et al. Five-lipoxygenase inhibitors can mediate apoptosis in human breast cancer cell lines through complex eicosanoid interactions. *FASEB J* 2001;15:2007–2009.

99. McCormick DL, Spicer AM. Nordihydroguaiaretic acid suppression of rat mammary carcinogenesis induced by N-methyl-N-nitrosourea. *Cancer Lett* 1987;37:139–146.

100. Kitagawa H, Noguchi M. Comparative effects of piroxicam and esculetin on incidence, proliferation, and cell kinetics of mammary carcinomas induced by 7,12-dimethylbenz[a]anthracene in rats on high- and low-fat diets. *Oncology* 1994;51:401–410.

101. Avis IM, Jett M, Boyle T, et al. Growth control of lung cancer by interruption of 5-lipoxygenase-mediated growth factor signaling. *J Clin Investig* 1996;97:806–813.

102. Kulkarni AP. Lipoxygenase—a versatile biocatalyst for biotransformation of endobiotics and xenobiotics. *Cell Mol Life Sci* 2001;58:1805–1825.

103. Chaudry A, McClinton S, Moffat LE, Wahle KW. Essential fatty acid distribution in the plasma and tissue phospholipids of patients with benign and malignant prostatic disease. *Br J Cancer* 1991;64:1157–1160.

104. Chaudry AA, Wahle KW, McClinton S, Moffat LE. Arachidonic acid metabolism in benign and malignant prostatic tissue in vitro: effects of fatty acids and cyclooxygenase inhibitors. *Int J Cancer* 1994;57:176–180.

105. Rose DP, Connolly JM. Effects of fatty acids and eicosanoid synthesis inhibitors on the growth of two human prostate cancer cell lines. *Prostate* 1991;18:243–254.

106. Anderson KM, Seed T, Ondrey F, Harris JE. The selective 5-lipoxygenase inhibitor A63162 reduces PC3 proliferation and initiates morphologic changes consistent with secretion. *Anticancer Res* 1994;14:1951–1960.

107. Liu XH, Connolly JM, Rose DP. The 12-lipoxygenase gene-transfected MCF-7 human breast cancer cell line exhibits estrogen-independent, but estrogen and omega-6 fatty acid-stimulated proliferation in vitro, and enhanced growth in athymic nude mice. *Cancer Lett* 1996;109:223–230.

108. Reddy N, Everhart A, Eling T, Glasgow W. Characterization of a 15-lipoxygenase in human breast carcinoma BT-20 cells: stimulation of 13-HODE formation by TGF alpha/EGF. *Biochem Biophys Res Commun* 1997;231:111–116.

109. Matsunaga K, Yoshimi N, Yamada Y, et al. Inhibitory effects of nabumetone, a cyclooxygenase-2 inhibitor, and esculetin, a lipoxygenase inhibitor, on N-methyl-N-nitrosourea-induced mammary carcinogenesis in rats. *Jpn J Cancer Res* 1998;89:496–501.

110. Djuric SW, Collins PW, Jones PH, et al. 7-[3-(4-acetyl-3-methoxy-2-propylphenoxy)propoxy]-3,4-dihydro-8-propyl-2H-1-benzopyran-2-carboxylic acid: an orally

active selective leukotriene B4 receptor antagonist. *J Med Chem* 1989;32:1145–1147.

111. Tsai BS, Keith RH, Villani-Price D, et al. The in vitro pharmacology of SC-51146: a potent antagonist of leukotriene B4 receptors. *J Pharmacol Exp Ther* 1994;268:1499–1505.

112. Liu B, Marnett LJ, Chaudhary A, et al. Biosynthesis of 12(S)-hydroxyeicosatetraenoic acid by B16 amelanotic melanoma cells is a determinant of their metastatic potential. *Lab Investig* 1994;70:314–323.

113. Anderson KM, Seed T, Jajeh A, et al. An in vivo inhibitor of 5-lipoxygenase, MK886, at micromolar concentration induces apoptosis in U937 and CML cells. *Anticancer Res* 1996;16:2589–2599.

114. Anderson KM, Levin J, Jajeh A, et al. Induction of apoptosis in blood cells from a patient with acute myelogenous leukemia by SC41661A, a selective inhibitor of 5-lipoxygenase. *Prostaglandins Leukot Essent Fatty Acids* 1993;48:323–326.

115. Snyder DS, Desforges JF. Lipoxygenase metabolites of arachidonic acid modulate hematopoiesis. *Blood* 1986;67:1675–1679.

116. Snyder DS, Castro R, Desforges JF. Antiproliferative effects of lipoxygenase inhibitors on malignant human hematopoietic cell lines. *Exp Hematol* 1989;17:6–9.

117. Lazarus SC, Lee T, Kemp JP, et al. Safety and clinical efficacy of zileuton in patients with chronic asthma. *Am J Manag Care* 1998;4:841–848.

118. Kelloff GJ, Boone CW, Steele VE, et al. Mechanistic considerations in chemopreventive drug development. *J Cell Biochem Suppl* 1994;20:1–24.

119. Jonat C, Rahmsdorf HJ, Park KK, et al. Antitumor promotion and antiinflammation: down-modulation of AP-1 (Fos/Jun) activity by glucocorticoid hormone. *Cell* 1990;62:1189–1204.

120. Wattenberg L. Chalcones, myo-inositol and other novel inhibitors of pulmonary carcinogenesis. *J Cell Biochem Suppl* 1995;22:162–168.

121. Wattenberg LW, Estensen RD. Studies of chemopreventive effects of budenoside on benzo[a]pyrene-induced neoplasia of the lung of female A/J mice. *Carcinogenesis* 1997;18:2015–2017.

122. Wattenberg LW, Wiedmann TS, Estensen RD, et al. Chemoprevention of pulmonary carcinogenesis by aerosolized budesonide in female A/J mice. *Cancer Res* 1997;57:5489–5492.

123. Wattenberg LW, Wiedmann TS, Estensen RD, et al. Chemoprevention of pulmonary carcinogenesis by brief exposures to aerosolized budesonide or beclomethasone dipropionate and by the combination of aerosolized budesonide and dietary myo-inositol. *Carcinogenesis* 2000;21:179–182.

124. Zhao Y, Agarwal VR, Mendelson CR, Simpson ER. Estrogen biosynthesis proximal to a breast tumor is stimulated by PGE2 via cyclic AMP, leading to activation of promoter II of the CYP19 (aromatase) gene. *Endocrinology* 1996;137:5739–5742.

125. Rao CV, Indranie C, Simi B, et al. Chemopreventive properties of a selective inducible nitric oxide synthase inhibitor in colon carcinogenesis, administered alone or in combination with celecoxib, a selective cyclooxygenase-2 inhibitor. *Cancer Res* 2002;62:165–170.

126. Torrance CJ, Jackson PE, Montgomery E, et al. Combinatorial chemoprevention of intestinal neoplasia. *Nat Med* 2000;6:1024–1028.

127. Reddy BS, Nayini J, Tokumo K, et al. Chemoprevention of colon carcinogenesis by concurrent administration of piroxicam, a nonsteroidal antiinflammatory drug with D,L-alpha-difluoromethylornithine, an ornithine decarboxylase inhibitor, in diet. *Cancer Res* 1990;50:2562–2568.

128. Rao CV, Tokumo K, Rigotty J, et al. Chemoprevention of colon carcinogenesis by dietary administration of piroxicam, alpha-difluoromethylornithine, 16 alpha-fluoro-5-androsten-17-one, and ellagic acid individually and in combination. *Cancer Res* 1991;51:4528–4534.

129. Fiorucci S, Meli R, Bucci M, Cirino G. Dual inhibitors of cyclooxygenase and 5-lipoxygenase. A new avenue in antiinflammatory therapy? *Biochem Pharmacol* 2001;62:1433–1438.

130. Williams JL, Borgo S, Hasan I, et al. Nitric oxide-releasing nonsteroidal anti-inflammatory drugs (NSAIDs) alter the kinetics of human colon cancer cell lines more effectively than traditional NSAIDs: implications for colon cancer chemoprevention. *Cancer Res* 2001;61:3285–3289.

131. Rigas B, Williams JL. NO-releasing NSAIDs and colon cancer chemoprevention: a promising novel approach (Review). *Int J Oncol* 2002;20:885–890.

132. Bak AW, McKnight W, Li P, et al. Cyclooxygenase-independent chemoprevention with an aspirin derivative in a rat model of colonic adenocarcinoma. *Life Sci* 1998;62:L-73.

133. Wechter WJ, Kantoci D, Murray ED Jr., et al. R-flurbiprofen chemoprevention and treatment of intestinal adenomas in the APC(Min)/+ mouse model: implications for prophylaxis and treatment of colon cancer. *Cancer Res* 1997;57:4316–4324.

134. Wechter WJ, Leipold DD, Murray ED Jr., et al. E-7869 (R-flurbiprofen) inhibits progression of prostate cancer in the TRAMP mouse. *Cancer Res* 2000;60:2203–2208.

135. Han S, Wada RK, Sidell N. Differentiation of human neuroblastoma by phenylacetate is mediated by peroxisome proliferator-activated receptor gamma. *Cancer Res* 2001;61:3998–4002.

136. Yoshimatsu K, Golijanin D, Paty PB, et al. Inducible microsomal prostaglandin E synthase is overexpressed in colorectal adenomas and cancer. *Clin Cancer Res* 2001;7:3971–3976.

137. Watanabe K, Kawamori T, Nakatsugi S, et al. Inhibitory effect of a prostaglandin E receptor subtype EP(1) selective antagonist, ONO-8713, on development of azoxymethane-induced aberrant crypt foci in mice. *Cancer Lett* 2000;156:57–61.

138. Kawamori T, Uchiya N, Nakatsugi S, et al. Chemopreventive effects of ONO-8711, a selective prostaglandin E receptor EP(1) antagonist, on breast cancer development. *Carcinogenesis* 2001;22:2001–2004.

139. Shureiqi I, Chen D, Lee JJ, et al. 15-LOX-1: a novel molecular target of nonsteroidal anti-inflammatory drug-induced apoptosis in colorectal cancer cells. *J Natl Cancer Inst* 2000;92:1136–1142.

140. Shureiqi I, Chen D, Lotan R, Yang P, Newman RA, Fischer SM, et al. 15-Lipoxygenase-1 mediates nonsteroidal anti-inflammatory drug-induced apoptosis independently of cyclooxygenase-2 in colon cancer cells. *Cancer Res* 2000;60:6846–6850.

141. Cormier RT, Hong KH, Halberg RB, et al. Secretory phospholipase Pla2g2a confers resistance to intestinal tumorigenesis. *Nat Genet* 1997;17:88–91.

142. Hong KH, Bonventre JC, O'Leary E, et al. Deletion of cytosolic phospholipase A(2) suppresses Apc(Min)-induced tumorigenesis. *Proc Natl Acad Sci* USA 2001;98:3935–3939.

143. Gately S. The contributions of cyclooxygenase-2 to tumor angiogenesis. *Cancer Metastasis Rev* 2000;19:19–27.

144. Williams CS, Tsujii M, Reese J, et al. Host cyclooxygenase-2 modulates carcinoma growth. *J Clin Investig* 2000;105:1589–1594.

145. Leung WK, To KF, Ng YP, et al. Association between cyclooxygenase-2 overexpression and missense p53 mutations in gastric cancer. *Br J Cancer* 2001;84:335–339.

146. Crosby CG, DuBois RN. The cyclooxygenase-2 pathway as a target for treatment or prevention of cancer. *Expert Opin Emerging Drugs* 2003;8:1–7.

147. Pai R, Szabo IL, Giap AQ, et al. Nonsteroidal anti-inflammatory drugs inhibit re-epithelialization of wounded gastric monolayers by interfering with actin, Src, FAK, and tensin signaling. *Life Sci* 2001;69:3055–3071.

148. Mann M, Sheng H, Shao J, et al. Targeting cyclooxygenase 2 and HER-2/neu pathways inhibits colorectal carcinoma growth. *Gastroenterology* 2001;120:1713–1719.

149. Howe LR, Subbaramaiah K, Patel J, et al. Celecoxib, a selective cyclooxygenase 2 inhibitor, protects against human epidermal growth factor receptor 2 (HER-2)/neu-induced breast cancer. *Cancer Res* 2002;62:5405–5407.

150. Sheng H, Shao J, DuBois RN. Akt/PKB activity is required for Ha-Ras-mediated transformation of intestinal epithelial cells. *J Biol Chem* 2001;276:14,498–14,504.

151. Miller C, Zhang M, He Y, et al. Transcriptional induction of cyclooxygenase-2 gene by okadaic acid inhibition of phosphatase activity in human chondrocytes: co-stimulation of AP-1 and CRE nuclear binding proteins. *J Cell Biochem* 1998;69:392–413.

152. Guo YS, Hellmich MR, Wen XD, Townsend CM, Jr. Activator protein-1 transcription factor mediates bombesin-stimulated cyclooxygenase-2 expression in intestinal epithelial cells. *J Biol Chem* 2001;276:22,941–22,947.

153. Subbaramaiah K, Cole PA, Dannenberg AJ. Retinoids and carnosol suppress cyclooxygenase-2 transcription by CREB-binding protein/p300-dependent and -independent mechanisms. *Cancer Res* 2002;62:2522–2530.

154. Subbaramaiah K, Lin DT, Hart JC, Dannenberg AJ. Peroxisome proliferator-activated receptor gamma ligands suppress the transcriptional activation of cyclooxygenase-2. Evidence for involvement of activator protein-1 and CREB-binding protein/p300. *J Biol Chem* 2001;276:12,440–12,448.

155. You Z, Saims D, Chen S, et al. Wnt signaling promotes oncogenic transformation by inhibiting c-Myc-induced apoptosis. *J Cell Biol* 2002;157:429–440.

156. Subbaramaiah K, Marmao TP, Dixon DA, Dannenberg AJ. Regulation of cyclooxygenase-2 mRNA stability by taxanes. Evidence for involvement of p38, MAPKAPK-2 and HuR@. *J Biol Chem* 2003.

157. Mukhopadhyay D, Houchen CW, Kennedy S, et al. Coupled mRNA stabilization and translational silencing of cyclooxygenase-2 by a novel RNA binding protein, CUGBP2. *Mol Cell* 2003;11:113–126.

158. Forman BM, Chen J, Evans RM. Hypolipidemic drugs, polyunsaturated fatty acids, and eicosanoids are ligands for peroxisome proliferator-activated receptors alpha and delta. *Proc Natl Acad Sci USA* 1997;94:4312–4317.

159. He TC, Chan TA, Vogelstein B, Kinzler KW. PPARdelta is an APC-regulated target of nonsteroidal anti-inflammatory drugs. *Cell* 1999;99:335–345.

160. Gupta RA, Tan J, Krause WF, et al. Prostacyclin-mediated activation of peroxisome proliferator-activated receptor delta in colorectal cancer. *Proc Natl Acad Sci USA* 2000;97:13,275–13,280.

161. Soslow RA, Dannenberg AJ, Rush D, et al. COX-2 is expressed in human pulmonary, colonic, and mammary tumors. *Cancer* 2000;89:2637–2645.

162. Nettelbeck DM, Rivera AA, Davydova J, et al. Cyclooxygenase-2 promoter for tumour-specific targeting of adenoviral vectors to melanoma. *Melanoma Res* 2003;13:287–292.

163. Denkert C, Kobel M, Berger S, et al. Expression of cyclooxygenase 2 in human malignant melanoma. *Cancer Res* 2001;61:303–308.

164. Uotila PJ, Erkkola RU, Klemi PJ. The expression of cyclooxygenase-1 and -2 in proliferative endometrium and endometrial adenocarcinoma. *Ann Med* 2002;34:428–433.

165. Tong BJ, Tan J, Tajeda L, et al. Heightened expression of cyclooxygenase-2 and peroxisome proliferator- activated receptor-delta in human endometrial adenocarcinoma. *Neoplasia* 2000;2:483–490.

166. Landen CN Jr., Mathur SP, Richardson MS, Creasman WT. Expression of cyclooxygenase-2 in cervical, endometrial, and ovarian malignancies. *Am J Obstet Gynecol* 2003;188:1174–1176.

167. Maitra A, Ashfaq R, Gunn CR, et al. Cyclooxygenase 2 expression in pancreatic adenocarcinoma and pancreatic intraepithelial neoplasia: an immunohistochemical analysis with automated cellular imaging. *Am J Clin Pathol* 2002;118:194–201.

168. Ding XZ, Tong WG, Adrian TE. Cyclooxygenases and lipoxygenases as potential targets for treatment of pancreatic cancer. *Pancreatology* 2001;1:291–299.

169. Furukawa F, Nishikawa A, Lee IS, et al. A cyclooxygenase-2 inhibitor, nimesulide, inhibits postinitiation phase of N-nitrosobis(2-oxopropyl)amine-induced pancreatic carcinogenesis in hamsters. *Int J Cancer* 2003;104:269–273.

170. Gunning WT, Kramer PM, Steele VE, Pereira MA. Chemoprevention by lipoxygenase and leukotriene pathway inhibitors of vinyl carbamate-induced lung tumors in mice. *Cancer Res* 2002;62:4199–4201.

171. Wenger FA, Kilian M, Achucarro P, et al. Effects of Celebrex and Zyflo on BOP-induced pancreatic cancer in Syrian hamsters. *Pancreatology* 2002;2:54–60.

6
Cyclooxygenase-2 Inhibitors and Colorectal Cancer Prevention

Raymond N. DuBois, MD, PhD

CONTENTS

1. INTRODUCTION

Colorectal cancer (CRC) causes approx 550,000 deaths worldwide each year, and is a major public health concern in most industrialized regions of the globe *(1)*. Once an individual is diagnosed with CRC, the disease is often advanced and treatment regimens are mostly ineffective and highly toxic. Alternative cytotoxic regimens are being developed which hold some promise for improved treatment responses *(2)*. Recently, selective cyclooxygenase-2 (COX-2) inhibitors have been evaluated for prevention or treatment of colorectal cancer. This chapter will review some of the key findings from both the laboratory and the clinic that have led to the hypothesis that COX-2 selective inhibitors may be useful in cancer prevention or treatment.

2. PRECLINICAL STUDIES

2.1. Cyclooxygenase Function and Biochemistry

The COX enzymes catalyze the enzymatic conversion of the endoperoxide intermediate prostaglandin $(PG)H_2$ from arachidonic acid (AA) *(3)*. PGH_2 is then converted to one of several structurally related PGs, including PGE_2, PGD_2, $PGF_2\alpha$, PGI_2, or Thromboxane A_2 (TXA_2), by specific PG synthases. The particular type of PG molecule produced by a cell is dependent on the predominant type of PG synthase isoform that is expressed. These bioactive lipids are lipid-soluble, and

can pass easily through lipid bilayer membranes. Specific PG transporters have been identified that presumably can facilitate transport of these molecules *(4)*. PGs act as local hormones near the site of their production, and are important in a broad number of physiological processes including blood clotting, ovulation, the initiation of labor, bone metabolism, nerve growth, development, wound healing, kidney function, blood vessel tone, and immune responses *(5)*. The importance of the COX pathway in human disease became obvious following the discovery in the 1970s that nonsteroidal antiinflammatory drugs (NSAIDs), a group of compounds used for more than a century in the treatment of various inflammatory disorders and fever, inhibited the activity of COX *(6)*.

2.2. Discovery of COX-2 and the Biochemistry of COX-2-Selective Inhibitors

Until recently, only one COX isoform (now known as COX-1) had been characterized. More than 10 years ago, two or three independent groups identified and cloned a second COX isoform, COX-2. Subsequent studies have brought forth a paradigm in which COX-1 is responsible for "housekeeping" PG biosynthesis, and is constitutively expressed in many tissues in the body *(7)*. COX-2, however, is not normally expressed in most tissues, but is induced by a variety of growth factors and pro-inflammatory cytokines in disease states. Based on this information, it was hypothesized

From: Cancer Chemoprevention, Volume 1: Promising Cancer Chemoprevention Agents
Edited by: G. J. Kelloff, E. T. Hawk, and C. C. Sigman © Humana Press Inc., Totowa, NJ

that the antiinflammatory and analgesic properties of traditional NSAIDs, which inhibit both COX-1 and COX-2, are most likely the result of their ability to inhibit COX-2 (8). In contrast, the gastric toxicity seen with chronic NSAID therapy may be caused by the inhibition of PG production mediated by COX-1. However, we now know that this was a gross oversimplification of the biological role of these enzymes, as COX-2 has been shown to play important roles in normal renal physiology (9).

Compounds that selectively inhibit the COX-2 isoform were developed by the pharmaceutical industry over a relatively short period of time. The best-known nonselective COX inhibitor, aspirin, inhibits COX enzymatic activity by covalent modification via acetylation of serine residue 530 in COX-1 and serine residue 516 in COX-2. In contrast, most other nonselective NSAIDs are competitive inhibitors that compete with the substrate—AA—for binding to the active site in both COX-1 and COX-2. Based on the availability of the three-dimensional structure of both COX-1 and COX-2, compounds that preferentially bind to the active site of COX-2 were synthesized (10). Currently available clinical evidence suggests that these COX-2-specific inhibitors (Coxibs) offer the therapeutic benefits of traditional NSAIDs, with a significant reduction in toxicity to the gastrointestinal mucosa (11,12). Finally, a new aspirin-like COX-2 inhibitor, APHS (o-(acetoxypheny)hept-2-ynyl sulfide), has been developed which is 21× more selective for COX-2 than COX-1 (13). Although this degree of selectivity is not as high as some of the other COX-2-selective inhibitors, APHS offers a unique advantage because it covalently modifies the enzyme, thus ensuring permanent inactivation of COX-2.

2.3. Effects of NSAIDs on Carcinogenesis

Early observational studies suggested that chronic use of NSAIDs might reduce cancer risk (see subheading 3). These observations led to a number of follow-up studies that examined the effects of these drugs in animal models of intestinal neoplasia (reviewed in ref. 14). One well-known murine model of colon cancer is the Min/+ mouse, which represents an animal model of the familial adenomatous polyposis (FAP) syndrome in humans. However, the mouse phenotype differs markedly from that seen in humans, since most of the adenomas in Min/+ mice occur in the small intestine instead of the colon. Several investigators have examined the ability of both nonselective

and COX-2-selective NSAIDs to inhibit polyposis using this model. Without exception, either nonselective or COX-2-selective inhibitors have proven to be potent suppressors of polyp formation in these mice. Another widely used animal model for colon cancer is the azoxymethane (AOM)-treated rat, in which the chemical carcinogen AOM induces preneoplastic colonic lesions known as aberrant crypt foci (ACF), which later progress to carcinomas. Both non-selective and COX-2-selective NSAIDs reduce the incidence, multiplicity, and size of colonic carcinomas in the AOM rat model.

2.4. Role of COX-2 in CRC Growth

The positive findings in animal models have restimulated additional research aimed at understanding the basic mechanism(s) by which NSAIDs inhibit CRC growth. Because the COX enzymes are the best-defined pharmacological targets of NSAIDs, one of the first considerations to emerge was the hypothesis that these drugs were inhibiting the presumed preneoplastic activity of either COX-1 and/or COX-2. This notion was supported by results that demonstrated increased levels of PGs in human colorectal tumors compared to normal adjacent colon (15) as well as in vitro experiments showing that some PGs can increase the growth of human CRC cells (16). In early attempts to examine the role of COX in CRC, several groups determined the levels of COX-1 and COX-2 in human colorectal adenomas and carcinomas (17,18). These results were consistent, and found that a comparison of neoplastic and adjacent normal tissue demonstrated little change in COX-1 expression, but increased levels of COX-2 in adenoma and adenocarcinoma tissue compared to the normal colonic mucosa.

This expression data suggested that NSAIDs suppress tumor growth via inhibition of COX-2. However, it could still be argued that elevated levels of COX-2 are simply a nonspecific result of the carcinogenic process, and that the enzyme has no direct role in promoting CRC growth. One way to determine the role of COX-2 in intestinal neoplasia is to use a genetic approach. Oshima et al. did this by evaluating the development of intestinal polyposis in Apc$^{\Delta 716}$ mice (a model similar to the Min/+ mouse) in a wild-type and homozygous null COX-2 genetic background (19). The number and size of polyps was reduced dramatically in the COX-2-null mice compared to COX-2 wild-type mice. In addition, treatment of the Apc$^{\Delta 716}$ COX-2 wild-type mice with a COX-2-selective inhibitor, MF tricyclic, reduced polyp numbers more significantly than sulindac. This experiment was one of the first to offer rigorous evidence in support of the hypothesis that NSAIDs inhibit tumor growth via inhibition of COX-2. More recent studies have confirmed a pro-oncogenic role for COX-2. For example, Liu et al. have demonstrated that overexpression of COX-2 alone is sufficient to induce cellular transformation (20). This group developed transgenic mice in which the murine mammary tumor virus (MMTV) promoter/enhancer directs COX-2 expression. Although virgin mice that overexpress COX-2 did not develop mammary tumors, multiparous mice showed significant increases in mammary gland carcinomas compared with age-matched controls. A related study by Neufang et al. has reported that transgenic expression of COX-2 in basal keratinocytes results in epidermal hyperplasia and dysplasia, suggesting a causal association between COX-2 expression and the development of preneoplastic lesions in the skin (21). However, Langenbach and colleagues have determined that lack of COX-1 can also reduce the number of adenomas in the Min/+ mouse model, indicating that in some situations, COX-1 can play a role in tumor promotion (22). Obviously, the precise role of COX-1 in carcinogenesis will require further investigation, but others have shown that COX-1 may not play a significant role in the process of tumor-associated angiogenesis (23,24).

2.5. COX-Independent Effects of NSAIDs

Many groups have now documented that high doses of NSAIDs can modify the biology of cultured cells independently of their ability to bind and inhibit COX-1 or COX-2. There is absolutely no doubt that NSAIDs can hit many other targets in the cell that can cause cell death. For example, transformed fibroblast-cell lines derived from wild-type, COX-1$^{-/-}$, COX-2$^{-/-}$, or COX-1$^{-/-}$/COX-2$^{-/-}$ mice all show comparable sensitivity to NSAID-induced cell death (25). Such results can be expected, since any xenobiotic agent is likely to have multiple targets, depending on the dose of the drug used. Non-COX cellular targets include IκB kinase β (26), the peroxisome proliferator-activated receptor (PPAR) family of nuclear hormone receptors (27,28), and the proapoptotic gene BAX (29). However, in all instances, "COX-independent" effects are seen at drug concentration(s) in the 50–1000 μM range. This is 10–200-fold higher than the serum concentration of celecoxib (approx 2–5 μM) required to inhibit tumor growth in animal models

of CRC (30). At these low concentrations, the best-characterized biochemical target of NSAIDs remains the COX enzymes, although it is likely that other unknown "high affinity" targets could be affected as well, and several groups are currently attempting to identify these targets.

2.6. COX-2: Mechanisms Underlying Neoplastic Effects

COX-2 protein has been found in both tumor epithelial cells and adjacent stromal cells. Thus, COX-2-derived PGs may be acting on the malignant epithelial cells or on the surrounding stromal cells, and there is evidence to support both effects.

Several studies suggest that forced expression of COX-2 in intestinal epithelial cell lines leads to changes in cellular pathways linked to carcinogenesis. For example, rat intestinal epithelial cells engineered to overexpress COX-2 have elevated levels of the anti-apoptotic protein Bcl-2 and exhibit increased resistance to apoptosis induced by sodium butyrate (31). In the Caco-2 cancer cell line, overexpression of COX-2 leads to an increase in cell migration and invasion that is associated with elevated levels of several members of the matrix metalloproteinase (MMP) family (32). This same cell line also secretes higher levels of several angiogenic factors compared with vector-transfected control cells, and promotes the formation of endothelial cell tubes when co-cultured with human umbilical-vein endothelial cells (33).

Several studies have suggested that COX-2 can also promote tumorigenesis through direct actions on the stromal compartment. These studies have largely centered on the ability of COX-2-derived PGs to stimulate tumor-associated angiogenesis. Using a model in which angiogenesis is evaluated in sponge implants injected with various growth factors, Majima et al. were one of the first groups to demonstrate that COX-2 inhibitors could block neovascularization (34,35). COX-2 inhibitors also blocked the migration of human microvascular endothelial cells and growth factor-induced corneal angiogenesis, effects that could be reconstituted with a TXA$_2$ agonist (36). A related study reported strong COX-2 immunoreactivity in tumor neovasculature in human colon, breast, prostate, and lung cancer biopsy tissue (23). In addition, corneal blood vessel formation in rats was potently suppressed by selective COX-2, but not COX-1, inhibitors. Jones et al. reported that both nonselective and COX-2-selective NSAIDs inhibit angiogenesis through direct actions on endothelial cells through both COX and non-COX mechanisms (37). Finally, a recent study provides genetic evidence that stroma-derived COX-2 can promote tumor growth through a landscaping mechanism (24). In this study, the growth of a lung cancer cell line was attenuated if engrafted onto COX-2$^{-/-}$ vs wildtype control mice. COX-2 expression within the stroma surrounding the tumor was localized primarily to fibroblasts, and cultured skin fibroblasts from the COX-2$^{-/-}$ mice exhibited defects in the basal secretion of several angiogenic growth factors. Collectively, this last set of experiments argues that COX-2 may modify tumor growth by limiting the ability of fibroblasts to support neovascularization within the microenvironment of a tumor. Recent experiments by Dormond et al. have helped to clarify the mechanism by which COX-2-derived PGs promote angiogenesis. Their studies demonstrated that COX-2-derived PGE$_2$ and PGI$_2$ play essential roles in αVβ3 integrin-mediated endothelial cell spreading and migration. Specifically, both PGs appear to be important in the activation of the small GTPases Cdc42/Rac that occurs following engagement of αVβ3 integrin with its substrate (38).

2.7. PG Receptors in CRC

The various classes of PGs exert their effects by binding to a G-protein-coupled cell-surface receptor that then leads to changes in the cellular levels of cyclic adenosine 3' 5' adenosine monophosphate and Ca^{2+} (for review, see ref. 39). In addition, studies increasingly suggest that PGs can also modulate cellular pathways by directly acting within the nucleus. For example, COX-2 has been localized to the perinuclear envelope (40) and the PGE$_2$ receptor (EP1) has been localized to the nuclear envelope in certain cell types, and activation of the receptor led to changes in nuclear levels of Ca^{2+} (41).

Studies on the role of specific PGs and PG receptors that act downstream of COX-2 during the progression of CRC have been limited. Several groups have reported elevated levels of the PG subtype PGE$_2$ in CRC biopsies compared with normal colonic mucosa (15,42). However, because many PGs are highly unstable, the physiological relevance of these studies is unclear. Furthermore, no systematic surveys have documented the expression of the known PG synthases and PG receptors in CRC tissues.

Several studies have reported a pro-carcinogenic effect of PGE$_2$ in cultured CRC cells. For example,

Sheng et al. reported a reduction in the basal apoptotic rate and increased levels of Bcl-2 after treatment of a human CRC cell line with PGE$_2$ (43). Exposure of a different colorectal cell line to PGE$_2$ led to an increase in cell proliferation and motility associated with activation of the phosphatidylinositol 3-kinase (PI3K)/Akt pathway, an effect probably caused by activation of the PGE$_2$-receptor subtype EP4 (44). A related study implicated PGE$_2$ in the ability of heregulin-beta1 to induce colon-cancer-cell migration and invasion (45). Genetic studies in mice suggest that PGE$_2$ promotes tumorigenesis at least in part by activating the EP1 receptor subtype. Mice with homozygous deletions in EP1, but not EP3, were partially resistant to AOM-mediated induction of ACF (46,47). Moreover, in AOM-treated wild-type mice, an EP1 receptor antagonist also decreased the incidence of ACF. Finally, Apc^{Min} mice treated with the same EP1 receptor antagonist had 57% fewer intestinal polyps than untreated mice. In contrast, Sonoshita et al. identified an important role for the EP2 receptor in CRC development. They examined the genetic role of all four PGE$_2$ receptors in the development of intestinal polyposis in Apc^{Δ716} mice. The number and size of intestinal polyps was significantly reduced only in mice that also harbored a homozygous deletion of the EP2 receptor (48).

3. NSAIDS AND CRC: CLINICAL RESEARCH

3.1. Observational Studies of CRC and NSAIDs

There are more than 14 published observational studies of the relationship between NSAID use and CRC incidence or mortality (49). This group of studies is remarkably consistent in demonstrating a protective effect of NSAIDs against the development of CRC. Only one of the studies failed to demonstrate a protective effect, and this study offered no methodological advantage over other studies in the group (50). The studies were carried out in three countries in a variety of settings (e.g., hospital-based, population-based, national surveys) utilizing various measures of aspirin and non-aspirin NSAID use (questionnaire and computerized pharmacy records).

Observational studies have demonstrated a protective effect for both aspirin and non-aspirin NSAIDs. The predominant theme to emerge from a comparison of the various studies is that consistent use of the drug is important to the achievement of statistically meaningful effects in cancer risk reduction (14). A second theme that emerges is that continual use of drug is also important, since attenuation of the chemopreventive effect is seen with as little as 1 yr of non-exposure. Most studies that have examined the duration of NSAID use have demonstrated increased risk reduction with more years of exposure. Finally, it should be noted that no large-scale observational studies have examined how the exposure to the new Coxib drugs affects CRC incidence.

3.2. Polyp Prevention in FAP Syndrome by Nonselective and COX-2-Selective NSAIDs

The first clinical observations of the effect of NSAIDs (sulindac) on adenoma formation occurred in groups of patients who had FAP syndrome. This disease is an autosomal dominant inherited condition marked by the development of hundreds to thousands of adenomatous polyps in the colon during early adulthood. Without an early colectomy, most of these patients will develop cancer in their 30s or 40s. In some centers, the patient undergoes a "subtotal colectomy," an operation that leaves behind the most distal colonic segment (rectum) in order to preserve normal rectal function. Because cancer may occur in this segment, these patients are usually followed with surveillance endoscopies during which polyps are identified and removed or biopsied.

Waddell noted a lack of polyps on a routine sigmoidoscopic surveillance exam in a single FAP patient who had received sulindac for other reasons (51). Subsequent randomized, controlled trials of polyp prevention in patients with FAP were carried out to determine whether NSAID use resulted in a significant clinical effect. The trial reported by Giardiello and colleagues is the most notable, and has served as a paradigm for subsequent studies (52). In this trial, sulindac or placebo was given to FAP patients who had previously undergone subtotal colectomy and who were engaged in a rectal screening program. Patients who received sulindac had a decrease in both the number and average size of their rectal polyps on exams at 3 and 6 mo. When the drug was stopped, the polyps increased in size and started to recur at the pretreatment rate. There were no such effects among those treated with placebo.

Recently the COX-2-selective drug, celecoxib, was tested as a potential chemopreventive agent in patients with FAP (53). This drug offers a potential advantage because it causes fewer serious GI side effects than traditional NSAIDs such as sulindac. The trial utilized celecoxib at two doses compared to placebo in cohorts of patients with FAP who were engaged in screening

regimens. There was a 28% reduction in polyp formation among those who took celecoxib at the higher dose (400 mg bid). Those who received celecoxib at the lower dose (100 mg bid) had a smaller (11%) nonsignificant decrease in the number of polyps at the follow-up endoscopy.

Thus, both traditional NSAIDs and at least one of the newer Coxib drugs decrease polyp formation in patients with FAP. It should be noted that authorities have recommended that NSAID therapy be considered only as a possible adjunct to established screening practices. The absolute decrease in polyps in the treatment groups is modest, and is not sufficient to replace standard screening practices and surgical intervention in FAP. Of some concern, there are case reports of cancer of the rectum occurring in patients with FAP who were on sulindac therapy (54) and the use of sulindac in preadolescents is not effective in reducing the polyp burden (55).

3.3. Future Clinical Studies of COX-2 Inhibitors and CRC

The current CRC chemoprevention trials underway are designed to test the efficacy of selective COX-2 inhibitors in preventing adenoma recurrence after polypectomy. These studies are not yet completed, and their design is similar to previously published studies of calcium carbonate in preventing polyp recurrence (56). In these studies, patients with sporadic polyps removed at an index colonoscopy are recruited from practices that provide screening colonoscopic examinations. The standard practice for most patients with adenomatous polyps would be to have a repeat colonoscopy in three years. Many of the chemoprevention studies incorporate a colonoscopy one year after the index exam to ensure that the colon has been "cleared" of polyps and that any polyps found on subsequent exams are "incident" polyps. Thus, the endpoint of interest is the recurrence rate of polyps at three or four years after the index date. The agents currently being tested in polyp prevention trials include aspirin and two of the COXIB drugs—celecoxib and rofecoxib.

No clinical data exists regarding the efficacy of COX-2 blockade therapy in the treatment of established CRCs. However, a number of clinical studies are underway to test the ability of COX-2 inhibitors to potentiate the effects of traditional anticancer regimens. There is emerging evidence from preclinical studies that combination therapy with COX-2 inhibitors and drugs that target other oncogenic pathways can lead to improved clinical outcomes. For example, two studies have recently reported enhanced antitumor efficacy in combination regimens consisting of an NSAID and an inhibitor that targets the ErbB/HER family of growth-factor receptors *(57,58)*.

4. SUMMARY

Although there is compelling evidence from both preclinical and clinical studies to suggest that targeted inhibition of COX-2 is a viable approach for CRC prevention and/or treatment, many questions remain unanswered. Future studies examining intestinal polyp susceptibility in mice with targeted deletions in specific PG synthases and receptors should help to clarify the mechanisms by which COX-2 promotes tumorigenesis. The precise signaling pathways and direct target genes that COX-2-derived PGs modulate in CRC cells are also largely unknown, and must be identified. Collectively, these experiments may lead to the discovery of novel and more potent inhibitors of CRC-cell growth.

ACKNOWLEDGMENTS

This work is supported in part from the United States Public Health Services Grants RO1DK 47279 (RND), P030 ES-00267-29 (RND), and P01CA-77839 (RND). RND is the Mina C. Wallace Professor. We also thank the T.J. Martell Foundation and the NCCRA for generous support. This chapter is an extensively modified and updated version of a review entitled "Colorectal Cancer Prevention and Treatment by Inhibition of Cyclooxygenase-2," *Nature Reviews Cancer* 1, 11–21 (2001).

REFERENCES

1. Greenlee RT, Murray T, Bolden S, Wingo PA. Cancer statistics, 2000. CA Cancer J Clin 2000;50:7–33.
2. Rothenberg ML. Irinotecan (CPT-11): recent developments and future directions—colorectal cancer and beyond. *Oncologist* 2001;6:66–80.
3. Smith WL, DeWitt DL, Garavito RM. Cyclooxygenases: structural, cellular, and molecular biology. *Annu Rev Biochem* 2000;69:145–182.
4. Kanai N, Lu R, Satriano JA, et al. Identification and characterization of a prostaglandin transporter. *Science* 1995;268:866–869.
5. DuBois RN, Abramson SB, Crofford L, et al. Cyclooxygenase in biology and disease. *FASEB J* 1998;12:1063–1073.
6. Vane JR. Inhibition of prostaglandin synthesis as a mechanism of action for aspirin-like drugs. *Nature* 1971;231:232–235.
7. Isakson P, Seibert K, Masferrer J, et al. Discovery of a better aspirin. *Adv Prostaglandins Thromboxane Leukot Res* 1995;23:49–54.
8. Masferrer JL, Zweifel BS, Manning PT, et al. Selective inhibition of inducible cyclooxygenase-2 in vivo is antiinflammatory and nonulcerogenic. *Proc Natl Acad Sci USA* 1994;91:3228–3232.
9. Harris RC, Breyer MD. Physiological regulation of cyclooxygenase-2 in the kidney. *Am J Physiol Renal Physiol* 2001;281:F1–F11.
10. Kurumbail RG, Stevens AM, Gierse JK, et al. Structural basis for selective inhibition of cyclooxygenase-2 by antiinflammatory agents. *Nature* 1996;384:644–648.
11. Silverstein FE, Faich G, Goldstein JL, et al. Gastrointestinal toxicity with celecoxib vs nonsteroidal antiinflammatory drugs for osteoarthritis and rheumatoid arthritis: the CLASS study: a randomized controlled trial. Celecoxib Long-term Arthritis Safety Study. *JAMA* 2000;284:1247–1255.
12. Bombardier C. An evidence-based evaluation of the gastrointestinal safety of coxibs. *Am J Cardiol* 2002;89:3D–9D.
13. Kalgutkar A, Crews B, Rowlinson S, et al. Aspirin-like molecules that covalently inactivate cyclooxygenase-2. *Science* 1998;280:1268–1270.
14. Smalley W, DuBois RN. Colorectal cancer and non steroidal antiinflammatory drugs. *Adv Pharmacol* 1997;39:1–20.
15. Rigas B, Goldman IS, Levine L. Altered eicosanoid levels in human colon cancer. *J Lab Clin Med* 1993;122:518–523.
16. Qiao L, Kozoni V, Tsioulias GJ, et al. Selected eicosanoids increase the proliferation rate of human colon carcinoma cell lines and mouse colonocytes in vivo. *Biochem Biophys Acta* 1995;1258:215–223.
17. Eberhart CE, Coffey RJ, Radhika A, et al. Up-regulation of cyclooxygenase-2 gene expression in human colorectal adenomas and adenocarcinomas. *Gastroenterology* 1994;107:1183–1188.
18. Kargman S, O'Neill G, Vickers P, et al. Expression of prostaglandin G/H synthase-1 and -2 protein in human colon cancer. *Cancer Res* 1995;55:2556–2559.
19. Oshima M, Dinchuk JE, Kargman SL, et al. Suppression of intestinal polyposis in APC$^{\Delta 716}$ knockout mice by inhibition of prostaglandin endoperoxide synthase-2 (COX-2). *Cell* 1996;87:803–809.
20. Liu HL, Chang SH, Narko K, et al. Over-expression of cyclooxygenase-2 is sufficient to induce tumorigenesis in transgenic mice. *J Biol Chem* 2001;276:18,563–18,569.
21. Neufang G, Furstenberger G, Heidt M, et al. Abnormal differentiation of epidermis in transgenic mice constitutively expressing cyclooxygenase-2 in skin. *Proc Natl Acad Sci USA* 2001;98:7629–7634.
22. Chulada PC, Thompson MB, Mahler JF, et al. Genetic disruption of Ptgs-1, as well as Ptgs-2, reduces intestinal tumorigenesis in Min mice. *Cancer Res* 2000;60:4705–4708.
23. Masferrer JL, Leahy KM, Koki AT, et al. Antiangiogenic and antitumor activities of cyclooxygenase-2 Inhibitors. *Cancer Res* 2000;60:1306–1311.
24. Williams CS, Tsujii M, Reese J, et al. Host cyclooxygenase-2 modulates carcinoma growth. *J Clin Investig* 2000;105:1589–1594.
25. Zhang X, Morham SG, Langenbach R, Young DA. Malignant transformation and antineoplastic actions of nonsteroidal antiinflammatory drugs (NSAIDs) on cyclooxygenase-null embryo fibroblasts. *J Exp Med* 1999;190:445–450.

26. Yin MJ, Yamamoto Y, Gaynor RB. The antiinflammatory agents aspirin and salicylate inhibit the activity of I(kappa)B kinase-beta. *Nature* 1998;396:77–80.

27. Lehmann JM, Lenhard JM, Oliver BB, et al. Peroxisome proliferator-activated receptors alpha and gamma are activated by indomethacin and other non-steroidal antiinflammatory drugs. *J Biol Chem* 1997;272:3406–3410.

28. Yamamoto Y, Yin MJ, Lin KM, Gaynor RB. Sulindac inhibits activation of the NF-kappaB pathway. *J Biol Chem* 1999;274:27,307–27,314.

29. Zhang L, Yu J, Park BH, et al. Role of BAX in the apoptotic response to anticancer agents. *Science* 2000;290:989–992.

30. Williams CS, Watson AJ, Sheng H, et al. Celecoxib prevents tumor growth in vivo without toxicity to normal gut: lack of correlation between in vitro and in vivo models. *Cancer Res* 2000;60:6045–6051.

31. Tsujii M, DuBois RN. Alterations in cellular adhesion and apoptosis in epithelial cells overexpressing prostaglandin endoperoxide synthase-2. *Cell* 1995;83:493–501.

32. Tsujii M, Kuwano S, DuBois RN. Cyclooxygenase-2 expression in human colon cancer cells increases metastatic potential. *Proc Natl Acad Sci USA* 1997;94:3336–3340.

33. Tsujii M, Kawano S, Tsuji S, et al. Cyclooxygenase regulates angiogenesis induced by colon cancer cells. *Cell* 1998;93:705–716.

34. Majima M, Isono M, Ikeda Y, et al. Significant roles of inducible cyclooxygenase (COX)-2 in angiogenesis in rat sponge implants. *Jpn J Pharmacol* 1997;75:105–114.

35. Majima M, Hayashi I, Muramatsu M, et al. Cyclo-oxygenase-2 enhances basic fibroblast growth factor-induced angiogenesis through induction of vascular endothelial growth factor in rat sponge implants. *Br J Pharmacol* 2000;130:641–649.

36. Daniel TO, Liu H, Morrow JD, et al. Thromboxane A$_2$ is a mediator of cyclooxygenase-2-dependent endothelial migration and angiogenesis. *Cancer Res* 1999;59:4574–4577.

37. Jones MK, Wang H, Peskar BM, et al. Inhibition of angiogenesis by nonsteroidal antiinflammatory drugs: insight into mechanisms and implications for cancer growth and ulcer healing. *Nat Med* 1999;5:1418–1423.

38. Dormond O, Foletti A, Paroz C, Ruegg C. NSAIDs inhibit alpha V beta 3 integrin-mediated and Cdc42/Rac-dependent endothelial-cell spreading, migration and angiogenesis. *Nat Med* 2001;7:1041–1047.

39. Sugimoto Y, Narumiya S, Ichikawa A. Distribution and function of prostanoid receptors: studies from knockout mice. *Prog Lipid Res* 2000; 39:289–314.

40. Morita I, Schindler M, Regier MK, et al. Different intracellular locations for prostaglandin endoperoxide H synthase-1 and -2. *J Biol Chem* 1995;270:10,902–10,908.

41. Bhattacharya M, Peri KG, Almazan G, et al. Nuclear localization of prostaglandin E2 receptors. *Proc Natl Acad Sci USA* 1998;95:15,792–15,797.

42. Giardiello FM, Spannhake EW, DuBois RN, et al. Prostaglandin levels in human colorectal mucosa: effect of sulindac in patients with familial adenomatous polyposis (FAP). *Gastroenterology* 1997;112:A568.

43. Sheng H, Shao J, Morrow J, et al. Modulation of apoptosis by prostaglandin treatment in human colon cancer cells. *Cancer Res* 1998;58:362–366.

44. Sheng H, Shao J, Washington MK, DuBois RN. Prostaglandin E2 increases growth and motility of colorectal carcinoma cells. *J Biol Chem* 2001;276:18,075–18,081.

45. Adam L, Mazumdar A, Sharma T, et al. A three-dimensional and temporo-spatial model to study invasiveness of cancer cells by heregulin and prostaglandin E2. *Cancer Res* 2001;61:81–87.

46. Watanabe K, Kawamori T, Nakatsugi S, et al. Inhibitory effect of a prostaglandin E receptor subtype EP(1) selective antagonist, ONO-8713, on development of azoxymethane-induced aberrant crypt foci in mice. *Cancer Lett* 2000;156:57–61.

47. Watanabe K, Kawamori T, Nakatsugi S, et al. Role of the prostaglandin E receptor subtype EP1 in colon carcinogenesis. *Cancer Res* 1999;59:5093–5096.

48. Sonoshita M, Takaku K, Sasaki N, et al. Acceleration of intestinal polyposis through prostaglandin receptor EP2 in ApcDelta716 knockout mice. *Nat Med* 2001;7:1048–1051.

49. DuBois RN, Giardiello FM, Smalley WE. Nonsteroidal antiinflammatory drugs, eicosanoids and colorectal cancer prevention. *Gastroenterol Clin N Am 1996;25:773–791.*

50. Paganini-Hill A, Hsu G, Ross RK, Henderson BE. Aspirin use and incidence of large-bowel cancer in a California retirement community. *J Natl Cancer Inst* 1991;83:1182–1183.

51. Waddell WR, Loughry RW. Sulindac for polyposis of the colon. *J Surg Oncol* 1983;24:83–87.

52. Giardiello FM, Hamilton SR, Krush AJ, et al. Treatment of colonic and rectal adenomas with sulindac in familial adenomatous polyposis. *N Engl J Med* 1993;328:1313–1316.

53. Steinbach G, Lynch PM, Phillips RKS, et al. The effect of celecoxib, a cyclooxygenase-2 inhibitor, in familial adenomatous polyposis. *N Engl J Med* 2000;342:1946–1952.

54. Matsuhashi N, Nakajima A, Shinohara K, et al. Rectal cancer after sulindac therapy for a sporadic adenomatous colonic polyp. *Am J Gastroenterol* 1998;93:2261–2266.

55. Giardiello FM, Yang VW, Hylind LM, et al. Primary chemoprevention of familial adenomatous polyposis with sulindac. *N Engl J Med* 2002;346:1054–1059.

56. Baron JA, Beach M, Mandel JS, et al. Calcium supplements for the prevention of colorectal adenomas. Calcium Polyp Prevention Study Group. *N Engl J Med* 1999;340:101–107.

57. Torrance CJ, Jackson PE, Montgomery E, et al. Combinatorial chemoprevention of intestinal neoplasia. *Nat Med* 2000;6:1024–1028.

58. Mann M, Sheng H, Shao J, et al. Targeting cyclooxygenase 2 and HER-2/neu pathways inhibits colorectal carcinoma growth. *Gastroenterology* 2001;120:1713–1719.

7 Lipoxygenases as Targets for Cancer Prevention

Susan M. Fischer, PhD
and Russell D. Klein, PhD

CONTENTS

1. LIPOXYGENASES

Although the cyclooxygenase (COX) metabolites of arachidonic acid (AA; 20:4; eicosatetraenoic acid) metabolism have received more attention than the metabolites of the lipoxygenases (LOX), there is growing evidence that inhibition of LOX offers an effective means of cancer (and other disease) prevention. As a family, LOX are dioxygenase enzymes that incorporate molecular oxygen into some polyunsaturated fatty acids, particularly AA and linoleic acid (LA; 18:2; octadecadienoic acid). LOX are widely distributed in plants, fungi, and mammals, but are absent in most bacteria and yeasts (1–3). The recognition that AA can be metabolized to COX and LOX products that are ligands for specific receptors has suggested their potential importance in regulating cell growth and/or differentiation. However, there is uncertainty regarding which metabolites are the most important or how they contribute to transformation, tumor growth, and metastases. It is the goal of this chapter to provide information on the known tissue distribution of the various LOX family members, their products, and the effect of inhibiting LOX in specific organ models of cancer.

1.1. Classification of Family Members

In animals, LOX enzymes are single polypeptides with a molecular mass of ~75–80 kDa, and contain a single non-heme iron in their large catalytic domains (1). Enzymatically, all LOX catalyze essentially the same three-step reaction. Only a limited number of polyunsaturated fatty acids can be utilized as substrates by LOX enzymes. For most—but not all—LOX, AA is the preferred substrate; LA (18:2) and eicosapentaenoic acid (20:5) can also be metabolized, although the V_{max} is generally less than that of AA (3). First, hydrogen is abstracted in a stereo-selective manner from double allelic methylene groups. Second, radical rearrangement occurs, which is accompanied by a Z,E-diene conjugation. Third, stereospecific (S- or R-) insertion of molecular dioxygen results in the formation of a hydroperoxy fatty acid—e.g., from AA, S- or R-hydroperoxyeicosatetraenoic acid (HPETE) is synthesized. HPETEs are reduced by cellular peroxidases to their corresponding hydroxyeicosatetraenoic acid (HETE). LA is metabolized to the S- or R-hydroperoxyoctadecadienoic acid that is reduced to hydroxyoctadecadienoic acid (HODE).

Most of the mammalian LOXs are S-LOX, although some R-LOX have been found (4). Detailed mechanisms of positional and enantiomeric specificity have been described (1,2,4–6). The particular carbon that is the site of oxygenation is determined by the particular LOX involved. LOX are categorized with respect to their positional specificity of AA oxygenation,—e.g., the 12-LOX produces 12-HETE, 8-LOX, 8-HETE, and so forth. However, positional specificity is not an absolute property because it depends on substrate structure and its alignment in the active site, as well as other conditions (4). To date, four LOX isoforms have been reported in mammals: 5-LOX, 8-LOX, the 12-LOXs, and the 15-LOXs. There is heterogeneity within

From: Cancer Chemoprevention, Volume 1: Promising Cancer Chemoprevention Agents
Edited by: G. J. Kelloff, E. T. Hawk, and C. C. Sigman © Humana Press Inc., Totowa, NJ

Table 1
Species-Specific Expression of Lipoxygenases

Position	Human	Mouse	Principal Product[a]
5	5(S)-LOX	5(S)-LOX	5-HETE
12	12(R)-LOX	12(R)-LOX	12(R)-HETE
	p12(S)-LOX	p12(S)-LOX	12-HETE
	[l12(S)-LOX]	l 12(S)-LOX	12-HETE
		e12(S)-LOX	12-HETE methyl esters
15	15(S)-LOX-1		13-HODE
	15(S)-LOX-2		15-HETE
8		8(S)-LOX	8-HETE

[a]The S- enantiomeric form, unless designated otherwise.

some isoform families, so that subclassification has been necessary. In mice, the 12(S)-LOX family is currently subdivided into platelet-type 12(S)-LOX, leukocyte-type 12(S)-LOX, and epidermis-type 12(S)-LOX. A 12(R)-LOX has also been identified in the murine and human epidermis. In humans, two 15(S)-LOX subfamilies have been found: the reticulocyte-type 15(S)-LOX, also referred to as 15-LOX-1; and the epidermis-type 15(S)-LOX, referred to as 15-LOX-2 (4).

LOX can be viewed as multifunctional enzymes because they occasionally oxygenate other carbons than the designated site—e.g., 15(S)-HETE can be synthesized by 12(S)-LOX. In addition, a particular stereospecific HPETE may serve as a substrate for a different LOX, resulting in two hydroperoxy groups—e.g., 15-HPETE can be oxygenated by 12(S)-LOX, resulting in di-HPETEs. 5(S)-LOX can transform its 5-HPETE product to an epoxide, a reaction that is required to synthesize leukotriene (LT) A_4, the precursor of the bioactive LTs: LTC_4 LTD_4, and LTE_4. Clearly, the multifunctional nature of LOX expands the repertoire of products considerably. What is not well understood is the extent to which this occurs in a given tissue or pathological condition, or what the biological functions of the various products are.

Not all mammals express the same families of LOX. As shown in Table 1, some LOX are expressed in humans but not mice, and others appear to be unique to mice (chosen for comparison here because of the extensive use of mice in experimental and preclinical studies). Because of differences in tissue distribution and in the function of many of the LOX products, an understanding of their role in cancer development requires an understanding of which LOX are preferentially expressed in a particular tissue, and how such expression is altered during neoplasia.

1.2. 5(S)-LOX

Of the four LOX subtypes, 5(S)-LOX has been the most extensively studied (reviewed in refs. 7–9). Of all the LOX family members only 5(S)-LOX is involved in the synthesis of LTs, which are mediators of anaphylactic and inflammatory disorders (2,10). LTs arise from the metabolism of 5-HPETE to LTA_4, the C-5 epoxide of AA, which can be converted to the peptidoleukotrienes, LTC_4, LTD_4, and LTE_4. The latter three molecules are components of the "slow reacting substance of anaphylaxis," and cause bronchial and vascular constriction during asthma attacks. They are also chemotactic for leukocytes, and thus play a major role in many inflammatory conditions (11).

5(S)-LOX is present in leukocytes, and in the lung, pancreas, small intestine, thymus, lymph nodes, spleen, and some parts of the brain. The levels of expression of 5(S)-LOX can be increased in at least some tissues by cytokines (5). 5(S)-LOX also differs from other LOXs because it must be activated through a process that involves calcium, adenosine 5' triphosphate (ATP), and a protein referred to as 5-lipoxygenase-activating protein (FLAP). It is currently hypothesized that nuclear membrane-bound FLAP mediates the transfer of AA to 5(S)-LOX; in the absence of FLAP, LTs cannot be synthesized, although 5-LOX is present. This implies that 5-LOX is inactive in the absence of FLAP, and that some type of inhibitory process is present that FLAP counteracts. The identity of this inhibitor is currently unknown (7–9). 5(S)-LOX activity can be pharmacologically inhibited by either direct inhibition of 5(S)-LOX or indirectly through inhibition of FLAP *(8)*.

Two types of receptors have been identified for LTs—plasma membrane and the nuclear peroxisome proliferator-activated receptors (PPARs). It has been suggested that activation of the plasma-membrane receptors is involved in paracrine effects of LTs, and that PPARs may mediate some of the autocrine effects *(8)*.

1.3. 12-LOXs

Several different 12-LOX genes (and thus enzymes) have been identified to date, which differ in stereospecificity and sometimes positional specificity. At least one form, the epidermal-type 12(S)-LOX (e12-LOX), is expressed in mice, but has not been found in humans (Table 1).

1.3.1. 12(S)-LOXs

12(S)-LOX occurs in three isoforms in mice—the platelet-, leukocyte-, and epidermis- types. In humans, the platelet-type or p12-LOX has been well-characterized *(12)*, and the leukocyte-type or l12(S)-LOX has been identified but not yet cloned *(1,10)*. The epidermis-type or e12(S)-LOX has not yet been found in humans. In mice, the three isoforms differ in tissue distribution, sequence homology, substrate affinity, and biological function. All three forms can metabolize AA into 12(S)-HPETE, which can be converted to either 12-HETE, hepoxillins, or lipoxins. Hepoxillins—monohydroxy epoxy forms of AA—play a role in releasing intracellular calcium and opening potassium channels. Lipoxins—trihydroxy forms of AA—are important in immune reactions. Many functions have been ascribed to 12-HETE, including chemotaxis, metastases, cell adhesion, and apoptosis *(11,13)*.

1.3.1.1. Platelet-Type 12(S)-LOX One of the primary functions of p12-LOX is regulation of thrombocyte activation, which involves translocation of adhesion molecules to the cell surface, resulting in platelet aggregation. The mechanisms are of interest because similar processes occur in tumor-cell metastasis. Autocrine motility-factor signaling results in p12(S)-LOX synthesis of 12-HETE, which activates protein kinase C (PKC), leading to translocation of cytoskeletal elements and eventually, to tumor-cell intravasation *(11,13)*.

p12(S)-LOX expression levels can be altered by transcriptional activation, as seen with epidermal growth factor (EGF) or transcriptional repression, as observed for the NFκB site in the human gene. In addition to platelets, p12(S)-LOX is expressed in epidermal keratinocytes and several epithelial tumor-cell lines *(14)*.

1.3.1.2. Leukocyte-Type 12(S)-LOX l12(S)-LOX has a rather broad tissue distribution, found in adrenal gland, pancreas, vascular smooth muscle, tracheal epithelium, and several regions of the brain, as well as other sites *(15)*. Little is known about the regulation of l12-LOX expression, except that in the mouse it can be induced by cytokines *(10)*. This LOX has a broad substrate affinity for C20, C18, and C22 fatty acids, unlike p12-LOX, which has a very strong preference for C20 fatty acids. Also unlike p12-LOX which prefers free fatty acid, l12-LOX can oxygenate AA that is esterified in membrane phospholipids. Thus, the biological outcome of p12-LOX and l12-LOX activity are probably very different *(11)*.

1.3.1.3. Epidermis-Type 12(S)-LOX This 12(S)-LOX differs from p12-LOX in substrate preference, because it has low affinities for LA and AA, but instead metabolizes the methyl esters of these fatty acids *(16)*. e12(S)-LOX is highly expressed in differentiated keratinocytes of the epidermis, in specific regions of the hair follicle, and in conjunctiva of the eyelid *(14)*, suggesting a role in differentiation. Unlike p12-LOX, e12(S)-LOX is not inducible by phorbol esters *(14–16)*.

1.3.2. 12(R)-LOX

In contrast to conventional LOXs, murine 12(R)-LOX uses methyl-AA, rather than free AA or LA, as a substrate. The products formed are both 12(R)-HETE-methyl ester and 12(R)-(HETE), which occurs as a result of hydrolysis *(17)*. Human 12(R)-LOX has also been cloned *(18)*; its expression is elevated in psoriasis and other proliferative disorders of the skin *(19)*. 12(R)-HETE has been reported to be a leukocyte chemotaxin with greater activity than 12(S)-HETE; however, it does not enhance cell adhesion like 12(S)-HETE (reviewed in ref. *20*).

1.4. 15(S)-LOXs

Like the family of 12-LOXs, the members of the 15(S)-LOX family differ in substrate preference, localization, and function. 15(S)-LOX have not been found in murine tissues, although they are expressed in rabbits and other mammals, including humans (reviewed in ref. *21*).

1.4.1. 15(S)-LOX-1

Unlike classical LOX, 15(S)-LOX-1 metabolizes LA to a much greater extent than AA. 15-LOX-1 has wide tissue distribution; it is expressed in the colon, skin, reticulocytes, liver, trachea, macrophages, and eosinophils (10,15,22–25). This enzyme was originally known as reticulocyte-type 15(S)-LOX because of its role in organelle degradation in the maturation of reticulocytes (26). This organelle-degrading activity has recently been extended to other tissues. In liver, 15(S)-LOX-1 is responsible for programmed degradation of peroxisomes (25). It is also associated with differentiation of tracheobronchial epithelial cells (24). 15(S)-LOX-1 is a highly regulated gene; expression is regulated at the transcriptional, translational, and post-translational levels, including calcium-mediated membrane association (15,21). Recently, 15(S)-LOX-1 was shown to be upregulated by nonsteroidal antiinflammatory drugs (NSAIDs) in a COX-2-independent manner. This upregulation of 15(S)-LOX-1 was further demonstrated to be responsible for NSAID-induced apoptosis in colon and esophageal cancer cells through the generation of the LA metabolite 13-HODE (27–28). In Balb/c 3T3 and Syrian hamster embryo cells, however, 13-HODE was reported to be necessary for growth factor-dependent mitogenesis (29).

1.4.2. 15(S)-LOX-2

15(S)-LOX-2 differs from 15(S)-LOX-1 because it has a distinct preference for AA, and LA is metabolized at one-third the efficiency of AA. In addition to carrying out its activities directly, 15-HETE can be selectively incorporated into phosphatidilinositol. Upon deacylation, it is converted to the 5,15-DiHETE, lipoxinA$_4$ and lipoxin B$_4$ (30). Also, unlike 15(S)-LOX-1, 15(S)-LOX-2 has limited tissue localization, with expression restricted to the lung, prostate, cornea, and skin; it is undetectable in the spleen, thymus, small intestine, colon, liver, kidney, or pancreas (31,32). The regulation of 15(S)-LOX-2 expression has only recently been examined. Membrane association is required for full activity, and occurs in a calcium-dependent manner. Splice variants of 15(S)-LOX-2 have been observed, and some of these have increased specific activities (33). 15-HETE, the major product of 15(S)-LOX-2, has been implicated as an antiinflammatory eicosanoid because of its ability to inhibit 5(S)-LOX production of LTs (34). 15-HETE has also been implicated in cell proliferation, although whether it enhances or inhibits appears to be dependent on cell type (35,36).

1.5. 8(S)-LOX

8-LOX is found in murine—but not human—epidermis, particularly in the suprabasal layers (1,37,38).

8(S)-LOX is highly inducible by phorbol esters in those strains of mice that produce a strong inflammatory response to phorbol esters (38,39). This LOX preferentially converts AA to 8-HETE, but can convert LA to 9-HODE, although at lower efficiency (40). Recently, at least one function of 8-HETE in keratinocytes was determined: the induction of keratin-1, a marker of keratinocyte differentiation. This occurs through 8-HETE activation of PPARα (41).

2. LOX INHIBITORS

Agents that inhibit one or more LOX can be classified either by target, (e.g., specific LOX that is inhibited) or by type of compound (e.g., flavonoids). As specific LOXs appear to be involved in particular types of cancer, it will probably be more valuable to consider inhibitors based on their specificity for a particular LOX. The reader is also referred to several excellent reviews of LOX inhibitors (42–45).

2.1. Nonselective Inhibitors of LOX and COX

A wide variety of plant products inhibit both LOXs and COXs. Inhibitory activity for most of these compounds is probably the result of their antioxidant characteristics. Nearly all have polyphenolic structures, and also inhibit oxidative stress (46). Thus, although they may be potent chemopreventive agents, assigning the mechanism to the inhibition of specific enzymes must be done carefully.

2.1.1. Tea

Black and green tea, and the polyphenols derived from them, have been studied extensively as cancer-prevention agents (reviewed in refs. 43,47–49). Many, but not all, epidemiology studies have indicated that black or green tea protects against cancers of the breast, colon, gallbladder, liver, lung, nasopharynx, pancreas, stomach, and uterus (43,49,50). In rodent models, protection was seen against cancers of skin, lung, esophagus, stomach, liver, duodenum, small intestine, pancreas, and mammary gland. Green and black tea (4.0 and 4.4 mg/mL tea solids in drinking water) reduced skin carcinomas by at least 80% (47), particularly in skin UV carcinogenesis. Green tea polyphenols (0.1% wt/vol) also significantly delayed tumor appearance and burden in the TRAMP model of spontaneous murine prostate cancer (51). As a result of the many positive preclinical studies, green tea and epigallocatechin-3-gallate (EGCG) are in clinical trials to test for a reduction in skin, head and neck, and colon cancers *(43)*.

The active ingredients in green tea are believed to be primarily the catechins, which include the polyphenols EGCG, epigallocatechin (EGC), and epicatechin-3-gallate (ECG), with EGCG as the most abundant *(52)*. Black tea, a fermented product, contains reduced levels of catechins because they have been converted to theaflavins and thearubigins. A number of different mechanisms have been proposed for the anticancer effects of tea, including inhibition of COX and LOX, ornithine decarboxylase activity, protein kinase C (PKC), and Akt signaling *(52)*. With regard to LOX and COX inhibition, all the polyphenols—e.g., EGCG, EGC, ECG, and the theaflavins and thearubigins, inhibited LOX and COX activity by 30–75% at 30 μg/mL doses. ECG was the most potent inhibitor of both LOX and COX. A recent study suggests that COX-2 may not be inhibited as strongly by tea polyphenols. Additionally, black tea theaflavins may enhance prostaglandin (PG) synthesis from COX-2, although the extent to which this affects tumor development is unknown *(52)*.

2.1.2. CURCUMIN AND DERIVATIVES

Curcumin, a polyphenolic phytochemical, is a yellow spice from turmeric that is often used to flavor curries and mustards. Turmeric has been used in Southeast Asia and in India to treat inflammation and skin wounds; this is a reflection of its antiinflammatory and antioxidant properties (reviewed in ref. *43*). Clinical trials are being conducted with curcumin to evaluate its effectiveness in preventing cancer of the oral cavity, colon, and breast. In experimental animal studies, curcumin has been shown to inhibit carcinogen adduct formation in phorbol ester promotion of tumors in skin *(43)*, and benzopyrene-induced forestomach and lung tumorigenesis *(53)*. Dietary doses of 0.5–2.0% curcumin were needed to achieve ~50% tumor inhibition *(53)*, and 2% dietary curcumin also reduced azoxymethane(AOM)-induced colon adenocarcinoma incidence by ~100% *(47)*.

Among its other activities, curcumin has been shown to reduce the formation of LOX and COX metabolites in colon and liver *(43)*. In mouse epidermal enzyme preparations, 3–10 μM curcumin inhibited 5- and 8-HETE synthesis by 40–60%; these same doses inhibited PG synthesis by ~20–70% *(54)*. Curcumin inhibits LOX through binding to the catalytic site *(55)*; the mechanism for inhibition of PG synthesis

is unknown. Curcumin is also a potent inhibitor of inducible nitric oxide synthase (iNOS), PKC, EGF-receptor tyrosine kinase, and IκB kinase *(47)*. It is unknown to what extent these or the LOX/COX-inhibitory activities of curcumin are responsible for its cancer-prevention efficacy.

Several structurally related derivatives of curcumin, chlorogenic acid, caffeic acid, and ferulic acid, have also been investigated. These derivatives were considerably less active than curcumin in inhibiting phorbol ester-induced ornithine decarboxylase (ODC) activity, edema, DNA synthesis, and skin-tumor promotion. With epidermal preparations, these derivatives had IC_{50} values of >100 μM for 5- and 8-HETE synthesis, which is very high compared to curcumin. The correlation between the ability of curcumin and its derivatives to reduce epidermal inflammation and LOX/COX activities suggest the importance of these eicosanoids in tumor promotion *(54)*. However, for caffeic acid, other studies have reported strong LOX-inhibitory activity, with an IC_{50} of 3.7–72 μM for 5-LOX and 5.1–30 μM for 15-LOX *(56,57)*.

2.1.3. RESVERATROL

Resveratrol (*trans*-3,4′,5-trihydroxystilbene) occurs in the skin of grapes and some other plants, and thus is present in red but not white wines (reviewed in ref. *58*). Epidemiological studies suggest that the consumption of red wine reduces the incidence of mortality from coronary heart disease. The protective effect has been linked to the polyphenols, particularly resveratrol *(59)*. Although little epidemiological evidence is available, studies in animals suggest that resveratrol has chemopreventive efficacy in several organ models. When topically applied, it significantly inhibited skin tumor development in the two-stage mouse model *(60)*. Resveratrol was also reported to inhibit the multiplicity of colorectal aberrant crypt foci (ACF) in rats fed 20 μg/kg/d *(61)*, to suppress invasion of hepatoma cells (100–200 μM) *(62)*, and to cause apoptosis of an ascites hepatoma *(63)*.

Inhibition of tumor-cell growth has been linked to the antioxidant activity of resveratrol and its ability to inhibit 5-LOX and COX-2 (IC_{50} of 4.5 μM for 5-LOX, 40 μM for 15-LOX, and 35 μM for COX) *(64)*. However, there is also evidence that resveratrol affects AP-1 activity and inhibits activation of the NFκB signaling pathway *(43)*. Because resveratrol displays numerous properties related to very different mechanisms of action, it is difficult to determine the extent to which inhibition of LOX plays a role in the efficacy of resveratrol *(65)*.

2.1.4. ACETYLENIC FATTY ACIDS AND OTHER COMPOUNDS

Several acetylenic fatty acids have been used as nonselective inhibitors of LOX and COX, although some have some selectivity for LOX. Eicosatetraynoic acid (ETYA) is an irreversible suicide inhibitor that inhibits all isoforms of LOX with an IC_{50} of 4 μM; the IC_{50} for COX-1 is 8 μM *(66)*. When applied topically, 100-μg doses of ETYA were shown to inhibit phorbol ester skin tumor promotion by 75% *(67)*. Recently, ETYA was also found to be a ligand for PPARs at a slightly higher IC_{50} (10 μM) *(68)*, which can make interpretation of its biological effects less than straightforward. 5,8,11-Eicosatriynoic acid (ETI) preferentially inhibits LOX over COX, with IC_{50}s of 24 μM for human p12-LOX and 340 μM for COX *(66)*. 5,6-dehydroarachidonic acid inhibits 5-LOX with IC_{50} values of 10–15 μM *(69)*, and 8,11,14-eicosatriynoic acid (EtriYA), which lacks the triple bond between C5 and C6, cannot inhibit 5-LOX, although it rapidly inactivates 12- and 15-LOX *(10)*. Interestingly, 15(S)-HETE can inhibit both 5- and 12-LOXs *(70)*.

The selenoorganic compound ebselen, a glutathione peroxidase mimic, is a scavenger of peroxynitrite *(71)*. It also inhibits LOX and COX, although this inhibition is lost in the presence of glutathione *(10)*. Another dual inhibitor, phenidone (1-phenyl-3-pyrazolidinone), has an IC_{50} of 24 μM for LOX and an IC_{50} of 11.8 μM for COX. When combined with COX inhibitors indomethacin or sulindac, phenidone reduced the number of lung metastases in the Lewis lung model *(72)*. Applied topically with phorbol esters, phenidone (100 μg) reduced murine skin-tumor incidence by 45% *(67)*.

2.2. Selective 12-LOX Inhibitors

2.2.1. BAICALEIN

Baicalein is a flavonoid isolated from *Scutellaria baicalenis* Georgy roots, one of the seven ingredients that makes up the Japanese herbal Sho-saiko-to *(45,73)*, widely used to treat chronic hepatitis. In addition to suppressing the growth of hepatocellular carcinoma cell lines, Sho-saiko-to was reported to inhibit growth and metastasis of a murine malignant melanoma. The active ingredient was shown to be baicalein *(73)*. In in vitro studies, baicalein was reported to have antiproliferative effects in bladder cancer cell lines *(74)*, prostate cancer cell lines *(75)*, and others at micromolar levels *(45,76)*.

Treatment of human prostate cancer cells Du145 and PC-3 with 25 μM baicalein decreased proliferation by 50% and resulted in apoptosis in 63% and 39% of the cells, respectively. Adding back 12-HETE, but not 5- or 15-HETE, prevented baicalein-induced apoptosis, indicating the specificity of the response *(77)*. Topical application of baicalein at micromolar levels to mouse skin significantly inhibited tumor development, as well as ODC activity and edema *(78)*. The IC_{50} of baicalein has been reported to be 0.12 μM for rat platelet 12-LOX, and >100 μM is needed for COX inhibition *(79)*. Baicalein has potent free-radical scavenging actions, however; its antiproliferative effects may not be completely caused by its 12-LOX inhibitory activity *(80)*.

2.2.2. HYDROXAMIC ACIDS

A number of hydroxamic acids have been studied and used as selective 12-LOX inhibitors. Hydroxamic acids were created as substrate analogs, containing an iron-chelating functionality. Several hydroxamic acids of AA have been shown to be inhibitors of 5-LOX, and others predominantly inhibit 12-LOX *(81)*. The hydroxyamic acids salicyl- and naphthyl-hydroxamate are effective 15-LOX inhibitors *(21)*. N-benzyl-N-hydroxy-5-phenylpentanamide (BHPP) was reported to inhibit 12-LOX at sub- to micromolar levels *(45)*. BHPP was also used to demonstrate a role for endothelial-cell 12-HETE in angiogenesis *(82)*. Mouse melanoma cells and Lewis lung carcinoma cells were used to show selective inhibition of 12-HETE synthesis by BHPP and an 80% reduction in cell adhesion at doses of $10^{-5}M$. In addition, 25–50 mg/kg oral doses inhibited lung colony formation by Lewis lung cells by 25–50% *(83)*. A novel synthetic cyclic hydroxamic compound, BMD188, was reported to inhibit the growth of PC-3 prostate cancer cell lines by 50% at doses of ~10 μM. Normal prostate epithelial cells demonstrated a two- to fivefold lower cytotoxicity to BMD188, indicating a desirable selectivity for tumor cells. However, the apoptotic effects of BMD188 were not caused by 12-LOX inhibition, since 12-LOX was not detected in PC-3 cells *(84)*. This finding suggests that care should be taken in interpreting data using BMD188, although it is potentially a useful chemopreventive agent via other mechanisms.

2.3. Selective 5-LOX Inhibitors

2.3.1. 5-LOX-ACTIVATING PROTEIN INHIBITORS

Inhibition of the 5-LOX pathway can be achieved by several mechanisms, including inhibition of FLAP, inhibition of 5-LOX itself, and interference with LT binding to its receptors. The FLAP inhibitor MK886, an indole originally identified as a potent inhibitor of LT synthesis, was reported to cause massive apoptosis at 10 μM in human prostate cancer cells. This effect could be inhibited by addition of 5-HETE, supporting the conclusion that the 5-LOX pathway is essential to prostate-cancer-cell survival (85). Oral administration of MK886 (0.08 mmol/kg body wt/d) was reported to reduce chemically induced lung cancer in A/J mice by approx 50% (42). Recently, MK886 was shown to cause apoptosis in several cell types through a FLAP-independent mechanism. AA886 was also reported to inhibit PPARα (but not PPAR β or δ), although this does not appear to be the mechanism by which it induces apoptosis (86). However, it is clear that the multiple activities of MK886 must be considered when evaluating the role of 5-LOX in cell survival or other behaviors.

2.3.2. SELECTIVE 5-LOX INHIBITORS

Selective inhibitors of 5-LOX include AA861 (docebenone or 2,3,5 trimethyl-6-(12-hydroxy-5,10-dodecadiynyl)-1,4-benzoquinone), which has been used to demonstrate a role for 5-HETE in the proliferation and vascular EGF expression of malignant mesothelial cells (87). Non-small-cell lung cancer cells (NSCLC) are also inhibited by AA861, with an IC_{50} of 7 μM. Another inhibitor, nordihydroguaiaretic acid (masoprocol, NDGA), which has IC_{50} values of 0.2, 30, and 30 μM for 5-, 12- and 15-LOX (88), has also been used as a 5-LOX inhibitor. Ten μM NDGA significantly reduced the clonogenicity of NSCLC cells and their growth as a xenograft in mice (89). When included in the diet at 1000 mg/kg diet, NDGA reduced chemically induced mammary cancer incidence and multiplicity in rats by 30–40% (90). However, whether this was a result of inhibition of 5-LOX or all the LOXs is unknown. NDGA has also been used to significantly reduce human actinic keratosis in a clinical setting (91). Based on recent studies showing that NDGA delays the growth of pancreatic and cervical tumors established in athymic mice, it was suggested that NDGA should be considered as a lead compound in the development of novel therapeutic agents for a variety of cancer types (92).

Gossypol, a polyphenolic pigment in cottonseed, is an inhibitor of both 5-LOX (IC_{50} = 0.3 μM) and 12-LOX (IC_{50} = 0.7 μM), and has been demonstrated to inhibit the growth of several types of malignant cells. Gossypol was reported to significantly inhibit the human prostate cancer cell line PC-3 at doses of 1–2 μM; the mechanism of growth arrest appears to involve an upregulation of transforming growth factor (TGF)β (93). Recently, it was shown that the (−) enantiomer of gossypol has much higher anticancer activity than the (+) enantiomer in regard to inhibiting breast cancer cell growth (94). Gossypol has been used in several clinical trials on advanced and/or metastatic cancers, although it was only effective in metastatic adrenal cancer (95–97). A potential side effect of using gossypol as a cancer prevention agent is its contraceptive activity in men (98).

A potent N-hydroxyurea 5-LOX inhibitor is zileuton ([N-(1-benzo[b]-thien-2yl)ethyl)-N-hydroxyurea]), which has shown efficacy in a number of human inflammatory conditions (99). In vitro studies showed growth-inhibitory activity for zileuton against murine adenocarcinomas, although it was less effective when these tumor cells were grown in vivo (100). Recently, zileuton was shown to reduce vinyl carbamate-induced lung tumors in mice by 28.1%, along with a reduction in tumor size and in the progression of adenomas to carcinoma. The 1200 mg/kg dose is comparable to human doses for treating asthma, suggesting the possible use of this drug (Zyflo, Abbott Laboratories) in human lung cancer prevention (101). Zileuton (28 mg daily) was also shown to reduce the incidence and size of established pancreatic cancers in Syrian hamsters (102); this suggests that zileuton may have therapeutic efficacy as well.

Newer N-hydroxyurea-containing 5-LOX inhibitors have a long duration of action. The most active of these is R(+)-N-[3-[5-(4-fluorophenoxy)-2-furanyl]-1-methyl-2-propynyl]-N-hydroxyurea (A79175; AT175), a selective 5-LOX inhibitor with an IC_{50} of 25 nM in human polymorphonuclear leukocytes. This compound also inhibited LT formation in the rat with oral ED_{50}s of 1–2 mg/kg (103). Although the use of this compound in cancer prevention has not been extensively studied, oral administration of 0.37 mmol/kg/d has been reported to inhibit carcinogen-induced lung tumor multiplicity in mice by 75% (42).

2.3.3. LT RECEPTOR ANTAGONISTS

For tumors in which LTs play a role in proliferation or other events, agents that are antagonists of LT receptors offer possible avenues of chemoprevention. Accolate (Zafirlukast; cyclopentyl 3-[2-methoxy-4-{[o-toylsulfonyl]benzyl}-1-methylindole-5-carbanate), orally administered at 540 mg/kg, reduced vinyl carbamate-induced lung tumors in mice by approx 30% *(101)*. SC41930, a competitive antagonist of LTB$_4$, abrogated the proliferative effects of LTB$_4$ in HT-29 human colon carcinoma cells *(104)*. However, in cell types such as MCF-7 human mammary cancer cells, LTB$_4$ is growth inhibitory *(105)*. This suggests that a better understanding of the function of LTs in various tissues is needed in order to determine the appropriateness of LT antagonists as chemopreventive agents

2.4. Selective 15-LOX Inhibitors

Studies of the role of either 15-LOX-1 or 15-LOX-2 have been hampered by the lack of selective inhibitors. One study used caffeic acid at 2.2 μM (IC$_{50}$ is 0.8 μM), which is at least fivefold less than the IC$_{50}$s for 5- or 12-LOX or the COXs, to prevent the apoptotic effect of upregulated 15-LOX-1 in colon-cancer cells *(106,107)*. PD 146 176, a selective 15-LOX inhibitor, was recently developed, but it has not been studied outside the atherosclerosis field *(108)*.

3. LOX INVOLVEMENT IN CANCER

3.1. Prostate Cancer

Recent studies indicate that LOX enzymes may play an important role in regulating prostate carcinogenesis. Several LOXs are reported to be expressed in human prostate tissue or cell lines, including 5(S)-LOX, platelet-type 12(S)-LOX, 15(S)-LOX-1, and 15(S)-L0X-2. The role of lipoxygenase in prostate cancer was recently reviewed by Nie et al. *(109)*.

In one study of 22 matched benign and malignant samples from radical prostatectomies, Gupta et al. *(110)* found increased 5-LOX expression in malignant tissues. 5-LOX mRNA was reported to be sixfold higher in malignant tissue as determined by RT-PCR, and protein expression and 5-HETE synthesis were significantly (*p* < 0.001) increased in malignant tissues: 2.6- and 2.2-fold, respectively. However, there is some question as to the validity of the RT-PCR data, as the reported size of the amplified product does not match the expected size *(109)*. In contrast to these results, no 5-LOX enzyme activity was detected in surgical specimens of benign or malignant prostate tissues tested by Shappell et al. *(111)*. Additionally, 5-LOX protein and RNA expression were found to be much higher in cultured normal prostate epithelial cells compared to prostate carcinoma cell lines *(112)*. Therefore, further studies are needed to confirm the overexpression of 5-LOX in malignant prostate tissue.

Selective inhibitors of 5-LOX or FLAP have been reported to inhibit growth *(113,114)* and induce apoptosis *(85,115)* of prostate cancer cell lines. The FLAP inhibitor MK886 caused apoptosis in all prostate cell lines tested, yet results with other 5-LOX selective inhibitors have been less consistent. Ghosh et al. *(114)* reported that AA861 reduced cell growth and induced apoptosis in PC-3 prostate carcinoma cells, but this inhibitor had virtually no effect on prostate cell death in studies by Tang et al. *(115)*. Another 5-LOX inhibitor, SC41661A, appeared to induce cell death by a different mechanism than MK886 in PC-3 cells *(114)*. The dose of MK886 required to induce apoptosis in PC-3 cells is far greater than the dose required to inhibit 5-LOX activity in other systems (reviewed in ref. *109*). In addition, the prostate cancer cell lines PC-3 and LNCaP express very low levels of FLAP or none at all *(115)*. It is therefore highly likely that MK886 induces apoptosis in prostate cancer cell lines through a mechanism other than FLAP inhibition, a possibility supported by the recent finding that MK886 is a PPARα antagonist *(86)*. The role of 5-LOX in protecting prostate cells from apoptosis clearly requires further study before inhibitors of 5-LOX enzyme activity can be recommended for clinical prevention trials.

Expression of p12-LOX was observed by Gao et al. *(116)* in a study of 122 matching normal and cancerous prostate tissue samples taken from radical prostatectomies. Elevation of 12-LOX RNA was present in 38% of cancerous tissue compared to matched normal tissue. In addition, elevated 12-LOX RNA correlated with advanced stage and a higher grade of prostate cancer among cases. However, Shappell et al. *(111)* did not detect 12-HETE from prostate cancer tissue homogenates incubated with exogenous AA, indicating a lack of 12-LOX activity. In addition, although Timar et al. *(117)* reported strong expression of p12-LOX protein by Western analysis in LNCaP, Du145, TSU, and PPC-1 prostate cancer-cell lines, Tang et al. *(112)* were unable to detect any p12-LOX protein in these cell lines. This contradiction could be the result of differences in immunoblotting protocols; however, the issue is currently unresolved. We have detected significant levels of 12-HETE in media from cultured Du145, LNCaP, and PC-3 cells, indicating the presence of 12-LOX activity in these cells (unpublished results). Further analysis of endogenous 12-HETE levels in prostate-cancer tissue is clearly necessary to determine the importance of this LOX product in prostate cancer progression.

The ability of 12-LOX to affect biological processes involved in the progression of prostate cancer has been tested in a number of cell-culture models. PC-3 cells stably transfected with p12-LOX grew faster and were more angiogenic when injected subcutaneously into athymic nude mice (118). Treatment of Du145 cells with the 12-LOX-specific inhibitor BHPP (117) prior to tail-vein injection into severe combined immuno-deficiency (SCID) mice significantly decreased lung colonization compared to untreated Du145 cells. Furthermore, treatment of PC-3 and Du145 cells with 12-LOX inhibitors baicalein or BHPP blocked cell-cycle progression and induced apoptosis. Cell-cycle inhibition and apoptosis induced by baicalein was attributed to a reduction in Rb phosphorylation and decreased Akt phosphorylation, respectively. The addition of 12-HETE to cultures prior to baicalein treatment protected Du145 cells from phospho-Rb reduction and apoptosis. Cell signaling induced by 12-HETE has been extensively reviewed (109), and includes activation of PKCα and PI-3-kinase and subsequent activation of the p42/p44 MAP kinase and Akt pathways.

15-LOX-1 and 15-LOX-2, two 15-LOX enzymes expressed in human prostate tissues, differ both in their substrate specificity and their expression patterns in prostate cancer development. Elevated expression of 15-LOX-1 protein, as determined by immunohisto-chemistry, has been reported in prostate carcinomas (118). In an analysis of 48 radical prostatectomies, 15-LOX-1 protein was elevated in 75% of cancers compared to their adjacent normal tissue, and 15-LOX-1 expression correlated positively with the presence of p53 mutations and higher Gleason grade scores. Spindler et al. (119) also reported an elevation of 13-HODE in prostate cancers compared to adjacent normal tissue, as determined by immunohistochemistry. Expression of 15-LOX-1 protein has also been observed in cultured prostate cancer cell lines (112,120,121), although expression does not appear to be elevated compared to normal prostate epithelial cell isolates (112).

13-(S)-Hydroxyoctadecanoic acid (13-HODE), is synthesized from LA, the preferred substrate for 15-LOX-1. There is substantial evidence that 13-HODE enhances cellular proliferation in a variety of cell types (reviewed in ref. 122). There are also reports that 13-HODE is proapoptotic in colon and esophageal cell lines (28,123), and therefore might be anticarcino-genic. Overexpression of 15-LOX-1 in PC-3 cells resulted in increased 13-HODE synthesis, in vitro pro-liferative index, and tumorigenicity, yet reduction of

15-LOX-1 in these cells by antisense RNA reduced all of these endpoints compared to mock-transfected controls (121). These results indicate that, at least in prostate tissue, the synthesis of 13-HODE by 15-LOX-1 may be protumorigenic.

Shappell et al. (111,124) determined that 15-LOX-2 protein was expressed in the secretory cells of benign prostatic epithelium within the peripheral zone of 18 radical prostatectomy samples. A loss of 15-LOX-2 expression within areas of adenocarcinoma was noted in 14 of 18 cases, and the ability of malignant tissue to synthesize 15-HETE in an in vitro assay was reduced more than 90% compared to benign tissue. In addition, the extent of 15-LOX-2 immunostaining correlated negatively with increasing grade (125). Tang et al. (112) recently reported that 15-LOX-2 was highly expressed in normal prostate epithelial isolates, but that expression was greatly reduced or lost in several prostate cancer cell lines. In addition, 15-LOX-2 expression in normal prostate cells inversely correlated with cell-cycle progression, and forced expression of 15-LOX-2 in prostate cancer cells (PPC-1) caused a partial inhibition of cell-cycle progression. In summary, it appears that 15-LOX-1 may play a protumorigenic role in the development of prostate cancer through the synthesis of 13-HODE from LA, and 15-LOX-2 may negatively regulate the progression of prostate cancer through the synthesis of 15-HETE from AA. In support of this hypothesis, it was recently reported that 13-HODE increases activation of MAP kinase and Akt signaling in PC-3 cells treated with EGF or IGF-1, and 15-HETE reduced signaling through these pathways (23). Phosphorylation of PPARγ was also increased by 13-HODE, inhibiting PPARγ activity, and 15-HETE treated cells had reduced levels of phosphorylated PPARγ. These studies present a possible mechanism by which these two 15-LOX enzymes can have opposing effects on prostate cancer development.

3.2. Colon Cancer

Until recently, research on LOX activity in colon tissues had focused primarily on 5-LOX and LT synthesis (reviewed in ref. 45). Synthesis of 5-HETE and LTs by colon cancer cell lines has been reported (126–128), as has expression of low levels of 5-LOX and FLAP RNA in cultured human intestinal cells. In vitro studies have provided support for a potential role of LTs in the development of colon cancer. LTB_4 is capable of stimulating proliferation in HT-29 and HCT-15 human colon cancer cell lines, and this stimulation is abrogated by co-treatment with the LTB_4 competitive antagonist SC41930 (104,129). In addition, Hussey and Tisdale (100) reported that a number of 5-LOX inhibitors inhibited proliferation in the murine colon cancer cell lines MAC13, MAC16, and MAC26, and that BWA4C reduced tumor-growth rate and volume of MAC16 and MAC26 colon tumor fragments transplanted into NMRI mice. It is important to note that not all of the 5-LOX inhibitors were equally effective in inhibiting growth in these studies, and that the doses required for growth inhibition were higher than the amount necessary to inhibit 5-LOX activity in other systems (130). There is limited evidence that 12-LOX could be involved in the development of colon cancer. The expression of p12-LOX RNA in the Clone A human colon cancer cell line has been reported (83), and treatment of these cells with exogenous 12-HETE decreased DCC and increased MDM2 gene expression (131). Further studies are needed to clarify the importance of 12-LOX enzyme activity in the development of colon cancer.

Recently, the role of 15-LOX-1 in colon carcinogenesis has received a great deal of attention. Ikawa et al. (132) analyzed 21 matched pairs of colorectal tumor and adjacent normal tissues for 15-LOX-1 expression by Western analysis. 15-LOX-1 was detected in tissues from 18 cases, and expression in tumor tissue was elevated compared to normal adjacent tissue in 14 of those cases. 15-LOX-1 protein was localized to epithelial cells within both tumor and normal tissues. The presence of 15-LOX-1 RNA was confirmed by RT-PCR and 15-LOX activity was confirmed in tissue homogenates by HPLC following incubation with exogenous AA. In a similar study, Shureiqi et al. (123) analyzed 18 matched pairs of colon cancer tissue and adjacent normal mucosa. A slight, nonsignificant increase in the levels of 15-LOX-1 protein in tumors compared to normal tissues was observed by Western analysis of tissue homogenates. In contrast, the authors report that analysis of tissues by immunohistochemistry revealed a significant decrease of 15-LOX-1 protein in tumor tissues compared to their normal matched tissue. In addition, 13-HODE levels in these tissues, as evaluated by enzyme-linked immunosorbent assay (ELISA) and immunohistochemistry, were significantly decreased (threefold) in tumors compared to normal tissue. The conflicting results from these two studies remain unresolved; however, it is clear that 15-LOX-1 is expressed in colon epithelium and that 13-HODE is synthesized in both normal and tumor tissue.

There is further controversy surrounding the effect of 13-HODE synthesis on colon cancer cell growth. Shureiqi et al. (123) reported that 13-HODE treatment (75–100 μM) inhibits growth and induces apoptosis in HT-29 colon cancer cells. In addition, treatment of RKO and HT-29 cells with the NSAIDs sulindac and NS398 was found to increase 15-LOX-1 protein expression and 13-HODE synthesis, and the increase in 13-HODE was found to be necessary for the induction of apoptosis by NSAIDs in these cell lines (106,107). However, Hsi et al. (22,23) determined that low doses of 13-HODE (<10 μM) increase MAP kinase phosphorylation in HCT-116 colon cancer cells and cause phosphorylation (inactivation) of PPARγ. This effect was diminished with doses above 10 μM of 13-HODE. Furthermore, stable transfection of these cells with a 15-LOX-1 expression vector resulted in increased MAP kinase and PPARγ phosphorylation. No data on the effect of low doses of 13-HODE or 15-LOX-1 transfection on cell growth or apoptosis was presented. In an attempt to reconcile these data, it has been proposed that at high concentrations, 13-HODE may exert a differentiating and/or apoptotic effect on colon cancer cells (possibly through activation of PPARγ), while at low concentrations it can be growth-promoting (possibly through inactivation of PPARγ) (122). This hypothesis has not yet been proven.

3.3. Breast Cancer

Expression analyses of LOX in human breast tissue have been quite limited. Natarajan et al. (133) analyzed cancerous breast tissue and adjacent normal tissue from six patients for expression of 12-LOX and 15-LOX. Cancerous breast tissue consistently expressed higher levels of 12-LOX RNA (3–33-fold) as compared to normal tissue by RT-PCR analysis. All tissues expressed 15-LOX RNA; however, there was no consistent change in expression between cancerous and noncancerous tissue. A more rigorous analysis of the expression and activity of LOX proteins in normal and neoplastic breast tissue is clearly needed.

The expression of 5-LOX and its activating protein FLAP has been demonstrated for several breast cancer cell lines (76), including MB231, H2380, SKBR3, T47D, ZR75, and MCF. A number of breast cancer cell lines have also been analyzed for their ability to synthesize 13-HODE (122). Only cell lines that were estrogen receptor-negative and overexpressed EGF receptor and/or erbB-2 synthesized 13-HODE. The cell lines SKBR3, BT-20, MDA-MB-453, and MDA-MB-468 synthesized the highest levels of 13-HODE. When the BT-20 cell was further analyzed, it was determined that 13-HODE synthesis was dependent on TGFα/EGF-stimulated 15-LOX-1 protein expression *(134)*.

The involvement of LOX enzymes, particularly 12-LOX, in breast cancer has been implicated by a number of in vitro and in vivo studies. Treatment of MDA-MB-435 cells with LA increased the secretion of 12- and 15-HETE and increased the invasive capacity of these cells *(135)*. This effect was blocked by the 5- and 12-LOX inhibitor esculetin. The addition of 0.1 μ*M* 12-HETE replicated the effect of LA on invasion. Furthermore, transfection of the estrogen-dependent breast cancer cell line MCF-7 with a 12-LOX expression vector rendered the cells able to grow in the absence of estrogen *(136)*. Transfected cells also became responsive to LA-induced proliferation, growing approximately threefold faster after LA treatment than parental cells. In addition to these studies which implicate a role for 12-LOX in breast cancer, it has recently been reported that selective inhibitors of 5-LOX increased apoptosis and decreased proliferation of several breast cancer cell lines, and that insulin-like growth factor (IGF)-1 and transferrin increased 5-HETE secretion by these cells *(137,138)*. These results must be interpreted with caution, considering the known nonspecific effects of 5-LOX inhibitors. Inhibition of 7,12-dimethylbenz[*a*]anthracene (DMBA) and methyl-nitrosourea-induced rat mammary-tumor development by nonselective LOX inhibitors has also been reported *(90,139–141)*, providing evidence that LOX inhibition can effect mammary-cancer development in an in vivo system.

3.4. Lung Cancer

Less is known about LOX expression patterns in lung cancer than in prostate, colon, and breast cancers. A comprehensive analysis of LOX expression patterns of normal and malignant lung tissues is needed. The expression of 5-LOX, FLAP, 12-LOX, and 15-LOX-1 RNA has been confirmed in several lung cancer cell lines by RT-PCR *(89,142)*. In addition, 5-LOX RNA was detected in primary lung cancers *(142)*, and 15-LOX-1 protein was detected by immunofluorescence in human tracheal and bronchial airway cells *(143)*. Treatment of lung cancer cell lines with growth factors induced 5-HETE synthesis, and treatment with exogenous 5-HETE stimulated cell growth in vitro *(142)*.

The general LOX inhibitor NDGA inhibits growth and clonogenic potential of human SCLC and NSCLC cell lines in culture *(89,144)*, as do selective inhibitors of the 5-LOX pathway *(89)*. In addition, NDGA inhibited the multiplicity of urethane-induced lung tumor in A/J mice and inhibited growth of NSCLC cells xenografted into athymic nude mice *(89)*. The 5-LOX inhibitor A79175 and FLAP inhibitor MK886 decrease 4-(methylnitrosamino)-1-(3-pyridyl)-1-butanone (NNK)-induced lung-tumor multiplicity and tumor volume in A/J mice, and A79175 also decreased tumor incidence by 20%. Inhibition of LT synthesis by feeding MK886, Accolate, or zileuton in the diet reduced tumor size, multiplicity, and conversion to carcinoma in female strain A mice injected with vinyl carbamate *(101)*. These studies provide evidence that LT pathway inhibitors may be useful chemopreventive agents for lung cancer. However, it is possible that these inhibitors are not acting solely through inhibition of LT synthesis. A careful comparison of the doses required to inhibit LT synthesis in these models and the doses necessary to inhibit tumorigenesis would help to clarify this issue.

3.5. Skin Cancer

LOXs have been reported to be expressed in the skin, including 5-LOX *(145)*, three types of 12-LOX *(16,146)*, 15-LOX-2 in human skin *(31)*, and 8-LOX in the mouse skin *(147)*. Most studies of LOX expression in skin cancer have been carried out in the DMBA and 12-*O*-tetradecanoylphorbol-13-acetate (TPA) mouse skin-tumor model. Many different compounds with LOX inhibitory activity have been reported to inhibit tumor formation in this model (reviewed in ref. *148)*, including NDGA, quercetin, morin, AA861, phenidone, and ETYA. Krieg et al. *(149)* reported that 12-HETE levels were greatly increased in papillomas and carcinomas arising from DMBA- and TPA-treated skin of NMRI mice. This increase was attributed primarily to the expression of p12-LOX. Genetic disruption of the p12-LOX gene in B6/129 Sv mice, but not in Sencar mice, reduced the conversion of DMBA/TPA-induced papillomas to carcinomas from 37.5% incidence in wild-type mice to 8.3% in p12-LOX–/– mice. No effect was observed on papilloma incidence, and no effect was observed on incidence of papillomas or carcinomas when a complete carcinogenic dose of DMBA was used to induce tumors *(150)*. Thus far, mechanistic roles for specific LOX products in skin carcinogenesis are not clearly defined; however, there is evidence that some could be involved in differentiation through activation of PPAR nuclear receptors *(41)*.

4. CONCLUSION AND PERSPECTIVES

For many reasons, LOX are often not considered when searching for good targets for cancer prevention. Unlike the COX family, in which two enzymes and a handful of product receptors have been identified and characterized, the LOX family has many members with diverse tissue expression. The functions of the many LOX products in normal or neoplastic tissues have not been well-characterized, partly because receptors have not been identified for most of the LOX products. There is concern that although some LOX products have protumorigenic activities, others may be anti-tumorigenic. Other complications in understanding the LOX-cancer relationship are differences in types of LOX enzymes expressed in humans and mice. Since many studies are carried out in mice, the function of some uniquely murine LOX are better characterized than human LOX. 8-LOX, expressed in murine but not human keratinocytes, is an example of the questions that differences in species raise (40). 8-HETE, an 8-LOX product, was shown to cause mouse keratinocyte differentiation through binding to and activating PPARα (41). In murine papillomas, highly differentiated benign tumors, 8-LOX is upregulated, suggesting that 8-HETE is a driving force in differentiation (151). The functional human equivalent is currently unknown. The reverse situation also occurs: 15-LOX-1 and 15-LOX-2, expressed in humans but not mice, have been linked to colon and prostate cancer (107,112), but proving a critical involvement experimentally is difficult. Current approaches introduce these genes into mice in a tissue-specific manner. It is highly likely that the outcome of these and related studies will be significant. Like the COX products, some of the LOX products are likely to be shown to directly contribute to neoplastic transformation.

The question of whether to inhibit specific LOX or all LOXs is not an easy one. The answer depends partially on what the target population is—general or high-risk. For example, because prostate cancer cells may require 5-HETE, at-risk or "watchful waiting" men could be a target for 5-LOX inhibitors, particularly some of the newly developed drugs that have received FDA approval (85). On the other hand, if prevention of all (or many) cancers is the goal, nonselective LOX inhibitors may be a better approach.

When considering general vs selective LOX inhibition, particularly with regard to use of agents such as resveratrol or tea polyphenols that are also antioxidants, cell-cycle inhibitors, etc., the issue is whether inhibiting multiple pathways can be better achieved through a combination of specific inhibitors or through the use of a single "multi-purpose" agent. The use of single "multi-purpose" agents may be a more realistic approach in cancer prevention in a general population. Combining LOX inhibitors with other types of inhibitors certainly deserves further consideration (and experimentation). One of the more logical combinations is LOX and COX inhibitors. Inhibition of COX metabolism of AA results in an increase in its availability for LOX metabolism to HETEs. It has recently been suggested that the gastrointestinal ulcerogenic activity of NSAIDs is not caused by reduced PGs but rather an increase in LTs, which are known to play an important role in the development of gastrointestinal ulcers. A new COX/5-LOX inhibitor, ML3000, is in Phase III clinical trials for chronic inflammation to test this approach (152). Such an approach may also apply to colon (and other) cancer prevention, given the gastrointestinal problems associated with NSAID use.

Considering all of these factors as a whole, along with the substantial number of preclinical studies showing that LOX inhibitors have significant cancer preventive activity, it is reasonable to anticipate that inhibition of LOX will be an effective approach to preventing human cancer. Additional studies are needed to increase our understanding of the function of human LOX products in normal and pathological conditions. Such studies should lead to the development of more efficacious agents and to new approaches to cancer prevention.

REFERENCES

1. Brash AR. Lipoxygenases: occurrence, functions, catalysis, and acquisition of substrate. *J Biol Chem* 1999;274:23,679–23,682.
2. Kuhn H, Borngraber S. Mammalian. 15-lipoxygenases. Enzymatic properties and biological implications. *Adv Exp Med Biol* 1999;447:5–28.
3. Yamamoto S. Enzymatic lipid peroxidation: reactions of mammalian lipoxygenase. *Free Radic Biol Med* 1991;10:149–159.
4. Kuhn H. Structural basis for the positional specificity of lipoxygenases. *Prostaglandins Other Lipid Mediat* 2000;62:255–270.
5. Yamamoto S. Mammalian lipoxygenases: molecular structures and functions. *Biochim Biophys Acta* 1992;1128:117–131.
6. Gaffney BJ. Lipoxygenases: structural principles and spectroscopy. *Annu Rev Biophys Biomol Struct* 1996;25:431–459.

7. Peters-Golden M. Cell biology of the 5-lipoxygenase pathway. *Am J Respir Crit Care Med* 1998;157:S227–S232.

8. Radmark OP. The molecular biology and regulation of 5-lipoxygenase. *Am J Respir Crit Care Med* 2000;161:S11–S15.

9. Kuhn H, Theile BJ. The diversity of the lipoxygenase family. Many sequence data but little information of biological significance. *FEBS Lett* 1999;449:7–11.

10. Dailey LA, Imming P. 12-Lipoxygenase: classification possible therapeutic benefits for inhibition and inhibitors. *Curr Med Chem* 1999;6:389–398.

11. Chen X-S, Funk CD. Structure-function properties of human platelet 12-lipoxygenase: chimeric enzyme and in vitro mutagenesis studies. *FASEB J* 1993;7:694–701.

12. Honn KV, Tang DG, Gao X, et al. 12-lipoxygenases and 12(S)-HETE: role in cancer metastasis. *Cancer Metastasis Rev* 1994;13:365–396.

13. Funk CD, Keeney DS, Oliw EH, et al. Functional expression and cellular localization of a mouse epidermal lipoxygenase. *J Biol Chem* 1996;271:23,338–23,344.

14. Funk CD. The molecular biology of mammalian lipoxygenases and the quest for eicosanoid functions using lipoxygenase-deficient mice. *Biochim Biophys Acta* 1996;1304:65–84.

15. Siebert M, Krieg P, Lehmann WD, et al. Enzymic characterization on epidermis-derived 12-lipogenzase isoenzymes. *J Biochem* 2001;355:97–104.

16. Krieg P, Siebert M, Kinzig A, et al. Murine 12(R)-lipoxygenase: functional expression, genomic structure and chromosomal localization. *FEBS Lett* 1999;446:142–148.

17. Sun D, McDonnill M, Chen X, et al. Human 12(R)-lipoxygenase and the mouse ortholog. *J Biol Chem* 1998;273:33,540–33,547.

18. Boeglin WE, Kim RB, Brash AL. A 12(R)-lipoxygenase in human skin: mechanistic evidence, molecular cloning, and expression. *Proc Natl Acad Sci USA* 1998;95:6744–6749.

19. Fretland DJ, Djuric SW. 12(R)-and 12(S)-Hydroxyeicosatetraenoic acids: chemistry, biology, and pharmacology. *Prostagladins Leukot Essent Fatty Acids* 1989;38:215–228.

20. Kuhn H, Heydeck D, Brinkman R, Trebus F. Regulation of cellular 15-lipoxygenase activity on pretranslational translational and postranslational levels. *Lipids* 1999;34:S273–S279.

21. Hsi LC, Wilson LC, Eling TE. Opposing effects of 15-lipoxygenase-1 and -2 metabolites on MAPK signaling in prostate: alteration in PPARgamma. *J Biol Chem* 2002;277:405–456.

22. Hsi LC, Wilson L, Nixon J, Eling TE. 15-lipoxygenase-1 metabolites down-regulate peroxisome proliferator-activated receptor γ via the MAPK signaling pathway. *J Biol Chem* 2001;276:34,545–34,552.

23. Hill EM. Eling T. Nettesheim P. Changes in expression of 15-lipoxygenase and prostaglandin-H synthase during differentiation of human tracheobronchial epithelial cells. *Am J Respir Cell Mol Biol* 1998;18:662–669.

24. Yokota S, Oda T, Fahimi HD. The role of 15-lipoxygenase in disruption of the peroxisomal membrane and in programmed degradation of peroxisomes in normal rat liver. *J Histochem Cytochem* 2001;49:613–621.

25. VanLeyen K, Duvoisin RM, Engelhardt H, Wiedmann M. A function for lipoxygenase in programmed organelle degradation. *Nature* 1998;395:392–395.

26. Shureiqi I, Chen D, Lotan R, et al. 15-Lipoxygenase-1 mediates nonsteroidal antiinflammatory drug-induced apoptosis independently of cyclooxygenase-2 in colon cancer cells. *Cancer Res* 2000;60:6846–6850.

27. Shureiqi I, Xu X, Chen D, et al. Nonsteroidal anti-inflammatory drugs induce apoptosis in esophageal cancer cells by restoring 15-lipoxygenase-1 expression. *Cancer Res* 2001;61:4879–4884.

28. Eling TE, Glasgow WC. Cellular proliferation and lipid metabolism: importance of lipoxygenases in modulating epidermal growth factor-dependent mitogenesis. *Cancer Metastases Rev* 1994;13:397–410.

29. Brezinski ME, Serhan CN. Selective incorporation of 15(S)-hydroxyeicosatetraenoic acid in phosphatidylinositol of human neutrophils: agonist-induced deacylation and transformation of stored hydroxyeicosanoids. *Proc Natl Acad Sci USA* 1990;87:6248–6252.

30. Brash AR, Boeglin WE, Chang MS. Discovery of a second 15S-lipoxygenase in humans. *Proc Natl Acad Sci USA* 1997;94:6148–6152.

31. Brash AR, Jisaka M, Boeglin WE, et al. Investigation of a second 15S-lipoxygenase in humans and its expression in epithelial tissues. *Adv Exp Med Biol* 1999;469:83–89.

32. Kilty I, Logan A, Vickers PJ. Differential characteristics of human 15-lipoxygenase isozymes and a novel splice variant of 15S-lipoxygenase. *Eur J Biochem* 1999;266:83–93.

33. Kang L, Vanderhoek JY. Characterization of specific subcellular 15-hydroxyeicosatetraenoic acid (15-HETE) binding sites on rat basophilic leukemia cells. *Biochim Biophys Acta* 1995;125:297–304.

34. Bailey M, Fletcher J, Vanderhoek Y, Makheya AN. Regulation of human T-lymphocyte proliferative responses by the lipoxygenase product 15-HETE. *Biochem Soc Trans* 1997;25:2475.

35. Postoak D, Nystuen L, King L, et al. 15-Lipoxygenase products of arachidonate play a role in proliferation of transformed erythroid cells. *Am J Physiol* 1990;259:C849–C853.

36. Fürstenberger G, Hagedorn H, Jacobi T, et al. Characterization of an 8-lipoxygenase activity induced by the phorbol-13-acetate in mouse skin in vivo. *J Biol Chem* 1991;266:15,738–15,745.

37. Huges MA, Brash AR. Investigation of the mechanism of biosynthesis of 8-hydroxyeicosatetraenoic acid in mouse skin. *Biochim Biophys Acta* 1991;1081:347–354.

38. Fischer SM, Baldwin JK, Jasheway DW, et al. Phorbol ester induction of 8-lipoxygenase in inbred SENCAR (SSIN) but not C57BL/6J mice correlated with hyperplasia, edema, and oxidant generation but not ornithine decarboxylase induction. *Cancer Res* 1988;48:658–664.

39. Jisaka M, Kim RB, Boeglin WE, et al. Molecular cloning and functional expression of a phorbol ester-inducible 8S-lipoxygenase form mouse skin. *J Biol Chem* 1997;272:24,410–24,416.

40. Muga SJ, Thuillier P, Pavone A, et al. 8S-Lipoxygenase activates peroxisome proliferator-activated receptor alpha and induces differentiation in murine keratinocytes. *Cell Growth Differ* 2000;11:447–454.

41. Rioux N, Castonguay A. Inhibitors of lipoxygenase: a new class of cancer chemopreventive agents. *Carcinogenesis* 1998;19:1393–1400.

42. Cuendet M, Pezzuto JM. The role of cyclooxygenase and lipoxygenase in cancer chemoprevention. *Drug Metabol Drug Interact* 2000;17:109–157.

43. Steele VE, Holmes CA, Hawk ET, et al. Potential use of lipoxygenase inhibitors for cancer chemoprevention. *Expert Opin Invest Drugs* 2000;9:2121–2138.

44. Steele VE, Holmes CA, Hawk ET, et al. Lipoxygenase inhibitors as potential cancer chemopreventives. *Cancer Epidemiol Biomarkers Prev* 1999;8:467–483.

45. Weisburger JH. Mechanisms of action of antioxidants as exemplified in vegetables, tomatoes and tea. *Food Chem Toxicol* 1999;37:943–948.

46. Conney AH, Lou YR, Xie JG, et al. Some perspectives on dietary inhibition of carcinogenesis: studies with curcumin and tea. *Proc Soc Exp Biol Med* 1997;216:739–743.

47. Yang CS, Wang Z-Y. Tea and cancer. *J Natl Cancer Inst* 1993;85:1038–1049.

48. Katiyar SK, Mukhtar H. Tea antioxidants in cancer chemoprevention. *J Cell Biochem Suppl* 1997;27:59–67.

49. Katiyar SK, Mukhtar H. Tea in chemoprevention of cancer: epidemiologic and experimental studies review. *Int J Oncol* 1996;8:221–238.

50. Gupta S, Hastak K, Ahmad N, Lewin JS, Mukhtar H. Inhibition of prostate carcinogenesis in TRAMP mice by oral infusion of green tea polyphenols. *Proc Natl Acad Sci USA* 2001;98:10,350–10,355.

51. Hong J, Smith TJ, Ho C, et al. Effects of purified green and black tea polyphenols on cyclooxygenase and lipoxygenase-dependent metabolism of arachidonic acid in human colon mucosa and colon tumor tissues. *Biochem Pharmacol* 2001;62:1175–1183.

52. Lin J, Lin-Shiav S. Mechanisms of cancer chemoprevention by curcumin. *Proc Natl Sci Counc Repub China* [B] 2001;25:59–66.

53. Huang M, Lysz T, Ferraro T, et al. Inhibitory effects of curcumin on in vitro lipoxygenase and cyclooxygenase activities in mouse epidermis. *Cancer Res* 1991;51:813–819.

54. Skrzypczak-Jakun E, McCake NP, Selman SH, Jankun J. Curcumin inhibits lipoxygenase by binding to its central cavity: theoretical and x-ray evidence. *Int J Mol Med* 2000;6:521–526.

55. Koshihara Y, Neichi T, Murota SI, et al. Caffeic acid is a selective inhibitor for leukotriene biosynthesis. *Biochem Biophys Acta* 1984;792:92–97.

56. Kohyama N, Nagata T, Fujimoto S. Inhibition of aracidonate activities by 2-(3,4-dihydroxy-phenyl) ethanol, a phenolic compound from olives. *Biosci Biotechnol Biochem* 1997;61:347–350.

57. Soleas GJ, Diamandis EP, Goldberg DM. Resveratrol: a molecule whose time has come? and gone? *Clin Biochem* 1997;30:91–113.

58. Das DK, Sato M, Ray PS, et al. Cardioprotection of red wine: role of polyphenolic antioxidants. *Drugs Exp Clin Res* 1999;25:115–120.

59. Jang M, Cai L, Udeani G, et al. Cancer chemopreventive activity of resveratrol, a natural product derived from grapes. *Science* 1997;275:218–220.

60. Tessitore L, Davit A, Sarotto I, Caderni G. Resveratrol depresses the growth of colorectal aberrant crypt foci by affecting bax and p21(CIP) expression. *Carcinogenesis* 2000;21:1619–1622.

61. Kozuki Y, Miura Y, Yagasaki K. Resveratrol suppresses hepatoma cell invasion independently of its anti-proliferative action. *Cancer Lett* 2001;167:151–156.

62. Carbo N, Costelli P, Baccino FM, et al. Resveratrol, a natural product present in wine, decreases tumour growth in a rat tumour model. *Biochem Biophys Res Commun* 1999;254:739–743.

63. MacCarrone M, Lorenzon T, Guerrieri P, Agro AF. Resveratrol prevents apoptosis in K562 cells by inhibiting lipoxygenase and cyclooxygenase. *Eur J Biochem* 1999;265:27–34.

64. Savouret JF, Quesne M. Resveratrol and cancer: a review. *Biomed Pharmacother* 2002;56:84–87.

65. Hammarström S. Selective inhibition of platelet n-8 lipoxygenase by 5,8,11-eicosatriynoic acid. *Biochim Biophys Acta* 1977;487:517–519.

66. Fischer SM, Mills GD, Slaga, TJ. Inhibition of mouse skin tumor promotion by several inhibitors of arachidonic acid metabolism. *Carcinogenesis* 1982;3:1243–1245.

67. Kliewer SA, Lenhard JM, Willson TM, et al. A prostaglandin J$_2$ metabolite binds peroxisome proliferator-activated receptor γ and promotes adipocyte differentiation. *Cell* 1995; 83:813–819.

68. Sok D-E, Han C-Q, Pai J-K, Sih CJ. Inhibition of leukotriene biosynthesis by acetylenic analogs. *Biochem Biophys Res Commun* 1982;107:101–108.

69. Vanderhoek JY, Bryant RW, Bailey JM. Inhibition of leukotriene biosynthesis by the leukocyte product 15-hydroxy-5,8,11,13-eicosatetraenoic acid. *J Biol Chem* 1980;255:10,064–10,065.

70. Masumoto H, Kissner R, Koppenol WH, Sies H. Kinetic study of the reaction of ebselen with peroxynitrite. *FEBS Lett* 1996;398:179–182.

71. Theicher BA, Korbut TT, Menon K, et al. Cyclooxygenase and lipoxygenase inhibitors as modulators of cancer therapies. *Cancer Chemother Pharmacol* 1994;33:151–522.

72. Kato M, Liu W, Yi H, et al. The herbal medicine sho-saiko-to inhibits growth and metastasis of malignant melanoma primarily developed in ret-transgenic mice. *J Investig Dermatol* 1998;111:640–644.

73. Ikemoto S, Sugimura K, Yoshida N, et al. Anti tumor effects of *Scutellariae radix* and its components baicalein, baicalin and wogonin on bladder cancer cell lines. *Urology* 2000;55:951–955.

74. Chen S, Raun S, Bedner E, et al. Effects of the flavonoid baicalin and its metabolite baicalein on androgen receptor expression, cell cycle progression and apoptosis of prostate cancer cell lines. *Cell Prolif* 2001;34:293–304.

75. Hong, SH, Avis I, Vos MD, et al. Relationship of arachidonic acid metabolizing enzyme expression in epithelial cancer cell lines to the growth effect of selective biochemical inhibitors. *Cancer Res* 1999;59:2223–2228.

76. Pidgeon GP, Kandouz M, Meram A, Honn KV. Mechanisms controlling cell arrest and induction of apoptosis after 12-lipoxygenase inhibition in prostate cancer cells. *Cancer Res* 2002;62:2721–2727.

77. Lee MJ, Wang CJ, Tsai YY, et al. Inhibitory effect of 12-*O*-tetradecanoylphorbol-13-acetate-caused tumor promotion in benz[*a*]pyrene-initiated CD-1 mouse skin by baicalein. *Nutr Cancer* 1999;34:185–191.

78. Sekiya K, Okuda H. Selective inhibition of platelet lipoxygenase by baicalein. *Biochem Biophys Res Commun* 1982;105:1090–1095.

79. Hamada H, Hiramatsu M, Edmatasu R, Mori A. Free radical scavenging action on baicalein. *Arch Biochem Biophys* 1993;306:261–266.

80. Huang F, Shoupe TS, Lin CJ, et al. Differential effects of a series of hydroxamic acid derivatives on 5-lipoxygenase and cyclooxygenase from neutrophils and 12-lipoxygenase from platelets and their in vivo effects on inflammation and anaphylaxis. *J Med Chem* 1989;32:1836–1842.

81. Nie D, Honn, KV. Cyclooxygenase, lipoxygenase and tumor angiogenesis. *Cell Mol Life Sci* 2002;59:799–807.

82. Chen YQ, Duniec SM, Liu B, et al. Endogenous 12(S)-HETE production by tumor cells and its role in metastasis. *Cancer Res* 1994;54:1574–1579.

83. Li L, Zhu S, Johsi B, et al. A novel hydroxamic acid compound, BMD188 demonstrates anti-prostate cancer effects by inducing apoptosis in in vitro studies. *Anticancer Res* 1999;19:51–60.

84. Ghosh J, Myers CE. Inhibition of arachidonate 5-lipoxygenase triggers massive apoptosis in human prostate cancer cells. *Proc Natl Acad Sci USA* 1998;95:13,182–13,187.

85. Kehrer JP, Biswal SS, La E, et al. Inhibition of peroxisome-proliferator-activated receptor (PPAR)α by MK886. *Biochem J* 2001;356:899–906.

86. Romano M, Catalano A, Nutini M, et al. 5-Lipoxygenase regulates malignant mesothelial cell survival: involvement of vascular endothelial growth factor. *FASEB J* 2001;15:2326–2336.

87. Hamasaki Y, Tai HH. Gossypol, a potent inhibitor of arachidonate 5- and 12-lipoxygenases. *Biochim Biophys Acta* 1985;834:37–41.

88. Moody TW, Leyton J, Martinez A, et al. Lipoxygenase inhibitors prevent lung carcinogenesis and inhibit non-small cell lung cancer growth. *Exp Lung Res* 1998;24:617–628.

89. McCormick DL, Spicer AM. Nordihydroguaiaretic acid suppression of rat mammary carcinogenesis induced by *N*-methyl-*N*-nitrosourea. *Cancer Lett* 1987;37:139–146.

90. Olsen EA, Abernethy ML, Kul-Shorten C, et al. A double-blind vehicle-controlled study evaluating masoprocol cream in the treatment of actinic keratoses on the head and neck. *J Am Acad Dermatol* 1991;24:738–743.

91. Seufferlein T, Seckl MJ, Schwarz E, et al. Mechanisms of nordihydroguaiaretic acid-induced growth inhibition and apoptosis in human cancer cells. *Br J Cancer* 2002;86:1188–1198.

92. Shidaifat F, Canatan H, Kulp SK, et al. Inhibition of human prostate *cancer cell* growth by gossypol is associated with stimulation of transforming growth factor-beta. *Cancer Lett* 1996;107:37–44.

93. Liu S, Kulp SK, Sugimoto Y, et al. The (−)–enantiomer of gossypol possesses higher anticancer potency than racemic gossypol in human breast cancer. *Anticancer Res* 2002;22:33–38.

94. Stein RC, Joseph AE, Matlin SA, et al. A preliminary clinical study of gossypol in advanced human cancer. *Cancer Chemother Pharmacol* 1992;30:480–482.

95. Van Poznak C, Seidman AD, Reidenberg MM, et al. Oral gossypol in the treatment of patients with refractory metastatic breast cancer: a Phase I/II clinical trial. *Breast Cancer Res Treat* 2001;66:239–248.

96. Flack MR, Pyle RG, Mullen NM, et al. Oral gossypol in the treatment of *metastatic adrenal cancer. J Clin Endocrinol Metab* 1993;76:1019–1024.

97. Qian SZ, Wang ZG. Gossypol: a potential antifertility agent for males. *Annu Rev Pharmacol Toxicol* 1984;24:329–360.

98. Garcia-Marcos L, Schuster A. Antileukotrienes in asthma: present situation. *Expert Opin Pharmacother* 2001;2:441–466.

99. Hussey HJ, Tisdale MJ. Inhibition of tumour growth by lipoxygenase inhibitors. *Br J Cancer* 1996;74:683–687.

100. Gunning WT, Kramer PM, Steele, VE, Pereira MA. Chemoprevention by lipoxygenase and leukotriene inhibitors of vinyl carbamate-induced lung tumors in mice. *Cancer Res* 2002;62:4199–4201.

101. Wenger FA, Kilian M, Achucarr P, et al. Effects of celebrex and zyflo on BOP-induced pancreatic cancer in Syrian hamsters. *Pancreatology* 2002;2:54–60.

102. Bell RL, Bouska JB, Malo PE, et al. Optimization of the potency and duration of action of N-hydroxyurea 5-lipoxygenase inhibitors. *J Pharmacol Exp Ther* 1995;272:724–731.

103. Bortuzzo C, Hanif R, Kashfi K, et al. The effect of leukotrienes B and selected HETEs on the proliferation of colon cancer cells. *Biochim Biophys Acta* 1996;1300:240–246.

104. Przylipiak A, Hafner J, Przylipiak J, et al. Influence of leukotrines on in vitro growth of human mammary carcinoma cell line MCF-7. *Eur J Obstet Gynecol Reprod Biol* 1998;77:61–65.

105. Shureiqi I, Chen D, Lee JJ, et al. 15-LOX-1: a novel molecular target of nonsteroidal anti-inflammatory drug-induced apoptosis in colorectal cancer cells. *J Natl Cancer Inst* 2000;92:1136–1142.

106. Shureiqi I, Chen D, Lotan R, et al. 15-Lipoxygenase-1 mediates nonsteroidal antiinflammatory drug-induced apoptosis independently of cyclooxygenase-2 in colon cancer cells. *Cancer Res* 2000;60:6846–6850.

107. Sendobry SM, Cornicelli JA, Welch K, et al. Attenuation of diet-induced atherosclerosis in rabbits with a highly selective 15-lipoxygenase inhibitor lacking significant antioxidant properties. *Br J Pharmcol* 1998;120:1199–1206.

108. Nie D, Che M, Grignon D, et al. Role of eicosanoids in prostate cancer progression. *Cancer Metastasis Rev* 2001;20:195–206.

109. Gupta S, Srivastava M, Ahmad N, et al. Lipoxygenase-5 is overexpressed in prostate adenocarcinoma. *Cancer* 2001;91:737–743.

110. Shappell SB, Boeglin WE, Olson SJ, et al. 15-lipoxygenase-2 (15-LOX-2) is expressed in benign prostatic epithelium and reduced in prostate adenocarcinoma. *Am J Pathol* 1999;155:235–245.

111. Tang S, Bhatia B, Maldonado CJ, et al. Evidence that arachidonate 15-lipoxygenase 2 is a negative cell-cycle regulator in normal prostate epithelial cells. *J Biol Chem* 2002;277:16,189–161,201.

112. Ghosh J, Myers CE. Arachidonic acid stimulates prostate cancer cell growth: critical role of 5-lipoxygenase. *Biochem Biophys Res Commun* 1997;235:418–423.

113. Anderson KM, Seed T, Vos M, et al. 5-Lipoxygenase inhibitors reduce PC-3 cell proliferation and initiate nonnecrotic cell death. *Prostate* 1998;37:161–173.

114. Tang DG, La E, Kern J, Kehrer JP. Fatty acid oxidation and signaling in apoptosis. *Biol Chem* 2002;383:425–442.

115. Gao X, Grignon DJ, Chbihi T, et al. Elevated 12-lipoxygenase mRNA expression correlates with advanced stage and poor differentiation of human prostate cancer. *Urology* 1995;46:227–237.

116. Timar J, Raso E, Dome B, et al. Expression, subcellular localization and putative function of platelet- type 12-lipoxygenase in human prostate cancer cell lines of different metastatic potential. *Int J Cancer* 2000;87:37–43.

117. Nie D, Hillman GG, Geddes T, et al. Platelet-type 12-lipoxygenase in a human prostate carcinoma stimulates angiogenesis and tumor growth. *Cancer Res* 1998;58:4047–4051.

118. Kelavkar UP, Cohen C, Kamitani H, et al. Concordant induction of 15-lipoxygenase-1 and mutant p53 expression in human prostate adenocarcinoma: correlation with Gleason staging. *Carcinogenesis* 2000;21:1777–1787.

119. Spindler SA, Sarkar FH, Sakr WA, et al. Production of 13-hydroxyoctadecadienoic acid (13-HODE) by prostate tumors and cell lines. *Biochem Biophys Res Commun* 1997;239:775–781.

120. Kelavkar UP, Nixon JB, Cohen C, et al. Overexpression of 15-lipoxygenase-1 in PC-3 human prostate cancer cells increases tumorigenesis. *Carcinogenesis* 2001;22: 1765–1773.

121. Kelavkar U, Glasgow W, Eling TE. The effect of 15-lipoxygenase-1 expression on cancer cells. *Curr Urol Rep* 2002;3:207–214.

122. Shureiqi I, Wojno KJ, Poore JA, et al. Decreased 13-S-hydroxyoctadecadienoic acid levels and 15-lipoxygenase-1 expression in human colon cancers. *Carcinogenesis* 1999;20:1985–1995.

123. Shappell SB, Manning S, Boeglin WE, et al. Alterations in lipoxygenase and cyclooxygenase-2 catalytic activity and mRNA expression in prostate carcinoma. *Neoplasia* 2001;3:287–303.

124. Jack GS, Brash AR, Olson SJ, et al. Reduced 15-lipoxygenase-2 immunostaining in prostate adenocarcinoma: correlation with grade and expression in high-grade prostatic intraepithelial neoplasia. *Hum Pathol* 2000;31:1146–1154.

125. Dias VC, Wallace JL, Parsons HG. Modulation of cellular phospholipid fatty acids and leukotriene B4 synthesis in the human intestinal cell (CaCo-2). *Gut* 1992;33:622–627.

126. Sjolander A, Schippert A, Hammarstrom S. A human epithelial cell line, intestine 407, can produce 5-hydroxyeicosatetraenoic acid and leukotriene B4. *Prostaglandins* 1993;45:85–96.

127. Cortese JF, Spannhake EW, Eisinger W, et al. The 5-lipoxygenase pathway in cultured human intestinal epithelial cells. *Prostaglandins* 1995;49:155–166.

128. Bortuzzo C, Hanif R, Kashi K, et al. The effect of leukotrienes B and selected HETEs on the proliferation of colon cancer cells. *Biochim Biophys Acta* 1996;1300:240–246.

129. Werz O, Schneider N, Brungs M, et al. A test system for leukotriene synthesis inhibitors based on the in vitro differentiation of the human leukemic cell lines HL-60 and Mono Mac 6. *Naunyn Schmiedebergs Arch Pharmacol* 1997;356:441–445.

130. Gao X, Porter AT, Honn KV. Involvement of the multiple tumor suppressor genes and 12-lipoxygenase in human prostate cancer. Therapeutic implications. *Adv Exp Med Biol* 1997;407:41–53.

131. Ikawa H, Kamitani H, Calvo BF, et al. Expression of 15-lipoxygenase-1 in human colorectal cancer. *Cancer Res* 1999;59:360–366.

132. Natarajan R, Esworthy R, Bai W, et al. Increased 12-lipoxygenase expression in breast cancer tissues and cells. Regulation by epidermal growth factor. *J Clin Endocrinol Metab* 1997;82:1790–1798.

133. Reddy N, Everhart A, Eling T,Glasgow W. Characterization of a 15-lipoxygenase in human breast carcinoma BT-20 cells: stimulation of 13-HODE formation by TGF alpha/EGF. *Biochem Biophys Res Commun* 1997;231:111–116.

134. Liu X H, Connolly JM, Rose DP. Eicosanoids as mediators of linoleic acid-stimulated invasion and type IV collagenase production by a metastatic human breast cancer cell line. *Clin Exp Metastasis* 1996;14:145–152.

135. Liu XH, Connolly JM, Rose DP. The 12-lipoxygenase gene-transfected MCF-7 human breast cancer cell line exhibits estrogen-independent, but estrogen and omega-6 fatty acid- stimulated proliferation in vitro, and enhanced growth in athymic nude mice. *Cancer Lett* 1996;109:232–230.

136. Avis I, Hong SH, Martinez A, et al. Five-lipoxygenase inhibitors can mediate apoptosis in human breast cancer cell lines through complex eicosanoid interactions. *FASEB J* 2001;15:2007–2009.

137. Tong W, Ding X, Adrian T. The mechanisms of lipoxygenase inhibitor-induced apoptosis in human breast cancer cells. *Biochem Biophys Res Commun* 2002;296:942–948.

138. Noguchi M, Kitagawa H, Miyazaki I, Mizukami Y. Influence of esculetin on incidence, proliferation, and cell kinetics of mammary carcinomas induced by 7,12-dimethylbenz[a] anthracene in rats on high- and low-fat diets. *Jpn J Cancer Res* 1993;84:1010–1014.

139. Kitagawa H, Noguchi M. Comparative effects of piroxicam and esculetin on incidence, proliferation, and cell kinetics of mammary carcinomas induced by 7,12-dimethylbenz[a]anthracene in rats on high- and low-fat diets. *Oncology* 1994;51:401–410.

140. Matsunaga K, Yoshimi N, Yamada Y, et al. Inhibitory effects of nabumetone, a cyclooxygenase-2 inhibitor, and esculetin, a lipoxygenase inhibitor, on N-methyl-N-nitrosourea-induced mammary carcinogenesis in rats. *Jpn J Cancer Res* 1998;89:496–501.

141. Avis IM, Jett M, Boyle T, et al. Growth control of lung cancer by interruption of 5-lipoxygenase-mediated growth factor signaling. *J Clin Investig* 1996;97:806–813.

142. Nadel JA, Conrad DJ, Ueki IF, et al. Immunocytochemical localization of arachidonate 15-lipoxygenase in erythrocytes, leukocytes, and airway cells. *J Clin Investig* 1991;87:1139–1145.

143. Soriano AF, Helfrich B, Chan DC, et al. Synergistic effects of new chemopreventive agents and conventional cytotoxic agents against human lung cancer cell lines. *Cancer Res* 1999;59:6178–6184.

144. Kowal-Bielecka O, Distler O, Neidhart M, et al. Evidence of 5-lipoxygenase overexpression in the skin of patients with systemic sclerosis: a newly identified pathway to skin inflammation in systemic sclerosis. *Arthritis Rheum* 2001;44:1865–1875.

145. Takahashi Y, Reddy GR, Ueda N, et al. Arachidonate 12-lipoxygenase of platelet-type in human epidermal cells. *J Biol Chem* 1993;268:16,443–16,448.

146. Krieg P, Kinzig A, Heidt M, et al. cDNA cloning of a 8-lipoxygenase and a novel epidermis-type lipoxygenase from phorbol ester-treated mouse skin. *Biochim Biophys Acta* 1998;1391:7–12.

147. Nakadate T. The mechanism of skin tumor promotion caused by phorbol esters: possible involvement of arachidonic acid cascade/lipoxygenase, protein kinase C and calcium/calmodulin systems. *Jpn J Pharmacol* 1989;49:1–9.

148. Krieg P, Kinzig A, Ress-Loschke M, et al. 12-Lipoxygenase isoenzymes in mouse skin tumor development. *Mol Carcinog* 1995;14:118–129.

149. Virmani J, Johnson EN, Klein-Szanto AJ, Funk CD. Role of 'platelet-type' 12-lipoxygenase in skin carcinogenesis. *Cancer Lett* 2001;162:161–165.

150. Bürger F, Kreig P, Kinzig, A, et al. Constitutive expression of 8-lipoxygenase in papillomas and clastogenic effects of lipoxygenase-derived arachidonic acid metabolites on keratinocytes. *Mol Carcinog* 1999;24:108–117.

151. Fiorucci S, Meli R, Bucci M, Cirino G. Dual inhibitors of cyclooxygenase and 5-lipoxygenase. A new avenue in anti-inflammatory therapy? *Biochem Pharmacol* 2001;62:1433–1438.

8 Inducible Nitric Oxide Synthase as a Target for Chemoprevention

Lorne J. Hofseth, PhD, Tomohiro Sawa, PhD, S. Perwez Hussain, PhD, and Curtis C. Harris, MD

CONTENTS

1. NITRIC OXIDE IN CARCINOGENESIS

Nitric oxide (NO$^•$) was first described as endothelium-derived relaxation factor (EDRF) in the 1980s *(1–5)*. Since then, it has been shown to be a key signaling molecule that mediates both physiological and pathological processes, including vasodilation *(6)*, neurotransmission *(7)*, host defense, *(8)*, platelet aggregation *(9,10)*, and iron metabolism *(11,12)*. Increasing evidence suggests that NO$^•$ is a pivotal mediator of inflammatory-associated carcinogenesis because of its impact on DNA damage, cell cycle, and modifications of cancer-related proteins *(13–18)*.

NO$^•$ is endogenously formed by a family of enzymes known as NO$^•$ synthases (NOS) utilizing L-arginine as a substrate and molecular oxygen and nicotinamide adenine dinucleotide phosphate (NADPH) as co-factors (Fig. 1; *19*). Two of the three isoforms of NOS—neuronal (NOS1) and endothelial (NOS3)—are Ca^{2+}-dependent and constitutively expressed, and the Ca^{2+}-independent isoform (NOS2 or iNOS) requires induction. Recently, however, NOS1 and NOS3 have been shown to be inducible *(20)*, and inducible NOS (iNOS) has been shown to be expressed constitutively in some tissues (e.g., bronchus and ileum) *(21,22)*. Ca^{2+}-dependent NOS1 and NOS3 isoforms produce low levels of NO$^•$ that range from pico- to nanomolar concentrations. In contrast, iNOS produces a sustained NO$^•$ concentration in the micromolar range *(23,24)*.

Although iNOS is easily induced and expressed in macrophages through host-defense mechanisms, many other cell types (including endothelial and epithelial cells) have also been shown to express iNOS (reviewed in *25*). An increased level of constitutive and iNOS expression and/or activity is also observed in a variety of human cancers *(26–34)*. Moreover, iNOS expression and/or nitrotyrosine accumulation in the mucosa of patients with chronic inflammatory diseases, including ulcerative colitis (UC) *(35–37)*, *Helicobacter pylori* (HP)-associated gastritis *(38–40)*, viral hepatitis *(41–44)*, Wilson's disease (WD) *(45)*, hemochromatosis (HC) *(45,46)*, and Barrett's esophagus *(47)*, indicate that NO$^•$ production and peroxynitrite formation may be involved in the pathogenesis of these diseases, and thus predispose these individuals to cancer *(48)*; (Table 1).

The induction of iNOS and the subsequent biological action of NO$^•$ is complex. The net effect is a result of its available concentration, interactions with reactive oxygen species (ROS), metal ions, and proteins. Recent studies have described the involvement of NO$^•$ in several biological processes in carcinogenesis. For example, an endothelial growth factor mediates tumor vascularization *(49,50)* and tumor blood flow *(51)*. Although high concentrations of NO$^•$ induce apoptosis

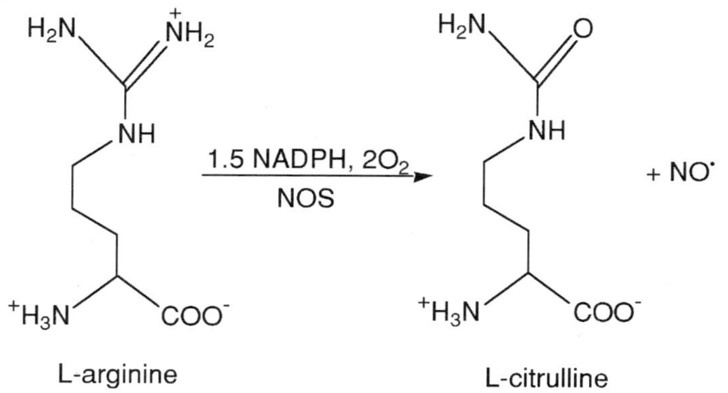

Fig. 1. Nitric oxide production from L-arginine catalyzed by nitric oxide synthase.

in susceptible cells (52), low concentrations can be anti-apoptotic (53). Billiar and colleagues have shown that both exogenously and endogenously produced NO• reduce the frequency of apoptosis by inhibiting caspases in cultured hepatocytes (54). NO•-induced apoptosis is both complex and dependent on NO• concentration, cell type, redox state, and the level of metal-ion complex within the cell (55,56). Because cytokines and hypoxia synergistically induce iNOS expression in stromal macrophages (57), the microenvironmental changes in premalignant and malignant tumor tissue may establish sustained and high NO• production, thereby supporting clonal selection of preneoplastic cells and tumor growth.

A high concentration of NO• production modifies DNA directly (58–60) and may inhibit DNA repair activities (61), such as human thymine-DNA glycosylase, which has been shown to repair G:T mismatches at CpG sites (62). Because NO• production also induces p53 accumulation and post-translational modification (63–65), the resulting growth inhibition provides additional selection pressure for the clonal expansion of cells with mutant p53. Therefore, NO• may act as both an endogenous initiator and promoter in human colon carcinogenesis. As described later, in this chapter, specific inhibitors of iNOS, demonstrated recently in animal tumor models (66–68), may have significant chemopreventive potential in human colorectal cancer (CRC).

NO• may also enhance tumor progression. To determine its role in tumor progression, we generated human cancer cell lines that constitutively produced NO• in an amount comparable to those found in human cancer. Cancer cells with wild-type p53 and iNOS expression showed increased induction of the G_1-S

cell-cycle checkpoint protein, $p21^{waf1}$, and reduced tumor growth and increased tumor necrosis as xenografts in athymic nude mice. However, those with mutated p53 had accelerated tumor growth associated with increased vascular endothelial growth factor (VEGF) expression and neovascularization (69). Other investigators have confirmed that NO• regulates VEGF (49,70–72). These data indicate that tumor-associated NO• production may promote cancer progression by providing both a selective growth advantage to tumor cells with mutant p53 and an angiogenic stimulus. As a protective mechanism from the constant barrage of NO•, wild-type p53 has been shown to trans-repress iNOS expression and NO• production in vitro (64). As predicted from these results, p53 knockout mice have increased basal and induced expression of iNOS (73). These studies show that tissues that undergo chronic inflammation in the absence of wild-type p53 may be more susceptible to cancer development because of a lack of negative regulation of iNOS, leading to increased NO• production.

NO• generated by iNOS may mutate p53 during human carcinogenesis (74–76). Recently, we have shown that patients with UC have elevated iNOS expression as well as high p53 codon 247 and 248 mutation frequencies, especially in inflamed lesional regions of the colon (75). Patients with WD or HC also have high expression of iNOS, as well as G:C to T:A transversions at codon 249, C:G to A:T transversions and C:G to T:A transitions at codon 250 (WD) and higher frequencies of G:C to T:A transversions at codon 249 (HC) (45). In spontaneous colon tumors, iNOS activity appears to be expressed throughout the tumorous colon; it is highest in adenomas, then declines with an advancing tumor stage, and is lowest in metastatic tumors

Table 1

Oxyradical Overload Diseases, iNOS Expression, and Human Cancer

Disease	Tissue iNOS Levels		Cancer Site	Relative Risk	Reference
	Preneoplastic	Neoplastic			
Inherited					
Hemochromatosis	↑	No change	Liver	219	*45,46,178*
Wilson's disease	↑	*	Liver	†	†
Crohn's disease	↑	*	Colon	3.4	*36,37,179–182*
Ulcerative colitis	↑	*	Colon	5.7	*36,37,75,180–184*
Acquired					
Viral					
Hepatitis B	↑	↑	Liver	88	*42,185,186*
Hepatitis C	↑	↑	Liver	30	*42,185–187*
Papillomavirus	*	*	Cervix	15.6	*188*
Bacterial					
Helicobacter pylori	↑	*	Gastric	10.4	*40,189,190*
Bladder Catheterization‡	↑	*	*Urinary Bladder	4.7–28	*191*
Cholecystitis‡	↑	↑	Gall Bladder	§	*192,193*
Parasitic					
Schistosoma hematobium	No Change	↑	Urinary Bladder	2–14	*194,195*
S. japonicum	*	*	Colon	1.2–5.7	*194*
Liver fluke/	↑	*	Liver	14.1	*196,197*
Opisthorchis viverrini			(Cholangiocarcinoma)		
Chemical/Physical					
Barrett's esophagus/	↑	↑	Esophageal	50–100	*47,198*
Acid reflux					
Asbestos	*	↑	Mesothelioma	8.1	*199,200*
Smoking	*	↑	Lung	4.3¶	*201,202*

*Indicates unknown, or evidence is not clear from the literature; † Indicates specific relative risk has not clearly been shown in the literature because of early death from complications other than primary hepatocellular carcinoma; ‡ Indicates other physical irritations such as that from the catheter (for bladder catheterization) or gallstones (for cholecystitis) are likely to play a role in the genesis of cancer; § Indicates the study has not been done; ¶ Indicates if smoked equivalent to 20 cigarettes/d for 20 yr. Oxyradical overload may contribute to other known mechanisms of increasing relative risk, e.g., multiple chemical carcinogens found in tobacco smoke.

(74,77). The decline in iNOS activity with an advancing tumor stage may be attributed to FAS-ligand-induced killing of tumor-associated mononuclear cells (TMC) in advanced tumors *(78)*. In colon tumors, *p53* mutations occur primarily in the evolutionarily conserved region of the gene, which contains about 85% of the *p53* mutations and all the mutational hotspots at CpG sites *(79,80)*. iNOS activity is positively correlated with G:C to A:T mutations at 5-methylcytosine sites in *p53*; and the rates of all other mutations vary inversely with iNOS activity *(74)*. Interestingly, G:C to A:T transition mutations are common in lymphoid, esophageal, head and neck, stomach, brain, and breast cancers *(79–81)*, and four of these cancers are known to have elevated iNOS expression *(27,77,82,83)*. Thus, the evidence that NO• and its derivatives mutate cancer-related genes (including *p53*) pro-

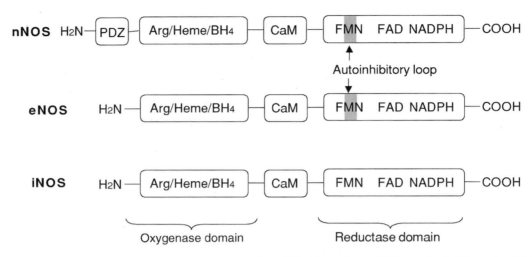

Fig. 2. Domain structure of human NOS. PDZ, PSD-95 discs large/ZO-1 homology; BH4, tetrahydrobiopterin; CaM, calmodulin.

2. NITRIC OXIDE SYNTHASES: STRUCTURE AND INHIBITION

vides a selection pressure for clonal expansion of mutated or aberrant cells, and promote angiogenesis, indicates that NO· can act as both an endogenous tumor initiator and progressor in human carcinogenesis.

The human iNOS gene was first cloned in 1993 *(84–86)*, and has a high homology among different animal species. For example, the overall nucleotide sequence identity between murine and human iNOS cDNA is 80% *(84)*. The iNOS gene is approx 37 kb in length, and is located on chromosome 17cen-q11.2 *(87,88)*. The protein contains 1203 amino acids (131 K_d).

NO· has been shown to be inducibly synthesized by lipopolysaccharide (LPS) *(89)* and by several molecules involved in the inflammatory process (e.g., cytokines *[89–91]*), by microbial products, e.g., LPS *(92)*, and by viral proteins, e.g., HBx *(93,94)*. In addition to transcriptional regulation of iNOS, NOS proteins can also be post-translationally regulated by phosphorylation, dimerization, protein-protein interactions, subcellular localization, and substrate availability and cofactor binding *(95–100)*.

Figure 2 represents the domain structures of human NOS isoforms *(101)*. All isoforms consist of two distinct domains, a so-called oxygenase domain and a reductase domain, connected by a calmodulin-binding domain. The oxygenase domain contains an L-arginine-binding site, heme, and (6R)-5,6,7,8-tetrahydrobiopterin (BH$_4$). The reductase domain of NOS shows at least 50% homology with other flavin mononu-

cleotide (FMN)-and flavin adenine dinucleotide (FAD)-containing reductases such as cytochrome P450 reductase. Electrons from NADPH are transferred through the reductase domain to heme iron, then utilized to activate oxygen and catalyze NO· synthesis. In endothelial NOS (eNOS) and neuronal NOS (nNOS), electron transfer from the reductase domain to heme is triggered by calmodulin binding, whereas binding of calmodulin to iNOS is essentially irreversible. This may explain the differential Ca^{2+}-dependency between eNOS/nNOS and iNOS. eNOS and nNOS have 40–50 amino acids inserted in the middle of the FMN-binding site, known as the autoinhibitory loop. This autoinhibitory loop is believed to play a role in the calmodulin sensitivity of nNOS and eNOS by destabilizing calmodulin binding at low Ca^{2+}*(102)*.

All NOS isoforms are homodimers in their active forms *(101)*. In iNOS, heme incorporation into non-heme enzyme accelerates dimerization and subsequent binding of BH$_4$ and L-arginine stabilize the dimer form. In this context, compounds such as substituted pyrimidine imidazoles that bind to the heme domain affect dimerization of NOS.

Most NOS inhibitors thus far discovered and developed are competitive inhibitors against the L-arginine-binding site *(103)*. These inhibitors include analogs of L-arginine, L-citrulline, or L-lysine, and derivatives of aminoguanidine, isothiourea, isoquinolinamine, and iminopyrrolidine (Fig. 3). Some of these compounds show reversible inhibition against NOS—e.g., N$^{\omega}$-cyclopropyl-L-arginine, but others irreversibly inactivate the enzymes in the presence of cofactors (NADPH) through the formation of reactive intermedi-

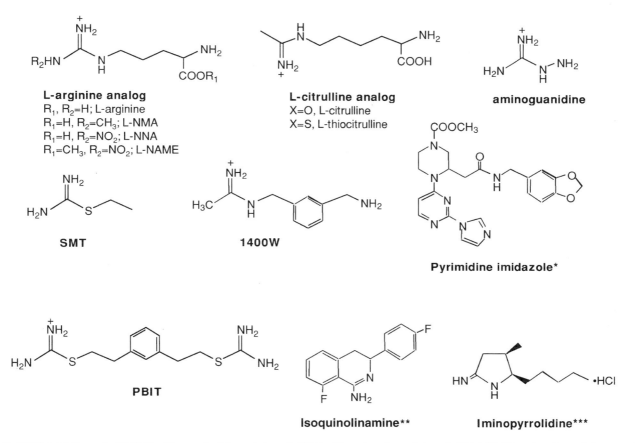

Fig. 3. NOS inhibitors. L-NMMA, Nw-methyl-L-arginine; L-NNA, Nw-nitro-L-arginine; L-NAME; Nw-nitro-L-arginine methyl ester; L-NIL, N6-(1-iminoethyl)-L-lysine; pyrimidine imidazole*, (N-[1,3-benzodioxol-5-yl)methyl]-1-[2-(1H-imidazol-1-yl)pyrimidin-4-yl]-4-(methoxycarbonyl)-piperazine-2-acetamide; PBIT, S,S'-(1,3-phenylenebis(1,2-ethanediyl))bisisothiourea; iso-quinolinamine**, 3-(4'-fluorophenyl)-3,4-dihydro-8-fluoro-1-isoquinolinamine; iminopyrrolidine***, (+)-cis-4-methyl-5-pentylpyrrolidin-2-imine, monohydrochloride.

ates. The latter inhibitors, such as aminoguanidine and L-NMMA, are called "mechanism-based inactivators (or suicide substrates)."

Another class of compounds inhibits NOS activity through inhibiting dimerization of the NOS monomer, which is a prerequisite for the enzyme to express full activity. Recently, McMillan et al. *(104)* reported a highly iNOS-selective inhibitor of this class by using a combinatorial chemistry approach. This substituted pyrimidine imidazole (Fig. 3) does not directly inhibit NOS activity, but very potently inhibits dimerization of iNOS during its synthesis and assembly. This compound was more than 1000-fold selective for iNOS vs eNOS dimerization. Therefore, this class of dimerization inhibitor has broad therapeutic potential in iNOS-mediated pathologies.

In the use of NOS inhibitors for chemoprevention, isoform selectivity of the inhibitors has considerable importance. Undesirable cardiovascular side effects

may occur from nonspecific systemic inhibition of eNOS by the treatment of NOS inhibitors. Table 2 summarizes isoform selectivity of NOS inhibitors. It should be noted that IC_{50} values can only be compared when they are determined under constant substrate concentration. As shown in Table 2, conventional and frequently used NOS inhibitors such as L-NMA and L-NNA are not selective for iNOS vs eNOS or nNOS. Aminoguanidine is partially selective for iNOS vs eNOS (11-fold), but not nearly as selective for iNOS vs nNOS (5.5-fold). Recent development of iNOS-selective inhibitors such as 1400W and derivatives of iminopyrrolidine and isoquinolinamine (Table 2) merits further investigation as chemopreventive agents.

3. INOS AS A TARGET FOR CHEMOPREVENTION

Strategies for preventing cancer in high-risk populations, such as those with chronic inflammation,

Table 2

Isoform Selectivity of NOS Inhibitors

Inhibitor	IC_{50} (μM) nNOS	INOS	eNOS	Reference
L-NMMA	4.9	6.6	3.5	203
L-NNA	0.29	3.1	0.35	101
L-NIL	37	1.6	49	101
Aminoguanidine	170	31	330	203
S-ethylisothiourea	0.015	0.02	0.28	204
1400W	7.3	0.23	1000 >	101
Iminopyrrolidine*	3.2	0.25	226	205
Isoquinolinamine**	16	0.16	100>	206

Abbreviations: L-NMMA, N^{ω}-methyl-L-arginine; L-NNA, N^{ω}-nitro-L-arginine; L-NIL, N^6-(1-iminoethyl)-L-lysine; isoquinolinamine*, 3-(4'-fluorophenyl)-3,4-dihydro-8-fluoro-1-isoquinolinamine; iminopyrrolidine**, (+)-cis-4-methyl-5-pentylpyrrolidine-2-imine, monohydrochloride.

include vaccination and/or eradication of the causative agent, gene therapy, behavioral changes, surveillance, screening, and prophylactic surgery. All approaches may be complemented by chemoprevention strategies that could significantly reduce the risk of cancer in high-risk tissues. Populations in which specific inhibitors of iNOS may reduce cancer risk include those with chronic inflammation.

Chronic inflammation can provide a microenvironment that drives tumorigenesis (reviewed in *105,106*). The production of cytokines and the activation of inflammatory cells with the subsequent generation of ROS and nitrogen oxide species (RNS) during chronic inflammation can alter a number of targets (DNA, proteins, and lipids) and pathways that are critical to normal tissue homeostasis (reviewed in ref. *107*). Mutations in oncogenes and tumor-suppressor genes or post-translational modifications of proteins by ROS and RNS are some key events that can increase the risk of developing cancer. In addition, oxidative/nitrosative stress can modulate cell growth and tumor promotion by activating signal-transduction pathways, resulting in the transcriptional induction of growth competence-related protooncogenes, chromatin remodeling, apoptosis, and cell cycle checkpoints *(108–113)*.

Table 1 summarizes how chronic inflammation can develop into chronic inflammatory disease that can have an etiology that is from several sources: inherited—e.g., HC, WD, UC, Crohn's disease (CD); acquired through viruses, e.g., hepatitis B or C viruses and liver cancer; human papillomavirus and cervical cancer; bacterial,

e.g., *H. pylori* and gastric cancer; long-term bladder catheterization and bladder cancer; cholecystitis and gall bladder cancer; parasites, e.g., *Schistosoma hematobium* and bladder cancer, *S. japonicum* and colon cancer; liver flukes/*Opisthorchis viverrini* and cholangiocarcinoma; or acquired through chemical induction, e.g., acid reflux in Barrett's esophagus and esophageal cancer; asbestos and mesothelioma; smoking and lung cancer. Although the specific mechanisms are still unclear, cancer susceptibility is frequently a pathological consequence of extensive oxidative and nitrosative stress-related damage in these diseases. The diversity of reactive species produced during chronic inflammation under various cellular microenvironments has impaired identification of a clear biomarker that identifies the involvement of a single reactive species in the carcinogenic process. However, as summarized in Table 1, many of these diseases are associated with an increase in iNOS expression and nitrosative stress in precancerous tissue. Based on these observations, along with evidence from animal models, one can hypothesize that chronic overexpression of iNOS and associated NO• production may contribute to tumorigenesis, and is thus an attractive target for chemoprevention. Evidence suggesting the effectiveness of targeting iNOS in chemoprevention comes from experiments in iNOS knockout mice, first generated in 1995 *(114)*. Some studies have shown extensive early-phase inflammation in iNOS$^{-/-}$ mice treated with trinitrobenzene sulphonic acid *(115)*. This is a well-established model of experimental colitis, which has an immunological component and is known to develop into

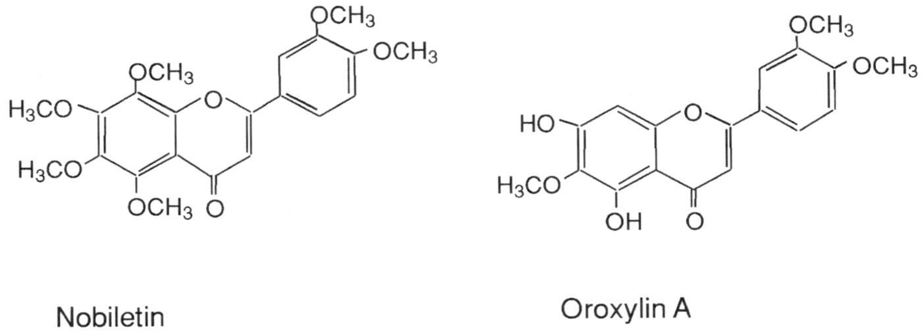

Nobiletin   Oroxylin A

Fig. 4. Naturally occurring polyphenols that inhibit iNOS expression through disruption of NFkB pathway.

a chronic intestinal inflammation approx 1 wk after the induction of colitis. Others have found these mice to have significant resistance to trinitrobenzene-induced lethality and colonic damage, as well as reduced nitrotyrosine formation and malondialdehyde concentrations *(116)*. When these mice are fed dextran sodium sulfate (DSS), they have reduced signs and symptoms of colitis compared with wild-type mice, indicating iNOS plays a critical role in the pathology of colitis *(117,118)*. The implications of this reduced inflammation on development of colon cancer in these mice have not been shown. A study by Konopka et al. *(119)* describes fewer tumors and lower VEGF expression in iNOS$^{-/-}$ mice injected with B16-F1 melanoma cells, indicating a role for iNOS in tumor progression. Cooper and colleagues found mice with a germline adenomatous polyposis coli (APC) gene mutation (*Min* mice) when fed DSS develop significantly accelerated colitis, dysplasia, and cancer compared with wild-type mice, indicating that this mutation may contribute to cancer associated with inflammatory bowel disease *(120)*. Finally, Ahn and Ohshima have shown a significant reduction in adenomas in *Min*/iNOS$^{-/-}$ mice compared with *Min* mice alone *(121)*, indicating that NO• plays a key role in promoting colon carcinogenesis in a background of APC mutation. The implications of these findings to human cancers have not yet been determined.

One strategy to target iNOS for chemoprevention is through the targeting of the NFκB pathway, because this pathway is central to iNOS induction. The therapeutic potential of NFκB pathway inhibition in the treatment of inflammation and cancer has been reviewed by Yamamoto and Gaynor *(122)*. Briefly, this pathway is the target of many antiinflammatory drugs, including degradation-resistant IκB proteins, glucocorticoids, nonsteroidal antiinflammatory drugs (NSAIDs), immunosuppressive agents, cyclopentenone

prostaglandins, proteasome inhibitors, and flavonoids (quercetin, resveratrol, and myricetin). Several laboratories have described NFκB sites in the promoter region of iNOS that are required for transcriptional activity. Therefore, it is not surprising to find that many drugs targeting NFκB also block iNOS gene expression and subsequent NO• production. Although these drugs reduce inflammation, studies are required to understand more fully their impact on carcinogenesis. Of the drugs that have been shown to reduce carcinogenesis, it is unclear whether the mechanism acts through iNOS expression and NO• production, or whether this is just coincidental. The evidence, indicating a critical role for iNOS and NO• in inflammation and carcinogenesis, has led to the development of drugs that specifically target these molecules.

We previously outlined the effect of genetic ablation of iNOS on carcinogenesis in animals. To date relatively few studies have examined the direct impact of iNOS inhibitors on carcinogenesis in animal models of human cancer, and thus far, no studies have been reported in humans. Exogenous administration of xenobiotics and transgenic mouse models that increase iNOS and NO• production have been used to examine NO• effects on inflammation and tumorigenesis. For example, SJL mice injected with superantigen-bearing RcsX (pre-B-cell lymphoma) cells generate large amounts of NO• with associated apoptosis, nitrotyrosine formation, etheno DNA adducts, mutagenesis, and tumor formation *(123–125)*. Although many other animal models of chronic inflammation show the induction of iNOS and NO• generation and increased tumorigenesis *(124,126–128)*, these models provide only indirect evidence that NO• drives tumorigenesis. Further direct evidence comes from the administration of iNOS and NO• inhibitors. For example, the inhibition of NO• synthesis has been shown to inhibit hepatitis

Table 3

Animal Studies Showing Inhibition of Inflammation and Tumorigenesis by iNOS Ablation or Inhibitors

Treatment	Regimen	Experimental Model	Observed Effect	Reference
iNOS KO	6 mg, anally	Trinitrobenzene-treated mice	Transiently increased inflammation from 24–72 h	115
iNOS KO	1 mg, anally	Trinitrobenzene-treated mice	Decreased inflammation from 3–7 d	116
iNOS KO	N/A	B16-BL6 and –F10 melanoma cells injected into iNOS mice	Decreased metastases	155,157
Aminoguanidine	10 mg/kg, ip	Concanavalin-treated mice	Reduced hepatitis	129
Aminoguanidine	20 mg/kg, sc	Serotonin-treated rats	Reduced gastritis	130
Aminoguanidine	1 g/L in drinking water	APC(Min/+) mice	Reduced adenoma	121
Aminoguanidine	1800 ppm, in food	AOM-treated mice	Reduced ACF	131
Aminoguanidine	1.5 μmol/kg/d, orally	Trinitrobenzene-treated rats	Reduced damage, myeloperoxidase activity, and serum nitrogen oxide	207
Aminoguanidine	10 mg/kg, ip	Trinitrobenzene-treated rats	Reduced colonic damage and myeloperoxidase activity	208
NMA	30 mM, in drinking water	SJL mice	Reduced nitrate/nitrite, mutation frequency, and etheno adducts	125,127
L-NAME	1g/L, in drinking water	Transplanted rat P22 carcinosarcoma cells into flank of rats	Reduced tumor blood flow	135
L-NNA	3 mg/kg, iv	Transplanted rat P22 carcinosarcoma cells into flank of rats	Reduced tumor blood flow	51,136
L-NAME	2 mM, in drinking water	A-431 explants onto rabbit cornea	Delayed angiogenic response	83
L-NAME	0.1 g/d, in drinking water	Rabbit cornea assay	Inhibited angiogenesis by the tachykinin, 'Substance P'	137

140

Agent	Dose/route	Model	Effect	Ref.
L-NAME	0.1–1 mg/mL, in drinking water	Transplanted C3-L5 mammary cancer cells	Reduce tumor growth and* metastases	138
L-NAME	80 mg/kg, ip	Renal subcapsular CC531 adenocarcinoma rat model or isolated limb perfusion model	Reduced tumor growth	209
L-NAME	10 mg/kg, iv	Implanted murine mammary and human colon cells	Reduced vessel diameter and* blood flow (sc) into mice	210
L-NAME	2 mg, ip	Breast cancer cells injected into mice	Reduced metastases	153
L-NAME	2 mM, osmotic minipumps	Murine breast cancer injected into mice	Reduced tumor size and metastases	211
L-NAME	100 ppm, in food	AOM-treated mice	Reduced ACF	133
L-NAME S-methyliso-thiourea sulphate	50 mg/kg	sc implant of hepatoma cells	Reduced tumor growth	134
SC-51	0–100 ppm in food	AOM-treated mice	Reduced ACF	131
PBIT	50 ppm in food	AOM-treated mice	Reduced ACF	132
1400W	2 mg/kg/d, ip	Trinitrobenzene-treated rats	Reduced damage score, iNOS activity and myeloperoxidase activity	212
1400W	12 mg/kg/h, continuous infustion	EMT6 murine mammary adenocarcinoma	Reduced tumor wt	66
1400W	6 mg/kg/h, continuous infustion	Human tumor xenograft (DLD-1 cells + iNOS)	Reduced tumor growth	66

Table 4

Animal Studies Showing No Effect or Enhancement of Inflammation and Tumorigenesis by iNOS Ablation or Inhibitors

Treatment	Regimen	Experimental Model	Observed Effect	Reference
iNOS KO	N/A	Pancreatic cells implanted into the pancreas of mice	Slight increase in liver metastases	156
iNOS KO	N/A	M5076 murine ovarian cells injected into mice	Increased metastases	156,157
L-NIL or Aminoguanidine	60 mg/kg/d, orally	Spontaneous monkey colitis	No impact on colitis	139
L-NAME Aminoguanidine	100 mg/kg/d, orally 400 mg/kg/d, orally	DSS-induced rat colitis	Worsened DSS-induced inflammation	140
L-NAME	10 mg/kg, in drinking water	AOM-treated rats	Promotes colon ACF	148
L-NAME	9.3 µmol, iv	Experimental pulmonary metastases	Promotes metastases	152
L-NAME Aminoguanidine	500 mg/L, in drinking water	Trinitrobenzene-treated rats	No impact on colitis	213
NMA	10 mg, injected twice daily	M5076 iv injected into mice for liver metastases	Inhibits anti-tumor effect of iNOS	160
NMA	20 mg, injected twice daily	iNOS transfected cells iv injected into mice	Inhibits anti-tumor effect of iNOS	163
L-NMMA	50 mg/kg, ip	Trinitrobenzene-treated rats	Increased colonic damage score	214
L-NNA	10 mg/kg, ip	Trinitrobenzene-treated rats	Aggravated colonic damage and myeloperoxidase activity	208

in animal models *(129)* and gastritis *(130)*. Ahn and Ohshima *(121)* found that administration of the iNOS inhibitor aminoguanidine (AG) in drinking water or an L-arginine-deficient diet to APC (*Min*/+) mice resulted in a significant decrease in adenoma development. Rao et al. *(131)* examined the impact of specific iNOS inhibitors alone or in combination with cyclooxygenase (COX)-2 inhibitors on the development of azoxymethane (AOM)-induced colonic aberrant crypt foci (ACF), a precursor of colonic cancer. They found a significant inhibition of ACF with the iNOS inhibitors L-*N*(6)-(1-iminoethyl)lysine tetra-zolamide (SC-51) and AG and an even greater reduction in the frequency of ACF with the co-administration of SC-51 and the COX-2 inhibitor, celecoxib. This study is an extension of earlier studies showing an inhibition of AOM-induced ACF formation by the iNOS-specific inhibitor PBIT *(132)*. Kawamori et al. *(133)* showed that l-*N*(G)-nitroarginine methyl ester (L-NAME) fed to rats inhibited AOM-induced ACF formation by 24–39%. Doi et al. *(134)* described a moderate suppression of experimental solid tumor (AH136 hepatoma)-cell growth in rats by L-NAME. Finally, Thomsen et al. *(66)* showed that the novel selective iNOS inhibitor 1400W significantly reduced tumor growth of EMT6 murine mammary adenocarcinomas and human tumor xenografts (colon adenocarcinoma DLD-1) that were genetically engineered to express iNOS constitutively.

We have described the impact of NO• on VEGF and angiogenesis *(49, 69–72)*. To further evaluate this connection, Tozer et al. *(135)* showed that coadministration of the tubulin-destabilizing agent disodium combretastatin A-4 3-*O*-phosphate (CA-4-P) with *N*(ω)-nitro-L-arginine (L-NNA) methyl ester dramatically reduces the established tumor vasculature, leading to the development of extensive tumor-cell necrosis. Similarly, the same investigation showed a reduction in tumor blood flow with the administration of L-NNA alone *(51,136)*. In independent studies using a rabbit cornea assay, Ziche et al. *(137)* and Gallo et al. *(83)* described the inhibition of NO•-induced angiogenesis by blocking NO• production, using L-NNA. Similarly, L-NAME treatment reduces tumor growth in adeno-carcinoma-bearing mice *(138)*. Finally, Jenkins and colleagues *(49)* showed an increase in vessel density and tumor growth in iNOS-transfected tumors.

In contrast to these studies, some studies have had no effect or have even exacerbated inflammation and tumorigenesis by NO• inhibition. In a Rhesus monkey model, Ribbons and colleagues found no effect of L-*N*6-(1-iminoethyl) (L-NIL) or AG on spontaneous colitis *(139)*. Yoshida et al. *(140)* showed that inhibition of NO• production by either L-NAME or AG worsened DSS-induced inflammation, suggesting a protective role for NO• in acute colitis. As described earlier, one explanation for this effect may be the observation that NO• acts as a ROS scavenger *(141)* and can inhibit induction of inflammation-associated genes *(142–147)*. Because NO• donors can also exaggerate inflammation, inflammation can be aggravated by either too much or too little NO•. Treatment of inflammatory diseases should therefore aim for maintenance of "appropriate" levels of NO• in the target tissue. Because of the inherent heterogeneity of NO• on normal and tumor cells, it is still unclear which levels are appropriate.

Using cancer as an endpoint, Schleiffer and colleagues *(148)* showed that L-NAME enhances AOM-induced ACF formation by 47%. Others have shown that immunomodulators can reduce tumor growth and metastasis through the activation of iNOS expression in macrophages *(149,150)*. The observation of an inverse correlation between expression of endogenous iNOS and NO• production and metastasis, indicates that NO• can reduce the metastatic potential of tumors (reviewed in *151*). This inhibition of metastases by NO• is supported with experiments by Yamamoto and colleagues, who showed increased experimental pulmonary metastasis by L-NAME *(152)*. However, Iwasaki et al. found that incidence and number of osteolytic bone metastases and the number of bones with metastasis is significantly reduced in L-NAME-treated mice *(153)*. Also, Edwards and colleagues described an augmentation of tumor growth and metastasis by NO• in mice injected with EMT-6 murine breast cancer cells *(154)*. Insight into these contradictory results has been presented by Xie's and Fiedler's groups through an elegant set of studies using iNOS ablation, iNOS inhibitors, iNOS induction, or NO• donors. They suggest that the effect of NO• on tumor growth and metastases depends on the levels of NO• delivered (high NO• levels often lead to cell death and therefore tumor ablation), genetic background, and cell type, which determine NO• sensitivity *(151,155–164)*.

Most studies on the impact of NO• on angiogenesis have established an exacerbation of angiogenesis by NO• (and a protective effect against angiogenesis by specific iNOS inhibitors). Although studies have mostly shown that iNOS inhibitors reduce inflammation, tumor promotion, and metastases, some have found opposite results (e.g., inhibition of inflammation and tumorigenesis by NO•). This apparent contradictory evidence in animals highlights the importance of careful scrutiny when using iNOS inhibitors as chemopreventive agents in humans. Studies have now also shown the value of using NO• as an adjuvant therapy, as it appears to sensitize cells to the effects of chemotherapy (165–167). The putative cytotoxic effects of NO• or its role in a negative feedback loop may also be exploited in the clinical setting to suppress the expression of genes involved in chronic inflammation, in addition to sending damaged cells into apoptosis. However, although NO• clearly induces DNA damage and can drive tumorigenesis, the impact of directly inhibiting tumorigenesis with iNOS inhibitors needs further evaluation. One can hypothesize that the opposing roles of NO• in tumorigenesis are a function of the complex chemistry of NO°, as well as NO• levels, the biologic phenotype and genetic makeup of the tumor cells, and the surrounding microenvironment (e.g., scavengers, hypoxia, or pH). NO• at high concentrations may damage cells extensively enough to initiate apoptosis. In contrast, because of their phenotype and genotype, some cells may resist NO•-driven apoptosis, or certain areas may produce a relatively low amount of NO• that provides a microenvironment conducive to cell survival, clonal expansion, and tumorigenesis (possibly through an interactive role with COX-2). The key role of genetic background is highlighted by the observation that cell response to NO• depends largely on p53 status (69,168). Because adenoma frequency is reduced in Min/ iNOS$^{-/-}$ mice compared with Min mice alone (121), NO• can also promote carcinogenesis in the genetic background of APC mutation.

These studies have allowed us to understand the potential responses of tissue and tumors to NO•-targeted treatments. Animal models must be carefully chosen to properly evaluate the efficacy of iNOS inhibitors in chemoprevention and tumorigenesis. Further studies are required to identify molecules that are better at targeting iNOS, to identify the efficacy and mechanisms of current and future iNOS-specific inhibitors in tumorigenesis/tumor protection, and to guide the use of these molecules as chemopreventive agents in humans. One way to monitor such use of these agents is through intermediate biomarkers. Ultimately, the most valid biomarkers are those that are mechanistically involved in carcinogenesis (e.g., DNA damage, proliferation, differentiation, and apop-

totic markers), properly predict cancer outcome, and can be measured in human tissue or surrogate biological fluids. Few promising markers fit into these categories. Many markers of internal dose (e.g., levels of reactive oxygen and nitrogen byproducts) and internal dose effect (e.g., levels of DNA or protein adducts/damage in target and/or surrogate tissue) and their use in chemoprevention trials, have been well-reviewed (169). Some specific markers used in monitoring nitrosative stress and chemoprevention of this stress include: N-nitrosoproline (NPRO), N-nitrosamino acid (NAA) and NO_3^- in urine or plasma; 8-oxodeoxyguanosine (8-oxodGuo), 8-nitrosoguanosine (8-nitroGua), exocyclic etheno- and malondialdehyde-DNA adducts in leukocytes or target tissue; and 3-nitrotyrosine protein adducts (169–172). The consequences of these effect markers on human carcinogenesis are unknown. Thus, more direct markers are aimed at the identification of molecular changes in genes or proteins directly associated with carcinogenesis. One such marker is a highly sensitive genotypic assay developed by Cerutti and colleagues. This has enabled the detection of low-frequency mutations in normal-appearing human tissues as well as in cells exposed to an environmental carcinogen (173–177). As described earlier, we have used this technique to detect p53 mutations in target tissue of patients with the oxyradical overload diseases UC (colon), HC (liver), and WD (liver) (45,75). Others have found specific DNA profiles (hotspots) associated with NO• exposure (59). The identification of these hotspots, the detection of specific mutations in cancer-causing genes, or the use of microarrays to detect patterns of gene expression and/or protein changes in normal-appearing tissue may help identify individuals at increased cancer risk and help in the evaluation of iNOS and NO• inhibitors in chemoprevention.

ACKNOWLEDGMENTS

We thank Drs. Gerald Wogan and Stefan Ambs for guidance in manuscript preparation, Ms. Dorothea Dudek for editorial assistance, and Mrs. Karen MacPherson for bibliographic assistance.

REFERENCES

1. Furchgott RF, Zawadzki JV. The obligatory role of endothelial cells in the relaxation of arterial smooth muscle by acetylcholine. *Nature* 1980;288:373–376.

2. Cherry PD, Furchgott RF, Zawadzki JV, Jothianandan D. Role of endothelial cells in relaxation of isolated arteries by bradykinin. *Proc Natl Acad Sci USA* 1982;79:2106–2110.

3. Ignarro LJ. Biological actions and properties of endothelium-derived nitric oxide formed and released from artery and vein. *Circ Res* 1989;65:1–21.

4. Murad F, Arnold WP, Mittal CK, Braughler JM. Properties and regulation of guanylate cyclase and some proposed functions for cyclic GMP. *Adv Cyclic Nucleotide Res* 1979;11:175–204.

5. Palmer RM, Ferrige AG, Moncada S. Nitric oxide release accounts for the biological activity of endothelium-derived relaxing factor. *Nature* 1987;327:524–526.

6. Furchgott RF, Jothianandan D. Endothelium-dependent and -independent vasodilation involving cyclic GMP: relaxation induced by nitric oxide, carbon monoxide and light. *Blood Vessels* 1991;28:52–61.

7. Sanders KM, Ward SM. Nitric oxide as a mediator of nonadrenergic noncholinergic neurotransmission. *Am J Physiol* 1992;262:G379–G392.

8. Nathan C, Shiloh MU. Reactive oxygen and nitrogen intermediates in the relationship between mammalian hosts and microbial pathogens. *Proc Natl Acad Sci USA* 2000;97:8841–8848.

9. Cheung PY, Salas E, Etches PC, et al. Inhaled nitric oxide and inhibition of platelet aggregation in critically ill neonates. *Lancet* 1998;351:1181–1182.

10. Salvemini D, de Nucci G, Gryglewski RJ, Vane JR. Human neutrophils and mononuclear cells inhibit platelet aggregation by releasing a nitric oxide-like factor. *Proc Natl Acad Sci USA* 1989;86:6328–6332.

11. Pantopoulos K, Weiss G, Hentze MW. Nitric oxide and oxidative stress (H_2O_2) control mammalian iron metabolism by different pathways. *Mol Cell Biol* 1996;16:3781–3788.

12. Domachowske JB. The role of nitric oxide in the regulation of cellular iron metabolism. *Biochem Mol Med* 1997;60:1–7.

13. Moncada S, Palmer RM, Higgs EA. Nitric oxide: physiology, pathophysiology, and pharmacology. *Pharmacol Rev* 1991;43:109–142.

14. Nathan C, Xie QW. Nitric oxide synthases: roles, tolls, and controls. *Cell* 1994;78:915–918.

15. Bredt DS, Snyder SH. Nitric oxide: a physiologic messenger molecule. *Annu Rev Biochem* 1994;63:175–195.

16. Hentze MW, Kuhn LC. Molecular control of vertebrate iron metabolism: mRNA-based regulatory circuits operated by iron, nitric oxide, and oxidative stress. *Proc Natl Acad Sci USA* 1996;93:8175–8182.

17. Tamir S, Tannenbaum SR. The role of nitric oxide (NO•) in the carcinogenic process. *Biochim Biophys Acta* 1996;1288:F31–F36.

18. Ambs S, Hussain SP, Harris CC. Interactive effects of nitric oxide and the p53 tumor suppressor gene in carcinogenesis and tumor progression. *FASEB J* 1997;11:443–448.

19. Marletta MA. Nitric oxide synthase: aspects concerning structure and catalysis. *Cell* 1994;78:927–930.

20. Forstermann U, Kleinert H. Nitric oxide synthase: expression and expressional control of the three isoforms. *Naunyn Schmiedebergs Arch Pharmacol* 1995;352:351–364.

21. Guo FH, De Raeve HR, Rice TW, et al. Continuous nitric oxide synthesis by inducible nitric oxide synthase in normal human airway epithelium in vivo. *Proc Natl Acad Sci USA* 1995;92:7809–7813.

22. Hoffman RA, Zhang G, Nussler NC, et al. Constitutive expression of inducible nitric oxide synthase in the mouse ileal mucosa. *Am J Physiol* 1997;272:G383–G392.

23. Beckman JS, Beckman TW, Chen J, et al. Apparent hydroxyl radical production by peroxynitrite: implications for endothelial injury from nitric oxide and superoxide. *Proc Natl Acad Sci USA* 1990;87:1620–1624.

24. Malinski T, Taha Z, Grunfeld S, et al. Diffusion of nitric oxide in the aorta wall monitored *in situ* by porphyrinic microsensors. *Biochem Biophys Res Commun* 1993;193:1076–1082.

25. Geller DA, Billiar TR. Molecular biology of nitric oxide synthases. *Cancer Metastasis Rev* 1998;17:7–23.

26. Thomsen LL, Lawton FG, Knowles RG, et al. Nitric oxide synthase activity in human gynecological cancer. *Cancer Res* 1994;54:1352–1354.

27. Thomsen LL, Miles DW, Happerfield L, et al. Nitric oxide synthase activity in human breast cancer. *Br J Cancer* 1995;72:41–44.

28. Cobbs CS, Brenman JE, Aldape KD, et al. Expression of nitric oxide synthase in human central nervous system tumors. *Cancer Res* 1995;55:727–730.

29. Koh E, Noh SH, Lee YD, et al. Differential expression of nitric oxide synthase in human stomach cancer. *Cancer Lett* 1999;146:173–180.

30. Mendes RV, Martins AR, de Nucci G, et al. Expression of nitric oxide synthase isoforms and nitrotyrosine immunoreactivity by B-cell non-Hodgkin's lymphomas and multiple myeloma. *Histopathology* 2001;39:172–178.

31. Wolf H, Haeckel C, Roessner A. Inducible nitric oxide synthase expression in human urinary bladder cancer. *Virchows Arch* 2000;437:662–666.

32. Baltaci S, Orhan D, Gogus C, et al. Inducible nitric oxide synthase expression in benign prostatic hyperplasia, low- and high-grade prostatic intraepithelial neoplasia and prostatic carcinoma. *BJU Int* 2001;88:100–103.

33. Vakkala M, Kahlos K, Lakari E, et al. Inducible nitric oxide synthase expression, apoptosis, and angiogenesis in *in situ* and invasive breast carcinomas. *Clin Cancer Res* 2000;6:2408–2416.

34. Tschugguel W, Schneeberger C, Unfried G, et al. Expression of inducible nitric oxide synthase in human breast cancer depends on tumor grade. *Breast Cancer Res Treat* 1999;56:145–151.

35. Singer II, Kawka DW, Scott S, et al. Expression of inducible nitric oxide synthase and nitrotyrosine in colonic epithelium in inflammatory bowel disease. *Gastroenterology* 1996;111:871–885.

36. Kimura H, Hokari R, Miura S, et al. Increased expression of an inducible isoform of nitric oxide synthase and the formation of peroxynitrite in colonic mucosa of patients with active ulcerative colitis. *Gut* 1998;42:180–187.

37. Dijkstra G, Moshage H, van Dullemen HM, et al. Expression of nitric oxide synthases and formation of nitrotyrosine and reactive oxygen species in inflammatory bowel disease. *J Pathol* 1998;186:416–421.

38. Mannick EE, Bravo LE, Zarama G, et al. Inducible nitric oxide synthase, nitrotyrosine, and apoptosis in Helicobacter pylori gastritis: effect of antibiotics and antioxidants. *Cancer Res* 1996;56:3238–3243.

39. Goto T, Haruma K, Kitadai Y, et al. Enhanced expression of inducible nitric oxide synthase and nitrotyrosine in gastric

mucosa of gastric cancer patients. *Clin Cancer Res* 1999;5:1411–1415.

40. Fu S, Ramanujam KS, Wong A, et al. Increased expression and cellular localization of inducible nitric oxide synthase and cyclooxygenase 2 in Helicobacter pylori gastritis. *Gastroenterology* 1999;116:1319–1329.

41. Kane JM III, Shears LL II, Hierholzer C, et al. Chronic hepatitis C virus infection in humans: induction of hepatic nitric oxide synthase and proposed mechanisms for carcinogenesis. *J Surg Res* 1997;69:321–324.

42. Majano PL, Garcia-Monzon C, Lopez-Cabrera M, et al. Inducible nitric oxide synthase expression in chronic viral hepatitis. Evidence for a virus-induced gene upregulation. *J Clin Investig* 1998;101:1343–1352.

43. Garcia-Monzon C, Majano PL, Zubia I, et al. Intrahepatic accumulation of nitrotyrosine in chronic viral hepatitis is associated with histological severity of liver disease. *J Hepatol* 2000;32:331–338.

44. Cuzzocrea S, Zingarelli B, Villari D, et al. Evidence for in vivo peroxynitrite production in human chronic hepatitis. *Life Sci* 1998;63:L25–L30.

45. Hussain SP, Raja K, Amstad PA, et al. Increased p53 mutation load in nontumorous human liver of Wilson Disease and hemochromatosis: oxyradical overload diseases. *Proc Natl Acad Sci USA* 2000;97:12,770–12,775.

46. Marrogi AJ, Khan MA, van Gijssel HE, et al. Oxidate stress and p53 mutations in the carcinogenesis of iron overload-associated hepatocellular carcinoma. *J Natl Cancer Inst* 2001;93:1652–1655.

47. Wilson KT, Fu S, Ramanujam KS, Meltzer SJ. Increased expression of inducible nitric oxide synthase and cyclooxygenase-2 in Barrett's esophagus and associated adenocarcinomas. *Cancer Res* 1998;58:2929–2934.

48. Ohshima H, Bartsch H. Chronic infections and inflammatory processes as cancer risk factors: possible role of nitric oxide in carcinogenesis. *Mutat Res* 1994;305:253–264.

49. Jenkins DC, Charles IG, Thomsen LL, et al. Roles of nitric oxide in tumor growth. *Proc Natl Acad Sci USA* 1995;92:4392–4396.

50. Maeda H, Noguchi Y, Sato K, Akaike T. Enhanced vascular permeability in solid tumor is mediated by nitric oxide and inhibited by both new nitric oxide scavenger and nitric oxide synthase inhibitor. *Jpn J Cancer Res* 1994;85:331–334.

51. Tozer GM, Prise VE, Chaplin DJ. Inhibition of nitric oxide synthase induces a selective reduction in tumor blood flow that is reversible with L-arginine. *Cancer Res* 1997;57:948–955.

52. Nicotera P, Bonfoco E, Brune B. Mechanisms for nitric oxide-induced cell death: involvement of apoptosis. *Adv Neuroimmunol* 1997;5:411–420.

53. Dimmeler S, Haendeler J, Nehls M, Zeiher AM. Suppression of apoptosis by nitric oxide via inhibition of interleukin-1β-converting enzyme (ICE)-like and cysteine protease protein (CPP)-32-like proteases. *J Exp Med* 1997;185:601–607.

54. Li J, Bombeck CA, Yang S, et al. Nitric oxide suppresses apoptosis via interrupting caspase activation and mitochondrial dysfunction in cultured hepatocytes. *J Biol Chem* 1999;274:17,325–17,333.

55. Chung HT, Pae HO, Choi BM, et al. Nitric oxide as a bioregulator of apoptosis. *Biochem Biophys Res Commun* 2001;282:1075–1079.

56. Kim PK, Zamora R, Petrosko P, Billiar TR. The regulatory role of nitric oxide in apoptosis. *Int Immunopharmacol* 2001;1:1421–1441.

57. Melillo G, Musso T, Sica A, et al. A hypoxia-responsive element mediates a novel pathway of activation of the inducible nitric oxide synthase promoter. *J Exp Med* 1995;182:1683–1693.

58. Zhuang JC, Wright TL, deRojas-Walker T, et al. Nitric oxide-induced mutations in the HPRT gene of human lymphoblastoid TK6 cells and in Salmonella typhimurium. *Environ Mol Mutagen* 2000;35:39–47.

59. Tretyakova NY, Burney S, Pamir B, et al. Peroxynitrite-induced DNA damage in the supF gene: correlation with the mutational spectrum. *Mutat Res* 2000;447:287–303.

60. Zhuang JC, Lin C, Lin D, Wogan GN. Mutagenesis associated with nitric oxide production in macrophages. *Proc Natl Acad Sci USA* 1998;95:8286–8291.

61. Wink DA, Hanbauer I, Grisham MB, et al. Chemical biology of nitric oxide: regulation and protective and toxic mechanisms. *Curr Top Cell Regul* 1996;34:159–87.

62. Sibghat-Ullah, Gallinari P, Xu YZ, et al. Base analog and neighboring base effects on substrate specificity of recombinant human G:T mismatch-specific thymine DNA-glycosylase. *Biochemistry* 1996;35:12,926–12,932.

63. Messmer UK, Brune B. Nitric oxide-induced apoptosis: p53-dependent and p53-independent signalling pathways. *Biochem J* 1996;319:299–305.

64. Forrester K, Ambs S, Lupold SE, et al. Nitric oxide-induced p53 accumulation and regulation of inducible nitric oxide synthase (NOS2) expression by wild-type p53. *Proc Natl Acad Sci USA* 1996;93:2442–2447.

65. Nakaya N, Lowe SW, Taya Y, Chenchik A, Enikolopov G. Specific pattern of p53 phosphorylation during nitric oxide-induced cell cycle arrest. *Oncogene* 2000;19:6369–6375.

66. Thomsen LL, Scott JM, Topley P, et al. Selective inhibition of inducible nitric oxide synthase inhibits tumor growth in vivo: studies with 1400W, a novel inhibitor. *Cancer Res* 1997;57:3300–3304.

67. DuBois RN. New paradigms for cancer prevention. *Carcinogenesis* 2001;22:691–692.

68. Gupta RA, DuBois RN. Combinations for cancer prevention. *Nat Med* 2000;6:974–975.

69. Ambs S, Merriam WG, Ogunfusika MO, et al. p53 and vascular endothelial growth factor regulate tumour growth of NOS2-expressing human carcinoma cells. *Nat Med* 1998;4:1371–1376.

70. Chin K, Kurashima Y, Ogura T, et al. Induction of vascular endothelial growth factor by nitric oxide in human glioblastoma and hepatocellular carcinoma cells. *Oncogene* 1997;15:437–442.

71. Frank S, Stallmeyer B, Kampfer H, et al. Differential regulation of vascular endothelial growth factor and its receptor FMS-like-tyrosine kinase is mediated by nitric oxide in rat renal mesangial cells. *Biochem J* 1999;338:367–374.

72. Papapetropoulos A, Garcia-Cardena G, Madri JA, Sessa WC. Nitric oxide production contributes to the angiogenic properties of vascular endothelial growth factor in human endothelial cells. *J Clin Investig* 1997;100:3131–3139.

73. Ambs S, Ogunfusika MO, Merriam WG, et al. Upregulation of NOS2 expression in cancer-prone p53 knockout mice. *Proc Natl Acad Sci USA* 1998;95:8823–8828.

74. Ambs S, Bennett WP, Merriam WG, et al. Relationship between p53 mutations and inducible nitric oxide synthase expression in human colorectal cancer. *J Natl Cancer Inst* 1999;91:86–88.

75. Hussain SP, Amstad P, Raja K et al. Increased p53 mutation load in noncancerous colon tissue from ulcerative colitis: a cancer-prone chronic inflammatory disease. *Cancer Res* 2000;60:3333–3337.

76. Umetani N, Sasaki S, Watanabe T, et al. Genetic alterations in ulcerative colitis-associated neoplasia focusing on APC, K-*ras* gene and microsatellite instability. *Jpn J Cancer Res* 1999;90:1081–1087.

77. Ambs S, Merriam WG, Bennett WP, et al. Frequent nitric oxide synthase-2 expression in human colon adenomas: implication for tumor angiogenesis and colon cancer progression. *Cancer Res* 1998;58:334–341.

78. Alleva DG, Burger CJ, Elgert KD. Tumor-induced regulation of suppressor macrophage nitric oxide and TNF-α production. Role of tumor-derived IL-10, TGF-β, and prostaglandin E$_2$. *J Immunol* 1994;153:1674–1686.

79. Hollstein M, Sidransky D, Vogelstein B, Harris CC. p53 mutations in human cancers. *Science* 1991;253:49–53.

80. Greenblatt MS, Bennett WP, Hollstein M, Harris CC. Mutations in the p53 tumor suppressor gene: clues to cancer etiology and molecular pathogenesis. *Cancer Res* 1994;54:4855–4878.

81. Levine AJ, Momand J, Finlay CA. The p53 tumour suppressor gene. *Nature* 1991;351:453–456.

82. Ellie E, Loiseau H, Lafond F, et al. Differential expression of inducible nitric oxide synthase mRNA in human brain tumours. *Neuroreport* 1995;7:294–296.

83. Gallo O, Masini E, Morbidelli L, et al. Role of nitric oxide in angiogenesis and tumor progression in head and neck cancer. *J Natl Cancer Inst* 1998;90:587–596.

84. Geller DA, Lowenstein CJ, Shapiro RA, et al. Molecular cloning and expression of inducible nitric oxide synthase from human hepatocytes. *Proc Natl Acad Sci USA* 1993;90:3491–3495.

85. Sherman PA, Laubach VE, Reep BR, Wood ER. Purification and cDNA sequence of an inducible nitric oxide synthase from a human tumor cell line. *Biochemistry* 1993;32:11,600–11,605.

86. Charles IG, Palmer RM, Hickery MS, et al. Cloning, characterization, and expression of a cDNA encoding an inducible nitric oxide synthase from the human chondrocyte. *Proc Natl Acad Sci USA* 1993;90:11,419–11,423.

87. Chartrain NA, Geller DA, Koty PP, et al. Molecular cloning, structure, and chromosomal localization of the human inducible nitric oxide synthase gene. *J Biol Chem* 1994;269:6765–6772.

88. Marsden PA, Schappert KT, Chen HS et al. Molecular cloning and characterization of human endothelial nitric oxide synthase. *FEBS Lett* 1992;307:287–293.

89. Stuehr DJ, Cho HJ, Kwon NS, et al. Purification and characterization of the cytokine-induced macrophage nitric oxide synthase: an FAD- and FMN-containing flavoprotein. *Proc Natl Acad Sci USA* 1991;88:7773–7777.

90. Markewitz BA, Michael JR, Kohan DE. Cytokine-induced expression of a nitric oxide synthase in rat renal tubule cells. *J Clin Investig* 1993;91:2138–2143.

91. Koide M, Kawahara Y, Tsuda T, Yokoyama M. Cytokine-induced expression of an inducible type of nitric oxide syn-

thase gene in cultured vascular smooth muscle cells. *FEBS Lett* 1993;318:213–217.

92. Lowenstein CJ, Alley EW, Raval P, et al. Macrophage nitric oxide synthase gene: two upstream regions mediate induction by interferon γ and lipopolysaccharide. *Proc Natl Acad Sci USA* 1993;90:9730–9734.

93. Amaro MJ, Bartolome J, Carreno V. Hepatitis B virus X protein transactivates the inducible nitric oxide synthase promoter. *Hepatology* 1999;29:915–923.

94. Elmore LW, Hancock AR, Chang SF, et al. Hepatitis B virus X protein and p53 tumor suppressor interactions in the modulation of apoptosis. *Proc Natl Acad Sci USA* 1997;94:14,707–14,712.

95. Dimmeler S, Fleming I, Fisslthaler B, et al. Activation of nitric oxide synthase in endothelial cells by Akt-dependent phosphorylation. *Nature* 1999;399:601–605.

96. Pan J, Burgher KL, Szczepanik AM, Ringheim GE. Tyrosine phosphorylation of inducible nitric oxide synthase: implications for potential post-translational regulation. *Biochem J* 1996;314:889–894.

97. Michel T, Li GK, Busconi L. Phosphorylation and subcellular translocation of endothelial nitric oxide synthase. *Proc Natl Acad Sci USA* 1993;90:6252–6256.

98. Cho HJ, Martin E, Xie QW, et al. Inducible nitric oxide synthase: identification of amino acid residues essential for dimerization and binding of tetrahydrobiopterin. *Proc Natl Acad Sci USA* 1995;92:11,514–11,518.

99. Kone BC. Protein-protein interactions controlling nitric oxide synthases. *Acta Physiol Scand* 2000;168:27–31.

100. Govers R, Rabelink TJ. Cellular regulation of endothelial nitric oxide synthase. *Am J Physiol Renal Physiol* 2001;280:F193–F206.

101. Alderton WK, Cooper CE, Knowles RG. Nitric oxide synthases: structure, function and inhibition. *Biochem J* 2001;357:593–615.

102. Salerno JC, Harris DE, Irizarry K, et al. An autoinhibitory control element defines calcium-regulated isoforms of nitric oxide synthase. *J Biol Chem* 1997;272:29,769–29,777.

103. Babu BR, Griffith OW. Design of isoform-selective inhibitors of nitric oxide synthase. *Curr Opin Chem Biol* 1998;2:491–500.

104. McMillan K, Adler M, Auld DS, et al. Allosteric inhibitors of inducible nitric oxide synthase dimerization discovered *via* combinatorial chemistry. *Proc Natl Acad Sci USA* 2000;97:1506–1511.

105. Balkwill F, Mantovani A. Inflammation and cancer: back to Virchow? *Lancet* 2001;357:539–545.

106. O'Byrne KJ, Dalgleish AG. Chronic immune activation and inflammation as the cause of malignancy. *Br J Cancer* 2001;85:473–483.

107. Christen S, Hagen TM, Shigenaga MK, Ames BN. Chronic inflammation, mutation, and cancer, in *Microbes and Malignancy: Infection as a Cause of Cancer*. Parsonnet J, Hornig S, eds. Oxford University Press, New York,1999, pp.35–88.

108. Adler V, Yin Z, Tew KD, Ronai Z. Role of redox potential and reactive oxygen species in stress signaling. *Oncogene* 1999;18:6104–6111.

109. Shackelford RE, Kaufmann WK, Paules RS. Oxidative stress and cell cycle checkpoint function. *Free Radic Biol Med* 2000;28:1387–1404.

110. Kyriakis JM, Avruch J. Mammalian mitogen-activated protein kinase signal transduction pathways activated by stress and inflammation. *Physiol Rev* 2001;81:807–869.

111. Cerutti PA, Trump BF. Inflammation and oxidative stress in carcinogenesis. Cancer Cells 1991;3:1–7.

112. Shalon D, Smith SJ, Brown PO. A DNA microarray system for analyzing complex DNA samples using two-color fluorescent probe hybridization. *Genome Res* 1996;6:639–645.

113. Cerutti PA. Prooxidant states and tumor promotion. *Science* 1985;227:375–381.

114. MacMicking JD, Nathan C, Hom G, et al. Altered responses to bacterial infection and endotoxic shock in mice lacking inducible nitric oxide synthase. *Cell* 1995;81:641–650.

115. McCafferty DM, Miampamba M, Sihota E, et al. Role of inducible nitric oxide synthase in trinitrobenzene sulphonic acid induced colitis in mice. *Gut* 1999;45:864–873.

116. Zingarelli B, Szabo C, Salzman AL. Reduced oxidative and nitrosative damage in murine experimental colitis in the absence of inducible nitric oxide synthase. *Gut* 1999;45:199–209.

117. Hokari R, Kato S, Matsuzaki K, et al. Reduced sensitivity of inducible nitric oxide synthase-deficient mice to chronic colitis. *Free Radic Biol Med* 2001;31:153–163.

118. Krieglstein CF, Cerwinka WH, Laroux FS, et al. Regulation of murine intestinal inflammation by reactive metabolites of oxygen and nitrogen: divergent roles of superoxide and nitric oxide. *J Exp Med* 2001;194:1207–1218.

119. Konopka TE, Barker JE, Bamford TL, et al. Nitric oxide synthase II gene disruption: implications for tumor growth and vascular endothelial growth factor production. *Cancer Res* 2001;61:3182–3187.

120. Cooper HS, Everley L, Chang WC, et al. The role of mutant *Apc* in the development of dysplasia and cancer in the mouse model of dextran sulfate sodium-induced colitis. *Gastroenterology* 2001;121:1407–1416.

121. Ahn B, Ohshima H. Suppression of intestinal polyposis in *Apc*$^{Min/+}$ mice by inhibiting nitric oxide production. *Cancer Res* 2001;61:8357–8360.

122. Yamamoto Y, Gaynor RB. Therapeutic potential of inhibition of the NFκB pathway in the treatment of inflammation and cancer. *J Clin Investig* 2001;107:135–142.

123. Tamir S, deRojas-Walker T, Gal A, et al. Nitric oxide production in relation to spontaneous B-cell lymphoma and myositis in SJL mice. *Cancer Res* 1995;55:4391–4397.

124. Gal A, Tamir S, Tannenbaum SR, Wogan GN. Nitric oxide production in SJL mice bearing the RcsX lymphoma: a model for in vivo toxicological evaluation of NO•. *Proc Natl Acad Sci USA* 1996;93:11,499–11,503.

125. Gal A, Wogan GN. Mutagenesis associated with nitric oxide production in transgenic SJL mice. *Proc Natl Acad Sci USA* 1996;93:15,102–15,107.

126. Ahn B, Han BS, Kim DJ, Ohshima H. Immunohistochemical localization of inducible nitric oxide synthase and 3-nitrotyrosine in rat liver tumors induced by N-nitrosodiethylamine. *Carcinogenesis* 1999;20:1337–1344.

127. Nair J, Gal A, Tamir S, et al. Etheno adducts in spleen DNA of SJL mice stimulated to overproduce nitric oxide. *Carcinogenesis* 1998;19:2081–2084.

128. Goldstein SR, Yang GY, Chen X, et al. Studies of iron deposits, inducible nitric oxide synthase and nitrotyrosine in a rat model for esophageal adenocarcinoma. *Carcinogenesis* 1998;19:1445–1449.

129. Okamoto T, Masuda Y, Kawasaki T, et al. Aminoguanidine prevents concanavalin A-induced hepatitis in mice. *Eur J Pharmacol* 2000;396:125–130.

130. Yasuhiro T, Korolkiewicz RP, Kato S, Takeuchi K. Role of nitric oxide in pathogenesis of serotonine-induced gastric lesions in rats. *Pharmacol Res* 1997;36:333–338.

131. Rao CV, Indranie C, Simi B, et al. Chemopreventive properties of a selective inducible nitric oxide synthase inhibitor in colon carcinogenesis, administered alone or in combination with celecoxib, a selective cyclooxygenase-2 inhibitor. *Cancer Res* 2002;62:165–170.

132. Rao CV, Kawamori T, Hamid R, Reddy BS. Chemoprevention of colonic aberrant crypt foci by an inducible nitric oxide synthase-selective inhibitor. *Carcinogenesis* 1999;20:641–644.

133. Kawamori T, Takahashi M, Watanabe K, et al. Suppression of azoxymethane-induced colonic aberrant crypt foci by a nitric oxide synthase inhibitor. *Cancer Lett* 2000;148:33–37.

134. Doi K, Akaike T, Fujii S, et al. Induction of haem oxygenase-1 nitric oxide and ischaemia in experimental solid tumours and implications for tumour growth. *Br J Cancer* 1999;80:1945–1954.

135. Tozer GM, Prise VE, Wilson J, et al. Combretastatin A-4 phosphate as a tumor vascular-targeting agent: early effects in tumors and normal tissues. *Cancer Res* 1999;59:1626–1634.

136. Tozer GM, Prise VE, Motterlini R, et al. The comparative effects of the NOS inhibitor, Nω-nitro-L-arginine, and the haemoxygenase inhibitor, zinc protoporphyrin IX, on tumour blood flow. *Int J Radiat Oncol Biol Phys* 1998;42:849–853.

137. Ziche M, Morbidelli L, Masini E, et al. Nitric oxide mediates angiogenesis in vivo and endothelial cell growth and migration in vitro promoted by substance P. *J Clin Investig* 1994;94:2036–2044.

138. Orucevic A, Lala PK. NG-nitro-L-arginine methyl ester, an inhibitor of nitric oxide synthesis, ameliorates interleukin 2-induced capillary leakage and reduces tumour growth in adenocarcinoma-bearing mice. *Br J Cancer* 1996;73:189–196.

139. Ribbons KA, Currie MG, Connor JR, et al. The effect of inhibitors of inducible nitric oxide synthase on chronic colitis in the rhesus monkey. *J Pharmacol Exp Ther* 1997;280:1008–1015.

140. Yoshida Y, Iwai A, Itoh K, et al. Role of inducible nitric oxide synthase in dextran sulphate sodium-induced colitis. *Aliment Pharmacol Ther* 2000;14 Suppl 1:26–32.

141. Wink DA, Hanbauer I, Krishna MC, et al. Nitric oxide protects against cellular damage and cytotoxicity from reactive oxygen species. *Proc Natl Acad Sci USA* 1993;90:9813–9817.

142. Peng HB, Rajavashisth TB, Libby P, Liao JK. Nitric oxide inhibits macrophage-colony stimulating factor gene transcription in vascular endothelial cells. *J Biol Chem* 1995;270:17,050–17,055.

143. Berendji-Grun D, Kolb-Bachofen V, Kroncke KD. Nitric oxide inhibits endothelial IL-1[β]-induced ICAM-1 gene expression at the transcriptional level decreasing Sp1 and AP-1 activity. *Mol Med* 2001;7:748–754.

144. De Caterina R, Libby P, Peng HB, et al. Nitric oxide decreases cytokine-induced endothelial activation. Nitric oxide selectively reduces endothelial expression of adhesion molecules and proinflammatory cytokines. *J Clin Investig* 1995;96:60–68.

145. Clancy R, Varenika B, Huang W et al. Nitric oxide synthase/COX cross-talk: nitric oxide activates COX-1 but inhibits COX-2-derived prostaglandin production. *J Immunol* 2000;165:1582–1587.

146. Stadler J, Harbrecht BG, Di Silvio M, et al. Endogenous nitric oxide inhibits the synthesis of cyclooxygenase products and interleukin-6 by rat Kupffer cells. *J Leukoc Biol* 1993;53:165–172.

147. Gurjar MV, DeLeon J, Sharma RV, Bhalla RC. Mechanism of inhibition of matrix metalloproteinase-9 induction by NO in vascular smooth muscle cells. *J Appl Physiol* 2001;91:1380–1386.

148. Schleiffer R, Duranton B, Gosse F, et al. Nitric oxide synthase inhibition promotes carcinogen-induced preneoplastic changes in the colon of rats. *Nitric Oxide* 2000;4:583–589.

149. Bruns CJ, Shinohara H, Harbison MT, et al. Therapy of human pancreatic carcinoma implants by irinotecan and the oral immunomodulator JBT 3002 is associated with enhanced expression of inducible nitric oxide synthase in tumor-infiltrating macrophages. *Cancer Res* 2000;60:2–7.

150. Shinohara H, Bucana CD, Killion JJ, Fidler IJ. Intensified regression of colon cancer liver metastases in mice treated with irinotecan and the immunomodulator JBT 3002. *J Immunother* 2000;23:321–331.

151. Xie K, Fidler IJ. Therapy of cancer metastasis by activation of the inducible nitric oxide synthase. *Cancer Metastasis Rev* 1998;17:55–75.

152. Yamamoto T, Terada N, Seiyama A, et al. Increase in experimental pulmonary metastasis in mice by L-arginine under inhibition of nitric oxide production by NG-nitro-L-arginine methyl ester. *Int J Cancer* 1998;75:140–144.

153. Iwasaki T, Higashiyama M, Kuriyama K, et al. NG-nitro-L-arginine methyl ester inhibits bone metastasis after modified intracardiac injection of human breast cancer cells in a nude mouse model. *Jpn J Cancer Res* 1997;88:861–866.

154. Edwards P, Cendan JC, Topping DB, et al. Tumor cell nitric oxide inhibits cell growth in vitro, but stimulates tumorigenesis and experimental lung metastasis in vivo. *J Surg Res* 1996;63:49–52.

155. Wang B, Xiong Q, Shi Q, et al. Genetic disruption of host nitric oxide synthase II gene impairs melanoma-induced angiogenesis and suppresses pleural effusion. *Int J Cancer* 2001;91:607–611.

156. Wang B, Xiong Q, Shi Q, et al. Intact nitric oxide synthase II gene is required for interferon-β-mediated suppression of growth and metastasis of pancreatic adenocarcinoma. *Cancer Res* 2001;61:71–75.

157. Shi Q, Xiong Q, Wang B, et al. Influence of nitric oxide synthase II gene disruption on tumor growth and metastasis. *Cancer Res* 2000;60:2579–2583.

158. Shi Q, Huang S, Jiang W, et al. Direct correlation between nitric oxide synthase II inducibility and metastatic ability of UV-2237 murine fibrosarcoma cells carrying mutant p53. *Cancer Res* 1999;59:2072–2075.

159. Juang SH, Xie K, Xu L, et al. Suppression of tumorigenicity and metastasis of human renal carcinoma cells by infection with retroviral vectors harboring the murine inducible nitric oxide synthase gene. *Hum Gene Ther* 1998;9:845–854.

160. Xie K, Huang S, Dong Z, et al. Direct correlation between expression of endogenous inducible nitric oxide synthase and regression of M5076 reticulum cell sarcoma hepatic metastases in mice treated with liposomes containing lipopeptide CGP 31362. *Cancer Res* 1995;55:3123–3131.

161. Xie K, Dong Z, Fidler IJ. Activation of nitric oxide synthase gene for inhibition of cancer metastasis. *J Leukoc Biol* 1996;59:797–803.

162. Dong Z, Staroselsky AH, Qi X, et al. Inverse correlation between expression of inducible nitric oxide synthase activity and production of metastasis in K-1735 murine melanoma cells. *Cancer Res* 1994;54:789–793.

163. Xie K, Huang S, Dong Z, et al. Transfection with the inducible nitric oxide synthase gene suppresses tumorigenicity and abrogates metastasis by K-1735 murine melanoma cells. *J Exp Med* 1995;181:1333–1343.

164. Xie K, Huang S, Dong Z, et al. Destruction of bystander cells by tumor cells transfected with inducible nitric oxide (NO·) synthase gene. *J Natl Cancer Inst* 1997;89:421–427.

165. Matthews NE, Adams MA, Maxwell LR, et al. Nitric oxide-mediated regulation of chemosensitivity in cancer cells. *J Natl Cancer Inst* 2001;93:1879–1885.

166. Janssens MY, Van den Berge DL, Verovski VN, et al. Activation of inducible nitric oxide synthase results in nitric oxide-mediated radiosensitization of hypoxic EMT-6 tumor cells. *Cancer Res* 1998;58:5646–5648.

167. Maccarrone M, Fantini C, Ranalli M, et al. Activation of nitric oxide synthase is involved in tamoxifen-induced apoptosis of human erythroleukemia K562 cells. *FEBS Lett* 1998;434:421–424.

168. Ho YS, Wang YJ, Lin JK. Induction of p53 and p21/WAF1/CIP1 expression by nitric oxide and their association with apoptosis in human cancer cells. *Mol Carcinog* 1996;16:20–31.

169. Bartsch H. Studies on biomarkers in cancer etiology and prevention: a summary and challenge of 20 years of interdisciplinary research. *Mutat Res* 2000;462:255–279.

170. Marnett LJ. Oxyradicals and DNA damage. *Carcinogenesis* 2000;21:361–370.

171. Burney S, Caulfield JL, Niles JC, et al. The chemistry of DNA damage from nitric oxide and peroxynitrite. *Mutat Res* 1999;424:37–49.

172. Marnett LJ, Plastaras JP. Endogenous DNA damage and mutation. *Trends Genet* 2001;17:214–221.

173. Aguilar F, Harris CC, Sun T, et al. Geographic variation of p53 mutational profile in nonmalignant human liver. *Science* 1994;264:1317–1319.

174. Aguilar F, Hussain SP, Cerutti P. Aflatoxin B1 induces the transversion of G—>T in codon 249 of the p53 tumor suppressor gene in human hepatocytes. *Proc Natl Acad Sci USA* 1993;90:8586–8590.

175. Hussain SP, Aguilar F, Amstad P, Cerutti P. Oxy-radical induced mutagenesis of hotspot codons 248 and 249 of the human p53 gene. *Oncogene* 1994;9:2277–2281.

176. Hussain SP, Aguilar F, Cerutti P. Mutagenesis of codon 248 of the human p53 tumor suppressor gene by *N*-ethyl-*N*-nitrosourea. *Oncogene* 1994;9:13–18.

177. Hussain SP, Kennedy CH, Amstad P, et al. Radon and lung carcinogenesis: mutability of p53 codons 249 and 250 to 238Pu alpha-particles in human bronchial epithelial cells. *Carcinogenesis* 1997;18:121–125.

178. Niederau C, Fischer R, Sonnenberg A, et al. Survival and causes of death in cirrhotic and in noncirrhotic patients with primary hemochromatosis. *N Engl J Med* 1985;313:1256–1262.

179. Gillen CD, Walmsley RS, Prior P, Andrews HA, Allan RN. Ulcerative colitis and Crohn's disease: a comparison of the colorectal cancer risk in extensive colitis. *Gut* 1994;35:1590–1592.

180. Guihot G, Guimbaud R, Bertrand V, et al. Inducible nitric oxide synthase activity in colon biopsies from inflammatory areas: correlation with inflammation intensity in patients with ulcerative colitis but not with Crohn's disease. *Amino Acids* 2000;18:229–237.

181. Boughton-Smith NK. Pathological and therapeutic implications for nitric oxide in inflammatory bowel disease. *J R Soc Med* 1994;87:312–314.

182. Leonard N, Bishop AE, Polak JM, Talbot IC. Expression of nitric oxide synthase in inflammatory bowel disease is not affected by corticosteroid treatment. *J Clin Pathol* 1998;51:750–753.

183. Ekbom A, Helmick C, Zack M, Adami HO. Ulcerative colitis and colorectal cancer. A population-based study. *N Engl J Med* 1990;323:1228–1233.

184. Iwashita E, Iwai A, Sawazaki Y, et al. Activation of microvascular endothelial cells in active ulcerative colitis and detection of inducible nitric oxide synthase. *J Clin Gastroenterol* 1998;27 Suppl 1:S74–S79.

185. Shin HR, Lee CU, Park HJ, et al. Hepatitis B and C virus, *Clonorchis sinensis* for the risk of liver cancer: a case-control study in Pusan, Korea. *Int J Epidemiol* 1996;25:933–940.

186. Kane JM III, Shears LL, Hierholzer C, et al. Chronic hepatitis C virus infection in humans: induction of hepatic nitric oxide synthase and proposed mechanisms for carcinogenesis. *J Surg Res* 1997;69:321–324.

187. Rahman MA, Dhar DK, Yamaguchi E, et al. Coexpression of inducible nitric oxide synthase and COX-2 in hepatocellular carcinoma and surrounding liver: possible involvement of COX-2 in the angiogenesis of hepatitis C virus-positive cases. *Clin Cancer Res* 2001;7:1325–1332.

188. Mitchell H, Drake M, Medley G. Prospective evaluation of risk of cervical cancer after cytological evidence of human papilloma virus infection. *Lancet* 1986;1:573–575.

189. Zhang ZF, Kurtz RC, Klimstra DS, et al. *Helicobacter pylori* infection on the risk of stomach cancer and chronic atrophic gastritis. *Cancer Detect Prev* 1999;23:357–367.

190. Tatemichi M, Ogura T, Nagata H, Esumi H. Enhanced expression of inducible nitric oxide synthase in chronic gastritis with intestinal metaplasia. *J Clin Gastroenterol* 1998;27:240–245.

191. Esrig D, McEvoy K, Bennett CJ. Bladder cancer in the spinal cord-injured patient with long-term catheterization: a causal relationship? *Semin Urol* 1992;10:102–108.

192. Kanoh K, Shimura T, Tsutsumi S, et al. Significance of contracted cholecystitis lesions as high risk for gallbladder carcinogenesis. *Cancer Lett* 2001;169:7–14.

193. Csendes A, Becerra M, Burdiles P, et al. Bacteriological studies of bile from the gallbladder in patients with carcinoma of the gallbladder, cholelithiasis, common bile duct stones and no gallstones disease. *Eur J Surg* 1994;160:363–367.

194. Rosin MP, Hofseth LJ. Schistosomiasis, bladder and colon cancer, in *Microbes and Malignancy: Infection as a Cause of Cancer*. Parsonnet J, Hornig S, eds Oxford University Press, New York, 1999, pp. 313–345.

195. Shochina M, Fellig Y, Sughayer M, et al. Nitric oxide synthase immunoreactivity in human bladder carcinoma. *Mol Pathol* 2001;54:248–252.

196. Jaiswal M, LaRusso NF, Shapiro RA, et al. Nitric oxide-mediated inhibition of DNA repair potentiates oxidative DNA damage in cholangiocytes. *Gastroenterology* 2001;120:190–199.

197. Haswell-Elkins MR, Mairiang E, Mairiang P, et al. Cross-sectional study of *Opisthorchis viverrini* infection and cholangiocarcinoma in communities within a high-risk area in northeast Thailand. *Int J Cancer* 1994;59:505–509.

198. Streitz JM Jr. Barrett's esophagus and esophageal cancer. *Chest Surg Clin N Am* 1994;4:227–240.

199. Marrogi A, Pass HI, Khan M, et al. Human mesothelioma samples overexpress both cyclooxygenase-2 (COX-2) and inducible nitric oxide synthase (NOS2): in vitro antiproliferative effects of a COX-2 inhibitor. *Cancer Res* 2000;60:3696–3700.

200. Bourdes V, Boffetta P, Pisani P. Environmental exposure to asbestos and risk of pleural mesothelioma: review and meta-analysis. *Eur J Epidemiol* 2000;16:411–417.

201. Stevens RG, Moolgavkar SH. Estimation of relative risk from vital data: smoking and cancers of the lung and bladder. *J Natl Cancer Inst* 1979;63:1351–1357.

202. Liu CY, Wang CH, Chen TC, et al. Increased level of exhaled nitric oxide and upregulation of inducible nitric oxide synthase in patients with primary lung cancer. *Br J Cancer* 1998;78:534–541.

203. Young RJ, Beams RM, Carter K, et al. Inhibition of inducible nitric oxide synthase by acetamidine derivatives of hetero-substituted lysine and homolysine. *Bioorg Med Chem Lett* 2000;10:597–600.

204. Wolff DJ, Gauld DS, Neulander MJ, Southan G. Inactivation of nitric oxide synthase by substituted aminoguanidines and aminoisothioureas. *J Pharmacol Exp Ther* 1997;283:265–273.

205. Hagen TJ, Bergmanis AA, Kramer SW, et al. 2-Iminopyrrolidines as potent and selective inhibitors of human inducible nitric oxide synthase. *J Med Chem* 1998;41:3675–3683.

206. Beaton H, Hamley P, Nicholls DJ, et al. 3,4-Dihydro-1-iso-quinolinamines: a novel class of nitric oxide synthase inhibitors with a range of isoform selectivity and potency. *Bioorg Med Chem Lett* 2001;11:1023–1026.

207. Nakamura H, Tsukada H, Oya M, et al. Aminoguanidine has both an antiinflammatory effect and a proliferative effect on colonic mucosal cells. *Scand J Gastroenterol* 1999;34:1117–1122.

208. Yamaguchi T, Yoshida N, Ichiishi E, et al. Differing effects of two nitric oxide synthase inhibitors on experimental colitis. *Hepatogastroenterology* 2001;48:118–122.

209. de Wilt JH, Manusama ER, van Etten B, et al. Nitric oxide synthase inhibition results in synergistic anti-tumour activity with melphalan and tumour necrosis factor alpha-based isolated limb perfusions. *Br J Cancer* 2000;83:1176–1182.

210. Fukumura D, Yuan F, Endo M, Jain RK. Role of nitric oxide in tumor microcirculation. Blood flow, vascular permeability, and leukocyte-endothelial interactions. *Am J Pathol* 1997;150:713–725.

211. Jadeski LC, Lala PK. Nitric oxide synthase inhibition by *N*(G)-nitro-L-arginine methyl ester inhibits tumor-induced angiogenesis in mammary tumors. *Am J Pathol* 1999;155:1381–1390.

212. Menchen LA, Colon AL, Moro et al. *N*-(3-(aminomethyl)benzyl)acetamidine, an inducible nitric oxide synthase inhibitor, decreases colonic inflammation induced by trinitrobenzene sulphonic acid in rats. *Life Sci* 2001;69:479–491.

213. Armstrong AM, Campbell GR, Gannon C, et al. Oral administration of inducible nitric oxide synthase inhibitors reduces nitric oxide synthesis but has no effect on the severity of experimental colitis. *Scand J Gastroenterol* 2000;35:832–838.

214. Hosoi T, Goto H, Arisawa T, et al. Role of nitric oxide synthase inhibitor in experimental colitis induced by 2,4,6-trinitrobenzene sulphonic acid in rats. *Clin Exp Pharmacol Physiol* 2001;28:9–12.

9 Chemoprevention of Cancer of the Respiratory Tract by Agents Delivered by Aerosol

Applications to Glucocorticoids and 5-Fluorouracil

Timothy S. Wiedmann, PhD and Lee W. Wattenberg, MD

CONTENTS

1. INTRODUCTION

Aerosol administration of chemopreventive agents has distinct advantages in chemoprevention of respiratory tract carcinogenesis. First, the agent is delivered directly to the target tissue. Another major advantage is the favorable ratio of agent concentration reaching the respiratory tract as compared to that reaching the systemic tissues. At the same dose, the initial agent concentration in the lung will be approx 30× greater when the compounds are given by aerosol than when administered orally *(1)*. This difference is further enhanced for agents that undergo metabolism in systemic tissues *(2)*.

Nevertheless, aerosol administration is much less common than oral or intravenous (iv) delivery. One major limitation is the necessity of using a delivery device and the problems associated with patient education *(3)*. In addition, some compounds that are irritating to the respiratory tract mucosa must be evaluated in initial toxicity studies *(4)*. However, significant improvements have been introduced into the design of aerosol-generating devices *(5,6)*. These have resulted in respiratory delivery systems that have largely overcome the problems experienced with the older devices. In fact, devices are now available that treat local diseases and may also meet the therapeutic demands of a systemic disease such as diabetes by providing reproducible delivery of insulin *(5)*. Clearly, it is time to fully exploit these technological advances in order to treat—and more importantly, to prevent—lung cancer.

The first part of this chapter states the pharmacological basis for the use of glucocorticoids and for 5-fluorouracil (5-FU) in chemoprevention. Thereafter, the basic requirements for aerosol administration are presented. The objective is to provide the theoretical and practical aspects of respiratory drug delivery, particularly for animal models, in order to stimulate future work in this promising field. The final sections discuss the successes of chemoprevention of carcinogenesis with aerosol delivery of glucocorticoids and 5-FU in the respiratory tract.

2. CHEMOPREVENTION WITH GLUCOCORTICOIDS

Several desirable attributes of candidates for chemopreventive compounds in lung carcinogenesis

From: Cancer Chemoprevention, Volume 1: Promising Cancer Chemoprevention Agents
Edited by: G. J. Kelloff, E. T. Hawk, and C. C. Sigman © Humana Press Inc., Totowa, NJ

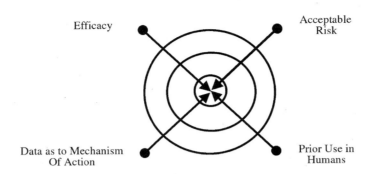

Fig. 1. Desirable attributes for candidate chemopreventive agents.

are presented in a diagrammatic form in Fig.1. First, it is essential for a compound to have efficacy. Secondly, the drug must have an acceptable risk. As shown here, aerosol delivery enhances efficacy and reduces toxicity by direct spatial placement of the drug at the target site. A third attribute is information regarding the mechanism of action. The fourth attribute is the prior use of a compound in human subjects, either as a medicinal or dietary constituent (natural or additive).

Although prior use in humans only occurs occasionally, it merits particular attention because of its important role in evaluating potential toxicity. Tamoxifen is a notable past example of an agent with this chemopreventive attribute. Currently, we are witnessing a vigorous effort in evaluating the chemopreventive capacities of cyclooxygenese (COX)-2 inhibitors. These compounds are effective chemopreventive agents in some in vivo studies, and have widespread use as antiinflammatory compounds in human populations. One major positive aspect of glucocorticoids is that they fall into the selective group of potential chemopreventive agents with widespread human use. These compounds have been extensively used in asthma patients. This historical perspective demonstrates that glucocorticoids can be used for chemoprevention in dose ranges that are safe in humans (7–10).

Glucocorticoids have several mechanisms of action that are particularly relevant to their role as chemopreventive agents for pulmonary carcinogenesis (Table 1). Particularly significant is their capacity to act as differentiating agents in pulmonary tissues of both humans and experimental animals. A striking example is their ability to induce differentiation of Type II alveolar cells in premature infants who otherwise would have developed a respiratory distress syndrome. In these infants, Type II alveolar cells have not differentiated, and do not produce the surfactant required for expansion of the lungs. Administration of glucocorticoids produces the required maturation of these cells (11).

Differentiation is a pleiotropic response that can bypass the manifestations of a malignant genotype. Many studies have examined the role of differentiation in control of the neoplastic process, which is briefly summarized in the references provided (12–18). Several other major consequences of glucocorticoid action are shown in Table 1. Each of these by itself has the potential to provide an inhibitory effect on carcinogenesis. The combination of these mechanisms (or possibly other mechanisms) that is responsible for the overall chemopreventive effects of glucocorticoids has not yet been established. This is an extraordinarily complex field.

2.1. Initial Chemoprevention Studies of Pulmonary Neoplasia With Glucocorticoids

The initial experiments with glucocorticoids involved oral administration of dexamethasone (9). In these studies, chemopreventive agents were sought that would be effective in the postinitiation period. At the beginning of these studies, protocols were used in which *myo*-inositol was found to have chemopreventive activity. However, high concentrations of *myo*-inositol in the diet were required to produce inhibition, and the inhibition was of a modest magnitude (19–21). In reviewing the literature, the use of dexamethasone appeared to be a plausible candidate for chemoprevention. This was based on two attributes. First, glucocorticoids, including dexamethasone, were shown to inhibit the promotion phase of tumorigenesis in the skin of the mouse (22,23). The second attribute was data showing that dexamethasone targeted the lung-producing maturation of Type II alveolar cells (11).

An initial experiment was carried out to determine whether dexamethasone would inhibit pulmonary carcinogenesis in the postinitiation period in the A/J strain

Table 1
Potential Protective Effects of Glucocorticoids Against Carcinogenesis

Differentiating agents

Decrease formation of prostaglandins (suppression of phospholipase A_2 activity and COX-2 synthesis)

Inhibition of cell proliferation by effects on nuclear transcription

Enhancement of cell–cell contacts

mouse model given benzo[a]pyrene (B[a]P) (24). Three oral doses of B[a]P were administered, and 1 wk later the mice were fed either 0.1 or 0.5 µg dexamethasone per g of diet. The higher dose of dexamethasone produced a 57% reduction in pulmonary adenoma formation. The lower dose of dexamethasone had no effect (19). In this experimental protocol, mice given B[a]P developed squamous-cell tumors of the forestomach in addition to pulmonary adenomas. The magnitude of inhibition of the forestomach tumor formation was similar to that of pulmonary adenoma formation. This finding was considered important because it provided evidence that glucocorticoids had the capacity to inhibit tumors of either squamous or glandular origin.

In a second study, the effect of dexamethasone in the diet on the occurrence of B[a]P-induced pulmonary carcinogenesis in the female A/J mouse and also on pulmonary carcinogenesis resulting from administration of the tobacco-specific carcinogen 4-methylnitrosamino-1-(3-pyridyl)-1-butanone (NNK) was studied (21). When dexamethasone, 0.5 µg/g of diet, was fed to the animals receiving B[a]P in the postinitiation period, an inhibition of approx 50% in the occurrence of pulmonary adenomas was found. In addition, the effect of feeding dexamethasone solely in the initiation period was studied. Under these conditions, a 20% inhibition of tumor formation occurred. Finally, an experiment in mice that received NNK, where dexamethasone was fed throughout the study, resulted in a 41% inhibition of the occurrence of pulmonary adenomas (21).

The findings of the inhibitory effects of dexamethasone given in the diet on B[a]P- and NNK-induced pulmonary tumor formation in the A/J mouse did not have encouraging implications for humans. Oral administration of dexamethasone at a dose that might have adverse side effects was a major difficulty. However, at that time, the aerosol administration of glucocorticoids was commonly used in the management of asthma with minimal side effects. Thus, in terms of application to chemoprevention of pulmonary

carcinogenesis, aerosol administration of glucocorticoids could provide agents that come into direct contact with the target tissue, and at a safe dose. Based on the properties of the various anti-asthmatic glucocorticoids, the second-generation compound, budesonide, was selected for investigation (7–9,25).

Before the initiation of work with aerosol budesonide, experiments were conducted in which budesonide was added to the diet (26). This work was performed in the A/J mouse pulmonary tumor model in the same manner as with dexamethasone in order to determine whether budesonide had chemopreventive efficacy at the oral dose required. Several experiments were done. The first showed that administration of a diet containing 1.5µg/g of budesonide would inhibit the occurrence of pulmonary adenoma formation in the A/J mouse when initial administration was given 1 wk after the last dose of B[a]P and continued for the duration of the study. Ninety percent inhibition of pulmonary adenoma formation was observed. In the second experiment, the diet containing budesonide was started at different time intervals following the last dose of B[a]P. If the feeding was started at 1 wk after carcinogen administration, an 80% inhibition occurred. If it was started 5 wk after the last dose of B[a]P, a 67% inhibition occurred. These studies indicated that budesonide had a chemopreventive effect against pulmonary carcinogenesis when given orally in the postinitiation period. Moreover, the inhibitory effect was maintained at a high level for up to 5 wk after the last dose of carcinogen.

As mentioned previously, myo-inositol, a hydrolysis product of inositol hexaphosphate (phytate), had been studied for its effect as a chemopreventive agent against pulmonary carcinogenesis in the A/J mouse (9,20,21). In an interesting series of studies, both inositol hexaphosphate and inositol inhibited carcinogen-induced neoplasia of the large bowel of rats and mice, and the inhibition occurred when the compounds were administered solely in the postinitiation period (27). When studied for its chemopreventive efficacy against pulmonary carcinogenesis in the mouse, *myo*-inositol was found to have activity. Although the mechanism of action is unknown, some of its biological effects have been identified.

Myo-inositol produces maturation of Type II alveolar cells, as manifested by surfactant synthesis. This capacity to enhance surfactant synthesis has been used clinically in premature infants in the treatment of pulmonary distress syndrome secondary to lung immaturity *(28)*. In vitro studies have shown that *myo*-inositol can produce differentiation in Clara-cell precursors *(29)*. Two additional attributes of *myo*-inositol are that it is an osmolyte and has effects on glucose metabolism *(30)*. However, studies conducted by a number of investigators have failed to define its precise mechanism of action as a chemopreventive agent against pulmonary carcinogenesis. Since the chemopreventive effect of *myo*-inositol is quite modest, the compound would probably be most useful in chemoprevention when administered in an agent combination. Studies of this type were carried out with the glucocorticoids, in which it was shown that the two compounds had an additive effect *(10,21)*. One particularly attractive attribute of *myo*-inositol is that it has extraordinarily few adverse effects.

3. CHEMOPREVENTION WITH 5-FU

5-FU is widely recognized for its effectiveness in chemotherapy. However, it also has been used as a chemopreventive agent. It was the first agent extensively used for chemoprevention of cancer in humans, where it prevented premalignant lesions of the skin from progressing to epidermal carcinomas *(31,32)*. A summary of the experience with this type of administration by Williams and Klein in 1970 described more than 700 subjects who were given topical applications of 5-FU to prevent progression of premalignant keratoses of the skin to cancer *(32)*. Experimental studies in animals also demonstrated chemoprevention of epidermal carcinogenesis by 5-FU *(33)*. Topical application is a special method of drug administration and the recognition of the fact that chemoprevention can be achieved by local administration has been largoly ignored except for skin.

5-FU is primarily administered via the intravenous (iv) route, since absorption from the gastrointestinal (GI) tract is unpredictable and incomplete. It has also been administered topically for treatment of recurrent superficial carcinoma of the urinary bladder *(34)*.

Tatsumura et al. *(35)* carried out experiments to determine whether 5-FU could be administered by aerosol for the treatment of lung cancer. Results of this study have a direct bearing on the possible use of 5-FU for chemoprevention of carcinogenesis of the respiratory tract. These investigators showed that aerosol administration of 5-FU to dogs resulted in accumulation of the compound in the trachea, bronchi, and regional lymph nodes. In contrast, the levels in other organs were very low *(35)*. Only a trace of 5-FU was found in the serum. Similar data on the distribution were obtained when human subjects with lung cancers were given the aerosol compound.

Based on this background data, these investigators carried out a treatment study on a group of ten human subjects with lung cancer. Several went into complete remission, others had partial remissions, and others did not respond. One important aspect of their work, which relates to the use of aerosol 5-FU for chemoprevention, is that they found very little toxicity. In view of the low toxicity and some responses with lung cancer, it seemed possible that aerosol 5-FU might be applicable to chemoprevention of respiratory-tract carcinogenesis, particularly in high-risk individuals. Accordingly, we conducted a study of its chemopreventive capacities in an animal model *(36)*. The inhalation studies of 5-FU, as well as budesonide *(37)*, are discussed following a brief description of the theoretical and practical aspect of aerosol drug delivery to the respiratory tract.

4. AEROSOL DELIVERY OF CHEMOPREVENTIVE AGENTS

4.1. Considerations of Bioavailability

The first issue to address in more detail is the value of aerosol drug delivery for chemoprevention. Administration of drugs to the lung for the prevention of lung cancer is preferred for its direct approach. However, drug delivery by inhalation is inherently more complicated, and thus more demanding *(3)*. How much better should respiratory drug delivery be relative to oral administration? For a first approximation, the concentration in the lung is given by the deposited dose divided by the lung volume. With the subsequent distribution to the systemic circulation, the blood concentration would rise to a level equal to the product of the lung-to-plasma volume ratio and the lung concentration *(38–41)*:

$$C_{lung} = Mass_{lung}/Volume_{lung} \rightarrow$$
$$Mass_{lung}/Volume_{systemic} = C_{systemic}$$

Table 2
Aerosol Characteristics for Particles Generated by a Jet Nebulizer and Counter Current Flowing Water

Solute	Concentration in soln (mg/mL)	Air Flow Rate (L/min)	Solute Output Rate (mg/min)	Aerosol Conc. (mg/L)	Dose (mg/kg)
Budesonide	0.1	1.6	7.4 ±0.8	4.6	5
	0.3	1.6	22.0 ± 2.1	14	15
	1.0	1.6	74.0 ± 7.3	46	50
	2.0	1.6	153 ± 12	96	100
	4.0	1.6	293 ± 18	183	190

Alternatively, to achieve the same lung concentration by oral delivery as was achieved by inhalation, the entire body must be raised to the lung concentration (assuming equal distribution). Thus, the advantage of respiratory drug delivery to oral drug delivery is approximated by the total body-to-lung volume ratio or about a factor of 30 (1). This is significant, and justifies the effort.

Another issue is the delivery of drug, which involves three considerations. The most obvious element is the dose. The dose is the mass of drug administered expressed as a ratio to body wt (e.g., mg/kg), although surface area is also used. The route of administration is also paramount because it dictates the spatial placement of the drug, and profoundly affects the availability of the drug. Drug bioavailability is easily defined, but relatively difficult to establish with confidence when there is non-zero but incomplete absorption. Bioavailability is most often established in the context of the drug concentration in blood. This represents a convenient site for measurement, although the blood is rarely the site of action, especially for chemopreventive agents. To characterize bioavailability properly, even when referenced to the blood, the measurement requires determination of the time dependence, which represents the final aspect of drug delivery. Thus, delivery of chemotherapeutic/preventive agents requires consideration of the spatial placement and temporal duration of a given dose that is ideally determined at the site of action.

A related aspect is drug-delivery efficiency, which is related to bioavailability. The intuitive definition of bioavailability is the fraction of the dose that reaches the site of action. For respiratory drug delivery, bioavailability may be determined in small animals with little difficulty if the delivery occurs within a short period. The general approach is to administer a bolus

dose of drug, immediately sacrifice the animal, and then determine the amount of drug in the lung by a reliable assay. Often, long exposure times are used to administer the desired dose, and therefore multiple time-points are needed to obtain the profile of the lung concentration as a function of time. Mathematical models are then used to calculate the amount of drug deposited in the lung. This is further complicated by the rapid distribution of the drug from the lung to the general circulation, which requires a correction for the background drug in the blood that is present in excised lung. Finally, long exposure times prevent measurement of the drug levels prior to completion of the entire dose, so there is also concern in the reliability of the early time-points.

An alternative approach is to collect urine samples, with the constraint that the drug must be largely excreted unchanged by the kidney (42). The obvious drawback is that no information about the drug concentration in the lung is obtained. With respiratory drug delivery, significant absorption from the GI tract is common, which can obscure the result. GI absorption can be blocked by co-administration of charcoal orally, which allows a relatively direct measure of the fraction of the dose made available from measurement of the total amount of drug excreted in the urine.

If drug levels in the lung are measured with time following administration by inhalation, it is possible to determine the area under the curve (AUC) of the drug concentration as a function of time plot. Although this reflects the amount of drug, it must be compared to the AUC when a known amount of drug has been administered, which can be accomplished with iv dosing, AUC_{iv}. The relative bioavailability in the lung, F_{lung}, is given as (42):

$$F_{lung} = AUC_{inhal}/AUC_{iv}$$

However, chemopreventive agents are rarely administered intravenously, since it is well-recognized that this route of administration would not be tolerated by patients as a long-term solution to prevent cancer. Thus, for comparison to the inhalation route, only data following oral administration is usually available. In this case, no estimate of the fraction of the drug absorbed is possible. It is possible to estimate the pharmacokinetic advantage, R_d, of inhalation relative to oral administration by a comparison of the AUCs as follows (42):

$$Rd=(AUCM_{lung}/AUC_{plasma})_{inhalation}$$
$$/(AUC_{lung}/AUC_{plasma})_{iv}$$

The use of this expression requires that the pharmacokinetics must be linear with concentration.

For respiratory drug delivery to humans, the current advanced technology of metered dose and dry powder inhalers would be used, which are capable of delivering the entire dose in just a few seconds. Again, patients would find drug administration times—which are often more than 30 min in animal studies—unacceptably long. Thus, there is a question of whether the nature of the drug concentration as a function of time profile affects the therapeutic activity. The answer to this is often unknown, as many of the target sites of compounds are uncertain. As such, administration of drug to animals may be better if it can be done in a short time period to provide a better predictor of the ultimate manner in which drug will be administered in humans.

4.2. Considerations of Lung Heterogeneity and Drug Clearance in Humans

Until to this point, there has been the implicit assumption that all drug delivered to the lung is the same. However, just as the type of cancer that is observed in the human lung varies with location, the disposition of drug following administration also depends on the site of deposition. The lung is divided according to function into the conducting and pulmonary regions with an intervening transitional zone (43). Thus, the conducting region consists of a dichotomous branched system that provides a pathway for air to reach the pulmonary region where gas exchange takes place. The physiological arrangement minimizes the deposition of microorganisms, dust, and importantly, carcinogens in the bronchioles and alveolar ducts and sacs of the pulmonary region of the lung. However, this poses a problem for efficient drug delivery to the lung, since it will only take place secondarily to particle deposition.

It is important to remember that deposition of carcinogen-laden particles is the primary cause of lung cancer and deposition of drug-laden particles is likely to occur at the same sites. Therefore, greater specificity can be achieved with aerosol delivery of chemopreventive agents for prevention of lung cancer. Notwithstanding, the drug deposited in the conducting region of the lung has no effective means to reach the pulmonary region. In addition, the drug deposited in the pulmonary region is only slowly transported to the conducting region of the lung.

From the conducting region of the lung, the mucociliary system is an important pathway for clearance of carcinogens as well as drugs (44–46). This system involves the activity of two cell types: goblet cells, which secrete mucus, and ciliated pseudostratified columnar cells, which transport the mucus. The movement of the cilia propels the mucus toward the pharynx, where it may be removed by coughing or swallowing. With mucociliary clearance, particles are removed relatively rapidly from the nasopharyngeal, laryngeal, tracheal, and bronchial regions. These clearance processes occur simultaneously with the solid particles going into solution, absorption of drug into lung tissue, and subsequent transfer to the blood or lymph supply. Recognition of the mucociliary clearance pathway provides a rationale for the high concentrations of 5-FU observed in the trachea (35).

For deposition in the pulmonary region of the lung, clearance of particles occurs through different mechanisms (47). Here, alveolar macrophages can translocate the particles on the mucociliary escalator or into hilar lymph nodes, interstitial spaces, or subpleural spaces. From the lymph nodes, macrophages enter lymphatic channels and ultimately are drained by the pulmonary lymphatic system. There is also evidence that particles may be translocated independently of alveolar macrophages (48). Clearance of particles by these mechanisms is much less efficient, and thus particles may be retained within the alveoli air space for an extended period, if they do not dissolve. This is reflected in the extremely long half-lives reported for clearance of insoluble particles from the lung.

Although dependent on the location of deposition, empirical mathematical expressions have been developed to describe drug clearance from the entire lung (40,41). In such studies, a biphasic response is often observed. Fitting the initial rapid phase of the insoluble particle clearance yields a half-life for clearance of 2–4 hours in humans (44). Indeed, less than 5% of the

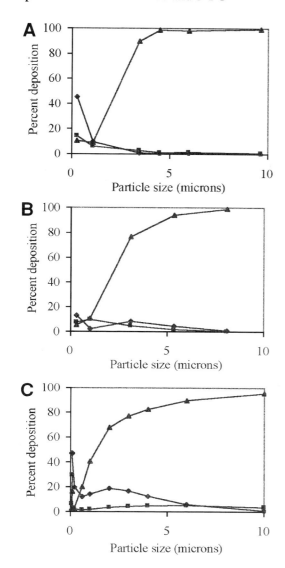

Fig. 2. Percent of mass deposited in (A) mice, (B) hamster and (C) human given as a function of particle size for the (▲) Nasopharyngeal, (■) Tracheal Bronchial, and (◆) Pulmonary Regions of the Lung (47,38).

monodispersed particles with a geometric diameter larger than 6 μm were observed in the lung 24 h following inhalation. The conclusion is that such large particles are essentially all deposited in the trachea and bronchi (TB) region of the lung, and are rapidly cleared by the mucociliary escalator.

In general, the clearance rate following deposition of insoluble particles in the alveoli is very slow, numbered in hundreds of days (44). In comparison, the rate at which carcinogens and drugs go into solution is relatively rapid. Therefore, the clearance from the pulmonary region of the lung is determined by the rate of dissolution and absorption into the lung tissue. In this case, the rate is determined by the physicochemical properties of the solutes.

Finally, it is important to consider the ultimate fate of the drug. Particles that are cleared by the mucociliary system are swallowed and thus enter the GI tract (40,41). From the GI tract, the drug may be absorbed and enter the general circulation. Particles cleared by macrophages usually reach systemic circulation via lymphatic circulation. These mechanisms are common to both humans and rodents, although their magnitudes appear to be quantitatively different.

4.3. Considerations for Drug Deposition in the Respiratory Tract

Considering that the conducting and pulmonary regions have unique clearance mechanisms and associated rates, the next question is: what determines the extent of particle deposition in these regions? The sites of particle deposition are generally defined as occurring in the naso- or oropharynx (NP region), (TB tracheo bronchial region), or pulmonary (P region) (49). The NP region includes the larynx, pharynx, and either the oral or nasal cavity, depending on the cavity through which the drug was inhaled. The percent deposition is defined as the percent of particles retained within the lung relative to the particles that are inhaled. Thus, just as a considerable portion of cigarette smoke is exhaled, drug bioavailability is also reduced by exhalation of particles.

The three primary mechanisms by which particles are deposited in the lung are inertial, sedimentational, and diffusional impaction. Many excellent discussions are available that provide the underlying physics of these processes (6,51). There are important differences in particle deposition in rodents and humans and principles that must be considered in relating safety and efficacy data between lower and higher species.

Beginning with rodents, Raabe et al. (50) conducted the seminal work in the late 1980s. In this study, the deposition of aluminosilicate particles labeled with ^{169}Yb was measured in five different animal species. These included CF1 mice, golden Syrian hamster, Fischer 344 rats, Hartley guinea pigs, and New Zealand rabbits. The near monodispersed particles were generated with a modified vibrating liquid stream generator, and were dried and concentrated in a centripeter stage, fused in a 1200°C furnace, and delivered in a nose-only exposure system. A total of eight to 20 animals were exposed for up to 45 min. One-half were sacrificed immediately after exposure, and one-half were sacrificed after 20 h to measure bronchial clearance. The difference in the lung loads immediately and after 20 h was used to estimate the pulmonary deposition.

Results from the mouse are given in Fig. 2A. Data from this study were pooled into three sites of P, TB, and larynx, nasopharyngeal, GI, and skull (NPL). The last category represents extrathoracic deposition. As can be seen for the mouse, the percent deposition is about 45% in the pulmonary region for particles with a diameter of 0.27 μm. As the particle size increases, the percent deposition decreases to less than 1% at a particle size of 3.45 μm. The combined deposition in the TB region is relatively small in comparison to the P region. At 0.27 μm, only 14% is deposited, and this decreases to about 2% at 3.45 μm. In contrast, the extrathoracic deposition is only about 10% at a particle size of 0.27 μm, but rises to near 90% at a particle size of 3.45 μm.

Data for the hamster is given in Fig. 2B. The overall features are similar to the mouse, although the percent deposition in the P region for 0.3 μm particles is only 7.5%. Thus, even with very small particles, it does not seem possible to deposit a significant fraction of the dose in the hamster. In addition, there is slightly more deposition in the TB region for intermediary-sized (1–5 μm) particles. This higher deposition in the TB region occurs concurrently with considerable deposition in the NPL region.

These results are readily understood within the context of the physiological aspects of rodents. Rodents are obligate nose-breathers. The nasal cavity is exceptionally efficient at trapping particles by inertial impaction, and therefore, only relatively small particles are able to pass through. Drug deposition in this region will be transported to the GI tract as a result of mucociliary clearance. Moreover, of the fraction that reaches the GI tract, a significant portion will reach the systemic circulation, although this depends on oral bioavailability. Because the drug reaching the systemic circulation is diluted by the blood volume, only a small amount has access to the site of action in the lung. Although it does not contribute to the therapeutic efficacy, there is also a comparably small contribution to side effects. In summary, delivery of relatively large particles to rodents has a minimal advantage over oral administration.

The continual rise in the deposition fraction with decreasing particle size that occurs in rodents indicates that diffusional impaction is the predominant mechanism, since inertial and sedimentational impaction efficiency decrease with decreasing particle size. Evidently, because of the relatively small size of the airways of the rodents coupled with the exposure that takes place with tidal breathing, sedimentation is not a significant mechanism for deposition of small particles. As such, drug delivery to rodents is improved with the use of small particles.

In Fig. 2C, the percentage of deposition of aerosol particles in humans is given as a function of aerodynamic particle size for the NP, TB, and P regions of the lung (51). These deposition studies were determined with mouth breathing, and thus, the extensive loss that occurs with nose breathing was avoided. Deposition was determined at one tidal volume and the inspiratory rate and breath-holding times were fixed. Thus, the first significant difference between human and rodent studies is that the breathing pattern can be controlled. This factor provides a powerful means to control the fraction of particles deposited at the site at which deposition occurs.

The deposition of particles between 0.1 and 10 μm is most important, since this is the size range relevant for aerosol formulations. For 10 μm particles, essentially all are deposited in the oropharyngeal area of the respiratory tract. As with rodents, these particles will first be diverted to the GI tract. Thereafter, the drug will reach the systemic circulation if there is appreciable oral bioavailability. As the particle size decreases, there is a drop in the fraction deposited in the NP simultaneous with a rise in the TB and P regions of the lung. The maximum observed with the TB region results in the diminishing efficiency of sedimentation and inertial particle impaction with decreasing particle size. This decreasing efficiency for impaction in the TB regions allows more particles to be deposited in the P region. The pulmonary deposition displays a maximum with decreasing particle size as the sedimentation becomes less efficient with smaller particles. The minimum in the deposition in the P region arises from the transition from a mechanism of sedimentation to diffusional impaction. The latter continues to increase with decreasing particle size.

For optimal drug delivery to humans, inhalation devices are developed to generate aerosols with a particle size in the range of 1–5 μm. With this size range and using the ventilation parameters of Fig. 2C, about

5% will deposit in the TB region, 20% in the P region, and about 60% will deposit in the NP region. For reference purposes, about 15% and 32% of budesonide were deposited in the human lung using a metered dose inhaler (MDI) and dry powder inhaler (DPI), respectively (52). The total fractions of the dose that gained access to the systemic circulation were 26% and 38% with the same devices. From this information, the devices are first seen to deliver the expected fraction of the dose when lung deposition is considered. Second, the deposition in humans exceeds the deposition that is typically observed with rodents. Although not directly evident in this data, oral bioavailability of budesonide has been measured at 6–11 %. Thus, a third point is that a considerable fraction of the dose reaches the GI tract.

With recent advances in aerosol-device technology, even greater deposition fractions are possible. In contrast, the use of the same device for delivery to the mouse would result in about 1% deposition in the lung and near 99% deposition in the NP region. The hamster is similar to the mouse, although even less drug would be expected to deposit in the lung. Overall, with the more rapid clearance and the lower deposition, respiratory delivery to rodents is much less efficient than what can be achieved in man.

4.4. Considerations of Aerosol Science

Although initially daunting, relatively few concepts related to the delivery are needed to be understood in order to undertake a chemopreventive study using aerosols. First and foremost is the particle size. Much has been said about particle size, but the nature of the measurement of the particle has not been addressed. The aerodynamic equivalent diameter is used for the measure of the particle size. A particle with this effective diameter will exhibit the same resistance to air as a spherical particle of the same diameter and unit density (53,54). That is, the aerodynamic equivalent diameter, d_{ae}, of a spherical particle can be expressed in terms of its true geometric diameter, d, density of the particle, ρ, and unit density, ρ_o, as follows:

$$d_{ae} \sim d(\rho/\rho_o)^{1/2}$$

A term, χ, may be added to correct for nonspherical shape as follows:

$$d_{ae} \sim d(\rho/\rho_o\chi)^{1/2}$$

Although it is difficult to relate the geometric characteristics of a particle to the aerodynamic size, it is relatively straightforward to measure.

The standard method for measuring the aerodynamic particle-size distribution is by means of a cascade impactor (53,54). This simple device allows the aerosol cloud to pass through a series of stages in which each subsequent stage traps a smaller range of particles. The method of capture relies on inertial impaction—the disparate motion of the particle relative to the flow of air. Thus, the capture of the particle depends on its aerodynamic property, and as such the calculated diameter is aerodynamically defined. Measurement of the mass on these stages directly yields a histogram of the particle mass as a function of the aerodynamic size. Rather than determining an arithmetic average, the usual parameter is the mass median aerodynamic diameter (MMAD). As the name implies, the distribution is based on the aerodynamic diameter of a mass distribution in which the median is chosen in preference to the mean.

Respiratory devices usually produce polydispersed aerosol clouds that yield log normal distributions. As such, a Gaussian curve is obtained when the cumulative mass of particles of a given diameter is plotted as a function of the logarithm of the particle diameter. For log normal distributions, the appropriate measure of the breadth of the distribution is the geometric standard deviation (GSD) rather than the typical standard deviation or standard error of the mean. The geometric standard deviation can be calculated as the ratio of the size at the 84 percentile and at the 50 percentile (or 50 and 16 percentile).

Other important terms of aerosol-generating devices are the output (mass) and output rate (mass/time). In examining commercial systems, the output is often given as the concentration of particles per unit volume. This is not very practical for drug delivery, since the mass of drug, which relates to the dose, will depend on the particle-size distribution. A better measure is the mass of drug in a given volume of air, which can be referred to as the aerosol concentration of drug. The advantage of this parameter is that there is a direct mathematically relationship between the aerosol concentration and the dose. That is, the dose to the animal (mass of drug/ kilogram body wt) is given by the following equation (36,55):

$$\text{Inhaled Dose} = [Aer]*RMV*t$$

where [Aer] is the concentration of solute in the aerosol (mass/volume of air), RMV is the respiratory minute volume calculated from Guyton's formula (volume of air inhaled/unit time/body wt), and t is the exposure time *(56)*. Guyton's formula provides the quantitative relationship between body wt and RMV, which is

$$RMV = a \, (\text{body wt})^b$$

where *a* and *b* are constants. From the calculated inhaled dose, the percent deposited in the lung or lung bioavailability may range from zero to over 50%. Of the deposited dose or bioavailability, only a fraction may reach the site of action, whether it is in the conducting or pulmonary regions of the lung.

The aerosol concentration is in turn determined by the output rate of the aerosol-generating device and the efficiency of delivering the particles to the animal. Specifically, the aerosol concentration is determined by the performance of the device as follows *(57)*:

$$[Aer] = C * Q_l * E / Q_a$$

where C is the solute concentration of the chemopreventive agent in the device (e.g., g/mL), Q_l is the output rate of solution in the form of aerosol droplets (mL/min), E is the particle transit efficiency through the tubing, and Q_a is the airflow rate (L/min or lpm). Thus, by combining these equations, the performance of the device may match the needed dose to the animal.

Aerosol output is readily determined by the filter capture method *(57)*. Microfibrile glass filters may be placed at the column outlet, and particles are collected with reduced pressure. The filters are extracted; and the solution is centrifuged and assayed for drug. Blank filters should also be extracted to correct for the background absorbance. The calculated mass divided by the collection time yields the output rate in g/min (although μg/min are often more convenient units).

Finally, most delivery systems developed for animals rely on the production of liquid droplets. However, the use of a carrier gas results in the partial or complete evaporation of the liquid. Thus, the particle size is dynamic. With complete evaporation of the solvent, there is a relationship between the initial droplet size, D_{wet}, and the final size of a dry solid particle, D_{dry}, as follows *(55)*:

$$D_{dry} \sim (\rho/c)^{1/3} \, D_{wet}$$

where ρ is the estimated true density of the solid particles typically near 1.2 g/mL, and c is the w/v concentration of the solution being nebulized.

Since initial droplets are often relatively large for deposition in rodents, drying is a means to further reduce the particle size to enhance deposition. Columns for removing solvent vapor or water are commercially available, but also are easily constructed *(58)*. The drying agent may be separated from the flow by screen mesh at the outer surface, which forms an annular ring. A vertical arrangement has the advantage of minimizing loss of particles from sedimentation. Drying agents may be charcoal for organic vapors and silica for removing water. The drying agent may be regenerated by placing the column in an oven or by heating the external surface of the column with heating tape while passing air through the column.

Considering the nature of deposition in animals, it becomes clear that optimal drug delivery to animals by inhalation requires strict attention to the particle size. Moreover, since rodents are obligate nose-breathers, deposition is increased by reducing the particle size. However, producing submicron-sized particles is technologically demanding. Nevertheless, a number of approaches can be adapted to deliver a wide range of compounds. In general, these methods have involved the initial production of liquid aerosol particles that can be dried to yield a smaller size that is more appropriate for deposition *(57)*. The rationale is that a tremendous amount of energy is required to generate submicron-sized particles from a coarse powder, since there is a significant contribution from creating interfacial area and curvature effects also become very important at 1 μ and below. Thus, dust generators have not been widely used to deliver particles to small rodents.

4.5. Considerations of Aerosol Generation Methods

Although the choices for devices for respiratory delivery in humans are numerous, relatively few are appropriate for chemopreventive studies in rodents. These include jet nebulization, ultrasonic atomization, and the vibrating orifice. All of these readily generate particle sizes in the 1–3-μm size range with simple aqueous or organic solvents, such as ethanol. For complex systems involving liposomes, genes, and proteins the strengths and limitation of these methods becomes critical. In this discussion, the focus will be on the delivery of simple organic compounds with reasonable solubility in aqueous or organic solutions.

The jet nebulizer generates aerosol particles by forcing an air stream past the top of a tube *(59)*. This "dip tube" descends into a reservoir containing an aqueous solution of drug. As a matter of physics, the flow of air reduces the pressure at the orifice of the dip

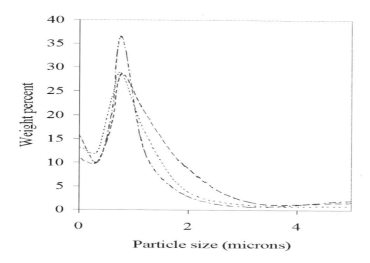

Fig. 3. Particle size distribution produced from jet nebulized budesonide at three different solution concentrations. The broader curves were determined at the higher concentrations.

tube and draws liquid up the tube. The liquid is blown clear from the tube to create the liquid-in-air dispersion. Directly in the path of the emanating droplets is a baffle that intercepts the large particles, and thereby reduces the particle-size and narrows the particle size distribution of the aerosol. It is the presence of the baffle that distinguishes a nebulizer from an atomizer. In the laboratory, pressured air tanks are used to provide the airflow for the nebulizer.

Jet nebulizers are also commonly used in hospitals and in homes for smaller children (≤ 4yr of age) who are unable to use MDIs or DPIs. Since many jet nebulizers are commercially available and require minimal ancillary equipment, they often are the device of choice. Problems can arise with foaming with compounds that are surface-active. With evaporation and associated concentration change, there is an increase in the dose with time of exposure. Finally, although 300 μL/min is typically the liquid output, the high flow rate of air results in a relatively small aerosol concentration of drug in the nebulizer. Therefore, long exposure times are needed unless the aerosol cloud is concentrated by a centripeter or cyclone concentrator. Nevertheless these have been successfully used to deliver genes and chemopreventive agents to rodents' lungs (59,60).

Budesonide has been delivered successfully with this approach in a chemoprevention study involving A/J mice (10,36). In this study (36), Mini-Heart nebulizers were initially tested for uniformity, since occasionally, a unit will not perform according to specifications. The jet nebulizer was driven by air at a flow rate between 1.6 and 2.2 lpm. The initial liquid droplets, which are about 3 μm, were entrained and passed through a wide-diameter, glass horizontal column. In the bottom half of the column, flowing water was used to remove the solvent. At the exit port of the column, a fixture was attached to enable the animal to be exposed to the aerosol.

Results from these studies are given in Table 1. Five different concentrations of budesonide were used, resulting in aerosol concentrations in the range of 4.6–183 μg/L. The results from characterization of the particle size are given in Fig. 3, in which the curves were smoothed to facilitate comparison. Although the jet nebulizer probably produces initial liquid droplets of approx 3 μm, increasing concentration led to an increase in the mean size of the dried particles. This is evidenced by the broadening of the particle distribution. Theoretically, an increase in concentration by a factor of 6.4 should lead to an increase in particle size by the cube root or 1.85. The actual ratio was only 1.2—the probable result of the lower efficiency of transit of the larger particles.

The second device is the ultrasonic atomizer (61). The driving force for particle generation is a piezo-electric crystal that is submerged within a conducting fluid and vibrates at a high frequency (≥ 1 MHz). A cup with a flexible bottom containing the solution to be atomized is placed at the optimal distance from the vibrating plate. A baffle system is attached to the cup to allow ancillary air to entrain the aerosol particles produced at the surface of the solution. The primary advantage of ultrasonic atomization is the high output, which is achieved without the use of a high airflow rate. Therefore, concentrated aerosol clouds are easily obtained, and are useful for delivering high doses of drug.

With ultrasonic atomization, the initial droplet diameter, D_i, is given by the following relationship (61,62):

$$D_i = 0.34(8\pi\gamma/\rho_l f^2)^{1/3}$$

where γ is the surface tension of the liquid, ρ_l is the density of the solution, and f is the frequency of the atomizer. The density and surface tension are easily measured, but these measurements are not often needed, as the range of possible values is rather limited. In addition, they enter the expression only as the cube root, and thereby have a minor impact on the overall result.

5. CHEMOPREVENTIVE ACTIVITY OF BUDESONIDE AEROSOL IN MICE

Following the promising work with glucocorticoids given in the diet, studies were initiated using budesonide administered by aerosol. To carry out these experiments, an aerosol delivery system had to be constructed that produced particle sizes that could reach the periphery of the lung and contain a concentration of the agent sufficient to produce efficacy for chemoprevention. A relatively simple apparatus was designed that contained a jet nebulizer and a column for removing the solvent. For the initial experiments, the same protocol as the one employed for dietary addition of glucocorticoids was carried out using the A/J mouse model.

Aerosol administrations of budesonide were begun 1 wk following three administrations of B[a]P. In the initial experiment, budesonide was given by aerosol for 1 min 6 d/wk for 16 wk. Three inhaled dose levels were administered: 23, 72, and 126 μg/kg body wt, as calculated from the aerosol concentration and respiratory minute volume. At the lowest doses, there was an 83% inhibition of pulmonary adenoma formation (36). There was a negligible difference in body wt (1 g) between these mice and those of the solvent control. However, a difference in splenic weight, (e.g., 42 mg as compared to 59 mg) occurred, most likely the result of stress.

Greater inhibition of pulmonary tumor formation occurred in mice that received the higher doses of budesonide, but there was also retardation of weight gain. In subsequent studies with budesonide, lower doses were used. One regimen used in several experiments entailed an inhaled dose of 25 μg/kg body wt administered over a period of 20 seconds 3×/wk. Under these conditions, a 60% reduction in pulmonary adenoma formation was produced (10). The body wts were essentially the same between the animals receiving solvent by aerosol and those receiving budesonide. However, there was a loss of splenic weight of about 25%.

In addition to budesonide, studies were carried out with beclomethasone diproprionate, a second glucocorticoid administered by aerosol. Like budesonide, this compound is also used in humans for control of symptoms of bronchial asthma. Beclomethasone diproprionate was slightly less potent than budesonide although in other respects, the two compounds behaved similarly (10). Dosage comparisons between small rodents and humans are imprecise. However, data showed that the calculated dose of approx 10 μg/kg body wt per d (25 μg 3 ×/wk), which produced a 60% reduction in pulmonary adenoma formation, is at the upper level of that recommended for treating moderately severe asthma. Moreover, an even lower dose in humans would be estimated if the difference in the aerosol deposition between human and rodent was considered.

Human studies of the effects of budesonide in smokers with bronchial dysplasia have been initiated by Dr. Stephen Lam and his colleagues. A Phase IIa study has been conducted to determine the potential effect of inhaled budesonide 800 μg twice daily (Pulmicort Turbuhaler) in smokers with bronchial lesions. The bronchial dysplasias were identified by fluorescence bronchoscopy and biopsied. The same areas were re-biopsied after 6 mo on budesonide medication. Changes in the histopathology grade of the biopsies were evaluated before and after treatment. New areas that were suspected to show dysplasia were also biopsied. Combined histopathology and nuclear morphometry were used as the primary endpoint. The results of this work are planned for publication in the near future.

6. CHEMOPREVENTIVE ACTIVITY OF 5-FU AEROSOL IN HAMSTER

The model chosen for determining the chemopreventive efficacy of 5-FU was squamous cell carcinoma of the upper respiratory tract (oropharynx, larynx and trachea) of the hamster induced by administering six doses of *N*-methyl-*N*-nitrosourea (MNU) intratracheally using a modification of previously used procedures *(36)*. In the protocol used, the animals were randomized by body wt into experimental groups 1 wk after the last dose of MNU, and aerosol administrations were begun. 5-FU was given 3×/wk for 16 wk and then stopped. The experiment was continued for an additional 4 wk, and the hamsters were subjected to euthanasia.

The following method was used to generate the aerosol particles of 5-FU. An ultrasonic atomizer equipped with a glass baffle that consisted of concentric glass cylinders was constructed. At the bottom of the baffle, a membrane (derivatized Teflon) was attached with a screw cap and O-ring assembly. This separated the solution containing solute from the piezoelectric transducer and conducting fluid. The conducting fluid was ice water to maintain a constant temperature and dissipate the heat generated by the ultrasonic atomizer.

The device produced initial aerosol droplets with diameters near 3 μm. 5-FU was added at concentrations of 28 and 46 mg/mL. Following drying, the particles had a MMAD ± GSD of 1.12 μm ± 1.9 and 1.13 μm ± 1.8, respectively. These distributions were narrower than those observed with the jet nebulizer. The corresponding doses for these concentrations were 1.45 mg/kg and 2.08 mg/kg body wt. In addition, an absolute (no aerosol) control and a solvent control, which was given as an aerosol of water with 3% NH_4OH (the solvent in which 5-FU was dissolved), were included to yield four groups of hamsters in the protocol.

5-FU administrations resulted in a decreased incidence of infiltrating squamous carcinomas in this experiment *(36)*. Both control groups showed about a 30% incidence of infiltrating squamous cell carcinomas. This incidence was reduced to 15% in the group receiving the lower dose of 5-FU and 10% in those receiving the higher dose of 5-FU. Thus, 5-FU was found to have an inhibitory effect on the occurrence of MNU-induced infiltrating squamous cell carcinoma of the upper respiratory tract when given subsequent to the carcinogen—e.g., in the post-initiation period.

Efficacy against squamous cell carcinogenesis of the respiratory tract is important because of its high incidence in this anatomic region and the poor response to available chemopreventive agents. The chemoprevention work described is in an early phase of its development. The magnitude of the inhibition that can be

obtained with aerosol 5-FU and the conditions in which it occurs remain to be established. An issue of importance with 5-FU is its safety; 5-FU is toxic when given parenterally or orally as is done for chemotherapy. In the limited aerosol administration to humans, toxicity was not encountered *(35)*. Further studies are required to confirm these data.

Aerosol administration provides an optimal delivery system to the respiratory tract and draws attention to the possibility of employing chemopreventive agents that could not be given by oral or parenteral means. It would be anticipated that the most likely chemoprevention application of 5-FU would be under supervision to selected high-risk individuals.

7. SUMMARY

Aerosol delivery has advantages for achieving chemoprevention of carcinogenesis of the respiratory tract. This direct delivery method produces a favorable ratio of the dose delivered to the target organ in relationship to systemic tissues. Details of the basic science and technology of aerosol delivery have been presented, indicating that studies may be readily carried out in rodents. The two essential features of aerosols are particle-size distribution and concentration of the compound. These determine the site of delivery and the dose level achieved. With the techniques and equipment employed, initial success has been obtained with two compounds, budesonide and 5-FU. The former has an excellent record of efficacy in preclinical animal models. Presently, budesonide has reached the stage in a Phase IIa clinical trial in humans aimed at evaluating its efficacy in reversing or preventing progression of bronchial dysplasias. The second compound, 5-FU, is in an early stage of preclinical development. It provides evidence that aerosol administration may broaden the range of potent chemopreventive agents that can be used, which would be too toxic if given by more conventional routes.

REFERENCES

1. Sharma S, White D, Imondi AR, et al. Development of inhalational agents for oncologic use. *J Clin Oncol* 2001;19:1839–1847.
2. Edsbacker S. Uptake, retention, and biotransformation of corticosteroids in the lung and airways. Schleimer RP, O'Byrne PM, Szefler SJ, Brattsand R, eds. in: *Inhaled Steroids in Asthma*: Marcel Dekker, Inc., New York, 2002, pp. 213–246.
3. Everard ML. Aerosol therapy past, present, and future: a clinician's perspective. *Respir Care* 2000;45:769–776.

4. Hickey AJ, Garcia-Contreras L. Immunological and toxico-logical implications of short-term studies in animals of pharmaceutical aerosol delivery to the lungs: relevance to humans. *Crit Rev Ther Drug Carrier Syst* 2001;18:387–431.

5. Gonda I. The ascent of pulmonary drug delivery. *J Pharm Sci* 2000;89:940–945.

6. Dalby RN, Hickey AJ, Tiano SL. Medical devices for the delivery of therapeutic aerosols to the lungs, in *Inhalation Aerosols. Physical and Biological Basis for Therapy.* Hickey AJ, ed. Marcel Dekker, Inc., New York, Inc., 1996,pp.441–473.

7. Guidelines for the Diagnosis and Management of Asthma: Expert Panel Report. Bethesda, MD National Heart, Lung and Blood Institute, 1997, pp.57–79.

8. Barnes PJ. Inhaled glucocorticoids for asthma. *N Engl J Med* 1997;332:868–875.

9. Pederson S, Hansen OR. Budesonide treatment of moderate and severe asthma in children: a dose-response study. *J Allergy Clin Immunol* 1994; 29–33.

10. Wattenberg LW, Wiedmann TS, Estensen RD, et al. Chemoprevention of pulmonary carcinogenesis by brief exposures to aerosolized budesonide or beclomethasone dipropionate and by the combination of aerosolized budesonide and dietary *myo*-inositol. *Carcinogenesis* 2000;21:179–182.

11. Bolt, RJ, van Weissenbruch MM, Lafeber HN, Delemarre-van de Waal HA. Glucocorticoids and lung development in the fetus and preterm infant. *Pediatr Pulmonol* 2001;32:76–91.

12. Pierce GB, Speers WC. Tumors as caricatures of the process of tissue renewal: prospects for therapy by directing differentiation. *Cancer Res* 1988;48:1996–2004.

13. Marks PA, Rifkind RA. Differentiating agents in cancer therapy, in *Cancer Chemotherapy and Biological Response Modifers Annual 12.* Pinedo HM, Longo DL, Chabner BA, eds. Elsevier Science Publishers, New York, 1991, pp.291–305.

14. Conley BA, Egorin MJ, Tait N, et al. Phase I study of the orally administered butyrate prodrug, tributyrin, in patients with solid tumors. *Clin Canc Res* 1998;4:629–634.

15. Cheson BD, Jasperse DM, Chun HG, Friedman MA. Differentiating agents in the treatment of human malignancies. *Cancer Treat Rev* 1986;13:129–145.

16. Mintz B, Illmensee K. Normal genetically mosaic mice produced from malignant teratocarcinoma cell. *Proc Natl Acad Sci USA* 1975;72:3585–3589.

17. Jones PA, Taylor SM. Cellular differentiation, cytidine analogs and DNA methylation. *Cell* 1980;20:85–93.

18. Sporn MB, Roberts AB. Role of retinoids in differentiation and carcinogenesis. *Cancer Res* 1983;43:3034–3040.

19. Estensen RD, Wattenberg LW. Studies of chemopreventive effects of *myo*-inositol on benzopyrene-induced neoplasia of the lung and forestomach of female A/J mice. *Carcinogenesis* 1993;14:1975–1977.

20. Wattenberg LW. Chalcones, *myo*-inositol and other novel inhibitors of pulmonary carcinogenesis. *J Cell Biochem Suppl* 1995;22:1162–1168.

21. Wattenberg LW, Estensen RD. Chemopreventive effects of *myo*-inositol and dexamethasone on benzo[a]pyrene and 4-(methyl-nitrosamino)-1-(3-pyridyl)-1-butanone-induced pulmonary carcinogenesis in female A/J mice. *Cancer Res* 1996;56:5132–5135.

22. Belman S, Troll W. The inhibition of croton oil-promoted mouse skin tumorigenesis by steroid hormones. *Cancer Res* 1972;32:450–454.

23. Verma AK, Garcia CT, Ashendel CL, Boutwell RK. Inhibition of 7-bromomethylbenz[a]anthracene-promoted mouse skin tumor formation by retinoic acid and dexamethasone. *Cancer Res* 1983;43:3045–3049.

24. Shimkin MB. Pulmonary tumors in experimental animals. *Adv Cancer Res* 1955;3:223–267.

25. Pederson S, Hansen OR. Budesonide treatment of moderate and severe asthma in children: a dose-response study. *J Allergy Clin Immunol* 1994;95:29–33.

26. Wattenberg LW, Estensen RD. Studies of chemopreventive effects of budesonide on benzopyrene induced neoplasia of the lung in female A/J mice. *Carcinogenesis (Lond)* 1997;18:2015–2017.

27. Ullah A, Shamsuddin AM. Dose-dependent inhibition of large intestinal cancer by inositol hexaphosphate in F344 rats. *Carcinogenesis* 1990;11:2219–2222.

28. Hallman M, Bry K, Hoppu K, Lappi M, Pohjavuori M. Inositol supplementation in premature infants with respiratory distress syndrome. *N Engl J Med* 1992;326:1233–1239.

29. Jyonouchi H., Sun S, Iijima K, et al. Effects of anti-7,8-dihydroxy-9,10-epoxy-7,8,9,10-tetrahydrobenzo[a]pyrene on human small airway epithelial cells and the protective effects of *myo*-inositol. *Carcinogenesis* 1999;20:139–145.

30. Yorek MA, Dunlap JA, Lowe WL Jr. Osmotic regulation of the NA$^+$/*myo*-inositol cotransporter and postinduction normalization. *Kidney Int* 1999;55:215–224.

31. Dillaha CJ, Jansen GT, Honeycutt WM, Holt GA. Further studies with topical 5-fluorouracil. *Arch Dermatol* 1965;92:410–417.

32. Williams AC, Klein E. Experiences with local chemotherapy and immunotherapy in premalignant and malignant skin lesions. *Cancer* 1970;24(2):450–462.

33. Olson PR, Wattenberg LW. Inhibition by 5-fluorouracil of the early stages of chemical carcinogenesis in mouse skin (34054). *Proc Soc Exp Biol Med* 1969;131:1135–1137.

34. Hugosson J, Bergdahl S, Carlsson G, et al. Effects of intravesical instillation of 5-fluorouracil and interferon in patients with recurrent superficial urinary bladder carcinoma. *Scand J Urol Nephrol* 1997;31:343–347.

35. Tatsumura T, Koyama S, Tsujimoto M, et al. Further study of nebulisation chemotherapy; a new chemotherapeutic method in the treatment of lung carcinomas: fundamental and clinical. *Br J Cancer* 1993;68:1146–1149.

36. Wiedmann TS, Wattenberg LW. Chemoprevention of infiltrating squamous cell carcinoma of the upper respiratory tract of the Syrian golden hamster by 5-fluorouacil delivered by aerosol. *Proc Am Assoc Cancer Res* 2002;43:307, abst no 1526.

37. Wattenberg LW, Wiedmann TS, Estensen RD, et al. Chemoprevention of pulmonary carcinogenesis by aerosolized budesonide in female A/J mice. *Cancer Res* 1997;57:5489–5492.

38. Mygind N. Upper airway: structure, function and therapy, in *Aerosols in Medicine.* Moren F, Newhouse M, Dolovich MB, eds. Elsevier, New York, 1985, pp.1–20.

39. Hochhaus G, Mollmann H, Derendorf H, Gonzalez-Rothi RJ. Pharmacokinetic/pharmacodynamic aspects of aerosol therapy using glucocorticoids as a model. *J Clin Pharmacol* 1997;37:881–892.

40. Byron PR. Prediction of drug residence times in regions of the human respiratory tract following aerosol inhalation. *J Pharm Sci* 1986;75:433–438.

41. Ghonda I. Drugs administered directly into the respiratory tract; modeling of the duration of effective drug levels. *J Pharm Sci* 1988;77:340–346.

42. Collins JM. Pharmacological rationale for regional drug delivery. *J Clin Oncol* 1984;2:498–504.

43. Mygind N, Dahl R. Anatomy, physiology and function of the nasal cavities in health and disease. *Adv Drug Delivery Rev* 1998;29:3–12.

44. Kreyling WG, Scheuch G. Clearance of particles deposited in the lungs, in *Lung Biology in Health and Disease, Vol. 143*. Gehr P, Heyder J, eds. Marcel Dekker, Inc., New York, 2000, pp. 323–376.

45. Gehr P, Hof VI, Geiser M, Schurch S. The fate of particles deposited in the intrapulmonary conducting airways. *J Aerosol Med* 1991;4:349–361.

46. Girod S, Zahm J-M, Plotkowski C, et al. Role of the physicochemical properties of mucus in the protection of the respiratory epithelium. *Eur Respir* J 1992;5:477–487.

47. Geiser M, Hof VI, Gehr P, Schurch S. Structural and interfacial aspects of particle retention, in *Lung Biology in Health and Disease, Vol. 143*. Gehr P, Heyder J, eds. Marcel Dekker, Inc., New York, 2000, pp. 291–321.

48. Ferin J, Oberdorster G, Penney DP. Pulmonary retention of ultrafine and fine particles in rats. *Am J Respir Cell Mol Biol* 1992;6:535–542.

49. Heyder J, Gebhart J, Rudolf G, et al. Deposition of particles in the human respiratory tract in the size range 0.005–15 μm. *J Aerosol Sci* 1986;17:811–825.

50. Raabe OG, Al-Bayati MA, Teague SV, Rasolt A. Regional deposition of inhaled monodispersed coarse and fine aerosol particles in small laboratory animals. *Ann Occup Hyg* 1988;32:53–65.

51. Swift DL. Use of mathematical aerosol deposition models in predicting the distribution of inhaled therapeutic aerosols, in Inhalation aerosols. Physical and biological basis for therapy, in. *Lung Biology in Health and Disease, Vol 94,* Hickey AJ, ed. Marcel Dekker, Inc., New York, 1996; pp. 51–81.

52. Edsbacker S, Szefler SJ, Glucocorticoid pharmacokinetics, in *Inhaled Glucocorticosteroids in Asthma.* Schleima RP, Busse WW, O'Byrne PM eds. Marcel Dekker, Inc., NY, 1997; pp.381–492.

53. Hickey AJ, Concessio NM. Descriptors of irregular particle morphology and powder properties. *Adv Drug Delivery Rev* 1997;26:29–40.

54. Washington C. Particle size analysis in inhalation therapy, in *Metered Dose Inhaler Technology*. Purewal TS, Grant DJW, eds. Interpharm Press, Inc., Buffalo Grove, IL, 1998, 117–146.

55. Phillips PR, Gonda I. Droplets produced by medical nebulizers. Some factors affecting their size and solute concentration. *Chest* 1990;97:1327–1332.

56. Guyton AC. Measurement of the respiratory volumes of laboratory animals. *Am J Physiol* 1947;150:7–77.

57. Wiedmann TS, Ravichandran A. Ultrasonic nebulization system for respiratory drug delivery. *Pharm Dev Technol* 2001;6:83–90.

58. Pham S, Wiedmann TS. A novel method for the rapid screening of poorly water soluble drugs for respiratory delivery. *Pharm Res* 1999;16:1857–1863.

59. Niven RW. Atomization and nebulizers in inhalation aerosols, in *Physical and Biological Basis for Therapy*. Hickey AJ, ed. Marcel Dekker, Inc., New York, 1996, pp. 273–312.

60. Greenspan BJ. Ultrasonic and electrohydrodynamic methods for aerosol generation, in *Physical and Biological Basis for Therapy*. Hickey AJ, ed. Marcel Dekker, Inc., New York,1996, pp.313–35.

61. Lang RJ. Ultrasonic atomization of liquids. *J Acoust Soc Am* 1962;34:6–8.

62. Taylor KMG, McCallion ONM. Ultrasonic nebulizers for pulmonary drug delivery. *Int J Pharm* 1997;153:93–104.

10 Chemoprevention of Cancer by Curcumin

Bandaru S. Reddy, DVM, PhD and Chinthalapally V. Rao, PhD

CONTENTS

INTRODUCTION
PRECLINICAL EFFICACY STUDIES
PRECLINICAL TOXICITY STUDIES
SUMMARY AND CONCLUSIONS
REFERENCES

1. INTRODUCTION

Cancer is a major cause of death throughout the world; in the developed world, it is generally exceeded only by cardiovascular disease. An estimated 10 million new cases and more than 7 million deaths from cancer occur annually *(1)*. Several epidemiological and preclinical studies suggest a relationship between colorectal cancer (CRC) and dietary factors *(1–4)*, thus, diet modification is a logical preventive strategy. There is increasing evidence that consumption of certain kinds of vegetables and fruits and intake of certain nonnutrients present in foods actually reduce the risk of colon cancer. There are many reasons why this is biologically plausible *(5)*. Although the protective mechanisms underlying the effects of fruit and vegetable consumption are complex, it is likely that many food items contain significant levels of phytochemicals, and some of these have chemopreventive potential. These include curcuminoids, carotenoids, terpenoids, tocopherols, isothiocyanates, allium compounds, and plant sterols, to cite a few. Phytochemicals are present in human diets in substantial quantities. They give little concern for toxicity and are relevant for primary prevention of colon cancer in the general population as well as for secondary prevention in patients with colonic polyps. As our understanding of the mechanism of carcinogenesis has increased, we envision more possibilities for intervening at multiple points along the multistep process of carcinogenesis,—namely during initiation, promotion, and/or progression. The concept of cancer prevention before the occurrence of clinically detectable tumors is receiving increasing attention as an attractive and plausible approach to cancer control *(6,7)*.

Notably, the use of medicinal plants or their crude extracts in the prevention and/or treatment of several chronic diseases has been traditionally practiced in various ethnic societies worldwide. In South and Southeast Asia (including India) turmeric, the powdered rhizome of *Curcuma longa* L., has been used extensively in food preparations and in the treatment of inflammatory conditions and chronic diseases; it is also known as a coloring and flavoring additive to foods *(8,9)*. Curcumin (diferuloylmethane; 1,7-*bis*-[4-hydroxy-3-methoxyphenyl]-1,6-heptadine-3,5-dione), the major pigment in turmeric, has both antiinflammatory and antioxidant properties *(Fig.1; 10–13)*. Antioxidant/antiinflammatory activities include scavenging of reactive electrophiles and oxygen radicals, modulation of eicosanoid production, and induction of apoptosis. Preclinical efficacy studies have demonstrated that dietary administration of curcumin inhibits carcinogen-induced tumors in the skin, colon, mammary gland, and oral cavity in model assays. The chemopreventive efficacy of curcumin is based on multiple mechanisms, including the inhibition of lipid peroxidation, free radical formation, lipoxygenase (LOX) and cyclooxygenase (COX), and protein kinase C (PKC).

This chapter focuses on the chemopreventive efficacy of curcumin in preclinical models of cancer prevention, with emphasis on cancer of the skin, colon, mammary gland, prostate, and oral cavity.

From: *Cancer Chemoprevention, Volume 1: Promising Cancer Chemoprevention Agents*
Edited by: G. J. Kelloff, E. T. Hawk, and C. C. Sigman © Humana Press Inc., Totowa, NJ

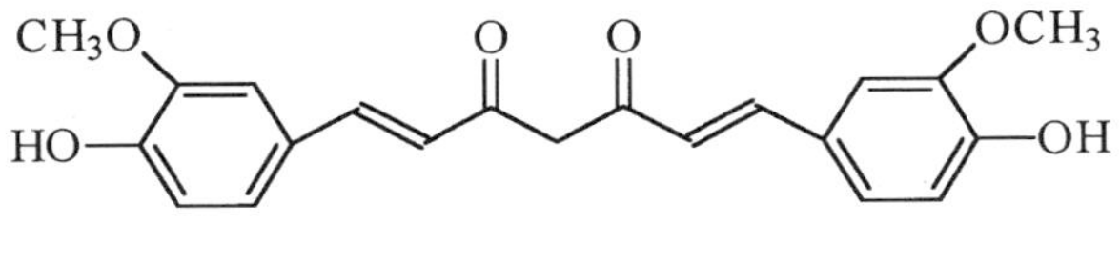

Fig. 1. Curcumin.

2. PRECLINICAL EFFICACY STUDIES

2.1. Skin Carcinogenesis

Earlier studies have indicated that antioxidants and antiinflammatory agents inhibit polycyclic aromatic hydrocarbon (PAH)-induced initiation as well as tumor promotion by 12-*O*-tetradecanoylphorbol-β-acetate (TPA) in mouse skin. For example, Huang et al. *(14–16)* conducted a series of studies in mice on the chemopreventive efficacy of curcumin against skin carcinogenesis. Topical application of 1, 2, or 10 μmol of curcumin together with TPA twice a week for 20 wk inhibited the number of skin tumors/CD mouse by 39, 77, and 98%, respectively, and reduced tumor incidence (percentage of animals with skin tumors) by 21%, 66%, and 82%. In another study, application of 10 μmol of curcumin 2×/wk for 19 wk completely inhibited 7,12-dimethylbenz[*a*]anthracene (DMBA)-induced and TPA-promoted skin tumor incidence and multiplicity. Furthermore, topical application of 3 or 10 μmol of curcumin prior to application of benzo[*a*]pyrene (B[*a*]P) or DMBA and TPA reduced skin tumor multiplicity by 58% and 62%, respectively. Soudamani and Kuttan *(17)* showed that topically applied curcumin significantly suppressed DMBA-induced and croton oil-promoted skin carcinogenesis in Swiss mice. These studies provide convincing evidence that topical application of curcumin is an effective inhibitor of skin tumorigenesis in preclinical models. In most of these studies, curcumin was found to be less than 85% pure. The mechanism by which curcumin inhibits skin carcinogenesis is not fully understood, but it is known that inhibition of skin tumorigenesis is associated with inhibition of TPA-induced DNA synthesis and ornithine decarboxylase (ODC) activity in the epidermis, and also with TPA- and arachidonic acid (AA)-induced edema of mouse ears *(18)*. It has also been shown that curcumin strongly inhibits epidermal COX and LOX activities in vitro *(19,20)*. This suggests that curcumin may inhibit the enzymes that metabolically activate B[*a*]P and DMBA. Thus, the chemopreventive properties of curcumin against skin carcinogenesis could be related to its potent inhibitory

effect on AA-induced inflammation and on AA metabolism through both the COX and LOX pathways in mouse epidermis *(19,20)*.

2.2. Forestomach Carcinogenesis

Curcumin has also been tested as a chemopreventive agent against chemically induced forestomach carcinogenesis in preclinical models *(21)*. Administration of commercial-grade curcumin at 0.5 or 2.0% in the diet during the initiation period (2 wk before, during, and for 1 wk after carcinogen treatment) suppressed B[*a*]P-induced forestomach tumors in A/J mice by 51–53% *(21)*. In the diet given at 0.5% and 2.0% levels during the postinitiation period (1 wk after carcinogen treatment), curcumin inhibited B[*a*]P-induced forestomach tumors in A/J mice by 47–67%. In these assays, dietary curcumin also reduced tumor size and multiplicity of papillomas and squamous cell carcinomas of the forestomach. Curcumin appears to influence the metabolic activation and detoxification of B[*a*]P and/or the metabolic activation of B[*a*]P to DNA adducts, and to inhibit AA metabolism via COX and LOX activities by inhibiting formation and preventing progression of tumors of the forestomach in this model assay *(19–22)*.

2.3. Colon Carcinogenesis

Curcumin has been tested as a chemopreventive agent against azoxymethane (AOM)-induced colon carcinogenesis in preclinical models, and dietary administration of curcumin inhibits the formation of aberrant crypt foci (ACF), putative preneoplastic lesions that occur in the colon of both animals and humans *(23)*. Lesions in humans resemble those induced in rodents with carcinogens. ACF express mutations in the adenomatous polyposis coli (APC) gene and *ras* oncogene that appear to be biomarkers of colon cancer development. Because ACF are induced specifically by carcinogens that predominately elicit colonic tumors, they are considered to be precursors of colon cancer. The multiplicity of ACF increases over time, and reliably predicts colon tumor outcome. We have shown that 0.2% curcumin in the diet significantly inhibits AOM-induced colonic ACF in rats *(23)*. Other investigators have reported that oral administration of 2% curcumin inhibited AOM-induced colonic ACF in rats *(24)* and AOM-induced focal areas of dysplasia in the colon in mice *(25)*. Also, dietary administration of 0.2% and 0.5% tetrahydrocurcumin, a derivative of curcumin, significantly inhibited 1,2-dimethylhydrazine-induced colonic ACF in mice *(26)*.

Bromodeoxyuridine (BrdU) labeling indices were also decreased in animals given curcumin (25).

The studies described here provided an impetus to investigate the chemopreventive efficacy of curcumin against colon carcinogenesis with tumors as the end point. We observed that dietary administration of curcumin during the initiation and postinitiation stage at 0.2% level significantly suppressed the incidence and multiplicity of AOM-induced adenocarcinomas (invasive and noninvasive) of the colon, and also reduced tumor volume in male F344 rats (27). The results of this study conducted with synthetic (99.9% pure) curcumin are of great interest because long-term dietary administration produced no gross changes in the liver, kidney, stomach, intestine, and lungs of F344 rats. Huang et al. (21) found that dietary administration of 0.2%, 2.0%, or 4.0% curcumin during initiation and/or postinitiation suppressed AOM-induced colon adenomas and adenocarcinomas in CF-1 mice by 50–66%. Pereira et al. (24) reported that 0.8% and 1.6% curcumin when administered in the diet during initiation and postinitiation stages inhibited both the incidence and multiplicity of adenomas in a dose-dependent manner.

All these studies clearly demonstrate the chemopreventive efficacy of curcumin during the initiation and postinitiation period of colon carcinogenesis. We have also evaluated the efficacy of curcumin during the promotion/progression stage when premalignant lesions would have developed (28), and found that 0.2% and 0.6% of curcumin in the diet given during promotion/progression period (14 wk after carcinogen treatment) inhibited AOM-induced colon tumors by 33–56%. This suggests that curcumin may effectively retard growth and/or development of existing neoplastic lesions in the colon, and bodes well for the potential use of this agent in secondary prevention of colon cancer in high-risk individuals, such as patients with colonic polyps.

In terms of the mechanism by which curcumin inhibits colon carcinogenesis, it is noteworthy that decreased activities of colonic mucosal and tumor phospholipase A_2 (PLA_2) (50%) and phospholipase $C\gamma1$ ($PLC\gamma1$) (40%) and levels of prostaglandin E_2 (PGE_2) (38%) have been observed (23,27). PLA_2 and $PLC\gamma1$ are dominant pathways for AA release. Thus, curcumin may exert its inhibitory effect by directly acting on the regulators of PLA_2 or $PLC\gamma1$, resulting in decreased levels of AA and its metabolites. Curcumin may not only modulate PLA_2 and $PLC\gamma1$ to alter the endogenous AA available as a substrate for production

of COX and LOX metabolites, but may also affect COX and LOX pathways. The formation of prostaglandins such as PGE_2, $PDG_{2\alpha}$, PGD_2, PGF_{1a}, and thromboxane B_2 through the COX system and the production of 5(S)-,8(S)-, 12(S)-, and 15(S)-hydroxyeicosatetraenoic acids (HETEs) via the LOX pathway from AA was reduced in the colonic mucosa and in tumors of animals fed curcumin as compared to those on control diet. The inhibition of colon tumorigenesis was also associated with increased apoptosis (29). Curcumin has also inhibited cell growth of colon carcinoma cells and induced apoptosis in humans (30). The precise mechanism by which curcumin inhibits colon tumorigenesis must be further elucidated; however, it is likely that the chemopreventive action may at least partly be related to the modulation of AA metabolism and increased apoptosis.

Molecular mechanisms underlying the chemopreventive activities of curcumin and related phytochemicals have been studied by several investigators. Curcumin has been shown to suppress activation of the transcription factor nuclear factor κB (NFκB), which is involved in the regulation of COX-2 and inducible nitric oxide synthase (iNOS) expression (31,32). Li et al. (33) demonstrated that curcumin is also a potent inhibitor of PKC, epidermal growth factor receptor (EGFR) tyrosine kinase, and IκB kinase. Curcumin also inhibits the expression of c-Jun, c-Fos, c-Myc and iNOS, suggesting that it may suppress tumor promotion by blocking signal-transduction pathways in the target cells.

2.4. Mammary Carcinogenesis

Dietary administration of 1% turmeric or 0.5% ethanolic extract of turmeric inhibited DMBA-induced mammary carcinogenesis during the initiation as well as the postinitiation phase (34). Singletary et al. (35) demonstrated that intraperitoneal(ip) administration of 100 and 200 mg curcumin/kg significantly inhibited the number of DMBA-induced mammary tumors in female rats. Inhibition of mammary tumors in this model system was associated with a decrease in the formation of mammary DMBA-DNA adducts. In radiation-induced mammary carcinogenesis, dietary administration of 1% curcumin to pregnant rats during the initiation phase significantly inhibited mammary adenocarcinomas (37). There was no change in litter size or in body wt of pups born from curcumin-fed pregnant rats, proving the lack of toxicity. Administration of 1% curcumin in the diet significantly inhibited radiation-induced mammary adenocarcinomas and estrogen receptor (ER) (+) and progesterone receptor (PGR) (+) tumors in rats during the promotion phase *(36)*. Mehta et al. *(38)* examined the antiproliferative effects of curcumin in several breast cancer cell lines, including hormone-dependent and -independent as well as multidrug-resistant (MDR) cell lines. All these cell lines were highly sensitive to curcumin. The growth-inhibiting effect of curcumin was linked to its inhibition of ODC activity, suggesting that curcumin is a potent antiproliferative agent in breast tumor cells. Another in vitro study of transformed human breast epithelial cells (MCF10A) showed that curcumin inhibits H-*ras*-induced invasive phenotype in these cells and downregulates matrix metalloproteinases (MMP) in a dose-dependent manner *(39)*. Curcumin-induced cell death in H-*ras* MCF10A cells was mainly caused by apoptosis in which downregulation of Bcl-2 and upregulation of BAX were involved, suggesting that curcumin inhibits invasion and induces apoptosis.

2.5. Prostate Cancer

Curcumin decreased the proliferative potential and induced apoptosis in both androgen-dependent and androgen-independent prostate cancer cells in vitro *(40,41)*. Dietary administration of 2% curcumin also caused a marked decrease in cell proliferation, a significant increase in apoptosis, and a significant decrease in angiogenesis in nude mice treated with LNCaP prostate-cancer cells *(40)*. Thus, curcumin could be a therapeutic anticancer agent and potentially prevent the progression of prostate cancer to its hormone-refractory state *(40)*. A study by Dorai et al. *(41)* showed that curcumin inhibits tyrosine kinase activity in EGFR, and can induce apoptosis in both androgen-dependent and androgen-independent prostate cancer cells.

2.6. Other Organs

There is evidence that curcumin inhibits esophageal and oral carcinogenesis. Inhibitory effects of curcumin administered during the initiation or postinitiation stage of *N*-nitrosomethylbenzylamine (NMBA)-induced esophageal carcinogenesis in male F344 rats were described by Ushida et al. *(42)*. Administration of 500 ppm curcumin in the diet significantly suppressed the incidence and multiplicity of NMBA-induced esophageal preneoplastic lesions and neoplasms during both the initiation and post-initiation phases of carcinogenesis. This inhibition was associated with suppression of NMBA-induced cell proliferation. Tanaka et al. *(43)* showed that dietary curcumin inhibits 4-nitroquinoline-1-oxide-induced oral carcinogenesis (primarily in the tongue) in rats. Also, curcumin at 0.1, 1.0, and 10-μM doses induced significant dose-dependent inhibition of both cell growth and cell proliferation of the human oral squamous carcinoma cell line, SCC-25 *(44)*. Curcumin was also effective against diethylnitrosamine (DEN)-induced murine hepatocarcinogenesis *(45)*. Administration of 0.2% curcumin in the diet 4 d before DEN treatment and until death—e.g., at 42 wk of age—suppressed the incidence (by about 62%) and multiplicity (by about 81%) of hepatocellular carcinomas. This inhibition of hepatocarcinogenesis was associated with the modulation of *ras p21* and proliferating cell nuclear antigen (PCNA).

3. PRECLINICAL TOXICITY STUDIES

There are limited preclinical toxicity studies on curcumin; however, extensive studies carried out as part of the National Toxicology Program (NTP) utilized turmeric oleoresin. The studies with curcumin mostly used the commercial grade (~75% curcumin) rather than the pure agent. In rats, the curcumin oral LD_{50} is >3500 mg/kg-bw. A single i.g. dose of curcumin between 1380 and 3500 mg/kg-bw produced no adverse effects in rats *(46)*. In another study, single i.g. doses of curcumin up to 5000 mg/kg-bw produced no clinical symptoms and did not affect relative organ weights in male and female rats *(47)*. In a 90-d rat study, curcumin at 1995 mg/kg-bw/d and above given by i.g. intubation to male rats decreased reticulocyte counts and increased corpuscular hemoglobin (MCH)—results that were not considered biologically significant *(46)*. In dogs, 250, 500, and 1000 mg curcumin/kg-bw/d in a gelatin capsule significantly increased MCH levels at higher doses, but these results were not considered biologically relevant because overt anemia was not detected *(46)*. The safe no observed adverse effects (NOAE) dose for curcumin appears to be < 1000 mg/kg-bw/d in male and female dogs. There are several short and long-term studies on curcumin in the literature that confirm the lack of significant toxic effects on body wt, hematology, serum chemistry, and histology of the gastrointestinal (GI) tract, liver, spleen, or kidney from this agent used as a food component *(48)*. Also, *per os* administration to rats of curcumin up to 1000 ppm mg/kg-bw/d for 3 mo, and to monkeys at doses up to 800 mg/kg bw for 3 mo, caused no evidence of adverse effects on growth, behavior, biochemical, and histopathological parameters *(49,50)*. Absorption, distribution, and metabolism studies using radiolabeled curcumin suggested poor GI absorption and very limited extrahepatic metabolism of this agent *(51,52)*. Curcumin addition of 2,000–50,000 ppm to the diet (2-yr NTP study) failed to show evidence of carcinogenesis in rats and mice *(53)*. Curcumin was not mutagenic in the Ames *Salmonella typhimurium* assay with or without metabolic activation or in the mouse dominant lethal assay *(54,55)*. In contrast, positive results were obtained in some assays of clastogenicity depending on the dose, length, and route of exposure to curcumin *(56)*. Overall, even at high dose levels, curcumin is free of adverse effects on growth, biochemical, histopathological, mutagenic, carcinogenic, and reproductive toxicities in preclinical studies.

4. SUMMARY AND CONCLUSIONS

Curcumin is a major pigment in turmeric, the powdered rhizome of *Curcuma longa Linn*, which has been widely used as a coloring and flavoring agent in foods and found to be effective for the treatment of certain inflammatory conditions and even chronic diseases. There is convincing evidence in preclinical model assays that dietary curcumin inhibits tumorigenesis in the oral cavity, skin, forestomach, colon, prostate, and mammary gland when administered during the initiation and postinitiation stages of carcinogenesis. Earlier studies have demonstrated that topical application of low doses of curcumin markedly inhibited skin carcinogenesis in mice. In the rat, dietary administration of curcumin during the promotion/progression stage of colon carcinogenesis led to growth retardation of existing preneoplastic lesions in the colon. Several studies have also provided strong evidence of modulation of AA metabolism through COX and LOX activities, and that the induction of apoptosis may be related to its chemopreventive efficacy. The inhibition of tumorigenesis by curcumin may be mediated through modulation of a signal-transduction pathway(s) associated with tumor promotion. Preclinical efficacy studies and the lack of toxicity and side effects, as well as the availability of curcumin as a natural product that has been used in population groups for several centuries, are compelling reasons to schedule this agent for human clinical trials for chemopreventive efficacy. Curcumin has several advantages over other synthetic agents with similar modes of action and efficacy that are already being tested in human clinical trials.

REFERENCES

1. American Cancer Society. Cancer Statistics 2001. *CA Cancer J Clin* 2000;51.
2. Wynder EL, Kajitani T, Ishidawa S, et al. Environmental factors in cancer of colon and rectum. *Cancer (Phila)* 1969;23:1210–1220.
3. Willett WC, Stampfer MJ, Colditz GA, et al. Relation of meat, fat and fiber intake to the risk of colon cancer in a prospective study among women. *N Engl J Med* 1990;323:1664–1672.
4. Reddy BS. Nutritional factors and colon cancer. *Crit Rev Food Sci Nutr* 1995;35:175–190.
5. Potter JD, Steinmatz K. Vegetables, fruits and phytoestrogens as preventive agents. *IARC Sci Publ* 1995;139:61–90.
6. Kelloff GJ, Boone CW, Malone WE, Steele VE. Recent results in preclinical and clinical drug development of chemopreventive agents at the National Cancer Institute, in *Cancer Chemoprevention*. Wattenberg LW, Lipkin CW, Boone CW, Kelloff GJ, eds. CRC Press, Boca Raton, FL, 1992, pp. 41–56.
7. Greenwald P, Kelloff GJ, Boone CW, McDonald SN. Genetic and cellular changes in colorectal cancer: proposed targets of chemopreventive agents. *Cancer Epidemiol Biomarkers Prev* 1995;4:691–702.
8. Ammon HPT, Wahl MA. Pharmacology of *Curcuma longa*. *Planta Med* 1991;57:1–7.
9. Nadkarani KM. Curcuma longa, in *India Materia Medica*. Nadkarani KM, ed. Popular Prakashan Publishing, Bombay, India, 1976:414–416.
10. Tonnesen HH. Chemistry of curcumin and curcuminoids, in *Phenolic Compounds in Food and their Effect on Health, Vol. 1: Analysis, Occurrence and Chemistry*. Ho C-T, Lee CY, Huang M-T, eds. ACS Symposium Series No. 506, American Chemical Society, Washington, DC, 1992, pp. 143–153.
11. Srimal RC, Dhawan BN. Pharmacology of diferuloylmethane (curcumin), a non-steroidal anti-inflammatory agent. *J Pharm Pharmacol* 1973;25: 447–452.
12. Satoskar RR, Shah SJ, Shenoy SG. Evaluation of antiinflammatory property of curcumin (diferuloylmethane) in patients with postoperative inflammation. *Int J Clin Pharmacol Ther Toxicol* 1986;24: 651–654.
13. Sharma OP. Antioxidant activity of curcumin and related compounds. *Biochem Pharmacol* 1976;25:1811–1812.
14. Huang M-T, Wang ZY, Georgiadis CA, et al. Inhibitory effects of curcumin on tumor initiation by benzo[*a*]pyrene and 7,12-dimethylbenz[*a*]anthracene. *Carcinogenesis* 1992;13:2183–2186.
15. Huang M-T, Ma W, Yen P, et al. Inhibitory effects of topical application of low doses of curcumin on 12-*O*-tetradecanoylphorbol-13-acetate-induced tumor promotion and oxidized DNA bases in mouse epidermis. *Carcinogenesis* 1997;18:83–88.
16. Huang M-T, Smart RC, Wong C-Q, Conney AH. Inhibitory effect of curcumin, chlorogenic acid, caffeic acid, and ferulic acid on tumor promotion in mouse skin by 12-*O*-tetradecanoylphorbol-13-acetate. *Cancer Res* 1988;48:5941–5946.

17. Soudamini KK, Kuttan R. Inhibition of chemical carcinogenesis by curcumin. *J Ethnopharmacol* 1989;27:227–233.

18. Huang M-T, Smart RC, Wong C-Q, Conney AH. Inhibitory effect of curcumin, chlorogenic acid, caffeic acid, and ferulic acid on tumor promotion in mouse skin by 12-*O*-tetradecanoylphorbol-13-acetate. *Cancer Res* 1988;48:5941–5946.

19. Huang M-T, Lysz T, Ferraro T, et al. Inhibitory effects of curcumin on in vitro lipoxygenase and cyclooxygenase activities in mouse epidermis. *Cancer Res* 1991;51:813–819.

20. Flynn DL, Rafferty MF, Boctor AM. Inhibition of 5-hydroxyeicosatetraenoic acid (5-HETE) formation in intact human neutrophils by naturally occurring diarylheptanoids: Inhibitory activities of curcuminoids and yakuchinones. *Leukotrienes Med* 1986;22:357–360.

21. Huang M-T, Lou Y-R, Ma W, et al. Inhibitory effects of dietary curcumin on forestomach, duodenal, and colon carcinogenesis in mice. *Cancer Res* 1994;54:5841–5847.

22. Singh SV, Hu X, Srivastava SK, et al. Mechanism of inhibition of benzo*[a]*pyrene-induced forestomach cancer in mice by dietary curcumin. *Carcinogenesis* 1998;19:1357–1360.

23. Rao CV, Simi B, Reddy BS. Inhibition by dietary curcumin of azoxymethane-induced ornithine decarboxylase, tyrosine protein kinase, arachidonic acid metabolism and aberrant crypt foci formation in the rat colon. *Carcinogenesis* 1993;14:2219–2225.

24. Pereira MA, Grubbs CJ, Barnes LH, et al. Effects of the phytochemicals, curcumin and quercetin, upon azoxymethane-induced colon cancer and 7,12-dimethylbenz*[a]*anthracene-induced mammary cancer in rats. *Carcinogenesis* 1996;17:1305–1311.

25. Huang MT, Deschner EE, Newmark HL, et al. Effect of dietary curcumin and ascorbyl palmitate on azoxymethanol-induced colonic epithelial cell proliferation and focal areas of dysplasia. *Cancer Lett* 1992;64:117–121.

26. Kim JM, Araki S, Kim DJ, et al. Chemopreventive effects of carotenoids and curcumins on mouse colon carcinogenesis after 1,2-dimethylhydrazine initiation. *Carcinogenesis* 1998;19: 81–85.

27. Rao CV, Rivenson A, Simi B, Reddy BS. Chemoprevention of colon carcinogenesis by dietary curcumin, a naturally occurring plant phenolic compound. *Cancer Res* 1995;55:59–266.

28. Kawamori T, Lubet R, Steele VE, et al. Chemopreventive effect of curcumin, a naturally occurring anti-inflammatory agent, during promotion/progression stages of colon cancer. *Cancer Res* 1999;59:597–601.

29. Samaha HS, Hamid R, El-Bayoumy K, et al. The role of apoptosis in the modulation of colon carcinogenesis by dietary fat and by the organoselenium compound 1,4-phenylenebis(methylene)selenocyanate. *Cancer Epidemiol Biomark Prev* 1997;6:699–704.

30. Chen H, Zhang ZS, Zhang YL, Zhou DY. Curcumin inhibits cell proliferation by interfering with the cell cycle and inducing apoptosis in colon carcinoma cells. *Anticancer Res* 1999;19:3675–3680.

31. Plummer SM, Holloway KA, Manson MM, et al. Inhibition of cyclo-oxygenase 2 expression in colon cells by the chemopreventive agent curcumin involves inhibition of NF-κB activation via the NIK/IKK signaling complex. *Oncogene* 1999;18:6013–6020.

32. Surh YJ, Chun KS, Chai HH, et al. Molecular mechanisms underlying chemopreventive activities of anti-inflammatory phytochemicals: down-regulation of COX-2 and iNOS through suppression of NF-κB activation. *Mutat Res* 2001;1:243–268.

33. Li JK, Lin-Shia SY. Mechanisms of cancer chemoprevention by curcumin. *Proc Natl Sci Counc Repub China* B 2001;25:59–66.

34. Deshpande SS, Ingle AD, Maru GB. Chemopreventive efficacy of curcumin-free aqueous turmeric extract in 7,12-dimethylbenz*[a]*anthracene-induced rat mammary tumorigenesis. *Cancer Lett* 1998;123:35–40.

35. Singletary K, MacDonald C, Wallig M, Fisher C. Inhibition of 7,12-dimethylbenz[a]anthracene (DMBA)-induced mammary tumorigenesis and DMBA-DNA adduct formation by curcumin. *Cancer Lett* 1996;103:137–141.

36. Inano H, Onoda M, Inafuku N, et al. Chemoprevention by curcumin during the promotion stage of tumorigenesis of mammary gland in rats irradiated with gamma-rays. *Carcinogenesis* 1999;20: 1011–1018.

37. Inano H, Onoda M, Inafuku N, et al. Potent preventive action of curcumin on radiation-induced initiation of mammary tumorigenesis in rats. *Carcinogenesis* 2000;21:1835–1841.

38. Mehta K, Pantazis P, McQueen T, Aggarwal BB. Antiproliferation effect of curcumin (diferuloylmethane) against human breast tumor cell lines. *Anticancer Drugs* 1997;8:470–478.

39. Kim MS, Kang HJ, Moon A. Inhibition of invasion and induction of apoptosis by curcumin in H-ras-transformed MCF10A human breast epithelial cells. *Arch Pharmacol Res* 2001;24:349–354.

40. Dorai T, Cao YC, Dorai B, et al. Therapeutic potential of curcumin in human prostate cancer. III. Curcumin inhibits proliferation, induces apoptosis, and inhibits angiogenesis of LNCaP prostate cancer cells in vivo. *Prostate* 2001;47:293–303.

41. Dorai T, Gehani N, Katz A. Therapeutic potential of curcumin in human prostate cancer. II. Curcumin inhibits tyrosine kinase activity of epidermal growth factor receptor and depletes the protein. *Mol Urol* 2000;4:1–6.

42. Ushida J, Sugie S, Kawabata K, et al. Chemopreventive effect of curcumin on N-nitrosomethylbenzylamine-induced esophageal carcinogenesis in rats. *Jpn J Cancer Res* 2000;91:893–898.

43. Tanaka T, Makita H, Ohnishi M, et al. Chemoprevention of 4-nitroquinoline 1-oxide-induced oral carcinogenesis by dietary curcumin and hesperidin: comparison with the protective effect of β-carotene. *Cancer Res* 1994;54:4653–4659.

44. Elattar TM, Virji AS. The inhibitory effect of curcumin, genistein, quercetin and cisplatin on the growth of oral cancer cells in vitro. *Anticancer Res* 2000;20:1733–1738.

45. Chuang SE, Kuo ML, Hsu CH, et al. Curcumin-containing diet inhibits diethylnitrosamine-induced murine hepatocarcinogenesis. *Carcinogenesis* 2000;21:331–335.

46. Kelloff GJ, Crowell JA, Hawk ET, et al. Clinical developmental plan: curcumin. *J Cell Biochem* 1996;26S:72–85.

47. Wahlstrom B, Blennow GA. Study on the fate of curcumin in the rat. *Acta Pharmacol Toxicol* 1978;43: 86–92.

48. Sambaiah K, Ratankumar S, Kamanna VS, et al. Influence of turmeric and curcumin on growth, blood constituents and serum enzymes in rats. *J Food Sci Technol* 1982;19:187–190.

49. Srimal RC. Curcumin. *Drugs Future* 1987;12: 331–333.

50. Govindarajan VS. Turmeric—chemistry, technology, and quality. *Crit Rev Food Sci Nutr* 1980;12:199–299.

51. Ravindranath F, Chandrasekhara N. Metabolism of curcumin—studies with [^{3}H]-curcumin. *Toxicol* 1981;22:337–344.

52. Holder GM, Plummer JL, Ryan AJ. The metabolism and excretion of curcumin (1,7-bis-(4-hydroxy-3methoxyphenyl)-1,6-heptadiene-3,5-dione) in the rat. *Xenobiotica* 1978;8:761–768.

53. National Toxicology Program (NTP). Toxicology and carcinogenesis studies of turmeric oleoresins (CAS No. 8024-37-1) (major component 79%–85% curcumin, CAS No. 458-37-7) in F344/N rats and B6C3F1 mice (feed studies). *NTP Technical Report Series,* No. 427, 1993.

54. Jensen NJ. Lack of mutagenic effect of turmeric oleoresin and curcumin in the salmonella/mammalian microsome test. *Mutat Res* 1982;105:393–396.

55. Vijayalaxmi. Genetic effects of turmeric and curcumin in mice and rats. Mutat Res 1980;79:125–132.

56. Ishidate M Jr, Harnois MC, Sofuni T. A comparative analysis of data on the clastogenicity of 951 chemical substances tested in mammalian cell cultures. *Mutat Res* 1988;195:151–213.

11 Prostacyclin and Lung Cancer Chemoprevention

Robert L. Keith, MD, York E. Miller, MD, Paul A. Bunn Jr., MD, Patrick Nana-Sinkam, MD, Raphael A. Nemenoff, PhD, and Mark W. Geraci, MD

CONTENTS

DESCRIPTION
MECHANISM OF ACTION
PREVIOUS EFFICACY/STUDIES
SAFETY
PHARMACODYNAMICS
POPULATIONS BENEFITING FROM INTERVENTION
CLINICAL STUDIES
PROMISING ENDPOINTS (BIOMARKERS)
REFERENCES

1. DESCRIPTION

1.1. Eicosanoids and Cancer

Eicosanoids are a family of bioactive lipid metabolites of arachidonic acid (AA). AA is hydrolyzed from membrane phospholipids through the action of phospholipase A_2 (PLA_2). Free AA can then be metabolized through three major pathways: cyclooxygenase (COX) to produce prostaglandins (PG) and thromboxane, lipoxygenase (LOX) to produce leukotrienes and hydroxy eicosatetraenoic acid (HETES), and cytochrome P-450 to produce epoxyeicosatrienoic acids (EETs). Most studies that have examined eicosanoids and cancer have focused on COX-2 in colon cancer. Elevated COX-2 expression was first demonstrated in colon cancer, in which colon tumors increased COX-2 expression compared to normal colon tissues (1). This has also been demonstrated in colon cancer cell lines (2), and is associated with constitutively high levels of prostaglandin E_2 (PGE_2) production. Inhibition of PG production by nonsteroidal antiinflammatory drugs (NSAIDs) such as sulindac sulfide, a potent COX inhibitor, decreases the size and number of rectal polyps and colonic tumors in humans (3). More selective COX inhibitors

block the growth of colon cancer cells (4) and H-*ras*-transformed intestinal epithelial cells (5). Epidemiological studies indicate that sustained use of aspirin or other NSAIDs reduces the risk of colon cancer (6). An important role for COX-2 in tumorigenesis was provided by experiments using COX-2(-/-) mice. Crossing adenomatous polyposis coli ($Apc^{\Delta716}$) geneknockout mice, a model for human familial adenomatous polyposis, with COX-2 knockout mice dramatically decreased the number of intestinal polyps (7). As a whole, these data strongly support a role for COX-2 in the development and/or progression of colon cancer. Importantly, transgenic mice that overexpress COX-2 under the control of the murine mammary tumor virus (MMTV) promoter developed mammary carcinomas, indicating that induction of COX-2 is *sufficient* to cause tumor development in certain tissue (8).

Eicosanoid production in the etiology of lung cancer is also important. Epidemiological studies demonstrate a protective effect of NSAIDs against the risk for developing lung cancer (9). Non-small-cell lung cancers (NSCLC) produce readily detectable levels of PGE_2 and 6 keto-$PGF_{2\alpha}$ (10,11). Thromboxane biosynthesis has been detected in several cell lines derived from human adenocarcinomas (12). No detectable

From: Cancer Chemoprevention, Volume 1: Promising Cancer Chemoprevention Agents
Edited by: G. J. Kelloff, E. T. Hawk, and C. C. Sigman © Humana Press Inc., Totowa, NJ

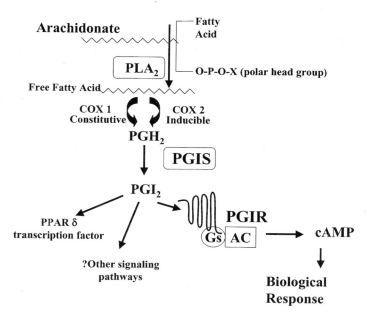

Fig. 1. Pathway of prostacyclin production and receptor activation. PLA2 and COX enzymes form the precursor substrate (PGH2) for prostacyclin, which can act through its membrane receptor (PGIR) or a nuclear receptor (PPAR for signaling effects δ).

prostaglandin production was observed in small-cell lung cancer (SCLC) lines in these studies, although no attempt was made to identify metabolites of either the LOX or cytochrome P-450 pathways in either SCLC or NSCLC. Some SCLC lines produce HETEs, which may contribute to their growth *(13)*. Consistent with increased eicosanoid production, COX-2 overexpression occurs within lung adenocarcinomas *(14–16)*. Our laboratory has reported that increased PGE_2 production and COX-2 expression occur in a subset of NSCLC that express gain-of-function mutations in *ras* *(17)*. COX-2 and COX-1 expression are increased in mouse lung tumors *(18)*. Inhibition of eicosanoid production by treatment with NSAIDs inhibits growth of NSCLC cell lines *(17,19)*, as well as growth of lung tumors in mice *(20)*.

Recent studies examined the role of cytosolic phospholipase A_2 ($cPLA_2$) in the development of chemically induced gastrointestinal (GI) cancer *(21,22)*. These studies demonstrated that $cPLA_2$ (-/-) mice were protected from developing tumors in the small intestine when crossed with the $Apc^{\Delta716}$ mouse. However, these animals were not protected from developing large-intestine tumors. This result suggests that the role of $cPLA_2$ in tumorigenesis is tissue-specific. This complexity is underscored by finding that disruption of the mouse group IIA secretory phospholipase A_2 locus (Pla2g2a), a potential source of AA for

COX-2, increases the incidence of tumors, despite the fact that the mutation was predicted to decrease PG production *(23)*.

Downstream enzymes in the eicosanoid pathway also contribute to tumorigenesis. NSCLC tumor samples and cell lines show increased expression of prostaglandin E synthase (PGES) *(24)*, the enzyme responsible for PGE_2 production. The mechanisms whereby prostaglandins mediate tumor growth remain poorly defined. Some studies have proposed direct mitogenic effects of eicosanoids. However, it is likely that additional effects that are not directly related to cell growth contribute to tumorigenesis. Overexpression of COX-2 in normal epithelial cells appears to make them more resistant to apoptosis *(25)*, and increases metastatic potential *(26)*. In at least some systems, increased production of PGE_2 has been linked to induction of vascular endothelial growth factor (VEGF), a critical angiogenic factor *(27)*.

1.2. The Biology of Prostacyclin

Prostacyclin (PGI_2) is a lipid mediator derived from the COX pathway. The cascade leading to the production of PGI_2 is shown in Fig. 1. PLA_2 cleaves AA from lipid bilayers to form free fatty acids. It is generally believed that rate-limiting steps in the AA cascade occur at both AA formation and the formation of prostaglandin H_2 (PGH_2) by prostaglandin H_2 synthase (otherwise known as COX) *(28)*. The two PGH synthase isozymes, COX-1 and COX-2, are each coded by a different gene *(29)*. COX-1 is a constitutive enzyme that is present in many cells. COX-2 *(30)* shares 60% amino acid homology with COX-1. PGI_2 is formed from the precursor PGH_2, in an isomerization reaction catalyzed by prostacyclin synthase (PGIS) *(31)*. PGI_2 expresses its biological actions via specific receptors *(32)*, G protein activation, and stimulation of adenyl cyclase and subsequent increase in intracellular cyclic adenosine 5' monophosphate (cAMP) concentration *(33)*; *see* Fig. 1.

PGI_2 is one of the main products of AA in all vascular tissues tested to date *(34)*. Once released from cells, PGI_2 acts as an autocrine and paracrine effector to regulate the function of various differentiated cells and platelets. PGI_2 has several important biologic effects. It is the most potent endogenous inhibitor of platelet aggregation yet discovered *(34)*, and as a product of the vascular wall endothelium and smooth-muscle cells, PGI_2 produces vasodilation of all vascular beds studied *(35)*. PGI_2 inhibits both proliferation and DNA synthesis of smooth-muscle cells *(36)*. Along with other prostaglandins, PGI_2 shares a cytoprotective activity that is not yet fully understood. For example, in models of myocardial infarction, PGI_2 reduces infarct size and oxygen demand *(37,38)*.

1.3. Prostacyclin and Lung Cancer

Lung cancer is the leading cause of cancer death in men and women in North America *(39)*. Although primary prevention of tobacco smoking and smoking cessation are the most potent interventions available, most lung cancers are diagnosed in former smokers *(39)*, underscoring the need for effective chemoprevention strategies. PGH_2, the product of the COX enzymes, is metabolized to a number of eicosanoids, and some of these may be chemopreventive. COX inhibition decreases the levels of PGH_2 and all downstream PGs and thromboxanes. COX manipulation has been investigated as a chemopreventive strategy. In a large US cohort, 32% fewer lung cancers developed in frequent aspirin users *(9)*. Mouse models of lung carcinogenesis display both histologic and molecular genetic similarities to adenocarcinoma *(40)*, the most common histologic type of human lung cancer. In these models, either nonselective COX-1 and COX-2 inhibition or selective COX-2 inhibition caused 34–52% reduction in lung tumor multiplicity and no significant change in incidence *(20,41)*. Chronic administration of

LOX inhibitors, which diminish leukotriene formation, decreases lung tumor multiplicity by 30% *(42)*. To date, large-scale interventional trials of COX inhibition in human lung cancer chemoprevention have not been performed.

The role of PGI_2 in carcinogenesis is under intense translational investigation by our group. Early studies focused on the physiological role of PGI_2, including suppression of inflammation *(43)*, platelet inhibition *(44)*, metastasis prevention *(45)*, and growth inhibition of established micrometastases *(46)*. PGI_2 can be administered by either continuous intravenous (iv) infusion or intermittent inhalation, but the short half-life of PGI_2 and difficulties controlling tissue levels have prevented animal studies testing PGI_2 as a cancer-chemopreventive agent. PGI_2 production in normal lung and human NSCLC has been examined. PGI_2 is the most abundant prostaglandin in the normal lung, but is produced in small amounts by human NSCLC *(47)*. Noting this discrepency, we examined NSCLC samples with immunohistochemistry using a polyclonal antibody to PGIS that we developed *(48)*. Figures 2–4 demonstrate the typical finding that NSCLC express very little PGIS compared to the surrounding normal lung. In contrast, PGE_2 is the predominant prostaglandin in NSCLC *(11)*. High levels of PGE_2 are observed in NSCLC containing Ki-*ras* mutations because these mutations induce constitutively high expression of $cPLA_2$ and COX-2 *(17)*. Based on these findings, we hypothesized that pulmonary-specific overexpression of PGIS in a transgenic mice model would confer protection. We demonstrated that the transgenic mice were heavily protected from the development of lung tumors in various tumorigenesis models *(49)*.

In the following section, we focus on PGI_2 and its potential role as a cancer chemopreventive agent.

2. MECHANISM OF ACTION

2.1. Prostacyclin Receptors

The PGI_2 receptor (PGIR) has been cloned and characterized *(50)*. The receptor has seven putative transmembrane domains and an amino acid sequence that is 30–40% identical to the transmembrane domains of the PGE-receptor subtypes and the thromboxane A_2 receptor *(50)*. When stimulated, cells transfected with PGIR respond with increased cAMP levels and inositol phosphate generation, indicating coupling to multiple signal-transduction pathways *(51)*.

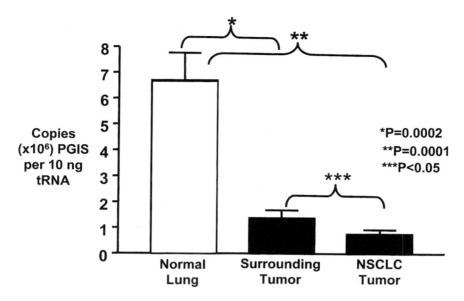

Fig. 2. Absolute quantitation of PGIS mRNA in the normal lung and in tumors. Quantitative real-time PCR was performed using primers and probes specific for PGIS. Absolute copy number was estimated from results of plasmid amplification. Histologically normal lung, more than 2 cm from the tumor, contains more mRNA for PGIS than paired tumor samples. Normal lung from non-cancer patients is shown for relative comparison.

The domains that confer ligand-binding specificity have been evaluated using chimeric receptors (52). The sixth to seventh transmembrane domain confers specificity of this receptor to its ligand. The receptor is both glycosylated and phosphorylated. Recent work suggests that the desensitization of the receptor following Iloprost (a synthetic PGI_2 analog) exposure requires protein kinase-C (PKC)-dependent phosphorylation of the receptor at Ser-328 (53). PGIR contains a conserved putative isoprenylation CAAX motif with the sequence CSLC. Isoprenylation is required for effective coupling to the effectors adenyl cyclase and phospholipase C (54).

Only one type of PGI_2 membrane receptor is present in the genome. This conclusion is drawn from the work of Professor Shuh Narumiya et al. in generating the PGIR knockout (PGIR KO) mouse (55). This animal has the phenotype of increased susceptibility to thrombosis, diminished inflammatory and pain response, and no vasodilatory response to exogenously administered PGI_2. In collaboration with Professor Narumiya, Department of Pharmacology, Kyoto University Faculty of Medicine, we have an established colony of PGIR KO mice (55) that have been bred into the FVB/N background. We have evaluated the susceptibility of these animals to hypobaric hypoxia. PGIR-deficient

mice develop more severe pulmonary hypertension than wild-type (wt) animals after chronic hypobaric hypoxia. Right ventricular hypertrophy and pulmonary vascular remodeling accompany this pulmonary hypertension (56). To evaluate the role of PGIR in murine lung tumorigenesis, we have transferred the PGIR KO locus to the FVB/N strain.

Several lines of evidence suggest that the effects of PGI_2 are mediated by PGI_2 activation of the nuclear hormone receptor peroxisome proliferator-activated receptor δ (PPARδ), demonstrating the first reported biologic function of this receptor-signaling pathway (57). The PPARs, ligand-dependent transcription activators, are members of the nuclear receptor (NR) superfamily (58,59). Three distinct PPAR isoforms (α, δ, and γ), have been isolated and characterized (60). Recently, Lim et al. presented several lines of evidence suggesting that PGI_2 was not signaling through the G-coupled membrane receptor (57). COX-2-deficient mice demonstrate multiple reproductive failures, including a defect in embryo implantation (61). The major PG subtype produced at the implantation site is PGI_2. High levels of PPARδ are produced at the implantation site, but no PGIR. Furthermore, administration of PGI_2 rescues the implantation defect, as does a PPARδ agonist. However, cicaprost, a PGI_2

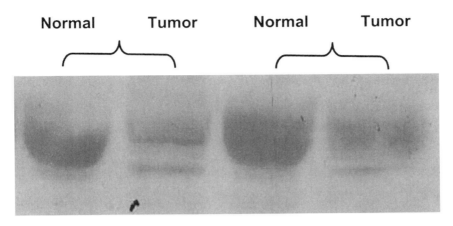

Fig. 3. Western analysis of NSCLC and surrounding paired normal lung. Immunoblots demonstrate decreased PGIS protein expression by Western analysis. Two examples of different tumors compared to the paired surrounding normal lung are demonstrated.

agonist that activates PGIR but not PPARδ, does not rescue the phenotype. These studies show presumptive evidence of PPARδ signaling.

Guided by our results from microarray experiments, in which we found upregulation of PPARγ and coordinated downregulation of both COX-2 and PPARδ, we began a collaboration with Dr. Ray DuBois at Vanderbilt University. Using transfection experiments, we were able to demonstrate that COX-2-derived PGI$_2$ transactivates the PPARδ promoter responsive element *(62)*. PPARδ expression increases in some human cancers, including colon and lung cancers *(63)*, and may play a critical role in malignant transformation. Precursors and products of eicosanoid metabolism are ligands for PPARδ *(64)*, and can modify PPAR activity. PPARδ is downregulated by the APC gene and upregulated by β-catenin *(65)*. APC expression is decreased during mouse lung tumorigenesis *(66)*. NSAIDs mimic the effects of APC by downregulating the transcriptional activity of PPARδ through disruption of DNA binding *(63)*. COX-2 overexpression is associated with colorectal and gastric cancer *(67)*, and contributes to tumor formation in the APC murine model of colon cancer *(7)*. COX-2 overexpression is associated with inhibition of apoptosis *(25)*, and can stimulate the production of angiogenic factors such as VEGF *(68)*. COX-2 expression is increased in mouse lung tumors. The finding that both PPARδ and COX-2 exhibit decreased expression in the chemoprotected transgenic mice may provide insight into signaling cascades affected by PGIS overexpression.

3. PREVIOUS EFFICACY/STUDIES

3.1. Prostacyclin Synthase Expression is Decreased in NSCLC Adenocarcinomas

We hypothesized that PGIS plays a protective role in the carcinogenesis process, and that NSCLC may be associated with decreased PGIS expression. We systematically assayed 10 adenocarcinoma specimens and 10 normal lung samples for PGIS expression by real-time quantitative PCR, and by Western analysis using an antibody specific for PGIS, which we had developed and previously characterized *(48)*. The results are shown in Fig. 2 and 3.

In Fig. 2, absolute copy number for PGIS was assessed using a TaqMan probe. Ten normal lung samples and 10 paired adenocarcinomas were analyzed. There was decreased PGIS mRNA in tumors compared to either surrounding normal lung, or normal lung from a non-cancer sample. In Fig. 3, Western analysis revealed that PGIS protein decreased in the tumors compared to the paired surrounding normal lung.

In order to further define the variability of PGIS expression in NSCLC, PGIS immunostaining was performed on a tissue array containing samples of NSCLC from the Specialized Programs of Research Excellence (SPORE) tissue bank at the University of Colorado Cancer Center. Results are shown in Fig. 4, which demonstrates the selective immunostaining of PGIS in NSCLC. As predicted, a variable level of expression for PGIS was detected in different tumors. We are currently seeking to correlate this

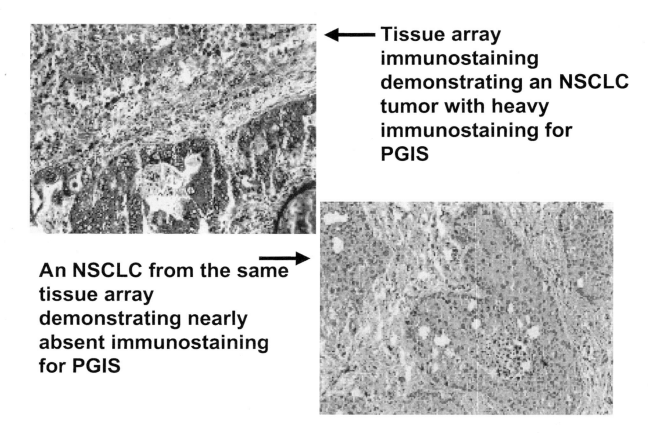

Fig. 4. Tissue-array immunostaining for PGIS in NSCLC. Immunostaining of several NSCLC tumor samples demonstrates a range of expression of this enzyme in tumors.

variable PGIS expression with selected clinical outcomes, as well as the expression of other enzymes and receptors in the pathway that modulates the action of PGI_2.

3.2. PGIS Overexpression Chemoprevents Murine Lung Tumors

Blocking the AA pathway by inhibiting COX activity decreases eicosanoid production and prevents lung cancer in some animal models. We tested the hypothesis that selective pulmonary PGIS overexpression would also protect against murine lung tumorigenesis. Transgenic mice with pulmonary PGIS overexpression were created using a construct of the human surfactant protein C (SPC) promoter and the rat PGIS cDNA (69). The human SPC promoter directs expression of transgenes to alveolar type II and Clara cells (70), the progenitors for human and mouse lung adenocarcinomas. To determine a gene-dosing effect, two different transgenic lines were exposed to carcinogens: low-expressing mice with a 50% increase in lung PGIS activity (exhibited by a 1.5-fold increase in 6-keto

$PGF_{1\alpha}$, the stable metabolic product of PGI_2, compared to wt littermates), and a high-expressing line with a threefold increase in lung 6-keto $PGF_{1\alpha}$.

Transgenic mice (Tg^+) and wt littermates (Tg^-), 8–12 wk of age, were subjected to two distinct lung carcinogenesis protocols. In the first model, urethane, a complete carcinogen that selectively induces pulmonary adenomas (71), was administered in a single dose. In an initiation/promotion model, 3-methylcholanthrene (MCA), a polycyclic aromatic hydrocarbon (PAH) found in tobacco smoke that exhibits dose-dependent initiation of murine lung tumors (72), was given as a single ip dose, followed by six weekly ip treatments with butylated hydroxytoluene (BHT), a tumor promoter that induces reversible pulmonary damage characterized by alveolar type I cell necrosis, selective pulmonary inflammation, and hyperplasia of alveolar type II cells (73). Controls for both models consisted of mice injected with vehicle alone. Experimental mice were sacrificed 14 wk following urethane and 20 wk after MCA/BHT; tumors were enumerated.

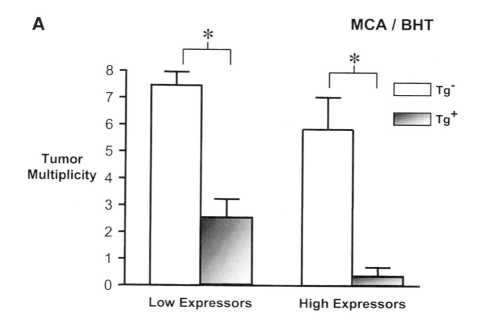

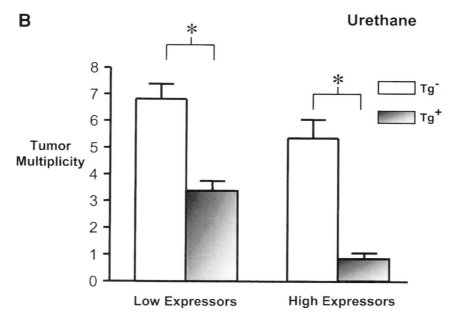

Fig. 5. Lung-tumor multiplicities following urethane (A) and MCA/BHT (B) protocols. **(A)** Following a single exposure to urethane, low-expressing transgenic animals ($n = 22$) demonstrated a 50% reduction in tumor number compared to transgene-negative littermates ($n = 17$) (3.4 vs 6.8 tumors per mouse, $*p < 0.0001$). High-expressing transgenic animals ($n = 18$) showed an 85% reduction in urethane-induced tumor multiplicity compared to transgene-negative littermates ($n = 11$) (0.8 vs 5.2 tumors/mouse, $**p < 0.0001$). **(B)** Following an initiation/promotion protocol, low-expressing transgenic mice ($n = 8$) have a 66% reduction in tumor number compared to transgene-negative littermates ($n = 11$) (2.5 vs 7.5 tumors/mouse, $*p < 0.0001$). High-expressing transgenic animals ($n = 5$) demonstrate a 92% reduction in tumor multiplicity compared to transgene-negative littermates ($n = 6$) (0.4 vs 5.2 tumors/mouse, $**p < 0.001$).

Transgenic overexpression of PGIS significantly decreased tumor multiplicity and incidence in both carcinogenesis models (Fig. 5A,B). Tg^+ mice that expressed low levels of PGIS exhibited a 50% reduction in urethane-induced tumor multiplicity (3.4 vs 6.8 tumors/mouse, $p < 0.001$) and a 66% reduction in the MCA/BHT model (2.5 vs 7.5 tumors/mouse, $p < 0.001$) (Fig. 5a, 5b). Untreated mice (both Tg^- and Tg^+) receiving either corn oil delivery vehicle or normal saline without carcinogen failed to develop tumors. Tg^+ mice that expressed high levels of PGIS exhibited even greater chemoprotection, demonstrating an 85% reduction in tumor multiplicity compared to Tg^- littermates (0.8 vs 5.2 tumors/mouse, $p < 0.0001$) (Fig. 5b). Most importantly,the incidence of lung tumors was also greatly decreased in these high-expressing mice, with 44% (8/18) of the Tg^+ mice remaining tumor-free as compared to the 100% incidence in Tg^- littermates ($P = 0.01$, Fisher's exact test). Protection by PGIS overexpression in distinct carcinogenesis models demonstrates the generality of this chemoprevention.

Chemoprotection in the PGIS overexpressors is not solely the result of alterations in PGE_2 levels. The beneficial effects of PGIS overexpression could be the result of either higher levels of PGI_2 or lower levels of PGE_2, as a result of depletion of the substrate PGH_2. To investigate whether, at the time of sacrifice, PGIS overexpression shifted the balance of PGH_2 metabolism in favor of PGI_2 and away from PGE_2 (a "steal" phenomenon), we determined the pulmonary levels of these metabolites. Baseline 6-keto $PGF_{1\alpha}$ levels were determined for both transgenic lines. In addition, at the termination of both carcinogenesis protocols, simultaneous 6-keto $PGF_{1\alpha}$ and PGE_2 levels were determined for both Tg^+ and Tg^- animals. In both carcinogenesis protocols, the significant elevations in 6-keto $PGF_{1\alpha}$ over baseline persisted at the time of sacrifice, with the same ratios of elevation (e.g., the low-expressing animals had a 50% increase and the high-expressing animals had a greater than 250% increase in 6-keto $PGF_{1\alpha}$, individual data in Fig. 6A and 6B). The MCA/BHT protocol showed no evidence of a "steal" phenomenon (Fig. 6A). Specifically, in the lower-expressing line there were no significant differences between the Tg^+ ($n = 8$) and Tg^- ($n = 10$) when PGE_2 levels were compared (162 vs 131 ng/g lung tissue, $p = 0.52$). The elevations in 6-keto $PGF_{1\alpha}$ were maintained, as Tg^+ ($n = 8$) demonstrated higher levels than Tg^- ($n = 10$)

(1665.6 vs 1325 ng/g lung tissue, $p < 0.05$). However, in the highest-expressing line, animals treated with urethane showed differences between Tg^+ and Tg^- with respect to PGE_2 levels. Tg^+ ($n = 17$) demonstrated the anticipated higher 6-keto $PGF_{1\alpha}$ levels than the Tg^- ($n = 11$) (6092 vs 2014 ng/g lung tissue, $p < 0.0001$). The Tg^+ ($n = 17$) displayed lower PGE_2 levels than their Tg^- ($n = 11$) littermates (97 vs 255 ng/g lung tissue, $p < 0.0001$). The individual data are shown in Fig. 6b. The inverse relationship (negative correlation) in Tg^+ animals between 6-keto $PGF_{1\alpha}$ and PGE_2 for the urethane-treated mice is significant (Pearson test, $r = -0.63$ at sacrifice [$p = 0.037$]).

Further studies into the chemoprotective mechanism consisted of microarray gene-expression analysis of Tg^+ and Tg^- lungs, revealing 37 genes increased more than twofold and 27 genes decreased more than twofold. Many genes implicated in carcinogenesis, for example, PPARδ and COX-2, exhibit decreased expression in Tg^+ mice and may provide insight into signaling cascades affected by PGIS overexpression. Manipulation of PG metabolism distal to COX produces more profound lung cancer reduction than COX inhibition, and could be the basis for new approaches to lung cancer chemoprevention.

4. SAFETY

Prostacyclin has been widely used to treat both primary and some forms of secondary pulmonary hypertension. Epoprostenol (Flolan) is administered by continuous infusion because of its short half-life. The drug has proven efficacious in extending the lives of patients with primary pulmonary hypertension. The main side effects are related to the chronic infusion and the presence of an indwelling vascular catheter. Patients also experience side effects related to epoprostenol's vasodilatory properties, including flushing, hypotension, lightheadedness, and jaw pain.

Considerable research efforts have focused on alternative prostacyclin preparations, particularly oral and aerosolized. Iloprost, a synthetic, long-acting PGI_2 analog, can be administered orally, parenterally, or by inhalation. The iv formulation has been extensively studied in patients with peripheral arterial occlusive disease (PAOD) *(43)*. In pooled data from eight large placebo-controlled trials in which Iloprost was infused at doses of 0.5–2 ng/kg/min or until the patient developed intolerable symptoms for up to 5 h/d for 30 d, the most frequent adverse events (AEs)

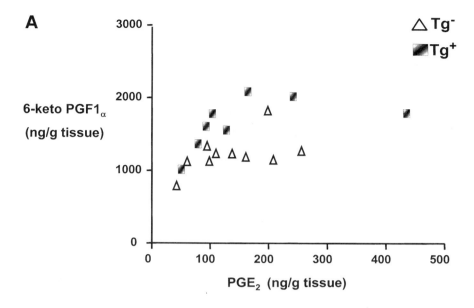

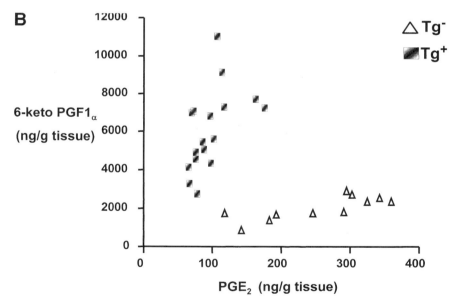

Fig. 6. Comparison of 6-keto PGF1a and PGE2 levels following MCA/BHT **(A)** and urethane **(B)** treatment. **(A)** Following MCA/BHT treatment, at the end of the experiment, the low-expressing line demonstrated no significant differences between the Tg+ ($n = 8$) and Tg- ($n = 10$) when PGE2 levels were compared (162 vs 131 ng/g lung tissue, $p = 0.52$). Elevations in 6-keto PGF1a were maintained, as Tg+ ($n = 8$) demonstrated higher levels than Tg- ($n = 10$) (1665.6 vs 1325 ng/g lung tissue, $p < 0.05$). Individual data are graphed. **(B)** Following urethane treatment, at the end of the experiment, Tg+ mice in the highest expression group showed higher 6-keto PGF1a levels and lower PGE2 levels than their Tg- littermates, Pearson r = –0.63, $p < 0.05$. Tg+ ($n = 17$) demonstrated higher 6-keto PGF1$_a$ levels than Tg- ($n = 11$) (6092 vs 2014 ng/g lung tissue, $p < 0.0001$. Tg+ ($n = 17$) displayed lower PGE$_2$ levels than Tg- ($n = 11$) littermates (97 vs 255 ng/g lung tissue, $p < 0.0001$). Individual data are graphed.

in the Iloprost group (n = 551 patients) were headache (71%), flushing (58%), nausea (40%), vomiting (24%), injection-site reaction (18%), sweating (14%), and abdominal discomfort/pain (14%). In the placebo group, (n = 493 patients) the most frequent events were headache (14%), flushing (13%), nausea (8%), vomiting (4%), injection-site reaction (4%), sweating (5%), and abdominal discomfort/pain (4%). Most AEs were transient and/or mild, and were easily controlled by dose reduction. Serious drug-related AEs were rare in a Raynaud's population (2/102 patients). Based on favorable experience with iv Iloprost, an extended-release (ER) oral formulation was developed to treat outpatients long-term.

The use of oral Iloprost has been investigated (oral doses of 50–300 µg administered twice daily were further explored). In early-phase studies, 89 patients were treated with varying doses and schedules. The most frequent AEs were similar to those seen with iv Iloprost, including headache, flushing, nausea, dizziness, pain, vomiting, and diarrhea. Most toxicity occurred with higher doses. Reversible liver-enzyme elevations were seen in six patients. The overall conclusion was that Iloprost at doses greater than 200 µg bid was not well-tolerated. In a prospective, randomized, placebo-controlled European study of 624 patients with severe PAOD, patients were randomized to three arms: placebo (n = 207); 50 µg iloprost bid (n = 210); or 50–150 µg iloprost bid (n = 207), for 12 mo. The most frequent AEs were headache (6.8%, 24.8%, 32.9%) flushing (7.2%, 16.7%, 31.9%), and nausea (9.2%, 13.8%, 17.9%), respectively. Overall, serious adverse events (SAEs) including stroke, myocardial infraction, and thrombotic events were reported in 37.2% of patients on the placebo group, 33.3% of patients in the low-dose Iloprost group, and 33.3% of patients in the high-dose Iloprost group. Discontinuation rates resulting from AEs were 19% in the placebo group, 21% in the low-dose Iloprost group, and 23% in the high-dose Iloprost group. The death rate from all causes was 6.3%, 7.1%, and 9.2%, respectively between groups. In conclusion, iloprost in doses of 50–150 µg bid was well-tolerated in 417 patients for >6 mo; patients receiving iloprost were more likely to reach the endpoints of no lesions, no rest pain, no death, and no major amputation. A subsequent randomized placebo-controlled trial with 800 PAOD patients who received 50 µg bid, 100–150 µg bid, or placebo for 6 mo has recently been completed. Trials using oral iloprost have been completed or are ongoing in patients with Raynaud's phenomenon secondary to systemic sclerosis, and patients with thromboangiitis obliterans. A definite clinical benefit has been seen, and toxicity profiles are similar to those observed in the trials mentioned here.

5. PHARMACODYNAMICS

Following oral administration of iloprost aqueous solution or ER tablets or capsules to healthy subjects, iloprost is rapidly absorbed from the gut. Peak plasma levels (C_{max}) are reached within 10–40 min. The time to reach C_{max} (t_{max}) was significantly delayed to 1.2–2.6 h after oral administration of the ER capsules, type I and M. Because of the extensive first-pass effect, the absolute bioavailability of iloprost after administration of ER capsules, type I and M, ranged from 16–19%. Food (normal hospital breakfast) did not increase the rate (+18%) and extent (+8%) of bioavailable iloprost released from the ER capsules.

The findings after oral administration of labeled iloprost given in a buffered solution were similar to the results after the iv administration. Recovery of total radioactivity was 70–90% after oral administration. The principal elimination route of total radioactivity was via renal excretion. The main metabolites cochromatographed with the four diastereoisomers of tetranor-iloprost, and sulfated and glucuronidated conjugates of tetranor-iloprost were also present. The elimination of the metabolites from the body was significantly slower than that of Iloprost.

In a study involving 25 PAOD patients (Fontaine Stages II–IV) who received ER capsules—type I and M—twice daily, the following pharmacokinetic parameters were obtained: peak iloprost levels were 178 and 184 pg/mL^{-1}, 249 and 237 mg/mL^{-1}, and 405 and 427 pg/mL^{-1} after first and second intake of 100, 150, and 300 µg iloprost, respectively. The second dose, given after a 6-h interval, did not lead to a higher peak concentration than the first dose. The values of area under the curve (AUC) (0–6) were 625, 870, and 1425 pg/mL^{-1}/h after first dose administration at levels of 100, 150, and 300 µg iloprost, respectively. Both peak plasma levels and AUC values displayed dose-proportionality. Plasma levels exceeding 50 pg/mL^{-1}, an anti-aggregatory effective concentration, were maintained for 5.8–6.9 h after oral doses in excess of 100 µg, and plasma levels exceeding the half maximum concentration were maintained for 4 h. The apparent terminal half-life of iloprost ranged from 2–3 h.

The inter- and intra-individual variations in the pharmacokinetics of iloprost were studied with ER capsules, type I and M, in 20 middle-aged or elderly hospitalized PAOD patients (16 males and 4 females) after repeated oral administrations of 150 μg iloprost. The intersubject coefficients of variation (CVs) for C_{max}, t_{max}, and AUC (0–8) were 48.2%, 33.1%, and 41.7%, respectively. Corresponding CVs were 38.6%, 28.4%, and 21.9%.

6. POPULATIONS BENEFITING FROM INTERVENTION

Mounting evidence supports a role for prostaglandins in carcinogenesis. COX inhibition induces dramatic regression of dysplastic colonic adenomas in patients with familial adenomatous polyposis coli (FAP) and daily aspirin use reduces the risk of developing lung and colon cancer. These findings probably result from a combination of decreased PGE_2 levels, improving the immune surveillance of tumors, and accelerated apoptotic rates induced by the COX inhibitors. Our preliminary data support a role for prostanoids in the development of lung cancer.

Adenocarcinoma is the most rapidly increasing type of lung cancer. Distinct from squamous-type lung cancer, adenocarcinomas arise from the distal lung. In mice, MCA/BHT and urethane carcinogenesis paradigms induce distal lung cancer with adenocarcinoma properties, including a high incidence of K-ras mutations. NSAIDs offer an exciting and promising therapeutic strategy for the treatment of human cancer. Based on encouraging results in the treatment of colon cancer, these findings should be extrapolated to lung cancer. Human epidemiologic studies, such as the Cancer Prevention Study II, found a significant decrease in death rates from colon and lung cancer among "frequent" aspirin users, attributed to COX inhibition (55,64). Animal models provide an excellent system to test the efficacy of new compounds developed by the pharmaceutical industry, and lead to new treatments in patients with lung cancer.

Although COX inhibition is attractive as a chemopreventive strategy, our findings involving PGIS suggest that manipulation of the AA pathway downstream from COX may prove to be even more promising. The observed decreases in tumor multiplicity are more impressive than those seen in studies of COX (20,41) or LOX (42) inhibition. In PGIS transgenic mice, chemoprotection in various carcinogenesis models confirms the generality of PGIS overexpression in lung cancer chemoprevention. The encouraging results observed in this transgenic mouse model, coupled with the current safe use of continuous intravenous or intermittent inhaled PGI_2 to treat pulmonary hypertension (74), have directly translated into our chemoprevention trial in individuals at high risk for lung cancer.

Improved success in decreasing lung cancer rates will rely not only on smoking prevention and cessation, but also on effective chemopreventive strategies. Huge populations of former smokers remain at risk for lung cancer, and altering PG production or metabolism may prove to be beneficial in certain populations.

7. CLINICAL STUDIES

Recently, the National Cancer Institute has funded the investigation of iloprost for lung cancer chemoprevention. This SPORE supplement (NCI 3 P50 CA58187-08S2, Assessment of Oral Iloprost in Prevention of Human Lung Cancer) has Dr. Robert Keith as Principal Investigator. Iloprost is a long-acting, orally available prostacyclin analog produced by Schering A-G in Berlin (Berlex in the United States). The long-term safety of oral iloprost has been established in more than 1000 subjects with various conditions, including primary pulmonary hypertension, scleroderma with Raynaud's phenomenon (75), peripheral vascular disease/atherosclerosis with lower-extremity ulceration, and Buerger's disease (thromboangiitis obliterans) (76) who have received the drug for 6 mo or longer. Our intervention will consist of iloprost or placebo administered to patients at high risk for lung cancer in a double-blind, randomized prospective trial of 6 mo duration. Subjects will be stratified according to enrollment center and smoking status (current or ex-smoker), and have at least a 20 pack-yr cigarette smoking history and sputum cytologic dysplasia of mild or worse. Laser-induced fluorescence emission (LIFE) and/or white light bronchoscopy will be performed at baseline and the end of the trial. Placebo and iloprost groups will be recruited from the University of Colorado and other participating institutions. The planned sample size is 152 patients with 76 patients per arm (iloprost vs placebo), including 38 smokers per arm and 38 ex-smokers per arm. Eligible patients will be randomly assigned to active treatment or placebo treatment within each stratum. Group sizes of 38 smokers per arm provide a chi-square test of at least 80% power to detect a difference in response rates of 35% (for any combination of responses rates yielding a difference of 35%) between iloprost and placebo-treated smokers. Similarly, group sizes of 38 ex-smokers per arm provide a chi-square test of at least 80% power to detect a difference in response rates of 35% (for any combination of responses rates) between iloprost- and placebo-treated ex-smokers. Measurement of response will include: histology pre- and post-treatment using the WHO classification for bronchial epithelium; Ki-67 labeling index (a secondary endpoint); and a panel of biomarkers including immunohistochemistry and quantitative polymerase chain reaction (qPCR) for PGIS, COX-2, PPARδ and γ, along with MCM2, *p53*, tyrosine kinase receptor proteins (EGFR, HER2/neu, ErbB3, ErbB4, Akt), and microvessel density. To date, thirty patients have been enrolled at the University of Colorado.

8. PROMISING ENDPOINTS (BIOMARKERS)

The exact mechanisms for the observed prostacyclin-mediated chemoprotection have not yet been elucidated. The beneficial effects of PGIS overexpression could result from either increased prostacyclin levels, decreased PGE_2 levels (through depletion of the common precursor, PGH_2), or both. Measurement of prostaglandin levels demonstrates that increases in prostacyclin, but not decreases in PGE_2, are associated with chemoprevention (49). Our studies into the chemoprotective mechanism have included microarray gene-expression analysis of Tg+ and Tg– lungs. In these experiments, PPARγ was upregulated, and PPARδ, along with COX-2, were reduced in expression. We have also shown that prostacyclin is the first naturally occurring ligand for PPARδ, and transactivates the PPARδ promoter only when cotransfection with PGIS and COX-2 is present, not COX-1 (62). Activation of this family of nuclear transcription factors could alter the expression of a number of genes to create a chemoprotective milieu. One concern is that the transgenic model, although providing a constant increase in the PGI_2 levels, may not be the same as a drug effect. However, our data comparing the transfection of PGIS vs addition of long-acting PGI_2 analogs to colon cancer-cell lines found a similar effect on PPARδ

activation with gene transfection or drug (62). This provides strong evidence that drug administration will be similar to transgene overexpression.

Considering these findings, we believe that expression of PGIS and/or its receptor confers protection. Therefore, loss of expression of either PGIS or PGIR should mark a more aggressive tumor. We are currently focusing on a panel of five markers we propose as excellent candidates for direct assessment of the effect of this enzyme system in lung carcinogenesis:

1. PGIS enzyme, to be assayed by immunohistochemistry. We have shown this enzyme to be decreased in lung tumors (Fig 2–4). We have generated a polyclonal anti-PGIS antibody against the peptide corresponding to amino acids 115–124 (C)NFNPSEEKAR] of the rat PGIS cDNA. Antibody specificity was confirmed by enzyme-linked immunosorbent assay (ELISA) using solid-phase immobilized antigen to capture the peptide-specific antibody. Following the optimization of this antibody for paraffin-embedded tissues, we have shown this enzyme to be decreased in pulmonary tissue from patients with severe pulmonary hypertension (48).

2. PGIR, to be assayed by immunohistochemistry. We have developed a polyclonal antibody that specifically decorates PGIR, utilizing the following peptide: [(C)HMYRQQRRHHGSFVPTSR-$_{COOH}$] corresponding to amino acids 241–258 of the rat PGIS cDNA. Antibody specificity was confirmed by ELISA using solid-phase immobilized antigen (0.1 μg/100 μl per microwell of peptide Cys-GGG) to capture the peptide-specific antibody. The antisera crossreacts with human and murine species, and has been optimized for paraffin-embedded tissues.

3. COX-2: We have demonstrated that COX-2 is elevated in human NSCLC, and in the murine models (18). Our microarray data demonstrate that animals with increased prostacyclin production have reduced COX-2. Furthermore, our microarray data demonstrate that cells stably transfected with PGIS demonstrate reduced expression of COX-2. Therefore, we believe that studying the interaction of COX-2 expression in relation to PGIS expression may provide important markers of lung tumorigenesis. We have optimized the goat polyclonal COX-2 antibody (Santa Cruz, C-20) for use in paraffin-embedded tissue (18).

4. PPARγ: PPARγ has tumor-suppressor effects. Our microarray data suggests that prostacyclin upregulates expression of PPARγ. Furthermore, cells that are stably transfected with PGIS demonstrate

increased PPARγ expression in lung cancer patients. In related studies, decreased PPARγ gene expression was correlated with poor clinical prognosis in patients with NSCLC (77). We are currently optimizing PPARγ antibodies.

5. PPARδ: We have shown that prostacyclin is a direct ligand for PPARδ, and acts to directly transactivate the PPARδ promoter-responsive element (62). Furthermore, COX-2 and PPARδ both show increased expression in human colon cancer (62). In related studies, others have demonstrated that PPARδ expression is increased in regions of head and neck squamous cell carcinoma that also demonstrate increased expression of VEGF and COX-2 (78). We are currently optimizing the PPARδ antibodies.

In conclusion, preclinical studies demonstrate that prostacyclin has chemopreventive properties in murine models of lung tumorigenesis. The efficacy of long-acting oral analogs are currently being tested in human lung-cancer chemoprevention trials.

REFERENCES

1. Kargman SL, O'Neill GP, Vickers PJ, et al. Expression of prostaglandin G/H synthase–1 and –2 protein in human colon cancer. *Cancer Res* 1995;55:2556–2559.
2. Kutchera W, Jones DA, Matsunami N, et al. Prostaglandin H synthase 2 is expressed abnormally in human colon cancer: evidence for a transcriptional effect. *Proc Natl Acad Sci USA* 1996;93:4816–4820.
3. Rao CV, Rivenson A, Simi B, et al. Chemoprevention of colon carcinogenesis by sulindac, a nonsteroidal anti-inflammatory agent. *Cancer Res* 1995;55:1464–1472.
4. Sheng H, Shao J, Kirkland SC, et al. Inhibition of human colon cancer cell growth by selective inhibition of cyclooxygenase-2. *J Clin Investig* 1997;99:2254–2259.
5. Sheng GG, Shao J, Sheng H, et al. A selective cyclooxygenase 2 inhibitor suppresses the growth of H-*ras*-transformed rat intestinal epithelial cells. *Gastroenterology* 1997;113:1883–1891.
6. Thun MJ. Aspirin, NSAIDs, and digestive tract cancers. *Cancer Metastasis Rev* 1994;13:269–277.
7. Oshima M, Dinchuk JE, Kargman SL, et al. Suppression of intestinal polyposis in Apc delta716 knockout mice by inhibition of cyclooxygenase 2 (COX-2). *Cell* 1996;87:803–809.
8. Liu CH, Chang SH, Narko K, et al. Overexpression of cyclooxygenase-2 is sufficient to induce tumorigenesis in transgenic mice. *J Biol Chem* 2001;276:18,563–18,569.
9. Schreinemachers DM, Everson RB. Aspirin use and lung, colon, and breast cancer incidence in a prospective study. *Epidemiology* 1994;5:138–146.
10. Hubbard MJ, Cohen P. On target with a new mechanism for the regulation of protein phosphorylation. *Trends Biochem Sci* 1993;18:172–177.
11. Lau SS, McMahon JB, McMenamin MG, et al. Metabolism of arachidonic acid in human lung cancer cell lines. *Cancer Res* 1987;47:3757–3762.
12. Hubbard WC, Alley MC, McLemore TL, Boyd MR. Evidence for thromboxane biosynthesis in established cell lines derived from human lung adenocarcinomas. *Cancer Res* 1988;48:2674–2677.
13. Avis IM, Jett M, Boyle T, et al. Growth control of lung cancer by interruption of 5-lipoxygenase-mediated growth factor signaling. *J Clin Investig* 1996;97:806–813.
14. Huang M, Stolina M, Sharma S, et al. Non-small cell lung cancer cyclooxygenase-2-dependent regulation of cytokine balance in lymphocytes and macrophages: up-regulation of interleukin 10 and down-regulation of interleukin 12 production. *Cancer Res* 1998;58:1208–1216.
15. Hida T, Yatabe Y, Achiwa H, et al. Increased expression of cyclooxygenase 2 occurs frequently in human lung cancers, specifically in adenocarcinomas. *Cancer Res* 1998;58:3761–3764.
16. Wolff H, Saukkonen K, Anttila S, et al. Expression of cyclooxygenase-2 in human lung carcinoma. *Cancer Res* 1998;58:4997–5001.
17. Heasley LE, Thaler S, Nicks M, et al. Induction of cytosolic phospholipase A2 by oncogenic *Ras* in human non-small cell lung cancer. *J Biol Chem* 1997;272:14,501–14,504.
18. Bauer AK, Dwyer-Nield LD, Malkinson AM. High cyclooxygenase 1 (COX-1) and cyclooxygenase 2 (COX-2) contents in mouse lung tumors. *Carcinogenesis* 2000;21:543–550.
19. Hida T, Leyton J, Makheja AN, et al. Non-small cell lung cancer cycloxygenase activity and proliferation are inhibited by non-steroidal antiinflammatory drugs. *Anticancer Res* 1998;18:775–782.
20. Duperron C, Castonguay A. Chemopreventive efficacies of aspirin and sulindac against lung tumorigenesis in A/J mice. *Carcinogenesis* 1997;18:1001–1006.
21. Takaku K, Sonoshita M, Sasaki N, et al. Suppression of intestinal polyposis in Apc(delta 716) knockout mice by an additional mutation in the cytosolic phospholipase A(2) gene. *J Biol Chem* 2000;275:34,013–34,016.
22. Hong KH, Bonventre JC, O'Leary E, et al. Deletion of cytosolic phospholipase A(2) suppresses Apc(Min)-induced tumorigenesis. *Proc Natl Acad Sci USA* 2001;98:3935–3939.
23. MacPhee M, Chepenik KP, Liddell RA, et al. The secretory phospholipase A2 gene is a candidate for the Mom1 locus, a major modifier of ApcMin-induced intestinal neoplasia. *Cell* 1995;81:957–966.
24. Yoshimatsu K, Altorki NK, Golijanin D, et al. Inducible prostaglandin E synthase is overexpressed in non-small cell lung cancer. *Clin Cancer Res* 2001;7:2669–2674.
25. Tsujii M, DuBois RN. Alterations in cellular adhesion and apoptosis in epithelial cells overexpressing prostaglandin endoperoxide synthase 2. *Cell* 1995;83:493–501.
26. Tsujii M, Kawano S, DuBois RN. Cyclooxygenase-2 expression in human colon cancer cells increases metastatic potential. *Proc Natl Acad Sci USA* 1997;94:3336–3340.
27. Casibang M, Purdom S, Jakowlew S, et al. Prostaglandin E2 and vasoactive intestinal peptide increase vascular endothelial cell growth factor mRNAs in lung cancer cells. *Lung Cancer* 2001;31:203–212.
28. Marnett LJ, Siedlik PH, Ochs RC, et al. Mechanism of the stimulation of prostaglandin H synthase and prostacyclin synthase by the antithrombotic and antimetastatic agent, nafazatrom. *Mol Pharmacol* 1984;26:328–335.

29. Kujubu DA, Herschman HR. Dexamethasone inhibits mitogen induction of the TIS10 prostaglandin synthase/cyclooxygenase gene. *J Biol Chem* 1992;267:7991–7994.

30. Kujubu DA, Fletcher BS, Varnum BC. TIS10, a phorbol ester tumor promoter-inducible mRNA from Swiss 3T3 cells, encodes a novel prostaglandin synthase/cyclooxygenase homologue. *J Biol Chem* 1991;266:12,866–12,872.

31. Hara S, Miyata A, Yokoyama C, et al. Isolation and molecular cloning of prostacyclin synthase from bovine endothelial cells. *J Biol Chem* 1994;269:19,897–19,903.

32. Shaul PW, Kinane B, Farrar MA, et al. Prostacyclin production and mediation of adenylate cyclase activity in the pulmonary artery. Alterations after prolonged hypoxia in the rat. *J Clin Investig* 1991;88:447–455.

33. Halushka PV, Mais DE, Morinelli TA. Thromboxane and prostacyclin receptors. *Prog Clin Biol Res* 1989;301:21–28.

34. Bunting S, Gryglewski R, Moncada S, Vane JR. Arterial walls generate from prostaglandin endoperoxides a substance (prostaglandin X) which relaxes strips of mesenteric and coeliac arteries and inhibits platelet aggregation. *Prostaglandins* 1976;12:897–913.

35. Moncada S, Vane JR. Pharmacology and endogenous roles of prostaglandin endoperoxides, thromboxane A2, and prostacyclin. *Pharmacol Rev* 1978;30:293–331.

36. Libby P, Warner SJ, Friedman GB. Interleukin 1: a mitogen for human vascular smooth muscle cells that induces the release of growth-inhibitory prostanoids. *J Clin Investig* 1988;81:487–498.

37. Jugdutt BI, Hutchins GM, Bulkley BH, Becker LC. Myocardial infarction in the conscious dog: three-dimensional mapping of infarct, collateral flow and region at risk. *Circulation* 1979;60:1141–1150.

38. Ribeiro LG, Brandon TA, Hopkins DG, et al. Prostacyclin in experimental myocardial ischemia: effects on hemodynamics, regional myocardial blood flow, infarct size and mortality. *Am J Cardiol* 1981;47:835–840.

39. Jemal A, Thomas A, Murray T, Thun M. Cancer statistics, 2002. *CA Cancer J Clin* 2002;52:23–47.

40. Malkinson AM. Molecular comparison of human and mouse pulmonary adenocarcinomas. *Exp Lung Res* 1998;24:541–555.

41. Rioux N, Castonguay A. Prevention of NNK-induced lung tumorigenesis in A/J mice by acetylsalicylic acid and NS-398. *Cancer Res* 1998;58:5354–5360.

42. Moody TW, Leyton J, Martinez A, et al. Lipoxygenase inhibitors prevent lung carcinogenesis and inhibit non-small cell lung cancer growth. *Exp Lung Res* 1998;24:617–628.

43. Vane JR. Prostacyclin: a hormone with a therapeutic potential. The Sir Henry Dale Lecture for 1981. *J Endocrinol* 1982;95:3P–43P.

44. Dusting GJ, Moncada S, Vane JR. Prostacyclin: its biosynthesis, actions, and clinical potential. *Adv Prostaglandin Thromboxane Leukot Res* 1982;10:59–106.

45. Honn KV, Cicone B, Skoff A. Prostacyclin: a potent antimetastatic agent. *Science* 1981;212:1270–1272.

46. Schirner M, Schneider MR. Inhibition of metastasis by cicaprost in rats with established SMT2A mammary carcinoma growth. *Cancer Detect Prev* 1997;21:44–50.

47. Hubbard WC, Alley MC, Gray GN, et al. Evidence for prostanoid biosynthesis as a biochemical feature of certain subclasses of non-small cell carcinomas of the lung as determined in established cell lines derived from human lung tumors. *Cancer Res* 1989;49:826–832.

48. Tuder RM, Cool CD, Geraci MW, et al. Prostacyclin synthase expression is decreased in lungs from patients with severe pulmonary hypertension. *Am J Respir Crit Care Med* 1999;159:1925–1932.

49. Keith RL, Miller YE, Hoshikawa Y, et al. Manipulation of pulmonary prostacyclin synthase expression prevents murine lung cancer. *Cancer Res* 2002;62:734–740.

50. Namba T, Oida H, Sugimoto Y, et al. cDNA cloning of a mouse prostacyclin receptor. Multiple signaling pathways and expression in thymic medulla. *Biol Chem* 1994;269:9986–9992.

51. Boie Y, Rushmore TH, Darmon-Goodwin A, et al. Cloning and expression of a cDNA for the human prostanoid IP receptor. *J Biol Chem* 1994;269:12,173–12,178.

52. Kobayashi T, Kiriyama M, Hirata T, et al. Identification of domains conferring ligand binding specificity to the prostanoid receptor. Studies on chimeric prostacyclin/prostaglandin D receptors. *J Biol Chem* 1997;272:15,154–15,160.

53. Smyth EM, Li WH, FitzGerald GA. Phosphorylation of the prostacyclin receptor during homologous desensitization. A critical role for protein kinase C. *J Biol Chem* 1998;273:23,258–23,266.

54. Hayes JS, Lawler OA, Walsh MT, Kinsella BT. The prostacyclin receptor is isoprenylated. Isoprenylation is required for efficient receptor-effector coupling. *J Biol Chem* 1999;274:23,707–23,718.

55. Murata T, Ushikubi F, Matsuoka T, et al. Altered pain perception and inflammatory response in mice lacking prostacyclin receptor. *Nature* 1997;388:678–682.

56. Hoshikawa Y, Voelkel NF, Gesell TL, et al. Prostacyclin receptor-dependent modulation of pulmonary vascular remodeling. *Am J Respir Crit Care Med* 2001;164:314–318.

57. Lim H, Gupta RA, Ma WG, et al. Cyclo-oxygenase-2-derived prostacyclin mediates embryo implantation in the mouse via PPAR delta. *Genes Dev* 1999;13:1561–1574.

58. Schmidt A, Endo N, Rutledge SJ, et al. Identification of a new member of the steroid hormone receptor superfamily that is activated by a peroxisome proliferator and fatty acids. *Mol Endocrinol* 1992;6:1634–1641.

59. Mangelsdorf DJ, Thummel C, Beato M, et al. The nuclear receptor superfamily: the second decade. *Cell* 1995;83:835–839.

60. Willson TM, Brown PJ, Sternbach DD, Henke BR. The PPARs: from orphan receptors to drug discovery. *J Med Chem* 2000;43:527–550.

61. Lim H, Paria BC, Das SK, et al. Multiple female reproductive failures in cyclooxygenase 2-deficient mice. *Cell* 1997;91:197–208.

62. Gupta RA, Tan J, Krause WF, et al. Prostacyclin-mediated activation of peroxisome proliferator-activated receptor delta in colorectal cancer. *Proc Natl Acad Sci USA* 2000;97:13,275–13,280.

63. He TC, Chan TA, Vogelstein B, Kinzler KW. PPARδ is an APC-regulated target of nonsteroidal anti-inflammatory drugs. *Cell* 1999;99:335–345.

64. Forman BM, Chen J, Evans RM. Hypolipidemic drugs, polyunsaturated fatty acids, and eicosanoids are ligands for peroxisome proliferator-activated receptors α and δ. *Proc Natl Acad Sci USA* 1997;94:4312–4317.

65. Vanden Heuvel JP. Peroxisome proliferator-activated receptors: a critical link among fatty acids, gene expression and carcinogenesis. *J Nutr* 1999;129:575–580.

66. Oreffo VI, Robinson S, You M. Decreased expression of the adenomatous polyposis coli (Apc) and mutated in colorectal cancer (Mcc) genes in mouse lung neoplasia. *Mol Carcinog* 1998;21:37–49.

67. DuBois RN, Abramson SB, Crofford L, et al. Cyclooxygenase in biology and disease *FASEB J* 1998;12:1063–1073.

68. Tsujii M, Kawano S, Tsuji S, et al. Cyclooxygenase regulates angiogenesis induced by colon cancer cells. *Cell* 1998;93:705–716.

69. Geraci MW, Gao B, Shepherd DC, et al. Pulmonary prostacyclin synthase overexpression in transgenic mice protects against development of hypoxic pulmonary hypertension. *J Clin Investig* 1999;103:1509–1515.

70. Korfhagen TR, Glasser SW, Wert SE, et al. *Cis*-acting sequences from a human surfactant protein gene confer pulmonary-specific gene expression in transgenic mice. *Proc Natl Acad Sci USA* 1990;87:6122–6126.

71. Mirvish SS. The carcinogenic action and metabolism of urethan and *N*-hydroxyurethan. *Adv Cancer Res* 1968;11:1–42.

72. Malkinson AM, Koski KM, Evans WA, Festing MF. Butylated hydroxytoluene exposure is necessary to induce lung tumors in BALB mice treated with 3-methylcholanthrene. *Cancer Res* 1997;57:2832–2834.

73. Witschi H, Malkinson AM, Thompson JA. Metabolism and pulmonary toxicity of butylated hydroxytolulene, in *Metabolic Activation and Toxicity of Chemical Agents to Lung Tissues and Cells.* 1st ed. Gram TE, ed. Pergamon Press, New York, 1993, pp.185–212.

74. Barst RJ, Rubin LJ, Long WA, et al. A comparison of continuous intravenous epoprostenol (prostacyclin) with conventional therapy for primary pulmonary hypertension. The Primary Pulmonary Hypertension Study Group. *N Engl J Med* 1996;334:296–302.

75. Black CM, Halkier-Sorensen L, Belch JJ, et al. Oral iloprost in Raynaud's phenomenon secondary to systemic sclerosis: a multicentre, placebo-controlled, dose-comparison study. *Br J Rheumatol* 1998;37:952–960.

76. Hildebrand M. Pharmacokinetics and tolerability of oral iloprost in thromboangiitis obliterans patients. *Eur J Clin Pharmacol* 1997;53:51–56.

77. Sasaki H, Tanahashi M, Yukiue H, et al. Decreased perioxisome proliferator-activated receptor gamma gene expression was correlated with poor prognosis in patients with lung cancer. *Lung Cancer* 2002;36:71–76.

78. Jaeckel EC, Raja S, Tan J, et al. Correlation of expression of cyclooxygenase-2, vascular endothelial growth factor, and peroxisome proliferator-activated receptor δ with head and neck squamous cell carcinoma. *Arch Otolaryngol Head Neck Surg* 2001;127:1253–1259.

III   NUCLEAR RECEPTOR SUPERFAMILY

12 Nuclear Receptor Superfamily

Targets for Chemoprevention

Julia A. Lawrence, DO and Kapil Dhingra, MBBS

CONTENTS

1. INTRODUCTION

The process of carcinogenesis is characterized by a loss of cellular growth control and a lack of differentiation of abnormally proliferating cells. This cellular disarray is partly a result of disruptions in the cellular and stromal environment crosscommunication that is mediated by paracrine signaling of cytokines and hormones *(1)*. The steroid hormones exert a variety of growth and differentiation effects relevant to normal physiology. Therefore, it is not surprising that these molecules are closely associated with the evolution of neoplasms, and provide useful targets for intervening in this process. Steroid hormones are produced mainly by the gonads (testes and ovary), adrenal cortex, and, to a lesser extent, other steroidogenic organs. The breast and prostate, other organs of sexual function that are dependent on steroids for development, are likewise affected by steroids during neoplastic transformation. In addition, a variety of other endogenous hormones (e.g., retinoids, vitamin D) exert biologic effects through receptors that share structural and functional homology with members of the steroid receptor family. These are collectively designated the nuclear receptor (NR) superfamily. The ubiquitous presence of tissue-specific actions of this receptor superfamily provides an opportunity to design agents with exquisitely selective cellular and organ-specific effects that could be harnessed to arrest or reverse carcinogenesis with modest adverse effects—the goal of ideal chemopreventive interventions. This receptor family and agents that target its members are discussed in this chapter and the following subchapters.

2. NR SUPERFAMILY

The NR superfamily consists of more than 150 members whose primary function is to regulate gene transcription following binding to the cognate ligand. It appeared early in the evolution of Metazoan life, approx 1000–800,000,000 years ago. Rexinoid receptor (RXR), chicken ovalbumin upstream promoter transcription factor (COUP-TF), and fushi tarazu transcription factor I (FTZ-FI) were present in the earliest organisms known to contain NRs—the jellyfish, hydra, and related phylogeny. It is believed that the first such receptors acted as monomers and in a ligand-independent fashion *(2)*. During the course of evolution, many of the receptors acquired the ability to bind to and be regulated by ligands and function as dimers, either homo- or heterodimers. The evolution in complexity in higher animals resulted in diversity and redundancy in transcriptional regulation to affect a far greater functional capability than that achieved in lower organisms. The transcriptional apparatus provides the cells/organisms with delicate yet robust

From: Cancer Chemoprevention, Volume 1: Promising Cancer Chemoprevention Agents
Edited by: G. J. Kelloff, E. T. Hawk, and C. C. Sigman © Humana Press Inc., Totowa, NJ

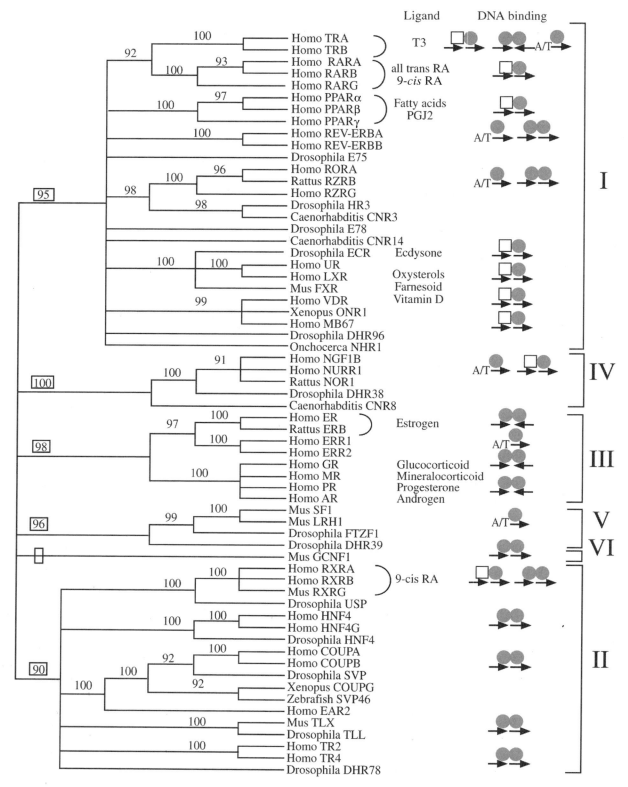

Fig. 1. Consensus Phylogenetic Tree of the NR Superfamily. The six subfamilies are identified by brackets. Bootstrap values of the branches are indicated. Bootstrap values that define the subfamilies are boxed. Subfamily VI has only one member, GCNF1, shown by a box along the branch. Selected ligands for each receptor are shown. A schematic representation of the ligand-binding and dimerization properties of the respective NR is shown in the columns at right. Arrows represent DRE motifs, which can be a single unit preceded by A/T-rich sequences (A/T →), a direct repeat (→→), or an inverted repeat (→←). Black circles represent the receptor; open squares represent RXR in the heterodimeric complexes. (Reproduced with minor modifications from Laudet *(4)* by kind permission of Prof. Vincent Laudet and the Society for Endocrinology, Bristol, UK.)

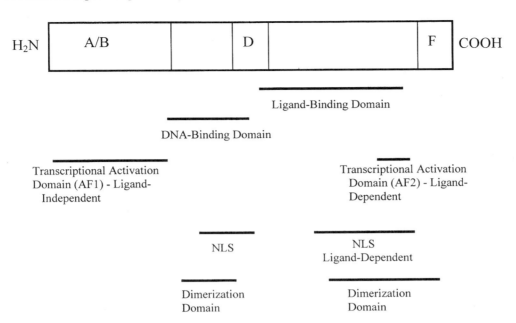

Fig. 2. Schematic Representation of the Consensus Structure of NR. Five distinct regions can be identified. Lines below the box indicate the receptor region responsible for the specific functional activities indicated.The sequence of DBD is highly conserved in the superfamily. NLS, nuclear localization signal.

homeostatic control of numerous physiologic processes involved in cell proliferation, differentiation, and organogenesis. Thus, perturbations of signaling mediated by these receptors underlie a variety of neoplastic events.

Based on DNA sequence homology, the NR superfamily is considered to include receptors for the steroid hormones (estrogen, progesterone, gluco- and mineralocorticoids), the retinoic acids (all-*trans*-retinoic acid [ATRA] and 9-*cis* retinoic acid [9-cRA]), thyroid hormone, fatty acids, leukotrienes, and prostaglandins, and a variety of orphan receptors with unidentified ligands (Fig. 1). A standardized nomenclature to replace their colloquial names has been published *(3)*. The superfamily can be grouped into six subfamilies *(4)*. The most relevant members for carcinogenesis are those from subfamilies I (retinoid acid receptor [RAR], vitamin D receptor [VDR]), II (RXR), and III (estrogen receptor [ER], progesterone receptor [PR], and androgen receptor [AR]). The phylogenetic position of a given NR within the tree generally correlates well with its DNA-binding and dimerization activity, but not with its ligand-binding.

2.1. Structure of NRs

NR superfamily members share a common structure (Fig. 2), consisting of five regions: A/B region or the N terminus with the ligand-independent transcriptional activation site (AF-1); C region or the DNA binding domain (DBD); D region; E region or the ligand-binding domain (LBD) with the second, ligand-dependent, transcriptional activation site (AF-2); and F region *(5)*. The two most critical determinants of receptor activity are the LBD and DBD. The core of the DBD is highly conserved (>90%) across the superfamily *(6)*. In contrast, the LBD of various NR subfamilies share limited sequence homology (<25%). However, performing crystal structure determinations of the ligand-bound LBDs of several receptors shows that they share a similar fold and common ligand-binding pocket, even when the sequence homology among them is modest *(7)*. The DBD is composed of two zinc fingers that fold into two α-helical domains upon coordination of a zinc atom to four cysteines and a third helix that extends from the zinc fingers *(8)*. It is believed that one helix determines DNA binding-site specificity, and is inserted into the major groove of the DNA response element while the remaining helices affect receptor dimerization.

2.2. Transcription Control by NRs

The primary function of NRs is to modulate gene transcription, although the specific modes of action vary among members of different subfamilies.Based on the nature of the dimerization partner and DNA-binding properties (c.f. phylogenetic classification described here and in Fig. 1), the NR family can be subdivided into four major classes *(9)*. Class I includes the steroid hormone receptors (glucocorticoid, ER, progesterone, mineralocorticoid, and AR). These receptors homodimerize following binding to the cognate ligand. The homodimers bind to the DNA response elements (DRE), called hormone response elements (HREs), which are inverted repeats (palindrome) of 5'-TGTTCT-3'-like sequences with three nucleotide spacers.

Class II NRs include thyroid hormone receptors (TRs), RARs, and VDRs. All of the ligand-dependent receptors, except the steroid hormone receptors, belong to this class. These receptors form heterodimers, often with RXRs, to exert their effects on transcription. The heterodimeric complexes bind to DNA elements composed of identical half sites or direct sequence repeats that are separated by one to five nucleotides, known as DR1 through DR5 *(10)*. The length of the intervening spacer sequence determines the heterodimer-DRE interaction specificity. For example, a DR separated by five nucleotides will most often be recognized by RXR-RAR, whereas a DR4 will bind RXR-TR. Class III includes RXRs, COUP, and hepatocyte nuclear factor 4 (HNF-4) receptors which function primarily by forming homodimers that bind to direct repeats. However, unlike the heterodimeric RXR complexes, RXR homodimers can bind only to DRs separated by one nucleotide, DR1. Class IV receptors, no growth factor (NGF)1-B, orphan receptors) generally bind to extended core sites as monomers.

The effect of NRs on transcription is modulated by a number of coregulatory proteins that may enhance (coactivators) or repress transcription (corepressors) without directly binding to the DRE. The conformational alteration produced by the interaction of the ligand with the cognate receptor leads to the recruitment of these coregulatory proteins that are likely to act as adaptor molecules during the assembly of transcriptional preinitiation complexes. Some of these are also capable of directly interacting with the basal transcriptional machinery. Some of these molecules also exhibit enzymatic activities that may play a role in gene regulation—e.g., histone acetyl transferase or deacetylase activities (11). The specific coregulatory proteins present in the cells of a particular organ and their relative abundance likely accounts for the tissue-selective agonist or antagonist effects of a ligand in different organs within the same organism.

3. NRS AND CARCINOGENESIS: PRECLINICAL EVIDENCE AND CLINICAL CHEMOPREVENTIVE STRATEGIES

3.1. Estrogen/Progesterone Receptors and Breast Cancer

The ovarian steroids estrogen and progesterone play a pivotal role in normal breast physiology throughout a woman's life, including the pubertal spurt in breast growth, cyclical changes in breast tissue during each menstrual cycle, pregnancy/lactation-related changes in breast tissue and their reversal following cessation of lactation, and the breast tissue atrophy associated with menopause. The influence of estrogen on epithelial proliferation is evident in the majority of invasive breast cancers, which often express a functional ER. Epidemiology-derived risk factors for breast cancer, including age at menarche and menopause, parity, and age at first live birth, are predominantly reflective of a woman's lifetime exposure to estrogen; incorporated into a statistical model, they reliably predict the risk of developing breast cancer *(12)*. Intact ovarian function or estrogen supplementation is required to induce tumors in rodent models of breast carcinogenesis. An extensive body of literature exists on the preclinical breast cancer chemopreventive efficacy of estrogen ablation/antiestrogens *(13)*.

Countering the effect of ovarian steroids on breast cancer cells has been a clinical therapeutic strategy since the nineteenth century, when Beatson performed oopherectomy to control breast cancer in premenopausal women. In modern times, this has been superseded by pharmacological approaches. More than 20 years of clinical experience with tamoxifen has proven the value of estrogen-signaling blockade in treating advanced as well as micrometastatic breast cancer. A serendipitous observation in these trials was a striking reduction in the incidence of new breast cancers in women who received tamoxifen after an initial diagnosis of breast cancer. These observations led to several prospective, randomized trials; the largest, Breast Cancer Prevention Trial (BCPT), included ~13,000 women and demonstrated a ~50% reduction in the incidence of breast cancer *(14)*. However, the effect of tamoxifen was restricted to the occurrence of ER$^+$ breast cancer and ER$^-$ breast cancers occured with a similar frequency in the two arms. The tamoxifen-mediated blockade of ER in breast epithelium at risk for disease may stabilize the epithelial cells by affecting the balance of proliferation and apoptosis, and/or regress early lesions of atypia and hyperplasia.

Table 1
Nuclear Receptor-Targeted Chemopreventive Agents

Agent	Target Receptor	Target Organ for Cancer Prevention	Evidence of Efficacy[#]		Comments
			Preclinical	Clinical	
SERMs					
Triphenylethylenes (e.g., tamoxifen, toremifene)	ER	Breast	+	+	Tamoxifen approved for prevention of breast cancer
Raloxifene	ER	Breast	+	+	Approved for prevention of osteoporsis; breast cancer prevention trial in progress
Others (e.g., Fulvestrant, SCH570050, CP336,156)	ER	Breast	+	−	Fulvestrant approved for treatment of breast cancer
Aromatase Inhibitors					
(e.g., Anastrozole, Letrozole, Exemestane, Vorazole)	ER, indirect inhibition of signaling by suppression of synthesis of ligand	Breast	−	+	Recent data from adjuvant trials of anastrozole suggest chemopreventive efficacy in postmenopausal women
Antiandrogens					
(e.g., Flutamide, Bicalutamide, Nilutamide)	AR	Prostate	+	−	Reduction in prostatic intraepithelial neoplasia
5-α Reductase Inhibitors					
(e.g., Finasteride)	AR, indirect inhibition of signaling by suppression of synthesis of ligand (DHT)	Prostate	+	−	Phase III trial of finasteride in progress
SARMs	AR	Prostate	+	−	Potential chemopreventive effect without antiandrogenic adverse effects *see refs. 37, 38, 41, 44–49.
Retinoids/Rexinoids**					
4-HPR	RXR	Breast, ovary, colon	+	−	Phase III secondary breast cancer prevention trial did not confirm efficacy
13-cRA	RAR	Upper aerodigestive tract, skin	+ +	±* ±**	*Secondary prevention efficacy in ex-/nonsmokers **see ref. 47

(continued)

199

Table 1 (continued)
Nuclear Receptor-Targeted Chemopreventive Agents

Agent	Target Receptor	Target Organ for Cancer Prevention	Evidence of Efficacy[#] Preclinical	Evidence of Efficacy[#] Clinical	Comments
Bexarotene	RXR	Upper aerodigestive tract, breast, others	+	–	
9-cRA	RAR/RXR	Upper aerodigestive tract, breast, colon	+	–	
Deltanoids	VDR	Colon, prostate, breast, skin, others	+	–	Hypercalcemia dose-limiting for most of the currently available agents
PPARγ Agonists (e.g., TZDs)	PPARγ	Breast	+	–	
SPARMs	PPAR	Breast	+	–	

'#' '+' indicates presence of evidence; '–' indicates absence of evidence or evidence of absence of effect

200

Interestingly, the most profound effect observed in the BCPT was in the subset of women with a prior diagnosis of atypical ductal hyperplasia (ADH). The 86% reduction in incidence of breast cancer in this subset suggests that tamoxifen may mediate an effect on other unidentified lesions of ADH. Other subsets of partially or completely extirpated premalignant lesions (DCIS, ductal carcinoma *in situ*, and LCIS, lobular carcinoma *in situ*) also derive a benefit from tamoxifen; a consistent reduction in the incidence of new breast cancers was seen in BCPT as well as in adjuvant trials of tamoxifen. However two other international trials reported at the same time as BCPT failed to demonstrate this chemopreventive benefit of tamoxifen. Potential reasons for these conflicting results have been discussed elsewhere *(15)*.

A second class of drugs known as aromatase inhibitors (e.g., anastrozole, letrozole, and exemestane), inhibit synthesis of estrogen. This class has recently shown significant activity against advanced breast cancer that equals or exceeds that of tamoxifen. Early results of an adjuvant therapy trial, ATAC (Arimidex, Tamoxifen Alone or in Combination), suggest a significant chemopreventive benefit of anastrozole, the first aromatase inhibitor to be tested in the adjuvant setting, in postmenopausal women *(16;* Table 1).

3.2. ER in Other Cancers

Epidemiological evidence supports a role for estrogens in the causation of endometrial, and possibly ovarian cancer in addition to breast cancer. Unopposed estrogenic stimulation leads to proliferative lesions of the endometrium, including endometrial cancer *(17)*. Most well-differentiated endometrial cancers contain ERα1, though recurrent/high-grade endometrial cancers generally lack it. Pharmacotherapy with systemic antiestrogens could be used to treat low-grade endometrial cancers and to prevent endometrial cancer in high-risk women. Anecdotal responses have been reported in endometrial cancer patients treated with tamoxifen. However, it is seldom used to treat or prevent endometrial lesions because of its known estrogen-like effects on the endometrium, especially in postmenopausal women. Novel and selective ER modulators (SERMs) that are known to be antiestrogenic on the uterus should be tested for prevention of endometrial cancer, provided their overall safety profile is acceptable for a chemopreventive application.

Approximately 30% of ovarian cancers also contain ERs *(18)*. However, a response to tamoxifen is observed in less than 10% of patients with advanced ovarian cancer *(19)*. Further investigation of the utility of novel SERMs in ovarian cancers is warranted.

Prostate carcinogenesis is considered to be primarily related to androgens rather than estrogens. However, the normal prostate gland contains ERα (stroma only) as well as ERβ (both epithelium and stroma). ERβ appears to be progressively lost during prostate carcinogenesis *(20)*. Even so, estrogens are highly effective in treating advanced prostate cancer. Antiestrogens have shown limited efficacy in the treatment of prostate cancer, and have shown chemopreventive efficacy in preclinical models of prostate cancer *(21)*. However, these agents can cause loss of libido, impotence, and in some cases, gynecomastia. Novel ER-targeting agents are needed to adequately test the relevance of ER as a target for prevention of prostate cancer.

3.3. SERMs: A Paradigm for Selective NR Modulators (SNRMs)

Cancer preventive agents are distinguished from cancer therapeutic agents primarily by the population to whom the drug is targeted. Cancer prevention agents are for populations that are unaffected by cancer yet have a risk of disease. The majority of individuals we can currently characterize as being at high risk for cancer will not develop it in their lifetime. Therefore, agents targeting this population must have a high therapeutic index with minimal toxicity to offer a compelling net clinical benefit without unintended adverse consequences. Although not necessarily unique to hormonal agents, this has been most vividly observed with agents targeting ER *(22)*.

Considering the widespread distribution of ER in normal tissues, it was not surprising that drugs that interfere with signaling through the ER are associated with beneficial as well as adverse effects in other organ systems. Somewhat surprising was the observation that the same drug, tamoxifen, could act as an estrogen in one organ while behaving as an antiestrogen in another organ. Tamoxifen acts as an estrogen-agonist on skeletal tissue, leading to preservation of bone-mineral density in postmenopausal women, although its effect is not as profound as estrogen. Like estrogen, it reduces LDL cholesterol; unlike estrogen, it does not increase HDL. These estrogenic effects are seen even as it exerts antiestrogenic effects on the breast and hypothalamic-pituitary axis. Tamoxifen acts as a weak estrogen on the uterus, especially in postmenopausal women. The full spectrum of clinical consequences of

Table 2
Attributes of Ideal Chemopreventive Agents that Target Nuclear Receptors

Agent/Class	Desirable Attributes of Currently Available Agents	Additional Desirable Attributes of Ideal Agents
SERMs	Antiestrogenic effect on breast tissue	Absence of hot flashes
	Prevention of osteoporosis	Absence of thromboembolic complications
	Reduction of cholesterol	Reduction of cardiovascular mortality
	Absence of uterine stimulation (some SERMs)	Estrogenic effect on CNS
		Antiosteoporotic activity equal to estrogens
		Antiestrogenic effect on uterus
		Absence of vaginal dryness
		Clinical chemopreventive efficacy against prostate cancer
SARMs	Antiandrogenic effect on prostate tissue	Androgenic effect on skeletal tissue
		No loss of libido
		No gynecomastia
Retinoids/Rexinoids	Chemopreventive effect in upper aerodigestive tract in ex-/nonsmokers	Chemopreventive efficacy in current smokers Absence of toxicity—skin dryness, mucositis, hyperlipidemia
		Absence of teratogenicity
Deltanoids	Chemopreventive efficacy (in preclinical models only thus far)	Absence of hypercalcemia at clinically efficacious doses
SPARMs	Chemopreventive efficacy (in preclinical models only thus far)	To be defined
	Favorable effects on glucose metabolism	

these diverse effects was realized in the BCPT *(14)*. In this trial, women randomized to receive tamoxifen demonstrated a ~twofold increase in the incidence of endometrial cancer as well as thromboembolic complications. In contrast, the incidence of fractures was reduced by ~20%. As breast cancer is predominantly a disease of postmenopausal women, the expectation is that a breast cancer chemoprevention agent would be offered to most women at a time in life when consideration is given to initiation of hormone replacement therapy (HRT). Therefore, the overall health benefits of such an intervention must be comparable to those generally considered, at least until recently, to be achievable from HRT. Of course, the recently observed adverse risk-benefit ratio of HRT has reignited a lot of old questions, which must be addressed carefully and scientifically as part of the ongoing debate on optimal interventions to preserve women's health *(23)*.

To optimize the overall health effects of a breast-cancer chemopreventive intervention, raloxifene— an agent for osteoporosis with minimal pro-estrogenic

effects on the uterus—has been tested. In clinical trials in osteoporotic women, this drug demonstrated a reduction in vertebral fracture risk. An incidental finding in this trial was reduced incidence of breast cancer. More importantly, the study demonstrated no excess of endometrial cancers *(24)*. A definitive trial to evaluate the comparative risk-benefit profile of raloxifene and tamoxifen (STAR) is ongoing.

The experience with raloxifene and tamoxifen shows that it is possible to design drugs that have agonist and antagonist profiles in selected target tissues. Both of these drugs act by binding to the LBD of ER; however, they induce different conformational changes in ER, leading to differential binding of coactivators and corepressors to the transcription initiation complex, which in turn leads to different phenotypic effects in the target tissue. This originated the concept of "ideal SERM" that has now been extended to other members of the NR superfamily (Table 2). The utility of SERMs may not be restricted to breast cancer, or even only to women *(25,26)*. Given the estrogen/SERM responsiveness of prostate cancer, SERMs could possibly be designed with efficacy against prostate cancer, but without the side effects commonly associated with antiandrogens.

3.4. Androgen Receptors and Prostate Cancer

Analogous to the role of estrogens in breast cancer, androgens are believed to play a major role in prostate carcinogenesis. However, without reliable derivations of lifetime sex-hormone exposure in men, as exist for women, causality is unproven. Epidemiologists have relied on determinations of discrete blood measurements as surrogates of long-term testosterone levels. These studies have revealed some correlation, although inconsistent, with a high risk of prostate cancer. Disparities in testosterone levels and risk for prostate cancer have been correlated with race, lifestyle, exercise, prior vasectomy, and the physical characteristic of male pattern baldness (27). Conversely, men born with a genetic deficiency of type II 5α-reductase and the inability to metabolize testosterone to the more potent androgen dihydrotestosterone (DHT) are protected from the development of prostate cancer.

Animal models of prostate carcinoma illustrate the role of androgens in the development of disease. Transgenic mice with insertion of SV40 T antigen specifically express the oncogene in the prostatic epithelium. With full expression of the oncogene, all of the transgenic mice develop prostatic intraepithelial neoplasia (PIN) within 8–12 wk of birth and progress to adenocarcinoma by 24–28 wk. Early androgen ablation, either medical or surgical, leads to a durable suppression of oncogene (SV40T antigen) expression in such models and significantly decreases development of prostate cancer (28,29). Similarly, antiandrogens have shown an ability to block progression of microscopic prostate carcinoma to macroscopic disease in a chemical carcinogenesis model (30).

Antiandrogenic therapy is the first option in the treatment of metastatic prostate cancer, producing durable remissions in the majority of patients. Neoadjuvant hormonal therapy in men with primary prostate cancer has been shown to reduce the incidence of PIN, considered to be a precursor of invasive prostate cancer (31). Finasteride, a 5α-reductase inhibitor that is widely used to treat benign prostatic hyperplasia, may decrease or reduce the rise of prostate-specific antigen (PSA) in men with prostate cancer, although it has no clinically meaningful activity against prostate cancer (32). 5α inhibitors have the advantage of not suppressing testosterone levels, thereby causing less

impotence and loss of libido. The Prostate Cancer Prevention Trial (PCPT), a randomized clinical trial of 18,000 men, is designed to test whether blockage of the testosterone activation pathway by finasteride leads to a decrease in the incidence of prostate cancer (33). Other agents in development may be more efficacious because of their ability to inhibit both type I and type II 5α-reductase enzymes, thereby more completely inhibiting conversion of testosterone to dihydrotestosterone.

Antiandrogens that bind to the AR have generally not been considered for chemoprevention because of their significant toxicities, although they are markedly more efficacious than finasteride against prostate cancer in both preclinical models and clinical settings. Key toxicities include hot flashes, gynecomastia, mastodynia, loss of muscle mass, and osteoporosis. Therefore, chemopreventive antiandrogens are currently evaluated only in very high-risk men, such as those with high-grade PIN. The success of SERMs for breast cancer has led to a similar effort to generate Selective Androgen Receptor Modulators (SARMs) (Table 2). Clinical evaluation of such agents is greatly anticipated.

3.5. Retinoid/Rexinoid Receptors

Based on experimental model systems, vitamin A (retinol) is important for maintaining epithelial integrity. Lack of this lipid-soluble vitamin induces cellular phenotypic changes consistent with metaplasia and dysplasia resembling precursor lesions of malignancy in animal models. Observations in humans to support the role of fat-soluble vitamins in carcinogenesis have been confounded by the ubiquitous supply of these vitamins in the diet. Many epidemiological studies of the association between vitamin supplements and cancer risk have found no direct beneficial effect of vitamin supplementation beyond that provided by the diet, although an effect is somewhat supported by studies of serum content of particular micronutrients, or dietary interrogations using well-validated questionnaires. Low dietary intake of carotenoids is associated with a risk of breast, bladder, ovarian, and lung cancer (34,35). The complexity of vitamin supplementation as a cancer prevention intervention was illustrated in three clinical trials of β-carotene supplementation that revealed an increased risk of cancer among current smokers who received β-carotene (36). The reason for the unexpected finding has not yet been determined. A large body of epidemiological data supported β-carotene's protective effect, but the reliability of such data is dependent on accurate reporting of smoking exposure. The possibility that β-carotene may act as a tumor promoter in the context of cigarette exposure has been demonstrated in some animal model systems. The outcome of these trials has brought caution to the field of chemoprevention in general, and to the use of retinoids in particular (37,38). However, compelling biological, mechanistic, and clinical evidence continues to support further evaluation of this class of drugs.

Receptors that mediate the pleiotropic effects of retinoids are widely distributed in tissue, reflecting their key role in the maintenance of epithelial cellular stability. Expression patterns across malignancies suggest that the receptors may play a critical role in the early stages of carcinogenesis. Studies of biopsies from stages of the neoplastic process ranging from normal to invasive disease found a comparative decrease in RARβ levels in early lesions of the head and neck, esophagus, and cervix. Loss of RARβ expression in carcinogenesis may be an important and obligatory step in the acquisition of a malignant phenotype. Re-introduction of RARβ into epithelial malignant cell lines can inhibit proliferation and activate apoptosis. Differences in expression patterns of other retinoid receptors have been identified in early premalignant lesions of the skin, breast, and prostate, suggesting a possible role for these receptors in early carcinogenesis. It has not yet been shown whether the events are causal or secondary to other events in the local environment influencing the hormonal milieu (39–41).

Mechanistic understanding, preclinical dose titration, and toxicity evaluations are critical to further successful development of retinoids for cancer prevention. Favorable drug efficacy results have been observed in numerous animal models of carcinogenesis using a variety of natural and synthetic retinoids. These include, among others, models that mimic carcinogenesis in the skin, breast, lung, oral cavity, prostate, bladder, colon, and liver (41–43). Efficacy has been observed in models of viral, chemical, and physical carcinogenesis. Systemic administration is efficacious in some models, and topical application is required in others.

Most efforts to evaluate the clinical chemopreventive potential of retinoids have focused on upper aerodigestive tract cancers. 13-cis-retinoic acid (13-cRA) was the first retinoid to demonstrate efficacy in regressing oral leukoplakia (44). However, although long-term maintenance therapy was associated with low rates of disease progression, the mucocutaneous toxicity associated with treatment was prohibitive. The efficacy of retinoids in the prevention of head and neck cancer

appears to be specific to time of intervention, supporting the idea that different processes critical for disease progression occur at different stages of disease. Retinoids have been effective when used to prevent second primary cancers or when given prior to the existence of a lesion identifiable by direct visualization (45). Once a premalignant lesion is established (moderate or severe dysplasia), retinoids are no longer effective at regression of lesions, but stabilization may occur.

Retinoids have been studied in various other clinical settings to determine their chemopreventive efficacy. In small studies, topical ATRA and systemic etretinate were found to reverse cutaneous actinic keratoses. In renal transplant patients with actinic keratoses, acitretin led to a reduction in the likelihood of progression to squamous cell carcinoma (46). However, results from larger trials are inconsistent (47). The only large, randomized clinical trial reported to evaluate cancer incidence in other organ systems used N-(4-hydroxyphenyl) retinamide (4-HPR) for secondary prevention of breast cancer. Overall cancer incidence did not decrease, although a subset analysis showed a trend toward cancer incidence reduction in premenopausal women (48). Polyprenic acid, an acyclic retinoid, was effective in preventing second primaries of hepatocellular carcinoma in a small, randomized clinical trial following surgical resection of an initial primary (49).

3.6. VDR and Deltanoids

Fat-soluble vitamin D is a primary regulator of calcium homeostasis. In the body, it is converted to $1,25(OH)_2D_3$, a dihydroxy active metabolite. Its receptor, VDR, is expressed in bone, intestine, skin, breast, prostate, and hematopoietic cells, among others. Ligand-bound VDR/RXR heterodimer binds to vitamin D response elements to modulate transcription of a variety of genes, including growth-regulatory genes such as $p21^{WAF1}$. The biologic consequences are inhibition of cellular proliferation, induction of differentiation, apoptosis, and mononuclear cell maturation, among others.

A significant body of epidemiological evidence suggests that vitamin D may play a physiological role in cancer prevention. Initial hints of this were gleaned from observing an inverse relationship between cancer incidence and the distance of a population from the equator. Cancer incidence in the northeastern United States is twice as high as that in the southern states. Ultraviolet B exposure, perhaps the most direct measure of a population's sun exposure, inversely correlated with frequency of breast, ovary, colon, prostate, bladder, esophageal, kidney, lung, pancreatic, rectal, stomach, and endometrium cancers, and non-Hodgkin's lymphoma. Four large epidemiological studies (Western Electric Employees study, Nurses Health study, Iowa Women's Health Study, and Health Professionals Follow-up Study) found an inverse association between total vitamin D intake and the incidence of colorectal cancer (CRC), although the effect was not significant in the latter two studies upon multivariate analysis. However, several case-control studies have not consistently confirmed this inverse correlation. Similarly, a study conducted in men living in northern California showed an inverse association between vitamin D_3 levels and prostate cancer; however, studies of men living in Maryland and Hawaii, and a study of US physicians, failed to confirm this. Several polymorphisms in the VDR gene are believed to have an impact on the risk of prostate cancer, but further studies are needed. The NIHANES1 epidemiological follow-up study has suggested an inverse correlation between sunlight exposure/vitamin D intake and the incidence of breast cancer. However, the evidence is inconclusive (reviewed in *50*).

VDR-knockout mice show a higher degree of proliferation in the descending colon (*51*) and a decrease in mammary ductal differentiation compared with wild-type mice. More direct evidence for a chemopreventive effect of vitamin D and analogs comes from preclinical models of carcinogenesis. Systemic administration is effective in models of chemical carcinogenesis in colon and stomach, APC^{Min} mouse model, N^1-methyl-N^1-nitrosourea (MNU) breast cancer model, and androgen-induced prostate cancer models, among others. Topical application of vitamin D is effective in preventing tumors in the hamster cheek pouch model, and 12-O-tetradecanoylphorbol-13-acetate (TPA)-promoted skin tumors. In addition, antitumor therapeutic efficacy of vitamin D and its analogs has been observed in several animal-tumor xenografts. In vitro, these compounds induce G_1 cell-cycle arrest accompanied by upregulation of CDK *p21*^{waf1} and *p27*^{kip1} in several human cancer cell lines (*21,43,50*).

Analogous to the steroid-receptor ligands, the study of vitamin D for chemoprevention has been hampered by widespread distribution of the cognate receptor, leading to undesirable mechanism-related side effects, most notably hypercalcemia. Therefore, numerous vitamin D analogs, collectively known as deltanoids, have been synthesized to discover those

that retain chemopreventive efficacy but are devoid of hypercalcemic effect (*52–55*). Although several deltanoids have shown efficacy at doses that do not produce hypercalcemia in preclinical studies, and some have undergone limited clinical exploration, the goal of developing an ideal selective VDR modulator remains elusive. For example, EB1089 showed broad anticancer activity in preclinical models without causing hypercalcemia, yet in the clinic, its dose-limiting toxicity was hypercalcemia (*56*). Compounds currently in the clinic are unlikely to have a sufficiently wide therapeutic index to be generally used for chemoprevention.

3.7. PPAR Agonists and Cancer Prevention

Peroxisome proliferator-activated receptors (PPARs) are the latest members of the NR superfamily discovered to play a role in carcinogenesis. Originally identified by their role in the terminal differentiation of adipocytes, the ligands for these receptors were subsequently shown to induce differentiation of breast cancer cells in vitro (*57*). Three distinct isoforms are known: α, β (δ), and γ (alternative splicing leads to two forms—γ1 and γ2). Expression of the three isoforms is tissue-specific. Thiazolidinediones (TZD), a class of drugs used to treat diabetes, act by binding to PPARγ.

Structural alterations (mutations and translocations) of these receptors are rare in cancer. However, loss of PPARγ-mediated signaling may be associated with carcinogenesis. A PAX8-PPARγ1 chimeric sequence present in follicular thyroid carcinomas can suppress rosiglitazone (a TZD)-induced transcription by the wild-type PPAR (*58*). Although PPARγ heterozygous mice demonstrate a marked increase in the risk of colonic neoplasia following exposure to azoxymethane, the constitutive expression of PPARγ has been shown to increase the risk of breast neoplasia in other rodent models. These seemingly paradoxical results have been attributed to potential dose-responsiveness of anticarcinogenic effects of PPAR signaling (*59*). Diabetes therapy with TZD has established the safety of PPAR agonists. These compounds have also demonstrated preclinical activity against several established human cancer cell lines from breast, colon, and prostate and chemopreventive efficacy in the MNU breast carcinogenesis model. However, in some models—e.g., Min mice—some members of this class seem to enhance carcinogenesis. The reasons for these discordant results remain to be elucidated. It has been suggested that at least some of the anticancer effects of

TZDs are mediated through mechanisms independent of their binding to PPAR (60).

As with other members of the NR superfamily, the effects of PPAR ligands are likely to depend on levels of expression of various members of the PPAR family and its heterodimeric partner, RXR; levels of various transcriptional coregulators of PPAR; and specificity of the ligand against specific members of the PPAR family. This has led to the concept of SPARMs, selective PPAR receptor modulators (59). Some interesting novel molecules have been identified (61). Clinical data on their biological effects are not yet available.

4. COMBINATION THERAPY WITH SNRMS

As discussed here, effective and safe chemopreventive intervention requires the development of selective modulators with tissue-specific desirable effects. Efforts thus far have generally focused on making drugs to fit a theoretical ideal profile that could be used as single agents (Table 2). Selectivity has been achieved at several levels—e.g., steroid vs retinoid receptors, RAR vs RXR, and RARα vs RARβ vs RARγ. It may not be possible to design small molecules with all the desirable features of an ideal SNRM when used as a single agent. Since many members of this family function as heterodimers, which can be activated by the ligands for either of the two partners, an alternative approach would combine drugs that target distinct receptors in a selective and specific fashion to achieve the desired profile. The concurrent presence of both ligands can result in a cooperative effect on the transactivation of target genes. For example, PPAR-RXR heterodimers can be activated by PPAR or RXR ligands. However, the two types of ligands recruit different coactivators to the heterodimer, which may explain their cooperative effects (62). The potential also exists for concurrent use of ligands for both receptors to lead to activation of genes that are not otherwise subject to regulation by either receptor alone. For example, the combination of RXR and PPAR can activate estrogen-responsive genes when activated by 9-cRA, even in the absence of ER (63). Some investigators have observed that RAR-RXR heterodimers can be activated only by RAR ligands because of allosteric inhibition of ligand binding to RXR by RAR (64). However, such an allosteric inhibition does not appear to be obligatory (65).

Preclinical data already show the additive/synergistic activity of combinations of SERMs + retinoids, SERMs + PPARγ agonists, SERMs + deltanoids, etc.

(55,59,66). It is possible that lower doses of individual agents could be used in such combinations, reducing dose-dependent toxicity without compromising efficacy (43). It may also be possible to modulate the toxicity of single agents by appropriately designed combinations. For example, certain RARα-mediated teratogenic effects in mice can be potentiated by RXR-selective agonists but reduced by RAR-selective agonists (67). Of course, the clinical development programs for evaluating such combinations can be quite challenging. Novel approaches incorporating surrogate biomarkers are needed, as discussed elsewhere in this book.

5. KEY CHALLENGES AND CONCLUSIONS

Important progress in realizing the chemopreventive potential of NR-targeted drugs has been made in the last three decades. First-generation drugs such as tamoxifen have already been incorporated into an integrated strategy for managing women at high risk for breast cancer. Second-generation drugs, such as raloxifene and aromatase inhibitors, have already yielded promising initial human data and are in advanced clinical trials to definitively evaluate their chemopreventive potential. Retinoids have been shown to prevent upper aerodigestive tract cancer in ex-/nonsmokers. Results of the first large prostate cancer prevention trial are expected soon. The most important lesson of the last 30 yr is to appreciate the complexity of NR signaling pathways. Negative surprises—e.g., the increased risk of uterine cancer with tamoxifen and the potentially increased risk of cancer in current smokers given β-carotene— required cautionary adjustments in clinical strategies and reassessment of the risk-benefit ratio. A variety of novel agents to target many of these receptors are on the horizon. It is important to carefully evaluate tissue-specific effects of these new agents in predictive preclinical models and in well-designed Phase I/II trials incorporating surrogate endpoints in relevant tissues/patient populations before initiating large-scale Phase III clinical trials. It is unlikely that efficacious agents that are completely devoid of toxicity will become available in the foreseeable future. However, the therapeutic index of these agents can be significantly improved through judicious patient selection using the complementary strategies of improving risk evaluation based on epidemiological, molecular genetic, and biochemical markers, and improving the predicted benefit from a specific chemopreventive intervention based on pharmacogenetic/ pharmacogenomic approaches. This requires a thoughtful multidisciplinary approach to the pursuit of chemopreventive strategies.

REFERENCES

1. Hong WK, Sporn MB. Recent advances in chemoprevention of cancer. *Science* 1997;278:1073–1077.
2. Owen GI, Zelent A. Origins and evolutionary diversification of the nuclear receptor superfamily. *Cell Mol Life Sci* 2000;57:809–827.
3. Comitee NR. A unified nomenclature system for the nuclear receptor superfamily. *Cell* 1999;97:161–163.
4. Laudet V. Evolution of the nuclear receptor superfamily: early diversification from an ancestral orphan receptor. *J Mol Endocrinol* 1997;19:207–226.
5. Kumar V, Green S, Stack G, et al. Functional domains of the human estrogen receptor. *Cell* 1987;51:941–951.
6. Rastinejad F. Structure and function of the steroid and nuclear receptor DNA binding domain, in *Molecular Biology of Steroid and Nuclear Hormone Receptors*. Freedman L, ed. Birkhauser, MA, Boston, 1998, pp.105–131.
7. Wurtz J-M, Bourget W, Renaud J-P, et al. A canonical structure for the ligand-binding domain of nuclear receptors. *Nat Struc Biol* 1996;3:87–94.
8. Schwabe JW, Chapman L, Finch JT, Rhodes D. The crystal structure of the estrogen receptor DNA-binding domain bound to DNA: how receptors discriminate between their response elements. *Cell* 1993;75:567–578.
9. Mangelsdorf DJ, Thummel C, Beato M, et al. The nuclear receptor superfamily: the second decade. *Cell* 1995;83:835–839.
10. Umesono K, Murakami KK, Thompson CC, Evans RM. Direct repeats as selective response elements for the thyroid hormone, retinoic acid, and vitamin D_3 receptors. *Cell* 1991;65:1255–1266.
11. Lee JW, Lee YC, Na S-Y, et al. Transcriptional coregulators of the nuclear receptor superfamily: coactivators and corepressors. *Cell Mol Life Sci* 2001;58:289–297.
12. Gail MH, Brinton LA, Byar DP, et al. Projecting individualized probabilities of developing breast cancer for white females who are being examined annually. *J Natl Cancer Inst* 1989; 81:1879–1885.
13. MacGregor JI, Jordan VC. Basic guide to the mechanisms of antiestrogen action. *Pharmacol Rev* 1998;50:151–196.
14. Fisher B, Costantino JP, Wickerham DL, et al. Tamoxifen for prevention of breast cancer: report of the National Surgical Adjuvant Breast and Bowel Project P-1 study. *J Natl Cancer Inst* 1998;90:1371–1388.
15. Pritchard KI. Is tamoxifen effective in prevention of breast cancer? *Lancet* 1998;352:80–81.
16. The ATAC (Arimidex, Tamoxifen Alone or in Combination) Clinical Trialists' Group.Anastrozole alone or in combination with tamoxifen versus tamoxifen alone for adjuvant treatment of postmenopausal women with early breast cancer: first results of the ATAC randomised trial. *Lancet* 2002;359:2131–2139.
17. Rose PG. Endometrial carcinoma. *N Engl J Med* 1996;335:640–649.
18. Danforth DN Jr. Hormone receptors in malignancy. *Crit Rev Oncol Hematol* 1992;12:91–149.
19. Marth C, Sorheim N, Kaern J, Trope C. Tamoxifen in the treatment of recurrent ovarian cancer. *Int J Gynecol Cancer* 1997;7:256–261.
20. Horvath LG, Henshall SM, Lee C-S, et al. Frequent loss of estrogen receptor-β expression in prostate cancer. *Cancer Res* 2001;61:5331–5335.
21. Lucia MS, Anzano MA, Slayter MV, et al. Chemopreventive activity of tamoxifen, N-(4-hydroxyphenyl) retinamide, and the vitamin D analogue Ro24-5531 for androgen-promoted carcinomas of the rat seminal vesicle and prostate. *Cancer Res* 1995;55:5621–5627.
22. Dhingra K. Selective estrogen receptor modulation: the search for an ideal hormonal therapy for breast cancer. *Cancer Investig* 2001;19:649–659.
23. Writing Group for the Women's Health Initiative Investigators.Risks and benefits of estrogen plus progestin in healthy postmenopausal women—principal results from the Women's Health Initiative Randomized Controlled Trial. *JAMA* 2002;288:321–333.
24. Cummings SR, Eckert S, Krueger KA, et al. The effect of raloxifene on risk of breast cancer in postmenopausal women—results from the MORE trial. *JAMA* 1999;281:2189–2197.
25. Resche-Rigon M, Gronemeyer H. Therapeutic potential of selective modulators of nuclear receptor action. *Curr Opin Chem Biol* 1998;2:501–507.
26. Dhingra K. Antiestrogens—tamoxifen, SERMs and beyond. *Investig New Drugs* 1999;17:285–311.
27. Brawley OW, Knopf K, Thompson I. The epidemiology of prostate cancer part II: the risk factors. *Semin Urol Oncol* 1998;16:193–201.
28. Eng MH, Charles LG, Ross BD. Early castration reduces prostatic carcinogenesis in transgenic mice. *Urology* 1999;54:1112–1119.
29. Raghow S, Kuliyev E, Steakley M, et al. Efficacious chemoprevention of primary prostate cancer by flutamide in an autochthonous transgenic model. *Cancer Res* 2000;60:4093–4097.
30. Tsukamoto S, Akaza H, Onozawa M, et al. A five-alpha reductase inhibitor or an antiandrogen prevents the progression of microscopic prostate carcinoma to macroscopic carcinoma in rats. *Cancer* 1998;82:531–537.
31. Balaji KC, Rabbani F, Tsai H, et al. Effect of neoadjuvant hormonal therapy on prostatic intraepithelial neoplasia and its prognostic significance. *J Urol* 1999;162:753–757.
32. Andriole G, Lieber M, Smith J, et al. Treatment with finasteride following radical prostatectomy for prostate cancer. *Urology* 1995;45:491–497.
33. Thompson IM Jr, Kouril M, Klein EA, et al. The Prostate Cancer Prevention Trial: current status and lessons learned. *Urology* 2001;57(Suppl 4A):230–234.
34. Peto R, Doll R, Buckley JD, Sporn MB. Can dietary beta-carotene materially reduce human cancer rates? *Nature* 1981;290:201–208.
35. Bertone ER, Hankinson SE, Newcomb PA, et al. A population-based case-control study of carotenoid and vitamin A intake and ovarian cancer (United States). *Cancer Causes Control* 2001;12:83–90.
36. Albanes D, Heinonen OP, Taylor PR, et al. Alpha-tocopherol and beta-carotene supplements and lung cancer incidence in the alpha-tocopherol, beta-carotene cancer prevention study:

effects of base-line characteristics and study compliance. *J Natl Cancer Inst* 1996;88:1560–1570.

37. Omenn GS. Chemoprevention of lung cancer: the rise and demise of beta-carotene. *Annu Rev Public* Health 1998;19:73–99.

38. Lippman SM, Lee JJ, Sabichi AL. Cancer chemoprevention: progress and promise. *J Natl Cancer Inst* 1998;90:1514–1528.

39. Xu XC, Mitchell MF, Silva E, et al. Decreased expression of retinoic acid receptors, transforming growth factor beta, involucrin, and cornifin in cervical intraepithelial neoplasia. *Clin Cancer Res* 1999;5:1503–1508.

40. Lawrence JA, Merino MJ, Simpson JF, et al. A high-risk lesion for invasive breast cancer, ductal carcinoma *in situ*, exhibits frequent overexpression of retinoid X receptor. *Cancer Epidemiol Biomark Prev* 1998;7:29–35.

41. Lotan R. Retinoids in chemoprevention. *FASEB J* 1996;10:1031–1039.

42. Sporn M, Dunlop N, Newton D, Smith J. Prevention of chemical carcinogenesis by vitamin A and its synthetic analogs (retinoids). *Fed Proc* 1976;35:1332–1338.

43. Cope MB, Steele VE, Eto I, et al. Prevention of methylnitrosourea-induced mammary cancers by 9-*cis*-retinoic acid and/or vitamin D_3. *Oncol Rep* 2002;9:533–537.

44. Hong WK, Endicott J, Itri LM, et al. 13-*cis*-Retinoic acid in the treatment of oral leukoplakia. *N Engl J Med* 1986;315:1501–1505.

45. Hong WK, Lippman SM, Itri LM, et al. Prevention of second primary tumors with isotretinoin in squamous-cell carcinoma of the head and neck. *N Engl J Med* 1990;323:795–801.

46. Bavinck JN, Tieben LM, van der Woude FJ, et al. Prevention of skin cancer and reduction of keratotic skin lesions during acitretin therapy in renal transplant recipients: a double-blind placebo-controlled study. *J Clin Oncol* 1995;13:1933–1938.

47. Moon TE, Levine N, Cartmel B, Bangert JL. Retinoids in prevention of skin cancer. *Cancer Lett* 1997;114:203–205.

48. Veronesi U, dePalo F, Marubini E, et al. Randomized trial of fenretinide to prevent second breast malignancy in women with early breast cancer. *J Natl Cancer Inst* 1999;91:1847–1856.

49. Muto Y, Moriwaki H, Ninomiya M, et al. Prevention of second primary tumors by an acyclic retinoid, polyprenoic acid, to patients with hepatocellular carcinoma. Hepatoma Prevention Study Group. *N Engl J Med* 1996;334:1561–1567.

50. Guyton KZ, Kensler TW, Posner GH. Cancer chemoprevention using natural vitamin D and synthetic analogs. *Annu Rev Pharmacol Toxicol* 2001;41:421–442.

51. Kallay E, Pietschmann P, Toyokuni S, et al. Characterization of a vitamin D receptor knockout mouse as a model of colorectal hyperproliferation and DNA damage. *Carcinogenesis* 2001;22:1429–1435.

52. Shiohara M, Uskokovic M, Hisatake J, et al. 24-Oxo metabolites of vitamin D_3 analogues: disassociation of their prominent antileukemic effects from their lack of calcium modulation. *Cancer Res* 2001;61:3361–3368.

53. Mathiasen IS, Colston RW, Binderup L. EB 1089, a novel vitamin D analogue, has strong antiproliferative and differentiation-inducing effects on cancer cells. *J Steroid Biochem Mol Biol* 1993;46:365–371.

54. Polek TC, Murthy S, Blutt SE, et al. Novel nonsecosteroidal vitamin D receptor modulator inhibits the growth of LNCaP xenograft tumors in athymic mice without increased serum calcium. *Prostate* 2001;49:224–233.

55. Anzano MA, Smith JM, Uskokovic MR, et al. 1 alpha, 25-Dihydroxy-16-ene-23-yne-26,27-hexafluorocholecalciferol (Ro24-5531), a new deltanoid (vitamin D analogue) for prevention of breast cancer in the rat. *Cancer Res* 1994;54:1653–1656.

56. Gulliford T, English J, Colston KW, et al. A phase I study of the vitamin D analogue EB 1089 in patients with advanced breast and colorectal cancer. *Br J Cancer* 1998;78:6–13.

57. Mueller E, Sarraf P, Tontonoz P, et al. Terminal differentiation of human breast cancer cells through PPARγ. *Mol Cell* 1998;1:465–470.

58. Kroll TG, Sarraf P, Pecciarini L, et al. PAX8-PPARγ1 fusion in oncogene human thyroid carcinoma. *Science* 2000;289:1357–1360.

59. Sporn MG, Suh N, Mangelsdorf DJ. Prospects for prevention and treatment of cancer with selective PPARγ modulators (SPARMs). *Trends Mol Med* 2001;7:395–400.

60. Palakurthi SS, Aktas H, Grubissich LM, et al. Anticancer effects of thiazolidinediones are independent of peroxisome proliferator-activated receptor γ and mediated by inhibition of translation initiation. *Cancer Res* 2001;61:6213–6218.

61. Suh N, Wang Y, Williams CR, et al. A new ligand for the peroxisome proliferator-activated receptor-γ (PPAR-γ), GW7845, inhibits rat mammary carcinogenesis. *Cancer Res* 1999;59:5671–5673.

62. Yang W, Rachez C, Freedman LP. Discrete roles for peroxisome proliferator-activated receptor γ and retinoid X receptor in recruiting nuclear receptor coactivators. *Mol Cell Biol* 2000;20:8008–8017.

63. Nunez SB, Medin JA, Braissant O, et al. Retinoid X receptor and peroxisome proliferator-activated receptor activate an estrogen responsive gene independent of the estrogen receptor. *Mol Cell Endocrinol* 1997;127:27–40.

64. Westin S, Kurokawa R, Nolte RT, et al. Interactions controlling the assembly of nuclear-receptor heterodimers and co-activators. *Nature* 1998;395:199–202.

65. Botling J, Castro DS, Oberg F, et al. Retinoic acid receptor retinoid X receptor heterodimers can be activated through both subunits providing a basis for synergistic transactivation and cellular differentiation. *J Biol Chem* 1997;272:9443–9449.

66. Ratko TA, Detrisac CJ, Dinger NM, et al. Chemopreventive efficacy of combined retinoid and tamoxifen treatment following surgical excision of primary mammary cancer in female rats. *Cancer Res* 1989;49:4472–4476.

67. Elmazar MA, Ruhl R, Reichert U, et al. RARα-mediated teratogenicity in mice is potentiated by an RXR agonist and reduced by an RAR antagonist: dissection of retinoid receptor-induced pathways. *Toxicol Appl Pharmacol* 1997;146:21–28.

A. ANTIANDROGENS

13 Prostate Cancer Chemoprevention

5α-Reductase Inhibitors

Jennifer E. Drisko, DVM, PhD and Siu-Long Yao, MD

CONTENTS

1. MECHANISM OF ACTION

5α-reductase is a nuclear membrane-bound NADPH-dependent δ-3-ketosteroid 5α-oxidoreductase. It is found in androgen-sensitive tissues, and catalyzes the conversion of testosterone to dihydrotestosterone (DHT). Two known isoenzymes of 5α-reductase have been identified: Type 1 predominates in peripheral tissues such as the skin and liver, and Type 2 is predominant in the prostate. Finasteride is a specific inhibitor of the Type 2 isoenzyme, and effectively blocks the Type 2-mediated conversion of testosterone to DHT, but does not inhibit the binding of DHT to the androgen receptor (AR) *(1)*.

Finasteride decreases serum prostate specific antigen (PSA) levels by approx 50% over the entire range of PSA values. PSA is a widely used screening tool for detecting prostate adenocarcinoma *(2)*. Finasteride does not affect the use of PSA as a marker of prostate cancer. PSA values should be double compared to normal ranges in untreated men *(1,3)*.

2. PHARMACOKINETICS OF FINASTERIDE

Finasteride is orally active and highly bioavailable (~80%). It is rapidly absorbed after oral administration, and peak plasma levels occur 1–2 h after drug intake; approx 90% of circulating finasteride is bound to plasma proteins *(4,5)*. Finasteride is the major component circulating in the plasma *(5)*. The serum $t_{1/2}$ of the drug is approx 6 h, although second-order kinetics are consistent with the formation of an irreversible complex, resulting in slow, gradual (several days) return of serum DHT to baseline after discontinuation of the drug.

After oral administration, finasteride is extensively metabolized in the liver by hydroxylation at the *tert*-butyl group (ω-hydroxyfinasteride), followed by further oxidation to the corresponding acid (finasteride-ω-oic acid), with ω-aldehyde finasteride as an intermediate. Each of the three steps of this oxidative pathway is mediated by cytochrome P450 3A4 *(6)*. The major metabolites, ω-hydroxyfinasteride and finasteride-ω-oic acid, possess minimal activity (<20%) as inhibitors of 5α-reductase, and are excreted mainly through bile *(4)*. Finasteride does not appear to affect the cytochrome P450-linked drug metabolism enzyme system.

3. PHARMACODYNAMICS OF FINASTERIDE

A single oral dose of finasteride (5 mg) markedly reduces serum DHT (~70% below baseline) in men within hours of dosing *(7)*. Further reduction of serum

From: Cancer Chemoprevention, Volume 1: Promising Cancer Chemoprevention Agents
Edited by: G. J. Kelloff, E. T. Hawk, and C. C. Sigman © Humana Press Inc., Totowa, NJ

DHT levels does not occur because of finasteride's specificity; Type 1 5α-reductase is not significantly affected. Daily dosing produces a similar and persistent suppression of serum DHT, and tachyphylaxis to the effects on DHT is not observed with chronic administration (8). In association with the marked reduction of DHT, a small (~15%) increase in serum testosterone is observed. Despite the significant changes in serum levels of DHT, serum levels of luteinizing hormone (LH) and follicle-stimulating hormone (FSH) increased slightly (~10%), but remained within normal limits with finasteride treatment, and the response of LH and FSH to gonadotropin-releasing hormone (GnRH) was not affected (9). No clinically relevant changes in serum-free testosterone or sex hormone-binding globulin were reported in men treated for 6 mo with finasteride (10). These findings indicate that finasteride does not affect the regulation of the hypothalamic-pituitary-testicular axis. Chronic administration of finasteride also had no effect on circulating levels of cortisol, prolactin, thyroid-stimulating hormone, or thyroxine. No effects on lipid profiles or glucose tolerance have been demonstrated.

4. PRECLINICAL SAFETY STUDIES

No evidence of mutagenicity has been observed in preclinical safety studies (1). These assays include in vitro bacterial and mammalian-cell mutagenesis assays, and an in vitro alkaline elution assay. In an in vitro chromosome aberration assay using Chinese hamster ovary cells, chromosome aberrations slightly increased at concentrations that corresponded to 4000–5000× peak plasma levels in men given a total dose of 5 mg. No treatment-related increase in chromosome aberrations was observed in an in vivo chromosome aberration assay in mice with finasteride at the maximum tolerated dose of 250 mg/kg/d (228× the human exposure), as determined in the carcinogenicity studies.

In sexually mature male rabbits treated with finasteride at 80 mg/kg/d (543× the human exposure) for up to 12 wk, no effect on fertility, sperm count, or ejaculate volume was seen. Sexually mature male rats treated with 80 mg/kg/d of finasteride (61× the human exposure) had no significant effects on fertility after 6 or 12 wk of treatment; however, treatment that continued for up to 24 or 30 wk apparently decreased fertility and fecundity, with an associated significant decrease in the weights of the seminal vesicles and prostate. This decrease in fertility in finasteride-treated rats is secondary to its effect on accessory sex organs (prostate and

seminal vesicles), resulting in a failure to form a seminal plug. The seminal plug is essential for normal fertility in rats, and is not relevant in man. All these effects were reversible within 6 wk of discontinuation of treatment. No drug-related effect on the testes or on mating performance has been seen in rats or rabbits.

There is no evidence of a tumorigenic effect in rats (1). Sprague-Dawley rats were treated for 24 mo with daily doses of finasteride up to 160 mg/kg in males and 320 mg/kg in females (111 and 274× the human exposure, respectively). Leydig-cell hyperplasia was observed in mice and rats at 23 and 39× the human exposure, correlating with mild, two- to threefold increases in LH levels, but this has not been shown to be clinically relevant. No drug-related Leydig-cell changes occurred in rats or dogs treated daily with finasteride for 1 yr at doses of 20 mg/kg and 45 mg/kg (30 and 350× the human exposure, respectively).

5. CLINICAL SAFETY

No clinically meaningful effects on sperm concentration, mobility, morphology, or pH were observed in healthy male volunteers treated with finasteride at 5 mg for 24 wk; however, there was a 0.6-mL (22.1%) median decrease in ejaculate volume with a concomitant reduction in total sperm per ejaculate (1). These parameters were within the normal range and were reversible upon discontinuation of therapy, with an average time to return to baseline of 84 wk.

Drug interactions of clinical importance have not been identified. Compounds tested in man have included antipyrine, digoxin, propranolol, theophylline, and warfarin; no clinically meaningful interactions were found. Finasteride was concomitantly used in clinical studies with acetaminophen, acetylsalicylic acid, α-blockers, angiotensin-converting enzyme (ACE) inhibitors, analgesics, anticonvulsants, β-adrenergic blocking agents, diuretics, calcium-channel blockers, cardiac nitrates, HMG-CoA reductase inhibitors, nonsteroidal antiinflammatory drugs (NSAIDs), benzodiazepines, H_2 antagonists, and quinolone anti-infectives, with no evidence of clinically significant adverse interactions. Finasteride has not been tested in men less than 18 yr of age, and is not indicated for use in women.

6. 5α-REDUCTASE INHIBITION AND RELATION TO PROSTATE CANCER

Among US men, prostate cancer is the most common non-skin cancer and the second most common cause of cancer death *(11)*. In the US alone, approximately one in six men will develop prostate cancer during his lifetime *(12)*. The prognosis and therapeutic options depend upon clinical stage at time of diagnosis. Older men with early stage, low Gleason score (well-differentiated) disease may be treated expectantly. Men with more aggressive cancer (higher Gleason scores) are probably best managed with surgery (radical prostatectomy) or radiation when tumors are confined to the prostate *(13)*. Hormonal treatment is often utilized once the cancer has spread beyond the capsule of the prostate. Although this is initially effective, all patients eventually develop hormonally resistant, androgen-insensitive disease, which can be rapidly progressive and is usually fatal *(14)*.

More than 60 yr of research have established that androgen deprivation decreases prostate tumor volume and slows disease progression (15–18). However, among the range of androgens, the role of DHT has been less clearly defined. A wealth of data accumulated over time suggests that DHT plays a central role in initiation and progression of prostate cancer. Several points illuminated by the data are discussed in the following paragraphs.

Males with a genetic deficiency of 5α-reductase have sparse facial and body hair, do not exhibit male pattern baldness, and have never been reported to develop prostate cancer *(19)*.

Although data conflict, some studies have suggested that men with relatively lower serum androgen levels have a decreased risk of developing carcinoma of the prostate *(20)*.

Analysis of human prostate cancer tissues has demonstrated that the DHT/DNA ratio is higher in more differentiated tumors *(21,22)*. If this is the case, a reduction of intraprostatic DHT may reduce its ability to serve as a promoter in the development of prostate cancer.

Many studies have demonstrated the dramatically increased risk of prostate cancer (both incidence and mortality) among US African-Americans and the significantly lower risk in Asian countries, especially China and Japan *(23,24)*. It has been postulated that this increased risk among US African-Americans is related to the relative increase in circulating testosterone in this group, estimated to be 10–15% higher than in US Caucasians *(20)*. Ross et al. conducted a study of US Caucasians and African-Americans as well as rural Japanese men to determine whether variations in 5α-reductase activity among these populations could explain the variability in the risk of prostate cancer

(25). Testosterone, sex hormone-binding-globulin-binding capacity (SHBG), as well as levels of 3α, 17β androstanediol glucuronide (A-diol-g), and androsterone glucuronide (A-g) (indirect measures of 5α reductase activity in serum), were measured in a group of 50 US Caucasian, 50 US African-American, and 54 Japanese young men. African-Americans had an 11% higher serum testosterone and a 9% higher SHBG level. Significantly higher levels of A-diol-g and A-g were detected in US African-Americans and Caucasians than in Japanese men. These data suggest that reduced 5α-reductase activity may be associated with a protective role in the development of prostate cancer in Japanese men *(25)*.

Finally, 5α-reductase inhibition causes a dose-dependent inhibition of two human prostate cancer cell lines in vitro *(26)*. Similar effects were also observed in in vivo models *(27,28)*.

Type 2 5α-reductase inhibitors produce long-term suppression of DHT formation, an important promoter of prostate growth, with minimal toxicity. It should be noted that the 80% decrease in intraprostatic DHT and the 10-fold increase in intraprostatic testosterone levels produced by finasteride therapy results in a net reduction in the overall intraprostatic androgen signal of approx 50% *(29)*.

7. CLINICAL STUDIES

In a double-blind, multicenter study, 28 asymptomatic men who presented with stage D prostate cancer were randomized to 6 wk of treatment with either finasteride 10 mg daily or placebo *(30,31)*. Men who relapsed after radical prostatectomy or surgery were excluded. After wk 3 and 6, the median percent change in PSA from baseline was significantly decreased by –22.9% and –15.1% respectively in the finasteride group compared with corresponding minor decreases of –2.9% and +9.9% for the placebo group. These declines were greater than would be expected if only benign tissue were affected *(32)*. Finasteride therapy markedly reduced DHT without affecting serum testosterone.

Although PSA declined more in the finasteride-treated patients, there was no apparent correlation between serum DHT, testosterone, and either prostatic acid phosphatase (PAP) or PSA. Effects were not different among men with positive or negative bone scans and quality of life, and Karnofsky performance status did not differ between the finasteride and placebo-treated patients. These results suggest that finasteride has an effect on established prostate cancer, although the effect was relatively modest compared with surgical or chemical castration *(32)*.

A subsequent study evaluated the effects of finasteride 10 mg once daily on PSA levels and prostate cancer recurrence rates in a 1-yr, randomized, double-blind, placebo-controlled study of 120 men who had undergone radical prostatectomy for prostate cancer within the past 10 yr. Some participants ($N = 84$) were also continued in a 1-year open-label extension study *(33,34)*. Patients had PSA levels between 0.6 and 10 ng/mL and no evidence of metastatic disease at enrollment. Finasteride ($N = 54$) significantly reduced serum DHT by 62% after 2 mo of therapy; the effect persisted throughout the study. PSA increased slowly and progressively in the placebo group from a median of 2.01 ng/mL at baseline to 3.8 ng/mL at 12 mo. In the finasteride group, PSA remained at or below the baseline level for 6 mo, then progressed more slowly than in the placebo group; a similar pattern was seen during the extension study, except that PSA decreased transiently in patients who had originally received placebo. By extrapolating data in the placebo group to 24 mo, it was estimated that finasteride delayed the increase in PSA by about 9 mo during the first year and by about 14 mo during the second year. During the first and second years of the study, respectively, prostate cancer recurrence rates as determined by development of positive bone scans or other signs of clinical progression (but not PSA criteria) were 7% and 12% in the finasteride group and 11% and 19% in the placebo group (patients on placebo received finasteride during the subsequent 12-mo extension component of the study). The overall effect of finasteride on PSA suggested a possible tumor-suppressing effect, further supported by reduced incidence of local and distant recurrences in the finasteride group *(33,34)*.

It is possible that the effects of finasteride may be greatest in men who are at risk for prostate cancer. Andriole et al. *(3)* evaluated the incidence of prostate cancer and PSA levels in over 3,000 men with benign prostatic hyperplasia (BPH) treated with either finasteride or placebo in the 4-yr placebo-controlled PLESS trial, and demonstrated that the overall incidence of prostate cancer in men treated with finasteride was similar to the placebo-treated group (4.7% on finasteride vs 5.1% on placebo, $p = 0.7$). However, the PLESS trial only biopsied a subset of patients, most with baseline PSA >4, and was not designed to evaluate prostate cancer prevention. An additional analysis of

the histologic grades of the prostate cancers detected no difference in metastatic or undifferentiated cancers.

Based on these and other considerations, the Prostate Cancer Prevention Trial (PCPT) was opened in October 1993 and enrolled 18,882 men aged ≥55 yr with normal digital rectal exams and PSA ≤3 ng/mL. The men were randomized to either finasteride 5 mg PO once a day or placebo over a period of 3 yr. Over time, 219 centers from the Southwest Oncology Group, the Eastern Cooperative Oncology Group, and the Cancer and Leukemia Group B contributed subjects. During the study, men were contacted by telephone every 3 mo, and annual PSAs and digital rectal exams were performed. Men with abnormal results at these interim visits would proceed to further evaluation (including biopsy, if necessary). After receiving treatment for 7 yr, individuals who did not develop cancer during the study will be biopsied in order to definitively determine the period prevalence of prostate cancer. The first biopsies were conducted in October 2000.

Several key assumptions are critical to successful completion and interpretation of PCPT study results. One potential problem is that men randomized to placebo would ultimately have higher PSAs, thus predisposing them to biopsy and a potentially higher rate of cancer (ascertainment bias). In order to avoid this potential confounding factor, an algorithm was employed in which PSA levels of men treated with finasteride would be adjusted so that the total number of biopsies would be approximately equal among the patients regardless of treatment, preserving the sensitivity and specificity of PSA testing; it was assumed that a simple mathematical adjustment would suffice. Other general statistical assumptions had to be maintained as well. For example, it was projected that total loss to various factors (e.g., death, follow-up, biopsy, nonadherence, crossover), would not exceed 55% of the study population. A data safety and monitoring committee continuously monitors the study results every 6 mo to ensure that these assumptions are reasonable and that changes to the protocol are not necessary. One final, critically important assumption is that end-of-study biopsies can be performed in a manner that will not oversample the smaller prostates of finasteride-treated men compared with the normal-sized prostates of men treated with placebo. Fortuitously, it appears that BPH and prostate cancer occur in different areas of the prostate (transition and peripheral zone, respectively). Finasteride is believed to predominantly affect the size of the transition zone and so directing biopsies laterally into the peripheral zone, where cancer is commonly found and finasteride is believed to have minimal volume effects, may be a potential solution to this confounder. It is hard to know, however, whether these assumptions will hold up; if they are inaccurate, it is likely that the null hypothesis will be unduly favored.

Despite the many assumptions and potential pitfalls, it is likely that the PCPT will provide as definitive an answer as is reasonably possible regarding the potential effect of finasteride in the prevention of prostate cancer. Regardless of the results, the successful completion of this trial will represent a historic step forward in the theory and practice of clinical trials in general and in chemoprevention in particular.

8. OTHER 5α-REDUCTASE INHIBITORS

8.1. Type 1 5α-Reductase Inhibitors

Several selective inhibitors of Type 1 5α-reductase have been studied (35–38). Early clinical studies with an orally active, selective Type 1 5α-reductase inhibitor, MK-386, demonstrated less suppression of serum DHT compared with the Type 2 inhibitor finasteride (22% vs 66%), but greater suppression of sebum DHT levels (49% vs 15%) (38). These findings are in keeping with type 1 5α-reductase being predominant in sebaceous glands (39–42). Expression of the Type 1 isozyme in the prostate is controversial. Some studies show Type 1 5α-reductase mRNA in both stroma and epithelial cells (43,44), in epithelial cells (45), and in stroma (46). Type 1 5α-reductase enzyme activity has been detected in some studies in prostate stroma (46) and in prostate homogenates (44, 47), but not detected at all in others (39,48). Immunolocalization of Type 1 5α-reductase is equally controversial (49,50). Regardless of the presence of Type 1 5α-reductase in the prostate, the clinical relevance of Type 1 5α-reductase inhibition in preventing prostate cancer has not been elucidated.

8.2. Nonselective (Type 1 and 2) 5α-Reductase Inhibitors

Inhibition of Type 1 and Type 2 5α-reductase may decrease serum and tissue DHT more than Type 2 inhibition alone, but clinical studies have not yet determined additional efficacy relative to specific Type 2 inhibition. A study in men treated with a combination of the selective Type 1 5α-reductase inhibitor MK-386 together with the specific Type 2 inhibitor finasteride

demonstrated nearly complete (90%) suppression of serum DHT (51). This study confirmed that both Type 1 and Type 2 isozymes of 5α-reductase contribute significantly to the pool of circulating DHT. Nonselective inhibitors, single compounds that inhibit both isoenzymes, appear to have the same effect (52–56). Dutasteride has been approved to treat BPH (55–57). Similarly to the combination of a Type 1 inhibitor and finasteride (51), dutasteride produced nearly complete (>90%) suppression of serum DHT in healthy male subjects (54–56).

8.3. Natural Products

Several natural products believed to possess 5α-reductase inhibitory activity have been used in treating androgenic disorders (57). Among the most common is Permixon®, a lipid-soluble extract from the fruit of *Serenoa repens* (also known as sabal serruta and saw palmetto berry) (58). The fatty acids found in the saponifiable fraction of this extract are believed to be responsible for its 5α-reductase inhibitory activity (59), although several other studies with Permixon® present data that do not reflect such inhibitory activity (60–63). However, these studies did not include any clinically relevant endpoints.

In vitro inhibition of human prostatic 5α-reductase by finasteride, Permixon®, and many other commercially available plant extracts believed to have 5α-reductase inhibitory activity (*Sabalis serrulatae*: Talso, Strogen Forte, Prostagutt, Remigeron; *Pygeum africanum*: Tadenan; *Radix urticae*: Bazoton; and *Hypoxis rooperi*: Harzol) have shown IC_{50} activity (ng/mL) that is 5600–500,000-fold greater than that of finasteride (1 ng/mg), indicating no activity compared to finasteride (64). This same study evaluated Permixon and Bazoton in a castrated rat model stimulated with testosterone or DHT, and showed that only finasteride inhibited testosterone-stimulated prostate growth.

Cactus flower extracts have shown 5α-reductase inhibition in vitro in cultured foreskin fibroblasts (1–100 μg/mL), and prostatic homogenates (0.05–1.3 mg/mL) (65). No clinical data have been presented to determine their efficacy in men. Cernilton®, a pollen extract, has also been reported to have an inhibitory effect on 5α-reductase activity (66).

Clinical trials are equally controversial (64,67–70). A 7-d clinical trial in men showed that finasteride and not Permixon decreased serum DHT (64). In contrast, a study that evaluated the effects of saw palmetto and finasteride on prostate androgen levels measured in biopsy samples showed that saw palmetto significantly reduced DHT levels by 32% and finasteride reduced DHT levels by 80% *(70)*. This result raises the question of whether saw palmetto has, at least, a mild 5α-reductase inhibitory effect. However, when Permixon® and finasteride were evaluated in a 6-mo, large, randomized non-placebo-controlled study in men with BPH, urinary symptoms and flow rate were comparable between groups, but only the finasteride group demonstrated a significant reduction from baseline in serum PSA and prostate size *(69)*. These data would suggest that Permixon® does not have a significant inhibitory effect on 5α-reductase.

In summary, the clinical efficacy of natural products that claim 5α-reductase inhibition in androgenic disorders has not yet been elucidated. Although some studies show in vitro efficacy, the clinical relevance of these products has not been established. In vivo studies in animal models have shown limited efficacy when using extremely high doses of plant extracts compared to finasteride at relatively low doses.

REFERENCES

1. US product circular Medical Economics Company, Inc., for PROSCAR® (finasteride 5 mg tablets), in *Physicians' Desk Reference 53rd ed.*, Montvale, NJ, 1999, pp.1880–1883.
2. Osterling JE. Prostate-specific antigen: a critical assessment of the most useful marker for adenocarcinoma of the prostate. *J Urol* 1991;145:907–923.
3. Andriole G, Guess HA, Epstein JI, et al. Treatment with finasteride preserves usefulness of prostate-specific antigen in the detection of prostate cancer: results of a randomized, double-blind, placebo-controlled clinical trial. PLESS Study Group. Proscar Long-Term Efficacy and Safety Study. *Urology* 1998;52:195–201.
4. Ohtawa M, Morikawa H, Shimazaki J. Pharmacokinetics and biochemical efficacy after single and multiple oral administration of N-(2-methyl-2-propyl)-3-oxo-4-aza-5α-androst-1-ene-17β-carboxamide, a new type of specific competitive inhibitor of testosterone 5α-reductase, in volunteers. *Eur J Drug Metab Pharmacokinet* 1991;16,15–21.
5. Carlin JR, Höglund P, Eriksson LO, et al. Disposition and pharmacokinetics of [14C] finasteride after oral administration in humans. *Drug Metab Dispos* 1992;20,148–155.
6. Huskey SW, Dean DC, Miller RR, et al. Identification of human cytochrome P450 isozymes responsible for the in vitro oxidative metabolism of finasteride. *Drug Metal Dispos* 1995;23,1126–1135.
7. Gormley GJ, Stoner E, Rittmaster RS, et al. Effects of finasteride (MK-906), a 5α-reductase inhibitor, on circulating androgens in male volunteers. *J Clin Endocrinol Metab* 1990;70,1136–1141.
8. Stoner E, the Finasteride Study Group. Three-year safety and efficacy data on the use of finasteride in the treatment of benign prostatic hyperplasia. *Urology* 1994;43,284–294.
9. Rittmaster RS, Lemay A, Zwicker H, et al. Effects of finasteride, a 5α-reductase inhibitor, on serum gonadotropins in normal men. *J Clin Endocrinol Metab* 1992;75,484–488.
10. Tenover JS, Zeitner ME, Plymate SR. Effects of 24-week administration of a 5α-reductase inhibitor (MK-906) on serum levels of testosterone (T), free T, and gonadotropins in men. Proceedings of 71st Annual Meeting of the Endocrine Society; *Program Abstr Endoc Soc Annu Meet* 1989;71:abst. S83.
11. Greenlee RT, Murray T, Bolden S, Wingo PA. Cancer statistics, 2000. *CA Cancer J Clin* 2000;50(1):7–33.
12. Gaddipati J, Ahmed T, Friedland M. Prostatic and bladder cancer in the elderly. *Clin Geriatr Med* 1987;3,649–667.
13. Smith PH, Armitage TG. Immediate vs deferred treatment for early prostatic cancer. *Postgrad Med J* 1987;63,1055–1060.
14. Isaacs JT, Coffey DS. Adaptation vs selection as the mechanism responsible for the relapse of prostatic cancer to androgen ablation therapy as studied in the Dunning R-3327-H adenocarcinoma. *Cancer Res* 1981;41,5070–5075.
15. Huggins C, Hodges CV. I. The effect of castration, of estrogen and of androgen injection on serum phosphatases in metastatic carcinoma of the prostate. *Cancer Res* 1941;1,293–297.
16. Huggins C, Stevens RE, Hodges CV. II. The effects of castration on advanced carcinoma of the prostate gland. *Arch Surg* 1943;43,209–223.
17. Melamed A. Current concepts in the treatment of prostate cancer. *Clin Pharm* 1987;21,247–253.
18. Smith J. New methods of endocrine management of prostatic cancer. *J Urol* 1987;137,1–10.
19. Trump DL, Waldstreicher JA, Kolvenbag G, et al. Androgen antagonists: potential role in prostate cancer prevention. *Urology* 2001;57 (Suppl 4A):64–67.
20. Ross RK, Bernstein L, Judd H, et al. Serum testosterone levels in healthy young black and white men. *J Natl Cancer Inst* 1976;76:45.
21. Bruun E, Frandsen H, Nielsen K, et al. Dihydrotestosterone measured in core biopsies from prostatic tissues. *Am J Clin Oncol* 1988 (Suppl 2):S27–S29.
22. Habib FK, Bissas A, Neill WA, et al. Flow cytometric analysis of cellular DNA in human prostate cancer: relationship to 5α-reductase activity of the tissue. *Urol Res* 1989;17:239–243.
23. Muir C, Waterhouse J, Mack T, et al. *Cancer Incidence in Five Continents, Vol. V*. IARC, Lyon, France, 1987.
24. SEER: *Cancer Incidence and Mortality in the United States*, 1973–1981. US Department of Health and Human Services, Public Health Service, National Institutes of Health, National Cancer Institute, Bethesda, MD, 1984.
25. Ross RK, Bernstein L, Lobo RA, et al. Evidence for reduced 5α-reductase activity in Japanese compared to US Caucasian and African-American males: implications for prostate cancer risk. *Lancet* 1992;339:887–889.
26. Bologna M, Muzi P, Biordi L et al. Antiandrogens and 5α-reductase inhibition of the proliferation rate in PC3 and DU145 human prostatic cancer cell lines. *Curr Ther Res* 1992;51:799–813.
27. Kadoham N, Karr JP, Murphy GP, Sandberg AA. Selective inhibition of prostatic tumor 5α-reductase by a 5-methyl-4-aza-steroid. *Cancer Res* 1984;44:4947–4954.
28. Petrow V, Padilla GM, Mukherji S, Marts SA. Endocrine dependence of prostatic cancer upon dihydrotestosterone

and not upon testosterone. *J Pharm Pharmacol* 1984;36:352–353.

29. McConnell JD, Wilson JD, George FW, et al. Finasteride, an inhibitor of 5α-reductase, suppresses prostatic dihydrotestosterone in men with benign prostatic hyperplasia. *Clin Endocrinol Metab* 1992;74,505–508.

30. Presti JC Jr, Fair WR, Andriole G,, et al. Multicenter, randomized, double blind, placebo controlled study to investigate the effect of finasteride (MK-906) on stage D prostate cancer. *J Urol* 1992;148:11,201–11,204.

31. Nacey JN, Meffan PJ, Delahunt B. The effect of finasteride on prostate volume, urinary flow rate and symptom score in men with benign prostatic hyperplasia. *N Z Med J* 1993;106:109–110.

32. Oesterling JE, Roy J, Agha A, et al. Finasteride PSA study group. Biologic variability of prostate-specific antigen and its usefulness as a marker for prostate cancer: effects of finasteride. *Urology* 1997;50:13–18.

33. Andriole G, Block N, Boake R, et al. Two years of treatment with finasteride after radical prostatectomy. *J Urol* 1994;151:435A.

34. Andriole G, Lieber M, Smith J, et al. Treatment with finasteride following radical prostatectomy for prostate cancer. *Urology* 1995;45:491–497.

35. Jones CD, Audia JE, Lawhorn DE, et al. Nonsteroidal inhibitors of human Type I steroid 5α-reductase. *J Med Chem* 1993;36:421–423.

36. Hirsch KS, Jones CD, Audia JE, et al. LY191704: a selective, nonsteroidal inhibitor of human steriod 5α-reductase Type 1. *Proc Natl Acad Sci USA* 1993;90:5277–5281.

37. Ellsworth K, Azzolina B, Baginsky W, et al. MK386: a potent, selective inhibitor of the human Type 1 5α-reductase. *J Steroid Biochem Mol Biol* 1996;58:377–384.

38. Schwartz JI, Tanaka WK, Wang DZ, et al. MK-386, an inhibitor of 5α-reductase Type 1, reduces dihydrotestosterone concentrations in serum and sebum without affecting dihydrotestosterone concentrations in semen. *J Clin Endocrinol Metab* 1997;82:1373–1377.

39. Harris G, Azzolina B, Baginsky W, et al. Identification and selective inhibition of an isozyme of steroid 5α-reductase in human scalp. *Proc Natl Acad Sci USA* 1992;89:10,787–10,791.

40. Russell DW, Wilson JD. Steroid 5α-reductase two genes/two enzymes. *Annu Rev Biochem* 1994;63:25–61.

41. Thigpen AE, Silver RI, Guileyardo JM, et al. Tissue distribution and ontogeny of steroid 5α-reductase isozyme expression. *J Clin Investig* 1993;92:903–910.

42. Thiboutot D, Harris G, Iles V, et al. Activity of the Type 1 5α-reductase exhibits regional difference in isolated sebaceous glands and whole skin. *J Invest Dermatol* 1995;105:209–214.

43. Pelletier G, Luu-The V, Huang XF, Lapointe H, Labrie F. Localization by the situ hybridization of steroid 5α-reductase isozyme gene expression in the human prostate and preputial skin. *J Urol* 1998;160:577–582.

44. Habib FK, Ross M, Bayne CW, et al. The localization and expression of 5α-reductase Type I and Type II mRNAs in human hyperplastic prostate and in prostate primary cultures. *J Endocrinol* 1998;156:509–517.

45. Iehlé C, Radvanyi F, Diez de Medina, SG, et al. Differences in steroid 5α-reductase iso-enzymes expression between normal and pathological human prostate tissue. *J Steroid Biochem Mol Biol* 1999;68:189–195.

46. Bruchovsky N, Sadar MD, Akakura K, et al. Characterization of 5α-reductase gene expression in stroma and epithelium of human prostate. *J Steroid Biochem* 1996;59:397–404.

47. Span PN, Benraad TJ, Sweep CGJ, Smals AGH. Kinetic analysis of steroid 5α-reductase activity of neutral pH in benign prostatic hyperplastic tissue: evidence for Type I isozyme activity in the human prostate. *J Steroid Biochem Mol Biol* 1996;57:103–110.

48. Smith CM, Ballard SA, Worman N, et al. 5α-reductase expression by prostate cancer cell lines and benign prostatic hyperplasia in vitro. *J Clin Endocrinol Metab* 1996;81:1361–1366.

49. Negri-Cesi P, Poletti A, Colciago A, et al. Presence of 5α-reductase isozymes and aromatase in human prostate cancer cells and in benign prostate hyperplastic tissue. *Prostate* 1998;34:283–291.

50. Silver RI, Wiley EL, Davis DL, et al. Expression and regulation of steroid 5α-reductase 2 in prostate disease. *J Urol* 1994;152:433–437.

51. Schwartz JI, Van Hecken A, De Schepper PJ, et al. Effect of MK-386, a novel inhibitor of Type 1 5α-reductase, alone and in combination with finasteride, on serum dihydrotestosterone concentrations in men. *J Clin Endocrinol Metab* 1996;81:2942–2947.

52. Bakshi RK, Rasmusson GH, Patel GF, et al. 4-Aza-3-oxo-5α-androst-1-ene-17 β-*N*-aryl-carboxamides as dual inhibitors of human Type 1 and Type 2 steroid 5α-reductases. Dramatic effect of N-aryl substituents on Type 1 and Type 2 5α-reductase inhibitory potency. *J Med Chem* 1995;38:3189–3192.

53. Kojo H, Nakayama O, Hirosumi J, et al. Novel steroid 5α-reductase inhibitor FK143: its dual inhibition against the two isozymes and its effect on transcription of the isozyme genes. *Mol Pharmacol* 1995;48:410–406.

54. Bramson HN, Hermann D, Batchelor KW, et al. Unique preclinical characteristics of GG745, a potent dual inhibitor of 5AR. *J Pharmacol Exp Ther* 1997;282:1496–1502.

55. Hermann DJ, Davis IM, Wilson TH. Effects of G1198745 (GG745), a novel 5α-reductase (5AR) inhibitor, on dihydrotestosterone (DHT). *Am Soc Clin Pharmacol Therapeut* 1996;59:162.

56. Hobbs S, Hermann DJ, Gabriel T, et al. Marked suppression of dihydrotestosterone in men by a novel 5α-reductase inhibitor, G1198745. *Fertil Steril* 1998;70:S455.

57. Dreikorn K, Borkowski A, Braeckman J, et al. Other medical therapies, in 4th International Consultation on Benign Prostatic Hyperplasia (BPH). Denis L, Griffiths, K, Cockett ATK, et al. eds. Plymouth, UK:Plymbridge Distributors Ltd., 1998, pp.635–659.

58. Délos S, Iehlé C, Martin PM. Inhibition of the activity of "basic" 5α-reductase (Type 1) detected in DU 145 cells and expressed in insect cells. *J Steroid Biochem Mol Biol* 1994;48:347–352.

59. Weisser H, Tunn S, Behnke B, Krieg M. Effects of the sabal serrulata extract IDS 89 and its subfractions on 5α-reductase activity in human benign prostatic hyperplasia. *Prostate* 1996;28:300–306.

60. Casarosa C, Coscio di Coscio M, Fratta M. Lack of effects of a lyposterolic extract of Seronoa repens on plasma levels of testosterone, follicle-stimulating hormone, and luteinizing hormone. *Clin Ther* 1988;5:585–588.

61. Strauch G, Perles P, Vergult G, et al. Comparison of finasteride (Proscar) and Serenoa repens (Permixon) in the inhibition of 5α-reductase in healthy male volunteers. *Eur Urol* 1994;26:247–252.

62. Braeckman J. The extract of Serenoa reopens in the treatment of benign prostatic hyperplasia: a multi-center open study. *Clin Ther Res* 1994;55:776–785.

63. Champault G, Patel JC, Bonnard A. A double-blind trial of an extract of the plant Serenoa repens in benign prostatic hyperplasia. *Br J Clin Pharmacol* 1984;18:461–462.

64. Rhodes L, Primka RL, Berman C, et al. Comparison of Finasteride (Proscar®), a 5α reductase inhibitor, and various commercial plant extracts in in vitro and in vivo 5α reductase inhibition. *Prostate* 1993;22:43–51.

65. Jonas A, Rosenblat G, Krapf D, et al. Cactus flower extracts may prove beneficial in benign prostatic hyperplasia due to inhibition of 5α-reductase activity, aromatase activity and lipid peroxidation. *Urol Res* 1998;26:265–270.

66. Tunn S, Krieg M. Alterations in the intraprostatic hormonal metabolism by the pollen extract Cernilton®, in *Benign Prostatic Disease*. Vahlensieck W, Rutishauser G, eds. Thieme Medical Publishers, New York, 1992:109–114.

67. Descotes JL, Rambeaud JJ, Deschaseaux P, Faure G. Placebo controlled evaluation of the efficacy and tolerability of Permixon® in benign prostatic hyperplasia after exclusion of placebo responders. *Clin Drug Investig* 1995;9:291–297.

68. Reece Smith H, Memon A, Smart CJ, Dewbury K. The value of Permixon in benign prostatic hypertrophy. *Br J Urol* 1986;58:36–40.

69. Carraro JC, Raynaud JP, Koch G, et al. Comparison of phytotherapy (Permixon) with finasteride in the treatment of benign prostate hyperplasia: a randomized international study of 1098 patients. *Prostate* 1996;29:231–224.

70. Marks LS, Partin AW, Epstein JI, et al. Effects of a saw palmetto herbal blend in men with symptomatic benign prostatic hyperplasia. *J Urol* 2000;163:1451–1456.

14 Searching For SARA

The Role Of Selective Androgen-Receptor Antagonists in Prostate Cancer

Mark S. Chapman, PhD, William Y. Chang, DVM, PhD, Andres Negro-Vilar, MD, PhD, and Jeffrey N. Miner, PhD

CONTENTS

1. INTRODUCTION

In the US, one in six men will develop prostate cancer during his lifetime *(1)*, and prostate cancer accounts for nearly 3% of all deaths in men over age 55 *(2)*. Since prostate cancer is primarily a malignancy of the aged, these numbers are likely to increase as the population ages. Primary treatment for prostate cancer typically involves radical prostatectomy, external beam radiation, or brachytherapy (seeding· the prostate with radioisotope). All these therapies lead to about a 30% rate of recurrence *(2a)*. Androgen ablation is most often used as second-line therapy, since prostate-derived cancers are, at least initially, androgen-dependent for growth. Androgen ablation is commonly achieved by surgical castration, the use of GnRH super-agonists to block LH release and thus inhibit testosterone synthesis, or the use of androgen antagonists alone or in combination with GnRH agonists.

This chapter provides an overview of the mechanism of androgen action, particularly how it relates to both prostate cancer and current therapies. We also discuss some relevant issues regarding androgen signaling in current prostate cancer treatments, and some strategies intended to develop selective androgen receptor antagonists (SARAs), improved antagonists of androgen-receptor action for prostate cancer.

2. THE ANDROGEN RECEPTOR/ANDROGEN RECEPTOR (AR) ACTION

Androgen action is required during embryogenesis to develop male sex organs, and at puberty to initiate spermatogenesis and enlargement of sex organs, including the prostate *(3)*. Throughout adulthood, males need androgens to maintain sexual function as well as bone and muscle mass. Androgens act primarily by altering gene expression via the androgen receptor (AR), which functions as a ligand-dependent transcription factor. Studies increasingly point to the non-genomic effects of androgens (as well as other steroids). For example, rapid responses to testosterone can occur through a calcium-signaling pathway, apparently utilizing a membrane-bound receptor *(4)*. However, the majority of cellular and organismal responses to androgens are mediated by AR. AR is a member of the nuclear receptor (NR) superfamily, which includes other steroid

From: Cancer Chemoprevention, Volume 1: Promising Cancer Chemoprevention Agents
Edited by: G. J. Kelloff, E. T. Hawk, and C. C. Sigman © Humana Press Inc., Totowa, NJ

receptors such as the estrogen receptor (ER) and the glucocorticoid receptor, receptors for nonsteroidal ligands such as the thyroid hormone receptor (TR), retinoic acid receptor (RAR), and vitamin D receptor (VDR), as well as orphan receptors, so named because their regulatory ligands have not been identified. NRs function as ligand-dependent transcription factors, typically binding to their cognate response elements in the promoter region of target genes and positively or negatively regulating gene expression. The structural organization of NRs is highly conserved and modular, consisting of a carboxyl-terminal ligand-binding domain (LBD) which contains a ligand-dependent transcriptional activation function (AF-2), a central highly conserved zinc-finger DNA-binding motif, and usually an amino-terminal ligand-independent transcriptional activation function AF-1. Typically, AF-1 is much longer in steroid receptors than the N-terminal domain of other NRs.

AR is believed to be mainly cytoplasmic in the absence of androgens or other ligands, where it is associated with a complex of chaperones, including heat shock protein 90. After interacting with ligand, AR undergoes a conformational change, releases the chaperone complex, and becomes competent for nuclear localization, homodimerization, and DNA binding to androgen response elements (AREs) in the promoter region of AR target genes. Thus, the sequence of events in AR action is: binding in the cytoplasm of the ligand to the AR LBD, nuclear localization, dimerization, and DNA binding, followed by activation (or repression) of the target genes (5). AR does not bind directly to the DNA of genes that are repressed by androgens, but rather to another DNA-binding protein (such as the transcription factor NFκB), inhibiting its transactivation (6). AR activates and represses transcription through interaction with a large number of coactivator and corepressor proteins. These factors, together with the receptor, mediate signaling between the androgen and gene.

Two major natural ligands for AR are testosterone and dihydrotestosterone (DHT) (5). Testosterone can be converted to DHT by 5α-reductases. Since many of the negative effects of androgens (such as prostate stimulation, acne, and male pattern baldness) have been attributed to DHT, attempts have been made to suppress the action of 5α-reductases. For example, finasteride, a 5α-reductase inhibitor, has been examined in a prospective study as a cancer-chemopreventive agent, but was not clearly shown to be effective (7), perhaps because testosterone remains as a strong AR agonist. Several synthetic AR agonists have been developed, and most

of these are structurally and functionally very similar to testosterone and DHT. Testosterone—and to a lesser extent, synthetic androgens—are used to treat hypogonadism (defined as low endogenous testosterone), a common condition, especially among aging men. Antagonists for AR, such as the artificial steroid cyproterone acetate or the nonsteroidal antagonists flutamide and casodex, bind with high affinity to AR but do not activate the receptor. As antagonists, they block or compete with agonists for AR binding. Thus, even in the presence of testosterone or DHT, these antagonists can block the proliferative effects of AR on prostate cells.

Cofactors (coactivators and corepressors) act as bridging proteins or adaptors between NRs and the basal transcription machinery (8). One well-studied class of cofactors, shown to interact with many NRs, is the LxxLL motif-containing family (where L denotes leucine and x any amino acid). The LxxLL sequence is critical for interaction with NRs via an α-helical portion of the NR LBD. Upon ligand binding, the LBD undergoes a conformational change that permits interaction between the LxxLL region of the cofactor and the NR (8).

A number of cofactors have been identified that interact with AR, including several containing LxxLL-motifs (9). Some cofactors appear to be restricted to specific tissues; this is believed to be one way in which tissue-specific gene expression is achieved. For example, the coactivator ARA55 is highly expressed in prostate but expressed at only very low levels in other tissues. Since ARA55 has been shown to coactivate AR (10), it may contribute to the prostate specificity of AR target gene expression for genes such as prostate-specific antigen (PSA). Thus, cell- or tissue-specific cofactor expression could provide a mechanism for androgens to exert different effects on different tissues even when AR expression and ligand availability do not vary between such cells or tissues. However, it is also clear that the tissue-selective expression of cofactors is only one of several mechanisms that contribute to tissue- and gene-specific effects of androgens and other steroid hormones. For example, varying levels of combinatorial recruitment of co-activators and release of co-repressors at different times in different cell or tissue contexts is also believed to play a major role in tissue-selective gene regulation by steroid hormones, including androgens.

Recruitment of cofactors to NRs can also be influenced by the nature of the ligand bound in the LBD. X-ray crystallographic analysis of the receptor has demonstrated that upon binding ligand, the LBD collapses in around the embedded ligand, incorporating the ligand into the internal structure of the liganded receptor *(11)*. The molecular structure of the ligand influences conformation of the LBD, and these changes are transmitted to the outer surface of the receptor. Such surface changes can influence the affinity and specificity of cofactors for the receptor, which in turn could modulate the effectiveness of AR regulation of a subset of genes. For example, if an AR ligand causes a conformational change that prevents a cofactor (for example, the cofactor GRIP1) from interacting with AR, genes that require GRIP1 for transactivation by AR will not be regulated in response to that ligand. In fact, ligands with this profile will act as antagonists on GRIP1-requiring genes when co-administered with a full agonist such as testosterone. Synthetic NR ligands are being developed to have increased selectivity in cofactor recruitment (compared to the natural ligand for the receptor or synthetic derivatives currently used as drugs), therefore regulating a desirable subset of the target genes. Selective estrogen receptor modulators (SERMs) such as tamoxifen may work in this way *(12)*. These molecular approaches have now been extended to search for other similar targets to obtain a beneficial therapeutic ratio from molecules displaying tissue selectivity. In particular, selective AR modulators (SARMs) that are currently in development provide novel agents for treating and preventing androgen-mediated disorders such as prostate cancer, benign prostatic hypertrophy, acne, hirsutism, and changes associated with hypogonadism—e.g., osteoporosis, sexual dysfunction, frailty, and cachexia *(13,14)*.

Unlike most nuclear receptors, the AR amino-terminal end can interact with a portion of the AR LBD in a ligand-dependent manner. Interestingly, an LxxLL-like motif, FxxLF (in which phenyalanines replace two of the leucines) in the amino-terminal portion of AR is required for this so-called *N–C* interaction *(15)*. He et al. have shown that this *N–C* interaction can inhibit recruitment of LxxLL-containing coactivators such as GRIP1 to the AR LBD *(16)*; however, the significance of the *N–C* interaction and its role in AR function is not fully understood. AR has been shown to undergo a number of posttranslational modifications, such as phosphorylation *(17,18)*, acetylation *(19)*, and sumoylation *(20)*. Phosphorylation of AR may in some cases result in receptor activation in the absence of ligand *(18,21)*.

A number of AR target genes have been identified. PSA is probably the best-known of these, because of its diagnostic value. PSA is used as an early marker of prostate cancer onset, and to evaluate disease progression. The regulatory region of the PSA gene contains several AREs, in addition to elements that confer a high degree of prostate specificity *(22)*. More recently, Nelson et al. used microarray technology to identify 146 genes that respond to androgens in the prostate cancer cell line LNCaP *(23)*; a subset of these are likely to be direct AR targets. Despite advances like these, it should be noted that the genetic program by which AR causes prostate-cell proliferation and its potential linkage to cancer progression are not fully understood.

3. THE PROSTATE: AN AR TARGET ORGAN

The prostate is a multifunctional glandular component of the male reproductive system located anterior to the rectum and just below the bladder. The primary function of the prostate is to contribute to seminal fluid, which transports sperm during ejaculation. Seventy percent (70%) of this organ is comprised of secretory tissue and supporting stroma. The prostate also contains approximately 30% smooth-muscle tissue; contraction of this gland during ejaculation helps to expel semen into the urethra *(24)*.

Men less than 40 yr of age rarely present with complications associated with the prostate; therefore, prostatic diseases are considered to be diseases of the aged. Men age 40 and over are more prone to development of benign prostatic hyperplasia (BPH), prostatitis, and prostate cancer. The incidence of prostate cancer in these men is 1 in 10 *(25)*. Since the prostate is a walnut-sized secretory gland that surrounds the urethra near the bladder neck, many prostate diseases can result in structural changes in the urethra and dysuria. BPH is a benign enlargement that occurs in the transitional zone, the region of the prostate immediately surrounding the urethra. Histologically present in 80% of men over 40, BPH's predilection for the transitional zone often results in signs of increased urinary frequency, urinary hesitancy, or urinary urgency. Prostatitis also occurs in the transitional zone of the prostate, but most frequently presents with dysuria resulting from local inflammation. Prostate cancer, however, usually occurs in the peripheral zone of the prostate; therefore, urinary symptoms do not usually present unless cancer is advanced *(26)*. Prostate cancer is more often diagnosed by elevated circulating PSA and digital rectal examination, with subsequent confirmation via biopsy.

Causes of these prostatic diseases are unknown, but circulating androgens are believed to be a contributing factor. Men who are castrated at a young age do not develop BPH and surgical castration has been shown to cause regression of prostate cancer. Currently, no known association exists between BPH and prostate cancer.

4. CLINICAL NEED: PROSTATE CANCER

AR antagonists have been widely used in the treatment of advanced prostate cancer. In the 1940s, Huggins and Hodges first proposed that prostate cancer is hormonally responsive when they demonstrated that surgical castration can reduce prostate size in prostate cancer patients (27). Since then, endocrine therapy targeting reduction in circulating levels of androgens and/or inhibition of androgenic effects has been the basis of therapeutics for prostate cancer. Prostatectomy with or without external beam irradiation is standard for localized tumors (28), but endocrine therapy is the treatment of choice for more advanced prostate cancer. GnRH analogs such as Lupron are used to reduce endogenous synthesis of testicular androgens as a form of medical castration. The major challenge in prostate cancer treatment, however, is progression of advanced prostate cancer to an androgen-independent state following 2–4 yr of endocrine therapy. Although initial experience with estrogen-insensitive breast cancers suggested that the hormone-insensitive state may be associated with a loss of steroid-receptor expression, in prostate cancer the AR has been detected immunohistochemically in hormonal-refractory cancers (29–33). Although mutations of AR have been identified that affect ligand activity, the majority of cancers contain wild-type AR. Retention of functional AR suggests that, even in an androgen-insensitive state, the receptor may still play a critical role in cancer progression, and may be a potential target for development of novel therapeutics against hormone-refractory prostate cancer.

5. ENDOCRINE THERAPY FOR PROSTATE CANCER

The current principles of therapy for prostate cancer still stem from the findings of Huggins and Hodges (27). Patients with locally advanced and metastatic prostate cancers are treated using GnRH analogs (e.g.,

Lupron) or surgical castration to abolish testicular androgens. Surgical castration by bilateral orchiectomy, although still practiced, has been largely replaced by chemical castration using GnRH analogs. A nonsteroidal antiandrogen (e.g., flutamide, bicalutamide, or nilutamide) can be given in combination with castration for a more complete ablation of androgen effects by blocking remaining adrenal androgens (combination androgen blockade, CAB) (25). Adrenal androgen synthesis inhibitors such as ketoconazole and hydrocortisone can be added. However, whether endocrine therapy is surgical or chemical, the drawback of endocrine therapy is tumor development to an androgen-independent state within 18–48 mo (26). Any SARA that initially targets androgen-responsive prostate cancer should have the potential to delay the progression of androgen independence and clinical trials of SARAs should assess this potential benefit (34).

The current recommended protocol for endocrine treatment of prostate cancer is undergoing more rigorous scrutiny. A recent Overview Consensus Statement by the Second International Conference on Newer Approaches to Androgen Deprivation Therapy (35) recommended that CAB using a GnRH agonist with a nonsteroidal androgen antagonist should not be considered standard therapy in asymptomatic patients with early prostate cancer. This recommendation was submitted in the absence of data that CAB had any clinically significant disease-free or overall survival advantage or significant quality-of-life advantage over antiandrogen monotherapy (35–37). Early results from a monotherapy study suggest that bicalutamide may even reduce objective progression of disease and PSA progression after a median follow-up of 3 yr (38). Antiandrogen monotherapy does have beneficial effects on PSA failure rates, but more studies are needed to evaluate its impact on disease-free and overall survival rates (35). In patients with advanced metastatic prostate cancer, medical or surgical castration still offers a better outcome than antiandrogen monotherapy (35). However, some studies suggest that survival time for locally advanced or metastatic prostate cancer was the same for 150 mg/d bicalutamide and castration (39). These recommendations may need to be revisited as more clinical data are accumulated.

6. SIDE EFFECTS OF ENDOCRINE THERAPY

Interest in new therapeutic regimens such as antiandrogen monotherapy and intermittent hormone therapy arose from the potential to provide improved quality of life compared to GnRH analog therapy. Quality-of-life concerns are growing increasingly more significant in men with prostate cancer, causing greater demand for better pharmaceutical approaches and/or regimens using currently available drugs *(39)*. Intermittent hormone therapy involves discontinuing GnRH analogs after 7 mo of treatment if the patient's PSA levels fall below 4 ng/dL, until PSA levels rise above 20 ng/dL *(40)*. In addition to reducing the impact of side effects associated with endocrine therapy, intermittent hormone therapy also seeks to reduce costs of medication and, theoretically, to prolong time to development of androgen independence. Antiandrogen monotherapy may also offer quality-of-life benefits while maintaining the same effectiveness as castration in treatment of early prostate cancer *(41,42)*. Some major side effects of clinical concern in androgen ablation therapy include the loss of bone and increased risk of fractures, reduced muscle mass and strength, breast pain and/or gynecomastia, and diminished sexual function. In theory, an optimal SARA would maintain full efficacy in prostate cancer growth inhibition without generating these side effects.

Loss of libido and erectile dysfunction are frequent concerns associated with androgen ablation therapy. In fact, concerns about the impact of endocrine therapy on sexual function are so significant that many patients are willing to trade survival time to maintain sexual function *(43,44)*. Although factors contributing to overall decline in sexual function may include the psychological impact of diagnosis and the disease process itself, the predominant factor is loss of libido resulting from ablation and/or blockade of androgens effected by the treatment regimen *(45)*. With advanced prostate cancer, medical or surgical castration alone or combined with an antiandrogen is used to reduce circulating androgen levels and to reduce the androgenic impact of residual androgens. Both approaches are associated with loss of libido and erectile function in more than 80% of patients *(39)*. Some scientists have advocated the use of antiandrogen monotherapy in an effort to preserve sexual function. The theoretical basis for this is built on the potential of antiandrogens to block negative feedback of testosterone on the hypothalamus and the pituitary gland, thus elevating or maintaining circulating LH and testosterone levels, while antagonizing the effects of androgens at target tissues *(39)*. Since sexual function is believed to be maintained by metabolites of testos-

terone, an antiandrogen may have no effect on these pathways *(46–48)*. Studies have shown that testosterone levels are maintained within normal ranges when using antiandrogen monotherapy, and estrogen levels are elevated because aromatase is still available *(49)*. In support of this theory, men treated with bicalutamide monotherapy maintained greater libido and erectile function than those treated with castration *(38,50,51)*. However, not all antiandrogens spared sexual function. Cyproterone acetate was reported to reduce libido and erectile potency, similarly to castration *(50)*. Inadequate androgen blockade, which is associated with lower doses of bicalutamide or flutamide, or questionable accuracy in reporting loss of sexual activity and the quality of the questionnaires used to evaluate libido, may have contributed to the persistence of sexual function in the previously mentioned studies. Further understanding of the actions of androgens and their metabolites in sexual motivation and function is essential to the continued development of antiandrogens with minimal or no detrimental effects.

Another side effect of concern in androgen ablation therapy is bone loss. Daniell reported an increased rate of osteoporotic fractures in men who were undergoing androgen ablation therapy *(53)*. In a retrospective study, the frequency of osteoporotic fractures in men after orchiectomy was 15% compared with 1% in men with prostate cancer who did not have androgen ablation therapy *(53)*. Similarly, medical castration using GnRH agonists has been shown to decrease bone-mineral density in prostate cancer patients *(54,55)*. It has been postulated that contributing factors include low initial bone-mineral density as a result of advanced age *(56,57)*, bone loss resulting from therapy *(56)*, and increased tendency to fall caused by muscle weakness, age, and impaired balance *(58)*. However, encouraging data suggests that bone loss could be minimized with synthetic compounds such as SARAs. In a study using age-matched controls, long-term (median duration 5.5 yr) bicalutamide monotherapy in men with prostate cancer had no effect on bone-mineral density in the lumbar spine, proximal femur, and total hip compared to age-matched controls *(59)*. In the same study, bone mineral density was lower in orchiectomized men *(59)*. These results suggest that an androgen antagonist could have diverse activity in certain tissue targets, such as bone.

The most common complaints associated with antiandrogen monotherapy are gynecomastia and breast pain. Complaints of gynecomastia and breast pain were reported in approx 40% of those taking bicalutamide monotherapy (38,42). This incidence of gynecomastia is higher than that of GnRH therapy (51). Although this complication is well-tolerated, it represents a side effect in which a synthetic antiandrogen may present a greater disadvantage than GnRH therapy. Hot flashes appear to be less prevalent in patients using bicalutamide monotherapy vs a GnRH analog; this result could also be caused by incomplete androgen blockade (42).

These data on current antiandrogens suggest that it is possible to develop androgen-receptor antagonists with reduced side-effect profiles. Successful development of SARAs with minimal complications is feasible with greater understanding of the processes that lead to side effects associated with antiandrogen therapy and the pivotal role of ARs in these processes.

7. PROSTATE CANCER PROGRESSION TO AN ANDROGEN-INSENSITIVE STATE

In order to understand the challenges involved in the development of a SARA for prostate cancer, this section reviews some theories behind the mechanisms through which prostate cancer develops androgen independence, and benefits and side effects of current nonsteroidal antiandrogens.

Several theories on the mechanism through which prostate cancer progresses to an androgen-independent state include: AR amplification, AR mutation, ligand-independent activation of the AR by growth factors, and interactions with coregulators (AR in the refractory state, reviewed in ref. 60). All of these mechanisms rely on the presence of AR, postulating a critical function for AR even in androgen-independent cells. Thus, although these tumors are termed androgen-independent, they are AR-dependent. Despite their independence from androgens, these tumors may still be viable targets for SARAs. And, as the diverse theories on progression to an androgen-independent state suggest, there may not be one "catch-all" SARA strategy for hormone-refractory prostate cancers, in which AR amplification and overexpression are common (61–65). Amplification and overexpression of wild-type AR allows prostate cancer cells to become hypersensitive to low circulating androgen levels, and may be favorable for the cancer to undergo clonal expansion in an androgen-deprived environment. To combat this phenomenon, clinicians have employed the therapeutic strategy of CAB, which uses GnRH analogs to block endogenous synthesis of testosterone

and antiandrogens to block residual activity on AR with or without blockers of adrenal androgen synthesis.

Another mechanism for progression to the androgen-independent state is mutation of the AR. Depending on the location and type of mutation, the receptor may develop hypersensitivity, promiscuity, or gain of function (66–75). One of the most frequently characterized mutations is the LNCaP mutation, in which the threonine at codon 877 is replaced with an alanine (76–78). The mutant receptor is no longer strictly androgen-dependent, but can function as a transcriptional activator by binding to ligands for other receptors such as cortisone and other glucocorticoids, as well as estrogenic and progestogenic steroids (79). Perhaps most disturbingly, the LNCaP mutant AR responds to nonsteroidal antiandrogens such as flutamide as though they were agonists (76–78). Such promiscuity of the AR as a result of a mutation in the coding sequence has been postulated to be the cause of antiandrogen withdrawal syndrome (80,81). In such cases, removal of antiandrogen can result in at least a transient inhibition of cancerous growth and transient decreases in PSA levels. Kelly et al. (82) and Scher and Kelly (83) first described prostate cancer patients on CAB (GnRH or castration with flutamide) who showed subsequent increases in PSA 12–28 mo following initial response to hormonal therapy. Consequent discontinuation of flutamide reduced PSA by 37–89%. One case with bone lesions even showed clinical improvement. This syndrome has also been described for bicalutamide (82,84,85) and nilutamide (86). Mutations such as the LNCaP mutation that allow activation of AR by hormones other than androgens may favor clonal expansion in an androgen-deprived environment (26,71,87). This theory is supported by the observation that the frequency of AR mutation is rare in localized prostate cancer (88), with increasing frequency in more advanced cancers. Subsequent acquisition of mutations following tumor progression suggests that mutation is not a causative factor of tumor initiation, but rather a result of androgen ablation therapy (26). The frequency of AR mutations in hormone-refractory prostate cancer is still not well-established, but it does not appear to occur in the majority of these cancers (63,69,89–92).

The polyglutamine region on the AR coding sequence is also associated with prostate cancer progression. Located on exon 1 of the AR, the polyglutamine region is encoded by CAG repeats and associated with androgen insensitivity *(93)*, prostate cancer risk *(94,95)*, and tumor aggressiveness *(96,97)*. Reported somatic contraction of the CAG repeat may give cells a growth advantage that promotes cancer progression *(63,98)*. The polyglutamine region may act as a regulator of AR transactivational activity, since length of the CAG repeat has been inversely correlated with the ability of AR to activate transcription *(99)*. The region's function in transactivational activity may be related to its role in regulating receptor mRNA stability, interacting with cofactors that bind to the *N*-terminus of AR, or interacting between *N*- and *C*-termini of AR *(100–105)*. Currently, the polyglutamine region's function has not been clearly established. Additional studies on the link between of CAG polymorphism and prostate cancer risk are needed to confirm this hypothesis.

In an androgen-deprived environment, ligand-independent activation of AR may become a critical signaling pathway for induction of transcriptional activity in hormone-refractory prostate cancer. Human AR has been shown to be activated in a non-ligand-mediated fashion by growth factors (e.g., EGF, IGF-I, KGF) in androgen-independent prostate cancer cells *(21,106,107)*. In fact, forskolin, an activator of protein kinase A, increases intracellular cyclic adenosine monophospate (cAMP) and can activate AR in a prostate cancer-cell line whose growth is androgen- independent *(21,107)*. These signals may reduce or eliminate the need for androgens in activation of the androgen-signaling pathways *(108)*. Ligand-independent activation of AR may play a role in the ability of prostate cells to maintain function and thrive in an androgen-deprived state.

Finally, transcriptional activity of AR is regulated by interaction with various coregulators *(109)*. For example, overexpression of some coactivators such as transcriptional intermediary factor-2 (TIF-2), steroid receptor coactivator-1 (SRC-1) and ARA_{70} may increase the activational activity of AR and make the receptor superactive *(64,109,110)*. This suggests the possibility that altered regulation or mutation of coregulators may produce aberrant prostate cancer growth.

8. DEVELOPMENT OF NOVEL ANTIANDROGENS

Since there are several mechanisms by which prostate cancer can become androgen-independent, many approaches can be taken to develop improved antiandrogens. Of course, the ideal drug should target the wild-type receptor in androgen-dependent prostate cancer as well as both mutant and wild-type receptors in androgen-independent prostate cancer.

In a subset of prostate cancers that fail therapy using existing AR antagonists (e.g., bicalutamide, flutamide, and nilutamide), AR has undergone a point mutation in the LBD that causes the antagonist to act as an agonist (reviewed in *60*). Since some of these point mutations frequently occur in prostate cancer, an AR antagonist that is resistant to specific LBD mutations could be developed (for example, a compound that still functions as an antagonist in LNCaP cells). This type of drug would be of specific value in patients who have failed treatment with existing AR antagonists as a result of the specific mutation. On average, it may also delay onset of androgen independence when used as the initial antiandrogen. However, in some cases, it is likely that selective pressure would eventually result in novel AR LBD mutations and subsequent clonal expansions, just as with existing antiandrogens.

More novel approaches to suppression of AR activity may result in a drug with a longer useful life in treating prostate cancer. In theory, any of the steps in androgen action could be targeted, including AR nuclear localization, dimerization, or DNA binding, AR protein post-translational modifications, AR-cofactor interactions, AR protein stability, or even specific AR target gene products. Intriguingly, certain polyphenolic flavonoids that have been effective in cancer treatment also decrease androgen-stimulated growth of prostate cancer-cell lines and reduce nuclear localization of AR in LNCaP cells *(111)*, suggesting that blocking AR from the nucleus may indeed be a viable pharmacologic approach. Furthermore, small molecules that specifically inhibit AR dimerization or DNA binding might be developed. The enzymes involved in posttranslational modifications of AR are also potential targets, although inhibition of such enzymes may affect other pathways as well. Drugs that specifically block interactions between AR and cofactors (or the AR *N-C* interaction) would be particularly attractive, especially if they involved prostate-specific cofactors. Clearly, further research is warranted in this area in order to realize the full potential of developing a truly novel SARA for chemopreventive and chemotherapeutic use.

REFERENCES

1. Potosky AL, Miller BA, Albertson PC, et al. The role of increasing detection in the rising incidence of prostate cancer. *JAMA* 1995;273:548–552.

2. Hanks GE, Myers CE, Scardino PT. Cancer of the prostate, in *Cancer: Principles and Practice of Oncology*, 4th ed. DeVita VT Jr, Hellman S, Rosenberg SA, eds. Philadelphia, PA, J.B. Lippincott Co. 1993, pp. 1073–1113.

2a. Feldman BJ, Feldman D. The development of androgen-independent prostate cancer. *Nat Rev Cancer* 2001;1:34–45.

3. Nef S, Parada LF. Hormones in male sexual development. *Genes Dev* 2000;14:3075–3086.

4. Guo Z, Benton WP, Krucken J, Wunderlich F. Nongenomic testosterone calcium signaling. Genotropic actions in androgen receptor-free macrophages. *J Biol Chem* 2002;277:29,600–29,607.

5. Beato M, Klug J. Steroid hormone receptors: an update. *Hum Reprod Update* 2000;6:225–236.

6. Keller ET, Chang C, Ershler WB. Inhibition of NFκB activity through maintenance of IκBα levels contributes to dihydrotestosterone-mediated repression of the interleukin-6 promoter. *J Biol Chem* 1996;271:26,267–26,275.

7. Irani J, Ravery V., Pariente JL, et al. Effect of nonsteroidal anti-inflammatory agents and finasteride on prostate cancer risk. *J Urol* 2002;168:1985–1988.

8. Glass CK, Rosenfeld MG. The coregulator exchange in transcriptional functions of nuclear receptors. *Genes Dev* 2000;14:121–141.

9. Beitel LK. http://ww2.mcgill.ca/androgendb/ARinteract.pdf. 2002.

9a. Sampson ER, Yeh SY, Chang HC, et al. Identification and characterization of androgen receptor associated coregulators in prostate cancer cells. *J Biol Regul Homeost Agents* 2001;15:123–129.

10. Fujimoto N, Yeh S, Kang HY, et al. Cloning and characterization of androgen receptor coactivator, ARA55, in human prostate. *J Biol Chem* 1999;274:8316–8321.

11. Weatherman RV, Fletterick RJ, Scanlan TS. Nuclear-receptor ligands and ligand-binding domains. *Annu Rev Biochem* 1999;68:559–581.

12. Shang Y, Hu X, DiRenzo J, et al. Cofactor dynamics and sufficiency in estrogen receptor-regulated transcription. *Cell* 2000;103:843–852.

13. Negro-Vilar A. Selective androgen receptor modulators (SARMs): a novel approach to androgen therapy for the new millennium. *J Clin Endocrinol Metab* 1999;84:3459–3462.

14. Reid P, Kantoff P, Oh W. Antiandrogens in prostate cancer. *Investig New Drugs* 1999;17:271–284.

15. He B, Kemppainen JA, Wilson EM. FXXLF and WXXLF sequences mediate the NH2-terminal interaction with the ligand binding domain of the androgen receptor. *J Biol Chem* 2000;275:22,986–22,994.

16. He B, Bowen NT, Minges JT, Wilson EM. Androgen-induced NH2- and COOH-terminal interaction inhibits p160 coactivator recruitment by activation function 2. *J Biol Chem* 2001;276:42,293–42,301.

17. Goueli SA, Holtzman JL, Ahmed K. Phosphorylation of the androgen receptor by a nuclear cAMP-independent protein kinase. *Biochem Biophys Res Commun* 1984;123:778–784.

18. Gioeli D, Ficarro SB, Kwiek JJ, et al. Androgen receptor phosphorylation. Regulation and identification of the phosphorylation sites. *J Biol Chem* 2002;277:29,304–29,314.

19. Gaughan L, Logan IR, Cook S, et al. Tip60 and histone deacetylase 1 regulate androgen receptor activity through changes to the acetylation status of the receptor. *J Biol Chem* 2002;277:25,904–25,913.

20. Nishida T, Yasuda H. PIAS1 and PIASxalpha function as SUMO-E3 ligases toward androgen receptor and repress androgen receptor-dependent transcription. *J Biol Chem* 2002;277:41,311–41,317.

21. Nazareth LV, Weigel NL. Activation of the human androgen receptor through a protein kinase A signaling pathway. *J Biol Chem* 1996;271:19,900–19,907.

22. Farmer G, Connolly ES Jr, Mocco J, Freedman LP. Molecular analysis of the prostate-specific antigen upstream gene enhancer. *Prostate* 2001;46:76–85.

23. Nelson PS, Clegg N, Arnold H, et al. The program of androgen-responsive genes in neoplastic prostate epithelium. *Proc Natl Acad Sci USA* 2002;99:11,890–11,895.

24. Pennefather JN, Lau WA, Mitchelson F, Ventura S. The autonomic and sensory innervation of the smooth muscle of the prostate gland: a review of pharmacological and histological studies. *J Auton Pharmacol* 2000;20:193–206.

25. Kolvenbag GJ, Iversen P, Newling DW. Antiandrogen monotherapy: a new form of treatment for patients with prostate cancer. *Urology* 2001;58:16–23.

26. Taplin ME, Ho SM. Clinical review 134: the endocrinology of prostate cancer. *J Clin Endocrinol Metab* 2001;86:3467–3477.

27. Huggins C, Hodges CV. The effect of castration, of oestrogen and of androgen injections on serum phosphatases in metastatic carcinoma of the prostate. *Cancer Res* 1941;1:293–297.

28. Bolla M, Gonzales D, Warde P, et al. Improved survival in patients with locally advanced prostate cancer treated with radiotherapy and goserelin. *N Engl J Med* 1997;337:295–300.

29. Culig Z, Hobisch A, Bartsch G, Klocker H. Androgen receptor—an update of mechanisms of action in prostate cancer. *Urol Res* 2000;28:211–219.

30. de Winter JA, Trapman J, Brinkmann AO, et al. Androgen receptor heterogeneity in human prostatic carcinomas visualized by immunohistochemistry. *J Pathol* 1990;160:329–332.

31. Baumann CT, Lim CS, Hager GL. Intracellular localization and trafficking of steroid receptors. *Cell Biochem Biophys* 1999;31:119–127.

32. Trapman J, Cleutjens KB. Androgen-regulated gene expression in prostate cancer. *Semin Cancer Biol* 1997;8:29–36.

33. van der Kwast TH, Schalken J, Ruizeveld de Winter JA, et al. Androgen receptors in endocrine-therapy-resistant human prostate cancer. *Int J Cancer* 1991;48:189–193.

34. Lieberman R. Androgen deprivation therapy for prostate cancer chemoprevention: current status and future directions for agent development. *Urology* 2001;58(Suppl 1):83–90.

35. Carroll PR, Kantoff PW, Balk SP, et al. Overview consensus statement. Newer approaches to androgen deprivation therapy in prostate cancer. *Urology* 2002;60(Suppl 1):1–6.

36. Eisenberger MA, Blumenstein BA, Crawford ED, et al. Bilateral orchiectomy with or without flutamide for metastatic prostate cancer. *N Engl J Med* 1998;339:1036–1042.

37. Caubet JF, Tosteson TD, Dong EW, et al. Maximum androgen blockade in advanced prostate cancer: a meta-analysis of

published randomized controlled trials using nonsteroidal antiandrogens. *Urology* 1997;49:71–78.

38. McLeod DG. Emerging role of adjuvant hormonal therapy. *Urology* 2002;60(Suppl 1):13–20.

39. Iversen P, Melezinek I, Schmidt, A. Nonsteroidal antiandrogens: a therapeutic option for patients with advanced prostate cancer who wish to retain sexual interest and function. *BJU Int* 2001;87:47–56.

40. Crook JM, Szumacher E, Malone S, et al. Intermittent androgen suppression in the management of prostate cancer. *Urology* 1999;53:530–534.

41. Tyrrell CJ, Kaisary AV, Iversen P, et al. A randomised comparison of 'Casodex' (bicalutamide) 150 mg monotherapy versus castration in the treatment of metastatic and locally advanced prostate cancer. *Eur Urol* 1998;33:447–456.

42. Iversen P, Tyrrell CJ, Kaisary AV, et al. Bicalutamide monotherapy compared with castration in patients with non-metastatic locally advanced prostate cancer: 6.3 years of followup. *J Urol* 2000;164:1579–1582.

43. Mazur DJ, Hickman DH. Patient preferences: survival vs quality-of-life considerations. *J Gen Intern Med* 1993;8:374–377.

44. Singer PA, Tasch ES, Stocking C, et al. Sex or survival: trade-offs between quality and quantity of life. *J Clin Oncol* 1991;9:328–334.

45. Eton DT, Lepore SJ. Prostate cancer and health-related quality of life: a review of the literature. *Psychooncology* 2002;11:307–326.

46. de Bruijn M, Broekman M, van der Schoot P. Sexual interactions between estrous female rats and castrated male rats treated with testosterone propionate or estradiol benzoate. *Physiol Behav* 1988;43:35–39.

47. Sodersten P, Eneroth P, Hansson T, et al. Activation of sexual behaviour in castrated rats: the role of oestradiol. *J Endocrinol* 1986;111:455–462.

48. Crews D, Morgentaler A. Effects of intracranial implantation of oestradiol and dihydrotestosterone on the sexual behaviour of the lizard *Anolis carolinensis*. *J Endocrinol* 1979;82:373–381.

49. Verhelst J, Denis L, Van Vliet P, et al. Endocrine profiles during administration of the new non-steroidal anti-androgen Casodex in prostate cancer. *Clin Endocrinol (Oxf)* 1994;41:525–530.

50. Chodak G, Sharifi R, Kasimis B, et al. Single-agent therapy with bicalutamide: a comparison with medical or surgical castration in the treatment of advanced prostate carcinoma. *Urology* 1995;46:849–855.

51. Boccardo F, Rubagotti A, Barichello M, et al. Bicalutamide monotherapy versus flutamide plus goserelin in prostate cancer patients: results of an Italian Prostate Cancer Project study. *J Clin Oncol* 1999;17:2027–2038.

52. Narayan P, Trachtenberg J, Lepor H, et al. A dose-response study of the effect of flutamide on benign prostatic hyperplasia: results of a multicenter study. *Urology* 1996;47:497–504.

53. Daniell HW. Osteoporosis after orchiectomy for prostate cancer. *J Urol* 1997;57:439–444.

54. Smith MR. Osteoporosis during androgen deprivation therapy for prostate cancer. *Urology* 2002;60(Suppl 1):79–86.

55. Ross RW, Small EJ. Osteoporosis in men treated with androgen deprivation therapy for prostate cancer. *J Urol* 2002;167:1952–1956.

56. Daniell HW, Dunn SR, Ferguson DW, et al. Progressive osteoporosis during androgen deprivation therapy for prostate cancer. *J Urol* 2000;163:181–186.

57. Wei JT, Gross M, Jaffe CA, et al. Androgen deprivation therapy for prostate cancer results in significant loss of bone density. *Urology* 1999;4:607–611.

58. Daniell HW. Osteoporosis due to androgen deprivation therapy in men with prostate cancer. *Urology* 2001;58(Suppl 1):101–107.

59. Iversen P. Antiandrogen monotherapy: indications and results. *Urology* 2002;60(Suppl 1):64–71.

60. Grossmann ME, Huang H, Tindall DJ. Androgen receptor signaling in androgen-refractory prostate cancer. *J Natl Cancer Inst* 2001;93:1687–1697.

61. Moul JW, Srivastava S, McLeod DG. Molecular implications of the antiandrogen withdrawal syndrome. *Semin Urol* 1995;13:157–163.

62. Visakorpi T, Hyytinen E, Koivisto P, et al. In vivo amplification of the androgen receptor gene and progression of human prostate cancer. *Nat Genet* 1995;9:401–406.

63. Wallen MJ, Linja M, Kaartinen K, et al. Androgen receptor gene mutations in hormone-refractory prostate cancer. *J Pathol* 1999;189:559–563.

64. Sadar MD, Hussain M, Bruchovsky N. Prostate cancer: molecular biology of early progression to androgen independence. *Endocr Relat Cancer* 1999;6:487–502.

65. Balk SP. Androgen receptor as a target in androgen-independent prostate cancer. *Urology* 2002;60(Suppl 1):132–139.

66. Crocitto LE, Henderson BE, Coetzee GA. Identification of two germline point mutations in the 5' UTR of the androgen receptor gene in men with prostate cancer. *J Urol* 1997;158:1599–1601.

67. Culig Z, Hobisch A, Cronauer MV, et al. Mutant androgen receptor detected in an advanced-stage prostatic carcinoma is activated by adrenal androgens and progesterone. *Mol Endocrinol* 1993;7:1541–1550.

68. Ingles SA, Ross RK, Yu MC, et al. Association of prostate cancer risk with genetic polymorphisms in vitamin D receptor and androgen receptor. *J Natl Cancer Inst* 1997;89:166–170.

69. Elo JP, Kvist L, Leinonen K, et al. Mutated human androgen receptor gene detected in a prostatic cancer patient is also activated by estradiol. *J Clin Endocrinol Metab* 1995;80:3494–3500.

70. Fenton MA, Shuster TD, Fertig AM, et al. Functional characterization of mutant androgen receptors from androgen-independent prostate cancer. *Clin Cancer Res* 1997;3:1383–1388.

71. Taplin ME, Bubley GJ, Shuster TD, et al. Mutation of the androgen-receptor gene in metastatic androgen-independent prostate cancer. *N Engl J Med* 1995;332:1393–1398.

72. Veldscholte J, Berrevoets CA, Mulder E. Studies on the human prostatic cancer cell line LNCaP. *J Steroid Biochem Mol Biol* 1994;49:341–346.

73. Zhao XY, Malloy PJ, Krishnan AV, et al. Glucocorticoids can promote androgen-independent growth of prostate cancer cells through a mutated androgen receptor. *Nat Med* 2000;6:703–706.

74. Gregory CW, Johnson RT Jr, Mohler JL, et al. Androgen receptor stabilization in recurrent prostate cancer is associated with hypersensitivity to low androgen. *Cancer Res* 2001;61:2892–2898.

75. Tan J, Sharief Y, Hamil GH, et al. Dehydroepiandrosterone activates mutant androgen receptors expressed in the andro-

gen-dependent human prostate cancer xenograft CWR22 and LNCaP cells. *Mol Endocrinol* 1997;11:450–459.

76. Veldscholte J, Ris-Stalpers C, Kuiper GG, et al. A mutation in the ligand binding domain of the androgen receptor of human LNCaP cells affects steroid binding characteristics and response to anti-androgens. *Biochem Biophys Res Commun* 1990;173:534–540.

77. Veldscholte J, Berrevoets CA, Brinkmann AO, et al. Anti-androgens and the mutated androgen receptor of LNCaP cells: differential effects on binding affinity, heat-shock protein interaction, and transcription activation. *Biochemistry* 1992;31:2393–2399.

78. Montgomery BT, Young CY, Bilhartz DL, et al. Hormonal regulation of prostate-specific antigen (PSA) glycoprotein in the human prostatic adenocarcinoma cell line, LNCaP. *Prostate* 1992;21:63–73.

79. Chang CY, Walther PJ, McDonnell DP. Glucocorticoids manifest androgenic activity in a cell line derived from a metastatic prostate cancer. *Cancer Res* 2001;61:8712–8717.

80. Culig Z, Hobisch A., Hittmair A, et al. Androgen receptor gene mutations in prostate cancer. Implications for disease progression and therapy. *Drugs Aging* 1997;10:50–58.

81. Wirth MP, Froschermaier SE. The antiandrogen withdrawal syndrome. *Urol Res* 1997;25:S67–S71.

82. Kelly WK, Slovin S, Scher HI. Steroid hormone withdrawal syndromes. *Pathophysiology* and clinical significance. *Urol Clin North Am* 1997;24:421–431.

83. Scher HI, Kelly WK. Flutamide withdrawal syndrome: its impact on clinical trials in hormone-refractory prostate cancer. *J Clin Oncol* 1993;11:1566–1572.

84. Nieh PT. Withdrawal phenomenon with the antiandrogen casodex. *J Urol* 1995;153:1070–1073.

85. Small EJ, Carroll PR. Prostate-specific antigen decline after casodex withdrawal: evidence for an antiandrogen withdrawal syndrome. *Urology* 1994;43:408–410.

86. Huan SD, Gerridzen RG, Yau JC, Stewart DJ. Antiandrogen withdrawal syndrome with nilutamide. *Urology* 1997;49:632–634.

87. Taplin ME, Bubley GJ, Ko YJ, et al. Selection for androgen receptor mutations in prostate cancers treated with androgen antagonist. *Cancer Res* 1999;59:2511–2515.

88. Marcelli M, Ittmann M, Mariani S, et al. Androgen receptor mutations in prostate cancer. *Cancer Res* 2000;60:944–949.

89. Suzuki H, Sato N, Watabe Y, et al. Androgen receptor gene mutations in human prostate cancer. *J Steroid Biochem Mol Biol* 1993;46:759–765.

90. Evans BA, Harper ME, Daniells CE, et al. Low incidence of androgen receptor gene mutations in human prostatic tumors using single strand conformation polymorphism analysis. *Prostate* 1996;28:162–171.

91. Suzuki H, Akakura K, Komiya A, et al. Codon 877 mutation in the androgen receptor gene in advanced prostate cancer: relation to antiandrogen withdrawal syndrome. *Prostate* 1996;29:153–158.

92. Watanabe M, Ushijima T, Shiraishi T, et al. Genetic alterations of androgen receptor gene in Japanese human prostate cancer. *Jpn J Clin Oncol* 1997;27:389–393.

93. Chamberlain NL, Driver ED, Miesfeld RL. The length and location of CAG trinucleotide repeats in the androgen receptor

N-terminal domain affect transactivation function. *Nucleic Acids Res* 1994;22:3181–3186.

94. Irvine RA, Yu, MC, Ross RK, Coetzee GA. The CAG and GGC microsatellites of the androgen receptor gene are in linkage disequilibrium in men with prostate cancer. *Cancer Res* 1995;55:1937–1940.

95. Sartor O, Zheng Q, Eastham JA. Androgen receptor gene CAG repeat length varies in a race-specific fashion in men without prostate cancer. *Urology* 1999;53:378–380.

96. Stanford JL, Just JJ, Gibbs M, et al. Polymorphic repeats in the androgen receptor gene: molecular markers of prostate cancer risk. *Cancer Res* 1997;57:1194–1198.

97. Giovannucci E, Stampfer MJ, Krithivas K, et al. The CAG repeat within the androgen receptor gene and its relationship to prostate cancer. *Proc Natl Acad Sci USA* 1997;94:3320–3323.

98. Schoenberg MP, Hakimi JM, Wang S, et al. Microsatellite mutation (CAG24-->18) in the androgen receptor gene in human prostate cancer. *Biochem Biophys Res Commun* 1994;198:74–80.

99. Hakimi JM, Rondinelli RH, Schoenberg MP, Barrack ER. Androgen-receptor gene structure and function in prostate cancer. *World J Urol* 1996;14:329–337.

100. Irvine RA, Ma H, Yu MC, et al. Inhibition of p160-mediated coactivation with increasing androgen receptor polyglutamine length. *Hum Mol Genet* 2000;9:267–274.

101. Hsiao PW, Lin DL, Nakao R, Chang C. The linkage of Kennedy's neuron disease to ARA24, the first identified androgen receptor polyglutamine region-associated coactivator. *J Biol Chem* 1999;274:20,229–20,234.

102. Beilin J, Ball EM, Favaloro JM, Zajac JD. Effect of the androgen receptor CAG repeat polymorphism on transcriptional activity: specificity in prostate and non-prostate cell lines. *J Mol Endocrinol* 2000;25:85–96.

103. Choong CS, Wilson EM. Trinucleotide repeats in the human androgen receptor: a molecular basis for disease. *J Mol Endocrinol* 1998;21:235–257.

104. Park JJ, Irvine RA, Buchanan G, et al. Breast cancer susceptibility gene 1 (BRCAI) is a coactivator of the androgen receptor. *Cancer Res* 2000;60:5946–5949.

105. Buchanan G, Greenberg NM, Scher HI, et al. Collocation of androgen receptor gene mutations in prostate cancer. *Clin Cancer Res* 2001;7:1273–1281.

106. Isaacs JT. The biology of hormone refractory prostate cancer. Why does it develop? *Urol Clin North Am* 1999;26:263–273.

107. Culig Z, Hobisch A, Cronauer MV, et al. Androgen receptor activation in prostatic tumor cell lines by insulin-like growth factor-I, keratinocyte growth factor, and epidermal growth factor. *Cancer Res* 1994;54:5474–5478.

108. Culig Z, Hobisch A, Hittmair A, et al. Expression, structure, and function of androgen receptor in advanced prostatic carcinoma. *Prostate* 1998;35:63–70.

109. Heinlein CA, Chang C. Androgen receptor (AR) coregulators: an overview. *Endocr Rev* 2002;23:175–200.

110. Navarro D, Luzardo OP, Fernandez L, et al. Transition to androgen-independence in prostate cancer. *J Steroid Biochem Mol Biol* 2002;81:191–201.

111. Zhu W, Zhang JS, Young CY. Silymarin inhibits function of the androgen receptor by reducing nuclear localization of the receptor in the human prostate cancer cell line LNCaP. *Carcinogenesis* 2001;22:1399–1403.

B. ANTIESTROGENS

15 Aromatase Inhibitors as Chemopreventives of Breast Cancer

Mitchell Dowsett, PhD and Judy E. Garber, MD

CONTENTS

1. MECHANISM OF ACTION

Aromatase is a cytochrome P450 enzyme present in the endoplasmic reticulum (ER) which is responsible for the synthesis of steroidal estrogens. It appears that a single aromatase gene codes for the enzyme in all tissues, but, as discussed here, the control of this gene is tissue-specific according to the usage of a number of different promoters *(1)*. Aromatase catalyzes the conversion of androstenedione (the preferred substrate) and testosterone to estrone, then to estradiol. The conversion of estrone to estradiol—the most potent estrogen—is reversible, and is catalyzed by the 17β hydroxysteroid-dehydrogenase enzyme system (Fig. 1).

In non-pregnant premenopausal women, the richest source of aromatase is in the granulosa cells of the ovarian follicle. In the ovary, androstenedione and testosterone are synthesized predominantly in thecal cells adjacent to the granulosa cells; their conversion to their respective estrogens is under the stimulatory control of luteinizing hormone (LH) and follicle-stimulating hormone (FSH) levels. This stimulation is subject to a subtle feedback control that results in the cyclical estrogen levels of the menstrual cycle.

Aromatase inhibitors have only been modestly investigated as estrogen suppressants in premenopausal women. The interruption of ovarian estrogen synthesis leads to increased gonadal stimulation which, in studies with early aromatase inhibitors, led to incomplete estrogen suppression *(2–4)*, and in animal studies, to development of multiple ovarian follicles and increases in ovarian weight *(5,6)*. This phenomenon of increased gonadal stimulation has recently been exploited as a means of ovulation induction in infertile women *(7)*.

At menopause, the ovary becomes devoid of follicles; despite increased gonadal stimulation, no aromatase is synthesized, and estrogen synthesis from the ovaries no longer occurs. Plasma estradiol levels are reduced about 10-fold to mean levels of about 25 pmol/L (8 pg/mL). This residual estrogen results from conversion by aromatase of circulating androgens that are released from the adrenals, and to a lesser extent the postmenopausal ovary. The conversion occurs in so-called peripheral tissues (such as the stromal cells of subcutaneous [sc] fat) so that there is a significant relationship between plasma estrogen levels and body mass index *(8)*. The control of estrogen synthesis in

From: Cancer Chemoprevention, Volume 1: Promising Cancer Chemoprevention Agents
Edited by: G. J. Kelloff, E. T. Hawk, and C. C. Sigman © Humana Press Inc., Totowa, NJ

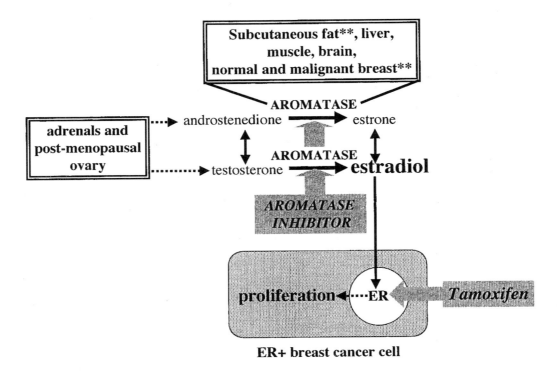

Fig. 1. Mechanisms of action of aromatase inhibitors and tamoxifen.

these peripheral tissues is not fully characterized, but there seems to be no significant role for gonadotrophins in these circumstances. Peripheral conversion increases in older women, but whether this is related to age or to the onset of menopause is unclear *(9)*.

Aromatase is also expressed in normal and malignant breast tissue *(10)*. In some breast carcinomas, aromatase levels are substantially higher than in local normal tissues. The relative importance of this local aromatase production, compared with the uptake of estrogen from the circulation, has been a subject of intense debate for many years. This question has been investigated through treatment of patients prior to surgical removal of a breast carcinoma with ^{3}H-androstenedione and ^{14}C-estrone *(11)*. These experiments confirm earlier studies in vitro, which indicated that aromatase activity in breast carcinomas was highly variable, and that the proportion of estrogen in tumors, which results from intratumoral aromatase, also varies markedly between tumors *(11–14)*. Overall, in about one-half of breast carcinomas, uptake is more important than synthesis; in the other half, the reverse is true *(11)*.

Epidemiological evidence increasingly supports a role for estrogen in the development and continued growth of breast carcinomas. Several reproductive

factors that increase the degree or extent of estrogen exposure are positively correlated with the risk of breast cancer *(15)*. For example, early menarche, late menopause, and the use of exogenous estrogens in the form of hormone replacement therapy are all related to an increased risk of breast cancer. The duration of menstrual activity prior to first pregnancy is also a risk factor, suggesting that estrogen exposure is most significant prior to the differentiation of the breast during pregnancy.

During the late 1970s and throughout the 1980s, many studies were conducted to establish whether breast cancer patients had higher plasma estrogen levels than normal matched controls. The data from these numerous studies was exceptionally varied, with some reports of positive associations but many reports of no association. A more recent series of studies that made prospective plasma collections consistently demonstrated an increased risk of breast cancer development in women with high plasma estradiol levels (reviewed in *16*). Significant but weaker relationships also exist with plasma androgen levels; an inverse relationship exists with sex hormone-binding globulin levels. Each of these observations is consistent with a mechanism in which androgens are converted to estrogens by aromatase, and these estrogens are the determinant of the

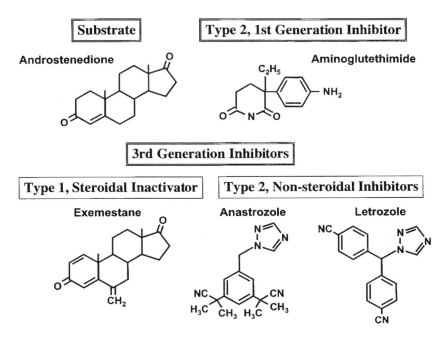

Fig. 2. Chemical structures of the main aromatase inhibitors.

higher risk of breast cancer. It is also notable that plasma androgen levels retain a significant—yet weaker—relationship after the adjustment for plasma estradiol. This may be explained by higher androgen levels leading to increased local estrogen synthesis. Data that supports the relationship between increased estrogen exposure and the risk of breast cancer were also provided by the inverse correlation between the incidence of breast cancer and osteoporotic fractures *(17)*: the latter was more common in women with lower estrogen levels. These relationships with plasma hormone levels may be useful for targeting prevention strategies.

Most data indicate that the major mechanism of action of estrogens in these circumstances is promoting growth of cells in which a carcinogen-induced mutation has occurred. However, it is argued, that estrogens may also play a role in causing such mutations, both indirectly and directly. They may act indirectly by promoting the proliferation of the normal breast epithelium, which decreases the efficiency of DNA repair mechanisms, thereby enhancing the likelihood of incorporating mutations. Data also indicate that certain estrogen metabolites might themselves be able to bind directly to DNA and lead to mutations *(18)*. In either of these circumstances, estrogen deprivation would lead to a reduced incidence of the earliest malignant changes.

During the last twenty years, a series of aromatase inhibitors have been synthesized and have entered clin-ical development. The prototype inhibitor was aminog-lutethimide, a nonsteroidal compound with clinical efficacy, which was also associated with significant non-specificity and clinical side effects such as somnolence and ataxia *(19)*. Second- and third-generation inhibitors may be separated into two main groups. Structures of the third-generation inhibitors with contemporary impor-tance are shown according to this grouping in Fig. 2.

Two steroidal substrate analogs—4-hydroxyan-drostenedione (formestane) and exemestane—have been used clinically. These are known as type 1 inhibitors, which act as irreversible enzyme inactivators *(20,21)* with the potential for exquisite selectivity for the enzyme target. They also have the potential for long-term effec-tiveness, because recovery of enzyme activity depends on the resynthesis of enzyme as much as on pharmacoki-netics of the drug. However, it was notable that orally administered formestane was followed by a relatively rapid rise in plasma estradiol levels after the cessation of treatment, suggesting that the aromatase enzyme was replaced in peripheral tissues within about 24 h *(22)*. Thus, this inactivation mechanism may not provide a clinically significant advantage over a reversible inhibitor. Minor androgenic activity has been observed on some clinical biochemical endpoints (notably sex hormone-binding globulin levels) with both formes-tane and exemestane, which could have significant consequences in long-term preventive usage *(22,23)*.

Nonsteroidal type 2 inhibitors have a basic nitrogen atom that allows them to interact with the iron atom in the heme prosthetic group of aromatase. The specific inhibition of the aromatase enzyme (as opposed to numerous other cytochrome P450 enzymes) is determined by other structural aspects of the drug and their close interaction with the substrate-binding site of the enzyme. A full understanding of these molecular interactions is restricted by the nonavailability of a crystallized aromatase preparation to allow crystallographic modeling, but comparisons with the known crystal structure of cytochrome P450(cam) has allowed visualization of the probable interaction of third-generation aromatase inhibitors anastrozole, letrozole, and vorozole with aromatase. The "fit" to the substrate-binding pocket was much closer than that with aminoglutethimide (24).

The potency of all of these drugs has been evaluated in vitro using human placental microsomal aromatase preparations, human breast fibroblasts, and/or aromatase-transfected human breast-cancer cells. Marginal differences have been observed between the acellular and cellular systems, suggesting that some of these compounds may be subject to differences in uptake by the cells (24,25).

2. PREVIOUS EFFICACY

2.1. Preclinical Models

Until recently, preclinical modeling of the use of aromatase inhibitors in established mammary tumors in rodents has been confined to model systems that are analogous to premenopausal women (e.g., with intact ovarian function). In these models, aromatase inhibitors have generally had good antitumor activity on carcinogen-induced mammary tumors (26–28). More recently, model systems have focused on the use of aromatase-transfected human MCF7 breast-cancer cells as xenografts in immune-deprived mice (29,30). These are more representative of the situation in postmenopausal women, but rely entirely on intratumoral aromatase activity as their source of estrogens.

The use of such models has made it possible to demonstrate the effectiveness of contemporary aromatase inhibitors and to make comparisons between them as well as with tamoxifen. In general, the inhibitors show greater efficacy than tamoxifen, and letrozole is more effective than anastrozole (20). However, the interpretation of these data depends on the comparative pharmacokinetics of the compounds

between the mouse and humans, and the degree to which the experimental tumor represents the range of biological characteristics of human breast cancer. For example, it is clear that the poorer efficacy of anastrozole compound with letrozole is at least partly the result of the more rapid metabolism of anastrozole seen in rodents (31,32).

Most models of mammary-cancer prevention used with aromatase inhibitors have evaluated their affect on inducibility of tumors using the carcinogens 7,12-dimethylbenz[a]anthracene (DMBA) or N-methyl-N-nitrosourea (MNU). Vorozole, for example, was able to significantly restrict such tumor development (33). Data indicating that fadrozole and letrozole both markedly reduced the incidence of spontaneous primary cancers developing in a strain of Sprague-Dawley rats with a high incidence of such spontaneous tumors (34,35) are of particular interest. It should be noted that all of these models used animals with intact ovarian function. Thus, the relevance of the results to the withdrawal of estrogens in postmenopausal women—the setting for the use of aromatase inhibitors in humans—is questionable.

Tekmal has developed a helpful transgenic mouse model in which aromatase is overexpressed through its control by a mouse mammary-tumor virus enhancer promoter (36). Letrozole was able to completely abrogate the preneoplastic and neoplastic changes that occur in the mammary glands of these animals (37).

2.2. Epidemiological Studies

Epidemiological studies of the use of aromatase inhibitors have not provided data on prevention. However, as noted here, the incidence of breast cancer is strongly related to estrogen exposure. In addition, studies in which oophorectomy has been performed prior to menopause found a reduced lifetime risk of developing breast cancer (38). Although these epidemiological studies are of interest, they have been subject to criticism because of the possible link between the cause of breast cancer and the need for oophorectomy. Data on the reduced incidence of contralateral breast cancer in patients treated with adjuvant oophorectomy are more relevant to prevention considerations. In a study by Nissen-Meyer (39), only two carcinomas developed in the contralateral breast of women treated with ovarian ablation, compared with 13 in the control group. However, it is important to remember that these data relate to the use of estrogen deprivation in premenopausal women.

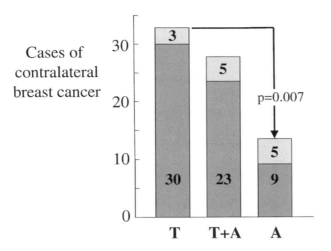

Fig. 3. Incidence of contralateral breast cancer after a median 33 months follow-up in the ATAC trial (T = tamoxifen; A = anastrozole).

2.3. Clinical Experience

Aromatase inhibitors are now widely used in advanced breast cancer, and studies are expanding our knowledge of their use in early breast cancer. In steroid receptor-positive advanced breast cancer, the third-generation compounds anastrozole, letrozole, vorozole and exemestane have shown significant clinical efficacy, with improved tolerability, and in some cases improved efficacy over established second-line hormonal agents such as megestrol acetate (40–43). More significantly, recent studies have demonstrated that anastrozole is at least as effective as tamoxifen in advanced breast cancer, and letrozole is more effective than tamoxifen (44,45). The superiority of letrozole over tamoxifen has been confirmed in a relatively large neoadjuvant study (46).

Recent results from the ATAC (anastrozole and tamoxifen, alone or combined) trial reported the first adjuvant trial of third-generation aromatase inhibitors (47). After a median follow-up of 33 mo, anastrozole treatment led to a lower incidence of relapse than tamoxifen or combination tamoxifen and anastrozole. Most significantly for the potential use of these compounds in prevention, the risk of contralateral breast cancer was reduced from 33 in patients treated with tamoxifen to 14 in those treated with anastrozole. Particularly remarkable was the reduction of incidence of invasive disease from 30 to 9 (Fig. 3). Previous studies indicated that tamoxifen reduces the incidence of contralateral breast cancer by about 50% (48), suggesting that in the absence of treatment, some 60 to 70 contralateral breast cancers would have been expected. This is consistent with predictions from the known

risk of developing a contralateral breast cancer of 0.7% per year (49). If confirmed by further follow-up, this indicates that aromatase inhibitors reduce the incidence of contralateral breast cancer, our best surrogate for breast cancer prevention, by approx 80%. Several other trials of aromatase inhibitors in early breast cancer are expected to confirm their advantage over tamoxifen.

3. PHARMACODYNAMICS

Measurement of whole-body aromatase activity in postmenopausal women treated with these compounds demonstrated that, although the prototype inhibitor aminoglutethimide reduced aromatase activity by a mean of about 90% at the high dose of 1000 mg/d (50), the third-generation compounds letrozole, anastrozole, and exemestane reduced aromatase activity by more than 95%, and letrozole provided the most complete aromatase inhibition at >99% (51,52). Available immunoassays have sufficient sensitivity to demonstrate that plasma levels of unconjugated estrogens are suppressed by >85% with these compounds, but cannot readily distinguish between the drugs (51). Plasma levels of estradiol are reduced to <3 pmol/L in a large proportion of patients. Plasma levels of estrone sulphate in postmenopausal women are much higher than estradiol or estrone, and its suppression by >90% can be demonstrated with the third-generation inhibitors (51). Maximal suppression of these estrogens occurs within the first few days of treatment; there is no indication of recovery of estrogen levels during continued treatment. Pharmacokinetic interactions between tamoxifen and anastrozole, and tamoxifen

Table 1

Incidence % of Prespecified Adverse Events in the Tamoxifen and Anastrozole Arms of the ATAC Trial (ATAC Trialists' Group)

Adverse Event	Anastrozole N = 3092	Tamoxifen N = 3093	P Values*
Hot flushes	34.3	39.7	<0.0001
Nausea and vomiting	10.5	10.2	0.7
Fatigue/tiredness	15.7	15.1	0.5
Mood disturbances	15.5	15.2	0.7
Musculoskeletal disorders	27.8	21.3	<0.0001
Vaginal bleeding	4.5	8.1	<0.0001
Vaginal discharge	2.8	11.4	<0.0001
Endometrial cancer	0.1	0.4	0.02
Fractures	5.8	3.7	<0.0001
Ischemic cardiovascular disease	2.5	1.9	0.14
Ischemic cerebrovascular event	1.0	2.1	0.0006
Venous thromboembolic events	2.1	3.5	0.0006
Deep vein thrombosis	1.0	1.7	0.02
Cataracts	3.5	3.7	0.6

and letrozole, result in lower levels of the aromatase inhibitors than when given as single agents, by 27% and 37%, respectively (53,54). These changes have not had a measurable impact on the effectiveness of estrogen suppression.

4. SAFETY

Data on the safety of aromatase inhibitors has been gathered from their use in advanced breast cancer. But the value of this information is limited by ongoing complications of disease and the effects of concomitant medication. Better data are available from the adjuvant ATAC trial (47), and from some pharmacological endpoints in presurgical studies.

Aminoglutethimide, the prototype aromatase inhibitor, was a relatively nonspecific cytochrome P450 inhibitor that suppressed the activity of several enzymes involved in glucocorticoid and mineralo-corticoid synthesis (55). This led to the use of aminoglutethimide in combination with replacement doses of glucocorticoid. The avoidance of this non-specificity was a focus for the development of the newer compounds. It has been reported that anastrozole has no effect on basal or adrenocorticotropic hormone (ACTH)-stimulated cortisol levels (56). Statistically

significant reductions in the response of cortisol and aldosterone during letrozole treatment have been reported, but these effects were minor, with no indication of an association with a significantly impaired response from individual patients (57). There are no reports of a link between adrenal insufficiency and third-generation aromatase inhibitors.

Minor changes in lipid levels have been reported for some, but not all, studies of aromatase inhibitors (58–60). Except for one case (61), these changes have been in patients with metastatic disease, making them difficult to interpret. The relationship between lipid changes and cardiovascular events is now uncertain. Thus, the impact of any effect of aromatase inhibitors is equally unclear. Increases in the level of urinary and serum markers of bone resorption with letrozole and vorozole indicate that the low estrogen levels in post-menopausal women retain some importance for the integrity of bone (58,62). These effects may be related to the relative increase in bone fractures seen in the ATAC trial.

Clinically, aromatase inhibitors are generally described as well-tolerated, with a very low incidence of serious short-term side effects. Most common are hot flushes, vaginal dryness, musculoskeletal pain, and headache, but these are rarely more than mild.

Comparative trials in advanced breast cancer have indicated the similarity in the nature and frequency of these side effects to those with tamoxifen (44,45).

Data from the ATAC trial are most informative, and are not confounded by tumor-related effects (47). However, it is important to recognize that even here the incidence is judged in relation to tamoxifen, as data on long-term side effects between aromatase inhibitor and placebo are not presently available. This can be valuable because choosing potential chemopreventives may lead to weighing advantages and disadvantages between tamoxifen and another agent. Data on the relative incidence of prespecified adverse events from the ATAC trial are shown in Table 1. It is particularly surprising that hot flushes were more common with tamoxifen than anastrozole. Endometrial cancer was more common with tamoxifen, although the absolute numbers were low. Deep vein thrombosis was also significantly lower with the aromatase inhibitor.

In contrast, fractures and musculoskeletal disorders were more frequent with anastrozole. The relative increase in fracture rate is probably caused by a reduction in fractures in the tamoxifen group because of the known bone-preserving effects of tamoxifen in postmenopausal women (64,67). However, as discussed previously, other aromatase inhibitors have been shown to increase the level of bone-resorption markers. Thus, some of this relative increase is likely to be the result of increased resorption caused by anastrozole treatment.

Overall, anastrozole's short-term tolerability appears to be better than tamoxifen, but in order for anastrozole or other aromatase inhibitors to be used as chemopreventives, some action will be needed to prevent these negative effects on bone, such as use of a bisphosphonate. There is concern that aromatase inhibitors may also have a negative impact on cognition; some studies associate use of estrogen replacement therapy with a reduced incidence of Alzheimer's disease (65). At present, no studies have examined this directly, but it will be a focus of future studies.

5. POTENTIAL POPULATIONS FOR BREAST CANCER PREVENTION WITH AROMATASE INHIBITORS

To date, aromatase inhibitors have been studied almost exclusively in postmenopausal women, in whom they block conversion of circulating androgens to estrogens in subcutaneous (sc) fat cells and normal breast tissue (22,66). The dominant role of ovarian estrogens and lack of data on adverse effects or efficacy in premenopausal women limits consideration of the clinical application of aromatase inhibitors as preventive agents to postmenopausal women for this discussion.

In the ATAC trial, anastrozole, a nonsteroidal aromatase inhibitor, was compared to tamoxifen and the combination of the two agents in adjuvant treatment of hormone receptor-positive breast cancers in postmenopausal women. Tamoxifen has repeatedly been shown to reduce the rate of primary contralateral breast cancer development, both invasive and ductal carcinoma in situ (67,68). When compared to tamoxifen and the combination, anastrozole further reduced the incidence of contralateral breast cancer (83% invasive) by 58% (47). The effects of both selective estrogen-receptor modulators (SERMS) and aromatase inhibitors in treating newly diagnosed and metastatic disease are limited to hormone receptor-positive breast cancers; risk-reducing effects of tamoxifen and raloxifene are also limited to hormone receptor-positive neoplasms. The ATAC trial report does not specifically address the hormone-receptor status of contralateral tumors (47).

Based on data presented earlier in the chapter and these clinical observations, aromatase inhibitors are expected to reduce the risk of hormone receptor-positive invasive and in situ carcinomas only. It would be particularly valuable to target prevention efforts using aromatase inhibitors to women with an increased risk of developing hormone receptor-positive tumors. This would be effective for trial design, and would protect women who are unlikely to benefit from the potential adverse effects of the aromatase inhibitors.

Several strategies should be considered for identication of a group of women with an elevated risk of developing breast cancer, particularly hormone-sensitive breast cancers. However, it is important to point out, that only the Gail model has been validated in a clinical trial.

The prevalence of estrogen receptor-positive tumors increases with advancing age (69). Older women are more often menopausal, and thus are appropriate for a prevention strategy targeting aromatase. However, age alone will not permit sufficiently precise identification of an appropriate cohort for a medical intervention to reduce risk that may have important adverse effects. Recent analyses of epidemiologic data suggest that established reproductive risk factors (age at menarche, age at first full-term pregnancy/nulliparity, and hormone replacement therapy) primarily increase the risk of hor-

Table 2

Definitive and Pilot Breast Cancer Prevention Trials Using Aromatase Inhibitors

Trial / Sponsor	Agents	Study Population	Trial Endpoints
IBIS II (Prevention) National funds from several European countries, Australia, and New Zealand	Anastrozole 1 mg vs placebo x 5 yr	6000 women Age 40–70 yr Postmenopausal increased risk based on genetic and epidemiologic risk factors	Breast cancer incidence
MAP1 NCIC CTG	Letrozole 2.5 mg vs placebo × 1 yr	137 women Postmenopausal No breast cancer history or ≥1 yr off adjuvant tamoxifen for ER+ breast cancer; mammographic density grade 4, 5, or 6	Change in mammographic density at 12 and 24 mo
MAP2 NCIC CTG	Exemestane 25 mg vs placebo × 1 yr	120 women Postmenopausal No breast cancer history; mammographic density ≥25%	Change in mammographic density at 12 and 24 mo; lipid profiles, menopausal symptoms
WISE NCI	Letrozole 2.5 mg vs placebo × 1 yr	110 Women Postmenopausal No breast cancer history Serum estradiol ≥12 pg/dL	Change in bone mineral density at 12 months; lipid profiles, menopause quality of life

mone-receptor-positive tumors (70,71). The multifactorial Gail model, which includes several reproductive factors, family history information, and breast biopsy results, was used to set eligibility for participation in the Breast Cancer Prevention Trial (BCPT) (tamoxifen vs placebo) and ongoing STAR (Study of Tamoxifen and Raloxifene) trial (72,73). Originally derived to estimate the incidence of breast cancer in populations, the model accurately estimated the number of breast cancers that developed in the placebo arm of the BCPT (73). It has also performed well when estimating the number of breast cancers in a cohort of women followed regularly with mammograms, such as the Nurses' Health Study cohort, although with some limitations (74). A recent analysis of the Nurses' Health Study longitudinal cohort, however, found that the Gail model did not clearly distinguish which individual women in the cohort would develop breast cancer during a follow-up period (75). As a whole, these data suggest that currently available multifactorial models based on epidemiologic risk factors should be useful in assembling chemoprevention study cohorts, although perhaps not as helpful for individual breast cancer risk prediction as clinicians would like.

One group of women who show excellent results in risk reduction with tamoxifen in the BCPT had histologic lesions associated with an increased risk of breast cancer. In fact, although a subset analysis, tamoxifen was shown to reduce the risk of breast cancer among women with atypical ductal hyperplasia (ADH), atypical lobular hyperplasia (ALH), or lobular carcinoma in situ (LCIS) by more than the 49% overall reduction observed for the overall study cohort (76). These lesions are associated with ER+ cells, and an increased risk of ER+ cancers in particular (77,78). Women with these lesions are often newly aware of their increased breast cancer risk, and often motivated to intervene to reduce that risk, as evidenced by their enrollment in the BCPT and STAR trials. Women with ADH, ALH, and LCIS are excellent candidates for risk-reducing intervention strategies.

It is possible that some women are more susceptible to a stimulatory effect of estrogen on breast tissue than others. Estrogen effect is a difficult thing to measure. One endpoint that has been shown to be associated with estrogen levels, and that appears to be affected by estrogen supplementation, blockade (tamoxifen), and withdrawal, is mammographic breast density *(79,80)*, which has itself been shown to be an independent risk factor for breast cancer *(81,82)*. Women with dense breast tissue measured using one of the standardized, validated approaches could be assigned to a risk group based on the density assessment, and may be considered for trial participation, in which the endpoint might be modulation of breast density, for example.

Recent studies have consistently observed an increase in the risk of breast cancer among postmenopausal women with higher circulating serum hormone levels. The most recent meta-analysis evaluated data from nine prospective studies of endogenous serum sex-hormone levels and the risk of breast cancer in postmenopausal women from regions around the world *(16)*. The analysis showed a statistically significant increase in the risk of breast cancer with increasing levels of free and total estradiol and estrone, as well as androgens *(16)*. A single postmenopausal hormone value is surprisingly stable in postmenopausal women over time *(83)*. However, the effect is markedly reduced in women who have used hormone replacement therapy *(16)*. Therefore, a carefully measured postmenopausal serum estrogen level could be used to determine eligibility for a prevention strategy employing estrogen modulation.

Finally, genetic markers of the risk of breast cancer are becoming increasingly important in distinguishing groups of women with similar probabilities of developing disease. The *CYP19* gene, which codes for the aromatase enzyme, is multi-allelic, with several of the identified polymorphisms hypothesized to alter aromatase activity *(84)*. It is logical to think that specific *CYP19* alleles would be associated with greater or lesser lifetime risk of breast cancer, and early studies were promising. However, a recent large, nested case-control study failed to observe an association between a previously implicated *CYP19* genotype and the risk of breast cancer, or elevated postmenopausal estrogen levels *(85)*.

6. CLINICAL TRIALS USING AROMATASE INHIBITORS FOR BREAST CANCER RISK REDUCTION

Building on experience with tamoxifen, the favorable therapeutic profile observed in metastatic disease studies, and early results from the adjuvant ATAC trial, pilot breast-cancer prevention trials are already in progress, and the initiation of definitive trials is imminent (Table 2). However, concerns about side effects anticipated from agents that are extremely effective in reducing circulating estrogen levels have prompted a number of pilot trials to begin to collect data on possible effects of aromatase inhibitors on bone density, lipid metabolism, and menopausal symptoms, including sexual function. Previous studies have shown that women will not tolerate the same level of side effects from an agent taken for prevention (tamoxifen) as they will for the same agent taken for adjuvant breast-cancer treatment, and will discontinue medication *(86)*. None of the current aromatase inhibitor studies in any setting has yet undertaken evaluation of possible effects of estrogen reduction on cognitive function.

Three pilot prevention trials have begun. The MAP1 study (Paul E. Goss, Principal Investigator) is conducted through the National Cancer Institute of Canada Clinical Trials Group (NCIC CTG). The study population will be 137 postmenopausal women with either no history of breast cancer or at least 1 yr off tamoxifen treatment for estrogen receptor-positive breast cancer, with sufficiently dense mammograms (percent mammographic density grade 4, 5, or 6 estimated using the methods of Boyd and Jaffe) randomized in a double-blind, placebo-controlled study of the nonsteroidal aromatase inhibitor letrozole (2.5 mg or placebo). Women will take medication for 1 yr. Breast density will be measured at the end of yr 1 and again 1 yr later, off medication. Bone density and lipid metabolism will also be monitored.

Another pilot trial using mammographic breast density both for an eligibility criterion and as a modulatable biomarker is MAP2 (Paul E. Goss, Principal Investigator), also coordinated by the NCIC CTG. This study is limited to 120 postmenopausal women with no personal history of breast cancer who have increased radiological density (≥25%) on routine mammogram. The double-blind trial compares the effect of the steroidal aromatase inhibitor exemestane 25 mg to placebo on mammographic breast density. Measurement is also at baseline, after 1 yr on the study drug, and after 1 yr without medication.

A third pilot trial (WISE: Women with Increased Serum Estradiol levels, Judy E. Garber, Principal Investigator) is underway at the Dana Farber/Harvard Cancer Center institutions in Boston, MA, evaluating letrozole (2.5 mg in a double-blind 2:1 randomization against placebo). The study is open to 110 postmenopausal women whose circulating estradiol levels are in the highest quartile (≥12 pg/mL). The study is powered for the effect of estrogen reduction on bone-mineral density as measured by DEXA scan, performed at baseline and 1 yr on study drug. Mammographic breast density, lipid levels, and menopause-specific quality of life are monitored, as in the MAP studies.

These pilot trials may be more important for the information they will provide about strategies to identify women at increased risk of breast cancer and potentially modulatable biomarkers than for their contribution to risk reduction, given their relatively small sample sizes. The first definitive trial evaluating an aromatase inhibitor for breast cancer risk reduction began in the summer of 2002, in Europe, under the direction of the International Breast Cancer Intervention Study (IBIS-II, Jack Cuzick, Principal Investigator). The study has two modules—one for prevention, the other for ductal carcinoma *in situ*. The prevention study will compare 5 yr of the nonsteroidal aromatase inhibitor anastrozole 1 mg daily to placebo in a double-blind study. The 6000 eligible women will be postmenopausal, with no history of breast cancer, ages 40–70 at enrollment, with increased risk of breast cancer based on genetic and epidemiologic risk factors used in IBIS-I, including participant age, family history, histologic lesions on biopsy, plus breast density (new in this trial).

Changes in bone-mineral density will be evaluated in associated sub-studies. Similar studies are under discussion in the United States and Canada. Questions from preclinical data raise the possibility that steroidal aromatase inhibitors may have less adverse effect on bone density—either because of an associated increase in androgen, or based on less clearly defined mechanisms.

Large studies comparing daily anastrozole 1 mg to tamoxifen 20 mg daily for 5 yr in women with ductal carcinoma *in situ* are in discussion at both the NSABP and IBIS groups. Data from clinical trials are eagerly awaited to assist women in choosing among agents that may have similar effects on the risk of breast cancer. The next chapter in breast cancer prevention trials, the aromatase inhibitors, will again provide important and interesting information about the prevention of breast cancer, as well as quality of life.

7. CONCLUSIONS

Aromatase inhibition has already proven to be an effective and well-tolerated approach to the treatment of hormone-sensitive breast cancers. The agents hold great promise in the chemoprevention of breast cancer. Their evaluation in this role has already begun. Results of clinical trials in both the adjuvant and prevention settings will provide important biological and clinical information for women at increased risk of breast cancer, and may also influence identification of women for hormonally mediated approaches to breast cancer risk reduction in the future.

REFERENCES

1. Simpson ER, Dowsett M. Aromatase and its inhibitors: significance for breast cancer therapy. *Recent Prog Horm Res* 2002;57:317–338.
2. Santen RJ, Samojlik E, Wells SA. Resistance of the ovary to blockade of aromatization with aminoglutethimide. *J Clin Endocrinol Metab* 1980;51:473–477.
3. Harris AL, Dowsett M, Jeffcoate SL, et al. Endocrine and therapeutic effects of aminoglutethimide in premenopausal patients with breast cancer. *J Clin Endocrinol Metab* 1982;55:718–722.
4. Stein RC, Dowsett M, Hedley A, et al. The clinical and endocrine effects of 4-hydroxyandrostenedione alone and in combination with goserelin in premenopausal women with advanced breast cancer. *Br J Cancer* 1990;62:679–683.
5. Sinha S, Kaseta J, Santner SJ, et al. Effect of CGS 20267 on ovarian aromatase and gonadotropin levels in the rat. *Breast Cancer Res Treat* 1998;48:45–51.
6. Shetty G, Krishnamurthy H, Krishnamurthy HN, et al. Effect of estrogen deprivation on the reproductive physiology of male and female primates. *J Steroid Biochem Mol Biol* 1997;61:157–166.
7. Mitwally MF, Casper RF. Aromatase inhibition for ovarian stimulation: future avenues for infertility management. *Curr Opin Obstet Gynecol* 2002;14:255–263.
8. Longcope C, Baker R, Johnston CC Jr. Androgen and estrogen metabolism: relationship to obesity. *Metabolism* 1986;35:235–237.
9. Hemsell DL, Grodin JM, Brenner PF, et al. Plasma precursors of estrogen. II Correlation of the extent of conversion of androstenedione to estrone with age. *J Clin Endocrinol Metab* 1974;38:476–479.
10. Miller WR, Dixon JM. Local endocrine effects of aromatase inhibitors within the breast. *J Steroid Biochem Mol Biol* 2001;79:93–102.
11. Miller WR. Importance of intratumoural aromatase and its susceptibility to inhibitors, in *Aromatase Inhibition—Then, Now and Tomorrow*. Dowsett M, ed., Partenon Publishing, London 1994, pp. 43–53.
12. Silva MC, Rowlands MG, Dowsett M, et al. Intratumoral aromatase as a prognostic factor in human breast carcinoma. *Cancer Res* 1989;49:2588–2591.
13. Lipton A, Santen RJ, Santner SJ, et al. Prognostic value of breast cancer aromatase. *Cancer* 1992;70:1951–1955.
14. Miller WR, Mullen P, Telford J, Dixon JM. Clinical importance of intratumoral aromatase. *Breast Cancer Res Treat* 1998;49 Suppl 1:S27–S32.
15. Feigelson HS, Henderson BE. Estrogens and breast cancer. *Carcinogenesis* 1996;17:2279–2284.
16. Endogenous Hormones and Breast Cancer Collaborative Group (EHBCCG). Endogenous sex hormones and breast cancer in postmenopausal women: reanalysis of nine prospective studies. *J Natl Cancer Inst* 2002;94:606–616.

17. Ettinger B, Black DM, Mitlak BH, et al. Reduction of vertebral fracture risk in postmenopausal women with osteoporosis treated with raloxifene: results from a 3-year randomized clinical trial. Multiple Outcomes of Raloxifene Evaluation (MORE) Investigators. *JAMA* 1999;282:637–645.

18. Liehr JG. Genotoxicity of the steroidal oestrogens oestrone and oestradiol: possible mechanism of uterine and mammary cancer development. *Hum Reprod Update* 2001;7:273–281.

19. Stuart-Harris RC, Smith IE. Aminoglutethimide in the treatment of advanced breast cancer. *Cancer Treat Rev* 1984;11:189–204.

20. Brodie A, Long B. Aromatase inhibition and inactivation. *Clin Cancer Res* 2001;12 Suppl:4343s–4349s.

21. Di Salle E, Giudici D, Ornati G, et al. 4-Aminoandrostenedione derivatives: a novel class of irreversible aromatase inhibitors. Comparison with FCE 24304 and 4-hydroxyandrostenedione. *J Steroid Biochem Mol Biol* 1990;37:369–374.

22. Dowsett M, Cunningham DC, Stein RC, et al. Dose-related endocrine effects and pharmacokinetics of oral and intramuscular 4-hydroxyandrostenedione in postmenopausal breast cancer patients. *Cancer Res* 1989;49:1306–1312.

23. Johannessen DC, Engan T, Di Salle E, et al. Endocrine and clinical effects of exemestane (PNU 155971), a novel steroidal aromatase inhibitor, in postmenopausal breast cancer patients: a Phase I study. *Clin Cancer Res* 1997;3:1101–1108.

24. Kao YC, Cam LL, Laughton CA, Zhou D, Chen S. Binding characteristics of seven inhibitors of human aromatase: a site-directed mutagenesis study. *Cancer Res* 1996;56:3451–3460.

25. Miller WR, Dixon JM. Antiaromatase agents: preclinical data and neoadjuvant therapy. *Clin Breast Cancer* 2000;1 Suppl 1:S9–S14.

26. Wing LY, Garrett WM, Brodie AM. Effects of aromatase inhibitors, aminoglutethimide, and 4-hydroxyandrostenedione on cyclic rats and rats with 7,12dimethylbenz(a)anthracene-induced mammary tumors. *Cancer Res* 1985;45:2425–2428.

27. Wilkinson JR, Williams JC, Singh D, et al. Response of nitrosomethylurea-induced rat mammary tumor to endocrine therapy and comparison with clinical response. *Cancer Res* 1986;46:4862–4865.

28. Schieweck K, Bhatnagar AS, Batzl C, Lang M. Anti-tumor and endocrine effects of non-steroidal aromatase inhibitors on estrogen-dependent rat mammary tumors. *J Steroid Biochem Mol Biol* 1993;44:633–636.

29. Lu Q, Yue W, Wang J, et al. The effects of aromatase inhibitors and antiestrogens in the nude mouse model. *Breast Cancer Res Treat* 1998;50:63–71.

30. Lee K, Macaulay VM, Nicholls JE, et al. An in vivo model of intratumoural aromatase using aromatase-transfected MCF7 human breast cancer cells. *Int J Cancer* 1995;62:297–302.

31. Dukes M. The relevance of preclinical models to the treatment of postmenopausal breast cancer. *Oncology* 1997;54 Suppl 2:6–10.

32. Liu XD, Xie L, Zhong Y, Li CX. Gender difference in letrozole pharmacokinetics in rats. *Acta Pharmacol Sinica* 2000;2:680–684.

33. Lubet RA, Steele VE, DeCoster R, et al. Chemopreventive effects of the aromatase inhibitor vorozole (R 83842) in the methylnitrosourea-induced mammary cancer model. *Carcinogenesis* 1998;19:1345–1351.

34. Gunson DE, Steele RE, Chau RY. Prevention of spontaneous tumours in female rats by fadrozole hydrochloride, an aromatase inhibitor. *Br J Cancer* 1995;72:72–75.

35. Gunson DE, Bell R, Sahota PS, Hsu HH. Inhibition of spontaneous mammary tumors by CGS 20267, an aromatase inhibitor, in female Sprague-Dawley rats. *Toxicol Pathol* 1996;24:789.

36. Tekmal RR, Ramachandra N, Gubba S, et al. Overexpression of int-5/aromatase in mammary glands of transgenic mice results in the induction of hyperplasia and nuclear abnormalities. *Cancer Res* 1996;56:3180–3185.

37. Mandava U, Kirma N, Tekmal RR. Aromatase overexpression transgenic mice model: cell type specific expression and use of letrozole to abrogate mammary hyperplasia without affecting normal physiology. *J Steroid Biochem Mol Biol* 2001;79:27–34.

38. Feinlieb M. Breast cancer and artificial menopause: a cohort study. *J Natl Cancer Inst* 1968;41:315–329.

39. Nissen-Meyer R. Primary breast cancer: the effect of primary ovarian irradiation. *Ann Oncol* 1991;2:343–346.

40. Dombernowsky P, Smith I, Falkson G, et al. Letrozole, a new oral aromatase inhibitor for advanced breast cancer: double-blind randomized trial showing a dose effect and improved efficacy and tolerability compared with megestrol acetate. *J Clin Oncol* 1998;16:453–461.

41. Kaufmann M, Bajetta E, Dirix LY, et al. Exemestane is superior to megestrol acetate after tamoxifen failure in postmenopausal women with advanced breast cancer: results of a Phase III randomized double-blind trial. The Exemestane Study Group. *J Clin Oncol* 2000;18:1399–1411.

42. Buzdar A, Jonat W, Howell A, et al. Anastrozole, a potent and selective aromatase inhibitor, versus megestrol acetate in postmenopausal women with advanced breast cancer: results of overview analysis of two Phase III trials. Arimidex Study Group. *J Clin Oncol* 1996;14:2000–2011.

43. Buzdar A, Douma J, Davidson N, et al. Phase III, multicenter, double-blind, randomized study of letrozole, an aromatase inhibitor, for advanced breast cancer versus megestrol acetate. *J Clin Oncol* 2001;19:3357–3366.

44. Bonneterre J, Buzdar A, Nabholtz JM, et al. Anastrozole is superior to tamoxifen as first-line therapy in hormone receptor positive advanced breast carcinoma. *Cancer* 2001;92:2247–2258.

45. Mouridsen H, Gershanovich M, Sun Y, et al. Superior efficacy of letrozole versus tamoxifen as first-line therapy for postmenopausal women with advanced breast cancer: results of a phase III study of the International Letrozole Breast Cancer Group. *J Clin Oncol* 2001;19:2596–2606.

46. Eiermann W, Paepke S, Appfelstaedt J, et al. Preoperative treatment of postmenopausal breast cancer patients with letrozole: a randomized double-blind multicenter study. *Ann Oncol* 2001;12:1527–1532.

47. ATAC Trialists' Group. Anastrozole alone or in combination with tamoxifen versus tamoxifen alone for adjuvant treatment of postmenopausal women with early breast cancer: first results of the ATAC randomised trial. *Lancet* 2002;359:2131–2139.

48. EBCTCG. Tamoxifen for early breast cancer: an overview of the randomised trials. Early Breast Cancer Trialists' Collaborative Group. *Lancet* 1998;351:1451–1467.

49. Peto J, Mack TM. High constant incidence in twins and other relatives of women with breast cancer. *Nat Genet* 2000;26:411–414.

50. MacNeill FA, Jones AL, Jacobs S, et al. The influence of aminoglutethimide and its analogue rogletimide on peripheral aromatisation in breast cancer. *Br J Cancer* 1992;66:692–697.

51. Geisler J, Haynes B, Anker G, et al. Influence of letrozole and anastrozole on total body aromatization and plasma estrogen levels in postmenopausal breast cancer patients evaluated in a randomized, cross-over study. *J Clin Oncol* 2002;20:751–757.

52. Geisler J, King N, Anker G, et al. In vivo inhibition of aromatization by exemestane, a novel irreversible aromatase inhibitor, in postmenopausal breast cancer patients. *Clin Cancer Res* 1998;4:2089–2093.

53. ATAC Trialists' Group. Pharmacokinetics of anastrozole and tamoxifen alone, and in combination, during adjuvant endocrine therapy for early breast cancer in postmenopausal women: a sub-protocol of the 'Arimidex and tamoxifen alone or in combination' (ATAC) trial. *Br J Cancer* 2001;85:317–324.

54. Dowsett M, Pfister C, Johnston SR, et al. Impact of tamoxifen on the pharmacokinetics and endocrine effects of the aromatase inhibitor letrozole in postmenopausal women with breast cancer. *Clin Cancer Res* 1999;5:2338–2343.

55. Stuart-Harris RC, Smith IE. Aminoglutethimide in the treatment of advanced breast cancer. *Cancer Treat Rev* 1984;11:189–204.

56. Plourde PV, Dyroff M, Dowsett M, et al. ARIMIDEX: a new oral, once-a-day aromatase inhibitor. *J Steroid Biochem Mol Biol* 1995;53:175–179.

57. Bajetta E, Zilembo N, Dowsett M, et al. Double-blind, randomised, multicentre endocrine trial comparing two letrozole doses, in postmenopausal breast cancer patients. *Eur J Cancer* 1999;35:208–213.

58. Harper-Wynne C, Ross G, Sacks N, et al. Effects of the aromatase inhibitor letrozole on normal breast epithelial cell proliferation and metabolic indices in postmenopausal women: a pilot study for breast cancer prevention. *Cancer Epidemiol. Biomark Prev* 2002;11:614–621.

59. Engan T, Krane J, Johannessen DC, et al. Plasma changes in breast cancer patients during endocrine therapy—lipid measurements and nuclear magnetic resonance (NMR) spectroscopy. *Breast Cancer Res Treat* 1995;36:287–297.

60. Elisaf MS, Bairaktari ET, Nicolaides C, et al. Effect of letrozole on the lipid profile in postmenopausal women with breast cancer. *Eur J Cancer* 2001;37:1510–1513.

61. Harper-Wynne CL, Sacks NP, et al. Comparison of the systemic and intratumoral effects of tamoxifen and the aromatase inhibitor vorozole in postmenopausal patients with primary breast cancer. *J Clin Oncol* 2002b;20:1026–1035.

62. Heshmati HM, Khosla S, Robins SP, et al. Role of low levels of endogenous estrogen in regulation of bone resorption in late postmenopausal women. *J Bone Mineral Res* 2002;17:172–178.

63. Fisher B, Costantino JP, Wickerham DL, et al. Tamoxifen for prevention of breast cancer: report of the National Surgical Adjuvant Breast and Bowel Project P-1 Study. *J Natl Cancer Inst* 1998;90:1371–1388.

64. Powles TJ, Hickish T, Kanis JA, et al. Effect of tamoxifen on bone mineral density measured by dual-energy x-ray absorptiometry in healthy premenopausal and postmenopausal women. *J Clin Oncol* 1996;14:78–84.

65. Tang MX, Jacobs D, Stern Y, et al. Effect of oestrogen during menopause on risk and age at onset of Alzheimer's disease. *Lancet* 1996;348:429–432.

66. Harper-Wynne C, Dowsett M. Recent advances in the clinical application of aromatase inhibitors. *J Steroid Biochem Mol Biol* 2001;760:179–186.

67. Fisher B, Dignam J, Bryant J, et al. Five versus more than five years of tamoxifen therapy for breast cancer patients with negative lymph nodes and estrogen receptor-positive tumors. *J Natl Cancer Inst* 1996;88:1529–1542.

68. Stewart HJ, Prescott RJ, Forrest AP. Scottish adjuvant tamoxifen trial: a randomized study updated to 15 years. *J Natl Cancer Inst* 2001;93:456–462.

69. Tarone RE, Chu KC. The greater impact of menopause on ER- than ER+ breast cancer incidence: a possible explanation (United States). *Cancer Causes Control* 2002;13:7–14.

70. Huang WY, Newman B, Millikan RC, et al. Hormone-related factors and risk of breast cancer in relation to estrogen receptor and progesterone receptor status. *Am J Epidemiol* 2000;151:703–714.

71. Ursin G, Tseng CC, Paganini-Hill A, et al. Does menopausal hormone replacement therapy interact with known factors to increase risk of breast cancer? *J Clin Oncol* 2002;20:699–706.

72. Gail MH, Brinton LA, Byar DP, et al. Projecting individualized probabilities of developing breast cancer for white females who are being examined annually. *J Natl Cancer Inst* 1989;81:1879–1886.

73. Costantino JP, Gail MH, Pee D, et al. Validation studies for models projecting the risk of invasive and total breast cancer incidence. *J Natl Cancer Inst* 1999;91:1541–1548.

74. Spiegelman D, Colditz GA, Hunter D, Hertzmark E. Validation of the Gail et al. model for predicting individual breast cancer risk. *J Natl Cancer Inst* 1994;86:600–607.

75. Rockhill B, Spiegelman D, Byrne C, et al. Validation of the Gail et al. model of breast cancer risk prediction and implications for chemoprevention. *J Natl Cancer Inst* 2001;93:358–366.

76. Fisher B, Costantino JP, Wickerham DL, et al. Tamoxifen for prevention of breast cancer: report of the National Surgical Adjuvant Breast and Bowel Project P-1 Study. *J Natl Cancer Inst* 1998;90:1371–1388.

77. Shaaban AM, Sloane JP, West CR, Foster CS. Breast cancer risk in usual ductal hyperplasia is defined by estrogen receptor-alpha and Ki-67 expression. *Am J Pathol* 2002;160:597–604.

78. Shoker BS, Jarvis C, Sibson DR, et al. Oestrogen receptor expression in the normal and pre-cancerous breast. *J Pathol* 1999;188:237–244.

79. Rutter CM, Mandelson MT, Laya MB, et al. Changes in breast density associated with initiation, discontinuation, and continuing use of hormone replacement therapy. *JAMA* 2001;285:171–176.

80. Chow CK, Venzon D, Jones EC, et al. Effect of tamoxifen on mammographic density. *Cancer Epidemiol Biomark Prev* 2000;9:917–921.

81. Byrne C, Schairer C, Wolfe J, et al. Mammographic features and breast cancer risk: effects with time, age, and menopause status. *J Natl Cancer Inst* 1995;87:1622–1629.

82. Boyd NF, Byng JW, Jong RA, et al. Quantitative classification of mammographic densities and breast cancer risk: results from the Canadian National Breast Screening Study. *J Natl Cancer Inst* 1995;87:670–675.

83. Hankinson SE, Willett WC, Manson JE, et al. Plasma sex steroid hormone levels and risk of breast cancer in post-menopausal women. *J Natl Cancer Inst* 1998;90:1292–1299.

84. Kristensen VN, Harada N, Yoshimura N, et al. Genetic variants of CYP19 (aromatase) and breast cancer risk. *Oncogene* 2000;19:1329–1333.

85. Haiman CA, Hankinson SE, Spiegelman D, et al. No association between a single nucleotide polymorphism in CYP19 and breast cancer risk. *Cancer Epidemiol Biomarkers Prev* 2002;11:215–216.

86. Day R, Ganz PA, Costantino JP, et al. Health-related quality of life and tamoxifen in breast cancer prevention: a report from the National Surgical Adjuvant Breast and Bowel Project P-1 Study. *J Clin Oncol* 1999;17:2659–2669.

16 Breast Cancer Chemoprevention by Selective Estrogen Receptor Modulators

Carolyn L. Smith, PhD

CONTENTS

1. INTRODUCTION

The link between estrogens and breast cancer has long been recognized. More than 100 yr ago, George Beatson demonstrated that, in some cases, removing the ovaries from premenopausal women with metastatic breast cancer led to disease regression and improved prognosis *(1)*. Subsequent demonstrations of estrogen acting as a promoter of breast cancer-cell growth were consistent with the hypothesis that blocking estrogen action would be beneficial in breast cancer therapy. More recently, aromatase inhibitors, which block the synthesis of estrogens, have also shown promising results in breast cancer treatment *(2)*. The identification of estrogen receptors (ER) provided a therapeutic target for controlling estrogen action. Later, discovery of the antiestrogen tamoxifen provided a pharmacological method to negatively regulate ER function. Importantly, tamoxifen was shown to block the proliferation of ER-positive MCF-7 human breast cancer cells in vitro *(3)*, and inhibited the induction and growth of tumors in a 7,12-dimethylbenz[a]anthracene-induced (e.g., carcinogen-induced) rat mammary carcinoma model *(4)*. These laboratory experiments revealed that an antiestrogen could block growth and progression of breast tumors, and were among the first demonstrations of the breast cancer-preventative potential of an ER ligand.

2. OVERVIEW OF ER ACTION

The effects of estrogens are mediated via their cognate nuclear receptors, members of a superfamily of ligand-regulated transcription factors. There are two estrogen receptors, ERα and ERβ; the latter was only recently identified *(5)*. It is well-established that estradiol binding to ERs is accompanied by a conformational change in the hormone-binding domain, inducing it to dimerize and bind to estrogen response elements (EREs) generally located in the promoter region of target genes *(6)*. There, the "activated," ligand-bound receptor interacts with coactivators to form a multiprotein complex that contacts the general transcriptional machinery and increases the expression of target genes through processes involving chromatin remodeling, formation of stable pre-initiation complexes, and enhanced rates of RNA polymerase II reinitiation *(7–11)*. Two distinct regions within ERα, apart from the centrally located DNA-binding domain, contribute to transcriptional activity: the constitutively active activation function-1 (AF-1), and the ligand-regulatable AF-2. Depending on the cell type and promoter examined, AF-1 and AF-2 can regulate estrogen-induced transcription independently or synergistically *(12,13)*. ERβ also has a ligand-regulatable AF-2 domain, but its AF-1 region is less active than the corresponding region in ERα, and appears to possess a repressive function *(14)*.

From: Cancer Chemoprevention, Volume 1: Promising Cancer Chemoprevention Agents
Edited by: G. J. Kelloff, E. T. Hawk, and C. C. Sigman © Humana Press Inc., Totowa, NJ

When evaluated on EREs, the activities of ERs can be inhibited by binding to antagonistic ligands, of which there are two types. Type I antiestrogens, such as tamoxifen or its biologically active metabolite 4-hydroxytamoxifen (4HT), are referred to as "partial agonists" or "mixed agonists/antagonists". Depending on the cell and promoter context examined, these agents exert varying degrees of agonist and antagonist potential with respect to ER transcriptional activity. This biology is also reflected in the ability of these agents to exert estrogen vs antiestrogen effects in a tissue-specific manner. For instance, tamoxifen inhibits ER activity in the normal breast, but exerts estrogen-like effects in the uterus, where it stimulates endometrial-cell growth. Agents of this class, including tamoxifen and raloxifene, are thus frequently referred to as selective ER modulators, or SERMs. For ERα, 4HT blocks the ligand-activated AF-2 domain, most likely by inducing structural changes in this region that prevent coactivator binding while leaving AF-1 free to initiate gene expression (15–17). The requirement of AF-1 and AF-2 activities for stimulating gene expression varies in a promoter- and cell type-specific manner (15,18), and the ability of 4HT to stimulate gene expression via AF-1 in some but not all environments contributes to the cell- and tissue-selective nature of SERM activity. Importantly, the ability of 4HT to either activate or inhibit gene expression in a context-specific manner indicates that intrinsic cellular differences in factors such as cell-signaling pathways, accessory transcription factors, coactivators, and/or corepressors, may account for the distinct interpretations of 4HT biocharacter (e.g., agonist vs antagonist activity).

For ERβ, 4HT also inhibits its AF-2 function, and because of the receptor's relatively poor AF-1 activity, this ligand generally blocks ERβ transcriptional activity measured on EREs (14). However, it should be noted that almost all studies with human ERβ thus far have been conducted with a 530-amino-acid protein that was considered to be full length (19). A recent report indicates that the full-length form of ERβ consists of 548 amino acids and has significantly greater transcriptional activity than the 530 amino acid receptor (20). Since these additional residues are at the extreme amino-terminus, it is possible that they alter the activity of the AF-1 domain; further examination is required to firmly establish whether this is the case. In contrast to 4HT, type II antiestrogens such as ICI 182,780 (ICI) are called "pure" antiestrogens, since in almost all contexts they inhibit ERα and ERβ transcriptional activity on EREs and their activities are not cell-type-dependent. Both type I and II antiestrogens bind to the ERs with high affinity (21–23) and induce conformational changes in the ligand-binding domain (LBD) distinct from that of estradiol (7,17,18,24–26).

In addition to the classical pathway of ER activation in which gene expression is dependent on the receptor that binds directly to DNA, both ERα and ERβ may indirectly influence target gene expression through their interaction with other DNA-binding transcription factors such as AP-1 (27) or Sp1 (28). In this mechanism of ER action, in which the receptor is tethered indirectly to the gene promoter via another protein, ligands typically defined as agonists or antagonists may take on a completely distinct biocharacter. In HeLa cells, for example, 4HT is an antagonist of ERβ action at an ERE, yet it is able to stimulate gene expression via the same receptor at an AP-1 response element (29).

2.1. Coactivators and ERα Action

Among the many coactivators that bind ER in a hormone-dependent manner is a family of coactivator proteins consisting of steroid receptor coactivator-1 (SRC-1; also known as NCoA-1), transcriptional intermediary factor 2 (TIF2; also known as GRIP1, SRC-2, or NCoA-2), and receptor-associated coactivator 3 (RAC3; also known as SRC-3, p/CIP, AIB1, ACTR, or TRAM-1), as well as the CREB-binding protein (CBP) and p300 with which they synergize. This family significantly stimulates (≥ three fold) ER-mediated transcription (30–37). SRC-1, TIF2, and RAC3 are large proteins (~ 160 kDa) with extensive homology (9), referred to as either "SRC family" or "p160" coactivators. Apart from their ability to bind to receptors and promote interaction with general transcription factors, SRC-1, RAC3, CBP, and p300 also possess histone acetyltransferase (HAT) activity, which is believed to contribute to steroid receptor-dependent gene expression by promoting the acetylation of histones within the promoter and thereby stimulating chromatin remodeling (36,38,39). However, recent work also implicates HAT activity in the disassembly of receptor-coactivator complexes, and this may lead to attenuation of gene transcription (40). Alternatively, it may contribute to the ability of ERα to cycle on and off a target gene promoter during the early course of estrogen treatment, as demonstrated by chromatin immunoprecipitation (ChIP) experiments (41). A recent report also has shown that SRC-1 and the DRIP205/TRAP220 coactivators cycle off and on the pS2 promoter in response to estradiol treatment, indicating that coactivator association with target gene promoters is also dynamic *(42)*. Although the p160s and CBP/p300 have been most intensively studied, a relatively large (>50) number of coactivators has been identified to date (reviewed in *10,43*). Apart from HAT activity, some of these coactivators have been shown to possess or be modified by arginine methyltransferase *(44,45)*, ubiquitin ligase *(46)*, or protein kinase *(47–51)* activities. Thus, the ability of the ERs to activate transcription is a product of the receptors' interaction with coactivators and other proteins required for gene expression, and their collective effects on the formation, function, and/or disassembly of the receptor-coactivator complex.

2.1. LIGAND REGULATION OF COACTIVATOR-ER INTERACTIONS

Partial proteolysis experiments first indicated that estrogens and antiestrogens induce distinct conformational changes in the receptor's LBD *(7,18,52)*. Subsequently, the crystal structures of the LBDs of ERα and ERβ complexed with various ligands, including the agonists diethylstilbestrol *(17)* and estradiol *(26)*, were solved, and like other members of the steroid-receptor superfamily, these regions were found to be composed of 12 α-helices. Moreover, it was determined that the position of the twelfth helix in relation to the remainder of the LBD differed substantially from the agonist-bound structure when a partial ER antagonist such as tamoxifen or raloxifene occupied the ligand-binding pocket *(17,26,53)*. Thus, ER ligands are determinants of the conformation of the receptor's LBD.

The hypothesized ability of coactivators to bind to steroid receptors such as ER in an agonist-dependent manner was exploited in the initial identification of SRC family coactivators; estradiol promoted ER-coactivator interactions and tamoxifen did not *(30)*. Subsequent analyses have defined the NR box motifs (LxxLL, where L=leucine and x is any amino acid) found within coactivators such as the p160s and CBP/p300 as critical for their ability to bind to steroid receptors *(54)*. The region within the ERα and ERβ LBDs to which the LxxLL-containing region of coactivators bind has also been identified. The structure of the co-crystal complex of the ER agonist diethylstilbestrol with the ERα LBD and a NR box-containing portion of the GRIP1 coactivator reveals that residues within helix 12, as well as within helices 3 and 5, are important for mediating interactions between ERs and coactivators *(17,26,55)*. Of these helices, helix 12—by virtue of the

ability of ER ligands to alter its position relative to the remainder of the LBD—plays a critical role in regulating coactivator interactions with the receptor's LBD *(17,56,57)*. Thus, agonists promote coactivator binding to ERs by inducing a LBD structure that is favorable for this interaction. The p160 and CBP/p300 coactivators each possess multiple LxxLL sequences, and can utilize these distinct NR box motifs to interact with different receptors *(58)*. Notably, ERα and ERβ exhibit preferences for different NR box motifs depending on the p160s and ligand *(59)*. However, it is important to note that steroid receptors and coactivators can utilize other regions within their structures to bind to one another. For example, SRC family coactivators, as well as CBP and p300, bind to the A/B domain of ERα and ERβ in a hormone-independent fashion (60–62); at least in the case of GRIP1, this interaction is not dependent on LxxLL motifs.

In contrast to the agonist-bound structures of ERα and ERβ, antagonists such as tamoxifen and raloxifene induce a LBD conformation in which helix 12 is reoriented to make contact with the coactivator binding groove, therefore enabling it to block AF2-dependent interactions with coactivators *(17,53)*. The conformation of ERβ LBD bound to the pure antiestrogen ICI 164,384 is also distinct as revealed by crystallography; helix 12 is disordered, and therefore does not appear in the structure *(25)*. However, ICI's bulky side chain extends out of the ligand binding pocket and makes contact with a portion of the coactivator-binding groove, therefore likely precluding productive LBD interaction with coactivators. Thus, both partial and pure antiestrogens induce receptor conformations that do not support LBD interactions with coactivators, undoubtedly a major determinant of their antagonistic activity. As noted here, ICI antiestrogens, unlike SERMs such as tamoxifen, do not possess partial agonist activity. Not a result of inhibition of DNA binding *(7,63)*, this pure antagonistic activity is believed to reside in the ability of ICI 164,384 and ICI 182,780 to inhibit ERα dimerization, promote a modest nuclear-to-cytoplasmic shuttling of ERα, and induce this receptor's degradation *(64–67)*. The potent antiestrogen activity of the ICI compounds therefore resides in their ability to block coactivator interactions as well as other aspects of receptor function required for transcriptional activity.

2.2. Corepressors and ERα Action

The retinoic acid receptor (RAR) and thyroid hormone receptor (TR) are also members of the nuclear receptor superfamily, sharing many structural and functional features with ERα and ERβ (6). Both RAR and TR repress basal transcription in the absence of their cognate ligands, and this function is mediated, at least in part, by two large (~ 270 kDa) nuclear proteins, silencing mediator of retinoid and thyroid hormone receptor (SMRT) and nuclear receptor corepressor (NCoR), that bind to receptors via their CoR box motifs (LxxxI/HIxxxI/L, where L = leucine, I = isoleucine, H = histidine, and x is any amino acid) (68–71). Like coactivators, corepressors also function as part of larger protein complexes that include histone deacetylases (HDACs) as well as the general repressor mSin3A (72,73). Receptors such as RAR and TR also interact with SRC-1 and TIF2 (33,34,70), and both coactivators and corepressors therefore contribute to the overall ability of these transcription factors to modulate gene expression. In the absence of ligand, SMRT and/or NCoR are bound to TR and RAR and repress these receptors' basal transcriptional activities. Upon hormone binding, the corepressors dissociate from receptor and enable TR and RAR to associate with coactivators and stimulate gene expression (70). Accordingly, the occupancy of the LBD, and therefore its conformation, dictates whether the receptor interacts with coactivators or corepressors, and thereby activates or represses transcription, respectively (74,75).

In contrast to TR or RAR, neither ERα or ERβ are able to actively repress basal transcription, in accordance with their inability to bind either SMRT or NCoR in the absence of ligand (41,61,70). However, both NCoR and SMRT interact with ERα in the presence of tamoxifen, but not estradiol, in in vitro assays (76), and ChIP assays reveal the presence of both corepressors at the promoters of the ER target genes pS2 and cathepsin D in tamoxifen-treated MCF-7 cells (41). Moreover, overexpression of either NCoR or SMRT selectively represses the partial agonist activity of 4HT, but does not affect estrogen action (76–78), suggesting that 4HT's antagonistic activity may result from blocking coactivator association and from promoting interactions between ERs and corepressors and their associated histone deacetylases. Consistent with this, injecting cells with antibodies to NCoR or SMRT that presumably block the functions of these corepressors strongly promotes the agonist activity of 4HT (61). As a whole, the data indicate that SMRT and NCoR are ERα corepressors, and that these proteins inhibit the partial agonist activity of antiestrogens such as tamoxifen. In addition to these relatively well-studied

proteins, other molecules with ER corepressor function include MTA1, REA, HET/SAF-B and SAP30; these are also likely to contribute to the antagonistic activity of type I antiestrogens (79–82).

2.3. Coactivator and Corepressor Action In Vivo

In contrast to the detailed studies of coregulators (e.g., coactivator and corepressor) by in vitro approaches and overexpression in transient transfection assays, relatively little is known about the biology of these coregulatory molecules in their endogenous setting (9–11). There is limited information on alterations in coactivator and corepressor expression in normal vs tumor tissues that suggests that changes in coregulator expression may occur during cancer progression (e.g., expression of TIF2 appears to be higher in intraductal carcinomas than normal mammary gland, but NCoR levels are lower in invasive vs intraductal carcinoma) (83). It has also been proposed that alterations in coregulator expression may be relevant to acquired tamoxifen resistance, in which breast cancer growth initially inhibited by tamoxifen therapy becomes resistant to and eventually stimulated by this antiestrogen. For instance, tamoxifen-resistant MCF-7 tumors in mice have lower levels of NCoR expression than tamoxifen-sensitive tumors (61); the relative lack of corepressor expression may contribute to the loss of tamoxifen antagonist activity in the resistant tumor.

At the molecular level, there is also evidence to support the role of coactivators and corepressors as determinants of the tissue-specific agonist and antagonist action of SERMs. In MCF-7 cells in which 4HT and raloxifene are antagonists, these ligands promote the recruitment of NCoR, SMRT, HDAC2, and HDAC4 to several ER target gene promoters (84). In contrast, 4HT exhibits agonist activity in Ishikawa uterine cells as evidenced by its stimulation of c-myc gene expression, and fails to recruit the previously mentioned corepressors or HDACs to this gene's promoter. However, it does stimulate the recruitment of several coactivators including SRC-1 and CBP. Thus, the cell- and gene-specific ability of 4HT and raloxifene to regulate gene expression in a positive or negative fashion correlates with the selective recruitment of coactivators and corepressors, respectively.

The characterization of knockout mice for the coactivators SRC-1 (85), TIF2 (86), RAC3 (87,88), and E6-AP (89), and the NCoR corepressor (78), also provides animal and cell models in which to examine the absolute and relative roles of these coregulatory proteins in vivo. For instance, SRC-1 knockout mice have a phenotype of generalized resistance to steroid hormone action, with the mammary glands of virgin SRC-1 null mice exhibiting decreased ductal growth and branching (85). However, TIF2, RAC3 and E6-AP are not required for virgin mammary gland development, although they are expressed in this tissue, indicating that coactivators may play tissue- and/or cell-specific roles in vivo (86–89). Evidence obtained from mouse embryonic fibroblasts (MEFs) derived from NCoR knockout embryos support the importance of this corepressor for tamoxifen's antagonist activity. In transient transfection assays, 4HT stimulated ERα-dependent expression of a reporter gene in NCoR null MEFs; 4HT lacked agonist activity in wild-type MEFs (78). Moreover, expression of exogenous NCoR in the corepressor-deficient MEFs shifted 4HT's activity from agonist to antagonist, consistent with the hypothesis that NCoR plays a key role in defining the antiestrogen properties of this SERM. Unfortunately, loss of NCoR expression results in embryonic lethality, so it is not possible to examine tamoxifen action in adult NCoR null mice.

2.4. Influence of Intracellular Signaling Pathways on SERM and Coregulator Activity

The ability of 4HT to regulate ERα function may be influenced by the activity of intracellular signaling pathways that are induced by extracellular factors (e.g., growth factors) that can cross-talk to ERα (90). Indeed, in MCF-7 cells, activation of the cyclic adenosine 5' monophosphate (AMP)/protein kinase A (cAMP/PKA) pathway increases the partial agonist activity of tamoxifen and decreases its antagonist activity (91). Similarly, in HeLa cells, both cAMP and dopamine, a neuromodulator that acts in part through the cAMP/PKA pathway, increase the partial agonist activity of 4HT (77,92). The coactivator SRC-1 stimulates ER transcriptional activity in cells treated with 4HT and forskolin, an activator of cAMP, suggesting that coactivators play a role in gene expression under these conditions (77). It should be noted that phosphorylation pathways may target either ERα (93) or coactivators such as SRC-1, GRIP1/TIF2, and AIB1/RAC3 (47,48,50,94) and increase their transcriptional activity. In addition, intracellular signal-transduction pathways increase the agonist activity of 4HT by altering the recruitment of corepressors. Both cAMP and epidermal growth factor inhibit 4HT-dependent interactions between NCoR and ERα (61). Interestingly, activation of MAPK-extracellular signal-regulated kinase-1

(MEK1) and MEKK1 signaling pathways also induces redistribution of SMRT to the cytoplasmic compartment (95). These findings suggest that the activity of intracellular signaling pathways plays a significant role in the ability of the cell to interpret 4HT as an agonist or antagonist of ER action.

3. TAMOXIFEN AS AN ADJUVANT FOR BREAST CANCER

Studies conducted during the last 10 yr have revealed much about the molecular mechanisms by which drugs such as tamoxifen and raloxifene regulate ER function in a cell- and tissue-specific manner. These advances, however, have not occurred in a vacuum. Observations leading to the recognition of antiestrogens as SERMs with organ-specific ER agonist and antagonist properties were a major development in the clinical applications of these agents.

Tamoxifen was approved in 1998 by the Food and Drug Administration (FDA) as a preventative agent for pre- and postmenopausal women at high risk of developing breast cancer, thereby making it the first chemotherapeutic drug to be approved for the prevention of cancer (96). However, the long clinical history of this drug started with its first approval by the FDA in 1977 for treatment of advanced breast cancer. It was subsequently approved as an adjuvant hormone therapy with chemotherapy in 1986, and then on its own in postmenopausal patients with axillary lymph node-positive breast cancer in 1988. Finally, tamoxifen was approved for use in pre- and postmenopausal, node-negative women with ER-positive breast cancer in 1990.

Examination of the incidence of contralateral breast cancer in patients who had received adjuvant tamoxifen therapy indicated that tamoxifen may prevent breast cancer. The Early Breast Cancer Trialists' Collaborative Group summarized clinical outcomes from randomized trials of adjuvant tamoxifen in women with early breast cancer; the principal events analyzed were recurrence and death (97). Of the 37,000 women in 55 trials, nearly 8000 had low to undetectable levels of ER in their primary tumor. In the remaining nearly 30,000 women with ER-positive or untested tumors, the proportional recurrence reductions during 10 yr of follow-up were 21%, 29%, and 47% for trials of 1 yr, 2 yr, and ~ 5 yr of adjuvant tamoxifen, respectively. When all women were studied (including those with ER-negative or poor tumors) the reductions in contralateral breast cancer were 13%,

26%, and 47% in trials of 1, 2, or ~5 yr of adjuvant tamoxifen. In the study, patients of all ages, both lymph node- negative or -positive, benefited from adjuvant therapy regardless of menopausal status or tamoxifen dose (97). However, this benefit extended primarily to patients with tumors that expressed ER, a finding consistent with tamoxifen exerting its protective effect via blocking ER action in the breast.

Although this data above suggests that tamoxifen reduces the risk of all contralateral breast cancer, there is also data supporting the possibility that tamoxifen influences the nature (e.g., ER status) of any tumors that do arise during or following antiestrogen treatment. In a retrospective epidemiological study of breast cancer patients (4654 tamoxifen users and 4327 non-users), 189 women were subsequently diagnosed with contralateral breast cancer (98). Strikingly, tamoxifen decreased the risk of developing an ER-positive contralateral tumor to 0.8 (95% confidence interval 0.5–1.1) in comparison to tamoxifen non-users, and the risk of developing an ER-negative tumor was 4.9× greater (95% confidence interval 1.4–17.4) in tamoxifen users vs non-users. In contrast to this finding, prospective randomized clinical studies evaluating tamoxifen (99) or raloxifene (100) in a preventative mode did not reveal an increase in ER-negative primary breast cancer in comparison to the placebo groups.

4. TAMOXIFEN AS A CHEMOPREVENTIVE AGENT

Four clinical trials address the value of tamoxifen in preventing primary breast cancer; three are complete and one is ongoing. It should be noted in the context of these studies that prevention indicates a reduction in the incidence of invasive breast cancer during study, as opposed to preventing the initiation of breast cancer or permanently eliminating tumors that develop during the course of the trials. Of the three completed studies, two European studies failed to detect a difference in the incidence of breast cancer between tamoxifen and placebo control groups (101,102). The Royal Marsden Hospital trial evaluated the effects of 20 mg/d tamoxifen in healthy women with an increased risk of breast cancer resulting from family history (101). This study, which enrolled the smallest number of participants (2471 women), has the longest medial follow-up of the three completed trials (70 mo). Overall breast cancer frequency was the same for women on tamoxifen or placebo (relative risk 1.06; 95% confidence interval

0.7–1.7). The likelihood that a high proportion of BRCA1 and BRCA2 carriers enrolled in this study has been suggested, which could influence the outcome, since tumors associated with BRCA mutations are generally hormone-unresponsive. The Italian trial assessing 3837 women also found no effect of tamoxifen (20 mg/d) on reducing the incidence of breast cancer incidence (102). However, participants in this study had been previously hysterectomized, 47% of them with bilateral oophorectomy before menopause. Thus, with greatly reduced endogenous estrogens, this group of women had a very low risk of breast cancer in comparison with those enrolled in the other two trials. The International Breast Cancer Intervention Study (IBIS), still uncompleted, was launched in 1992 as a result of the favorable compliance and lack of unexpected toxicities in the Royal Marsden Hospital trial (103). It has mainly enrolled subjects with a greater than twofold risk for breast cancer as a result of family history.

The largest of the three completed studies, the National Surgical Adjuvant Breast and Bowel Project (NSABP) P-1 trial, evaluated 13,388 women at high risk for breast cancer because they were: 60 yr of age or older, had a history of lobular carcinoma in situ, or were 35–59 yr of age with a 5-yr predicted risk for breast cancer of at least 1.66% according to the Gail model, which considers age, age at menarche, number of first-degree relatives with breast cancer, children after the age of thirty, no children, number of breast biopsies, and pathologic diagnosis of atypical hyperplasia (99). Trial participants received 20 mg/d tamoxifen or placebo for 5 yr. Data analyses showed a 49% reduction in the incidence of invasive breast cancer in the tamoxifen-treated group (risk ratio 0.51 [95% confidence interval 0.39–0.66]) and a 50% reduced risk of noninvasive breast cancer (risk ratio 0.50 [95% confidence interval 0.33–0.77)]). Overall, tamoxifen prevention was especially beneficial for women with a history of atypical ductal hyperplasia (who had an 86% decrease in their incidence of invasive cancer) or lobular carcinoma in situ, Gail risk >5, or with two or more first-degree relatives diagnosed with breast cancer (99). Clearly there is a difference between the results of the three completed studies, and it is important to note that the three trials differ in study design, eligibility criteria, and participant characteristics.

A recent study examined the cost-effectiveness of tamoxifen as a chemopreventive agent in a hypothetical group of women (104) and concluded that the best overall increase in survival (e.g., number of days)

should be obtained for high-risk women with atypical hyperplasia. Initiating tamoxifen chemoprevention for these women at 35, 50, or 60 yr of age would prolong the average survival of a cohort member by 202, 89, and 45 days, respectively, and the average survival of all cohort members should be extended by 70, 42, and 27 d for tamoxifen treatment initiated at the same respective ages. Tamoxifen was found to be cost-effective in women starting treatment at ≤50 yr of age based on calculations of the financial cost of prevention vs the gain in life years, and almost cost-effective for women starting tamoxifen at ≥60 years of age who had atypical hyperplasia or Gail model risk greater than five *(104)*. In general, benefits appear to be greater when tamoxifen prevention is initiated before age 50. It should be noted that the model used to examine cost effectiveness assumed that the benefit of tamoxifen chemoprevention did not extend beyond the 5-yr period of tamoxifen treatment *(104)*. This may, however, be a conservative assumption since the Oxford Overview Analysis indicated that the benefits of adjuvant tamoxifen with respect to reducing the incidence of contralateral breast cancer extended long after the conclusion of treatment *(97)*.

The health-related quality of life component of the NSABP P-1 trial reported that the frequency of weight gain and depression, two problems associated anecdotally with tamoxifen use, were not increased in this trial of healthy women *(105)*. However, tamoxifen use has been associated with increases in vasomotor, gynecologic, and sexual function symptoms, although the latter was not associated with a change in the overall rate of sexual activity. In another recent study of 43 patients who were candidates for tamoxifen treatment because of their increased risk for breast cancer, only two women elected to start tamoxifen, even after education on its associated risks and benefits *(106)*. Fear of side effects (e.g., menopausal symptoms) and concern about safety issues, such as endometrial cancer and thromboembolic events were the most commonly cited reasons *(106)*. Thus, despite the apparent effectiveness of tamoxifen, there is a significant reluctance to employ this drug for primary breast cancer prevention, and it is not widely used as a chemopreventive agent.

4.1. Tamoxifen Safety

In addition to tamoxifen's ability to reduce the incidence of breast cancer, this drug affects many other organ systems; some of these effects are beneficial and others are not. On the positive side, adjuvant tamoxifen administration to postmenopausal women preserves bone mineral density in the axial skeleton *(107,108)*. In the NSABP P-1 trial, tamoxifen produced a near significant 19% reduction in the combined risk of hip, lower radius, and spine fractures (relative risk 0.81; 95% confidence interval 0.63–1.05) *(99)*. In addition, tamoxifen use is associated with a reduction in low-density lipoproteins *(109,110)*. Moreover, there have been no increases in cancers, other than endometrial in either the Early Breast Cancer Trialists' Collaborative Group adjuvant overview *(97)* or in the NSABP P-1 prevention study *(99)*. This has relieved concerns arising from early reports that suggest links between tamoxifen administration and liver tumors in rats *(111)* and colorectal cancer in humans receiving 40 mg/d tamoxifen *(112)*.

Although it has benefits, tamoxifen use has not been without concerns. For instance, the NSABP P-1 study reported a small increase in the risk of ischemic heart disease in the tamoxifen-treated group, but this was not significant *(99)*. However, this is balanced by analysis of the NSABP Breast Cancer Prevention Trial results on cardiovascular events in women with and without heart disease, which failed to detect an association between tamoxifen use and cardiovascular heart disease *(113)*. Similar to raloxifene *(100)* and hormone replacement therapy *(114)*, tamoxifen *(99)* is associated with an increase in the incidence of vascular events in postmenopausal women, including stroke (risk ratio 1.59; 95% confidence interval 0.93–2.77), pulmonary emboli (risk ratio 3.01; 95% confidence interval 1.15–9.27), and deep vein thrombosis (risk ratio 1.60; 95% confidence interval 0.91–2.86). The Italian prevention trial also reported an increased risk of vascular events *(102)*. It is therefore generally recommended that women with a history of clotting disorders avoid both estrogen and SERM therapy. Tamoxifen use also is associated with an increased risk of endometrial cancer. Early experimental work demonstrated that tamoxifen stimulated the growth of human endometrial cancer in athymic mice *(115)*, and several large randomized clinical trials have reported a two- to threefold increase in endometrial cancer risk in tamoxifen-treated postmenopausal women *(97,99,116)*. This probably arises from the relative ER agonist activity of tamoxifen in the uterus.

Considering the risks and benefits, it is apparent that tamoxifen therapy is not suitable for all women, and the development of other agents for the prevention of breast cancer is therefore desirable. Certainly, fear of tamoxifen side effects contributes to the low number of women who use this drug as a chemopreventive agent *(106)*. This includes fears of weight gain and depression, even though these are not born out in controlled studies, and concerns regarding vasomotor and gynecological symptoms *(99,101)*. However, on balance it should be noted that tamoxifen is relatively well-tolerated, and that in the NSABP P-1 trial, similar numbers of women in the tamoxifen and placebo groups (23.7% and 19.7%, respectively) prematurely left the study *(99)*.

5. RALOXIFENE AS A CHEMOPREVENTIVE AGENT

Like tamoxifen, raloxifene also inhibits growth of mammary cancers in animal models, but has also been shown to antagonize the mitogenic effects of either estrogen or tamoxifen in uterine cell cultures and the rodent uterus (117–120). The MORE (Multiple Outcomes of Raloxifene Evaluation) trial was a multicenter, randomized, double-blind, clinical trial with an initial follow-up of up to 40 mo designed to evaluate the effects of raloxifene on bone-mineral density and vertebral fracture incidence in postmenopausal women with osteoporosis *(121)*. The study demonstrated a decreased risk of vertebral fracture (for the 60-mg group, risk ratio 0.7; 95% confidence interval 0.5–0.8), as well as increased bone mineral density in the spine and femoral neck of 2.6% and 2.1%, respectively. Although there was an increased incidence of thromboembolic disease (risk ratio 3.1; 95% confidence interval 1.5–6.2) *(121)*, there was no increased risk of endometrial cancer (risk ratio 0.8; 95% confidence interval 0.2–2.7) *(100)*. The latter is a particularly attractive feature of raloxifene in comparison to tamoxifen. Raloxifene, like tamoxifen, is associated with a reduction of low-density lipoproteins *(122)*. Currently, raloxifene is FDA-approved for the prevention and treatment of postmenopausal osteoporosis.

MORE study participants were also monitored for incidence of breast cancer as a secondary endpoint. The number of cases of breast cancer in the raloxifene-treated group in comparison to the placebo group was significantly reduced for all breast cancer (risk ratio 0.35; 95% confidence interval 0.21–0.58) and invasive cancer (risk ratio 0.24; 95% confidence interval 0.13–0.44) (100). As expected, raloxifene effects were primarily reflected in reductions in ER-positive cancer (relative risk 0.10; 95% confidence interval 0.04–0.24), and ER-negative tumors were reduced by

only 12% *(100)*. The 4-yr follow-up data from the MORE trial reported that raloxifene reduced the risk of invasive breast cancer by 72% (risk ratio 0.28; 95% confidence interval 0.17–0.46), and that this was still a reflection of the large (84%) reduction in ER-positive breast cancer incidence *(123)*. These findings suggested that raloxifene may be efficacious in reducing the incidence of breast cancer, and the lack of increased endometrial cancer risk suggests an improved safety profile.

Although the NSABP P-1 trial has established tamoxifen as the standard of care for chemoprevention of breast cancer in high-risk women, the MORE results have prompted the question of whether raloxifene may be more advantageous as a chemopreventive agent than tamoxifen. Issues related to the relative profile of side effects of raloxifene vs tamoxifen also remain to be addressed. In July 1999, the STAR (Study of Tamoxifen and Raloxifene) trial (NSABP P-2) was initiated at nearly 500 centers in North America *(124)*. This Phase III, double-blind study randomized postmenopausal women (≥35 yr of age) to either tamoxifen (20 mg/d) or raloxifene (60 mg/d) treatment groups. The intent was to recruit ~22,000 women at increased risk of breast cancer by Gail criteria and follow them for 5 years, evaluating the two drugs for their ability to prevent invasive and noninvasive breast cancer, and monitoring patients for cardiovascular disease, endometrial cancer, bone fracture, vascular events, and general toxicities. Results are expected in 2006. Also ongoing is the RUTH (Raloxifene Use in The Heart) trial to examine incidence of cardiovascular events and invasive breast cancer in postmenopausal women at risk of coronary events *(125)*. Women are to receive 60 mg/d raloxifene or placebo. Enrollment of >10,000 women is complete and results are expected no earlier than 2005.

6. OUTLOOK ON BREAST CANCER CHEMOPREVENTION

Although tamoxifen is efficacious as a chemopreventive agent, there is room for improvement. A drug with good bioavailability, an optimal tissue-specificity profile (including lack of uterine stimulation) and minimal side effects (cardiovascular, thromboembolic, and vasomotor) in conjunction with breast cancer chemoprevention has not yet been developed. Based on its lack of uterine stimulation, raloxifene may well bring us at least one step closer to this goal and the

STAR trial results are eagerly awaited for information on the relative chemopreventive abilities of these two SERMs. In the meantime, other SERMs have been identified and are in various stages of study. These include arzoxifene *(126,127)*, EM-652 *(128,129)*, CP-336,156 *(130,131)*, and GW7604 *(132)*. An important aspect of each of these agents is that they do not stimulate breast or uterine-cell growth. Several have been evaluated and show promise in animal models of breast cancer *(127,128,131)*. When and/or if these agents are ultimately studied in clinical trials as breast cancer chemopreventives, it will be interesting to see how well they compare to tamoxifen.

REFERENCES

1. Beatson GT. On the treatment of inoperable cases of the carcinoma of the mamma: suggestions for a new method of treatment with illustrative cases. *Lancet* 1896;2:104–107.
2. Simpson ER, Dowsett M. Aromatase and its inhibitors: significance for breast cancer therapy. *Recent Prog Horm Res* 2002;57:317–338.
3. Lippman ME, Bolan G. Oestrogen-responsive human breast cancer in long term tissue culture. *Nature* 1975;256:592–593.
4. Jordan VC. Effect of tamoxifen (ICI 46,474) on initiation and growth of DMBA-induced rat mammary carcinomata. *Eur J Cancer* 1976;12:419–424.
5. Kuiper GG, Enmark E, Pelto-Huikko M, et al. Cloning of a novel estrogen receptor expressed in rat prostate and ovary. *Proc Natl Acad Sci USA* 1996;93:5925–5930.
6. Tsai M-J, O'Malley BW. Molecular mechanisms of action of steroid/thyroid receptor superfamily members. *Annu Rev Biochem* 1994;63:451–486.
7. Beekman JM, Allan GF, Tsai SY, et al. Transcriptional activation by the estrogen receptor requires a conformational change in the ligand binding domain. *Mol Endocrinol* 1993;7:1266–1274.
8. Fritsch M, Leary CM, Furlow JD, et al. A ligand-induced conformational change in the estrogen receptor is localized in the steroid binding domain. *Biochemistry* 1992;31:5303–5311.
9. McKenna NJ, Lanz RB, O'Malley BW. Nuclear receptor coregulators: cellular and molecular biology. *Endocr Rev* 1999;20:321–344.
10. Robyr D, Wolffe AP, Wahli W. Nuclear hormone receptor coregulators in action: diversity for shared tasks. *Mol Endocrinol* 2000;14:329–347.
11. Glass CK, Rosenfeld MG. The coregulator exchange in transcriptional functions of nuclear receptors. *Genes Dev* 2000;14:121–141.
12. Tora L, White JH, Brou C, et al. The human estrogen receptor has two independent nonacidic transcriptional activation functions. *Cell* 1989;59:477–487.
13. Tzukerman MT, Esty A, Santiso-Mere D, et al. Human estrogen receptor transactivational capacity is determined by both cellular and promoter context and mediated by two functionally distinct intramolecular regions. *Mol Endocrinol* 1994;8:21–30.
14. Hall JM, McDonnell DP. The estrogen receptor β-isoform (ERβ) of the human estrogen receptor modulates ERα transcriptional activity and is a key regulator of the cellular response to estrogens and antiestrogens. *Endocrinology* 1999;140:5566–5578.
15. Berry M, Metzger D, Chambon P. Role of the two activating domains of the oestrogen receptor in the cell-type and promoter-context dependent agonistic activity of the anti-oestrogen 4-hydroxytamoxifen. *EMBO J* 1990;9:2811–2812.
16. Webster NJG, Green S, Jin J-R, Chambon P. The hormone-binding domains of the estrogen and glucocorticoid receptors contain an inducible transcription activation function. *Cell* 1988;54:199–207.
17. Shiau AK, Barstad D, Loria PM, et al. The structural basis of estrogen receptor/coactivator recognition and the antagonism of this interaction by tamoxifen. *Cell* 1998;95:927–937.
18. McDonnell DP, Clemm DL, Hermann T, et al. Analysis of estrogen receptor function in vitro reveals three distinct classes of antiestrogens. *Mol Endocrinol* 1995;9:659–669.
19. Ogawa S, Inoue S, Watanabe T, et al. The complete primary structure of human estrogen receptor β (hERβ) and its heterodimerization with ERα in vivo and in vitro. *Biochem Biophys Res Comm* 1998;243:122–126.
20. Wilkinson HA, Dahllund J, Liu H, et al. Identification and characterization of a functionally distinct form of human estrogen receptor β. *Endocrinology* 2002;143:1558–1561.
21. Jordan VC. Biochemical pharmacology of antiestrogen action. *Pharmacol Rev* 1984;36:245–276.
22. Kuiper GG, Carlsson B, Grandien K, et al. Comparison of the ligand binding specificity and transcript tissue distribution of estrogen receptors α and β. *Endocrinology* 1997;138:863–870.
23. Kuiper GGJM, Lemmen JG, Carlsson B, et al. interaction of estrogenic chemicals and phytoestrogens with estrogen receptor β. *Endocrinology* 1998;139:4252–4263.
24. Paige LA, Christensen DJ, Gron H, et al. Estrogen receptor modulators each induce distinct conformational changes in ERα and ERβ. *Proc Natl Acad Sci USA* 1999;96:3999–4004.
25. Pike AC, Brzozowski AM, Walton J, et al. Structural insights into the mode of action of a pure antiestrogen. *Structure* 2001;9:145–153.
26. Brzozowski AM, Pike AC, Dauter Z, et al. Molecular basis of agonism and antagonism in the oestrogen receptor. *Nature* 1997;389:753–758.
27. Kushner PJ, Agard DA, Greene GL, et al. Estrogen receptor pathways to AP-1. *J Steroid Biochem Mol Biol* 2000;74:311–317.
28. Porter W, Saville B, Hoivik D, Safe S. Functional synergy between the transcription factor Sp1 and the estrogen receptor. *Mol Endocrinol* 1997;11:1569–1580.
29. Paech K, Webb P, Kuiper GG, et al. Differential ligand activation of estrogen receptors ERα and ERβ at AP-1 sites. *Science* 1997;277:1508–1510.
30. Halachmi S, Marden E, Martin G, et al. Estrogen receptor-associated proteins: Possible mediators of hormone-induced transcription. *Science* 1994;264:1455–1458.
31. Onate SA, Tsai SY, Tsai M-J, O'Malley BW. Sequence and characterization of a coactivator for the steroid hormone receptor superfamily. *Science* 1995;270:1354–1357.

32. Smith CL, Onate SA, Tsai M-J, O'Malley BW. CREB binding protein acts synergistically with steroid receptor coactivator-1 to enhance steroid receptor-dependent transcription. *Proc Natl Acad Sci USA* 1996;93:8884–8888.

33. Voegel JJ, Heine MJS, Zechel C, et al. TIF2, a 160 kDa transcriptional mediator for the ligand-dependent activation function AF-2 of nuclear receptors. *EMBO J* 1996;15:3667–3675.

34. Hong H, Kohli K, Garabedian MJ, Stallcup MR. GRIP1, a transcriptional coactivator for the AF-2 transactivation domain of steroid, thyroid, retinoid, and vitamin D receptors. *Mol Cell Biol* 1997;17(5):2735–2744.

35. Li H, Gomes PJ, Chen JD. RAC3, a steroid/nuclear receptor-associated coactivator that is related to SRC-1 and TIF2. *Proc Natl Acad Sci USA* 1997;94:8479–8484.

36. Chen H, Lin RJ, Schiltz RL, et al. Nuclear receptor coactivator ACTR is a novel histone acetyltransferase and forms a multimeric activation complex with P/CAF and CBP/p300. *Cell* 1997;90:569–580.

37. Hanstein B, Eckner R, DiRenzo J, et al. p300 is a component of an estrogen receptor coactivator complex. *Proc Natl Acad Sci USA* 1996;93:11,540–11,545.

38. Spencer TE, Jenster G, Burcin MM, et al. Steroid receptor coactivator-1 is a histone acetyltransferase. *Nature* 1997;389:194–198.

39. Ogryzko VV, Schlitz RL, Russanova V, et al. The transcriptional coactivators p300 and CBP are histone acetyltransferases. *Cell* 1996;87:953–959.

40. Chen H, Lin RJ, Xie W, et al. Regulation of hormone-induced histone hyperacetylation and gene activation via acetylation of an acetylase. *Cell* 1999;98:675–686.

41. Shang Y, Hu X, DiRenzo J, et al. Cofactor dynamics and sufficiency in estrogen receptor-regulated transcription. *Cell* 2000;103:843–852.

42. Burakov D, Crofts LA, Chang C-PB, Freedman LP. Reciprocal recruitment of DRIP/mediator and p160 coactivator complexes *in* vivo by estrogen receptor. *J Biol Chem* 2002;277:14,359–14,362.

43. Hermanson O, Glass CK, Rosenfeld MG. Nuclear receptor coregulators: multiple modes of modification. *Trends Endocrinol Metab* 2002;13:55–60.

44. Chen D, Huang S-M, Stallcup MR. Synergistic, p160 coactivator-dependent enhancement of estrogen receptor function by CARM1 and p300. *J Biol Chem* 2000;275:40,810–40,816.

45. Chen D, Ma H, Hong H, et al. Regulation of transcription by a protein methyltransferase. *Science* 1999;284:2174–2177.

46. Nawaz Z, Lonard DM, Smith CL, et al. The Angelman syndrome-associated protein, E6-AP, is a coactivator for the nuclear hormone receptor superfamily. *Mol Cell Biol* 1999;19:1182–1189.

47. Font de Mora JF, Brown M. AIB1 is a conduit for kinase-mediated growth factor signaling to the estrogen receptor. *Mol Cell Biol* 2000;20:5041–5047.

48. Wu R-C, Qin J, Hashimoto Y, Wong J, et al. Regulation of SRC-3 (pCIP/ACTR/AIB-1/RAC-3/TRAM-1) coactivator activity by IκB kinase. *Mol Cell Biol* 2002;22:3549–3561.

49. Yuan LW, Gambee JE. Phosphorylation of p300 at serine 89 by protein kinase C. *J Biol Chem* 2000;275:40,946–40,951.

50. Lopez GN, Turck CW, Schaufele F, et al. Growth factors signal to steroid receptors through mitogen-activated protein kinase regulation of p160 co-activator activity. *J Biol Chem* 2001;276:22,177–22,182.

51. Rowan BG, Garrison N, Weigel NL, O'Malley BW. 8-bromo-cyclic AMP induces phosphorylation of two sites in SRC-1 that facilitate ligand-independent activation of the chicken progesterone receptor and are critical for functional cooperation between SRC-1 and CREB binding protein. *Mol Cell Biol* 2000;20:8720–8730.

52. Van den G-JCM, Kuiper GGJM, Pols HAP, Van Leeuwen JPTM. Distinct effects on the conformation of estrogen receptor α and β by both the antiestrogens ICI 164,384 and ICI 182,780 leading to opposite effects on receptor stability. *Biochem Biophys Res Comm* 1999;261:1–5.

53. Pike AC, Brzozowski AM, Hubbard RE, et al. Structure of the ligand-binding domain of oestrogen receptor beta in the presence of a partial agonist and a full antagonist. *EMBO J* 1999;18:4608–4618.

54. Heery DM, Kalkhoven E, Hoare S, Parker MG. A signature motif in transcriptional co-activators mediates binding to nuclear receptors. *Nature* 1997;387:733–736.

55. Mak HY, Hoare S, Henttu PMA, Parker MG. Molecular determinants of the estrogen receptor-coactivator interface. *Mol Cell Biol* 1999;19:3895–3903.

56. Danielian PS, White R, Lees JA, Parker MG. Identification of a conserved region required for hormone dependent transcriptional activation by steroid hormone receptors. *EMBO J* 1992;11:1025–1033.

57. Henttu PM, Kalkhoven E, Parker MG. AF-2 activity and recruitment of steroid receptor coactivator 1 to the estrogen receptor depend on a lysine residue conserved in nuclear receptors. *Mol Cell Biol* 1997;17:1832–1839.

58. McInerney EM, Rose DW, Flynn SE, et al. Determinants of coactivator LXXLL motif specificity in nuclear receptor transcriptional activation. *Genes Dev* 1998;12:3357–3368.

59. Bramlett KS, Wu Y, Burris TP. Ligands specify coactivator nuclear receptor (NR) box affinity for estrogen receptor subtypes. *Mol Endocrinol* 2001;15:909–922.

60. Webb P, Nguyen P, Shinsako J, et al. Estrogen receptor activation function 1 works by binding p160 coactivator proteins. *Mol Endocrinol* 1998;12:1605–1618.

61. Lavinsky RM, Jepsen K, Heinzel T, et al. Diverse signaling pathways modulate nuclear receptor recruitment of N-CoR and SMRT complexes. *Proc Natl Acad Sci USA* 1998;95:2920–2925.

62. Kobayashi Y, Kitamoto T, Masuhiro Y, et al. p300 mediates functional synergism between AF-1 and AF-2 of estrogen receptor α and β by interacting directly with the N-terminal A/B domains. *J Biol Chem* 2000;275:15,645–15,651.

63. Reese JC, Katzenellenbogen BS. Examination of the DNA-binding ability of estrogen receptor in whole cells: implications for hormone-independent transactivation and the actions of antiestrogens. *Mol Cell Biol* 1992;12:4531–4538.

64. Dauvois S, Danielian S, White R, Parker MG. Antiestrogen ICI 164,384 reduces cellular estrogen receptor content by increasing its turnover. *Proc Natl Acad Sci USA* 1992;89:4037–4041.

65. Fawell SE, White R, Hoare S, et al. Inhibition of estrogen receptor-DNA binding by the "pure" antiestrogen ICI 164,384 appears to be mediated by impaired receptor dimerization. *Proc Natl Acad Sci USA* 1990;87:6883–6887.

66. Htun H, Holth LT, Walker D, et al. Direct visualization of the human estrogen receptor α reveals a role for ligand in the nuclear distribution of the receptor. *Mol Biol Cell* 1999;10:471–486.

67. Dauvois S, White R, Parker MG. The antiestrogen ICI 182780 disrupts estrogen receptor nucleocytoplasmic shuttling. *J Cell Sci* 1993;106:1377–1388.

68. Perissi V, Staszewski LM, McInerney EM, et al. Molecular determinants of nuclear receptor-corepressor interaction. *Genes Dev* 1999;13:3198–3208.

69. Chen D, Umesono K, Evans RM. SMRT isoforms mediate repression and anti-repression of nuclear receptor heterodimers. *Proc Natl Acad Sci USA* 1996;93:7567–7571.

70. Kurokawa R, Soderstrom M, Horlein A, et al. Polarity-specific activities of retinoic acid receptors determined by a co-repressor. *Nature* 1995;377:451–454.

71. Horlein AJ, Naar AM, Heinzel T, et al. Ligand-independent repression by the thyroid hormone receptor mediated by a nuclear receptor co-repressor. *Nature* 1995;377:397–404.

72. Nagy L, Kao HY, Chakravarti D, et al. Nuclear receptor repression mediated by a complex containing SMRT, mSin3A, and histone deacetylase. *Cell* 1997;89:373–380.

73. Heinzel T, Lavinsky RM, Mullen T-M, et al. A complex containing N-CoR, mSin3 and histone deacetylase mediates transcriptional repression. *Nature* 1997;387:43–48.

74. Schulman IG, Juguilon H, Evans RM. Activation and repression by nuclear hormone receptors: Hormone modulates an equilibrium between active and repressive states. *Mol Cell Biol* 1996;16:3807–3813.

75. Leng X, Tsai SY, O'Malley BW, Tsai M-J. Ligand-dependent conformational changes in thyroid hormone and retinoic acid receptors are potentially enhanced by heterodimerization with retinoic X receptor. *J Steroid Biochem Mol Biol* 1993;46:643–661.

76. Jackson TA, Richer JK, Bain DL, et al. The partial agonist activity of antagonist-occupied steroid receptors is controlled by a novel hinge domain-binding coactivator L7/SPA and the corepressors N-CoR or SMRT. *Mol Endocrinol* 1997;11:693–705.

77. Smith CL, Nawaz Z, O'Malley BW. Coactivator and corepressor regulation of the agonist/antagonist activity of the mixed antiestrogen, 4-hydroxytamoxifen. *Mol Endocrinol* 1997;11:657–666.

78. Jepsen K, Hermanson O, Onami TM, et al. Combinatorial roles of the nuclear receptor corepressor in transcription and development. *Cell* 2000;102:753–763.

79. Mazumdar A, Wang R-A, Mishra SK, et al. Transcriptional repression of oestrogen receptor by metastasis-associated protein 1 corepressor. *Nat Cell Biol* 2001;3:30–37.

80. Delage-Mourroux R, Martini PGV, Choi I, et al. Analysis of estrogen receptor interaction with a repressor of estrogen receptor activity (REA) and the regulation of estrogen receptor transcriptional activity by REA. *J Biol Chem* 2000;275:35,848–35,856.

81. Laherty CD, Billin AN, Lavinsky RM, et al. SAP30, a component of the mSin3 corepressor complex involved in N-CoR-mediated repression by specific transcription factors. *Mol Cell* 1998;2:33–42.

82. Oesterreich S, Zhang Q, Hopp T, et al. Tamoxifen-bound estrogen receptor (ER) strongly interacts with the nuclear matrix protein HET-SAF-B, a novel inhibitor of ER-mediated transactivation. *Mol Endocrinol* 2000;14:369–381.

83. Kurebayashi J, Otsuki T, Kunisue H, et al. Expression levels of estrogen receptor-alpha, estrogen receptor-beta, coactivators, and corepressors in breast cancer. *Clin Cancer Res* 2000;6:512–518.

84. Shang Y, Brown M. Molecular determinants for the tissue specificity of SERMs. *Science* 2002;295:2465–2468.

85. Xu J, Qiu Y, DeMayo FJ, et al. Partial hormone resistance in mice with disruption of the steroid receptor coactivator-1 (SRC-1) gene. Science 1998;279:1922–1925.

86. Gehin M, Mark M, Dennefeld C, et al. The function of TIF2/GRIP1 in mouse reproduction is distinct from those of SRC-1 and p/CIP. *Mol Cell Biol* 2002;22:5923–5937.

87. Xu J, Liao L, Ning G, et al. The steroid receptor coactivator SRC-3 (p/CIP/RAC3/AIB1/ACTR/TRAM-1) is required for normal growth, puberty, female reproductive function, and mammary gland development. *Proc Natl Acad Sci USA* 2000;97:6379–6384.

88. Wang A, Rose DW, Hermanson O, et al. Regulation of somatic growth by the p160 coactivator p/CIP. *Proc Natl Acad Sci USA* 2000;97:13,549–13,554.

89. Smith CL, DeVera DG, Lamb DJ, et al. Genetic ablation of the steroid receptor coactivator/ubiquitin ligase, E6-AP, results in tissue-selective steroid hormone resistance and defects in reproduction. *Mol Cell Biol* 2002;22:525–535.

90. Smith CL. Cross-talk between peptide growth factor and estrogen receptor signaling pathways. *Biol Reprod* 1998;58:627–632.

91. Fujimoto N, Katzenellenbogen BS. Alteration in the agonist/antagonist balance of antiestrogens by activation of protein kinase A signaling pathways in breast cancer cells: Antiestrogen selectivity and promoter dependence. *Mol Endocrinol* 1994;8:296–304.

92. Smith CL, Conneely OM, O'Malley BW. Modulation of the ligand-independent activation of the human estrogen receptor by hormone and antihormone. *Proc Natl Acad Sci USA* 1993;90:6120–6124.

93. Coleman KM, Smith CL. Intracellular signaling pathways: nongenomic actions of estrogens and ligand-independent activation of estrogen receptors. *Front Biosci* 2001;6:D1379–D1391.

94. Rowan BG, Weigel NL, O'Malley BW. Phosphorylation of steroid receptor coactivator-1. Identification of the phosphorylation sites and phosphorylation through the mitogen-activated protein kinase pathway. *J Biol Chem* 2000;275:4475–4483.

95. Hong S-H, Privalsky ML. The SMRT corepressor is regulated by a MEK-1 kinase pathway: inhibition of corepressor function is associated with SMRT phosphorylation and nuclear export. *Mol Cell Biol* 2000;20:6612–6625.

96. Jordan VC, Morrow M. Chemoprevention of breast cancer: a model for change. *J Clin Oncology* 2002;20:1–3.

97. Early Breast Cancer Trialist Collaborative Group. Tamoxifen for early breast cancer: an overview of the randomized trials. *Lancet* 1998;351:1451–1467.

98. Li CI, Malone KE, Weiss NS, Daling JR. Tamoxifen therapy for primary breast cancer and risk of contralateral breast cancer. *J Natl Cancer Inst* 2001;93:1008–1013.

99. Fisher B, Costantino JP, Wickerham DL, et al. Tamoxifen for prevention of breast cancer: report of the National Surgical Adjuvant Breast and Bowel Project P-1 study. *J Natl Cancer Inst* 1998;90:1371–1388.

100. Cummings SR, Eckert S, Krueger KA, et al. The effect of raloxifene on risk of breast cancer in postmenopausal women. Results from the MORE randomized trial. *JAMA* 1999;281:2189–2197.

101. Powles T, Eeles R, Ashley S, et al. Interim analysis of the incidence of breast cancer in the Royal Marsden Hospital

tamoxifen randomised chemoprevention trial. *Lancet* 1998;352:98–101.

102. Veronesi U, Maisonneuve P, Costa A, et al. Prevention of breast cancer with tamoxifen: preliminary findings from the Italian randomised trial among hysterectomised women. *Lancet* 1998;352:93–97.

103. Cuzick J. A brief review of the current breast cancer prevention trials and proposals for future trials. *Eur J Cancer* 2000;36:1298–1302.

104. Hershman D, Sundararajan V, Jacobson JS, et al. Outcomes of tamoxifen chemoprevention for breast cancer in very high-risk women: a cost-effectiveness analysis. *J Clin Oncol* 2002;20:9–16.

105. Day R, Ganz PA, Costantino JP, et al. Health-related quality of life and tamoxifen in breast cancer prevention: a report from the National Surgical Adjuvant Breast and Bowel Project P-1 study. *J Clin Oncol* 1999;17:2659–2669.

106. Port ER, Montgomery LL, Heerdt AS, Borgen PI. Patient reluctance toward tamoxifen use for breast cancer primary prevention. *Ann Surg Oncol* 2001;8:580–585.

107. Love RR, Mazess RB, Barden HS, et al. Effects of tamoxifen on bone mineral density in postmenopausal women with breast cancer. *N Engl J Med* 1992;326:852–856.

108. Kristensen B, Ejlertsen B, Dalgaard P, et al. Tamoxifen and bone metabolism in postmenopausal low-risk breast cancer patients: a randomized study. *J Clin Oncol* 1994;12:992–997.

109. Love RR, Newcomb PA, Wiebe DA, et al. Effects of tamoxifen therapy on lipid and lipoprotein levels in postmenopausal patients with node-negative breast cancer. *J Natl Cancer Inst* 1990;82:1327–1332.

110. Bagdade JD, Wolter J, Subbaiah PV, Ryan W. Effects of tamoxifen treatment on plasma lipids and lipoprotein lipid composition. *J Clin Endocrinol Metab* 1990;70:1132–1135.

111. Greaves P, Goonetilleke R, Nunn G, et al. Two-year carcinogenicity study of tamoxifen in Alderley Park Wistar-derived rats. *Cancer Res* 1993;53:3919–3924.

112. Rutqvist LE, Johansson H, Signomklao T, et al. Adjuvant tamoxifen therapy for early stage breast cancer and second primary malignancies. Stockholm Breast Cancer Study Group. *J Natl Cancer Inst* 1995;87:645–651.

113. Reis SE, Costantino JP, Wickerham DL, et al. Cardiovascular effects of tamoxifen in women with and without heart disease: breast cancer prevention trial. National Surgical Adjuvant Breast and Bowel Project Breast Cancer Prevention Trial Investigators. *J Natl Cancer Inst* 2001;93:16–21.

114. Hulley S, Grady D, Bush T, et al. Randomized trial of estrogen plus progestin for secondary prevention of coronary heart disease in postmenopausal women. Heart and Estrogen/Progestin Replacement Study (HERS) Research Group. *JAMA* 1998;280:605–613.

115. Gottardis MM, Robinson SP, Satyaswaroop PG, Jordan VC. Contrasting actions of tamoxifen on endometrial and breast tumor growth in the athymic mouse. *Cancer Res* 1988;48:812–815.

116. Fisher B, Costantino JP, Redmond CK, et al. Endometrial cancer in tamoxifen-treated breast cancer patients: findings from the National Surgical Adjuvant Breast and Bowel Project (NSABP) B-14. *J Natl Cancer Inst* 1994;86:527–537.

117. Gottardis MM, Jordan VC. Antitumor actions of keoxifene and tamoxifen in the N-nitrosomethylurea-induced rat mammary carcinoma model. *Cancer Res* 1987;47:4020–4024.

118. Anzano MA, Peer CW, Smith JM, et al. Chemoprevention of mammary carcinogenesis in the rat: combined use of raloxifene and 9-cis-retinoic acid. *J Natl Cancer Inst* 1996;88:123–125.

119. Sato M, Rippy MK, Bryant HU. Raloxifene, tamoxifen, nafoxidine, or estrogen effects on reproductive and nonreproductive tissues in ovariectomized rats. *FASEB J* 1996;10:905–912.

120. Kleinman D, Karas M, Danilenko M, et al. Stimulation of endometrial cancer cell growth by tamoxifen is associated wtih increased insulin-like growth factor (ICF)-I induced tyrosine phosphorylation and reduction in IGF binding proteins. *Endocrinology* 1996;137:1089–1095.

121. Ettinger B, Black DM, Mitlak BH, et al. Reduction of vertebral fracture risk in postmenopausal women with osteoporosis treated with raloxifene: results from a 3-year randomized clinical trial. Multiple Outcomes of Raloxifene Evaluation (MORE) Investigators. *JAMA* 1999;282:637–645.

122. Delmas PD, Bjarnason NH, Mitlak BH, et al. Effects of raloxifene on bone mineral density, serum cholesterol concentrations, and uterine endometrium in postmenopausal women. *N Engl J Med* 1997;337:1641–1647.

123. Cauley JA, Norton L, Lippman ME, et al. Continued breast cancer risk reduction in postmenopausal women treated with raloxifene: 4-year results from the MORE trial. Multiple Outcomes of Raloxifene Evaluation. *Breast Cancer Res Treat* 2001;65:125–134.

124. Dunn BK, Ford LG. From adjuvant therapy to breast cancer prevention: BCPT and STAR. *Breast J* 2001;7:144–157.

125. Mosca L, Barrett-Connor E, Wenger NK, et al. Design and methods of the Raloxifene Use for The Heart (RUTH) study. *Amer J Cardiol* 2002;88:392–395.

126. Munster PN, Buzdar A, Dhingra K, et al. Phase I study of a third-generation selective estrogen receptor modulator, LY353381.HCL, in metastatic breast cancer. *J Clin Oncol* 2001;19:2002–2009.

127. Suh N, Glasebrook AL, Palkowitz AD, et al. Arzoxifene, a new selective estrogen receptor modulator for chemoprevention of experimental breast cancer. *Cancer Res* 2001;61:8412–8415.

128. Labrie F, Labrie C, Belanger A, et al. EM-652 (SCH57068), a pure SERM having complete antiestrogenic activity in the mammary gland and endometrium. *J Steroid Biochem Mol Biol* 2001;79:213–225.

129. Gutman M, Couillard S, Roy J, et al. Comparison of the effects of EM-652 (SCH57068), tamoxifen, toremifene, droloxifene, idoxifene, GW-5638 and raloxifene on the growth of human ZR-75-1 breast tumors in nude mice. *Int J Cancer* 2002;99:273–278.

130. Ke HZ, Paralkar VM, Grasser WA, et al. Effects of CP-336,156, a new, nonsteroidal estrogen agonist/antagonist, on bone, serum cholesterol, uterus and body composition in rat models. *Endocrinology* 1998;139:2068–2076.

131. Cohen LA, Pittman B, Wang CX, et al. LAS, a novel selective estrogen receptor modulator with chemopreventive and therapeutic activity in the N-nitroso-N-methylurea-induced rat mammary tumor model. *Cancer Res* 2001;61:8683–8688.

132. Bentrem D, Dardes R, Liu H, et al. Molecular mechanism of action at estrogen receptor alpha of a new clinically relevant antiestrogen (GW7604) related to tamoxifen. *Endocrinology* 2001;142:838–846.

C. NATURAL VITAMIN D AND SYNTHETIC ANALOGS

17 Chemopreventive Efficacy of Natural Vitamin D and Synthetic Analogs

Kathryn Z. Guyton, PhD, DABT, Thomas W. Kensler, PhD, DABT, and Gary H. Posner, PhD

CONTENTS

INTRODUCTION
MECHANISMS OF ACTION
EFFICACY
DELTANOID SAFETY
CONSIDERATIONS FOR AGENT SELECTION
CLINICAL TARGETS FOR THE DEVELOPMENT OF DELTANOIDS AS CHEMOPREVENTIVES
SUMMARY AND PERSPECTIVES
ACKNOWLEDGMENTS
REFERENCES

1. INTRODUCTION

The activities of vitamin D and synthetic vitamin D analogs (deltanoids) are primarily mediated through binding to vitamin D receptors (VDRs), members of the steroid/thyroid receptor superfamily. Chemopreventive properties of this class of compounds include in vitro and in vivo antiproliferative, pro-apoptotic, pro-differentiating, and anti-angiogenic activities. Natural vitamin D and a number of deltanoids have shown chemopreventive efficacy in preclinical studies. Although also supported by substantial epidemiologic data, the development of natural vitamin D as a cancer chemopreventive has been hindered by dose-limiting hypercalcemic effects. Unfortunately, these same safety concerns also apply to many deltanoids, including those approved for treatment of secondary hyperparathyroidism in patients with end-stage renal disease. However, several new synthetic deltanoids have recently shown promise in preclinical safety and chemopreventive efficacy studies. Potential clinical targets for clinical chemoprevention studies include the colon—which is most strongly supported by epidemiologic and preclinical efficacy studies, as well as the prostate and breast. Ongoing efforts will further elucidate the molecular mechanisms through which vitamin D and synthetic deltanoids affect gene expression and cellular fate. These studies suggest proliferation and apoptotic indices as probable candidate endpoint biomarkers.

2. MECHANISMS OF ACTION

Figure 1 provides an overview of the metabolism and mechanisms of action of vitamin D that pertain to its chemopreventive potential. To attain biological activity, vitamin D must undergo two hydroxylation steps following cutaneous production or intestinal absorption from dietary sources. Vitamin D is first transported to the liver via serum vitamin D-binding protein, where hydroxylation at the 25 position yields 25-hydroxyvitamin D_3 (25(OH)D_3). This major circulating metabolite, which has a 19-d half-life, undergoes a second hydroxylation step in the kidney to produce the hormonally active metabolite $1\alpha,25$-Dihydroxyvitamin D_3 ($1\alpha,25(OH)_2D_3$). The mitochondrial 1α-hydroxylase enzyme that catalyzes this second hydroxylation step is also present in many target tissues that are relevant for chemoprevention, such as the colon (1). The activity of $1\alpha,25(OH)_2D_3$ is predominantly mediated through binding to VDRs, members of the steroid/thyroid receptor superfamily (2). $1\alpha,25(OH)_2D_3$ enhances

From: Cancer Chemoprevention, Volume 1: Promising Cancer Chemoprevention Agents
Edited by: G. J. Kelloff, E. T. Hawk, and C. C. Sigman © Humana Press Inc., Totowa, NJ

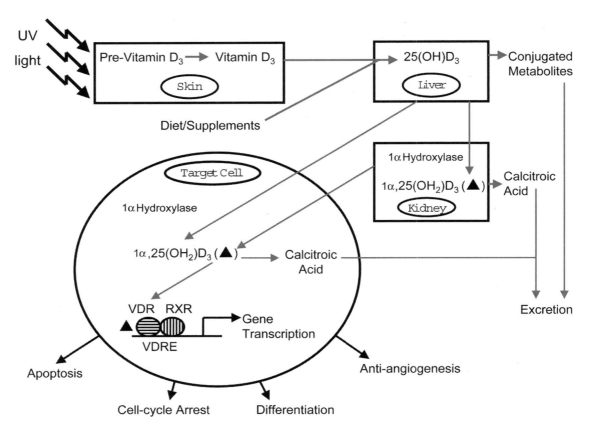

Fig. 1. $1\alpha,25(OH)_2D_3$ biosynthesis and function.

VDR expression *(3)*, and $1\alpha,25(OH)_2D_3$ binding increases the half-life and transcriptional potency of the receptor *(4)*. The ligand-VDR complex heterodimerizes with the retinoid X receptor and binds, in turn, to the specific DNA sequences that constitute vitamin D-response elements. More than 50 genes are regulated by VDRs. VDRs are expressed in the bone and intestine in addition to approximately 30 other tissues including the mammary glands, colon, prostate, hematopoietic cells, and skin *(5)*. This wide tissue distribution of VDRs underscores the ability of vitamin D to exert pleiotropic actions throughout the body. Well-known to function in regulation of calcium homeostasis, $1\alpha,25(OH)_2D_3$ also exerts effects that are comparable to steroid hormones on a number of cellular processes such as mononuclear-cell maturation and cytokine production. $1\alpha,25(OH)_2D_3$ also appears to act through non-genomic mechanisms that are independent of VDR-mediated gene transcription *(6)*.

More than 2,000 deltanoids have been designed and synthesized, and most contain structural changes in the C,D-ring and the side-chain region *(7)*. Promising examples include the following: Leo Pharmaceutical Company's KH1060, EB1089 *(8)*, and C18-attached side-chain analogs *(9)*; Hoffmann-La Roche's 16-ene-23-yne and 16,23-diene series *(10)*; Chugai Pharmaceutical Company's 22-oxa series *(11)*; the Riverside group's arocalciferols *(12)*; the Belgian C- and D-ring nor analogs *(13)* and 14-epi analogs *(3)*; and 24-ethyl analog 1α-hydroxyvitamin D_5 *(14)*. Prominent examples of deltanoids with structural modification exclusively in the A-ring region include the following: the Madison *(15)*, the Riverside *(16)*, and the Providence *(17)* 3-epi analogs, DeLuca's 19-nor analogs *(18)*, the Austrian aromatic analogs *(19)*, and the Johns Hopkins University 1-hydroxyalkyl series *(20)*. Structural changes in both the A-ring and also the C,D-ring side-chain regions have produced transcriptionally potent, noncalcemic hybrid analogs *(21)*. Figure 2 shows examples of the following structural modifications associated with chemopreventive activity: an extra ethyl group at position-24 [1α-hydroxyvitamin D_5,$1\alpha(OH)D_5$], an extra oxygen atom at position-22 (Chugai-OCT) plus

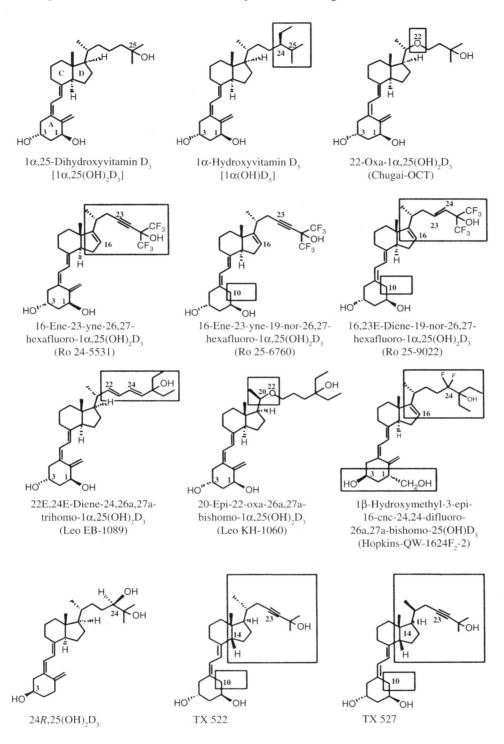

Fig. 2. Deltanoids discussed in this chapter.

20-epimerization (KH1060), 16- and 23-unsaturation with (Ro 24-5531) or without (Ro 25-9022 and Ro 25-6760) a 19-methylene group; an A-ring calcemia-lowering modification plus a side-chain-potentiating group (Hopkins QW-1624F2-2); a side-chain conjugated 22, 24-diene (EB1089); 14-epimerization without a 19-methylene group (TX 522 and TX 527); and 24-hydroxylation (24R,25-dihydroxyvitamin D_3 (24R,25-$(OH)_2D_3$)).

Vitamin D and synthetic deltanoids possess a number of prominent chemoprevention-related actions, including antiproliferative, pro-differentiating, pro-apoptotic, and anti-angiogenic effects (reviewed in ref.22). These activities have been observed in a variety of tissues and cell lines. For example, members of this class of agents inhibit the growth of cancer-cell lines derived from the skin, breast, endometrium, head and neck, lung, prostate, colon, and hematopoietic lineages (reviewed in ref. 2). As reviewed in Kelloff et al. (23), mechanisms through which vitamin D may achieve these effects on cellular fate include modulation of signal transduction and oncogene expression, and inhibition of ODC induction, DNA synthesis, lipid peroxidation, and transforming growth factor (TGF)β expression. Vitamin D appears to target an expanding number of genes involved in cell growth and differentiation, including cytokines, interleukins IL-1β, IL-2, IL-8, IL-12, (granulocyte macrophage colony-stimulating factor (GM-CSF), transcription factors, and tumor-suppressor genes (BRCA1 and E-cadherin) (reviewed in 2). Although some actions are independent of the receptor—for example, changes in PKC isoform expression by Ro 24-5531 in azoxymethane (AOM)-treated rat colon (24)—VDR appears to play a prominent role in mediating the chemopreventive effects of vitamin D and deltanoids. VDRs are expressed in numerous human malignancies, including colon, prostate, and breast cancers; VDR levels in breast cancers may be positively related to disease-free survival (reviewed in ref. 25).

The vitamin and synthetic deltanoids appear to enhance VDR expression and to directly affect VDR half-life and transcriptional activity. For example, the rate of VDR transcription as well as VDR protein levels were doubled or tripled by 1α,25$(OH)_2D_3$ or TX 522 and TX 527, respectively (3). KH1060 increased by three fold the half-life of VDR in human osteoblastic sarcoma MG-63 cells; EB1089 maintained VDR levels for a longer time than 1α,25$(OH)_2D_3$, although each doubled the half-life from 5 to 10 h (4). EB1089

may achieve this effect by stabilizing the high-affinity ligand-binding conformation of VDR (26). 1α,25$(OH)_2D_3$ and the deltanoid Chugai-OCT may increase the transactivation capacity of VDR by enhancing the efficiency with which the receptor binds other components of the transcriptional machinery, particularly the VDR-interacting protein coactivator complex (27). Upon ligand binding, the VDR may assume a conformation that is permissive of transcriptional activation, yet prevents binding of proteins that mediate degradation (4). In human skin 1α,25$(OH)_2D_3$ binding blocks ubiquitination of VDR and thereby retards receptor degradation via the ubiquitin/proteasome pathway (28). Structure-activity analyses have provided insight into the VDR residues at which certain deltanoids may bind to achieve enhanced VDR stabilization and activation. For example, Peleg et al. (29) demonstrated that some hybrid analogs with an unnatural 1-hydroxymethyl substituent do not interact with the transcription activation function 2 domain of the VDR, but do exhibit increased ability to stabilize and transcriptionally activate the receptor.

The antiproliferative effects of 1α,25$(OH)_2D_3$ and a number of deltanoids (e.g., EB1089, Ro 24-5531, Ro 25-6760, TX 522 and TX 527) appear to be mediated by the induction of arrest of cell-cycle progression at the G_0/G_1 phase (3,30–32). The growth arrest is associated with upregulation of the cyclin-dependent kinase inhibitors $p21^{waf1}$ and $p27^{kip1}$, decreased cyclin-dependent kinase activity, hypophosphorylation of retinoblastoma (RB) protein and repressed E2F transcriptional activity in several cell types; as the $p21^{waf1}$ gene promoter contains a VDR-response element, this effect may in part be VDR-dependent (3,33–38). $TGFβ_1$ induction may also play a role in the induction of these genes and the resulting growth arrest (39). 1α,25$(OH)_2D_3$ also enhances the expression of HoxA10, a homeobox protein that causes G_1 arrest (35). In breast cancer cells, vitamin D may also abrogate estrogen responsiveness; for example, EB1089 downregulates the expression of estrogen receptor in MCF-7 breast cancer cells and limits the mitogenic effect of 17β-estradiol (25). 1α,25$(OH)_2D_3$ likewise downregulates the estrogen receptor and suppresses estrogen action in MCF-7 breast cancer cells (40).

The ability of vitamin D and analogs to induce apoptosis has been investigated in vivo and in several cell types in vitro. For example, apoptosis was detected in prostate sections of EB1089-treated rats, an effect associated with increased expression of IGF-binding proteins −2, −3, −4, and −5 and of IGF-I mRNA (41). EB1089 and $1\alpha,25(OH)_2D_3$ also promote apoptosis of prostate cancer cells (32) and breast cancer cells in vitro, and enhance the sensitivity of breast cancer cells to antiestrogens and radiation (42,43) as well as $TNF\alpha$ (44). Vitamin D and EB1089 induce apoptosis in colon and breast cancer cells via a mechanism that is independent of p53 (45,46). Forced overexpression of bcl-2 renders MCF-7 breast cancer cells resistant to $1\alpha,25(OH)_2D_3$ and EB1089 (45). The BAK protein was suggested to mediate apoptosis in colon cancer cells (46). In MCF-7 breast cancer cells, $1\alpha,25(OH)_2D_3$ triggers generation of reactive oxygen species (ROS) (47), translocation of the pro-apoptotic protein BAX to the mitochondria, and induction of apoptosis in a caspase-independent manner (48,49). In murine squamous-cell carcinoma cells, $1\alpha,25(OH)_2D_3$ stimulates caspase-dependent cleavage of mitogen-activated protein kinase (MEK), resulting in greatly diminished MEK expression and signaling (50).

Vitamin D and deltanoids inhibit angiogenesis and metastasis in xenograft and transgenic mouse models, and limit the invasiveness of several cell types in vitro. For example, $1\alpha,25(OH)_2D_3$ (0.5 or 1 μg/kg/d) significantly reduced angiogenesis of human tumor-cell xenografts (cervical, vulval, and breast) in immunosuppressed Balb/c mice (51). In a separate study $1\alpha,25(OH)_2D_3$ (12.5 pmol/d for 5 wk) decreased tumor vascularity, as evaluated by vessel counts, in a MCF-7 breast-cancer-cell xenograft model; the vitamin also blocked vascular endothelial growth factor-induced endothelial-cell sprouting and elongation in vitro (52). 1α-hydroxyvitamin D_3 ($1\alpha(OH)D_3$) (0.1 or 1 μg/kg/d for 2 wk) also abrogated the growth and metastasis of Dunn murine osteosarcoma xenografts (53). Vitamin D (0.025 or 0.05 μg 5×/wk for 5 wk) inhibited angiogenesis, as evidenced by decreased vessel counts, in murine RB transgenic mice (54). Both $1\alpha,25(OH)_2D_3$ and EB1089 (1.0 μg/kg every other d) blocked prostate cancer-cell metastasis in the rat Dunning MAT LyLu model (55). In this study, treatment with $1\alpha,25(OH)_2D_3$ or EB1089 significantly reduced lung-tumor foci development; although EB1089 was significantly less calcemic than $1\alpha,25(OH)_2D_3$, both agents elevated serum calcium levels, and $1\alpha,25(OH)_2D_3$ also induced severe weight loss. In in vitro bioassays of cell invasion, $1\alpha,25(OH)_2D_3$ inhibited the invasiveness of human prostate cancer DU 145 cells (56) and mouse melanoma B16 cells (57). In both cases, reduced invasion was associated with a decrease

in secreted levels, of type IV collagenases. In vivo treatment with $1\alpha,25(OH)_2D_3$ (0.5 μg/kg) for 28 d reduced the formation of lung metastases in mice that were inoculated with B16 cells (57).

3. EFFICACY

3.1. Epidemiologic Evidence of Cancer-Preventive Activity

The potential for vitamin D in cancer prevention was first suggested by observations in the 1930s and 1940s of the inverse association between sun exposure, which enables cutaneous production of the vitamin, and cancer rates. Rates of skin and internal cancers were found to be inversely related, as were overall cancer death rates and distance from the equator (58,59). Enhanced sunlight exposure has since been associated with lower prostate, breast, and colon cancer death rates, and the historical geographic distribution of rickets parallels that for these cancer deaths (60–65). Furthermore, certain risk factors for prostate cancer, including advanced age and African-American ethnicity, are associated with reduced vitamin D levels (66). As detailed in the following paragraphs, a number of epidemiologic studies have sought to determine whether high intake or serum vitamin D levels are predictive of or associated with reduced colon, breast, or prostate cancer risk. Although many studies have supported the hypothesis that the vitamin is inversely associated with risk, this finding has not been definitively elucidated.

The strongest epidemiologic evidence supporting a protective role for the vitamin is from prospective studies of dietary or total (dietary and supplemental) vitamin D intake and colorectal cancer (CRC) development. Four such studies have reported inverse associations for vitamin D intake and colon or CRC, with relative risks ranging from 0.33–0.74 (reviewed in step 67). A 19-yr prospective study of 2,107 Western Electric employees found a significant association between reported dietary vitamin D intake and subsequent development of CRC (68). The Iowa Women's Health Study and the Health Professionals Follow-Up Study each found an inverse association between total vitamin D and the risk of colon cancer, but these findings were not significant after multivariate adjustment (69–71). An inverse correlation between total vitamin D intake and CRC risk was also suggested in a prospective study of 89,448 female nurses (72). The analysis based intake upon dietary questionnaires conducted in 1980, 1984 and 1986, and found relative risks for CRC of 0.72 and 0.42 for highest vs lowest intake categories for dietary and total vitamin D, respectively.

Results from case-control studies have been inconsistent regarding the association between vitamin D intake and CRC risk. A case-control study in Sweden found that increasing levels of dietary vitamin D were inversely associated with CRC, but only after adjustment for age, sex, and total caloric and protein intake (73). The associations found in this Swedish cohort were stronger for women. However a case-control study of Wisconsin women found that although higher vitamin D intake was weakly associated with reduced CRC risk, a consistent, dose-responsive effect was lacking (74). A French case-control study found that vitamin D was inversely related to the risk of small adenomas in women; no such association was found for men, and no significant correlation with CRC risk was noted (75).

Several recent studies have demonstrated an inverse association between serum $1\alpha,25(OH)_2D_3$ or $25(OH)D_3$ levels on biomarkers of the development of colon cancer. For example, a case-control study nested in the prospective Nurses' Health Study found an increased risk (OR = 1.58, 95% CI, 1.03–2.40) of distal colorectal adenomas for women with below normal plasma $1\alpha,25(OH)_2D_3$ levels (e.g., <26 pg/mL) (76). The association was stronger for large or villous adenomas. A separate case-control study found an inverse association of serum $25(OH)D_3$ and colorectal adenomas (77). Adenoma risk decreased by 26% (OR = 0.74, 95% CI 0.6–0.92) with each 10 ng/mL increase of serum $25(OH)D_3$. A third study found a significant inverse correlation between fasting serum $25(OH)D_3$ levels and colonic epithelial-cell proliferation, as measured by the crypt-labeling index and the size of the proliferative compartment (78).

Evidence of a potentially protective effect of vitamin D intake on the risk of breast cancer development is limited but intriguing. For example, the National Health and Nutrition Examination Survey (NHANES I) Epidemiologic Follow-up Study examined the effect of sunlight exposure and vitamin D intake on the risk of breast cancer in a multivariate analysis that controlled for age, education, age at menarche, age at menopause, body mass index, alcohol consumption, and physical activity (79). Several measures of sunlight exposure and dietary vitamin D intake each correlated with reduced risk of breast cancer risk. The association was strongest for women living in regions of high solar radiation, for whom relative risks were 0.35–0.75; no

risk reductions were found for women who resided in regions of low solar radiation. Although limited by small case numbers, the study suggested a dependency of the protective effect of sun and dietary vitamin D intake against breast cancer on high residential solar radiation.

Several epidemiological studies have demonstrated an inverse association between serum $1\alpha,25(OH)_2D_3$ or $25(OH)D_3$ levels and the risk of prostate cancer, but this finding has not been universally confirmed. For example, in a northern California cohort of European or African-American ethnicity, the 181 men who subsequently developed clinical prostate cancer had 1.8 pg/mL lower serum levels of total $1\alpha,25(OH)_2D_3$ than age-matched controls. This inverse association between prediagnostic serum $1\alpha,25(OH)_2D_3$ levels and clinical prostate cancer was strongest in men ≥57 yr of age (80). However, Braun et al. conducted a similar study in Maryland and observed no association with either $1\alpha,25(OH)_2D_3$ or $25(OH)D_3$ in 61 men diagnosed with prostate cancer (81). A nested case-control study in a cohort of 3737 Japanese-American Hawaiian men also failed to find a strong association between serum vitamin D levels and the subsequent development of prostate cancer (82). After a surveillance period of 23 yr, the serum levels of $25(OH)D_3$ and $1\alpha,25(OH)_2D_3$ among 136 incident cases of prostate cancer were comparable to those of age-matched controls. Likewise, Gann et al. reported in 1996 that the 232 diagnosed cases of prostate cancer in a cohort of 14,916 US physicians were not associated with significantly lower serum $1\alpha,25(OH)_2D_3$, $25(OH)D_3$ or vitamin D binding protein (83). Nonetheless a nonsignificant inverse association for $1\alpha,25(OH)_2D_3$ was present for older men with low $25(OH)D_3$ levels.

A number of studies have attempted to determine whether particular VDR polymorphisms are associated with increased risk of prostate cancer risk. For example, further study of the same cohort of US physicians described here found that 3' polymorphisms BsmI and TaqI (which do not affect receptor structure or function but may influence stability of VDR mRNA) are not strong, independent predictors of prostate cancer risk. Interestingly, for men with plasma $25(OH)D_3$ levels below the median, risk was reduced for those who were homozygous for the absence of the BsmI site (84). Increased risk of advanced prostate cancer in African-Americans was associated with a haplotype in which the BsmI site is absent and a long poly-A microsatellite is present *(85)*. A separate study found that men homozygous for the presence of the TaqI site were shown to have one-third the risk of developing prostate cancer requiring prostatectomy compared to men who were heterozygotes or homozygous for its absence *(86)*. Similarly, the genotype for homozygous absence of the TaqI site was statistically higher among Japanese patients with either locally advanced or metastatic prostate cancer (OR = 2.52; 95% CI, 1.21–5.27; p = 0.009) or poorly differentiated adeno-carcinoma of the prostate (OR = 5.38; 95% CI, 1.57–18.5; p = 0.002) compared to age-matched non-cancerous controls *(87)*. However, in a study of Austrian Caucasians, no association of the TaqI poly-morphism with the risk of prostate cancer risk was found *(88)*.

Emerging evidence suggests that 3' VDR polymor-phisms may affect the risk of other cancers as well. In two case-control studies of breast cancer risk, the VDR polymorphism BsmI was significantly associated with an increased risk of breast cancer The risk in a UK Caucasian population was 2.32 (95% CI, 1.23–4.39) *(89)*, and that in US Latinas was 2.2 (95% CI, 1–4.7) *(90)*. The 5' VDR polymorphism FokI, which may result in an altered translation start site, has also been associated with increased risk of certain cancers and cancer biomarkers. A hospital-based case-control study found that the homozygous FokI polymorphism was associated with a poor prognosis in patients with malignant melanoma *(91)*. Although a study of 373 colorectal adenoma cases and 394 controls found no significant association between the FokI polymor-phism and colorectal adenoma risk, risk of large (>1 cm) adenomas decreased in heterozygotes (OR = 0.70; 95% CI 0.44–1.41) and those that were homozygous for FokI absence (OR = 0.32; 95% CI 0.11–0.91). The FokI polymorphism genotype was more strongly relat-ed to large adenoma risk among subjects with low dietary calcium intake, low dietary vitamin D intake, or dark skin color *(92)*. In a case-control study, homozygous absence of the 3' BsmI polymorphism was likewise more strongly associated with lower risk of col-orectal adenoma development in the lowest tertile of vitamin D or calcium intake *(93)*. These intriguing find-ings suggest that calcium and vitamin D status may influence the effect of these VDR polymorphism geno-types on colorectal adenoma development. As noted previously for prostate cancer risk, there is some evi-dence that certain VDR 3' polymorphisms may also interact to affect risk. For example, a population-based case-control study in a mostly Caucasian population found that homozygous absence of the BsmI polymor-phism, presence of short poly-A microsatellite and presence of TaqI polymorphism were associated with reduced risk of colon cancer (OR = 0.5, 95% CI, 0.3–0.9) *(94)*.

3.2. Preclinical Evidence of Chemopreventive Efficacy of Vitamin D

Vitamin D has demonstrated chemopreventive effi-cacy in several experimental models of carcinogenesis, with the strongest evidence for colon cancer prevention. In various models, vitamin D_3 and its metabolites $1\alpha(OH)D_3$ or $1\alpha,25(OH)_2D_3$ were effective against carcinogenesis in the colon/intestine, and most stud-ies showed a 50% reduction in tumor burden and/or multiplicity. For example, concurrent and post-car-cinogen treatment with $1\alpha(OH)D_3$ (0.04 µg ig 3×/wk) reduced by one-half the formation of *N*-methyl-*N'*-nitro-*N*-nitrosoguanidine (MNNG)-induced tubular adenocarcinomas of the small intestine in male Wistar rats *(95)*. Serum calcium was significantly elevated by treatment. Concomitant administration of $1\alpha(OH)D_3$ (0.04 µg ig 3×/wk) abrogated the tumor-promoting effects of lithocholic acid on *N*-methyl-*N*-nitrosourea (MNU)-initiated colon tumorigenesis in female F344 rats *(96)*. $1\alpha(OH)D_3$ (0.12 µg/kg ip every other d) or $1\alpha,25(OH)_2D_3$ (0.06 µg/kg ip every other d) were also effective against AOM-induced colon carcinogenesis when administered post-carcinogen *(97)*. $1\alpha,25(OH)_2D_3$ (400ng/rat sc once/wk) reduced tumor multiplicity by half when given 1 wk before 1,2-dimethylhydrazine (DMH) to CD rats, but was ineffective when administered post-carcinogen, or concurrently with carcinogen *(98)*. The chemopre-ventive effect was associated with a reduction in ODC levels. Elevated serum calcium levels were observed in treated animals. In a separate study, $1\alpha,25(OH)_2D_3$ (3.0 nmol/kg-diet) blocked DMH-induced colon carcinogenesis in Sprague-Dawley rats when administered before and during carcinogen treatment *(99)*. Vitamin D_3 (2000 IU/kg-diet) inhibit-ed DMH-initiated and high fat diet-promoted colon carcinogenesis in male F344 rats *(100)*.

A chemopreventive effect of vitamin D and its metabolites has also been observed in models of the cheek pouch, stomach/intestine, skin, and mammary gland carcinogenesis. In addition, $1\alpha,25(OH)_2D_3$ (0.025 or 0.05 µg/mouse) inhibited retinoblastoma (RB) formation in transgenic SV40 T-antigen mice, although significant toxicity was manifested by hypercalcemia, weight loss, and death (101). Topical administration of vitamin D_3 or D_2 (approx 0.2 mL of a 0.8% solution) significantly inhibited cheek pouch tumors induced by 7,12-dimethylbenz[a]anthracene (DMBA); 13/20 male Syrian golden hamsters administered DMBA for 8–10 wk developed carcinomas as compared with 2/12 or 1/10 animals co-administered vitamin D_2 or D_3, respectively (102). The 1-α-hydroxylated metabolite (0.04 μg) also inhibited gastrointestinal (GI) tumorigenesis in female Wistar rats when administered for 24 wk after treatment with MNNG (95). $1\alpha(OH)D_3$ significantly reduced tumor incidence from 53% to 27%, and tumor multiplicity from 16 to 8, in the stomach and small intestine of carcinogen-treated animals. Topical $1\alpha,25(OH)_2D_3$ (1 μg/wk) also inhibited the multiplicity and enhanced the latency of skin tumors promoted by 12-O-tetradecanoylphorbol-13-acetate (TPA) alone, or TPA and mezerin, in DMBA-initiated female Sencar mice (103,104). However, dietary administration of vitamin D (200–4000 IU/kg-diet) did not affect DMBA-initiated, TPA-promoted skin-tumor carcinogenesis (105). Finally, $1\alpha,25(OH)_2D_3$ (105 ng ip 3×/wk) reduced the size of DMBA-induced mammary adenomas and carcinomas when administered concurrently with, or after, carcinogen to Sprague-Dawley rats (106).

3.3. Preclinical Chemopreventive Activity of Synthetic Deltanoids

Chemopreventive efficacy of synthetic deltanoids has been demonstrated in models of colon, breast, stomach, prostate, and skin cancer. Synthetic deltanoids with colon cancer chemopreventive efficacy in published reports include $24R,25-(OH_2)D_3$, Chugai-OCT, Ro 26-9114, Ro 25-5317, Ro 25-9022, and Ro 24-5531. Although it did not affect tumor number, a non-calcemic dose of Ro 26-9114 (5 μg ip 3 ×/wk) decreased the overall tumor load in Apc^{min} mice (107). Ro 25-5317 and Ro 25-9022 were efficacious against DMH-induced colon cancer development and metastases in Sprague-Dawley rats (99). Tumor incidence was reduced by 16%, 32%, and 28%, respectively, with Ro 25-5317 (3.5 nmol/kg-diet) or Ro 25-9022 (3.0 or 3.5 nmol/kg-diet). Ro 25-5317 completely abrogated the development of metastases, as did the higher Ro 25-9022 dose, and the lower Ro 25-9022 dose significantly reduced metastases. No undesirable lowering of animal weight gain, nor increase in serum calcium, was observed with either deltanoid. In a separate study, administration of Ro 24-5531 (2.5 nmol/kg-diet) before and during carcinogen treatment reduced AOM-induced colonic tumor incidence in F344 rats by 70%, and abolished adenocarcinoma development (24). $24R,25-(OH_2)D_3$ (5 ppm in diet) reduced tumor incidence in the large intestine by about one-third when administered post-initiation in a multi-organ, multi-carcinogen model in F344 rats (108). In the study, $24R,25-(OH_2)D_3$ had no effect on carcinogenesis in the esophagus, lung, or spleen, although tumor incidence was low in these target organs. In a separate multi-organ, multi-carcinogen study, Chugai-OCT (30 μg/kg ip 3×/wk) reduced aberrant crypt foci (ACF) number by half, completely blocked carcinoma formation in the small intestine, and reduced large intestine carcinoma incidence by one-third (109). Although tumor incidence was low in these target organs, Chugai-OCT was not effective against cancer of the urinary bladder, lung, kidney, or thyroid gland. Body wt gain was unaffected by Chugai-OCT, but plasma calcium concentrations were significantly elevated above those in controls (11.7 ± 0.6 vs 9.9 ± 0.4 mg/dL), as was also noted in rats that received only 3 μg/kg body wt of Chugai-OCT.

Chugai-OCT is approved in Japan for treatment of secondary hyperparathyroidism associated with chronic renal failure. As reviewed in Brown and Slatopolsky (110), this deltanoid is less calcemic than $1\alpha,25(OH)_2D_3$. Chugai-OCT (1.0 μg/kg-body wt). significantly inhibited the growth of established DMBA-induced mammary tumors in female Sprague-Dawley rats (111). However, the deltanoid did not induce regression of the tumors. No elevation of serum calcium levels was noted, but Chugai-OCT did slightly retard weight gain.

$1\alpha(OH)D_5$ has also demonstrated efficacy in preclinical models of breast cancer. In an in vitro cancer chemoprevention study, $1\alpha(OH)D_5$ inhibited the development of DMBA-induced preneoplastic lesions in mouse mammary organ culture; this effect was dose-related (0.01–10.0 μM) and had no observed toxicity (112). Although the natural hormone $1\alpha,25(OH)_2D_3$ was 10–100-fold more potent than $1\alpha(OH)D_5$ at preventing preneoplastic lesion development, it induced significant toxicity at concentrations of 1.0 μM or higher. Efficacy of both agents was associated with dramatically enhanced expression of both VDR and $TGF\beta_1$. $1\alpha(OH)D_5$ also reduced the incidence of MNU-induced rat mammary tumors from 80%–53% (25 μg/kg-diet) or 47% (50 μg/kg-diet)

(113). Tumor multiplicity was also reduced, although the effect was not statistically significant. A calcemic effect was not observed. Although this novel deltanoid is considerably less potent than Ro 24-5531 at inhibiting growth of U1S0-BC-4 human breast cancer cells in vitro *(14)*, $1\alpha(OH)D_5$ may deserve further preclinical evaluation in a chemoprevention model of breast cancer.

Like Chugai-OCT and $1\alpha(OH)D_5$, Ro 24-5531 may also have potential in breast cancer chemoprevention. Ro 24-5531 (1.25 or 2.5 nmol/kg-diet) significantly reduced the incidence as well as the multiplicity of mammary carcinomas induced by a single injection of MNU in female Sprague-Dawley rats *(114)*. The latency of palpable tumor incidence was also extended by deltanoid treatment, which began 1 wk post carcinogen and continued for 32 wk thereafter. No effect on either body wt or serum calcium levels was observed with Ro 24-5531. The chemopreventive effect was synergistic with tamoxifen.

Few studies have examined the efficacy of deltanoids against gastric or prostate cancer. $24R,25$-$(OH_2)D_3$ (2.5 or 5 ppm diet) reduced the incidence of gastric proliferative lesions induced by MNNG and NaCl in male Wistar rats from 66% to 38% or 21%, respectively *(115)*. Lesion multiplicity was also decreased by 45% or 74%, respectively, with 2.5 or 5 ppm dietary $24R,25$-$(OH_2)D_3$. When considered alone, the inhibitory effects in the fundus (but not the pylorus) were statistically significant. The deltanoid Ro 24-5531 (1.25 or 2.5 nmol/kg-diet) was only moderately effective in inhibiting the development of carcinogen-initiated and androgen-promoted carcinomas of the seminal vesicle and anterior prostate of Lobund-Wistar rats *(116,117)*.

Although oral administration of the natural vitamin was not efficacious in similar skin-cancer chemoprevention studies *(105)*, the hybrid deltanoid QW-1624F2-2 inhibited skin cancer development in female CD-1 mice initiated with DMBA and promoted twice wkly for 20 wk with TPA *(118)*. Topical application of QW-1624F2-2 (3 µg/mouse) 30 min before each TPA application significantly enhanced tumor latency in addition to reducing tumor incidence by 28% and tumor multiplicity by 63%. Unlike natural $1\alpha,25(OH)_2D_3$ at this dose, QW-1624F2-2 did not adversely affect body wt gain in these animals. Moreover, no increase in urinary calcium excretion was observed following QW-1624F2-2 treatment.

4. DELTANOID SAFETY

The primary dose-limiting toxicity associated with acute or long-term administration of excessive amounts of vitamin D is alterations in calcium metabolism (reviewed in *119*). In humans, vitamin D stimulates an increase in calcium absorption from the intestines and bone that results in elevated blood calcium levels. At pharmacological doses, the most common adverse effects are hypercalcemia and hypercalciurea; soft-tissue calcification and nephrocalcinosis also occur. Such effects have limited dose escalation in Phase II clinical trials of $1\alpha,25(OH)_2D_3$ for chemotherapy of advanced prostatic cancer, despite some evidence of efficacy *(120,121)*. Hypercalcemia has also been noted in clinical trials of $1\alpha,25(OH)_2D_3$ in myelodysplastic syndromes, early recurrent prostate cancer, non-Hodgkins lymphoma, and in patients with solid tumors (reviewed in *23*). Unfortunately, these calcemic effects have been noted at doses required to achieve chemopreventive efficacy

Many synthetic deltanoids share the calcemic properties of natural vitamin D. For example, although the calcemic effects of Ro 24-5531 following acute administration were only 6.7–10.4% of those engendered by the natural vitamin *(122)*, a separate study revealed Ro 24-5531 to be significantly calcemic *(123)*. In a long-term (55-wk) study, Ro 24-5531 actually enhanced bone properties in Balb/c mice *(124)*. Despite the immunosuppression (as evidenced by a profound decrease in serum IL-2) and decreased body weight seen in animals treated with either Ro 24-5531 or Ro 25-6760, the analogs were fairly well-tolerated at weekly doses of 0.0125 µg/mouse. However, a 50% dose reduction was necessitated at 16 wk by hypercalcemia, which nevertheless redeveloped near study end. Blood chemistries and gross organ pathology were otherwise normal. The hybrid 19-nor deltanoid Ro 25-6760 has been shown in a separate study to exhibit slightly higher calcemic activity than $1\alpha,25(OH)_2D_3$ *(123)*.

Synthetic deltanoid $1\alpha(OH)D_5$, which lacks the 25-hydroxyl group believed to be essential for effective ligand binding to the VDR, is only weakly calcemic. $1\alpha(OH)D_5$ (0.042 µg/kg/d) was 4× less calcemic in vitamin D-deficient Sprague-Dawley rats than $1\alpha,25(OH)_2D_3$ *(112)*. Some toxicity (e.g., decreased body wt gain) was observed in Balb/c athymic mice injected 3×/wk at a dose of 200 ng, but not 100 ng or less, of $1\alpha(OH)D_5$ *(14)*.

Two novel 14-epi deltanoids, TX 527 and TX 522, may also have non-calcemic potential. Both exhibited antiproliferative activity against MCF-7 breast cancer cells in vitro and in a xenograft model (3). Although TX 527 (25 μg/kg every other d) significantly increased serum calcium, TX 522 (80 μg/kg every other d) did not; however, both deltanoids decreased tibia calcium content. Nonetheless, $1\alpha,25(OH)_2D_3$ (5 μg/kg/d) decreased tibia calcium and elevated serum calcium to a greater extent than either deltanoid.

The efficacious oral dose of QW-1624F2-2 in a skin chemoprevention study was non-calcemic (118). This result is consistent with two earlier observations of this deltanoid's noncalcemic activity. In the first study, no hypercalcemia was observed in F344 rats administered daily doses up to 10 mg/kg (125). A separate experiment found no in vivo calcemic activity even when QW-1624F2-2 was administered to rats at a dose 100-fold higher (20 mg/kg body wt) (D. Somgen, A. Kaye and G. Posner, unpublished data) than that at which CB1093 caused significant weight loss (126).

Despite promising preclinical findings, several deltanoids have also induced hypercalcemia in clinical trials. 1αZHydroxyvitamin $D_2(1\alpha(OH)D_2$; Hectorol™; doxercalciferol) is an FDA-approved drug indicated for treatment of secondary hyperparathyroidism in patients with end-stage renal disease who are undergoing dialysis. $1\alpha(OH)D_2$ is a precursor of the active vitamin D_2 hormone, 1α,25-Dihydroxyvitamin D_2. This active hormone is formed upon hepatic 25-hydroxylation of $1\alpha(OH)D_2$. $1\alpha(OH)D_2$ does not require activation in the kidney, the normal site of 1α-hydroxylation, and thus can be used in patients with limited kidney function. In clinical trials in patients with renal failure, oral or iv $1\alpha(OH)D_2$ effectively reduced parathyroid hormone (PTH) levels. For example, in the oral study, 91 of 99 hemodialysis patients with initial intact PTH levels of 400 pg/mL showed greater than 50% suppression (127). Lesser increases in both serum calcium and phosphorus with equivalent suppression of PTH were achieved with iv administration. In particular, the incidence of hypercalcemia and hyperphosphatemia were 15% and 17%, respectively, with oral administration, and 8% and 14%, respectively, for iv administration (128). Preclinical studies support a lower toxicity (LD_{50}) of $1\alpha(OH)D_2$ vs vitamin D_3 compounds (129); however, $1\alpha(OH)D_2$ had the same potency as 1α-hydroxyvitamin D_3 for elevating serum calcium and phosphorus and reducing intact PTH levels in an ovariectomized rat model (130). In

a Phase I trial in 25 patients with metastatic hormone-refractory prostate cancer published in abstract form, reversible hypercalcemia (3 grade 1, and 2 each grade 2 and 3 events at 15 μg/d) and frequent hypercalciuria were observed (131). In an ongoing Phase II trial with a starting dose of 12 μg/d, frequent hypercalcemia was observed prompting dose reduction per protocol. Two of 11 patients have had stable disease >6 mo (131). Two metabolites of $1\alpha(OH)D_2$ under preclinical development may also have potential; LR 103, a metabolite of $1\alpha(OH)D_2$ in late-stage preclinical development, exhibits similar potency but less toxicity than $1\alpha(OH)D_2$. LR 103 inhibits skin, breast, and colon cancer-cell growth. A second compound, BCI 201, is metabolized to LR 103. BCI 201 is an oral deltanoid in preclinical development for potential treatment of psoriasis.

In a Phase I clinical trial in healthy volunteers, EB1089 (5–40 μg/d) increased intestinal absorption of calcium and caused hypercalcemia in 2 of 13 subjects (132). Severe hypercalcemia following EB1089 administration (≥ 0.45 μg/m^2/d) was observed in one-third of 36 patients with advanced breast or CRC; no antitumor effects were observed (133). The maximum tolerated dose was estimated at 7 μg/m^2/d. In a study of 10 patients with previously treated blastic myelodysplastic syndromes or acute myeloid leukemia in remission, the highest tolerated dose of EB1089 was 30 μg/d; hypercalcemia nonetheless developed after 21 d at this dose. In ongoing Phase II trials in 27 CRC patients and 22 hepatocellular carcinoma patients, dose-escalation was likewise limited by hypercalcemia (reviewed in 132). Two patients achieved complete response in the hepatocellular carcinoma study, although 17 withdrew because of disease progression. No objective responses were observed in a recent Phase II trial of EB1089 in advanced pancreatic cancer (134).

5. CONSIDERATIONS FOR AGENT SELECTION

The selection of a lead candidate for clinical development from among the numerous available synthetic deltanoids would be greatly facilitated by a series of preclinical cancer chemopreventive studies involving direct, side-by-side comparative performance. Of primary concern is relative calcemic activity, as this has limited dose-escalation in clinical trials with marketed deltanoids. Establishing comparative chemopreventive efficacy among candidate deltanoids is also important; tissue-specific activity should also be compared. The following combination treatment experiment, although in tumor-growth inhibition, illustrates such a side-by-side assessment. Combination of a deltanoid with paclitaxel (Taxol) has been reported to be efficacious in inhibiting the growth of MCF-7 human breast cancer cells in BNX nude mice when administered for 9 wk after inoculation *(126)*. EB1089, Ro 25-6760 or natural $1\alpha,25(OH)_2D_3$, administered alone or with Taxol, resulted in statistically smaller tumors than controls. The potency of EB1089 exceeded that of Ro 25-6760, which in turn was more potent than natural $1\alpha,25(OH)_2D_3$. Furthermore, EB1089 plus Taxol suppressed tumor growth more than either drug alone, causing a 30–50% reduction in average tumor weight compared to controls. No elevation in serum calcium levels was observed, and there was no statistically significant reduction in animal weight gain, by combined EB1089 and Taxol treatment. As noted here, EB1089 has been evaluated in a Phase I clinical trial of advanced breast and CRC; although less calcemic than $1\alpha,25(OH)_2D_3$, hypercalcemia limited the tolerable dose of EB1089 to 7 $\mu g/m^2/d$ *(133)*.

One deltanoid with considerable promise for chemopreventive development is QW-1624F2-2. This hybrid deltanoid has not only the calcemia-ablating $1\beta\text{-}CH_2OH$ group but also the potentiating C,D-ring 16-unsaturation and side-chain 24,24-difluorination and 26,27-homologation. Although conventional wisdom has required the presence of both the 1α-OH and the 25-OH groups for the high and diverse biological activities of $1\alpha,25(OH)_2D_3$ *(7)*, replacement of the natural 1α-OH group by a $1\beta\text{-}CH_2OH$ unit has produced antiproliferative analogs with diminished calcemic activity. The additional incorporation of potentiating side-chain structural modifications along with the 1β-CH_2OH moiety yields hybrid analogs that are antiproliferatively and transcriptionally potent but noncalcemic *(125)*. Despite the absence of the natural 1α-OH in hybrid QW-1624F-2-2, its vitamin D receptor-mediated transcriptional activity (ED_{50} = 5 × $10^{-11}M$) in rat osteosarcoma ROS 17/2.8 cells exceeds that of the natural hormone $1\alpha,25(OH)_2D_3$ (ED_{50} = $3\times10^{-10}M$) *(125)*. This compound is currently being tested in a preclinical rat mammary-cancer chemoprevention model. In addition, the NCI RAPID program will soon complete scale-up synthesis of the deltanoid, and thereafter the hybrid analog will be available to the general scientific community for further preclinical evaluation.

6. CLINICAL TARGETS FOR THE DEVELOPMENT OF DELTANOIDS AS CHEMOPREVENTIVES

The strongest evidence supporting the potential of vitamin D and synthetic deltanoids in cancer prevention comes from studies of colon cancer prevention. In various models, vitamin D_3 and its metabolites $1\alpha\text{-}(OH)D_3$ or $1\alpha,25\text{-}(OH_2)D_3$ were effective against colon carcinogenesis. Most studies of this type found a 50% reduction in tumor burden and/or multiplicity. Synthetic deltanoids with comparable colon cancer chemopreventive efficacy include $24R,25\text{-}(OH_2)D_3$, Chugai-OCT, Ro 26-9114, Ro 25-5317, Ro 25-9022, and Ro 24-5531. Supporting epidemiologic data include four prospective studies that showed inverse associations for vitamin D intake and colon or CRC development, with relative risks ranging from 0.33–0.74 *(67)*. Additional epidemiologic studies have found an association between serum levels of vitamin D metabolites and colon cancer biomarkers, including adenomatous polyps *(76,77)*. Collectively, these data support the application of deltanoids in colon cancer chemoprevention. Potential clinical studies could include tests of efficacy in adenoma prevention and against biomarkers of proliferation and apoptosis.

Epidemiologic and preclinical efficacy studies also support the potential of deltanoids in hormone-dependent cancers, and other important clinical targets for deltanoids include the prostate and breast. Only limited studies to date have tested the efficacy of deltanoids in preclinical prostate cancer chemoprevention models, but this merits further exploration. The few clinical studies of deltanoids in prostate cancer patients suggest the potential for efficacy. For example, in an ongoing Phase II clinical trial of the deltanoid $1\alpha(OH)D_2$ in metastatic hormone-refractory prostate cancer, two of 11 patients have had stable disease >6 mo *(131)*. It is possible that deltanoid intervention earlier in the disease process (e.g., in patients with prostatic intraepithelial neoplasia [PIN]) would engender greater success, since important determinants of response to deltanoids, including VDR polymorphisms, may be altered in metastatic disease. In support of this view, $25(OH)D_3\text{-}1\alpha$-hydroxylase activity is deficient in some human prostate cancer cells *(135)*; this enzyme, which metabolically activates the natural vitamin and other deltanoids lacking the 1α-OH moiety, is expressed in normal prostate tissue. Interestingly, this 1α-hydroxylase enzyme was shown to be expressed in malignant as well as adjacent normal colon tissue *(136)*.

Possible clinical endpoint biomarkers in breast cancer chemoprevention studies include markers of apoptosis, proliferation, and angiogenesis. A number of in vitro and in vivo studies have supported the ability of vitamin D metabolites and deltanoids to modulate such biomarkers in breast tissue or breast cancer-cell lines. Further support for the application of deltanoids in breast cancer chemoprevention comes from preclinical efficacy studies. In particular, $1\alpha,25\text{-}(OH)_2D_3$ as well as the deltanoids Chugai-OCT, $1\alpha(OH)D_5$ and Ro 24-5531 were efficacious in preclinical mammary-gland models. Emerging evidence also suggests that deltanoids may be able to modulate the mitogenic effects of estrogen and synergize with antiestrogens. For example, tamoxifen acts synergistically with vitamin D in the inhibition of breast cancer-cell growth in vitro and (137), and, tamoxifen synergistically enhances the chemopreventive efficacy of Ro 24-5531 against carcinogen-induced rat mammary carcinogenesis (114). Further exploration of the strategy of combining deltanoids with antiestrogens in preclinical models is needed.

7. SUMMARY AND PERSPECTIVES

This chapter reviews the substantial epidemiologic, mechanistic, and preclinical and clinical efficacy and safety data supporting the chemopreventive development of vitamin D and its synthetic analogs. Prominent clinical targets for chemopreventive application of deltanoids include the colon, prostate, and breast. Several deltanoids with considerable promise as chemopreventives in these target organs are presented here. The major obstacle to the clinical development of deltanoids has been hypercalcemic side effects. Although most are less potent than natural vitamin D at inducing hypercalcemia, many deltanoids (e.g., Ro 24-5531 and Ro 25-6760) do mediate such effects in a dose-dependent manner. One possible strategy for using a non-calcemic deltanoid dose in a chemoprevention setting is to administer deltanoids in combinations that would engender synergistic efficacy. The VDR heterodimerizes with the retinoid X receptor to control transcription of target genes, and therefore retinoids constitute one agent class that could be considered for combination chemopreventive interventions with deltanoids. In support of this approach, retinoids have been shown to synergize with vitamin D and synthetic deltanoids to inhibit the growth and promote the differentiation of human myeloid leukemia, and prostate and breast cancer cells in culture (137). Synergism with the

antiestrogen tamoxifen has also been suggested in both in vitro and in vivo studies. Selection of an appropriately safe and effective deltanoid for development, either in a single or combination chemopreventive regimen, would be facilitated by direct comparative analyses of candidate compounds.

ACKNOWLEDGMENTS

We thank the NIH for financial support (CA-44530), Barbara Gress for expert technical assistance, and Qiang Wang for help with Figures 1 and 2.

REFERENCES

1. Zehnder D, Bland R, Williams MC, et al. Extrarenal expression of 25-hydroxyvitamin d($_3$)-1α-hydroxylase. *J Clin Endocrinol Metab* 2001;86:888–894.
2. Segaert S, Bouillon R. Vitamin D and regulation of gene expression. *Curr Opin Clin Nutr Metab Care* 1998;1:347–354.
3. Verlinden L, Verstuyf A, Van Camp M, et al. Two novel 14-epi-analogues of 1,25-Dihydroxyvitamin D_3 inhibit the growth of human breast cancer cells in vitro and in vivo. *Cancer Res* 2000;60:2673–2679.
4. Jaaskelainen T, Ryhanen S, Mahonen A, et al. Mechanism of action of superactive vitamin D analogs through regulated receptor degradation. *J Cell Biochem* 2000;76:548–558.
5. Minghetti PP, Norman AW. 1,25(OH)2-vitamin D_3 receptors: gene regulation and genetic circuitry. *FASEB J* 1988;2:3043–3053.
6. Norman AW, Bishop JE, Bula CM, et al. Molecular tools for study of the genomic and rapid signal transduction responses initiated by 1-α,25-dihidroxyvitamin D_3. *Steroids* 2002;67:457–466.
7. Bouillon R, Okamura WH, Norman AW. Structure-function relationships in the vitamin D endocrine system. *Endocr Rev* 1995;16:200–257.
8. Mathiasen IS, Colston KW, Binderup L. EB1089, a novel vitamin D analogue, has strong antiproliferative and differentiation inducing effects on cancer cells. *J Steroid Biochem Mol Biol* 1993;46:365–371.
9. Grue-Sorensen G, Hansen CM. New 1 α,25-dihydroxy vitamin D_3 analogues with side chains attached to C-18: synthesis and biological activity. *Bioorg Med Chem* 1998;6:2029–2039.
10. Uskokovic MR, Studzinski GP, Gardner JP, et al. The 16-ene vitamin D analogues. *Curr Pharm Des* 1997;3:99–123.
11. Abe J, Nakano T, Nishii Y, et al. A novel vitamin D_3 analog, 22-oxa-1,25-dihydroxyvitamin D_3, inhibits the growth of human breast cancer in vitro and in vivo without causing hypercalcemia. *Endocrinology* 1991;129:832–837.
12. Figadere B, Norman AW, Henry HL, et al. Arocalciferols: synthesis and biological evaluation of aromatic side-chain analogues of 1 α,25-Dihydroxyvitamin D_3(1a). *J Med Chem* 1991;34:2452–2463.
13. Zhu G-D CY, Zhou X, Vanderwalle M, et al. Synthesis of C,D-ring modified 1,25-dihydroxyvitamin D analogues: C-ring analogues. *Bioorg Med Chem Lett* 1996;6:1703–1708.

14. Mehta RR, Bratescu L, Graves JM, et al. Differentiation of human breast carcinoma cells by a novel vitamin D analog: 1α-hydroxyvitamin D$_5$. *Int J Oncol* 2000;16:65–73.

15. Paaren HE, Mellon WS, Schnoes HK, DeLuca HF. Ring A-stereoisomers of 1-hydroxyvitamin D$_3$ and their relative binding affinities for the intestinal 1α, 25-dihydroxyvitamin D$_3$ receptor protein. *Bioorg Chem* 1985;13:62–75.

16. Muralidharan KR, De Lera AR, Isaeff SD, et al. Studies on the A-ring diastereomers of 1-α,25-dihydroxyvitamin D$_3$. *J Org Chem* 1993;58:1895–1899.

17. Reddy S. Synthesis and activity of 3-epi-vitamin D$_3$ compounds for use in treatment of disorders involving aberrant activity of hyperproliferative skin, parathyroid, and bone cells. PCT Int. Patent Appl. WO 98 51,663. *Chem Abstr* 1999;130:25,229X.

18. Perlman KL SR, Schnoes HK, DeLuca HF. 1-α,25-Dihydroxy-19-nor-vitamin D$_3$, a novel vitamin D-related compound with potential therapeutic activity. *Tetrahedron Lett* 1990;31:1823–1824.

19. Kanzler S HS, Van de Velde JP, Reischl W. A novel class of vitamin D analogs: synthesis and preliminary biological evaluation. *Bioorg Med Chem Lett* 1996;6:1865–1868.

20. Posner G, Dai H. 1-(Hydroxyalkyl)-25-hydroxyvitamin D$_3$ analogs of calcitriol.1. Synthesis. *Bioorg Med Chem Lett* 1993;3:1829–1834.

21. Posner GH, Lee JK, White MC, et al. Antiproliferative hybrid analogs of the hormone 1α,25-dihydroxyvitamin D$_{(3)}$: design, synthesis, and preliminary biological evaluation. *J Org Chem* 1997;62:3299–3314.

22. Guyton KZ, Kensler TW, Posner GH. Cancer chemoprevention using natural vitamin D and synthetic analogs. *Annu Rev Pharmacol Toxicol* 2001;41:421–442.

23. Kelloff GJ, Johnson JR, Crowell JA, et al. Approaches to the development and marketing approval of drugs that prevent cancer. *Cancer Epidemiol Biomark Prev* 1995;4:1–10.

24. Wali RK, Bissonnette M, Khare S, et al. 1 α,25-Dihydroxy-16-ene-23-yne-26,27-hexafluorocholecalciferol, a noncalcemic analog of 1 α,25-dihydroxyvitamin D$_3$, inhibits azoxymethane-induced colonic tumorigenesis. *Cancer Res* 1995;55:3050–3054.

25. Colston KW, Mork HC, Hansen C. Mechanisms implicated in the growth regulatory effects of vitamin D in breast cancer. *Endocr Relat Cancer* 2002;9:45–59.

26. Quack M, Mork HC, Binderup E, et al. Metabolism of the vitamin D$_3$ analog EB1089 alters receptor complex formation and reduces promoter selectivity. *Br J Pharmacol* 1998;125:607–614.

27. Yang W, Freedman LP. 20-Epi analogues of 1,25-dihydroxyvitamin D$_3$ are highly potent inducers of DRIP coactivator complex binding to the vitamin D$_3$ receptor. *J Biol Chem* 1999;274:16,838–16,845.

28. Li XY, Boudjelal M, Xiao JH, et al. 1,25-Dihydroxyvitamin D$_3$ increases nuclear vitamin D$_3$ receptors by blocking ubiquitin/proteasome-mediated degradation in human skin. *Mol Endocrinol* 1999;13:1686–1694.

29. Peleg S, Nguyen C, Woodard BT, et al. Differential use of transcription activation function 2 domain of the vitamin D receptor by 1,25-dihydroxyvitamin D$_3$ and its A ring-modified analogs. *Mol Endocrinol* 1998;12:525–535.

30. Fioravanti L, Miodini P, Cappelletti V, DiFronzo G. Synthetic analogs of vitamin D$_3$ have inhibitory effects on breast cancer cell lines. *Anticancer Res* 1998;18:1703–1708.

31. Pettersson F, Colston KW, Dalgleish AG. Differential and antagonistic effects of 9-*cis*-retinoic acid and vitamin D analogs on pancreatic cancer cells in vitro. *Br J Cancer* 2000;83:239–245.

32. Blutt SE, Polek TC, Stewart LV, et al. A calcitriol analogue, EB1089, inhibits the growth of LNCaP tumors in nude mice. *Cancer Res* 2000;60:779–782.

33. Liu M, Lee MH, Cohen M, et al. Transcriptional activation of the Cdk inhibitor p21 by vitamin D$_3$ leads to the induced differentiation of the myelomonocytic cell line U937. *Genes Dev* 1996;10:142–153.

34. Campbell MJ, Elstner E, Holden S, et al. Inhibition of proliferation of prostate cancer cells by a 19-nor-hexafluoride vitamin D$_3$ analogue involves the induction of p21[waf1], p27[kip1] and E-cadherin. *J Mol Endocrinol* 1997;19:15–27.

35. Rots NY, Liu M, Anderson EC, Freedman LP. A differential screen for ligand-regulated genes: identification of HoxA10 as a target of vitamin D$_3$ induction in myeloid leukemic cells. *Mol Cell Biol* 1998;18:1911–1918.

36. Jensen SS, Madsen MW, Lukas J, et al. Inhibitory effects of 1α,25-dihydroxyvitamin D$_3$ on the G$_1$-S phase-controlling machinery. *Mol Endocrinol* 2001;15:1370–1380.

37. Prudencio J, Akutsu N, Benlimame N, et al. Action of low calcemic 1α,25-dihydroxyvitamin D$_3$ analogue EB1089 in head and neck squamous cell carcinoma. *J Natl Cancer Inst* 2001;93:745–753.

38. Wang QM, Chen F, Luo X, et al. Lowering of p27[kip1] levels by its antisense or by development of resistance to 1,25-dihydroxyvitamin D$_3$ reverses the G$_1$ block but not differentiation of HL60 cells. *Leukemia* 1998;12:1256–1265.

39. Segaert S, Garmyn M, Degreef H, Bouillon R. Retinoic acid modulates the anti-proliferative effect of 1,25-dihydroxyvitamin D$_3$ in cultured human epidermal keratinocytes. *J Investig Dermatol* 1997;109:46–54.

40. Swami S, Krishnan AV, Feldman D. 1α,25-Dihydroxyvitamin D$_3$ down-regulates estrogen receptor abundance and suppresses estrogen actions in MCF-7 human breast cancer cells. *Clin Cancer Res* 2000;6:3371–3379.

41. Nickerson T, Huynh H. Vitamin D analog EB1089-induced prostate regression is associated with increased gene expression of insulin-like growth factor binding proteins. *J Endocrinol* 1999;160:223–229.

42. Sundaram S, Chaudhry M, Reardon D, et al. The vitamin D$_3$ analog EB1089 enhances the antiproliferative and apoptotic effects of adriamycin in MCF-7 breast tumor cells. *Breast Cancer Res Treat* 2000;63:1–10.

43. Sundaram S, Gewirtz DA. The vitamin D$_3$ analog EB1089 enhances the response of human breast tumor cells to radiation. *Radiat Res* 1999; 152:479–486.

44. Pirianov G, Colston KW. Interaction of vitamin D analogs with signaling pathways leading to active cell death in breast cancer cells. *Steroids* 2001;66:309–318.

45. Mathiasen IS, Lademann U, Jaattela M. Apoptosis induced by vitamin D compounds in breast cancer cells is inhibited by Bcl-2 but does not involve known caspases or p53. *Cancer Res* 1999;59:4848–4856.

46. Diaz GD, Paraskeva C, Thomas MG, et al. Apoptosis is induced by the active metabolite of vitamin D$_3$ and its analogue EB1089 in colorectal adenoma and carcinoma cells: possible implications for prevention and therapy. *Cancer Res* 2000;60:2304–2312.

47. Koren R, Hadari-Naor I, Zuck E, et al. Vitamin D is a proox-idant in breast cancer cells. *Cancer Res* 2001;61:1439–1444.

48. Narvaez CJ, Zinser G, Welsh J. Functions of 1α,25-dihydroxy-vitamin D(₃) in mammary gland: from normal development to breast cancer. *Steroids* 2001;66:301–308.

49. Narvaez CJ, Welsh J. Role of mitochondria and caspases in vitamin D-mediated apoptosis of MCF-7 breast cancer cells. *J Biol Chem* 2001;276:9101–9107.

50. McGuire TF, Trump DL, Johnson CS. Vitamin D(₃)-induced apoptosis of murine squamous cell carcinoma cells. Selective induction of caspase-dependent MEK cleavage and up-regu-lation of MEKK-1. *J Biol Chem* 2001;276:26,365–26,373.

51. Majewski S, Skopinska M, Marczak M, et al. Vitamin D₃ is a potent inhibitor of tumor cell-induced angiogenesis. *J Investig Dermatol Symp Proc* 1996;1:97–101.

52. Mantell DJ, Owens PE, Bundred NJ, et al. 1 α,25-Dihydroxyvitamin D(₃) inhibits angiogenesis in vitro and in vivo. *Circ Res* 2000;87:214–220.

53. Hara K, Kusuzaki K, Takeshita H, et al. Oral administration of 1 α hydroxyvitamin D₃ inhibits tumor growth and metas-tasis of a murine osteosarcoma model. *Anticancer Res* 2001;21:321–324.

54. Shokravi MT, Marcus DM, Alroy J, et al. Vitamin D inhibits angiogenesis in transgenic murine retinoblastoma. *Investig Ophthalmol Vis Sci* 1995; 36:83–87.

55. Lokeshwar BL, Schwartz GG, Selzer MG, et al. Inhibition of prostate cancer metastasis in vivo: a comparison of 1,23-dihydroxyvitamin D (calcitriol) and EB1089. *Cancer Epidemiol Biomark Prev* 1999;8:241–248.

56. Schwartz GG, Wang MH, Zang M, et al. 1 α,25-Dihydroxyvitamin D (calcitriol) inhibits the invasiveness of human prostate cancer cells. *Cancer Epidemiol Biomark Prev* 1997;6:727–732.

57. Yudoh K, Matsuno H, Kimura T. 1α,25-Dihydroxyvitamin D₃ inhibits in vitro invasiveness through the extracellular matrix and in vivo pulmonary metastasis of B16 mouse melanoma. *J Lab Clin Med* 1999;133:120–128.

58. Apperly F. The relation of solar radiation to cancer mortality in North America. *Cancer Res* 1941;1:191–195.

59. Peller S, Stephenson C. Skin irritation and cancer in the United States Navy. *Am J Med Sci* 1937;194:326–333.

60. Garland CF, Garland FC. Do sunlight and vitamin D reduce the likelihood of colon cancer? *Int J Epidemiol* 1980;9:227–231.

61. Garland FC, Garland CF, Gorham ED, Young JF. Geographic variation in breast cancer mortality in the United States: a hypothesis involving exposure to solar radiation. *Prev Med* 1990;19:614–622.

62. Gorham ED, Garland FC, Garland CF. Sunlight and breast cancer incidence in the USSR. *Int J Epidemiol* 1990;19:820–824.

63. Hanchette CL, Schwartz GG. Geographic patterns of prostate cancer mortality. Evidence for a protective effect of ultraviolet radiation. *Cancer* 1992;70:2861–2869.

64. Emerson JC, Weiss NS. Colorectal cancer and solar radiation. *Cancer Causes Control* 1992;3:95–99.

65. Garland CF, Garland FC, Gorham ED. Calcium and vitamin D. Their potential roles in colon and breast cancer prevention. *Ann NY Acad Sci* 1999;889:107–119.

66. Schwartz GG, Hulka BS. Is vitamin D deficiency a risk factor for prostate cancer? (Hypothesis). *Anticancer Res* 1990;10:1307–1311.

67. Martinez ME, Willett WC. Calcium, vitamin D, and col-orectal cancer: a review of the epidemiologic evidence. *Cancer Epidemiol Biomark Prev* 1998;7:163–168.

68. Garland C, Shekelle RB, Barrett-Connor E, et al. Dietary vita-min D and calcium and risk of colorectal cancer: a 19-year prospective study in men. *Lancet* 1985;1:307–309.

69. Bostick RM, Potter JD, Sellers TA, et al. Relation of calcium, vitamin D, and dairy food intake to incidence of colon can-cer among older women. The Iowa Women's Health Study. *Am J Epidemiol* 1993;137:1302–1317.

70. Kearney J, Giovannucci E, Rimm EB, et al. Calcium, vitamin D, and dairy foods and the occurrence of colon cancer in men. *Am J Epidemiol* 1996;143:907–917.

71. Zheng W, Anderson KE, Kushi LH, et al. A prospective cohort study of intake of calcium, vitamin D, and other micronutrients in relation to incidence of rectal cancer among postmenopausal women. *Cancer Epidemiol Biomark Prev* 1998;7:221–225.

72. Martinez ME, Giovannucci EL, Colditz GA, et al. Calcium, vitamin D, and the occurrence of colorectal cancer among women. *J Natl Cancer Inst* 1996;88:1375–1382.

73. Pritchard RS, Baron JA, de Verdier MG. Dietary calcium, vitamin D, and the risk of colorectal cancer in Stockholm, Sweden. *Cancer Epidemiol Biomark Prev* 1996;5:897–900.

74. Marcus PM, Newcomb PA. The association of calcium and vitamin D, and colon and rectal cancer in Wisconsin women. *Int J Epidemiol* 1998;27:788–793.

75. Boutron MC, Faivre J, Marteau P, et al. Calcium, phosphorus, vitamin D, dairy products and colorectal carcinogenesis: a French case-control study. *Br J Cancer* 1996;74:145–151.

76. Platz EA, Hankinson SE, Hollis BW, et al. Plasma 1,25-dihydroxy- and 25-hydroxyvitamin D and adenomatous polyps of the distal colorectum. *Cancer Epidemiol Biomark Prev* 2000;9:1059–1065.

77. Peters U, McGlynn KA, Chatterjee N, et al. Vitamin D, calcium, and vitamin D receptor polymorphism in colorec-tal adenomas. *Cancer Epidemiol Biomark Prev* 2001;10:1267–1274.

78. Holt PR, Arber N, Halmos B, et al. Colonic epithelial cell proliferation decreases with increasing levels of serum 25-hydroxy vitamin D. *Cancer Epidemiol Biomark Prev* 2002;11:113–119.

79. John EM, Schwartz GG, Dreon DM, Koo J. Vitamin D and breast cancer risk: the NHANES I Epidemiologic follow-up study, 1971–1975 to 1992. National Health and Nutrition Examination Survey. *Cancer Epidemiol Biomark Prev* 1999;8:399–406.

80. Corder EH, Guess HA, Hulka BS, et al. Vitamin D and prostate cancer: a prediagnostic study with stored sera. *Cancer Epidemiol Biomark Prev* 1993;2:467–472.

81. Braun MM, Helzlsouer KJ, Hollis BW, Comstock GW. Prostate cancer and prediagnostic levels of serum vitamin D metabolites (Maryland, United States). *Cancer Causes Control* 1995;6:235–239.

82. Nomura AM, Stemmermann GN, Lee J, et al. Serum vitamin D metabolite levels and the subsequent development of prostate cancer (Hawaii, United States). *Cancer Causes Control* 1998;9:425–432.

83. Gann PH, Ma J, Hennekens CH, et al. Circulating vitamin D metabolites in relation to subsequent development of prostate cancer. *Cancer Epidemiol Biomark Prev* 1996;5:121–126.

84. Ma J, Stampfer MJ, Gann PH, et al. Vitamin D receptor polymorphisms, circulating vitamin D metabolites, and risk of prostate cancer in United States physicians. *Cancer Epidemiol Biomark Prev* 1998;7:385–390.

85. Ingles SA, Coetzee GA, Ross RK, et al. Association of prostate cancer with vitamin D receptor haplotypes in African-Americans. *Cancer Res* 1998;58:1620–1623.

86. Taylor JA, Hirvonen A, Watson M, et al. Association of prostate cancer with vitamin D receptor gene polymorphism. *Cancer Res* 1996;56:4108–4110.

87. Hamasaki T, Inatomi H, Katoh T, et al. Clinical and pathological significance of vitamin D receptor gene polymorphism for prostate cancer which is associated with a higher mortality in Japanese. *Endocr J* 2001;48:543–549.

88. Gsur A, Madersbacher S, Haidinger G, et al. Vitamin D receptor gene polymorphism and prostate cancer risk. *Prostate* 2002;51:30–34.

89. Bretherton-Watt D, Given-Wilson R, Mansi JL, et al. Vitamin D receptor gene polymorphisms are associated with breast cancer risk in a UK Caucasian population. *Br J Cancer* 2001;85:171–175.

90. Ingles SA, Garcia DG, Wang W, et al. Vitamin D receptor genotype and breast cancer in Latinas (United States). *Cancer Causes Control* 2000;11:25–30.

91. Hutchinson PE, Osborne JE, Lear JT, et al. Vitamin D receptor polymorphisms are associated with altered prognosis in patients with malignant melanoma. *Clin Cancer Res* 2000;6:498–504.

92. Ingles SA, Wang J, Coetzee GA, et al. Vitamin D receptor polymorphisms and risk of colorectal adenomas (United States). *Cancer Causes Control* 2001;12:607–614.

93. Kim HS, Newcomb PA, Ulrich CM, et al. Vitamin D receptor polymorphism and the risk of colorectal adenomas: evidence of interaction with dietary vitamin D and calcium. *Cancer Epidemiol Biomark Prev* 2001;10:869–874.

94. Slatter ML, Yakumo K, Hoffman M, Neuhausen S. Variants of the VDR gene and risk of colon cancer (United States). *Cancer Causes Control* 2001;12:359–364.

95. Kawaura A, Tanida N, Nishikawa M, et al. Inhibitory effect of 1α-hydroxyvitamin D_3 on *N*-methyl-*N'*-nitro-*N*-nitrosoguanidine-induced gastrointestinal carcinogenesis in Wistar rats. *Cancer Lett* 1998;122:227–230.

96. Kawaura A, Tanida N, Sawada K, et al. Supplemental administration of 1α-hydroxyvitamin D_3 inhibits promotion by intrarectal instillation of lithocholic acid in *N*-methyl-*N*-nitrosourea-induced colonic tumorigenesis in rats. *Carcinogenesis* 1989;10:647–649.

97. Iseki K, Tatsuta M, Uehara H, et al. Inhibition of angiogenesis as a mechanism for inhibition by 1α-hydroxyvitamin D_3 and 1,25-dihydroxyvitamin D_3 of colon carcinogenesis induced by azoxymethane in Wistar rats. *Int J Cancer* 1999;81:730–733.

98. Belleli A, Shany S, Levy J, et al. A protective role of 1,25-dihydroxyvitamin D_3 in chemically induced rat colon carcinogenesis. *Carcinogenesis* 1992;13:2293–2298.

99. Evans SR, Shchepotin EI, Young H, et al. 1,25-Dihydroxyvitamin D_3 synthetic analogs inhibit spontaneous metastases in a 1,2-dimethylhydrazine-induced colon carcinogenesis model. *Int J Oncol* 2000;16:1249–1254.

100. Pence BC, Buddingh F. Inhibition of dietary fat-promoted colon carcinogenesis in rats by supplemental calcium or vitamin D_3. *Carcinogenesis* 1988;9:187–190.

101. Albert DM, Marcus DM, Gallo JP, O'Brien JM. The antineoplastic effect of vitamin D in transgenic mice with retinoblastoma. *Investig Ophthalmol Vis Sci* 1992;33:2354–2364.

102. Rubin D, Levij IS. Suppression by vitamins D_2 and D_3 of hamster cheek pouch carcinoma induced with 9,10-dimethyl-1,2-benzanthracene with a discussion of the role of intracellular calcium in the development of tumors. *Pathol Microbiol (Basel)* 1973;39:446–460.

103. Wood AW, Chang RL, Huang MT, et al. 1α, 25-Dihydroxyvitamin D_3 inhibits phorbol ester-dependent chemical carcinogenesis in mouse skin. *Biochem Biophys Res Commun* 1983;116:605–611.

104. Chida K, Hashiba H, Fukushima M, et al. Inhibition of tumor promotion in mouse skin by 1 α,25-dihydroxyvitamin D_3. *Cancer Res* 1985;45:5426–5430.

105. Pence BC, Richard BC, Lawlis RS, Kuratko CN. Effects of dietary calcium and vitamin D_3 on tumor promotion in mouse skin. *Nutr Cancer* 1991;16:171–181.

106. Saez S, Falette N, Guillot C, et al. 1,25(OH)2D$_3$ modulation of mammary tumor cell growth in vitro and in vivo. *Breast Cancer Res Treat.* 1993;27:69–81.

107. Huerta S, Irwin RW, Heber D, et al. 1α,25-(OH)(2)-D$_{(3)}$ and its synthetic analogue decrease tumor load in the Apc(min) Mouse. *Cancer Res* 2002;62:741–746.

108. Taniyama T, Wanibuchi H, Salim EI, et al. Chemopreventive effect of 24R,25-dihydroxyvitamin D$_{(3)}$ in *N*, *N'*-dimethyl-hydrazine-induced rat colon carcinogenesis. *Carcinogenesis* 2000;21:173–178.

109. Otoshi T, Iwata H, Kitano M, et al. Inhibition of intestinal tumor development in rat multi-organ carcinogenesis and aberrant crypt foci in rat colon carcinogenesis by 22-oxa-calcitriol, a synthetic analogue of 1α, 25-dihydroxyvitamin D$_3$. *Carcinogenesis* 1995;16:2091–2097.

110. Brown AJ, Slatopolsky E. Vitamin D analogs: perspectives for treatment. *Miner Electrolyte Metab* 1999;25:337–341.

111. Oikawa T, Yoshida Y, Shimamura M, et al. Antitumor effect of 22-oxa-1 α,25-dihydroxyvitamin D_3, a potent angiogenesis inhibitor, on rat mammary tumors induced by 7,12-dimethylbenz[*a*]anthracene. *Anticancer Drugs* 1991;2:475–480.

112. Mehta RG, Moriarty RM, Mehta RR, et al. Prevention of preneoplastic mammary lesion development by a novel vitamin D analogue, 1α-hydroxyvitamin D$_5$. *J Natl Cancer Inst* 1997;89:212–218.

113. Mehta R, Hawthorne M, Uselding L, et al. Prevention of *N*-methyl-*N*-nitrosourea-induced mammary carcinogenesis in rats by 1α-hydroxyvitamin D$_{(5)}$. *J Natl Cancer Inst* 2000;92:1836–1840.

114. Anzano MA, Smith JM, Uskokovic MR, et al. 1α,25-Dihydroxy-16-ene-23-yne-26,27-hexafluorocholecalciferol (Ro24-5531), a new deltanoid (vitamin D analogue) for prevention of breast cancer in the rat. *Cancer Res* 1994;54:1653–1656.

115. Ikezaki S, Nishikawa A, Furukawa F, et al. Chemopreventive effects of 24R,25-dihydroxyvitamin D$_3$, a vitamin D$_3$ derivative, on glandular stomach carcinogenesis induced in rats by *N*-methyl-*N'*-nitro-*N*-nitrosoguanidine and sodium chloride. *Cancer Res* 1996;56:2767–2770.

116. Lucia MS, Anzano MA, Slayter MV, et al. Chemopreventive activity of tamoxifen, *N*-(4-hydroxyphenyl)retinamide, and the vitamin D analog Ro24-5531 for androgen-promoted

carcinomas of the rat seminal vesicle and prostate. *Cancer Res* 1995;55:5621–5627.

117. Sporn MB. New agents for chemoprevention of prostate cancer. *Eur Urol* 1999;35:420–423.

118. Kensler TW, Dolan PM, Gange SJ, et al. Conceptually new deltanoids (vitamin D analogs) inhibit multistage skin tumorigenesis. *Carcinogenesis* 2000;21:1341–1345.

119. Norman AW. The vitamin D endocrine system: manipulation of structure-function relationships to provide opportunities for development of new cancer chemopreventive and immunosuppressive agents. *J Cell Biochem Suppl* 1995;22:218–225.

120. Konety BR, Johnson CS, Trump DL, Getzenberg RH. Vitamin D in the prevention and treatment of prostate cancer. *Semin Urol Oncol* 1999;17:77–84.

121. Miller GJ. Vitamin D and prostate cancer: biologic interactions and clinical potentials. *Cancer Metastasis Rev* 1998;17:353–360.

122. Bikle DD. Clinical counterpoint: vitamin D: new actions, new analogs, new therapeutic potential. *Endocr Rev* 1992;13:765–784.

123. Pakkala S, de Vos S, Elstner E, et al. Vitamin D_3 analogs: effect on leukemic clonal growth and differentiation, and on serum calcium levels. *Leuk Res* 1995;19:65–72.

124. Smith EA, Frankenburg EP, Goldstein SA, et al. Effects of long-term administration of vitamin D_3 analogs to mice. *J Endocrinol* 2000;165:163–172.

125. Posner GH, Lee JK, Wang Q, et al. Noncalcemic, antiproliferative, transcriptionally active, 24-fluorinated hybrid analogs of the hormone 1α, 25-dihydroxyvitamin D_3. Synthesis and preliminary biological evaluation. *J Med Chem* 1998;41:3008–3014.

126. Koshizuka K, Koike M, Asou H, et al. Combined effect of vitamin D_3 analogs and paclitaxel on the growth of MCF-7 breast cancer cells in vivo. *Breast Cancer Res Treat* 1999;53:113–120.

127. Frazao JM, Elangovan L, Maung HM, et al. Intermittent doxercalciferol (1α-hydroxyvitamin $D_{(2)}$) therapy for secondary hyperparathyroidism. *Am J Kidney Dis* 2000;36:550–561.

128. Maung HM, Elangovan L, Frazao JM, et al. Efficacy and side effects of intermittent intravenous and oral doxercalciferol (1α-hydroxyvitamin $D_{(2)}$) in dialysis patients with secondary hyperparathyroidism: a sequential comparison. *Am J Kidney Dis* 2001;37:532–543.

129. Sjoden G, Smith C, Lindgren U, DeLuca HF. 1α-Hydroxyvitamin D_2 is less toxic than 1α-hydroxyvitamin D_3 in the rat. *Proc Soc Exp Biol Med* 1985;178:432–436.

130. Weber K, Goldberg M, Stangassinger M, Erben RG. 1α-Hydroxyvitamin D_2 is less toxic but not bone selective relative to 1α-hydroxyvitamin D_3 in ovariectomized rats. *J Bone Mineral Res* 2001;16:639–651.

131. Bailey HH, Ripple G., Horvath, D, et al. Phase I and II trials of 1-hydroxyvitamin D_2 in patients with metastatic hormone-refractory prostate cancer. *Clin Cancer Res* 2000;6:4488s, abst no 112.

132. Hansen CM, Hamberg KJ, Binderup E, Binderup L. Seocalcitol (EB1089): a vitamin D analogue of anti-cancer potential. Background, design, synthesis, pre-clinical and clinical evaluation. *Curr Pharm Des* 2000;6:803–828.

133. Gulliford T, English J, Colston KW, et al. A Phase I study of the vitamin D analogue EB1089 in patients with advanced breast and colorectal cancer. *Br J Cancer* 1998;78:6–13.

134. Evans TR, Colston KW, Lofts FJ, et al. A Phase II trial of the vitamin D analogue Seocalcitol (EB1089) in patients with inoperable pancreatic cancer. *Br J Cancer* 2002;86:680–685.

135. Hsu JY, Feldman D, McNeal JE, Peehl DM. Reduced 1α-hydroxylase activity in human prostate cancer cells correlates with decreased susceptibility to 25-hydroxyvitamin D_3-induced growth inhibition. *Cancer Res* 2001;61:2852–2856.

136. Tangpricha V, Flanagan JN, Whitlatch LW, et al. 25-Hydroxyvitamin D-1α-hydroxylase in normal and malignant colon tissue. *Lancet* 2001;357:1673–1674.

137. Koga M, Sutherland RL. Retinoic acid acts synergistically with 1,25-dihydroxyvitamin D_3 or antioestrogen to inhibit T-47D human breast cancer cell proliferation. *J Steroid Biochem Mol Biol* 1991;39:455–460.

D. RETINOIDS

18 The Retinoids and Cancer Chemoprevention

Sutisak Kitareewan, PhD, Ian Pitha-Rowe, BA, Yan Ma, BM, Sarah J. Freemantle, PhD, and Ethan Dmitrovsky, MD

CONTENTS

I. INTRODUCTION

The retinoids—natural and synthetic derivatives of vitamin A—play a role in cancer therapy and prevention. Their role in chemoprevention has been highlighted through the results of clinical and epidemiological studies in conjunction with basic research on retinoid mechanisms of action, advances in genomic information, novel organic synthesis of retinoid analogs, and availability of reliable model systems. This chapter focuses on the results of recent retinoid clinical cancer therapy and chemoprevention trials, reviews the current understanding of the molecular mechanism of retinoid action, discusses in vitro models used to study retinoid chemoprevention, and summarizes information on retinoid target genes. An understanding of the convergence of clinical and basic scientific advances in the retinoid field should lead to improved strategies to use these pharmacological agents in cancer therapy or chemoprevention.

2. RETINOID CLINICAL ACTIVITIES

Retinoids have clinical activity in cancer therapy and prevention, as summarized in Table 1. They also play a role in vision, fertility, immune function, normal cellular homeostasis, and non-neoplastic diseases, as reviewed elsewhere *(1–4)*. The teratogenic effects of retinoids limit their use in women in their childbearing years *(1,2,5)*.

Retinoid receptors are of interest to both basic and clinical scientists. There are links between the expression or induction of certain retinoid receptors and a clinical response to retinoids. For example, in acute promyelocytic leukemia (APL), expression of the t(15;17) fusion product, PML/RARα, predicts response to all-*trans*-retinoic acid (ATRA) treatment *(6)*. In oral leukoplakia, induction of retinoic acid (RA) receptor-β (RARβ) is associated with a clinical response to 13-*cis*-retinoic acid (13cRA) *(7)*. Preclinical studies indicate that RARα regulates retinoid response in certain acute myeloid leukemic cells *(8)* and RARγ regulates growth and differentiation response in cultured male germ-cell tumors *(9)*. Ongoing work is focused on identifying target genes that are activated or repressed by retinoids to signal growth or maturation effects in a particular cellular context.

Clinical activity of the retinoids has been reported in neuroblastoma *(10)*, APL, mycosis fungoides, and juvenile chronic myelogenous leukemia (as reviewed in ref. 5). Clinical retinoid activity has also been reported in the treatment of preneoplastic diseases including oral leukoplakia *(11)*, xeroderma pigmentosum *(12)*, and cervical dysplasia *(13)*, among others (discussed in ref. 5). Combining 13cRA with interferon α2A produces

From: Cancer Chemoprevention, Volume 1: Promising Cancer Chemoprevention Agents
Edited by: G. J. Kelloff, E. T. Hawk, and C. C. Sigman © Humana Press Inc., Totowa, NJ

Table 1
Retinoid Clinical Activities in Cancer Therapy
and Prevention

Categories	Diseases/Conditions
Premalignancy	Oral leukoplakia
	Cervical dysplasia
	Xeroderma pigmentosum
	Actinic keratosis
Malignancy	Acute promyelocytic leukemia
	Juvenile chronic myelogenous leukemia
	Mycosis fungoides
	Neuroblastoma
Combination therapy	Squamous-cell cervical cancer
	Squamous-cell skin cancer
	Kidney cancer
Chemoprevention	Second primary head and neck cancers
	Second primary liver cancers
	Second primary breast cancers

The retinoids have activity in several clinical settings that include the treatment of certain premalignant or malignant diseases and in the prevention of some second primary cancers, as shown in this Table. When combined with interferon α2A, 13-cis-retinoic acid has reported activity in the treatment of several epithelial malignancies, as noted here under the category of combination therapy.

major clinical responses in patients with squamous-cell cancer, cervical cancer, and late-stage renal-cell carcinoma (as reviewed in refs. 1,2,5). Certain retinoids have been reported to reduce the incidence of second primary cancers in patients with prior cancers of the head and neck (14), breast (15), or liver (16).

Studies of retinoids used in the chemoprevention of primary or second primary cancers have been promising. The rationale for such use was first reported in 1925 by Wolbach and Howe (17), who found that vitamin A deficiency in experimental rodent models caused squamous metaplasia at diverse epithelial sites including the trachea, where the changes were similar to those found in the bronchial epithelium of smokers. When the deficiency was corrected, the metaplastic epithelial changes were reversed (17).

Evidence for a retinoid role in cancer chemoprevention has come from epidemiological studies (2) as well as from experiments performed in carcinogen-exposed animal models (4) and carcinogen-treated epithelial cells (18), where it has been shown that retinoids can prevent or inhibit carcinogenic transformation. Epidemiological evidence has shown an inverse relationship between serum β-carotene levels and the incidence of certain epithelial malignancies (as reviewed in 2). Nutritional intervention studies conducted in China reported a reduction in the incidence of specific epithelial malignancies (19), and Phase II trials have demonstrated a reduction in the risk of second cancers in retinoid-treated patients with prior cancers of the head and neck, lung, or liver (20,21).

In contrast to these promising results, large Phase III randomized clinical trials of β-carotene did not reduce the risk of lung cancers in high-risk individuals (22–24); in fact, the risk increased in smokers. A randomized intergroup study of 13cRA to reduce second cancers in patients with previously resected stage I lung cancer also showed negative effects in active smokers, although some potential benefit was shown in nonsmokers (25). These results highlight the value of confirming favorable results from Phase I or Phase II trials with Phase III randomized, placebo-controlled clinical chemopreventive trials to elucidate any negative interactions between smoking (or other factors) and treatment with retinoids.

As a single agent, the classical retinoid 13cRA may not be effective in the prevention of lung cancer because RARβ repression is common in epithelial carcinogenesis (7). Recent evidence indicates that methylation-induced silencing could contribute to this repression. Although treatment with a classical retinoid alone may not overcome this repression (26), treatment with a demethylation agent has been reported to restore RARβ expression (26). Perhaps a regimen combining an optimal retinoid with a demethylation agent could restore RARβ induction after RA-treatment. Future clinical trials should address this possibility.

Clinical treatments with classical retinoids have often been limited by toxicity (1,2,5). Receptor-selective retinoids were developed to reduce or eliminate such toxicities while retaining the desired biological effects (27,28). These and other non-classical retinoids could be evaluated for activity in future therapeutic or chemopreventive clinical trials. Retinoid X receptor (RXR) agonists (also known as rexinoids) are agents that activate the RXR pathway. These might overcome problems with transcriptional repression of the classical RAR pathway. Rexinoid activity has been observed in preclinical animal models of breast cancer chemoprevention *(29)*. The rexinoid bexarotene is being successfully used in the treatment of cutaneous T-cell lymphoma *(30)*. Clinical activity in lung cancer (which often exhibits RARβ repression) has been reported when a rexinoid is combined with chemotherapy *(31)*. The bifunctional ligand 9-*cis*-retinoic acid (9-*cis*-RA) can activate both the RAR and RXR pathways *(32,33)*, and is under active clinical investigation.

Other therapeutic strategies may reduce or eliminate retinoid-induced toxicity. Aerosolized delivery may limit systemic toxicity while directly targeting preneoplastic lung cells *(34)*. This approach should be considered in future clinical trials. Another therapeutic strategy to evaluate is the use of combination regimens that preferentially target pathways that would cooperate with the retinoids. Recent evidence has shown that cyclin D_1 is a common downstream target of both epidermal growth factor receptor (EGFR) and retinoid signaling pathways *(35)*. This suggests combining an EGFR inhibitor with an appropriate retinoid as a chemopreventative strategy.

Some retinoids exert their effects through receptor-independent pathways. The synthetic retinoid *N*-(4-hydroxyphenyl) retinamide (4-HPR or fenretinide) can induce apoptosis in responsive cells, including those resistant to classical retinoids *(36,37)*. 4-HPR triggers its biological effects in part through promotion of apoptosis that may be secondary to the generation of reactive oxygen species (ROS) *(38–40)*. 4-HPR has reported activity in the prevention of breast cancer *(15)*, and its clinical actions in other neoplastic or preneoplastic settings should be explored. CD437 and TAC101, other retinoids under study, have receptor-dependent activity for RARs, but also receptor-independent apoptogenic activity. Other retinoids can inhibit transcription factor AP-1, a key regulator of cellular growth and differentiation *(41)*. The clinical role of these and other non-classical retinoids has not been fully explored. Future studies should emphasize the clinical role of non-classical retinoids in cancer therapy and chemoprevention. These retinoids may also have synergy with other pharmacological agents.

3. MECHANISMS OF RETINOID ACTIONS

Metabolism and distribution of vitamin A (retinol) is tightly controlled by intracellular and extracellular binding proteins and by enzymes *(42)*. Predominant active forms of retinoids include ATRA and 9-*cis*-RA. When

Table 2
Ligands and Their Selectivities Toward RARs and RXRs

Retinoids	*Receptor Specificity*
Physiological retinoids	
All-*trans*-retinoic acid	RARs
9-*cis*-retinoic acid	RARs and RXRs
Synthetic retinoids: receptor-dependent activity	
Targretin/bexarotene *(30,45)*	RXRs
Synthetic retinoids: receptor-dependent and independent activity	
4-HPR /fenretinide *(36,46,47)*	RARγ, RARβ
CD437/6-[3-(1-adamantyl)-4-hydroxyphenyl]-2-naphthalene carboxylic acid (AHPN) *(48)*	RARγ
TAC-101 *(49,50)*	RARα

these molecules enter the nucleus, they bind to RARs *(43,44)*. Six genes encode retinoid receptors: RARα, β, and γ and RXRα, β, and γ. Each gene produces multiple receptor isoforms through alternate usage of splice sites and promoters. The ligand (receptor)-binding domains of RARs and RXRs are quite distinct, and therefore, can be targeted separately (Table 2). For RA to activate transcription, RARs must heterodimerize with RXRs. RXRs also heterodimerize with other nuclear receptors (NRs), including the thyroid hormone receptors (TRs), vitamin D receptor (VDR), and peroxisomal proliferator-activated receptor (PPAR), among others (as discussed in *44*). RXR ligands do not by themselves activate TR or RAR, but they can activate PPARγ *(45)*.

Several direct retinoid target genes have been reported, including genes involved in the retinoic acid signaling pathway (RARβ, cellular retinol binding protein [CRBP] II, and retinoic acid-binding protein [CRABP] II) and transcription factors or cofactors (organic cation transporter [Oct]3/4, Hoxa1, Hoxb4). Other genes are also RA targets *(51)*; initial microarray data have identified many new potential target genes and verified the expected differences in RA target genes between cell types *(52,53)*. Microarray technology should help reveal the diversity of retinoid-regulated mRNAs.

RAR-RXR heterodimers bind to specific DNA sequences called retinoic acid response elements

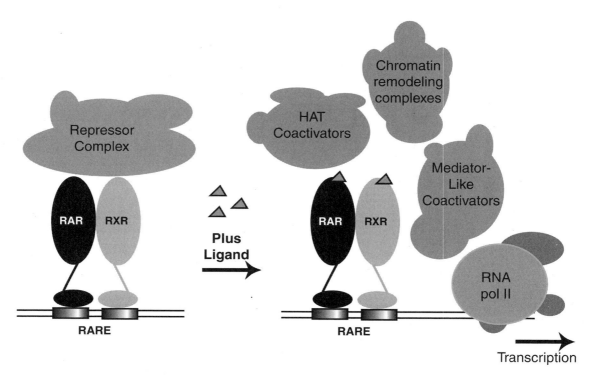

Fig. 1. Model for nuclear-receptor transcriptional activation through ligand-mediated displacement of corepressors and interaction with coactivators. Unliganded RAR actively represses transcription through interactions with repressor complexes (including SMRT and NCoR), which also contain histone deacetylase components. Histone acetyltransferase-containing coactivator complexes (including CBP/p300, SRC-1, and p/CAF) are believed to acetylate nucleosomes to open chromatin, making it accessible to other transcription factors. ATP-dependent chromatin remodeling complexes (including SWI/SNF and PBAF) are associated with activated nuclear receptors, and may also be involved in facilitating transcription. Coactivator complexes also link receptor activation to the basal transcriptional machinery that includes RNA polymerase II.

(RAREs), which are characterized by two half-sites with the consensus AGGTCA. The RARE is generally arranged as direct repeats separated by two or five nucleotides. Other RXR heterodimers bind the same half sites with different preferences for spacing and orientation *(43)*. Retinoid receptors can interact with inhibitory co-repressor or stimulatory co-activator proteins that affect transcriptional activities.

In the absence of ligand, the RXR-RAR heterodimers are bound to DNA in complex with corepressors—including the silencing mediator of RAR and TR (SMRT) and nuclear-receptor corepressor (NCoR) *(54,55)* which actively repress transcription (Fig. 1). Repression seems to occur primarily through the recruitment of histone deacetylases that prevent the opening of the chromatin structure associated with acetylation of nucleosomes and other coactivators (for review, *see 56–58)*. Change in the methylation state of chromatin can also affect retinoid-mediated transcriptional activity *(26,58)*. When the ligands bind, the corepressors are released and the coactivators can then bind to

activate transcription. CREB-binding protein and p300 both bind nuclear receptors in a ligand-dependent manner, and both have intrinsic histone acetyltransferase (HAT) activity. The p160 family of coactivators also bind ligand-activated receptors and has been shown to enhance transcription. Recently, a novel arginine methyltransferase (CARM1) was found to be associated with p160 coactivators; CARM1 can methylate histone H3 and other coactivators *(59)*. Several in-depth reviews have been published recently on coactivator function *(60–62)*.

The T_3R-receptor-associated protein/vitamin D receptor interacting protein (TRAP/DRIP) complex consists of at least nine proteins and, unlike the previously discussed coactivators, is devoid of HAT activity *(63)*. The ligand-dependent binding of this complex occurs through a single subunit (DRIP205/TRAP220). TRAP/DRIP also contains part of the "mediator complex," which is known to interact directly with the basal transcription machinery, including RNA polymerase II.

Complexes with ATP-dependent chromatin remodeling activity bind to NRs in a ligand-dependent manner *(64)*. Several distinct complexes have been isolated, and a recent study *(65)* indicated that a specific remodeling complex is required for receptor-mediated transcription. Other complexes were able to remodel the chromatinized template used in this study but only one, polybromo- and BRG_1-associated factor-containing complex (PBAF), could also activate transcription. This suggests that PBAF has a function beyond the chromatin remodeling seen with the other complexes, and that this function is essential for transcriptional activation.

4. RETINOIDS AND CANCER CHEMOPREVENTION MODELS

The fact that clinical studies have shown the negative effect of certain classical retinoids on lung-cancer prevention in smokers emphasizes the need for additional basic research to refine retinoid chemoprevention mechanisms. In vitro cellular models should prove useful in this regard. Several in vitro models are often used for mechanistic retinoid studies. These include the immortalized human bronchial-epithelial cell line BEAS-2B and its derived subclones, the NB4 APL cell line and the multipotent human embryonal carcinoma cell line NTERA-2 clone D1 (NT2/D1). For each of these cell lines, retinoid-resistant subclones have also been derived.

4.1. Bronchial-Epithelial Chemoprevention Model

To establish this chemoprevention model, BEAS-2B immortalized human bronchial-epithelial cells were transformed after independent exposure to the tobacco-derived carcinogens 4-(methylnitrosamino)-1-(3-pyridyl)-1-butanone (NNK) or cigarette smoke condensate (CSC). RA-treatment prevented NNK or CSC-dependent carcinogenic transformation *(18)*. RARβ or RXR agonists preferentially caused growth suppression in normal, immortalized, and carcinogen-transformed human bronchial-epithelial cells *(66)*. RA triggered G_1 cell-cycle arrest, concomitant growth suppression, and a decline in expression of G_1 cyclin proteins (18,66,67). A posttranslational mechanism was involved in regulating G_1 cyclin expression. Proteasome inhibitors prevented the decline in expression of cyclin D_1 *(66,67)*, indicating that proteolysis of cyclin D_1 can occur via the ubiquitin-dependent degradation pathway. Cyclin D_1 repression caused G_1 cell-cycle arrest that was hypothesized to permit repair of carcinogen-damaged DNA *(67)*. G_1 arrest after RA treatment appears to be a general mechanism of retinoid action, often mediated by cyclin D_1 degradation *(68)*.

An RA-resistant cell line was recently established to reveal important RA resistance mechanisms in bronchial-epithelial cells *(69)*. The BEAS-2B-R1 clonal cell line was derived from repeated passage of BEAS-2B cells in increasing ATRA dosages. This cell line is resistant to RA-signaled growth suppression, and is useful in identifying critical pathways involved in retinoid response. For example, RA treatment of BEAS-2B-R1 cells does not repress cyclin D_1 or cyclin E expression, which indicates how defects in the cyclin degradation may directly explain RA resistance *(69)*. These data are also consistent with the view of cyclin D_1 as an intermediate marker for clinical retinoid response: overexpression of cyclin D_1 *(70,71)* and cyclin E *(71)* occurs frequently in preneoplastic bronchial lesions. Correction of this aberrant expression by targeting the proteolysis pathway through retinoid treatment may be an effective lung cancer prevention strategy.

Recent work has revealed that RA-treatment prevents the increase in EGFR-expression that occurs after carcinogenic exposure of BEAS-2B cells *(72)*. EGFR activation promotes cellular growth and transformation, as well as other biological effects *(73)*. Overexpression of EGFR is often observed in non-small cell lung cancer (NSCLC) and bronchial preneoplasia *(74)*. Overexpression of EGFR ligand(s) and changes in EGFR-associated tyrosine kinase activity or receptor turnover, as well as expression of mutant receptor *(75)*, may play roles in altering angiogenesis *(76)* or tumorigenesis *(73)* through EGFR-dependent pathways. RA directly represses EGFR mRNA expression through a transcriptional mechanism *(72)*. In human bronchial-epithelial cells treated with epidermal growth factor (EGF), RA also prevented the induction of mitogenesis and cyclin D_1 expression *(72)*. Considering the importance of activation of the EGFR pathway, it is notable that retinoids can overcome effects of EGFR overexpression through transcriptional and posttranscriptional modulation. Combining an optimal retinoid with an EGFR antagonist would be an attractive regimen to consider for clinical cancer chemoprevention.

Other retinoid chemopreventive mechanisms have been identified in human bronchial-epithelial cells.

Retinoids degrade CDK_4 through the ubiquitin-protea-some pathway, which causes G_1 cell-cycle arrest *(77)*. Certain retinoids can also repress expression of telom-erase reverse transcriptase *(78)*. Microarray analysis of retinoid-treated vs untreated cells could discover additional mechanisms involved in retinoid chemo-preventive response. The retinoid-resistant cell lines derived could be used to search for defects in a high-lighted pathway.

4.2. Acute Promyelocytic Leukemia Differentiation Models

APL cases that contain a t(15;17) translocation express the fusion protein PML/RARα *(5)*, which typ-ically predicts complete remission in APL following ATRA differentiation therapy *(6)*. Variant translocations may also exist such as the t(11;17) rearrangement, which results in the promyelocytic leukemia zinc finger (PLZF)/RARα-fusion protein. PLZF/RARα-expressing APL cases are not clinically responsive to ATRA therapy *(79)*.

Derivation of the NB4 APL cell line, which contains the t(15;17) rearrangement *(80)*, has proven useful to study mechanisms of RA dependent differentiation of leukemic cells. Uncovered mechanisms are relevant to other tumor-cell contexts. RA treatment causes mor-phologic, immunophenotypic, and functional myeloid differentiation of NB4 APL cells *(80,81)*. Derived RA-resistant cells often have acquired mutations of PML/RARα, underscoring the protein's critical role in regulating RA response in APL *(81–84)*.

PML/RARα inhibits the PML and RARα pathways *(5)*; its expression in transgenic mice impaired myelopoiesis or triggered leukemogenesis *(85–88)*. Leukemogenesis may be triggered by functional dis-ruption of the PML or its associated pathways. PML can induce apoptosis, growth suppression, and cellular senescence upon oncogenic transformation (as reviewed in 89). Transgenic coexpression of PML/RARα with RARα/PML has been reported to increase the incidence of leukemogenesis, underscor-ing how genetic events in addition to PML/RARα expression contribute to leukemogenesis *(90)*. In NB4 APL cells, engineered overexpression (relative to PML/RARα) of RARα *(91)*, PML *(91,92)*, or RXRα *(81)* antagonized PML/RARα effects and caused growth suppression of transfectants. Targeting of PML/RARα expression by homologous recombination *(84)* or ribozyme-mediated inactivation *(84,93,94)* induced apoptosis with no evidence of leukemic-cell

maturation. These studies indicate that PML/RARα acts as an anti-apoptotic transcription factor. ATRA can overcome these anti-apoptotic effects by releasing the co-repressor complex from association with PML/RARα and recruiting a co-activator complex with histone acetylase activity *(95,96)*, which opens chromatin to stimulate transcription.

In contrast, PLZF/RARα contains two NcoR-binding sites. One is RA-sensitive and maps within the CoR box of RARα; the other maps to the *N*-terminal region of PLZF and forms a stable complex with co-repres-sors, resulting in retinoid resistance *(95,96)*. In APL cases that express the PLZF/RARα protein, there may be therapeutic benefits from combining RA with agents that affect methylation *(97)* or inhibit histone deacetylases to restore gene expression. Another hallmark of ATRA response in APL is the protea-some-dependent degradation of PML/RARα *(98)*. Recent microarray analyses have highlighted the ubiq-uitin activating-enzyme E1-like protein (UBE1L), which triggers the degradation of PML/RARα, as a potential RA target gene *(98)*. Other candidate retinoid target genes are discussed elsewhere in this chapter.

Several RA-resistant NB4 APL cell lines have been derived to explore mechanisms of retinoid resistance, and can identify key pathways involved in retinoid response *(81,82,99–101)*. Reported defects in such cells include persistent telomerase activity, nuclear body dis-organization *(81)*, mutations within the ligand-binding domain of the RAR portion of PML/RARα *(82–84)*, and deregulation of UBE1L *(98)*, among others. Future work will determine the clinical relevance of these or other observed defects in APL cellular responses to ATRA treatment. These models may provide clues to strategies to overcome clinical retinoid resistance.

4.3. Human Embryonal Carcinoma Differentiation Model

The NT2/D1 human embryonal carcinoma cell is a multipotent cell line that induces a neuronal phenotype and other lineages after RA treatment *(102)*, which can repress NT2/D1 tumorigenicity through induction of tumor-cell differentiation *(103)*. Retinoid-resistant NT2/D1 cells were derived through mutagenization and selective passage in increasing RA dosages *(104)*. These cells and a spontaneously retinoid-resistant embryonal carcinoma-cell line aberrantly expressed RARγ *(104,105)*. Cooperation between RARγ and RXRβ is required to trigger the full retinoid response in human embryonal carcinoma cells *(9,104,105)*.

Retinoid targets downstream of retinoid NRs have been identified in NT2/D1 cells. Repression of cyclin D_1 following RA treatment has been linked to the accumulation of hypophosphorylated RB protein and G_1 cell-cycle arrest. Repression of cyclin D_1 appears to play a key role in the induction of embryonal carcinoma differentiation (68). In NT2/D1 cells, RA-dependent repression of cyclin D_1 occurs through a ubiquitin-dependent cyclin D_1 proteolysis, and potentially the repression of cyclin D_1 transcription. These mechanisms may cooperate to trigger G_1 arrest (68).

Recent microarray work in NT2/D1 cells has revealed a novel candidate RA target gene that induces the receptor interacting protein 140 (RIP140) (53,106), which may be a direct RAR target that acts as a NR co-repressor. A feedback model has been proposed in which the binding of RA to its receptor induces RIP140 expression. This in turn would repress RAR-mediated gene expression (106). Whether RIP140 or other candidate retinoid target genes discovered in NT2/D1 cells play a role in regulating differentiation beyond human embryonal carcinoma is the subject of current studies.

5. RETINOID TARGETS

Retinoid treatment of BEAS-2B, APL, and NT2/D1 cell lines causes marked changes in growth and differentiation. Using these cell lines, research has described retinoid regulation of diverse differentiation, proteolytic, cell-cycle, or apoptotic pathways. Many retinoid actions downstream of retinoid NR signaling, have not yet been defined. An understanding of these processes should translate into clinical benefit in several ways. Specific retinoid targets could act as surrogate end-point biomarkers for clinical trials. Knowledge of the precise mechanisms of retinoid action would facilitate development of novel retinoids for use in cancer chemoprevention. Mechanistic insights may also lead to strategies to overcome *de novo* or acquired retinoid resistance. One approach that may elucidate important mechanisms involved in retinoid response is to reveal target genes that reproduce retinoid effects downstream of retinoid receptor signaling.

Several experimental approaches have been used to identify retinoid targets, including microarray analysis (52,53,107), differential or subtractive cDNA expression studies, and functional screens. Functional screens of drug action have been conducted using hammerhead ribozymes (84,93), genetic suppressor elements (108), technical knockout methods (109), or homologous recombination strategies (84). The recent development and use of small-inhibitory RNA in mammalian cellular models (110) should facilitate the functional analysis of target genes. Candidate target gene identification is an important step in revealing the precise mechanisms of retinoid action and developing novel therapeutics in cancer chemoprevention.

Although microarray analyses have the potential to identify many retinoid targets, any microarray screen has certain limitations. A candidate is highlighted because it is either induced or repressed by retinoid treatment. However, this regulation may not be a direct transcriptional effect, and auxiliary species may be required. It is important to validate that functional, retinoid-responsive motifs are evident in the promoter of the regulated gene. Also, a retinoid-regulated species in one cell type may not be affected by retinoid treatment in another cell-type; reported differences between NB4 APL (52,107) and NT2/D1 (53) microarray analyses have confirmed this point. In addition, even the most complex microarray chips display only a subset of potential candidate targets. A critical putative target may be absent from an individual chip, or a network of signals may be involved in retinoid response, but only some members of the network are on the chip. Also, changes in mRNA expression do not always accurately reflect changes in protein expression. Functional interactions between relevant protein species should certainly be examined. For example, proteolytic pathways are activated by retinoid treatment that affects the stability of PML/RARα (111–114) and G_1 cyclin proteins (18,66,67). These effects would not be apparent in a DNA microarray experiment, since this examines changes in expressed mRNA. The eventual development of reliable proteomic screens should address this limitation.

Microarray analyses produce many candidate retinoid target genes, and it can be daunting to choose candidates for an in-depth study. Attractive targets have been chosen based on the assumptions that a direct retinoid target gene would contain retinoid-responsive elements in its promoter and that its regulation would not typically require *de novo* protein synthesis. Retinoid regulation of a target gene is often aberrantly affected in retinoid-resistant cells. Development of retinoid-resistant cells should be useful in studying the retinoid response in cancer chemoprevention. Ultimately, engineered overexpression of a candidate retinoid target gene could reproduce retinoid biological effects, even without retinoid treatment.

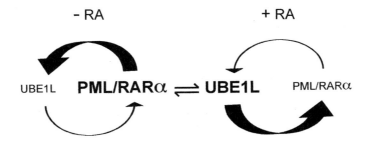

Fig. 2. An antagonistic relationship exists between UBE1L and PML/RARα. In APL cells in the absence of RA treatment, PML/RARα represses UBE1L transcription. Addition of RA induces UBE1L expression and triggers PML/RARα degradation, thereby overcoming the dominant-negative effects of PML/RARα. In this figure, lettering size depicts the relative abundance of each species. Arrow size conveys which relationships predominate before and after RA treatment.

Previously recognized biological or biochemical effects of a candidate target gene might account for its response to retinoids. It also is helpful to place the gene product(s) in the context of known retinoid actions. Retinoid-regulated species involved in cellular transcription are also candidate target genes. They could be involved in potentiating and modifying the upstream events of retinoid-dependent growth and differentiation signals. CREBPε and RIP140 are examples of such candidate target genes. CREBPε is an RA-regulated, nuclear-transcription factor that has been implicated in cellular differentiation of leukemic cells *(115)*; RIP140, as previously discussed, is a transcriptional repressor that has been identified as a potential retinoid target *(106)*.

UBE1L has a role in the retinoid-induced proteolytic pathway in APL cells *(98)*. Its expression is induced by ATRA treatment of differentiation-sensitive (but not differentiation-resistant) APL cells *(52,98)*. This regulation was observed at the mRNA and protein levels of UBE1L expression *(98)*. The UBE1L promoter was capable of mediating a transcriptional response to RA in a retinoid-receptor-selective manner, and the expression of PML/RARα inhibited UBE1L reporter activity *(98)*.

Exogenous expression studies have shown that overexpression of UBE1L in both transient and stable transfection experiments mimicked critical aspects of retinoid response. Cotransfection of UBE1L and PML/RARα in non-APL cells caused PML/RARα degradation, but transfected E1 did not trigger such degradation. Retroviral transduction of UBE1L into APL cells led to cellular apoptosis, but not maturation *(98)*. Previous studies have demonstrated that specifically targeting PML/RARα for degradation results in cellular apoptosis *(84,93)*. These results directly implicated UBE1L in RA-induced degradation of

PML/RARα, and are consistent with an antagonistic relationship between UBE1L and PML/RARα, as summarized in Fig. 2.

Retinoid targets may act in concert with other species to elicit a response. Recent work has placed UBE1L in the ISG15 conjugation pathway *(116)*. ISG15, a ubiquitin homolog, becomes conjugated to intracellular substrates after interferon treatment *(117,118)*. The role of retinoids in regulating this pathway is under active investigation, as is the pathway's role in PML/RARα degradation and whether retinoids regulate other members of the pathway.

An in-depth examination of these and other putative target genes may elucidate mechanisms of retinoid response or resistance. The development of validated preclinical models has increased opportunities to explore whether mechanistic studies are biologically relevant. Information about candidate target genes, and pathways should lead to the development of surrogate markers and an understanding of mechanisms of retinoid resistance, and perhaps to strategies to overcome this resistance. Conceivably, studies of retinoid target genes may reveal cancer therapy and prevention pathways that could represent novel pharmacological targets.

6. SUMMARY AND FUTURE DIRECTIONS

Basic and clinical research has shown that the retinoids are an attractive class of agents for cancer chemoprevention. This chapter reviews clinical findings that indicate an evolving role for the retinoids in cancer chemoprevention. Most clinical studies to date have emphasized the use of classical retinoids in cancer therapy and prevention; future work should explore the clinical use of non-classical retinoids, such as those that appear to act through retinoid-receptor-independent pathways and those that activate the RXR pathway. Future clinical studies should also explore combination chemopreventive therapy, using agents that cooperate with retinoids. These studies are especially relevant in lung cancer prevention, since negative clinical interactions have been reported in smokers entered in chemoprevention trials.

Here, we have summarized current knowledge of the mechanisms that signal retinoid response at the level of the retinoid receptors and their co-regulators. This understanding has been enhanced by in-depth studies of candidate target genes through analyses of established in vitro models. Retinoids produce diverse and pleiotropic effects, and are especially useful for discovering mechanistic pathways for cancer therapy and prevention that may in turn be targeted by other pharmacological agents. Identification of retinoid target genes downstream of NRs is the next step in understanding the retinoids in the context of cancer therapy and prevention. Future studies in retinoid cancer chemoprevention should exploit the convergence of basic and clinical findings in this field. In this way, it will become possible to learn when retinoids should be used to treat or prevent cancers, especially in those at high risk for primary or second primary cancers.

ACKNOWLEDGMENTS

We thank Ms. Ann Frost and Ms. Nancy Volkers for expert assistance in the preparation of this manuscript. We thank Dr. Michael Spinella for helpful discussions. This work was supported by National Institutes of Health Grants RO1-CA62275 (E.D.) and RO1-CA87546 (E.D.) as well as by a Lance Armstrong Award (S.J.F.), the Samuel Waxman Foundation Award (E.D.), and the Oracle Giving Fund (E.D.)

REFERENCES

1. Dmitrovsky E, Sporn MB. Pharmacology of cancer chemoprevention. Encyclopedia of Cancer. Academic Press, San Diego, CA, 2002, pp.449–456.
2. Hong WK, Itri LM. Retinoids and human cancer, in *The Retinoids: Biology, Chemistry, and Medicine, 2nd ed.* Sporn MB, Roberts AB, Goodman DS, eds. Raven Press Ltd, New York, NY, 1994, pp.597–630.
3. Gudas LJ, Sporn MB, Roberts AB. Cellular biology and biochemistry of retinoids, in *The Retinoids: Biology, Chemistry, and Medicine, 2nd ed.* Sporn MB, Roberts AB, Goodman DS, eds. Raven Press Ltd, New York, NY, 1994, pp.443–520.
4. Moon RC, Mehta RG, Rao KVN. Retinoids and cancer in experimental animals, in *The Retinoids: Biology, Chemistry,* *and Medicine, 2nd ed.* Sporn MB, Roberts AB, Goodman DS, eds. Raven Press Ltd, New York, NY, 1994, pp.573–595.
5. Nason-Burchenal K, Dmitrovsky E. The retinoids: cancer therapy and prevention mechanisms, in *Retinoids. The Biochemical and Molecular Basis of Vitamin A and Retinoid Action: Handbook of Experimental Pharmacology, vol. 139.* Nau H, Blaner W, eds. Springer-Verlag, Berlin, Heidelberg, 1999, pp.301–322.
6. Miller WH Jr, Kakizuka A, Frankel SR, et al. Reverse transcription polymerase chain reaction for the rearranged retinoic acid receptor α clarifies diagnosis and detects minimal residual disease in acute promyelocytic leukemia. *Proc Natl Acad Sci USA* 1992;89:2694–2698.
7. Lotan R, Xu XC, Lippman SM, et al. Suppression of retinoic acid receptor-β in premalignant oral lesions and its up-regulation by isotretinoin. *N Engl J Med* 1995;332:1405–1410.
8. Collins SJ, Robertson KA, Mueller L. Retinoic acid-induced granulocytic differentiation of HL-60 myeloid leukemia cells is mediated directly through the retinoic acid receptor (RAR-α). *Mol Cell Biol* 1990;10:2154–2163.
9. Spinella MJ, Kitareewan S, Mellado B, et al. Specific retinoid receptors cooperate to signal growth suppression and maturation of human embryonal carcinoma cells. *Oncogene* 1998;16:3471–3480.
10. Matthay KK, Villablanca JG, Seeger RC, et al. Treatment of high-risk neuroblastoma with intensive chemotherapy, radiotherapy, autologous bone marrow transplantation, and 13-*cis*-retinoic acid. Children's Cancer Group. *N Engl J Med* 1999;341:1165–1173.
11. Hong WK, Endicott J, Itri LM, et al. 13-*cis*-retinoic acid in the treatment of oral leukoplakia. *N Engl J Med* 1986;315:1501–1505.
12. Kraemer KH, DiGiovanna JJ, Moshell AN, et al. Prevention of skin cancer in xeroderma pigmentosum with the use of oral isotretinoin. *N Engl J Med* 1988;318:1633–1637.
13. Meyskens FL Jr, Surwit E, Moon TE, et al. Enhancement of regression of cervical intraepithelial neoplasia II (moderate dysplasia) with topically applied all-*trans*-retinoic acid: a randomized trial. *J Natl Cancer Inst* 1994;86:539–543.
14. Hong WK, Lippman SM, Itri LM, et al. Prevention of second primary tumors with isotretinoin in squamous-cell carcinoma of the head and neck. *N Engl J Med* 1990;323:795–801.
15. Veronesi U, De Palo G, Marubini E, et al. Randomized trial of fenretinide to prevent second breast malignancy in women with early breast cancer. *J Natl Cancer Inst* 1999;91:1847–1856.
16. Muto Y, Moriwaki H, Ninomiya M, et al. Prevention of second primary tumors by an acyclic retinoid, polyprenoic acid, in patients with hepatocellular carcinoma. Hepatoma Prevention Study Group. *N Engl J Med* 1996;334:1561–1567.
17. Wolbach SB, Howe PR. Tissue changes following deprivation of fat-soluble vitamin A. *J Exp Med* 1925;42:753–777.
18. Langenfeld J, Lonardo F, Kiyokawa H, et al. Inhibited transformation of immortalized human bronchial epithelial cells by retinoic acid is linked to cyclin E down-regulation. *Oncogene* 1996;13:1983–1990.
19. Blot WJ, Li JY, Taylor PR, et al. Nutrition intervention trials in Linxian, China: supplementation with specific vitamin/mineral combinations, cancer incidence, and disease-specific mortality in the general population. *J Natl Cancer Inst* 1993;85:1483–1492.

20. Dragnev KH, Stover D, Dmitrovsky E. Lung cancer prevention: the guidelines. *Chest* 2003;123:60S–71S.

21. Pastorino U, Infante M, Maioli M, et al. Adjuvant treatment of stage I lung cancer with high-dose vitamin A. *J Clin Oncol* 1993;11:1216–1222.

22. The Alpha-Tocopherol, Beta-Carotene Cancer Prevention Study Group. The effect of vitamin E and β-carotene on the incidence of lung cancer and other cancers in male smokers. *N Engl J Med* 1994;330:1029–1035.

23. Hennekens CH, Buring JE, Manson JE, et al. Lack of effect of long-term supplementation with β-carotene on the incidence of malignant neoplasms and cardiovascular disease. *N Engl J Med* 1996;334:1145–1149.

24. Omenn GS, Goodman GE, Thornquist MD, et al. Effects of a combination of β carotene and vitamin A on lung cancer and cardiovascular disease. *N Engl J Med* 1996;334:1150–1155.

25. Lippman SM, Lee JJ, Karp DD, et al. Randomized Phase III intergroup trial of isotretinoin to prevent second primary tumors in stage I non-small-cell lung cancer. *J Natl Cancer Inst* 2001;93:605–618.

26. Virmani AK, Rathi A, Zochbauer-Muller S, et al. Promoter methylation and silencing of the retinoic acid receptor-β gene in lung carcinomas. *J Natl Cancer Inst* 2000;92:1303–1307.

27. Lehmann JM, Dawson MI, Hobbs PD, et al. Identification of retinoids with nuclear receptor subtype-selective activities. *Cancer Res* 1991;51:4804–4809.

28. Lehmann JM, Jong L, Fanjul A, et al. Retinoids selective for retinoid X receptor response pathways. *Science* 1992;258:1944–1946.

29. Gottardis MM, Bischoff ED, Shirley MA, et al. Chemoprevention of mammary carcinoma by LGD1069 (Targretin): an RXR-selective ligand. *Cancer Res* 1996;56:5566–5570.

30. Heald P. The treatment of cutaneous T-cell lymphoma with a novel retinoid. *Clin Lymphoma Suppl* 2000;1:S45–S49.

31. Khuri FR, Rigas JR, Figlin RA, et al. Multi-institutional phase I/II trial of oral bexarotene in combination with cisplatin and vinorelbine in previously untreated patients with advanced non-small-cell lung cancer. *J Clin Oncol* 2001;19:2626–2637.

32. Heyman RA, Mangelsdorf DJ, Dyck JA, et al. 9-*cis* retinoic acid is a high affinity ligand for the retinoid X receptor. *Cell* 1992;68:397–406.

33. Levin AA, Sturzenbecker LJ, Kazmer S, et al. 9-*cis* retinoic acid stereoisomer binds and activates the nuclear receptor RXR alpha. *Nature* 1992;355:359–361.

34. Dahl AR, Grossi IM, Houchens DP, et al. Inhaled isotretinoin (13-*cis* retinoic acid) is an effective lung cancer chemopreventive agent in A/J mice at low doses: a pilot study. *Clin Cancer Res* 2000; 6:3015–3024.

35. Lonardo F, Dragnev KH, Freemantle SJ, et al. Evidence for the epidermal growth factor receptor as a target for lung cancer prevention. *Clin Cancer Res* 2002;8:54–60.

36. Kitareewan S, Spinella MJ, Allopenna J, et al. 4HPR triggers apoptosis but not differentiation in retinoid sensitive and resistant human embryonal carcinoma cells through an RARγ independent pathway. *Oncogene* 1999;18:5747–5755.

37. Delia D, Aiello A, Lombardi L, et al. *N*-(4-hydroxyphenyl)retinamide induces apoptosis of malignant hemopoietic cell lines including those unresponsive to retinoic acid. *Cancer Res* 1993;53:6036–6041.

38. Oridate N, Suzuki S, Higuchi M, et al. Involvement of reactive oxygen species in *N*-(4-hydroxyphenyl)retinamide-induced apoptosis in cervical carcinoma cells. *J Natl Cancer Inst* 1997;89:1191–1198.

39. Fanjul AN, Delia D, Pierotti MA, et al. 4-Hydroxyphenyl retinamide is a highly selective activator of retinoid receptors. *J Biol Chem* 1996;271:22,441–22,446.

40. Delia D, Aiello A, Meroni L, et al. Role of antioxidants and intracellular free radicals in retinamide-induced cell death. *Carcinogenesis* 1997;18:943–948.

41. Fanjul A, Dawson MI, Hobbs PD, et al. A new class of retinoids with selective inhibition of AP-1 inhibits proliferation. *Nature* 1994;372:107–111.

42. Blaner WS, Piantedosi R, Sykes A, Vogel S. Retinoic acid synthesis and metabolism, in *Retinoids. The Biochemical and Molecular Basis of Vitamin A and Retinoid Action: Handbook of Experimental Pharmacology, vol. 139.* Nau H, Blaner W, eds. Springer-Verlag, Berlin, Heidelberg, 1999, pp.117–152.

43. Mangelsdorf DJ, Evans RM. Retinoid receptors as transcription factors, in *Transcriptional Regulation.* McKnight SL, Yamamoto KR, eds. Cold Spring Harbor Laboratory Press, New York, 1992, pp.1137–1167.

44. Piedrafita FJ, Pfahl M. Nuclear retinoid receptors and mechanisms of action, in *Retinoids. The Biochemical and Molecular Basis of Vitamin A and Retinoid Action: Handbook of Experimental Pharmacology, vol. 139.* Nau H, Blaner W, eds. Springer-Verlag, Berlin, Heidelberg, 1999, pp.153–184.

45. Mukherjee R, Davies PJ, Crombie DL, et al. Sensitization of diabetic and obese mice to insulin by retinoid X receptor agonists. *Nature* 1997;386:407–410.

46. Torrisi R, Decensi A. Fenretinide and cancer prevention. *Curr Oncol Rep* 2000;2:263–270.

47. Wu JM, DiPietrantonio AM, Hsieh TC. Mechanism of fenretinide (4-HPR)-induced cell death. *Apoptosis* 2001;6:377–388.

48. Schadendorf D, Kern MA, Artuc M, et al. Treatment of melanoma cells with the synthetic retinoid CD437 induces apoptosis via activation of AP-1 in vitro, and causes growth inhibition in xenografts in vivo. *J Cell Biol* 1996;135(6Pt2):1889–1898.

49. Murakami K, Sakukawa R, Sano M, et al. Inhibition of angiogenesis and intrahepatic growth of colon cancer by TAC-101. *Clin Cancer Res* 1999;5:2304–2310.

50. Oikawa T, Murakami K, Sano M, et al. A potential use of a synthetic retinoid TAC-101 as an orally active agent that blocks angiogenesis in liver metastases of human stomach cancer cells. *Jpn J Cancer Res* 2001;92:1225–1234.

51. MaCaffery P, Drager UC. Regulation of retinoic acid signaling in the embryonic nervous system: a master differentiation factor. *Cytokine Growth Factor Rev* 2000;11:233–249.

52. Tamayo P, Slonim D, Mesirov J, et al. Interpreting patterns of gene expression with self-organizing maps: methods and application to hematopoietic differentiation. *Proc Natl Acad Sci USA* 1999;96:2907–2912.

53. Freemantle SJ, Kerley JS, Olsen SL, et al. Developmentally-related candidate retinoic acid target genes regulated early during neuronal differentiation of human embryonal carcinoma cells. *Oncogene* 2002;25:2880–2889.

54. Chen JD, Evans RM. A transcriptional co-repressor that interacts with nuclear hormone receptors. *Nature* 1995;377:454–457.

55. Horlein AJ, Naar AM, Heinzel T, et al. Ligand-independent repression by the thyroid hormone receptor mediated by a nuclear receptor co-repressor. *Nature* 1995;377:397–404.

56. Xu L, Glass CK, Rosenfeld MG. Coactivator and corepressor complexes in nuclear receptor function. *Curr Opin Genet Dev* 1999;9:140–147.

57. Urnov FD, Wolffe AP, Guschin D. Molecular mechanisms of corepressor function. *Curr Top Microbiol Immunol* 2001;254:1–33.

58. Privalsky ML. Regulation of SMRT and N-CoR corepressor function. *Curr Top Microbiol Immunol* 2001;254:117–136.

59. Xu W, Chen H, Du K, Asahara H, et al. A transcriptional switch mediated by cofactor methylation. *Science* 2001;294:2507–2511.

60. Rosenfeld MG, Glass CK. Coregulator codes of transcriptional regulation by nuclear receptors. *J Biol Chem* 2001;276:36,865–36,868.

61. Naar AM, Lemon BD, Tjian R. Transcriptional coactivator complexes. *Annu Rev Biochem* 2001;70:475–501.

62. Rachez C, Freedman LP. Mediator complexes and transcription. *Curr Opin Cell Biol* 2001;13:274–280.

63. Rachez C, Lemon BD, Suldan Z, et al. Ligand-dependent transcription activation by nuclear receptors requires the DRIP complex. *Nature* 1999;398:824–828.

64. Wallberg AE, Neely KE, Hassan AH, et al. Recruitment of the SWI-SNF chromatin remodeling complex as a mechanism of gene activation by the glucocorticoid receptor tau1 activation domain. *Mol Cell Biol* 2000;20: 2004–2013.

65. Lemon B, Inouye C, King DS, Tjian R. Selectivity of chromatin-remodelling cofactors for ligand-activated transcription. *Nature* 2001;414:924–928.

66. Boyle JO, Langenfeld J, Lonardo F, et al. Cyclin D1 proteolysis: a retinoid chemoprevention signal in normal, immortalized, and transformed human bronchial epithelial cells. *J Natl Cancer Inst* 1999;91:373–379.

67. Langenfeld J, Kiyokawa H, Sekula D, et al. Posttranslational regulation of cyclin D$_1$ by retinoic acid: a chemoprevention mechanism. *Proc Natl Acad Sci USA* 1997;94:12,070–12,074.

68. Spinella MJ, Freemantle SJ, Sekula D, et al. Retinoic acid promotes ubiquitination and proteolysis of cyclin D$_1$ during induced tumor cell differentiation. *J Biol Chem* 1999;274:22,013–22,018.

69. Dragnev KH, Pitha-Rowe IP, Ma Y, et al. Specific chemopreventive agents target proteasomal degradation of G$_1$ cyclins: implications for combination therapy. *Clin Cancer Res,* in Press.

70. Brambilla E, Gazzeri S, Moro D, et al. Alterations of Rb pathway (Rb-p16INK4-cyclin D$_1$) in preinvasive bronchial lesions. *Clin Cancer Res* 1999;5:243–250.

71. Lonardo F, Rusch V, Langenfeld J, et al. Overexpression of cyclins D$_1$ and E is frequent in bronchial preneoplasia and precedes squamous cell carcinoma development. *Cancer Res* 1999;59:2470–2476.

72. Lonardo F, Dragnev KH, Freemantle SJ, et al. Evidence for the epidermal growth factor receptor as a target for lung cancer prevention. *Clin Cancer Res* 2002;8:54–60.

73. Salomon DS, Brandt R, Ciardiello F, Normanno N. Epidermal growth factor-related peptides and their receptors in human malignancies. *Crit Rev Oncol Hematol* 1995;19:183–232.

74. Rusch V, Mendelsohn J, Dmitrovsky E. The epidermal growth factor receptor and its ligands as therapeutic targets in human tumors. *Cytokine Growth Factor Rev* 1996;7:133–141.

75. Ciardiello F, Tortora G. A novel approach in the treatment of cancer: targeting the epidermal growth factor receptor. *Clin Cancer Res* 2001;7:2958–2970.

76. Rak J, Yu JL, Klement G, Kerbel RS. Oncogenes and angiogenesis: signaling three-dimensional tumor growth. *J Investig Dermatol Symp Proc* 2000;5:24–33.

77. Sueoka N, Lee HY, Walsh GL, et al. Posttranslational mechanisms contribute to the suppression of specific cyclin: CDK complexes by all-trans retinoic acid in human bronchial epithelial cells. *Cancer Res* 1999;59:3838–4438.

78. Soria JC, Moon C, Wang L, et al. Effects of N-(4-Hydroxyphenyl)retinamide on hTERT expression in the bronchial epithelium of cigarette smokers. *J Natl Cancer Inst* 2001;93:1257–1263.

79. Melnick A, Licht JD. Deconstructing a disease: its fusion partners, and their roles in the pathogenesis of acute promyelocytic leukemia. *Blood* 1999;3167–3215.

80. Lanotte M, Martin-Thouvenin V, Najman S, et al. NB4, a maturation inducible cell line with t(15;17) marker isolated from a human acute promyelocytic leukemia (M3). *Blood* 1991;77:1080–1086.

81. Nason-Burchenal K, Maerz W, Albanell J, et al. Common defects of different retinoic acid resistant promyelocytic leukemia cells are persistent telomerase activity and nuclear body disorganization. *Differentiation* 1997;61:321–331.

82. Shao W, Benedetti L, Lamph WW, et al. A retinoid-resistant acute promyelocytic leukemia subclone expresses a dominant negative PML-RARα mutation. *Blood* 1997;89:4282–4289.

83. Kitamura K, Kiyoi H, Yoshida H, et al. Mutant AF-2 domain of PML-RARα in retinoic acid-resistant NB4 cells: differentiation induced by RA is triggered directly through PML-RARα and its down-regulation in acute promyelocytic leukemia. *Leukemia* 1997;11:1950–1956.

84. Nason-Burchenal K, Allopenna J, Begue A, et al. Targeting of PML/RARα is lethal to retinoic acid-resistant promyelocytic leukemia cells. *Blood* 1998;92:1758–1767.

85. Early E, Moore MA, Kakizuka A, et al. Transgenic expression of PML/RARα impairs myelopoiesis. *Proc Natl Acad Sci USA* 1996;93:7900–7904.

86. Grisolano JL, Wesselschmidt RL, Pelicci PG, Ley TJ. Altered myeloid development and acute leukemia in transgenic mice expressing PML-RARα under control of cathepsin G regulatory sequences. *Blood* 1997;89:376–387.

87. Brown D, Kogan S, Lagasse E, et al. A PMLRARα-transgene initiates murine acute promyelocytic leukemia. *Proc Natl Acad Sci USA* 1997;94:2551–2556.

88. He LZ, Tribioli C, Rivi R, et al. Acute leukemia with promyelocytic features in PML/RARα transgenic mice. *Proc Natl Acad Sci USA* 1997;94:5302–5307.

89. Salomoni P, Pandolfi PP. The role of PML in tumor suppression. *Cell* 2002;108:165–170.

90. Pollock JL, Westervelt P, Kurichety AK, et al. A bcr-3 isoform of RARα-PML potentiates the development of PML-RARα-driven acute promyelocytic leukemia. *Proc Natl Acad Sci USA* 1999;96:15,103–15,108.

91. Ahn MJ, Nason-Burchenal K, Moasser MM, Dmitrovsky E. Growth suppression of acute promyelocytic leukemia cells having increased expression of the non-rearranged alleles: RAR alpha or PML. *Oncogene* 1995;10:2307–2314.

92. Mu ZM, Chin KV, Liu JH, et al. PML, a growth suppressor disrupted in acute promyelocytic leukemia. *Mol Cell Biol* 1994;14:6858–6867.

93. Nason-Burchenal K, Takle G, Pace U, et al. Targeting the PML/RARα translocation product triggers apoptosis in promyelocytic leukemia cells. *Oncogene* 1998;17:1759–1768.

94. Pace U, Bockman JM, MacKay BJ, et al. A ribozyme which discriminates in vitro between PML/RARα, the t(15;17)-associated fusion RNA of acute promyelocytic leukemia, and PML and RARα, the transcripts from the nonrearranged alleles. *Cancer Res* 1994;54:6365–6369.

95. Lin RJ, Nagy L, Inoue S, et al. Role of the histone deacetylase complex in acute promyelocytic leukaemia. *Nature* 1998;391:811–814.

96. Grignani F, De Matteis S, Nervi C, et al. Fusion proteins of the retinoic acid receptor-α recruit histone deacetylase in promyelocytic leukaemia. *Nature* 1998;391:815–818.

97. Di Croce L, Raker VA, Corsaro M, et al. Methyltransferase recruitment and DNA hypermethylation of target promoters by an oncogenic transcription factor. *Science* 2002;295:1079–1082.

98. Kitareewan S, Pitha-Rowe I, Sekula D, et al. UBE1L is a retinoid target that triggers PML/RARα degradation and apoptosis in acute promyelocytic leukemia. *Proc Natl Acad Sci USA* 2002;99:3806–3811.

99. Duprez E, Ruchaud S, Houge G, et al. A retinoid acid 'resistant' t(15;17) acute promyelocytic leukemia cell line: isolation, morphological, immunological, and molecular features. *Leukemia* 1992;6:1281–1287.

100. Dermime S, Grignani F, Clerici M, et al. Occurrence of resistance to retinoic acid in the acute promyelocytic leukemia cell line NB4 is associated with altered expression of the pml/RAR alpha protein. *Blood* 1993;82:1573–1577.

101. Ruchaud S, Duprez E, Gendron MC, et al. Two distinctly regulated events, priming and triggering, during retinoid-induced maturation and resistance of NB4 promyelocytic leukemia cell line. *Proc Natl Acad Sci USA* 1994;91:8428–8432.

102. Andrews PW, Damjanov I, Simon D, et al. Pluripotent embryonal carcinoma clones derived from the human teratocarcinoma cell line Tera-2. Differentiation in vivo and in vitro. *Lab Invest* 1984;50:147–162.

103. Dmitrovsky E, Moy D, Miller WH Jr, et al. Retinoic acid causes a decline in TGF-alpha expression, cloning efficiency, and tumorigenicity in a human embryonal cancer cell line. *Oncogene Res* 1990;5:233–239.

104. Moasser MM, Khoo KS, Maerz WJ, et al. Derivation and characterization of retinoid-resistant human embryonal carcinoma cells. *Differentiation* 1996;60:251–257.

105. Moasser MM, Reuter VE, Dmitrovsky E. Overexpression of the retinoic acid receptor gamma directly induces terminal differentiation of human embryonal carcinoma cells. *Oncogene* 1995;10:1537–1543.

106. Kerley JS, Olsen SL, Freemantle SJ, Spinella MJ. Transcriptional activation of the nuclear receptor corepressor RIP140 by retinoic acid: a potential negative-feedback regulatory mechanism. *Biochem Biophys Res Commun* 2001;285:969–975.

107. Liu TX, Zhang JW, Tao J, et al. Gene expression networks underlying retinoic acid-induced differentiation of acute promyelocytic leukemia cells. *Blood* 2000;96:1496–1504.

108. Gudkov AV, Zelnick CR, Kazarov AR, et al. Isolation of genetic suppressor elements, inducing resistance to topoisomerase II-interactive cytotoxic drugs, from human topoisomerase II cDNA. *Proc Natl Acad Sci USA* 1993;90:3231–3235.

109. Deiss LP, Kimchi A. A genetic tool used to identify thioredoxin as a mediator of a growth inhibitory signal. *Science* 1991;252:117–120.

110. Elbashir SM, Harborth J, Lendeckel W, et al. Duplexes of 21-nucleotide RNAs mediate RNA interference in cultured mammalian cells. *Nature* 2001;411:494–498.

111. Nervi C, Ferrara FF, Fanelli M, et al. Caspases mediate retinoic acid-induced degradation of the acute promyelocytic leukemia PML/RARα fusion protein. *Blood* 1998;92:2244–2251.

112. Raelson JV, Nervi C, Rosenauer A, et al. The PML/RARα oncoprotein is a direct molecular target of retinoic acid in acute promyelocytic leukemia cells. *Blood* 1996;88:2826–2832.

113. Yoshida H, Kitamura K, Tanaka K, et al. Accelerated degradation of PML-retinoic acid receptor alpha (PML-RARA) oncoprotein by all-trans-retinoic acid in acute promyelocytic leukemia: possible role of the proteasome pathway. *Cancer Res* 1996;56:2945–2948.

114. Zhu J, Gianni M, Kopf E, et al. Retinoic acid induces proteasome-dependent degradation of retinoic acid receptor α (RARα) and oncogenic RARα fusion proteins. *Proc Natl Acad Sci USA* 1999;96:14,807–14,812.

115. Chih DY, Chumakov AM, Park DJ, et al. Modulation of mRNA expression of a novel human myeloid-selective CCAAT/enhancer binding protein gene (C/EBPϵ). *Blood* 1997;90:2987–2994

116. Yuan W, Krug RM. Influenza B virus NS1 protein inhibits conjugation of the interferon (IFN)-induced ubiquitin-like ISG15 protein. *EMBO J* 2001;20:362–371.

117. Loeb KR, Haas AL. The interferon-inducible 15-kDa ubiquitin homolog conjugates to intracellular proteins. *J Biol Chem* 1992;267:7806–7813.

118. Narasimhan J, Potter JL, Haas AL. Conjugation of the 15-kDa interferon-induced ubiquitin homolog is distinct from that of ubiquitin. *J Biol Chem* 1996;271:324–330.

E. DEHYDROEPIANDROSTERONE AND STRUCTURAL ANALOGS

19 Biologic and Therapeutic Effects of Dehydroepiandrosterone and Structural Analogs

Arthur G. Schwartz, PhD and Laura L. Pashko, PhD

1. INTRODUCTION

Dehydroepiandrosterone (DHEA) is a major adrenal cortical steroid in humans *(1,2)*. The plasma levels of DHEA and its sulfated ester rise early in life, reaching a maximum in the second decade, and decline thereafter throughout adult life, whereas cortisol levels rise linearly with age *(3)*. DHEA and related steroids are potent, non-competitive inhibitors of mammalian glucose-6 phosphate dehydrogenase (G6PDH), the rate-limiting enzyme of the pentose phosphate pathway, which is a major source of five-carbon sugars as well as nicotinamide adenine dinucleotide phosphate (NADPH), a critical modulator of cellular redox potential. NADPH supplies reducing equivalents for several reactions that generate oxygen-free radicals, which, in addition to their mutagenicity, act as intermediate messengers that stimulate mitogenesis and upregulate inflammation. In experimental animals, the DHEA steroids produce antiinflammatory, anti-hyperplastic, cancer-preventive, and anti-atherosclerotic effects, which are at least partially

mediated, through the inhibition of G6PDH and the pentose phosphate pathway. Preliminary epidemiological studies on male Sardinians carrying the Gd-Mediterranean allele for G6PDH deficiency suggest that these individuals experience an enhanced longevity. The DHEA steroids also produce biologic effects that are apparently not mediated through G6PDH inhibition, which antagonize various deleterious responses produced by excess glucocorticoid action. Excess glucocorticoid activity, in part produced by the enzyme 11β-hydroxysteroid dehydrogenase type 1, which interconverts active cortisol (corticosterone in the mouse) and their inert 11-keto forms, contributes to the development of the metabolic syndrome, characterized by visceral obesity, insulin resistance, and hypertriglyceridemia. The DHEA analog, 16α-fluoro-5-androsten-17-one, is highly effective in reducing hyperglycemia and hypertriglyceridemia in diabetic mice. In Phase II clinical trials, this compound significantly lowered fasting plasma triglyceride levels in hypertriglyceridemic patients.

From: Cancer Chemoprevention, Volume 1: Promising Cancer Chemoprevention Agents
Edited by: G. J. Kelloff, E. T. Hawk, and C. C. Sigman © Humana Press Inc., Totowa, NJ

2. OCCURRENCE OF DHEA

The adrenal cortex in humans secretes three classes of steroid hormone: the glucocorticoid (cortisol), the mineralocorticoid (aldosterone), and DHEA *(1)*. Although the physiologic effects of the first two steroids are well-characterized, the biologic significance of DHEA—aside from its role as a precursor to androgens and estrogens in peripheral tissue—is less clear. DHEA and its sulfate ester are secreted in approximately equal quantities by the adrenal glands, but DHEA-sulfate, because of its very low metabolic clearance rate (MCR), is the predominant circulating form in human plasma *(1,2)*.

The sulfated ester of DHEA is present in enormously high concentrations in human plasma, exceeding that of all other steroids except cholesterol *(3)*. Plasma levels of DHEA and its sulfate ester rise early in life and reach a maximum in the second decade, and thereafter decline profoundly throughout adult life *(3)*. Cortisol levels, by contrast rise linearly with age, leading to marked age-related changes in the cortisol-DHEA ratio *(4)*.

3. G6PDH INHIBITION AND EFFECTS OF DHEA ON CULTURED CELLS

DHEA is a potent noncompetitive inhibitor (with respect to $NADP^+$ and glucose-6-phosphate) of various mammalian G6PDHs, but does not inhibit spinach or yeast enzyme *(5–7)*. In an extensive study of structure-activity relationships, Raineri and Levy found that steroids in both the androstane and pregnane series were active inhibitors *(6)*. In the androstane steroids, a 17-keto group was required for inhibition and the β-OH group and β-carbonyl group at C-17 were unable to replace the keto group. Introduction of a Br atom in the 16α position markedly enhanced inhibition. In the pregnane series, a 20-keto group appeared to serve the same function as the 17-keto group did in the androstane series.

G6PDH is the rate-limiting enzyme of the pentose phosphate pathway *(8)*. This pathway is an important source of ribose-5-phosphate, which is required for nucleic acid synthesis, as well as that of extra-mitochondrial NADPH, which is utilized in specific reductive biosyntheses as well as in various reactions that generate oxygen-free radicals.

4. PROTECTION AGAINST CARCINOGENS

In 1975, we demonstrated that DHEA protected cultured rat-liver epithelial-like cells and embryonic fibroblasts against aflatoxin B_1- and 7,12dimethyl-benz[a]anthracene (DMBA)-induced cytotoxicity and transformation, whereas related steroids such as testosterone and etiocholanolone provided significantly less protection *(9)*. Treatment with DHEA also inhibited the rate of metabolism of [^{3}H]DMBA to water-soluble products by the cultured liver cells, and epiandrosterone, a more powerful G6PDH inhibitor than DHEA, was also more active in suppressing [^{3}H] DMBA metabolism. We hypothesized that DHEA protected cultured cells against carcinogen-induced cytotoxicity and transformation through inhibition of carcinogen activation by specific cytochrome P450s (which require NADPH as a cofactor) as a result of reducing NADPH levels. Lee et al. found that treatment of cultured rat tracheal-epithelial cells with DHEA or epiandrosterone decreased intracellular NADPH levels and protected the cells against toxicity by the herbicide paraquat *(10)*. The mechanism of paraquat toxicity is believed to result from the generation of oxygen free radicals through a redox reaction between paraquat and molecular oxygen *(11)*. NADPH is a source of reducing equivalents for several enzymes that generate oxygen free radicals, such as the leukocyte NADPH oxidase *(12)* and its more widely distributed homolog Mox1 *(13)*, nitric oxide synthase (NOS) *(14)*, and the Fenton reaction of iron-mediated catalysis of hydroxyl radical formation from H_2O_2 *(15)*. Thus, a reduction in the supply of NADPH may have a profound effect on oxygen free-radical formation.

5. INHIBITION OF CELL GROWTH AND DIFFERENTIATION

Two important consequences of inhibition of G6PDH and the pentose phosphate pathway are a reduction in the supply of ribose-5-phosphate required for nucleotide synthesis as well as in the availability of NADPH, which is utilized in specific reductive biosyntheses as well as in various reactions that generate oxygen-free radicals. Protection against carcinogen- and paraquat-induced cytotoxicity, as described previously, very likely results from a restriction in the supply of NADPH. However, in the work of Dworkin et al. *(16)* and Gordon et al. *(17)*, in which exogenous mixtures of deoxyribonucleosides or ribonucleosides overcame the inhibitory effect of DHEA steroids on growth and differentiation of cells in vitro, a restriction in the supply of pentose phosphate was probaly critical. Shantz et al. provided direct evidence that treatment of cultured 3T3 pre-adipocytes with DHEA and structural analogs resulted in an inhibition of G6PDH, leading to a block in differentiation to adipocytes *(18)*. These investigators found that treatment of 3T3-L1 cells with the potent G6PDH inhibitor, 16α-bromo-epiandrosterone, reduced the intracellular levels of 6-phosphogluconate and other products of the pentose phosphate pathway. Introduction of 6-phosphogluconate in liposomes into the cells raised the levels of 6 phosphogluconate and other pentose-phosphate-pathway sugar phosphates, and partially relieved the steroid-induced block in growth and differentiation.

Other investigators have found that treatment of various cultured cell lines with DHEA produces antiproliferative effects that are not reversed by exogenous mixtures of ribonucleosides or deoxyribonucleosides. Tian et al. determined the effect of DHEA on [³H] thymidine incorporation following growth stimulation with serum, platelet-derived growth factor (PDGF), or epidermal growth factor (EGF) in serum-starved cells of various cell lines *(19)*. They found that DHEA suppressed growth-factor stimulation in [³H] thymidine incorporation or cellular growth and that a mixture of deoxyribonucleosides or ribonucleosides did not reverse the growth inhibition. Treatment of cells with growth-inhibitory concentrations of DHEA for 24 h also reduced the NADPH/NADP⁺ level by about twofold. Similarly, Dashtaki et al. reported that DHEA and 16α-bromo-epiandrosterone dramatically reduced proliferation in primary cultures of rat tracheal smooth-muscle cells stimulated with fetal bovine serum or PDGF, and that a mixture of deoxyribonucleosides or ribonucleosides could not overcome the steroid-induced inhibition in growth *(20)*.

There is increasing evidence that growth-factor stimulation of mitogenesis is mediated, at least in part, by oxygen free radicals that act as intracellular second messengers *(21)*. An important source of oxygen free radicals activated by growth factors is the phagocyte NADPH oxidase and its homolog Mox 1, found in non-phagocytic cells *(13,21)*. We have previously shown that DHEA and 16α-bromo-epiandrosterone inhibit 12-*O*-tetradecanoylphorbol-13-acetate (TPA)-stimulated superoxide radical (O_2^-) formation in human neutrophils, very likely by inhibiting G6PDH and restricting the supply of NADPH *(22)*. Thus, it is a possibility that DHEA steroids may inhibit growth factor-stimulated mitogenesis by reducing NADPH-dependent oxygen free-radical formation. Experiments demonstrating that NADPH-liposome treatment reverses DHEA-analog suppression of TPA-induced

epidermal hyperplasia in mouse skin, as described here, support this hypothesis *(23)*.

6. CANCER PREVENTION

We first demonstrated that oral administration of DHEA (450 mg/kg 3×/wk) to C3H-A^vy (obese) and C3H-A/A (non-obese) mice inhibited spontaneous mammary-tumor development *(24,25)*. Dietary administration of DHEA (0.2–0.6%) inhibits tumor development in mice and rats in numerous carcinogen-induced, radiation-induced, and spontaneous models. A partial listing includes *N*-methyl-*N*-nitrosourea (MNU)-induced and radiation-induced mammary cancer in rats *(26,27)*, diethylnitrosamine-induced persistent liver nodules in rats subjected to the resistant hepatocyte protocol *(28)*, DMBA- and urethan-induced lung tumors in mice *(29)*, 1,2-dimethylhydrazine-induced colon tumors in mice *(30)*, MNU-induced prostate cancer in rats *(31)*, and spontaneous lymphomas and testicular Leydig-cell tumors in *p53*-deficient mice and aging F344 rats, respectively *(32,33)*. Also, topical application of either DHEA or various synthetic analogs on the backs of CD-1 mice inhibits DMBA-initiated and TPA-promoted skin papilloma development at both the initiation and promotion stages *(34)*, and suppresses the formation of skin papillomas and carcinomas produced by multiple applications of DMBA *(35)*.

6.1. Mechanism of Cancer Prevention

Topical application of DHEA or the synthetic steroid 3β-methyl-5-androsten-17-one to mouse skin inhibits the binding of [³H] DMBA to epidermal DNA, probably by reducing carcinogen activation by NADPH-dependent mixed-function oxidases *(34)*. This mechanism may explain the inhibition in DMBA-induced papilloma and carcinoma development produced by topical treatment with DHEA or 3β-methyl-5-androsten-17-one.

DHEA and two synthetic analogs, 3β-methyl-5-androsten-17-one and 16α-fluoro-5-androsten-17-one, also inhibit TPA-induced skin papilloma formation when applied topically before each application of TPA *(34,36)*. TPA, a protein kinase C (*PKC*) agonist, induces acute inflammation and epidermal hyperplasia in mouse skin *(37)*. Both the inflammatory and hyperplastic responses to TPA are suppressed by treatment with 16α-fluoro-5-androsten-17-one *(23)*. This steroid is a potent G6PDH inhibitor, with a K_i of 0.5 μ*M* vs 17 μ*M* for DHEA *(38)*.

Garcea et al. determined the effect of DHEA treatment on preneoplastic liver foci formation induced in rats by treatment with an initiating dose of diethylnitrosamine, followed 15 d later by a 15-d feeding of diet containing 0.03% 2-acetylaminofluorene with a partial hepatectomy at the feeding midpoint, and then by a 15-d treatment with 0.05% phenobarbital. Phenobarbital treatment greatly stimulated the development and [³H] thymidine-labeling indices of preneoplastic liver (γ-glutamyltranspeptidase positive) foci, and simultaneous treatment with DHEA (0.6% in the diet) abolished the effect of phenobarbital (39). DHEA treatment also greatly reduced pentose phosphate shunt activity in isolated hepatocytes. Importantly, these investigators found that intraperitoneal (ip) injections of a mixture of the four deoxyribonucleosides or ribonucleosides during the period of phenobarbital treatment completely overcame the inhibitory effect of DHEA on focus formation and on the [³H] thymidine-labeling index. We also found that treatment with a mixture of the four deoxyribonucleosides in the drinking water of CD-1 mice completely reversed 16α-fluoro-5-androsten-17-one-induced inhibition of TPA stimulation of epidermal hyperplasia and promotion of skin papillomas (36).

These experiments suggest that DHEA steroids inhibit tumor development through the inhibition of nucleic acid synthesis as a result of reducing the supply of five-carbon sugars. However, this mechanism may only partly account for the inhibition in tumor promotion. We have found that dosages of 16α-fluoro-5-androsten-17-one in rats as high as 12× the dose needed to inhibit TPA-stimulated epidermal hyperplasia produce no apparent toxicity and do not suppress mitogenesis in rapidly proliferating tissues, such as the bone marrow and GI tract (40). More importantly, using a mixture of NADPH and cationic liposomes to facilitate, uptake of the normally impenetrable dinucleotide, we found that intradermal injections of NADPH-liposomes completely reversed the antiinflammatory and antihyperplastic effects of 16α-fluoro-5-androsten-17-one in TPA-treated mouse skin (23). In contrast, similar injections of NADPH-liposomes had no effect on the antiinflammatory and anti-hyperplastic effects of corticosterone. We have also found that deoxyribonucleoside treatment reverses the antiinflammatory as well as the antihyperplastic effect of 16α-fluoro-5-androsten-17-one in TPA-treated skin (unpublished data). One possible interpretation of these data is that treatment with deoxyribonucleosides not only replaces depleted nucleotide pools, but also changes the redox state of the cells since NADPH is no longer needed for ribonucleotide and deoxyribonucleotide synthesis.

Thus, the antiproliferative effect of 16α-fluoro-5-androsten-17-one may be directly linked to its antiinflammatory action, and be more a result of inhibition in oxygen free-radical formation than reduction in deoxyribonucleotide synthesis. There is increasing evidence that oxygen free radicals—in part produced by the leukocyte NADPH oxidase and its homolog Mox 1—act as intermediate messengers that stimulate mitogenesis and upregulate the inflammatory response (13,21,41,42).

7. ANTI-ATHEROSCLEROTIC EFFECT

DHEA inhibits the development of experimentally induced atherosclerosis in rabbits. Gordon et al. produced severe atherosclerosis in rabbits by treatment with a balloon catheter to produce aortic endothelial injury followed by feeding a 2% cholesterol diet for 12 wk. DHEA treatment (0.5% in the diet) produced an almost 50% reduction in plaque size, and markedly reduced fatty infiltration of the heart and liver (43). These beneficial effects of DHEA were not attributable to differences in body wt gain, food intake, or plasma cholesterol levels. Arad et al. found that DHEA reduced aortic-fatty streak development by 30–40% in cholesterol-fed rabbits without vascular injury (44). Eich et al. studied the effect of DHEA in a hypercholesterolemic rabbit model of heterotropic cardiac transplantation that mimics the accelerated atherosclerosis seen in heart transplantation patients (45). In this model, hearts were transplanted heterotropically into recipient rabbits, and the animals then received a 1% cholesterol diet with or without 0.5% DHEA. The animals were sacrificed 5 wk later and the coronary arteries and myocardium were prepared for histological examination. DHEA treatment reduced the number of diseased arterial branches, the severity of luminal stenoses, and the intimal content of lipid-laden foam cells.

In these three studies, DHEA treatment inhibited atherosclerosis and fatty-streak development without any apparent effect on plasma lipids. Other biological agents, such as the probucol analog, MDL 29,311, and the angiotensin-converting enzyme (ACE) inhibitor enlapril, also inhibit atherosclerosis development in the Watanabe and cholesterol-fed rabbits, respectively, without reducing plasma cholesterol levels (46,47). Probucol is believed to act as an antioxidant, and may reduce the oxidative modification of LDL that is critical for lesion formation. Angiotensin II activates the NADPH-dependent membrane oxidase in vascular tissue, and may promote atherosclerosis by two redox-dependent mechanisms: increasing the oxidative modification of LDL and activating NFκB and inducing the expression of redox-sensitive gene products that upregulate the inflammatory response in the arterial wall (48). In a clinical trial involving 9,297 cardiovascular high-risk patients, treatment with the ACE inhibitor ramipril for a mean of 5yr significantly reduced the rates of death, myocardial infarction, and stroke (49). Only a small part of the benefit could be attributed to blood-pressure reduction, since the majority of patients were not hypertensive.

DHEA and structural analogs inhibit TPA-stimulated O_2^- production in human neutrophils and suppress TPA-stimulated inflammatory and hyperplastic effects in mouse skin, very probably by restricting the supply of NADPH (22,23). It is thus possible that DHEA inhibits experimentally induced atherosclerosis, at least in part, by reducing NADPH production and subsequent oxidative stress.

8. G6PDH DEFICIENCY

The human gene encoding G6PDH is located in the telomeric region of the long arm of the X chromosome, and more than 34 polymorphs have been identified that contain point mutations in the base sequence of this gene (50). The Gd-Mediterranean allele, which affects about 12–15% of the general Sardinian male population, is associated with erythrocyte-enzyme activity levels that are undetectable with routine methods (51,52). Non-erythrocyte cells—such as neutrophils, cultured fibroblasts, cultured lymphocytes, and lung tissue—also have very low levels of enzyme activity, on the order of 8–15% of normal (53–56). Feo et al. found that cultured fibroblasts and lymphocytes from G6PDH-deficient male Sardinians were less sensitive to the toxic and transforming effects of the carcinogen benzo[a]pyrene (B[a]P) than normal cells (53,54). The deficient cells also showed a marked reduction in the NADPH/NADP$^+$ ratio as well as a reduced capacity to produce B[a]P-water-soluble and mutagenic metabolites. DHEA treatment of normal cells in vitro mimicked the effect of G6PDH deficiency. Also, neutrophils from G6PDH-deficient individuals, when stimulated with TPA, produced 60% less O_2^- than stimulated normal neutrophils (55).

Numerous studies with DHEA and structural analogs strongly suggest that G6PDH inhibition, with a consequent reduction in NADPH availability and oxygen free-radical formation, mechanistically contributes to the inhibition of experimentally induced cancers and atherosclerosis. There is a growing awareness that endogenous production of oxygen free radicals is a major source of DNA damage and mutagenesis (57), and may be linked to the development of many age-related diseases, such as cancer (58), atherosclerosis (59), and neurodegenerative diseases (60), as well as the basic aging process (61).

Epidemiological studies suggest that male Sardinians bearing the Gd-Mediterranean allele experience a significantly reduced age-related mortality. In a 10-yr study in a cohort of 1756 G6PDH-deficient male Sardinians, using the general Sardinian male population as a reference, Cocco et al. found significantly fewer deaths from all causes in the deficient individuals, primarily the result of a fourfold reduction in deaths from cardiovascular and cerebrovascular disease (62). However, since the study cohort was not a random sample of the general Sardinian male population, selection bias could not be ruled out.

Very interesting recent epidemiological data suggest that male Sardinians experience a substantially lower age-related mortality than males elsewhere, whereas female mortality is essentially the same as elsewhere (63). There appears to be a larger proportion of male Sardinians who live past the age of 100 than males in any other country with reliable statistics, leading to a female:male ratio of centenarians of 2:1 instead of the usual 5:1. Passarino et al. found no correlation between the frequency of Y-chromosome-binary markers and longevity in a study involving 40 male Sardinian centenarians, suggesting that the high frequency of males among Sardinian centenarians is the result of gene(s) shared by women (64). The hypothesis that G6PDH deficiency may contribute to the enhanced longevity of male Sardinians is currently under investigation (65).

9. ANTI-OBESITY EFFECT

Yen et al. reported that DHEA treatment of VY-A^{vy}/$_a$ (genetically obese) mice markedly reduced weight gain (66). DHEA was administered orally in a suspension of sesame oil 3×/wk at a dose of 500 mg/kg. DHEA-treated mice consumed the same amounts of food as the controls, suggesting that the steroid-reduced weight gain by reducing metabolic efficiency.

Hepatic lipogenesis rates were reduced in the DHEA-treated animals, and the authors hypothesized that this may have resulted from G6PDH inhibition and reduction in the level of NADPH, which is required for fatty acid biosynthesis.

Many investigators have confirmed the anti-obesity action of DHEA in mice and rats bearing various obesity-producing mutations (ob, db, and fa) as well as in some non-obese strains *(67,68)*. In some strains of mice and rats, DHEA—when administered in the diet at dosages greater than 0.2%—may produce some suppression in food consumption that is frequently transient. However, pair-fed mice weigh more than their DHEA-treated counterparts, indicating that DHEA treatment reduces metabolic efficiency. The mechanism of the anti-obesity effect is unknown, and is probably not a result of G6PDH inhibition. Coleman et al. reported that 16α-bromo-epiandrosterone, a much more potent G6PDH inhibitor than DHEA *(6)*, failed to reduce weight gain or lower blood glucose in BKS.Cg-m$^+$/$_+$ Lepr^{db} mice when fed in the diet at 0.4% *(67)*. In contrast, DHEA administration at 0.4% of the diet markedly reduced blood glucose levels in diabetic mice and reduced weight gain in similar mutant strains.

10. ANTI-GLUCOCORTICOID ACTION

DHEA exerts important biological effects that are apparently not mediated by G6PDH inhibition, and which share the common property of antagonizing certain responses produced by the glucocorticoids *(69)*. Since these glucocorticoid-induced physiologic responses are deleterious, and since cortisol levels in humans rise with age, resulting in a marked decline in the DHEA-cortisol ratio, this has led to speculation that DHEA steroids could be used to treat certain age-related conditions that may be caused at least partially by excess cortisol action.

10.1. Immunosenescence

The glucocorticoids are potent immunosuppressive agents, and produce thymic atrophy when administered in high doses to laboratory mice. Blauer et al. reported that subcutaneous(sc) pretreatment of male Balb/c mice with 60 mg/kg DHEA for 3d significantly protected against thymic and splenic involution produced 24 h after a single injection of dexamethasone *(70)*. DHEA pretreatment for 3d in vivo also antagonized the marked suppression of in vitro blastogenic responses seen in T- and B-lymphocytes after a single injection of dexamethasone.

DHEA treatment protects mice against acute-lethal infection with several different viruses *(71,72)*, but does not demonstrate anti-viral activity in vitro *(71)*. Viral infections are known to elevate glucocorticoid levels, and treatment with DHEA at dosages that protected mice against West Nile virus infection also arrested the involution of thymus and spleen observed in these animals *(72)*. There is evidence that DHEA may produce immunostimulatory effects, independent of antiglucocorticoid action, in preserving immunocompetence in thermally injured mice *(73)*.

With aging, there is an increasing vulnerability to infectious diseases, and it has been suggested that DHEA steroids may be useful in potentiating immunocompetence in the elderly *(71)*.

10.2. Hippocampal Atrophy

Prolonged exposure to elevated glucocorticoid levels has been linked to hippocampal pathology in older rats *(74)*. Also, aged humans with significantly prolonged elevated plasma cortisol levels demonstrate reduced hippocampal volume and memory deficits when compared to normal cortisol controls *(75)*. DHEA treatment in vitro protected primary-rat-hippocampal cultures against toxicity induced by N-methyl-D-aspartic acid (NMDA), and, importantly, treatment in vivo markedly reduced NMDA-induced hippocampal toxicity *(76)*.

11. TYPE 2 DIABETES AND THE METABOLIC SYNDROME

The metabolic syndrome, consisting of visceral obesity, insulin resistance, and hypertriglyceridemia, is a common abnormality in humans *(77)*. Individuals with this condition experience a high incidence of cardiovascular disease *(78)*. There is considerable evidence that excess glucocorticoid exposure plays a critical role in the etiology of this syndrome *(77)*. Adrenalectomy reverses the hyperinsulinemia, hyperglycemia, hypertriglyceridemia, and obesity that are found in ob/ob mice and fa/fa Zucker rats, and daily injections of hydrocortisone in adrenalectomized fa/fa Zucker rats restore the hyperinsulinemia and hypertriglyceridemia *(79)*. Individuals with Cushing's disease, who experience excess-systemic-glucocorticoid exposure, develop the metabolic syndrome *(77)*.

There is recent evidence that glucocorticoid activity on target tissue depends on circulating levels of steroid as well as on intracellular enzymes, 11β-hydroxysteroid dehydrogenase type 1 (11β-HSD-1) and

11β-hydroxysteroid dehydrogenase type 2 (11β-HSD-2), which interconvert active cortisol (corticosterone in the mouse) and their inert 11-keto forms. 11β-HSD-2 is believed to function in vivo as a dehydrogenase, and inactivates glucocorticoids in the kidney, thus allowing aldosterone access to mineralocorticoid receptors *(80)*. In contrast, 11β-HSD-1, which is expressed in classical glucocorticoid-responsive tissues, regenerates active cortisol and corticosterone from inert 11-keto forms. Mice that are homozygous for a targeted deletion of the 11β-HSD-1 gene show reduced activation of glucocorticoid-sensitive hepatic gluconeogenic enzymes in response to stress or high-fat diet and develop a diabetes-resistant phenotype *(81)*. Interestingly, transgenic mice that overexpress 11β-HSD-1 selectively in adipose tissue have increased adipose tissue levels of corticosterone and develop visceral obesity and pronounced insulin-resistant diabetes and hypertriglyceridemia, providing strong evidence that target-organ glucocorticoid excess can produce the metabolic syndrome *(82)*.

DHEA and 16α-fluoro-5-androsten-17-one markedly reduce hyperglycemia, hyperinsulinemia, and hypertriglyceridemia in mice or rats that bearing either the ob, db, or fa mutations *(68,83,84)*. Although the mechanism of this effect is unknown, it is consistent with the anti-glucocorticoid action of the DHEA steroids. Treatment of cultured human skeletal myoblasts with DHEA inhibited the activity of 11β-HSD-1, and this may contribute to the anti-glucocorticoid activity of the steroid *(85)*. Clearly, further studies are needed to establish the mechanism of the anti-glucocorticoid action of the DHEA steroids, which could have substantial clinical significance.

12. CLINICAL TRIALS WITH 16α-FLUORO-5-ANDROSTEN-17-ONE

In numerous studies in laboratory animals in which DHEA treatment produced cancer-preventive, anti-atherosclerotic, anti-obesity, and anti-diabetic effects, the steroid was administered orally at high dosages in the range of 125 mg/kg–500 mg/kg *(86)*. Approximately bioequivalent dosages in the human would be on the order of 1000 mg–2000 mg daily *(87)*. In a double-blind placebo-controlled crossover study in which DHEA was administered orally at 1600 mg daily to six postmenopausal women for 4wk, plasma testosterone and dihydrotestosterone levels increased ninefold and 20-fold, respectively *(88)*. Plasma HDL levels decreased by 20–30%. Peak insulin levels during a 3-h glucose tolerance test were significantly higher, and

were associated with a 50% increase in the integrated insulin response. Thus, significant metabolism of DHEA into potent androgens may greatly limit the use of high-dose oral DHEA therapy. In addition to sex-hormonal side effects, DHEA is a peroxisome proliferator in mice and rats, and long-term administration to rats induces a high incidence of hepatocellular carcinoma *(89,90)*.

We have developed the synthetic steroid, known as 16α-fluoro-5-androsten-17-one, which in mice and rats does not demonstrate the androgenic, estrogenic, or peroxisomal-proliferating effects of DHEA, yet has retained the antiproliferative, cancer-preventive, anti-obesity, and antidiabetic activity of the native steroid *(27,36,38,83,91)*. In addition to cancer chemoprevention, 16α-fluoro-5-androsten-17-one may have important application in the treatment of type 2 diabetes and the prevention of atherosclerosis. In early Phase II clinical trials, 16α-fluoro-5-androsten-17-one, when administered orally in capsules at a daily dose of 1200 mg, significantly lowered fasting plasma triglycerides in individuals with hypertriglyceridemia (>200 mg/dL) (JP Kane et al., unpublished results). The drug appears to be particularly effective in obese individuals with a body mass index greater than 30. As more clinical data become available on safety and dosage, cancer prevention trials are anticipated. Based on preclinical models, target organs could include the prostate, breast, and colon, with proliferation and differentiation surrogate efficacy markers used in Phase II trials.

REFERENCES

1. VandeWiele RL, MacDonald PC, Gurpide E, Lieberman S. Studies on the secretion and interconversion of the androgens. *Recent Prog Horm Res* 1963;19:275–310.
2. Parker CR Jr. Dehydroepiandrosterone and dehydroepiandrosterone sulfate production in the human adrenal during development and aging. *Steroids* 1999;64:640–647.
3. Orentreich N, Brind JL, Rizer RL. Age changes and sex differences in serum dehydroepiandrosterone sulfate concentrations throughout adulthood. *J Clin Endocrinol Metab* 1984;59:551–555.
4. Lauglin GA, Barrett-Connor E. Sexual dimorphism in the influence of advanced aging on adrenal hormone levels: the Rancho Bernardo study. *J Clin Endocrinol Metab* 2000;85:3561–3568.
5. Marks PA, Banks J. Inhibition of mammalian glucose-6-phosphate dehydrogenase by steroids. *Proc Natl Acad Sci USA* 1960;46:447–452.
6. Raineri R, Levy HR. On the specificity of steroid interaction with mammary gland glucose-6-phosphate dehydrogenase. *Biochemistry* 1970;9:2233–2243.
7. Gordon GB, MacKow MC, Levy HR. On the mechanism of interaction of steroids with human glucose-6-phosphate dehydrogenase. *Arch Biochem Biophys* 1995;318:25–29.

8. Kletzien RF, Harris PK, Foellmi LA. Glucose-6-phosphate dehydrogenase: a "housekeeping" enzyme subject to tissue-specific regulation by hormones, nutrients, and oxidant stress. *FASEB J* 1994;8:174–181.

9. Schwartz AG, Perantoni A. Protective effect of dehydroepiandrosterone against aflatoxin B_1- and 7,12-dimethylbenz(*a*)anthracene-induced cytotoxicity and transformation in cultured cells. *Cancer Res* 1975;35:2482–2487.

10. Lee T-C, Lai G-J, Kao S-L, et al. Protection of a rat tracheal epithelial cell line from paraquat toxicity by inhibition of glucose-6-phosphate dehydrogenase. *Biochem Pharmacol* 1993;45:1143–1147.

11. Misra, HP, Gorsky LD. Paraquat and NADPH-dependent lipid peroxidation in lung microsomes. *J Biol Chem* 1981;256:9994–9998.

12. Babior BM. NADPH-oxidase: an update. *Blood* 1999;93:1464–1476.

13. Suh Y-A, Arnold RS, Lasegue B. et al. Cell transformation by the superoxide-generating oxidase, MOX 1. *Nature* 1999;401:79–82.

14. Marletta MA. Nitric acid synthase: aspects concerning structure and catalysis. *Cell* 1994;78:927–930.

15. Imlay JA, Linn S. DNA damage and oxygen radical toxicity. *Science* 1988;240:1302–1309.

16. Dworkin CR, Gorman SD, Pashko LL, et al. Inhibition of growth of HeLa and WI-38 cells by dehydroepiandrosterone and its reversal by ribo- and deoxyribonucleosides. *Life Sci* 1988;38:1451–1457.

17. Gordon GB, Shantz LM, Talalay P. Modulation of growth, differentiation and carcinogenesis by dehydroepiandrosterone. *Adv Enzyme Regul* 1987;26:355–382.

18. Shantz LM, Talalay P, Gordon GB. Mechanism of inhibition of growth of 3T3-L1 fibroblasts and their differentiation to adipocytes by dehydroepiandrosterone and related steroids: role of glucose-6-phosphate dehydrogenase. *Proc Natl Acad Sci USA* 1989;86:3852–3856.

19. Tian WN, Braunstein LD, Pang J, et al. Importance of glucose-6-phosphate dehydrogenase activity for cell growth. *J Biol Chem* 1998;273:10,609–10,617.

20. Dashtaki R, Wharton AR, Murphy TM, et al. Dehydroepiandrosterone and analogs inhibit DNA binding of AP-1 and airway smooth muscle proliferation. *J Pharmacol Exp Ther* 1998;285:876–883.

21. Irani K, Xi Y, Zweier JL, et al. Mitogenic signaling mediated by oxidants in *ras*-transformed fibroblasts. *Science* 1997;275:1649–1652.

22. Whitcomb JM, Schwartz AG. Dehydroepiandrosterone and 16α-Br epiandrosterone inhibit 12-*O*-tetradecanoylphorbol-13-acetate stimulation of superoxide radical production by human polymorphonuclear leukocytes. *Carcinogenesis* 1985;6:333–335.

23. Schwartz AG, Pashko LL. Suppression of 12-*O*-tetradecanoylphorbol-13-acetate-induced epidermal hyperplasia and inflammation by the dehydroepiandrosterone analog 16α-fluoro-5-androsten-17-one and its reversal by NADPH-liposomes. *Cancer Lett* 2001;168:7–14.

24. Schwartz AG. Inhibition of spontaneous breast cancer formation in female C3H-A^{vy}/A mice by long-term treatment with dehydroepiandrosterone. *Cancer Res* 1979;39:1129–1132.

25. Schwartz A, Hard G, Pashko L, et al. Dehydroepiandrosterone: an anti-obesity and anti-carcinogenic agent. *Nutr Cancer* 1981;3:46–53.

26. Inano H, Ishii-Ohba H, Suzuki K, et al. Chemoprevention by dietary dehydroepiandrosterone against promotion/progression phase of radiation-induced mammary tumorigenesis in rats. *J Steroid Biochem Mol Biol* 1995;54:47–53.

27. Ratko TA, Detrisac CJ, Mehta RG, et al. Inhibition of rat mammary gland chemical carcinogenesis by dietary dehydroepiandrosterone or a fluorinated analog of dehydroepiandrosterone. *Cancer Res* 1991;51:481–486.

28. Simile M, Pascale RM, DeMiglio MR, et al. Inhibition by dehydroepiandrosterone of growth and progression of persistent liver nodules in experimental rat liver carcinogenesis. *Int J Cancer* 1995;62:210–215.

29. Schwartz AG, Tannen RH. Inhibition of 7,12-dimethylbenz(*a*)anthracene- and urethan-induced lung tumor formation in A/J mice by long-term treatment with dehydroepiandrosterone. *Carcinogenesis* 1981;2:1335–1338.

30. Nyce JW, Magee PN, Hard GC, Schwartz AG. Inhibition of 1,2-dimethylhydrazine-induced colon tumorigenesis in Balb/c mice by dehydroepiandrosterone. *Carcinogenesis* 1984;5:57–62.

31. Rao KV, Johnson WD, Bosland MC, et al. Chemoprevention of rat prostate carcinogenesis by early and delayed administration of dehydroepiandrosterone. *Cancer Res* 1999;59:3084–3089.

32. Hursting SD, Perkins SN, Phang JM. Chemoprevention of spontaneous tumorigenesis in p53-knockout transgenic mice. *Proc Am Assoc Cancer Res* 1995;36:588.

33. Rao MS, Subbarao V, Yeldani AV, Reddy JK. Inhibition of spontaneous testicular Leydig cell tumor development in F-344 rats by dehydroepiandrosterone. *Cancer Lett* 1992;65:123–126.

34. Pashko LL, Rovito RJ, Williams JR, et al. Dehydroepiandrosterone (DHEA) and 3β-methylandrost-5-en-17-one: inhibitors of 7,12-dimethylbenz(*a*)anthracene (DMBA)-initiated and 12-*O*-tetradecanoylphorbol-13-acetate (TPA)-promoted skin papilloma formation in mice. *Carcinogenesis* 1984;5:463–466.

35. Pashko LL, Hard GC, Rovito RJ, et al. Dehydroepiandrosterone and 3β-methylandrost-5-en-17-one inhibit 7,12-dimethylbenz(*a*)anthracene-induced skin papillomas and carcinomas in mice. *Cancer Res* 1985;45:164–166.

36. Pashko LL, Lewbart ML, Schwartz AG. Inhibition of 12-*O*-tetradecanoylphorbol-13-acetate-promoted skin tumor formation in mice by 16α-fluoro-5-androsten-17-one and its reversal by deoxyribonucleosides. *Carcinogenesis* 1991;12:2189–2192.

37. Lee WY, Locknisar MF, Fischer SM. Interleukin-1α mediates phorbol-ester-induced inflammation and epidermal hyperplasia. *FASEB J* 1994;8:1081–1087.

38. Schwartz AG, Lewbart ML, Pashko LL. Novel dehydroepiandrosterone analogues with enhanced biological activity and reduced side-effects in mice and rats. *Cancer Res* 1988;48:4817–4822.

39. Garcea R, Daino L, Frassetto S, et al. Reversal by ribo- and deoxyribonucleosides of dehydroepiandrosterone-induced inhibition of enzyme altered foci in the liver of rats subjected to the initiation-selection process of experimental carcinogenesis. *Carcinogenesis* 1988;9:931–938.

40. Pallman J, Ackerman LJ. 28-Day Oral Toxicity Study in Rats, Pharmakon, USA.

41. Schreck R, Rieber P, Baeuerle PA. Reactive oxygen intermediates as apparently widely used messengers in activation of

NFκB transcription factor and HIV-1. *EMBO J* 1991;10:2247–2258.

42. Satriano JA, Shuldiner M, Hora K, et al. Oxygen radicals as second messengers for expression of the monocyte chemoattract protein, JE/MCP-1, and the monocyte colony-stimulating factor, CSF-1, in response to tumor necrosis factor-α and immunoglobulin G. Evidence for involvement of reduced nicotinamide adenine dinucleotide phosphate (NADPH)-dependent oxidase. *J Clin Investig* 1993;92:1564–1571.

43. Gordon GB, Bush DE, Weisman HF. Reduction of atherosclerosis by administration of dehydroepiandrosterone. *J Clin Invest* 1988;82:712–720.

44. Arad Y, Badimon JJ, Badimon L, et al. Dehydroepiandrosterone: feeding prevents aortic fatty streak formation and cholesterol accumulation in cholesterol-fed rabbit. *Arteriosclerosis* 1989;9:159–166.

45. Eich DM, Nestler JE, Johnson DE, et al. Inhibition of accelerated atherosclerosis with dehydroepiandrosterone in the heterotropic rabbit model of cardiac transplantation. *Circulation* 1993;87:261–269.

46. Mao SJ, Rates MT, Parker RA, et al. Attenuation of atherosclerosis in a modified strain of hypercholesterolemic Watanabe rabbits with use of a probucol analog (MDL 29,311) that does not lower serum cholesterol. *Arterioscler Thromb* 1991;11:1266–1275.

47. Schuh JR, Blehm DJ, Frierdich GE, et al. Differential effects of renin-angiotensin system blockade on atherogenesis in cholesterol-fed rabbits. *J Clin Invest* 1993;91:1453–1458.

48. Munzel T, Keaney JF Jr. Are ACE inhibitors a "magic bullet" against oxidative stress. *Circulation* 2001;104:1571–1574.

49. Yusuf S, Sleight P, Pogue J, et al. Effects of an angiotensin-converting-enzyme inhibitor, ramipril, on cardiovascular events in high-risk patients. The Heart Outcomes Prevention Evaluation Study Investigators. *N Engl J Med* 2000;342:145–153.

50. Luzzato L, Mehta A. Glucose-6-phosphate dehydrogenase deficiency, in *The Metabolic Basis of Inherited Diseases*, 6th ed. Scriver CR, Baudot AL, Sly WS, Valle D, eds McGraw Hill, New York 1989, pp.2237, 4517.

51. Siniscalo M, Bernini L, Latte B, Motulski AG. Favism and thalassemia and the relationship to malaria. *Nature* 1961;190:1179–1180.

52. Beutler E. G6PD deficiency. *Blood* 1994;84:3613–3636.

53. Feo F, Pirisi L, Pascale R, et al. Modulatory effect of glucose-6-phosphate dehydrogenase deficiency on benzo(a)pyrene toxicity and transforming activity for in vitro-cultured human skin fibroblasts. *Cancer Res* 1984;44:3419–3425.

54. Feo F, Pirisi L, Pascale R, et al. Modulatory mechanisms of chemical carcinogenesis: the role of the NADPH pool in benzo(a)pyrene activation. *Toxicol Pathol* 1984;12:261–268.

55. Pascale R, Garcea R, Ruggiu ME, et al. Decreased stimulation by 12-O-tetradecanoylphorbol-13-acetate of superoxide radical production by polymorphonuclear leukocytes carrying the Mediterranean variant of glucose-6-phosphate dehydrogenase. *Carcinogenesis* 1987;8:1567–1570.

56. Dessi S, Batetta B, Cherchi R, et al. Hexose monophosphate shunt enzymes in lung tumors from normal and glucose-6-

phosphate-dehydrogenase-deficient subjects. *Oncology* 1988;45:287–291.

57. Marnett LJ. Oxyradicals and DNA damage. *Carcinogenesis* 2000;361–370.

58. Cerutti P. Oxy-radicals and cancer. *Lancet* 1994;344:862–863.

59. Barry-Lane PA, Patterson C, van der Merwe M, et al. P47phox is required for atherosclerotic lesion progression in ApoE(-/-) mice. *J Clin Investig* 2001;108:1513–1522.

60. Jenner P. Oxidative damage in neurodegenerative disease. *Lancet* 1994;344:796–798.

61. Adelman R, Saul RL, Ames BN. Oxidative damage to DNA: relation to species metabolic rate and life span. *Proc Natl Acad Sci USA* 1988;85:2706–2708.

62. Cocco P, Todde P, Fornera S, et al. Mortality in a cohort of men expressing the glucose-6-phosphate dehydrogenase deficiency. *Blood* 1998;91:706–709.

63. Koenig R. Sardinia's mysterious male Methusalehs. *Science* 2001;291:2074–2076.

64. Passarino G, Underhill PA, Cavalli-Sforza LL, et al. Y chromosome binary markers to study the high prevalence of males in Sardinian centenarians and the genetic structure of the Sardinian population. *Hum Hered* 2001;52:136–139.

65. Cavalli-Sforza L, De Benedictis G. Personal communication.

66. Yen TT, Allan JV, Pearson DV, et al. Prevention of obesity in A^{vy}/a mice by dehydroepiandrosterone. *Lipids* 1977;12:401–413.

67. Coleman DL, Schwizer RW, Leiter EH. Effect of the genetic background on the therapeutic effects of dehydroepiandrosterone (DHEA) in diabetes-obesity mutants and in aged normal mice. *Diabetes* 1984;33:26–32.

68. Gansler TS, Muller S, Cleary MP. Chronic administration of dehydroepiandrosterone reduces pancreatic β-cell hyperplasia and hyperinsulinemia in genetically obese Zucker rats. *Proc Soc Exp Biol Med* 1985;180:155–162.

69. Kalimi M, Shafagoj Y, Loria R, et al. Anti-glucocorticoid effects of dehydroepiandrosterone (DHEA). *Mol Cell Biochem* 1994;131:99–104.

70. Blauer KL, Poth M, Rogers WM, Benton EW. Dehydroepiandrosterone antagonizes the suppressive effects of dexamethasone on lymphocyte proliferation. *Endocrinology* 1991;129:3174–3179.

71. Loria RM, Inge TH, Cook SS, et al. Protection against acute lethal viral infections with the native steroid dehydroepiandrosterone (DHEA). *J Med Virol* 1988;26:301–314.

72. Ben-Nathan D, Lachmi B, Lustig S, Feuerstein G. Protection by dehydroepiandrosterone in mice infected with viral encephalitis. *Arch Virol* 1991;120:263–271.

73. Araneo B, Daynes R. Dehydroepiandrosterone functions as more than an antiglucocorticoid in preserving immunocompetence after thermal injury. *Endocrinology* 1995;136:393–401.

74. Sapolsky RM. A mechanism for glucocorticoid toxicity in the hippocampus: increased neuronal vulnerability to metabolic insults. *J Neurosci* 1985;5:1228–1232.

75. Lupien SJ, de Leon M, de Santi S, et al. Cortisol levels during human aging predict hippocampal atrophy and memory deficits. *Nat Neurosci* 1998;1:69–73.

76. Kimonides VG, Khatibi NH, Svendsen CN, et al. Dehydroepiandrosterone (DHEA) and DHEA-sulfate

(DHEAS) protect hippocampal neurons against excitatory amino acid-induced neurotoxicity. *Proc Natl Acad Sci USA* 1998;95:1852–1857.

77. Pecke PM, Chrousos GP. Hypercortisolism and obesity. *Ann NY Acad Sci* 1995;771:665–676.

78. Sprecher DL, Pearce GL. How deadly is the "Deadly Quartet"? A post-CABG evaluation. *J Am Coll Cardiol* 2000;36:1159–1165.

79. Freedman MR, Horwitz BA, Stern JS. Effect of adrenalectomy and glucocorticoid replacement on development of obesity. *Am J Physiol* 1986;250:R595–R607.

80. Edwards CRW, Stewart PM, Burt D, et al. Localisation of 11β-hydroxysteroid dehydrogenase-tissue specific protector of the mineralocorticoid receptor. *Lancet* 1988;ii:986–989.

81. Kotelevtsev Y, Holmes MC, Burchell A, et al. 11beta-Hydroxysteroid dehydrogenase type 1 knockout mice show attenuated glucocorticoid-inducible responses and resist hyperglycemia obesity or stress. *Proc Natl Acad Sci USA* 1997;94:14,924–14,929.

82. Masuzaki H, Paterson J, Shinyama H, et al. A transgenic model of visceral obesity and the metabolic syndrome. *Science* 2001;294:2166–2170.

83. Pashko LL, Schwartz AG. Antihyperglycemic effect of the dehydroepiandrosterone analogue 16α-fluoro-5-androsten-17-one in diabetic mice. *Diabetes* 1993;42:1105–1108.

84. Coleman, DL, Leiter EH, Schwizer RW. Therapeutic effects of dehydroepiandrosterone (DHEA) on diabetic mice. *Diabetes* 1982;31:830–833.

85. Whorwood CB, Donovan SJ, Wood PJ, Phillips DI. Regulation of glucocorticoid receptor alpha and beta isoforms and type I 11beta-hydroxysteroid dehydrogenase expression in human skeletal muscle cells: a key role in the pathogenesis of insulin resistance? *J Clin Endocrinol Metab* 2001;86:2296–2308.

86. Svec F, Porter JF. The actions of exogenous dehydroepiandrosterone in experimental animals and humans. *Proc Soc Exp Biol Med* 1998;218:174–191.

87. Freireich EJ, Gehan EA, Rall DP, et al. Quantitative comparison of toxicity of anticancer agents in mouse, rat, hamster, dog, monkey and man. *Cancer Chemother Rep* 1966;50:219–244.

88. Mortola JF, Yen SSC. The effects of oral dehydroepiandrosterone on endocrine-metabolic parameters in postmenopausal women. *J Clin Endocrinol Metab* 1990;71:696–704.

89. Frenkel RA, Slaughter CA, Orth K, et al. Peroxisome proliferation and induction of peroxisomal enzymes in mouse and rat liver by dehydroepiandrosterone feeding. *J Steroid Biochem* 1990;35:333–342.

90. Rao MS, Subbarao V, Yeldani AV, Reddy JK. Hepatocarcinogenicity of dehydroepiandrosterone in the rat. *Cancer Res* 1992;52:2977–2979.

91. Perkins SN, Hursting SD, Haines DC, et al. Chemoprevention of spontaneous tumorigenesis in nullizygous p53-deficient mice by dehydroepiandrosterone and its analog, 16α-fluoro-5-androsten-17-one. *Carcinogenesis* 1997;18:989–994.

IV SIGNAL TRANSDUCTION MODULATORS

20 ras Oncogene Inhibitors

Nancy E. Kohl, PhD

1. RAS AND CANCER

The mammalian *ras* genes, N-, Ha- and Ki-*ras*, encode four highly homologous 21-K_d proteins— N- and Ha-Ras, and the splice variants Ki4A- and Ki4B-Ras—that function as molecular switches in the regulation of cell proliferation, survival, and differentiation. Situated at the inner surface of the plasma membrane, these proteins transmit extracellular signals from membrane-localized receptor tyrosine kinases to the nucleus. Typical of guanosine 5' triphosphate (GTP)-binding proteins, Ras cycles between the active, GTP-bound and inactive, guanosine 5' diphosphate (GDP)-bound states through the action of its intrinsic GTPase activity, together with the action of guanine nucleotide exchange factors and GTPase-activating proteins (GAPs). Constitutively activated forms of Ras with compromised GTPase activity that are capable of deregulated cell growth are encoded by *ras* genes with point mutations in codons 12, 13, or 61 *(1)*. Activation of Ras by mutation is a frequent finding in human tumors, with an overall incidence of 30%. Such oncogenic mutations are most commonly found in the Ki-*ras* gene, particularly in cancers of the colon, lung, and pancreas, and the N-*ras* gene, notably in neuroblastomas and various leukemias. Oncogenic mutations in the Ha-*ras* gene occur at a lower frequency in human cancers, and are most commonly associated with bladder and head and neck cancer *(2,3)*.

Substantial evidence suggests that oncogenically activated Ras plays an important role in tumorigenesis. Genetic disruption of the mutant *ras* gene in human colon cancer-cell lines *(4)* as well as a human fibrosarcoma cell line *(5)* leads to impairment of the transformed phenotype, despite the presence of additional genetic alterations in these cells. Furthermore, downregulation of Ras expression by ribozyme or antisense technologies in human tumor cells that harbor oncogenically mutated *ras.* genes abrogates the transformed phenotype *(6–10)*. Finally, expression of oncogenic alleles of Ki-*ras* in mice through spontaneous recombination in the whole animal predisposes the mice to a range of tumor types, predominantly early-onset lung cancer *(11)*. Thus, the importance and prevalence of oncogenically mutated Ras in human cancers suggests that this protein is an excellent target for the development of new cancer-therapeutic agents as well as preventive strategies.

2. INHIBITION OF RAS FUNCTION

Several strategies have been employed to inhibit the function of Ras, including inhibition of protein synthesis, restoration of GTPase activity to mutant Ras, and prevention of posttranslational processing. Each of these methods is discussed here, and its value in cancer chemoprevention is evaluated. Strategies that do not target Ras itself, such as inhibition of upstream or downstream members of the pathway, are not considered.

2.1. Inhibition of Ras Protein Synthesis

Ha- and Ki-*ras* oncogene expression in transformed cells has been suppressed using a variety of techniques, including antisense RNA and oligonucleotides, and ribozymes. Ribozymes and oligonucleotides targeted to the region of Ha-*ras* mRNA that contains the oncogenic point mutation selectively inhibit mutant Ha-*ras*

From: Cancer Chemoprevention, Volume 1: Promising Cancer Chemoprevention Agents
Edited by: G. J. Kelloff, E. T. Hawk, and C. C. Sigman © Humana Press Inc., Totowa, NJ

mRNA expression without affecting expression of wild type Ha-*ras* or other *ras* isoforms. Expression of these agents in transformed cells that harbor an activated Ha-*ras* gene results in inhibition of anchorage-dependent and anchorage-independent cell growth and reversion of the transformed morphology *(6,8)*. Expression of an anti-Ha-*ras* ribozyme in tumor cells abrogates the ability of the cells to form tumors in nude mice *(8)*. Antisense constructs containing wild-type Ki-*ras* sequences capable of hybridizing to both mutant and wild-type Ki-*ras* mRNAs were able to inhibit the growth and revert the transformed morphology of human pancreatic cell lines that harbored mutant Ki-*ras* genes. Interestingly, these constructs had no effect on the growth of human pancreatic tumor lines with wild-type Ki-*ras* genes, presumably because these cells are less dependent on Ki-*ras* for growth *(9,10)*. Administration of Ki-*ras* antisense constructs—either in a liposome complex or as a retrovirus—to mice that harbor human tumor cells significantly inhibited tumor growth *(7,9)*.

ISIS-2503, a 20-mer oligonucleotide that binds to the translation initiation region of human Ha-*ras* mRNA, is currently being tested in humans *(12–14)*. Despite its selective downregulation of Ha-Ras in vitro, ISIS-2503 shows broad antiproliferative activity in in vivo cancer models, inhibiting the growth of tumors that harbor either mutant Ki-*ras* or wild type *ras*. In a Phase I trial in patients with advanced cancer, no dose-limiting toxicity was observed when the oligonucleotide was administered by continuous 14-d infusion at doses up to 10 mg/kg/d. No objective responses were reported, but reduction in Ha-*ras* mRNA was observed in peripheral-blood mononuclear cells at the lowest doses *(12)*. ISIS 2503 is currently being tested in combination with gemcitabine *(13)* and as monotherapy in patients with advanced non-small-cell lung cancer (NSCLC) *(14)*.

Ribozymes and antisense constructs offer the opportunity to develop exquisitely selective agents. In the case of the *ras* genes, these strategies allow discrimination between *ras* alleles as well as between wild-type and mutant genes. Thus, such therapies might be expected to have minimal effects on normal cells. However, these agents have limitations that might affect their use as chemopreventive agents. Most significantly, all of these agents must currently be administered parenterally, a liability of any agent that will be administered to relatively healthy individuals over long periods of time.

2.2. Restoration of GTPase Activity

Mutant forms of Ras associated with human tumors are constitutively active because of point mutations—most commonly at codon 12 or 61—that impair the GTPase activity of the protein, even in the presence of GAP. Thus, a molecule that could restore the GTPase activity of oncogenic Ras may be effective in preventing and treating Ras-dependent human cancers. A GTP analog was identified that does just that *(15)*. Diaminobenzophenone-phosphonoamidate-GTP (DABP-GTP) is hydrolyzed by oncogenic Ras to yield GDP-bound, inactive Ras and DABP-Pi. Although this analog is hydrolyzed by wild-type Ras, it is hydrolyzed more efficiently by Ras mutants, particularly those proteins with a mutation at codon 12. The results with DABP-GTP demonstrate that oncogenic mutation does not irreversibly damage the catalytic ability of the protein, and provide the basis for further efforts to identify a candidate drug with similar properties.

These results are encouraging, yet there is much work to be done in this area. The reported experiments were performed in vitro using purified recombinant Ha-Ras protein. It has not yet been demonstrated that similar efficacy and selectivity can be achieved in a cell in the context of different Ras isoforms and other GTP-binding proteins. Indeed, DABP-GTP has previously been shown to be a substrate for both the mutant and wild-type G-protein, GS_α *(16)*. Ultimately, for use as a cancer chemopreventive agent, a compound must be identified that is active in cells and is amenable to systemic administration.

2.3. Inhibition of Ras Posttranslational Processing

The strategy that currently holds the most promise for development of an anticancer agent that targets Ras is inhibition of its posttranslational processing. Several compounds with this activity are currently in clinical trials, and appear to be well tolerated. However, issues such as identifying the mechanism of action of these compounds must be addressed in order to evaluate their utility as chemopreventive agents.

2.3.1. FARNESYL PROTEIN TRANSFERASE BIOCHEMISTRY

The Ras proteins are initially synthesized as cytoplasmic precursors that translocate to the inner surface of the plasma membrane and acquire full biological activity following a series of posttranslational modifications *(17*; Fig. 1). The first and obligatory step in this

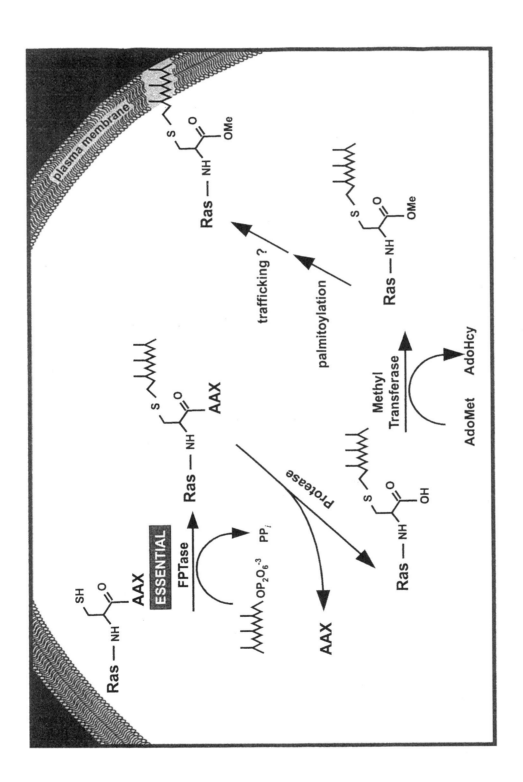

Fig. 1. Posttranslational modification of Ras. The 15-carbon isoprenoid farnesyl is added to the cysteine residue at four amino acids from the C-terminus of the protein in a reaction catalyzed by FPTase. This is followed by proteolytic cleavage of the AAX residues and methylation of the farnesylcysteine. In the case of the Ras proteins—except Ki4B-Ras—palmitate groups are then added to cysteine residues upstream of the farnesylated cysteine. These modifications increase the hydrophobicity of the protein and facilitate its localization to the inner surface of the plasma membrane, where it is biologically active.

sequence is the addition of a 15-carbon farnesyl isoprenoid to the cysteine residue at four amino acids from the C-terminus of the protein in a reaction catalyzed by the enzyme farnesyl protein transferase (FPTase). The modified cysteine is part of the CAAX tetrapeptide, in which C is cysteine, A is usually an aliphatic amino acid, and X is any amino acid. The X residue of the CAAX motif determines the selectivity of the protein substrate for modification by FPTase; for FPTase substrates, X is usually serine, methionine, glutamine, or alanine. The farnesyl group is derived from farnesyl pyrophosphate, an intermediate in the cholesterol biosynthetic pathway. Following farnesylation, AAX is proteolytically cleaved, and the now resulting C-terminal farnesylcysteine is methylated. In the case of all of the Ras proteins except Ki4B-Ras, palmitate groups are then added to cysteine residues upstream of the farnesylated cysteine. Although all of these posttranslational modifications contribute to the membrane-binding of Ras, studies demonstrating that only the farnesylation step is essential for the transforming ability of the Ras oncoproteins (18–21) spurred the development of inhibitors of FPTase to treat Ras-dependent cancers.

FPTase is one of a family of prenyltransferases found in mammalian cells. Two other enzymes, geranylgeranyl protein transferase (GGPTase) types I and II, catalyze the addition of a 20-carbon isoprenoid, geranylgeranyl, to the C-terminal cysteine residue(s) of substrate proteins (17). GGPTase-I preferentially recognizes CAAX-containing proteins in which X is leucine or phenylalanine. However, the specificity of FPTase and GGPTase-I is not absolute. For example, proteins that are preferentially farnesylated, such as N-Ras, Ki4A-Ras, and Ki4B-Ras, in which the X residue is methionine, can be substrates for geranylgeranylation by GGPTase-I (22–24). Indeed, it has been shown that Ki-Ras and N-Ras are geranylgeranylated in mammalian cells in which FPTase activity has been pharmacologically ablated (25,26). GGPTase-II transfers the geranylgeranyl group to both cysteines of proteins that have C-terminal sequences CXC, CC, or CCXX via an enzymatic mechanism that differs from that of the other two prenyltransferases (17).

2.3.2. DEVELOPMENT OF FPTASE INHIBITORS

The first FPTase inhibitors were CAAX tetrapeptides that derived from the observation that the CAAX motif contains all of the determinants required for interaction of the protein substrate with the enzyme (27). Minor

modifications to the Ras CAAX motifs rendered the tetrapeptides non-substrate inhibitors (28,29). Since both the peptide nature and the presence of a thiol group in the tetrapeptides were considered to be liabilities for cellular and in vivo application, subsequent efforts focused on identifying more stable and cell-permeable molecules with thiol replacements. This work ultimately yielded cell-active, protein-competitive FPTase inhibitors (reviewed in 30). The other substrate of the reaction, FPP, also served as a template for the development of FPTase inhibitors. Similarly, bisubstrate inhibitors mimicking the transition state were also developed. Finally, additional FPTase inhibitors were identified by screening compound collections and natural products (31).

2.3.3. PRECLINICAL BIOLOGY OF FPTASE INHIBITORS

Cell-permeable FPTase inhibitors have been shown to inhibit the prenylation of farnesylated proteins such as Ha-Ras in intact cells (32–40). Generally, these compounds have shown selectivity for inhibition of FPTase vs the closely related prenyltransferase GGPTase-I in cell prenylation assays. This selectivity was believed to be a desirable factor that prevented possible unwanted toxicity, a hypothesis that has recently been tested. Inhibition of signaling from Ras through the mitogen-associated protein (MAP) kinase pathway has also been demonstrated for several of these compounds (41–44).

The biological consequences of FPTase inhibition in cells have been evaluated in a variety of assays. In cell-culture models, selective cell-active FPTase inhibitors block both the anchorage-dependent (33,36,44–46) and anchorage-independent (34,35,39,40,44,47–52) growth of transformed cells. Importantly, these compounds are much less effective in inhibiting the growth of non-transformed cells (33,44,45,49). FPTase inhibitors also revert the transformed morphology of Ha-ras-transformed cells (33,36,39–41,45,46,52,53) and restore actin cables in these cells (36,45). In all these assays, the lack of inhibitory effect of FPTase inhibitors on cells transformed by a downstream, prenylation-independent gene such as v-raf, or a farnesylation-independent form of Ha-ras such as myristoylated Ha-ras, suggests that the effect of these compounds is not the result of nonspecific toxicity.

FPTase inhibitors show antitumor efficacy in rodent models of cancer. These compounds dose-dependently inhibit the growth of Ha-ras-transformed rodent fibroblasts in a nude mouse xenograft model

(35,37–39,46,47,50,52,54–57); in some cases this tumor-growth inhibition has been shown to correlate with inhibition of Ras processing in the tumor (35,54). These compounds also inhibit tumor growth in xenograft models using human tumor cell lines that harbor either a mutant or wild-type *ras* gene (37,38,40,46,50,52,57–59). Importantly, antitumor efficacy is achieved in these models in the absence of any gross or microscopic toxicity.

FPTase inhibitors also show antitumor activity in *ras* transgenic mouse models. Both MMTV-v-Ha-*ras* mice and wap-*ras* mice develop mammary and salivary tumors as a result of expression of an activated Ha-*ras* transgene. Treatment of these mice with an FPTase inhibitor leads to rapid tumor regression, partly due to an increase in tumor cell apoptosis *(50,60,61)*. In the case of the MMTV-v-Ha-*ras* mice, the antitumor effects of the FPTase inhibitor were independent of the *p53* status, since tumor regression was equally efficient in a p53-null or p53-wild-type background *(61)* . In the MMTV-v-Ha-*ras* mice, the regressed phenotype persists during treatment. However, soon after treatment is discontinued, tumor regrowth is evident, suggesting the need for continuous inhibition of FPTase for maintenance of the regressed tumor phenotype. In contrast to the tumor regression observed in the FPTase inhibitor-treated Ha-*ras* transgenic mice, treatment with a FPTase inhibitor resulted in tumor stasis in MMTV-N-*ras* and MMTV-Ki-*ras*B mice, which develop mammary tumors because of overexpression of wild-type N-*ras* or mutant Ki-*ras*, respectively *(62,63)*.

The cytostatic effects of FPTase inhibitors on transformed cells in culture and tumors in animals can be partly attributed to the inhibition of proliferation. In one study, a G_1 pause was observed in cells that harbored mutant Ha-*ras*, although in all other transformed cells that were sensitive to the growth inhibitory effects of the compounds, a G_2/M block was noted *(64,65)*. Interestingly, a human tumor cell line resistant to the effects of the FPTase inhibitor failed to show accumulation in the G_2/M phase. Another study showed that a subset of cell lines sensitive to the growth-inhibitory effect of the FPTase inhibitor exhibited a G_1 block *(66)*. In some situations, an increase in the level of apoptosis may contribute to the FPTase inhibitor-mediated growth inhibition. FPTase inhibitors have been shown to cause an induction of apoptosis when transformed cells are grown in low serum *(67)* or deprived of a substratum *(68)*. The latter situation is applicable to anchorage-independent growth

experiments and to tumor growth in animals. Although treatment of MMTV-v-Ha-*ras* mice with a FPTase inhibitor led to the disappearance of palpable tumors, small nodules of transformed cells were found at the site of the original, regressed tumor in mice necropsied at termination of treatment *(60)*. The central portion of the tumor, essentially growing in the absence of substratum, likely regressed as a result of induction of apoptosis, and the cells forming the outer portion of the tumor failed to undergo apoptosis because of attachment to the matrix. FPTase inhibitors may induce apoptosis by inhibiting activation of the phosphatidyl inositol-3-kinase (PI3K)/AKT pathway *(69,70)*. Interestingly, Ha-Ras has been shown to preferentially signal the PI3K pathway, and Ki-Ras favors the MAPK pathway *(71)*. This preference may be reflected in the tumor regression observed in both the wap-*ras* and MMTV-v-Ha-*ras* transgenic mice *(50,60)*.

2.3.4. MECHANISM OF ACTION OF FPTASE INHIBITORS

Studies that have evaluated the effect of FPTase inhibitors on the growth of a large number of human tumor cells have demonstrated no correlation between *ras* genotype and sensitivity to the inhibitor *(44,65)*. Thus, cells harboring mutant N- or Ki-*ras* genes are often as sensitive to the growth-inhibitory effect of the compounds as cells with a mutant Ha-*ras* genotype, although FPTase inhibitors do not inhibit the function of proteins encoded by these *ras* alleles, owing to prenylation by GGPTase-I. The geranylgeranylated forms of Ki- and N-Ras remain associated with the cellular membrane fraction. Furthermore, forms of oncogenic Ha-Ras and Ki-RasB engineered to be substrates for GGPTase I by modification of the CAAX motif retain the ability to transform rodent fibroblasts *(21,72)*. In addition, cells with wild-type *ras* genes are often as sensitive as cells with mutant *ras* genes to the inhibitors. These observations have led to the hypothesis that farnesylated proteins other than just Ras are responsible for the biological effects of the FPTase inhibitors.

Similar observations have been made when FPTase inhibitors have been used in in vivo tumor models. In xenografts of human tumor cell lines, tumor-growth inhibition has been observed for lines with a mutant N- or Ki-ras genotype as well as for lines with wild-type *ras* genes *(35,40,46,50,51)*. Furthermore, tumor-growth inhibition by a FPTase inhibitor was observed

Table 1

Faresyl Protein Transferase Inhibitors in Clinical Trials

Compound(Source)	In vitro IC$_{50}$ nM (substrate)		Preclinical Biological Profile	Clinical Trials		References
	FPTase	GGPTase-1		Indication	Toxicities	
R115777(Janssen Pharmaceutica)	0.86 (lamin B) 7.9 (Ki-RasB)	>50,000	Growth inhibitory in cell culture and in in vivo xenograft models using Ha-*ras* transformed rodent fibroblasts and human tumor-cell lines	PI: <u>monotherapy</u> solid tumors- acute leukemias- <u>combination</u> gemcitabine gemcitabine/cisplatin 5FU/LV capecitabine docetaxel irinotecan topotecan trastuzumab PII: Advanced breast cancer PIII: N/A	Fatigue, neuropathy and myelosuppression (neutropenia, thrombocytopenia)	*46,59,83,84, 87,90,94, 96–100, 115–120*
SCH 66336 (Schering Plough)	1.9 (Ha-Ras) 2.8 (N-Ras) 5.2 (Ki-Ras)	>50,000	Inhibited anchorage-independent growth of Ha- and Ki-*ras*-transformed fibroblasts and human tumor-cell lines in culture and of same cells in xenograft models; caused tumor regression in wap-*ras* mice	PI: <u>monotherapy</u> solid tumors <u>combination</u> gemcitabine paclitaxel PII: Metastatic pancreatic Metastatic transitional cell carcinoma of urothelial tract	GI toxicity (vomiting, diarrhea), fatigue, myelosuppression (neutropenia, thrombocytopenia), neurotoxicity	*50, 85, 91–93, 121–124*
L-778,123 (Merck)	2	100	Inhibited anchorage-independent growth of Ki-*ras*-transformed cells and tumors in Ki-*ras* transgenic mice; caused tumor regression in MMTV-Ha-*ras*B transgenic mice	PI: <u>Monotherapy</u> Solid tumors <u>Combination</u> Paclitaxel Radiation	Myelosuppression - (neutropenia - thrombocytopenia), fatigue, neuropathy, QTc prolongation	*80–82, 86, 107, 125, 126*

Compound	IC50	Activity	Clinical status	Toxicity	Ref
BMS 214662 (Bristol Meyers Squibb)	1.3 (Ha-Ras) 8.4 (Ki-Ras) / 1300 (Ha-Ras-CVLL) 2300 (Ki-Ras)	Inhibited anchorage-independent growth of Ha-and Ki-ras transformed rodent fibroblasts and human tumor-cell lines and caused tumor regression/cures in human tumor-cell line xenografts; potent inducer of apoptosis	PII: Solid tumors Development discontinued; PI: Monotherapy solid tumors Combination Paclitaxel Cisplatin PII: N/A	GI toxicity (vomiting, diarrhea)	40, 88, 89, 95 127–131
ABT-839 (Abbott)			PI: N/A		132
AZD-3409 (Astra Zeneca)			PI: N/A		133
OSI-754/CP-609,754 (OSI/Pfizer)			PI: N/A		133

309

in N-and Ki-*ras* transgenic mouse models *(62,63)*. Although FPTase was clearly inhibited in the treated Ki-*ras* transgenic mouse tumors, as evidenced by inhibition of prenylation of the exclusively farnesylated endogenous mouse protein HDJ2, there was no evidence of inhibition of Ki-Ras processing. It should be noted that the method of analysis used in these prenylation studies cannot distinguish between farnesylated and geranylgeranylated Ki-Ras, leaving open the possibility that the Ki-Ras in the treated tumor was modified by a geranylgeranyl group.

In these and other studies *(35,40,46)*, cells that harbor mutant Ha-*ras* are the most sensitive to the FPTase inhibitors. This sensitivity can be explained by the ability of the compounds to completely inhibit farnesylation, and therefore membrane localization and function of Ha-Ras. Furthermore, the cytoplasmic oncogenic Ha-Ras that accumulates following treatment with an FPTase inhibitor can still bind to its downstream effector Raf, resulting in the buildup of inactive Ras/Raf complexes in the cytoplasm *(43,73)*. Although biochemistry of Ha-Ras prenylation supports a central role for this protein in mediating the effects of FPTase inhibitors in cells transformed by Ha-*ras*, biological data that suggests a more complex scenario must be considered *(45)*. In Ha-*ras*-transformed cells, the kinetics of morphological reversion do not correlate with the kinetics of inhibition of Ha-*ras* farnesylation. Thus, although morphological reversion is observed within 18 h following initiation of treatment with a FPTase inhibitor, Ha-Ras processing is only partially inhibited at that time. Furthermore, although the reverted phenotype persists for several days following removal of the inhibitor, farnesylation of the accumulated unprocessed Ha-Ras occurs within a period of hours. It is possible that morphological reversion requires that only a portion of the cellular Ha-Ras be unprocessed, and that once this threshold level of unprocessed Ras has been reached, Ha-Ras is no longer required to maintain the reverted phenotype.

If Ras is not the sole biological effector of inhibition of FPTase, what protein(s) would be? Within a mammalian cell there are,— in addition to the Ras proteins— at least 20 other substrates of FPTase, including the nuclear lamins, the peroxisomal protein Pxf, the cell-regulatory phosphatases PTP1 and PTP2, two members of the rho family, RhoB and RhoE, and the centromere-associated proteins CENP-E and CENP-F *(74,75)*. Of these known farnesylated proteins, much attention has been given to RhoB and to CENP-E and CENP-F as critical mediators of FPTase biology. RhoB, an immediate early protein involved in regulation of cell shape, adhesion, and motility, is both farnesylated and geranylgeranylated in cells *(76)*. In FPTase inhibitor-treated cells, there is a loss of farnesylated RhoB and a corresponding gain in geranylgeranylated RhoB. Similar to treatment with FPTase inhibitors, expression of geranylgeranylated RhoB in *ras*-transformed cells leads to reversion of the transformed phenotype *(77,78)*; thus, RhoB has been proposed as principal mediator of the anticancer effects of FPTase inhibitors. However, another group has reported that forms of RhoB that are engineered to be either exclusively farnesylated or geranylgeranylated inhibit oncogenic signaling and suppress transformation in human tumor cells *(79)*, calling into question a critical role for RhoB in mediating the biological effects of FPTase inhibitors. More recently, CENP-E and CENP-F have been evaluated as targets of FPTase inhibition *(75)*. Both of these strictly farnesylated proteins are involved in the transition from the G_2 phase of the cell cycle to mitosis. Thus, their inhibition may contribute to the G_2/M cell-cycle block observed in many human tumor cells that are sensitive to the effects of FPTase inhibitors.

2.3.5. CLINICAL TRIALS OF FPTASE INHIBITORS

Three FPTase inhibitors—R115777 from Janssen Pharmaceutica, SCH66336 from Schering Plough, and BMS-214662 from Bristol Meyers Squibb—are currently in clinical trials (Table 1). Another compound, L-778,123 from Merck, was discontinued following Phase II testing *(80)*. Three additional compounds, ABT-839 from Abbott, CP-609,754 from Pfizer/OSI, and AZD-3409 from AstraZeneca, are rumored to be in human testing, but very little has been reported in the literature about these compounds. The four inhibitors for which information is available are all potent inhibitors of FPTase with selectivity relative to GGPTase-I. Merck's L-778,123 is the least selective of the inhibitors, with a FPTse vs GGPTase-I selectivity ratio of 50 *(81)*. All four compounds are kinetically competitive with the protein substrate in the prenylation reaction. The preclinical profiles of three of these compounds—R115777, SCH66336, and L-778,123— are similar, and all of the compounds show cytostatic growth-inhibitory effects against *ras*-transformed rodent fibroblasts or monkey cells and human tumor-cell lines with either a mutant or wild-type *ras* genotype in cell-culture models and in vivo tumor models

(46,50,59,82). In contrast, treatment of *ras*-transformed rodent fibroblasts and human tumor cells in culture with BMS-214662 leads to the induction of apoptosis. In in vivo tumor models, BMS-214662 can induce complete tumor regression. The ability of this compound to induce apoptosis is probably not related to its ability to inhibit Ras processing, as induction of apoptosis has been observed in cells transformed by oncogenes that are FPTase-independent, including v-*raf*, myristoylated Ha-*ras*, and Ha-*ras*-CVLL, a form of Ha-*ras* engineered to be an exclusive substrate of GGPTase I *(40)*. These data suggest that BMS-214662 may have a dual mechanism of action.

R115777 and SCH66336 are administered to patients orally, L-778,123 is administered by continuous intravenous (iv) infusion, and BMS-214662 is administered either by bolus iv infusion or orally. All these compounds have shown some indication of efficacy in Phase I trials. Notably, R115777 showed objective responses in 29% of patients with refractory acute leukemia in a Phase I trial *(83)*, including a complete response in 6% of the patients and a partial response in 24% of the patients. Significant antitumor efficacy has also been reported for R115777 in a Phase II trial of patients with advanced breast cancer. In this trial, 26% of the patients exhibited a partial response and 35% of the patients exhibited stable disease at the 9-mo evaluation point *(84)*.

In many of the trials with these compounds, pharmacodynamic assays have been employed to evaluate biochemical efficacy. These assays fall into three categories: measurement of inhibition of FPTase activity, measurement of inhibition of farnesylation of a marker protein—either prelamin A or the chaperone HDJ—or measurement of inhibition of Ras-pathway signaling. Cells for these assays have been obtained from peripheral blood, tumor biopsies, bone marrow, or buccal mucosa. In trials using one or more of these assays, inhibition of the target has been demonstrated, and in some cases, the inhibition has been shown to be dose-dependent *(85–98)*. What remains to be demonstrated is a correlation between inhibition of the surrogate marker and antitumor efficacy.

In general, the FPTase inhibitors achieved antitumor effects in animal models in the absence of gross or microscopic toxicity. In clinical trials across all four compounds, four toxicities have been prevalent: myelosuppression (neutropenia and thrombocytopenia); fatigue; neuropathy; and gastrointestinal (GI) toxicity (vomiting, diarrhea, and nausea). Each of these toxicities

has been dose-limiting for more than one of the compounds. In some cases, the occurrence of the toxicity is schedule- and dose-dependent. For example, no significant myelosuppression was observed when R115777 was administered intermittently at high doses *(99)*. In contrast, myelosuppression was the dose-limiting toxicity when the compound was administered at lower doses on a more chronic schedule *(100)*. QTc prolongation was a dose-limiting toxicity for L-778,123 *(86)*, but was not observed for any of the other compounds, suggesting that it is related to structure and not to the class of inhibitors.

Experiments performed in preclinical models have demonstrated additivity or synergy between FPTase inhibitors and selected cancer cytotoxics *(50,101–104)*. These results have been used to guide clinical trials combining a FPTase inhibitor with one or more of the cytotoxics (Table 1). In general, toxicities seen with the combinations have not been significantly different than those observed with either of the agents alone. Furthermore, no pharmacokinetic interactions between the compounds have been reported. Indications of efficacy have been noted in some of these combination trials. Based on preclinical data—which indicate that FPTase inhibitors increase the radiosensitivity of Ha-*ras*-transformed fibroblasts and that inhibition of Ras prenylation correlates with increased radiosensitivity in human tumor cell lines harboring oncogenically activated Ras *(105,106)*—, a trial of L-778,123 in combination with radiotherapy was initiated in patients with either pancreatic, head and neck, or NSCLC *(107)*. The combination treatment was well-tolerated, and several responses were reported.

2.3.6. FPTASE INHIBITORS: POTENTIAL CHEMOPREVENTIVE AGENTS?

Several studies have used FPTase inhibitors prophylactically. In one, SCH66336 was administered to wap-*ras* transgenic mice at an early age, prior to the onset of palpable tumor formation *(50)*. Treatment increased tumor latency and reduced the average number of tumors per mouse and the average tumor weight per animal. In another set of experiments, a CAAX peptidomimetic was administered to A/J mice that had received an initiating dose of 4-(methylnitrosamino)-1-(3-pyridyl)-1-butanone, which leads to development of lung tumors, the vast majority of which harbor Ki-*ras* mutations *(108)*. The percentage of mice with lung tumors was significantly lower in the treated group than the control group (58% vs 100%, $p< 0.01$). Furthermore, FPTase inhibitor treatment significantly reduced the number of tumors per mouse and total tumor volume. Finally, a preliminary report has been made that examines the preventive efficacy of BMS-214662 in three different mouse carcinogenesis models: skin tumors induced by 7,12-dimethylbenz[*a*]anthracene/12-*O*-tetradecanoylphorbol-13-acetate; lung tumors induced in the A/J mouse with *N*-methyl-*N*-nitrosourea; and colon tumors induced in CF-1 mice by azoxymethane. Although chronic administration of low doses of BMS-214662 resulted in efficacy in the skin-tumor model, fewer responses were observed in the lung-tumor and colon-tumor models *(109)*.

Preclinical data cited here support the use of FPTase inhibitors as cancer-chemopreventive agents, but issues that have arisen from the development of these compounds as cancer therapeutics must also be considered. Clearly, inhibition of FPTase does not lead to selective inhibition of Ras. Although Ha-Ras is one of the prenylated proteins with membrane localization and function that is inhibited, the function of many other farnesylated proteins is also blocked. This lack of selectivity for Ras could lead to unwanted side effects. Indeed, data from clinical trials showing common toxicities for four structurally diverse FPTase inhibitors suggest that these toxicities may be mechanism-based. Eliciting such toxicities as myelosuppression, neuropathy, fatigue, vomiting, and diarrhea may be unacceptable in a relatively healthy population. These toxicities may be eliminated by altering the compound dose and schedule of administration.

Although the inhibition of FPTase is an effective strategy for inhibiting the function of Ha-Ras, it is less effective for inhibiting the function of Ki-Ras, the most prevalent of the Ras oncoproteins in human cancer. In light of the resistance of Ki-Ras to FPTase inhibitors caused by subsequent prenylation by GGPTase-I, several groups have explored the possibility of combining inhibitors of FPTase and GGPTase-I or using dual prenyltransferase inhibitors, compounds that are inhibitory toward both prenyltransferases, to treat Ki-*ras*-transformed cells *(110–112)*. Inhibition of both FPTase and GGPTase-I leads to inhibition of Ki-Ras prenylation. However, inhibition of both prenyltransferases does not lead to improved antitumor activity, either in a xenograft model or in a *ras* transgenic mouse model. Furthermore, one group has reported that inhibition of GGPTase-I to the extent necessary to inhibit Ki-Ras processing when FPTase is completely inhibited is lethal *(112)*. Thus, it seems unlikely that

inhibition of Ki-Ras function can be safely achieved by inhibition of its posttranslational modification.

Another important consideration in the use of FPTase inhibitors as cancer chemopreventive agents is the ability of cells to develop resistance to these agents. A variant Ha-*ras*-transformed cell line that is resistant to inhibitor-induced morphological reversion was isolated following exposure to high levels of an FPTase inhibitor *(113)*. Resistance correlated with a reduction in the susceptibility of FPTase in the intact cells to drug inhibition. Although the mechanism of this reduced susceptibility remains unknown, it is not altered by drug accumulation or a change in enzyme structure. The FPTase in these resistant cells was not altered, yet it is clear from in vitro studies that a single amino acid change in the enzyme can lead to mutant forms of the enzyme that are resistant to FPTase inhibitors *(114)*. With the knowledge that resistance to FPTase inhibitors can be generated in preclinical models, it will be important to determine whether it can develop in humans. Relevant data may be derived from the ongoing human clinical trials.

3. CONCLUSION

Of the three strategies described here for inhibiting the function of oncogenically activated Ras, only inhibition of its posttranslational prenylation via development of inhibitors of the enzyme FPTase has yielded potent, cell-active, orally available compounds. Issues related to these compounds, such as mechanism-based toxicity and development of resistance, must be addressed to ensure their successful development as chemopreventive agents. Some of the answers may come from the continuing development of these compounds as cancer-therapeutic agents.

REFERENCES

1. Barbacid M. *ras* Genes. *Annu Rev Biochem* 1987;56:779–827.
2. Bos JL. The *ras* gene family and human carcinogenesis. *Mutat Res* 1988;195:255–271.
3. Bos JL. *ras* oncogenes in human cancer: a review. *Cancer Res* 1989;49:4682–4689.
4. Shirasawa S, Furuse M, Yokoyama N, Sasazuki T. Altered growth of human colon cancer cell lines disrupted at activated Ki-ras. *Science* 1993;260:85–88.
5. Plattner R, Anderson MJ, Sato KY, et al. Loss of oncogenic ras expression does not correlate with loss of tumorigenicity in human cells. *Proc Natl Acad Sci USA* 1996;93:6665–6670.
6. Saison-Behmoaras T, Tocque B, Rey I, et al. Short modified antisense oligonucleotides directed against Ha-ras point

mutation induce selective cleavage of the mRNA and inhibit T24 cells proliferation. *EMBO J* 1991;10:1111–1118.

7. Georges RN, Mukhopadhyay T, Zhang Y, et al. Prevention of orthotopic human lung cancer growth by intratracheal instillation of a retroviral antisense K-ras construct. *Cancer Res* 1993;53:1743–1746.

8. Kashani-Sabet M, Funato T, Florenes VA, et al. Suppression of the neoplastic phenotype in vivo by an anti-*ras* ribozyme. *Cancer Res* 1994;54:900–902.

9. Aoki K, Yoshida T, Sugimura T, Terada M. Liposome-mediated in vivo gene transfer of antisense K-*ras* construct inhibits pancreatic tumor dissemination in the murine peritoneal cavity. *Cancer Res* 1995;55:3810–3816.

10. Aoki K, Yoshida T, Matsumoto N, et al. Suppression of Ki-ras p21 levels leading to growth inhibition of pancreatic cancer cell lines with Ki-*ras* mutation but not those without Ki-*ras* mutation. *Mol Carcinog* 1997;20:251–258.

11. Johnson L, Mercer K, Greenbaum D, et al. Somatic activation of the K-*ras* oncogene causes early onset lung cancer in mice. *Nature* 2001;410:1111–1116.

12. Dorr A, Bruce J, Monia B, et al. Phase I and pharmacokinetic trial of ISIS 2503, a 20-mer antisense oligonucleotide against H-RAS, by 14-day continuous infusion (CIV) in patients with advanced cancer. *Proc Am Soc Clin Oncol* 1999;18:157a.

13. Adjei AA, Erlichman C, Sloan JA, et al. A Phase I trial of ISIS 2503, an antisense inhibitor of H-*ras* in combination with gemcitabine in patients with advanced cancer. *Proc Am Soc Clin Oncol* 2000;19:186a.

14. Dang T, Johnson D, Kelly K, et al. Multicenter Phase II trial of an antisense inhibitor of H-*ras* (ISIS-2503) in advanced non-small cell lung cancer (NSCLC). Proc *Am Soc Clin Oncol* 2001;20:332a.

15. Ahmadian MR, Zor T, Vogt D, et al. Guanosine triphosphatase stimulation of oncogenic Ras mutants. *Proc Nat Acad Sci USA* 1999;96:7065–7070.

16. Zor T, Bar-Yaacov M, Elgavish S, et al. Rescue of a mutant G-protein by substrate-assisted catalysis. *Eur J Biochem* 1997;249:330–336.

17. Zhang FL, Casey PJ. Protein prenylation: molecular mechanisms and functional consequences. *Annu Rev Biochem* 1996;65:241–269.

18. Willumsen BM, Norris K, Papageorge AG, et al. Harvey murine sarcoma virus p21 *ras* protein: biological and biochemical significance of the cysteine nearest the carboxy terminus. *EMBO J* 1984;3:2581–2585.

19. Hancock JF, Magee AI, Childs JE, Marshall CJ. All *ras* proteins are polyisoprenylated but only some are palmitoylated. *Cell* 1989;57:1167–1177.

20. Jackson JH, Cochrane CG, Bourne JR, et al. Farnesol modification of Kirsten-ras exon 4B protein is essential for transformation. *Proc Natl Acad Sci USA* 1990;87:3042–3046.

21. Kato K, Cox AD, Hisaka MM, et al. Isoprenoid addition to Ras protein is the critical modification for its membrane association and transforming activity. *Proc Natl Acad Sci USA* 1992;89:6403–6407.

22. Moores SL, Schaber MD, Mosser SD, et al. Sequence dependence of protein isoprenylation. *J Biol Chem* 1991;266:14,603–14,610.

23. James G, Goldstein JL, Brown MS. Resistance of K-RasBV12 proteins to farnesyltransferase inhibitors in Rat1 cells. *Proc Natl Acad Sci USA* 1996;93:4454–4458.

24. Zhang FL, Kirschmeier P, Carr D, et al. Characterization of Ha-Ras, N-Ras, Ki-Ras4A, and Ki-Ras4B as in vitro substrates for farnesyl protein transferase and geranylgeranyl protein transferase type I. *J Biol Chem* 1997;272:10,232–10,239.

25. Whyte DB, Kirschmeier P, Hockenberry TN, et al. K- and N-Ras are geranylgeranylated in cells treated with farnesyl protein transferase inhibitors. *J Biol Chem* 1997;272:14,459–14,464.

26. Rowell CA, Kowalczyk JJ, Lewis MD, Garcia AM. Direct demonstration of geranylgeranylation and farnesylation of Ki-Ras in vivo. *J Biol Chem* 1997;272:14,093–14,097.

27. Reiss Y, Goldstein JL, Seabra MC, et al. Inhibition of purified *p21*^ras farnesyl:protein transferase by Cys-AAX tetrapeptides. *Cell* 1990;62:81–88.

28. Goldstein JL, Brown MS, Stradley SJ, et al. Nonfarnesylated tetrapeptide inhibitors of protein farnesyltransferase. *J Biol Chem* 1991;266:15,575–15,578.

29. Pompliano DL, Rands E, Schaber MD, et al. Steady-state kinetic mechanism of Ras farnesyl:protein transferase. *Biochemistry* 1992;31:3800–3807.

30. Omer CA, Kohl NE. CAAX-competitive inhibitors of farnesyltransferase as anti-cancer agents. *Trends Pharmacol Sci* 1997;18:437–444.

31. Koblan KS, Kohl NE. Farnesyltransferase inhibitors: agents for the treatment of human cancer, in *G Proteins, Cytoskeleton and Cancer*. Maruta H, Kohama K, eds. RG Landes Co., Georgetown, TX, 1998, pp.291–302.

32. Garcia AM, Rowell C, Ackermann K, et al. Peptidomimetic inhibitors of Ras farnesylation and function in whole cells. *J Biol Chem* 1993;268:18,415–18,418.

33. James GL, Goldstein JL, Brown MS, et al. Benzodiazepine peptidomimetics: potent inhibitors of Ras farnesylation in animal cells. *Science* 1993;260:1937–1942.

34. Kohl NE, Mosser SD, deSolms SJ, et al. Selective inhibition of *ras*-dependent transformation by a farnesyltransferase inhibitor. *Science* 1993;260:1934–1937.

35. Nagasu T, Yoshimatsu K, Rowell C, et al. Inhibition of human tumor xenograft growth by treatment with the farnesyl transferase inhibitor B956. *Cancer Res* 1995;55:5310–5314.

36. Manne V, Yan N, Carboni JM, et al. Bisubstrate inhibitors of farnesyltransferase: a novel class of specific inhibitors of Ras transformed cells. *Oncogene* 1995;10:1763–1779.

37. Njoroge FG, Vibulbhan B, Rane DF, et al. Structure-activity relationship of 3-substituted *N*-(pyridinylacetyl)-4-(8-chloro-5,6-dihydro-11H-benzo[5,6]cyclohepta[1,2-b]pyridin-11-ylidene)-piperidine inhibitors of farnesyl-protein transferase: design and synthesis of in vivo active antitumor compounds. *J Med Chem* 1997;40:4290–4301.

38. Njoroge FG, Vibulbhan B, Pinto P, et al. Potent, selective, and orally bioavailable ticyclic pyridyl acetamide *N*-oxide inhibitors of farnesyl protein transferase with enhanced in vivo antitumor activity. *J Med Chem* 1998;41:1561–1567.

39. Ding CZ, Batorsky R, Bhide R, et al. Discovery and structure-activity relationships of imidazole-containing tetrahydrobenzodiazepine inhibitors of farnesyltransferase. *J Med Chem* 1999;42:5241–5253.

40. Rose WC, Lee FYF, Fairchild CR, et al. Preclinical antitumor activity of BMS-214662, a highly apoptotic and novel farnesyltransferase inhibitor. *Cancer Res* 2001;61:7507–7517.

41. Cox AD, Garcia AM, Westwick JK, et al. The CAAX peptidomimetic compound B581 specifically blocks farnesylated, but not geranylgeranylated or myristylated, oncogenic Ras signaling and transformation. *J Biol Chem* 1994;269:19,203–19,206.

42. James GL, Brown MS, Cobb MH, Goldstein JL. Benzodiazepine peptidomimetic BZA-5B interrupts the MAP kinase activation pathway in H-Ras-transformed Rat-1 cells, but not in untransformed cells. *J Biol Chem* 1994;269:27,705–27,714.

43. Lerner EC, Qian Y, Blaskovich MA, et al. Ras CAAX peptidomimetic FTI-277 selectively blocks oncogenic Ras signaling by inducing cytoplasmic accumulation of inactive Ras-Raf complexes. *J Biol Chem* 1995;270:26,802–26,806.

44. Sepp-Lorenzino L, Ma Z, Rands E, et al. A peptidomimetic inhibitor of farnesyl:protein transferase blocks the anchorage-dependent and -independent growth of human tumor cell lines. *Cancer Res* 1995;55:5302–5309.

45. Prendergast GC, Davide JP, deSolms SJ, et al. Farnesyltransferase inhibition causes morphological reversion of *ras*-transformed cells by a complex mechanism that involves regulation of the actin cytoskeleton. *Mol Cell Biol* 1994;14:4193–4202.

46. End DW, Smets G, Todd AV, et al. Characterization of the antitumor effects of the selective farnesyl protein transferase inhibitor R115777 in vivo and in vitro. *Cancer Res* 2001;61:131–137.

47. Kohl NE, Wilson FR, Mosser SD, et al. Farnesyltransferase inhibitors block the growth of ras-dependent tumors in nude mice. *Proc Natl Acad Sci USA* 1994;91:9141–9145.

48. Patel DV, Gordon EM, Schmidt RJ, et al. Phosphinyl acid-based bisubstrate analog inhibitors of ras farnesyl protein transferase. *J Med Chem* 1995;38:435–442.

49. Hunt JT, Lee VG, Leftheris K, et al. Potent, cell active, non-thiol tetrapeptide inhibitors of farnesyltransferase. *J Med Chem* 1996;39:353–358.

50. Liu M, Bryant MS, Chen J, et al. Antitumor activity of SCH 66336, an orally bioavailable tricyclic inhibitor of farnesyl protein transferase, in human tumor xenograft models and Wap-ras transgenic mice. *Cancer Res* 1998;58:4947–4956.

51. Njoroge FG, Taveras AG, Kelly J, et al. (+)-4-[2-[4-(8-chloro-3,10-dibromo-6,11-dihydro-5*H*-benzo[5,6]cyclohepta[1,2-*b*]-pyridin-11(R)-yl)-1-piperidinyl]-2-oxo-ethyl]-1-piperidinecarboxamide (SCH-66336): a very potent farnesyl protein transferase inhibitor as a novel antitumor agent. *J Med Chem* 1998;41:4890–4902.

52. Hunt JT, Ding CZ, Batorsky R, et al. Discovery of (R)-7-cyano-2,3,4,5-tetrahydro-1-(1*H*-imidazol-4-ylmethyl)-3-(phenylmethyl)-4-(2-thienylsulfonly)-1*H*-1,4-benzodiazepine (BMS-214662), a farnesyltransferase inhibitor with potent preclinical antitumor activity. *J Med Chem* 2000;43:3587–3595.

53. Bishop WR, Bond R, Petrin J, et al. Novel tricyclic inhibitors of farnesyl protein transferase. *J Biol Chem* 1995;270:30,611–30,618.

54. Sun J, Qian Y, Hamilton AD, Sebti SM. Ras CAAX peptidomimetic FTI 276 selectively blocks tumor growth in nude mice of a human lung carcinoma with K-*ras* mutation and p53 deletion. *Cancer Res* 1995;55:4243–4247.

55. Williams TM, Ciccarone TM, MacTough SC, et al. 2-Substituted piperazines as constrained amino acids. Application to the synthesis of potent, non carboxylic acid inhibitors of farnesyltransferase. *J Med Chem* 1996;39:1345–1348.

56. Leftheris K, Kline T, Vite GD, et al. Development of highly potent inhibitors of Ras farnesyltransferase possessing cellular and in vivo activity. *J Med Chem* 1996;39:224–236.

57. Liu M, Bryant MS, Chen J, et al. Effects of SCH 59228, an orally bioavailable farnesyl protein transferase inhibitor, on the growth of oncogene-transformed fibroblasts and a human colon carcinoma xenograft in nude mice. *Cancer Chemother Pharmacol* 1999;43:50–58.

58. Mallams AK, Njoroge FG, Doll RJ, et al. Antitumor 8-chlorobenzocycloheptapyridines: a new class of selective, nonpeptidic, nonsulfhydryl inhibitors of Ras farnesylation. *Bioorg Med Chem* 1997;5:93–99.

59. Kelland LR, Smith V, Valenti M, et al. Preclinical antitumor activity and pharmacodynamic studies with the farnesyl protein transferase inhibitor R115777 in human breast cancer. *Clin Cancer Res* 2001;7:3544–3550.

60. Kohl NE, Omer CA, Conner MW, et al. Inhibition of farnesyltransferase induces regression of mammary and salivary carcinomas in ras transgenic mice. *Nat Med* 1995;1:792–797.

61. Barrington RE, Subler MA, Rands E, et al. A farnesyltransferase inhibitor induces tumor regression in transgenic mice harboring multiple oncogenic mutations by mediating alterations in both cell cycle control and apoptosis. *Mol Cell Biol* 1998;18:85–92.

62. Mangues R, Corral T, Kohl NE, et al. Antitumor effect of a farnesyl transferase inhibitor in mammary and lymphoid tumors overexpressing N-ras in transgenic mice. *Cancer Res* 1998;58:1253–1259.

63. Omer CA, Chen Z, Diehl RE, et al. Mouse mammary tumor virus-Ki-*ras*B transgenic mice develop mammary carcinomas that can be growth-inhibited by a farnesyl:protein transferase inhibitor. *Cancer Res* 2000;60:2680–2688.

64. Miquel K, Pradines A, Sun J, et al. GGTI-298 induces G_0-G_1 block and apoptosis whereas FTI-277 causes G_2-M enrichment in A549 cells. *Cancer Res* 1997;57:1846–1850.

65. Ashar HR, James L, Gray K, et al. The farnesyl transferase inhibitor SCH 66336 induces a G_2/M or G_1 pause in sensitive human tumor cell lines. *Exp Cell Res* 2001;262:17–27.

66. Sepp-Lorenzino L, Rosen N. A farnesyl-protein transferase inhibitor induces p21 expression and G_1 block in p53 wild type tumor cells. *J Biol Chem* 1998;273:20,243–20,251.

67. Suzuki N, Urano J, Tamanoi F. Farnesyltransferase inhibitors induce cytochrome c release and caspase 3 activation preferentially in transformed cells. *Proc Natl Acad Sci USA* 1998;95:15,356–15,361.

68. Lebowitz PF, Sakamur D, Prendergast GC. Farnesyl transferase inhibitors induce apoptosis of ras-transformed cells denied substratum attachment. *Cancer Res* 1997;57:708–713.

69. Du W, Liu A, Prendergast GC. Activation of the PI3'K-AKT pathway masks the proapoptotic effects of farnesyltransferase inhibitors. *Cancer Res* 1999;59:4208–4212.

70. Jiang K, Coppola D, Crespo NC, et al. The phosphoinositide 3-OH kinase/AKT2 pathway as a critical target for farnesyltransferase inhibitor-induced apoptosis. *Mol Cell Biol* 2000;20:139–148.

71. Yan J, Roy S, Apolloni A, et al. Ras isoforms vary in their ability to activate *raf*-1 and phosphoinositide 3-kinase. *J Biol Chem* 1998:24,052–24,056.

72. Cox AD, Hisaka MM, Buss JE, Der CJ. Specific isoprenoid modification is required for function of normal, but not oncogenic, Ras protein. *Mol Cell Biol* 1992;12:2606–2615.

73. Miyake M, Mizutani S, Koide H, Kaziro Y. Unfarnesylated transforming Ras mutant inhibits the Ras-signaling pathway by forming a stable Ras-Raf complex in the cytosol. *FEBS Lett* 1996;378:15–18.

74. Gibbs JB, Oliff A. The potential of farnesyltransferase inhibitors as cancer chemotherapeutics. *Annu Rev Pharmacol Toxicol* 1997;37:143–166.

75. Ashar HR, James L, Gray K, et al. Farnesyl transferase inhibitors block the farnesylation of CENP-E and CENP-F, and alter the association of CENP-E with the microtubules. *J Biol Chem* 2000;275:30,451–30,457.

76. Adamson P, Marshall CJ, Hall A, Tilbrook PA. Post-translational modifications of p21rho proteins. *J Biol Chem* 1992;267:20,033–20,038.

77. Du W, Lebowitz PF, Prendergast GC. Cell growth inhibition by farnesyltransferase inhibitors is mediated by gain of geranylgeranylated RhoB. *Mol Cell Biol* 1999;19:1831–1840.

78. Du W, Prendergast GC. Geranylgeranylated RhoB mediates suppression of human tumor cell growth by farnesyltransferase inhibitors. *Cancer Res* 1999;59:5492–5496.

79. Chen A, Sun J, Pradines A, et al. Both farnesylated and geranylgeranylated RhoB inhibit malignant transformation and suppress human tumor growth in nude mice. *J Biol Chem* 2000;275:17,974–17,978.

80. Bell IA. Inhibitors of protein prenylation 2000. *Expert Opin Ther Patents* 2000;10:1813–1831.

81. Huber HE, Robinson RG, Watkins A, et al. Anions modulate the potency of geranylgeranyl-protein transferase I inhibitors. *J Biol Chem* 2001;276:24,457–24,465.

82. Kohl NE, Buser C, deSolms SJ, et al. L-778123 is an inhibitor of both farnesyl protein transferase and geranylgeranyl protein transferase type I that inhibits tumor growth in ras transgenic mice. *Clin Cancer Res* 2001;7:3829S.

83. Karp JE, Lancet JE, Kaufmann SH, et al. Clinical and biologic activity of the farnesyltransferase inhibitor R115777 in adults with refractory and relapsed acute leukemias: a Phase 1 clinical-laboratory correlative trial. *Blood* 2001;97:3361–3369.

84. Johnston SR, Ellis PA, Houston S, et al. A Phase II study of the farnesyl transferase inhibitor R115777 in patients with advanced breast cancer. *Proc Am Soc Clin Oncol* 2000;19:83a.

85. Adjei AA, Erlichman C, Davis JN, et al. A Phase I trial of the farnesyl transferase inhibitor SCH66336: evidence for biological and clinical activity. *Cancer Res* 2000;60:1871-1877.

86. Britten CD, Rowinsky EK, Soignet S, et al. A Phase I and pharmacological study of the farnesyl protein transferase inhibitor L-778,123 in patients with solid malignancies. *Clin Cancer Res* 2001;7:3894–3903.

87. Patnaik A, Izbicka E, Eckhardt SG, et al. Inhibition of HDJ2 protein farnesylation in peripheral blood mononuclear cells as a pharmacodynamic endpoint in a Phase I study of R115777 and gemcitabine. *Proc Am Assoc Cancer Res* 2001;42:488.

88. Sonnichsen D, Damle B, Manning J, et al. Pharmacokinetics (PK) and pharmacodynamics (PD) of the farnesyltransferase (FT) inhibitor BMS-214662 in patients with advanced solid tumors. *Proc Am Soc Clin Oncol* 2000;19:178a.

89. Tabernero J, Sonnichsen D, Albanell J, et al. A Phase I pharmacokinetic (PK) and serial tumor and PBMC pharmacodynamic (PD) study of weekly BMS-214662, a farnesyltransferase (FT) inhibitor, in patients with advanced solid tumors. *Proc Am Soc Clin Oncol* 2001;20:77a.

90. Holden SN, Echhardt S, Fisher S, et al. A Phase I pharmacokinetic (PK) and biological study of the farnesyl transferase inhibitor (FTI) R115777 and capecitabine in patients (PTS) with advanced solid malignancies. *Proc Amer Soc Clin Oncol* 2001;20:80a.

91. Hurwitz HI, Colvin OM, Petros WP, et al. Phase I and pharmacokinetic study of SCH66336, a novel FPTI, using a 2-week on, 2-week off schedule. *Proc Am Soc Clin Oncol* 1999;18:156a.

92. Hurwitz HI, Amado R, Prager D, et al. Phase I pharmacokinetic trial of the farnesyl transferase inhibitor SCH66336 plus gemcitabine in advanced cancers. *Proc Am Soc Clin Oncol* 2000;19:185a.

93. Kies MS, Clayman GL, El-Naggar AK, et al. Induction therapy with SCH 66336, a farnesyltransferase inhibitor, in squamous cell carcinoma (SCC) of the head and neck. *Proc Amer Soc Clin Oncol* 2001;20:225a.

94. Liebes L, Hochster H, Speyer J, et al. Enhanced myelosuppression of topotecan when combined with the farnesyl transferase inhibitor, R115777: a Phase I and pharmacodynamic study. *Proc Am Soc Clin Oncol* 2001;20:81a.

95. Mackay HJ, Hoekstra R, Eskens F, et al. A Phase I dose escalating study of BMS-214662 in combination with cisplatin (C) in patients with advanced solid tumors. *Proc Am Soc Clin Oncol* 2001;20:80a.

96. Nakagawa K, Yamamoto N, Nishio K, et al. A Phase I, pharmacokinetic (PK) and pharmacodynamic (PD) study of the farnesyl transferase inhibitor (FTI) R115777 in Japanese patients with advanced non-hematological malignancies. *Proc Am Soc Clin Oncol* 2001;20:80a.

97. Schwartz G, Rowinsky EK, Rha SY, et al. A Phase I, pharmacokinetic, and biologic correlative study of R115777 and Trastuzumab (Herceptin) in patients with advanced cancer. *Proc Am Soc Clin Oncol* 2001;20:81a.

98. Widemann BC, Salzer WL, Arceci RJ, et al. Phase I trial of R115777, an oral farnesyltransferase (FTase) inhibitor, in children with refractory solid tumors and neurofibromatosis type I (NFI). *Proc Am Soc Clin Oncol* 2001;20:368a.

99. Zujewski J, Horak ID, Bol CJ, et al. Phase I and pharmacokinetic study of farnesyl protein transferase inhibitor R115777 in advanced cancer. *J Clin Oncol* 2000;18:927–941.

100. Schellens J, Klerk Gd, Swart M, et al. Phase I and pharmacologic study with the novel farnesyltransferase inhibitor (FTI) R115777. *Proc Am Soc Clin Oncol* 2000;19:184a.

101. Moasser MM, Sepp-Lorenzino L, Kohl NE, et al. Farnesyl transferase inhibitors cause enhanced mitotic sensitivity to taxol and epothilones. *Proc Natl Acad Sci USA* 1998;95:1369–1374.

102. Sun J, Blaskovich MA, Knowles D, et al. Antitumor efficacy of a novel class of non-thiol-containing peptidomimetic inhibitors of farnesyltransferase and geranylgeranyltransferase I: combination therapy with the cytotoxic agents cisplatin, taxol, and gemcitabine. *Cancer Res* 1999;59:4919–4926.

103. Shi B, Yaremko B, Hajian G, et al. The farnesyl protein transferase inhibitor SCH66336 synergizes with taxanes in

vitro and enhances their antitumor activity in vivo. *Cancer Chemother Pharmacol* 2000;46:387–393.

104. Adjei AA, Davis JN, Bruzek LM, et al. Synergy of the protein farnesyltransferase inhibitor SCH66336 and cisplatin in human cancer cell lines. *Clin Cancer Res* 2001;7:1438–1445.

105. Bernhard EJ, Kao G, Cox AD, et al. The farnesyltransferase inhibitor FTI-277 radiosensitizes H-ras-transformed rat embryo fibroblasts. *Cancer Res* 1996;56:1727–1730.

106. Bernhard EJ, McKenna WG, Hamilton AD, et al. Inhibiting Ras prenylation increases the radiosensitivity of human tumor cell lines with activating mutations of ras oncogenes. *Cancer Res* 1998;58:1754–1761.

107. Hahn SM, Kiel K, Morrison BW, et al. Phase I trial of the farnesyl protein transferase (FPTase) inhibitor L-778123 in combination with radiotherapy. *Proc Am Soc Clin Oncol* 2000;19:231a.

108. Lantry LE, Zhang Z, Yao R, et al. Effect of farnesyltransferase inhibitor FTI-276 on established lung adenomas from A/J mice induced by 4-(methylnitrosamino)-1-(3-pyridyl)-1-butanone. *Carcinogenesis* 2000;21:113–116.

109. Bol DK, Dell J, Ho CP, et al. A comparison of the therapeutic and preventive efficacy of a novel Ras farnesyltransferase inhibitor in endogenous mouse carcinogenesis models. *Proc Am Assoc Cancer Res* 2000;41:220.

110. Lerner EC, Zhang T-T, Knowles DB, et al. Inhibition of the prenylation of K-Ras, but not H- or N-Ras, is highly resistant to CAAX peptidomimetics and requires both a farnesyltransferase and a geranylgeranyltransferase I inhibitor in human tumor cell lines. *Oncogene* 1997;15:1283–1288.

111. Sun J, Qian Y, Hamilton AD, Sebti SM. Both farnesyltransferase and geranylgeranyltransferase I inhibitors are required for inhibition of oncogenic K-Ras prenylation but each alone is sufficient to suppress human tumor growth in nude mouse xenografts. *Oncogene* 1998;16:1467–1473.

112. Lobell RB, Omer CA, Abrams MT, et al. Evaluation of farnesyl:protein transferase and geranylgeranyl:protein transferase inhibitor combinations in preclinical models. *Cancer Res* 2001;61:8758–8768.

113. Prendergast GC, Davide JP, Lebowitz PF, et al. Resistance of a variant Ras-transformed cell line to phenotypic reversion by farnesyl transferase inhibitors. *Cancer Res* 1996;56:2626–2632.

114. Villar KD, Urano J, Guo L, Tamanoi F. A mutant form of human protein farnesyltransferase exhibits increased resistance to farnesyltransferase inhibitors. *J Biol Chem* 1999;274:27,010–27,017.

115. Hudes GR, Schol J. Phase I trial of oral R115777 in patients with refractory solid tumors, in *Farnesyltransferase Inhibitors in Cancer Therapy.* Sebti SM, Hamilton AD, eds. Humana Press, Inc., Totowa, NJ, 2000, pp. 251–254.

116. Punt CJ, van Maanen L, Bol CJ, et al. Phase I and pharmacokinetic study of the orally administered farnesyl transferase inhibitor R115777 in patients with advanced solid tumors. *Anticancer Drugs* 2001;12:193–197.

117. Adjei AA, Erlichman C, Marks RS, et al. A Phase I trial of the farnesyltransferase inhibitor R115777, in combination with gemcitabine and cisplatin in patients with advanced cancer. *Proc Am Soc Clin Oncol* 2001;20:81a.

118. Verslype C, Steenbergen WV, Humblet Y, et al. Phase I trial of 5-FU/LV in combination with the farnesyltransferase inhibitor (FTI) R115777. *Proc Am Soc Clin Oncol* 2001;20:171a.

119. Piccart-Gebhart MJ, Branle F, Valeriola DD, et al. A Phase I, clinical and pharmacokinetic (PK) trial of the farnesyl transferase inhibitor (FTI) R115777 + docetaxel: a promising combination in patients (PTS) with solid tumors. *Proc Am Soc Clin Oncol* 2001;20:80a.

120. Verweij J, Kehrer D, Planting A, et al. Phase I trial of irinotecan in combination with the farnesyl transferase inhibiitor (FTI) R115777. *Proc Am Soc Clin Oncol* 2001;20:81a.

121. Eskens FA, Awada A, Cutler DL, et al. Phase I and pharmacokinetic study of the oral farnesyl transferase inhibitor SCH 66336 given twice daily to patients with advanced solid tumors. *J Clin Oncol* 2001;19:1167–1175.

122. Lersch C, Cutsem EV, Amado R, et al. Randomized Phase II study of SCH 66336 and gemcitabine in the treatment of metastatic adenocarcinoma of the pancreas. *Proc Am Soc Clin Oncol* 2001;20:153a.

123. Kim ES, Glisson BS, Meyers ML, et al. A Phase I/II study of the farnesyl transferase inhibitor (FTI) SCH66336 with paclitaxel in patients with solid tumors. *Proc Am Assoc Cancer Res* 2001;42:488.

124. Winquist E, Morre MJ, Chi K, et al. NCIC CTG IND.128: a Phase II study of a farnesyl transferase inhibitor (SCH 66336) in patients with unresectable or metastatic transitional cell carcinoma of the urothelial tract failing prior chemotherapy. *Proc Am Soc Clin Oncol* 2001;20:197a.

125. Rubin E, Abbruzzese JL, Morrison BW, et al. Phase I trial of the farnesyl protein transferase (FPTase) inhibitor L-778123 on a 14 or 28-day dosing schedule. *Proc Am Soc Clin Oncol* 2000;19:178a.

126. Sharma S, Britten C, Spriggs D, et al. A Phase I and PK study of farnesyl transferase inhibitor L-778,123 administered as a seven day continuous infusion in combination with paclitaxel. *Proc Am Soc Clin Oncol* 2000;19:185a.

127. Ryan DP, Eder JP, Supko JG, et al. Phase I clinical trial of the farnesyltransferase (FT) inhibitor BMS-214662 in patients with advanced solid tumors. *Proc Am Soc Clin Oncol* 2000;19:185a.

128. Voi M, Tabernero J, Cooper MR, et al. A Phase I study of the farnesyltransferase (FT) inhibitor BMS-214662 administered as a weekly 1-hour infusion in patients (Pts) with advanced solid tumors: clinical findings. *Proc Am Soc Clin Oncol* 2001;20:79a.

129. Camacho LH, Soignet SL, Pezzulli S, et al. Dose escalation study of oral farnesyl transferase inhibitor (FTI) BMS-214662 in patients with solid tumors. *Proc Am Soc Clin Oncol* 2001;20:79a.

130. Kim KB, Shin DM, Summey CC, et al. Phase I study of farnesyl transferase inhibitor, BMS-214662 in solid tumors. *Proc Am Soc Clin Oncol* 2001;20:79a.

131. Bailey HH, Marnocha R, Arzoomanian R, et al. Phase I trial of weekly paclitaxel and BMS214662 in patients with advanced solid tumors. *Proc Am Soc Clin Oncol* 2001;20:79a.

132. Gibbs RA, Zahn TJ, Sebolt-Leopold JS. Non-peptidic prenyltransferase inhibitors: diverse structural classes and surprising anti-cancer mechanisms. *Curr Med Chem* 2001;8:1437–1465.

133. Prendergast GC, Rane N. Farnesyltransferase inhibitors: mechanism and applications. *Expert Opin Invest Drugs* 2001;10:2105–2116.

21 The Potential of EGFR-Targeted Agents in Cancer Prevention

Steven D. Averbuch, MD and Fadlo R. Khuri, MD

CONTENTS

1. INTRODUCTION

The prevention of cancer and its recurrence in high-risk individuals has become an increasingly realistic goal with the introduction of targeted therapies. Like other therapies intended to prevent morbidity and mortality in populations at risk, such as lipid-lowering agents and antihypertensives, cancer-prevention agents are intended for use in generally healthy individuals, and therefore must be well-tolerated. Other challenges associated with the use of agents in cancer prevention, rather than treatment, include the identification of an appropriate dose (the optimal biological dose for advanced disease may not be the optimal dose for early disease or for use in chemoprevention); similarly, the most appropriate schedule and form of administration must be determined. For example, preclinical models of lung cancer chemoprevention suggest that the use of inhaled formulations of retinoids may reduce the systemic side effects associated with chronic oral administration *(1)*.

It is generally accepted that the toxicity of cytotoxic chemotherapy agents routinely used in patients with cancer precludes their use in chemoprevention; therefore, alternative active treatments have been sought. Targeted therapy with the antiestrogen tamoxifen has demonstrated a decrease in the incidence of breast cancer in women defined by an established quantitative model as at risk *(2,3)*. Recent research has shown that the epidermal growth factor receptor (EGFR) signaling pathway may play a role in the genesis, proliferation, and survival of cancer cells, and is therefore a prime target for both cancer chemoprevention and drug development. In this chapter, the rationale for targeting EGFR and the potential for EGFR-targeted agents are discussed, with particular reference to two groups that are prime candidates for chemoprevention: tobacco smokers at high risk for epithelial respiratory (mainly lung) cancer and women at high risk of developing breast cancer or those with ductal carcinoma *in situ* (DCIS).

2. RATIONALE FOR TARGETING EGFR

EGFR belongs to a family of four closely related cell-surface receptors: EGFR (HER1 or erbB1), erbB2 (HER2 or neu), erbB3 (HER3), and erbB4 (HER4). EGFR is a transmembrane glycoprotein comprised of an extracellular ligand-binding domain, a transmembrane domain, and an intracellular tyrosine kinase domain. EGFR tyrosine kinase is activated when a ligand such as epidermal growth factor (EGF), transforming growth factor α (TGFα), or amphiregulin binds to the external domain. This causes the receptor to combine with another EGFR to form a homodimer, or with another receptor family member (e.g., erbB2) to form a heterodimer. Receptor dimerization activates intracellular autophosphorylation of specific tyrosine residues, initiating a cascade of intracellular signaling reactions (Fig. 1; *4*). The *ras*/mitogen-activated protein (MAP) kinase cascade is important in tumorigenesis, leading to increased mitogenesis via induction of

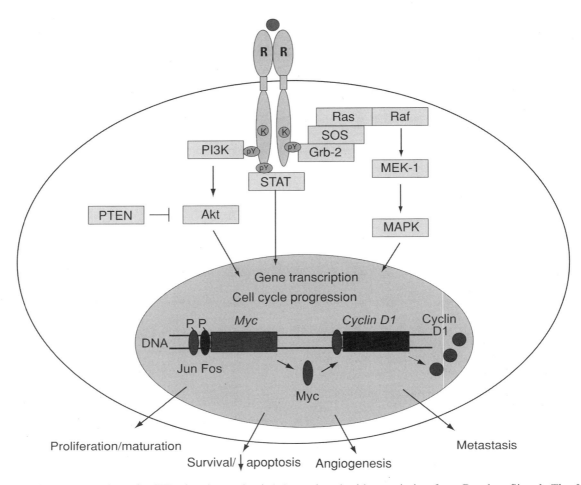

Fig. 1. Schematic representation of EGFR signal transduction (reproduced with permission from Baselga, Signal: *The Journal of EGFR-Targeted Cancer Therapy*, Copyright of Adis International Ltd.) *(4)*.

cyclin D1. EGFR is also implicated in the control of tumor-cell apoptosis, via the phosphatidylinositol-3-kinase (PI3K) pathway, angiogenesis, and metastasis *(5)*. Further studies have shown that EGFR activation can promote the release of vascular endothelial growth factor (VEGF) *(6,7)*, a key promoter of angiogenesis, and subsequently, metastasis. The involvement of EGFR in a range of processes involved in tumor development and growth suggests that EGFR-targeted agents have potential across the continuum of cancer development: prevention at the premalignant stage, prevention and delayed progression at the localized stage, and improvements in outcome for locally advanced disease or metastatic disease.

EGFR is expressed in tissues of epithelial, mesenchymal, and neuronal origin, and plays a key role in processes such as proliferation, regeneration, differentiation, and development *(8)*. It is therefore not surprising that high expression of EGFR, and presum-

ably activation of this pathway, is present in an extensive range of human cancers *(9)*, and has been correlated in many cases with a poor prognosis *(10–13)*. In addition to high expression of EGFR, the EGFR signaling pathway may also be activated by other mechanisms, such as EGFR mutations, increased expression of ligands or coexpression of receptor and ligands, and ligand/autocrine stimulation loops (Fig. 2; *14*). For example, a mutant form of the receptor EGFRvIII, in which the extracellular ligand-binding domain is lacking but the tyrosine kinase is constitutively activated, is found in a number of human tumors, often at high levels of expression *(15)*. EGFR signaling may also be affected by the level of expression of other members of the erbB-receptor family. When expression of erbB2 is low, homodimers of EGFR that result in only weak signaling are likely to form, whereas in the presence of high expression of erbB2, heterodimers of EGFR and

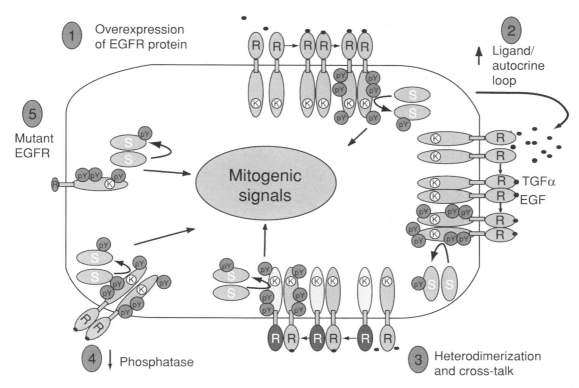

Fig. 2. Mechanisms of increased EGFR activation: 1) overexpression of the EGFR on the cell surface; 2) increased levels of receptor ligands with coexpression of one or more ligands resulting in activation of an autocrine system; 3) heterodimerization increases EGF-binding affinity and expands the repertoire of receptor-associated substrates and signaling responses; 4) decreased phosphatase leads to increased phosphorylation of the EGFR and, consequently, increased signaling; 5) mutant EGFRs can be constitutively active receptors that are not downregulated by endocytosis and are potently transforming.

erbB2, which result in potent signaling, preferentially form *(16)*. Furthermore, EGFR has been found to be involved in signaling networks activated by stimuli that do not directly interact with this receptor *(17)*. Thus, the level of expression of EGFR is not always an accurate indication of the activity of this signaling pathway.

There is no standard method used to analyze EGFR expression, and the variety of methods used in different laboratories makes it difficult to compare the results from different studies. Although immunohistochemistry is generally used to evaluate EGFR protein levels, various antibodies and techniques are used, and there is no consensus on the cut-off points for non-expression, expression, and high expression.

The evaluation of phosphorylated (activated) EGFR or markers downstream of EGFR, such as MAP kinase or the proliferation marker Ki-67, may provide an indication of the activation of the EGFR pathway. In a clinical study on the pharmacodynamic effects of the EGFR-targeted agent ZD1839 ("Iressa") on the skin, Albanell et al. showed that ZD1839 affected a range of signaling, proliferation, and maturation

markers, including EGFR phosphorylation and MAP kinase activation *(18)*. Limited data on these downstream markers from human tumors are also available *(19)*.

3. EGFR-TARGETED AGENTS

The clear potential of EGFR-targeted agents in the treatment of a variety of tumor types across the cancer continuum has prompted the development of a number of inhibitors, including the EGFR tyrosine kinase inhibitors (EGFR-TKIs) ZD1839, OSI-774, CI-1033, GW2016, EKB-569, and PKI-166, and the monoclonal antibodies (MAbs) IMC-C225, ABX-EGF, EMD72000, and trastuzumab. EGFR-TKIs are small-molecule, orally active inhibitors of the tyrosine kinase activity of the intracellular domain of the erbB receptors. ZD1839 and OSI-774 are selective for EGFR, PKI-166, GW2016, and EKB-569 inhibit EGFR and erbB2, and CI-1033 inhibits all of the erbB receptors. The monoclonal antibodies IMC-C225, ABX-EGF, and EMD72000 target the extracellular domain of EGFR and trastuzumab targets erbB2.

Since these EGFR-targeted agents act upon pathways that may be differentiated between malignant and normal cells, high therapeutic indices are expected with substantially less toxicity at clinically effective doses compared with nonspecific cytotoxic agents *(20)*. These basic differences between novel target-based anticancer therapies and cytotoxic agents bring challenges in the assessment of the clinical efficacy of EGFR-targeted agents; established endpoints for safety and antitumor activity may not be the most appropriate. For example, in Phase I evaluation, dose-limiting toxicities (DLTs) for EGFR-targeted agents may not be evident at doses that maximally inhibit EGFR phosphorylation; therefore, the maximum tolerated dose (MTD) may be much higher than the optimal biological dose. This separation of biological from toxicological endpoints is evident with ZD1839, which has a wide therapeutic margin. In Phase I studies, the MTD was 700–1000 mg/d ZD1839 *(21,22)*, whereas clinical pharmacodynamic studies using a range of doses from 150–1000 mg/d showed that doses ≥150 mg/d appeared to provide optimal receptor inhibition *(18)*. The recommended dose, confirmed in Phase II studies in patients with advanced non-small-cell lung cancer (NSCLC), is 250 mg/d *(23)*.

Long-term tolerability is paramount for chemopreventive agents. Clinical trials in patients with NSCLC have shown that the EGFR-TKIs ZD1839 and OSI-774 are well-tolerated *(23–26)*. In these patients, the most common adverse events (AE) associated with oral EGFR-targeted agents were mild, reversible-grade 1/2 diarrhea and skin rash, with grade 3/4 drug-related AE occurring in less than 10% of patients at the recommended doses (23–25). Although this safety profile is favorable compared with most cytotoxic chemotherapy agents, it has not been established whether or not the level of toxicity observed would be justifiable or acceptable for use in generally healthy yet high-risk individuals.

3.1. EGFR-Targeted Agents in Lung Cancer Chemoprevention

Lung cancer is the leading cause of cancer death worldwide, with an estimated 1.1 million lung-cancer-related deaths in the year 2000 *(27)*. In the United States alone, an estimated 154,900 deaths were anticipated from lung cancer in the year 2002, surpassing the combined death rates from breast, prostate, and colon cancers *(28)*. Although recent education campaigns in some countries have led to a substantial reduction in the

percentage of adults who smoke, lung cancer in former smokers still poses a substantial long-term health threat. The past 10 years have produced promising chemoprevention results in the reduction of mortality associated with some common epithelial cancers; however, the results of lung cancer chemoprevention trials, including those using β-carotene, α-tocopherol, and retinoids, have found either no effect or possible harmful effects in the chemoprevention of NSCLC (29–32); therefore, new approaches are needed.

EGFR is expressed or highly expressed in a high percentage of lung tumors *(33,34)*: EGFR expression has been identified in 81–93% of NSCLC samples, with high expression in 45–70% of tumors *(35)*. Many studies have associated increased tumor levels of EGFR with advanced disease, development of metastases, and poor clinical prognosis. In patients with NSCLC, EGFR expression has been correlated with poor prognosis in patients, with high coexpression of p53 *(36)* or erbB2 *(37)*.

The presence of EGFR expression in early bronchial neoplasia has been explored extensively in recent years. Kurie et al. showed that EGFR expression was higher in metaplastic biopsies than in normal bronchial epithelium in biopsies of 69 active smokers enrolled in a chemoprevention trial of retinoic acid vs placebo; high intensity EGFR antibody staining was observed in 81% of metaplastic biopsies compared with 67% of normal biopsies ($p = 0.02$) *(38)*. Reversal of bronchial metaplasia following treatment with retinoic acid or placebo was associated with decreased EGFR expression. EGFR expression decreased in 50% of the biopsy sites that reverted from metaplastic to normal during the study compared with only 20% of the biopsy sites that remained metaplastic ($p = 0.004$). Although univariate analysis revealed that both smoking cessation and histological change were statistically significant predictors of reduced EGFR expression ($p = 0.01$ and 0.04, respectively), multivariate analysis suggested that the effect of smoking cessation on EGFR expression was dependent on reversal of bronchial metaplasia. Thus, EGFR expression alone did not predict metaplasia reversal in response to retinoic acid, demonstrating that the level of expression of EGFR may not be a direct indicator of response.

Rusch et al. have also shown that high EGFR expression is frequently present in early bronchial neoplasia *(39)*. In this retrospective review of 34 patients with NSCLC, the expression of EGFR and p53 was evaluated in tissue from invasive NSCLC and its

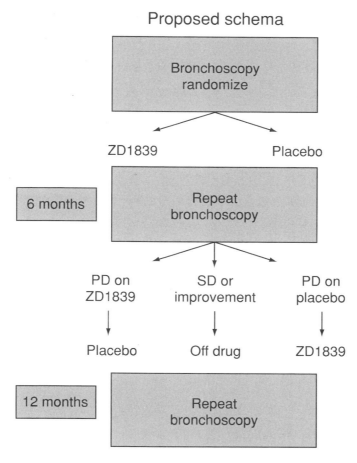

Fig. 3. Proposed schema for SPORE Phase IIB/III trial of ZD1839 vs placebo in former/current smokers (reproduced with permission from Averbuch, *Clin Cancer Res*).

associated bronchial lesions. Abnormal EGFR immunostaining was observed in 48% of the bronchial premalignant lesions (staining in the superficial layers of the bronchial epithelium as well as positivity of the basal-cell layer), with positive staining for EGFR in 53% of the invasive carcinomas. Furthermore, coexpression of *p53* and EGFR appeared to precede and predict development of squamous-cell carcinoma.

Perhaps most compelling is evidence that EGFR and TGFα coexpression appear to be independent of *ras* mutations in lung adenocarcinoma, suggesting that mutations of k-*ras* and increased expression of EGFR proceed through alternate pathways *(40)*. To test the hypothesis that these mechanisms proceed through independent pathways, the expression of EGFR and TGFα was studied in primary NSCLC. EGFR-TGFα coexpression was found in 73% of squamous-cell cancers, a type that rarely develops *ras* mutations. In contrast, EGFR-TGFα coexpression occurred with equal frequency in adenocarcinomas with either the wild-type

or the mutant *ras* genotype. These results indicate that the EGFR autocrine loop activity in adenocarcinoma might have alternative signaling activities aside from the activation of the *ras*/MAP kinase pathway, and therefore may be a viable target for chemopreventive strategies.

The potential importance of EGFR as a chemoprevention target in lung cancer has also been demonstrated by Lonardo et al. *(41,42)*. Using an in vitro model of human bronchial carcinogenesis, all-*trans*-retinoic acid (ATRA) blocked the cellular phenotypic change of increased EGFR expression and signal activation resulting from transformation with the carcinogen *N*-nitrosamine-4-(methylnitrosamino)-1-(3 pyridyl)-1-butanone. This decrease in EGFR expression was caused by the transcriptional downregulation of EGFR expression by ATRA. This study further suggests that ATRA-inhibited cyclin D_1 regulation of mitogenesis occurs through two independent mechanisms: posttranscriptional proteasome-dependent proteolysis *(43,44)*, and decreased EGFR transcription leading to reduced cyclin D_1 expression.

Thus, there is indirect evidence from clinical specimens and preclinical models that EGFR may be an important target for a chemoprevention approach with an EGFR-TKI. Indeed, these findings have provided the rationale for a multi-institutional SPORE trial of ZD1839 vs placebo in former/current smokers with a previous history of cancer as a pilot trial of lung cancer prevention (Fig. 3). Trial start-up was scheduled for late 2002, and over 15 premiere lung cancer institutions have been designated to participate. Target accrual is 150 patients, with a 2:1 randomization favoring the active agent in this randomized, double-blind, Phase IIb trial.

3.2. EGFR-Targeted Agents in Breast Cancer Chemoprevention

Breast cancer ranks second among cancer deaths in women, with an estimated 370,000 breast-cancer-related deaths worldwide in the year 2000 (27). In the United States, an estimated 39,600 deaths were anticipated from breast cancer in women in the year 2002 (28). Increased use of mammography screening has led to increased detection of DCIS, the earliest presentation in breast cancer. In the United States, an estimated 54,300 new cases of in situ breast cancer were expected to occur among women during 2002, of which approx 88% would have been DCIS. Unless treated effectively, this preinvasive lesion develops into invasive breast cancer in 25–30% of patients (45). Therefore, there is an opportunity to intervene with chemoprevention at an early stage of breast cancer development.

The balance of evidence from previous chemoprevention studies has shown that the antiestrogen tamoxifen is effective in the prevention of breast cancer in individuals at high risk of developing the disease (46,47). In these studies, women at high risk for breast cancer were randomized to treatment with either placebo or tamoxifen for 5 yr. Tamoxifen reduced the risk of invasive breast cancer by 30–40% (47) as a result of a reduced risk of estrogen receptor (ER)-positive tumors. However, there was no difference in the occurrence of ER-negative tumors, indicating that alternative approaches are required to prevent their development. In addition, most DCIS specimens are of the comedo subtype, which is ER-negative.

The members of the EGFR family are important in the normal development of breast tissue (48), and are highly expressed in breast tumors. In a review of 40

different series of patients, 48% of 5232 breast tumor samples were found to be positive for EGFR, and an inverse relationship between EGFR and ER expression was found in 28 of 31 studies (49). In a single study of 100 patient samples, 36%, 27%, 26%, and 82% of breast cancer tumors were positive for EGFR, erbB2, erbB3 and erbB4, respectively, and coexpression of EGFR and erbB2 was associated with a worse prognosis (50). Similarly, of 40 cases of DCIS, 48% were immunoreactive for EGFR, 63% for erbB2, 78% for erbB3, and 95% for erbB4 (51). Furthermore, receptors with the type III EGFR mutation (EGFRvIII) have been detected in 78% of breast carcinomas, but not in normal breast tissue (52).

EGFR-TKIs have been shown to provide a potential chemopreventive approach in patients at high risk for breast cancer, including invasive breast cancer of DCIS origin. In transgenic mice engineered to be highly susceptible to spontaneous breast cancer development, blockade of the EGFR tyrosine kinase markedly delayed tumor formation (53). This delay correlated with inhibition of EGFR and HER2/neu signaling, a reduction of downstream markers such as cyclin-dependent kinase 2 (CDK2), and MAP kinase activities, and a corresponding increase in levels of the CDK inhibitor p27^{Kip1}. Chan et al. have shown that the EGFR-TKI ZD1839 can reduce epithelial proliferation and increase apoptosis in EGFR-positive DCIS (54). Breast tissue from 16 women undergoing surgery for DCIS was implanted into immunosuppressed mice and treated with ZD1839 for 14–28 d, commencing 2 wk after implantation. Overall, a 56% reduction in epithelial proliferation was seen with ZD1839 in EGFR-positive DCIS compared with controls. Similar reductions in epithelial proliferation occurred in both ER-negative/EGFR-positive and ER-positive/EGFR-positive DCIS. ZD1839 also reduced epithelial proliferation and increased epithelial apoptosis in at-risk normal breast epithelial tissue adjacent to DCIS. In a similar study, ZD1839 significantly inhibited the proliferation of DCIS tissue implanted into immunosuppressed mice compared with controls, whereas the MAG trastuzumab did not (55).

4. CONCLUSION

EGFR plays an important role in tumor biology, and is an attractive target for cancer chemoprevention. EGFR-targeted agents such as ZD1839 and OSI-774 have been well-tolerated in clinical trials, indicating that they may be considered acceptable as long-term chemopreventive agents. Particular potential has been shown in the chemoprevention of tobacco-smoking-related lung cancer and breast cancer; however, for these tumors and others, many questions remain regarding dose, schedule, trial designs, and endpoints. Future basic and clinical studies designed to further investigate these possibilities are awaited with keen anticipation.

REFERENCES

1. Dahl AR, Grossi IM, Houchens DP, et al. Inhaled isotretinoin (13-*cis* retinoic acid) is an effective lung cancer chemopreventive agent in A/J mice at low doses: a pilot study. *Clin Cancer Res* 2000;6:3015–3024.

2. King MC, Wieand S, Hale K, et al. Tamoxifen and breast cancer incidence among women with inherited mutations in BRCA1 and BRCA2: National Surgical Adjuvant Breast and Bowel Project (NSABP-P1) Breast Cancer Prevention Trial. *JAMA* 2001;86:2251–2256.

3. Salih AK, Fentiman IS. 14. Breast cancer prevention. *Int J Clin Pract* 2002;56:267–271.

4. Baselga J. New technologies in epidermal growth factor receptor-targeted cancer therapy. *Signal* 2000;1:12–21.

5. Woodburn JR. The epidermal growth factor receptor and its inhibition in cancer therapy. *Pharmacol Ther* 1999;82:241–250.

6. Clarke K, Smith K, Gullick WJ, Harris AL. Mutant epidermal growth factor receptor enhances induction of vascular endothelial growth factor by hypoxia and insulin-like growth factor-1 via a PI3 kinase dependent pathway. *Br J Cancer* 2001;84:1322–1329.

7. Maity A, Pore N, Lee J, et al. Epidermal growth factor receptor transcriptionally up-regulates vascular endothelial growth factor expression in human glioblastoma cells via a pathway involving phosphatidylinositol 3'-kinase and distinct from that induced by hypoxia. *Cancer Res* 2000;60:5879–5886.

8. Olayioye MA, Neve RM, Lane HA, Hynes NE. The ErbB signaling network: receptor heterodimerization in development and cancer. *EMBO J* 2000;19:3159–3167.

9. Salomon DS, Brandt R, Ciardiello F, Normanno N. Epidermal growth factor-related peptides and their receptors in human malignancies. *Crit Rev Oncol Hematol* 1995;19:183–232.

10. Fontanini G, Vignati S, Bigini D, et al. Epidermal growth factor receptor (EGFr) expression in non-small cell lung carcinomas correlates with metastatic involvement of hilar and mediastinal lymph nodes in the squamous subtype. *Eur J Cancer* 1995;31A:178–183.

11. Mukaida H, Toi M, Hirai T, et al. Clinical significance of the expression of epidermal growth factor and its receptor in esophageal cancer. *Cancer* 1991;68:142–148.

12. Neal DE, Mellon K. Epidermal growth factor receptor and bladder cancer: a review. *Urol Int* 1992;48:365–371.

13. Sainsbury JR, Farndon JR, Needham GK, et al. Epidermal-growth-factor receptor status as predictor of early recurrence of and death from breast cancer. *Lancet* 1987;1:1398–1402.

14. Voldborg BR, Damstrup L, Spang-Thomsen M, Poulsen HS. Epidermal growth factor receptor (EGFR) and EGFR mutations, function and possible role in clinical trials. *Ann Oncol* 1997;8:1197–1206.

15. Moscatello DK, Holgado-Madruga M, Godwin AK, et al. Frequent expression of a mutant epidermal growth factor receptor in multiple human tumors. *Cancer Res* 1995;55:5536–5539.

16. Yarden Y, Sliwkowski MX. Untangling the ErbB signalling network. *Nat Rev Mol Cell Biol* 2001;2:127–137.

17. Carpenter G. Employment of the epidermal growth factor receptor in growth factor-independent signaling pathways. *J Cell Biol* 1999;146:697–702.

18. Albanell J, Rojo F, Averbuch S, et al. Pharmacodynamic studies of the epidermal growth factor receptor inhibitor ZD1839 in skin from cancer patients: histopathologic and molecular consequences of receptor inhibition. *J Clin Oncol* 2002;20:110–124.

19. Goss GD, Stewart DJ, Hirte H, et al. Initial results of Part 2 of a Phase I/II pharmacokinetic (PK), pharmacodynamic (PD) and biological activity study of ZD1839 (Iressa): NCIC CTG IND.122. *Proc Am Soc Clin Oncol* 2002;21:16a, abst 59.

20. Rowinsky EK. The pursuit of optimal outcomes in cancer therapy in a new age of rationally designed target-based anticancer agents. *Drugs* 2000;60 (Suppl 1):1–14.

21. Herbst RS, Maddox A-M, Rothenberg ML, et al. The selective oral epidermal growth factor receptor tyrosine kinase inhibitor ZD1839 ('Iressa') is generally well tolerated and has activity in non-small-cell lung cancer and other solid tumors: results of a Phase I trial. *J Clin Oncol* 2002;20:3815–3825.

22. Ranson M, Hammond LA, Ferry D, et al. ZD1839, a selective oral epidermal growth factor receptor-tyrosine kinase inhibitor, is well tolerated and active in patients with solid, malignant tumors: results of a Phase I trial. *J Clin Oncol* 2002;20:2240–2250.

23. Fukuoka M, Yano S, Giaccone G, et al. Final results from a Phase II trial of ZD1839 ('Iressa') for patients with advanced non-small-cell lung cancer (IDEAL 1). *Proc Am Soc Clin Oncol* 2002;21:298a, abst 1188.

24. Kris MG, Natale RB, Herbst RS, et al. A Phase II trial of ZD1839 ('Iressa') in advanced non-small-cell lung cancer (NSCLC) patients who had failed platinum- and docetaxel-based regimens (IDEAL 2). *Proc Am Soc Clin Oncol* 2002;21:292a, abst 1166.

25. Perez-Soler R, Chachoua A, Huberman M, et al. A Phase II trial of the epidermal growth factor receptor (EGFR) tyrosine kinase inhibitor OSI-774, following platinum-based chemotherapy, in patients (pts) with advanced, EGFR-expressing, non-small cell lung cancer (NSCLC). *Proc Am Soc Clin Oncol* 2001;20:310a, abst1235.

26. Hidalgo M, Siu LL, Nemunaitis J, et al. Phase I and pharmacologic study of OSI-774, an epidermal growth factor receptor tyrosine kinase inhibitor, in patients with advanced solid malignancies. *J Clin Oncol* 2001;19:3267–3279.

27. Ferlay J, Bray F, Pisani P, Parkin DM. GLOBOCAN 2000: Cancer Incidence, Mortality and Prevalence Worldwide, Version 1.0. IARC CancerBase No. 5. Lyon, FR: IARCPress, 2001. Limited version available from http://www-dep.iarc.fr/globocan/globocan.html 2001; last updated 03/02/2001.

28. Ries LAG, Eisner MP, Kosary CL, et al. SEER *Cancer Statistics Review* 1973–1999 Bethesda, MD: National Cancer Institute, 2002. http://seer.cancer.gov/csr/1973–1999/, 2002.

29. Lippman SM, Lee JJ, Karp DD, et al. Randomized Phase III intergroup trial of isotretinoin to prevent second primary tumors in stage I non-small-cell lung cancer. *J Natl Cancer Inst* 2001;93:605–618.

30. Hennekens CH, Buring JE, Manson JE, et al. Lack of effect of long-term supplementation with beta carotene on the incidence of malignant neoplasms and cardiovascular disease. *N Engl J Med* 1996;334:1145–1149.

31. Omenn GS, Goodman GE, Thornquist MD, et al. Effects of a combination of beta carotene and vitamin A on lung cancer and cardiovascular disease. *N Engl J Med* 1996;334:1150–1155.

32. The effect of vitamin E and beta carotene on the incidence of lung cancer and other cancers in male smokers. The Alpha-Tocopherol, Beta Carotene Cancer Prevention Study Group. *N Engl J Med* 1994;330:1029–1035.

33. Rusch V, Klimstra D, Venkatraman E, et al. Overexpression of the epidermal growth factor receptor and its ligand transforming growth factor alpha is frequent in resectable non-small cell lung cancer but does not predict tumor progression. *Clin Cancer Res* 1997;3:515–522.

34. Fontanini G, De Laurentiis M, Vignati S, et al. Evaluation of epidermal growth factor-related growth factors and receptors and of neoangiogenesis in completely resected stage I-IIIA non-small-cell lung cancer: amphiregulin and microvessel count are independent prognostic indicators of survival. *Clin Cancer Res* 1998;4:241–249.

35. Rusch V, Baselga J, Cordon-Cardo C, et al. Differential expression of the epidermal growth factor receptor and its ligands in primary non-small cell lung cancers and adjacent benign lung. *Cancer Res* 1993;53 (10 Suppl):2379–2385.

36. Ohsaki Y, Tanno S, Fujita Y, et al. Epidermal growth factor receptor expression correlates with poor prognosis in non-small cell lung cancer patients with p53 overexpression. *Oncol Rep* 2000;7:603–607.

37. Brabender J, Danenberg KD, Metzger R, et al. Epidermal growth factor receptor and HER2-*neu* mRNA expression in non-small cell lung cancer is correlated with survival. *Clin Cancer Res* 2001;7:1850–1855.

38. Kurie JM, Shin HJ, Lee JS, et al. Increased epidermal growth factor receptor expression in metaplastic bronchial epithelium. *Clin Cancer Res* 1996;2:1787–1793.

39. Rusch V, Klimstra D, Linkov I, Dmitrovsky E. Aberrant expression of p53 or the epidermal growth factor receptor is frequent in early bronchial neoplasia and coexpression precedes squamous cell carcinoma development. *Cancer Res* 1995;55:1365–1372.

40. Hsieh ET, Shepherd FA, Tsao MS. Co-expression of epidermal growth factor receptor and transforming growth factor-alpha is independent of *ras* mutations in lung adenocarcinoma. *Lung Cancer* 2000;29:151–157.

41. Lonardo F, Dragnev KH, Freemantle SJ, et al. Evidence for the epidermal growth factor receptor as a target for lung cancer prevention. *Clin Cancer Res* 2002;8:54–60.

42. Averbuch SD. Lung cancer prevention: retinoids and the epidermal growth factor receptor—a phoenix rising? *Clin Cancer Res* 2002;8:1–3.

43. Langenfeld J, Kiyokawa H, Sekula D, et al. Posttranslational regulation of cyclin D_1 by retinoic acid: a chemoprevention mechanism. *Proc Natl Acad Sci USA* 1997;94:12,070–12,074.

44. Boyle JO, Langenfeld J, Lonardo F, et al. Cyclin D_1 proteolysis: a retinoid chemoprevention signal in normal, immortalized, and transformed human bronchial epithelial cells. *J Natl Cancer Inst* 1999;91:373–379.

45. Price P, Sinnett HD, Gusterson B, et al. Duct carcinoma *in situ:* predictors of local recurrence and progression in patients treated by surgery alone. *Br J Cancer* 1990;61:869–872.

46. Fisher B, Costantino JP, Wickerham DL, et al. Tamoxifen for prevention of breast cancer: report of the National Surgical Adjuvant Breast and Bowel Project P-1 Study. *J Natl Cancer Inst* 1998;90:1371–1388.

47. Cuzick J. Update on new studies in Europe. *Eur J Cancer* 2002;38 (Suppl 3):abst 20.

48. Normanno N, Ciardiello F. EGF-related peptides in the pathophysiology of the mammary gland. *J Mammary Gland Biol Neoplasia* 1997;2:143–151.

49. Klijn JG, Berns PM, Schmitz PI, Foekens JA. The clinical significance of epidermal growth factor receptor (EGF-R) in human breast cancer: a review on 5232 patients. *Endocr Rev* 1992;13:3–17.

50. Suo Z, Risberg B, Kalsson MG, et al. EGFR family expression in breast carcinomas. c-erbB-2 and c-erbB-4 receptors have different effects on survival. *J Pathol* 2002;196:17–25.

51. Suo Z, Bjaamer A, Ottestad L, Nesland JM. Expression of EGFR family and steroid hormone receptors in ductal carcinoma in situ of the breast. *Ultrastruct Pathol* 2001;25:349–356.

52. Pedersen MW, Meltorn M, Damstrup L, Poulsen HS. The type III epidermal growth factor receptor mutation. Biological significance and potential target for anti-cancer therapy. *Ann Oncol* 2001;12:745–760.

53. Lenferink AE, Simpson JF, Shawver LK, et al. Blockade of the epidermal growth factor receptor tyrosine kinase suppresses tumorigenesis in MMTV/Neu + MMTV/TGF-alpha bigenic mice. *Proc Natl Acad Sci USA* 2000;97:9609–9614.

54. Chan KC, Knox WF, Gee JM, et al. Effect of epidermal growth factor receptor tyrosine kinase inhibition on epithelial proliferation in normal and premalignant breast. *Cancer Res* 2002;62:122–128.

55. Chan KC, Knox WF, Gandhi A, et al. Blockade of growth factor receptors in ductal carcinoma *in situ* inhibits epithelial proliferation. *Br J Surg* 2001;88:412–418.

22 Pharmacological Intervention With Multistep Oncogenesis

Potential Role for HSP90 Molecular Chaperone Inhibitors

Paul Workman, PhD

CONTENTS

1. INTRODUCTION

The first part of this chapter reviews current challenges involved in attacking multistep oncogenesis and discusses the consequences for therapeutic and chemopreventive strategies, highlighting in particular the probable need to inhibit multiple oncogenic targets in a combinatorial fashion to obtain therapeutic benefit in the majority of cancers. The second part of the chapter will describe the potential role of inhibitors of the heat shock protein (HSP90) molecular chaperone.

2. THE CHALLENGE OF PHARMACOLOGICAL INTERVENTION IN MULTISTEP ONCOGENESIS

The progressive elucidation of the genomic pathology of human cancer's multiple forms provides a conceptual framework within which to approach pharmacological intervention in a rational way at the molecular level (1–3). The genes and pathways that are hijacked in malignant progression offer a range of molecular targets against which to develop new designer drugs for the treatment and prevention of cancer. In the laboratory and clinic, we are currently testing the hypothesis that by intervening with the precise mechanisms that drive tumorigenesis, we will develop new molecular therapeutic agents that are more effective against cancer and have less severe side effects than the majority of currently used agents, which are broadly cytotoxic and antiproliferative in nature. These future preventive and therapeutic agents may be targeted to the precise genetic profile of the patient's tumor and its potential or actual malignancy (1,2). Selection of the most effective therapies could be based on gene-expression profiling, or even eventually on whole-genome sequencing.

Human genome sequencing has greatly enhanced identification of all 30,000–40,000 genes. The essentially complete sequence, although already published in draft form (4,5), was essential complete in spring 2003 on the fiftieth anniversary of the publication of the double helix structure of DNA by Watson and Crick. During the next five years, the Cancer Genome Project will build on the main human sequencing project to identify essentially all cancer genes responsible for the majority of human malignancies (6). This will accelerate us toward the goal of obtaining a complete molecular

From: Cancer Chemoprevention, Volume 1: Promising Cancer Chemoprevention Agents
Edited by: G. J. Kelloff, E. T. Hawk, and C. C. Sigman © Humana Press Inc., Totowa, NJ

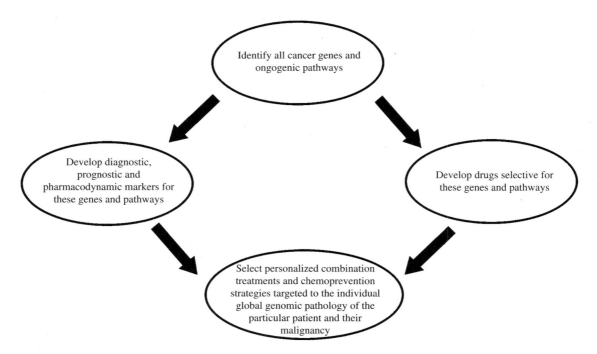

Fig. 1. The postgenomic approach to exploitation of cancer's molecular pathology in development and selection of personalized, combinatorial strategies for chemoprevention and treatment of individual cancers.

description of every type of human cancer, and facilitate our deployment of molecular therapeutics, most probably in combination, to treat any given cancer based on its genomic pathology. Since prevention and treatment strategies will ideally be tailored to the particular molecular pathology profile of the individual concerned, it will be necessary to develop both a series of molecular therapeutics and the corresponding molecular diagnostic/prognostic reagents. The overall strategy is shown schematically in Fig. 1.

This individualized, targeted, mechanism-based treatment scenario may have appeared to be futuristic as little as five years ago. However, a number of molecular therapeutic agents are now emerging from the laboratory, entering clinical trials, and obtaining regulatory approval at a rate that suggests that the end game may be about to begin (7). Successes with Gleevec, Herceptin, and Iressa established proof of principle and clinical validation for the molecular therapeutic approach (7). Because of their central importance in malignancy, drugs that act on the receptor tyrosine kinase (RTK)→Ras →Raf→ERK1/2 MAP kinase signaling pathway and also those hitting the phosphoinositide-3 kinase (PI3K)/molecular target of rapamycin (mTOR) pathway have been prominent among the first wave of molecular therapeutics (7,8).

The recent discovery that activating mutations in B-*raf* are extremely common in human malignant melanoma, and are also present at a lower incidence in colorectal, ovarian, and other cancers, has suggested that drugs targeting the kinase encoded by the mutant B-*raf* oncogene may offer particular promise for treating tumors that harbor this activated oncogene (6).

Most cancers develop as a result of the accumulation of a series of molecular abnormalities, both genetic and epigenetic, leading to an increasingly malignant phenotype. Epidemiological data indicate that most cancers appear to acquire at least 4–6 critical oncogenic defects during their natural history. Chromosomal translocations, deletions, and amplifications have revealed that many human solid tumors contain far more genetic abnormalities (9). Genes involved in multistep oncogenesis of human malignancy have been particularly well-characterized in colorectal cancer (10), and the elucidation of the molecular pathology of all human cancers is now an achievable goal. Over one hundred oncogenes and thirty tumor-suppressor genes have already been defined, and it is likely that many more will be discovered. Despite the large number of cancer genes, it is clear that the majority of them are on so-called mission-critical pathways that regulate cell proliferation, cell-cycle transit, and cell survival/apoptosis (11).

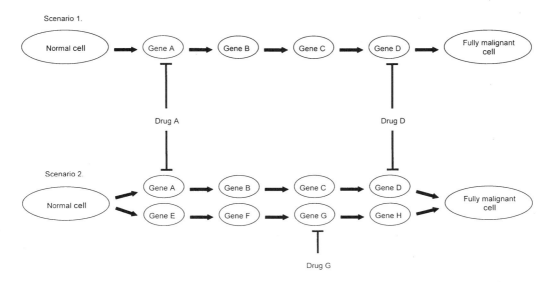

Fig. 2. Two scenarios of multistep oncogenesis with different outcomes in terms of the value of single agent vs combinatorial molecular therapeutics. Note that pathways involving genes A through D and E through H are biochemical—e.g., receptor tyrosine kinasea→RAS→RAF→MEK→ERK1/2 or receptor tyrosine kinase→PI3 kinase→ PDK1→AKT/PKB. They do not represent biochemically independent genes like those commonly depicted in the now-classic model of multistep oncogenesis of colorectal cancer *(9)*. For full details, see text.

Considering that most cancers have accumulated—and may therefore be driven by—a number of genomic and other molecular abnormalities, combining several different targeted pharmacological agents might provide optimal treatment or prevention. However, a significant body of evidence suggests that genetic correction of a single molecular abnormality within the context of a cancer cell harboring many genomic defects can bring about therapeutically valuable cell-cycle arrest and apoptosis *(12)*. For example, reintroduction of wild-type p53 or replacement of the mutant K-*ras* oncogene with the normal form by homologous recombination leads to beneficial effects in human colon cancer cells that harbor multiple genetic abnormalities. Such effects are consistent with a view of malignancy known as oncogene addiction or tumor-suppressor gene hypersensitivity *(12)*. This model postulates that, through selection for the malignant phenotype, cancer cells may become addicted or dependent upon a particular oncogenic pathway that has been switched on by activation of an oncogene or inactivation of a suppressor gene. These changes may become effectively hard-wired into the genome of the cancer cell. Based on this model, the correction of such a key abnormality by a pharmacological agent or by gene therapy might be anticipated to result in highly effective treatment. Similarly, chemopreventive treatments could be developed that target intervention with a key cancer-causing gene at an early stage in the natural history of malignant transformation.

An optimistic view is that malignancy is built of—and indeed is dependent upon—a series of discrete oncogenic abnormalities. Blocking any one of the underpinning genomic drivers of malignancy would completely disrupt the malignant phenotype.

A more pessimistic perspective would be that although cell-cycle arrest and apoptosis can be obtained in experimental models by correction of a single oncogenic defect, this will not necessarily translate into durable responses or cures. In fact, cancer cells may develop a degree of redundancy around the several oncogenic pathways that they routinely hijack. Such redundancy could mean that correction of a single defect may be insufficient to maintain a truly impressive therapeutic effect over a prolonged period. Redundancy may be present at the outset. Or it may be selected for or even induced by the treatment. Resistance to a single-agent strategy could also develop through mutation or altered expression of the target, or by an activation event further downstream in the oncogenic pathway. According to such bleaker scenarios, combinations of agents would be needed that target several—or even all—of the oncogenic abnormalities that drive the particular cancer to achieve a more effective and durable remission, or potentially, a cure of the disease.

To illustrate this discussion, two of many possible oncogenic scenarios are depicted as a model in Fig. 2. In the upper scenario (number 1) the normal cell develops into a fully malignant cell through genetic or epigenetic deregulation of a single mission-critical oncogenic pathway, typically a biochemical signaling pathway that in this case contains the products of four genes, A through D. The oncogenic signaling pathway might be activated by mutation or altered expression of any one of these genes (but not usually more than one in a given pathway). Depending on where the pathway is activated, blockade of that signaling trunk route by a single molecular therapeutic, such as Drug A or Drug B, could inhibit the pathway and block malignancy. For example, if the pathway is activated at the top of the signaling cascade (e.g., at Gene A, which might encode an RTK), then Drug A or B would each be active on its own. Conversely, if the pathway is activated further downstream at Gene D, then Drug D would be active but Drug A would not. Consider now the lower scenario (Fig. 2, number 2), in which the particular malignancy is driven by two oncogenic mission-critical signaling pathways. The first one is the same as that already described. The second one comprises the products of Genes E through H. Let us suppose that we have Drug G, which acts at the level of Gene G in the pathway. This will block the pathway if it is activated at Genes E, F, or G, but not if it is activated at Gene H. If there is no redundancy and both mission-critical pathways are essential to maintain the malignant state, then blocking either pathway A→D or pathway E→H will be sufficient to inhibit the tumor. If malignancy can be maintained by either pathway, then both oncogenic trunk routes will need to be blocked for sustained therapeutic success. Clearly, a combination of Drug G with either Drug A or Drug B would be much more efficacious than any one agent alone.

Of course, this illustration is a deliberately simplistic approach. Many more pathways are usually involved; moreover, cross-communication, feedback loops, and the like provide further complexity. Nevertheless, the overall message remains the same: although hitting a single molecular target could be useful in some cases, in other instances a combinatorial therapeutic attack on several targets is required.

Clearly, there are many possible scenarios. Although it is useful to conduct "thought experiments" of the type described here, it is also important to test our theoretical therapeutic "what if?" models against the emerging clinical data. So, what have we learned from our clinical experience with molecular therapeutics about the probable value of targeting a single oncogenic lesion vs multiple cancer-causing loci in human cancer?

Gleevec may be seen as a role model for molecular cancer therapeutics (13). Its inhibitory activity against the tyrosine kinases encoded by the bcr-abl and kit oncogenes clearly accounts for its undoubted therapeutic activity against chronic myeloid leukemia (CML) and gastrointestinal stromal tumors (GIST), respectively. On the other hand, although Gleevec has excellent activity against the early form of CML, it is much less active in the acute and blast phases of the disease. Evidence suggests that, perhaps unusually, bcr-abl may be the sole genetic abnormality that drives early-phase CML, whereas additional oncogenic defects participate in the later phases. In addition, acquired resistance is also being reported in patients treated with Gleevec, often because of mutation of the active site of the kinase enzyme (13). In both cases, combination treatments could offer significant advantages over single-agent Gleevec.

The humanized MAb Herceptin clearly provides therapeutic value in a subset of breast cancer patients by targeting the product of the erbB2 oncogene that is overexpressed in approx 30% of patients (14). Its activity is especially impressive when used in combination with cytotoxic chemotherapy. However, the improved responses are limited, and the cardiotoxicity of anthracycline-based treatments is increased by Herceptin. Additional oncogenic abnormalities are likely to contribute to malignancy in breast cancer, and targeting these genomic abnormalities alongside Herceptin therapy would offer greater patient benefit.

The third example is Iressa, a small-molecule inhibitor of tyrosine kinase activity of the epidermal growth factor receptor (EGFR), the product of the erbB1 oncogene that is overexpressed in a range of human cancers and mutated in some of them (14). Iressa has shown significant single-agent activity in such tumors, including head and neck, hormone-refractory prostate, and non-small-cell lung cancer (NSCLC). However, randomized trials with Iressa in combination with cytotoxic chemotherapy in NSCLC show no advantage for the inclusion of Iressa (15,16). There are many possible reasons for the disappointing results of the combination trials. However, as with Herceptin, it seems likely that targeting additional genes involved in driving the malignant phenotype would offer further therapeutic benefit.

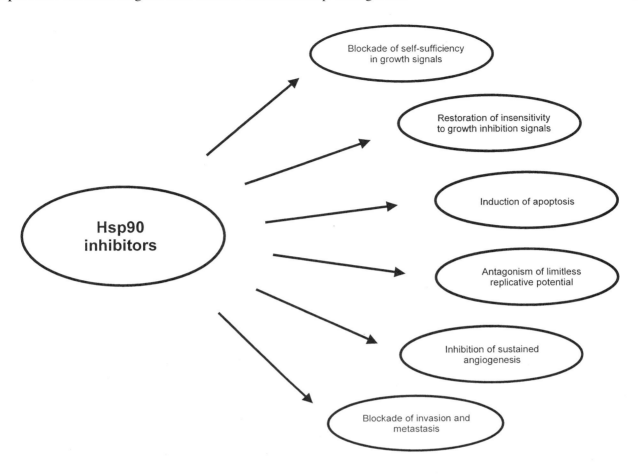

Fig. 3. HSP90 inhibitors have the potential to provide simultaneous pharmacological modulation of all six hallmark traits of the malignant phenotype, as defined by Hanahan and Weinberg *(19)*.

In summary, although there are many potential explanations and insufficient mechanistic data, the emerging clinical results with the first generation of molecular therapeutics suggests that combination treatments that attack different oncogenic targets could offer greater therapeutic utility compared to monotherapy with such agents or to combinations involving molecular-targeted monotherapy plus cytotoxic drugs.

If this thesis is correct, optimal combinatorial therapies of the future must await a complete molecular pathological description of cancer and development of agents that target every significant oncogenic abnormality, which will take some time. For now, clinicians will combine the emerging molecular therapeutics with each other, or with cytotoxics, in cocktails based to some degree on our existing understanding of multistep oncogenesis, or based on empirical combination

data from preclinical models that may or may not be predictive of the clinic. Perhaps more often, such combinations may be selected for even more pragmatic clinical reasons, such as lack of overlapping toxicities.

3. HSP90 INHIBITORS: KILLING MULTIPLE ONCOGENIC BIRDS WITH ONE THERAPEUTIC STONE

HSP90 is a molecular chaperone whose biological role involves maintaining the correct folding, conformation, and functional activity of a finite range of proteins known as clients *(17,18)*. Ubiquitously expressed and representing about 1–2% cellular protein, HSP90 may not at first seem to be an obvious target for anticancer agents in the new millennium. It does not appear to be an oncogene *per se*. But, in fact, its role in the biology of a range of oncogene products confers upon HSP90

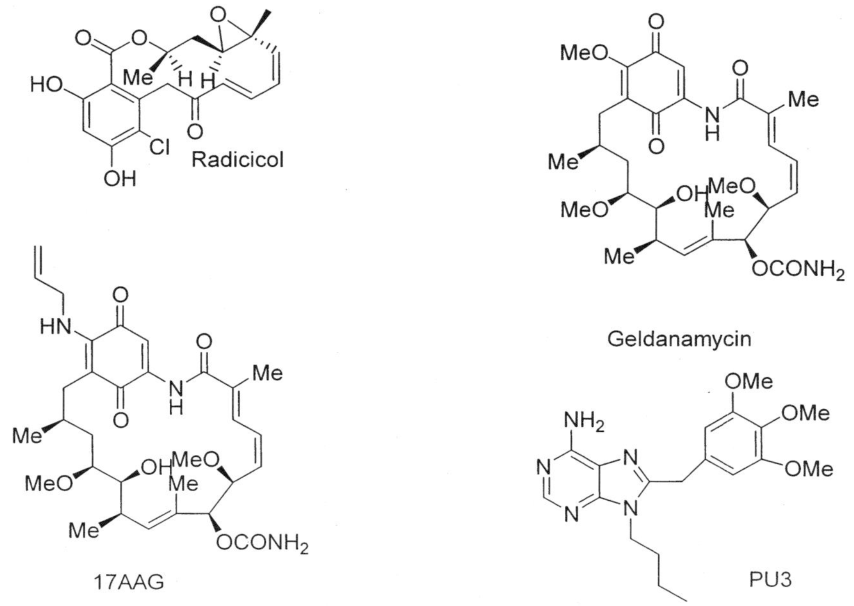

Fig. 4. Chemical structures of selected HSP90 inhibitors.

inhibitors the potential to blockade most key oncogenic signaling routes in cancer cells, including the mission-critical pathways (17,18). Thus, HSP90 inhibition could provide a means of killing multiple oncogenic birds with one therapeutic stone, and could potentially block six hallmark traits of malignancy (19) across a broad range of cancers (17); (Fig. 3).

The HSP90 family comprises four members: HSP90α, HSP90β, the endoplasmic reticulum counterpart GRP94, and the mitochondrial homolog TRAP1 (17). Although HSP90 is a stress-response protein, it plays a key role in the cell under normal physiological conditions, and does not act as a generic chaperone. Instead, it is involved in the relatively late stages of folding proteins, including a large number of oncogene products—particularly kinases associated with malignancy (17), most notably including ErbB2, Raf-1, CDK4, Polo-1, and Met. Additional HSP90 clients include mutant p53; HIF-1α; estrogen, androgen, and glucocorticoid receptors; and last but not least, the catalytic component of telomerase hTERT. Inhibition of HSP90 results in incomplete folding and stabilization of client proteins, leading to their elimination from the cell by the ubiquitin proteasome degradation pathway.

This simultaneous depletion of many important oncogenic client proteins confers upon HSP90 inhibitors the potential—as a downstream consequence—to provide a combinatorial blockade of multistep oncogenesis

although they act quite selectively on a single proximal molecular target. Interestingly, the groundbreaking work of Lindquist and colleagues in yeast, flies, and *Aridopsis* has shown that HSP90 acts as a capacitor of morphological evolution and phenotypic variation by preventing or buffering the phenotypic expression of mutations in the absence of stress conditions. Inhibition of HSP90 by genetic or pharmacological means removes the buffer and allows the mutations to be expressed phenotypically (20,21). Thus, one may speculate that treatment of cancer cells with an HSP90 inhibitor might reveal multiple mutations that could otherwise be hidden in the cells. Furthermore, such mutations expressed in combination with others may be damaging to the cancer cell, an effect known as synthetic lethality. Since the presence of chromosomal damage is probably the major feature that distinguishes cancer cells from normal cells, the induction of synthetic lethal effects has been seen as a highly desirable potential therapeutic approach to tumor-selective therapy (3).

3.1. 17-AAG: The First-in-Class HSP90 Inhibitor

Experience has shown that not all attractive targets are actually pharmaceutically amenable to therapeutic modulation by a small drug-like molecule. Confidence that a target is likely to be amenable to small-molecule intervention can sometimes be provided by natural products. In the case of HSP90, two classes of natural product that were already known to be bioactive, and indeed to have anticancer activity, turned out to act primarily as HSP90 inhibitors. These were the ansamycin antibiotics, such as the herbimycins and geldanamycin, and the structurally different compound radicicol (17). The chemical structures of some geldanamycins and of radicicol are shown in Fig. 4.

Geldanamycin was isolated from actinomycete broths more than thirty years ago (22). It was subsequently shown to reverse morphological transformation induced in fibroblasts by introduction of the v-*src* oncogene (23), as a result of which it was believed to act as a tyrosine kinase inhibitor. However, subsequent studies showed that the primary cellular target of geldanamycin was indeed HSP90 (24). This was confirmed by X-ray crystallography studies, which determined that geldanamycin binds to the *N*-terminal domain of the chaperone and docks into the nucleotide-binding pocket normally occupied by adenosine 5' triphosphate/adenosine 5' diphosphae (ATP/ADP) (25,26). This leads to inhibition of the ATPase activity that is essential for the chaperone function of HSP90 (27).

Geldanamycin has exhibited anticancer activity in cell culture and animal models, and was under investigation as a potential clinical development candidate (28,29). Development was halted because it exhibited liver toxicity with an insufficient therapeutic index (29). A large number of geldanamycin analogs have been evaluated (30,31). For reasons that are not clear, the analog 17-allylamino, 17-demethoxygeldanamycin (17-AAG; Fig. 3) is less hepatotoxic, but retains the same mechanism of action (32) and shows good antitumor activity in human tumor xenografts at doses that are well-tolerated (33).

17-AAG has undergone formulation and toxicity studies under the auspices of the US National Cancer Institute (NCI), and subsequently entered clinical trials as the first-in-class HSP90 inhibitor sponsored by the NCI and Cancer Research UK (formerly Cancer Research Campaign). These trials are discussed later in this chapter.

3.1.1. CELLULAR EFFECTS OF 17-AAG

A number of studies have shown that 17-AAG causes depletion of client proteins (e.g., 32–37). For example, our own work has demonstrated depletion of Raf-1 and also of the Akt/protein kinase B (PKB), leading to simultaneous blockade of both the ERK1/2 MAP kinase pathway and the PI3K pathway, as measured by

reduced phosphorylation of ERK1/2 and Akt/PKB in the cell (37). Thus, two of the mission-critical pathways that cancer cells require for proliferation and survival are blocked in a combinatorial manner. In addition, the cyclin-dependent kinase CDK4 is also depleted, thereby affecting cell-cycle control. Interestingly, the dependence on time of exposure and concentration of 17-AAG varies fairly consistently between the different client proteins, presumably reflecting, at least in part, the rate of degradation and resynthesis of each individual client. Some differences can also be noted when comparing results in various cell lines (36,37).

There is also some consistent variation between different cell lines in terms of the cellular outcome of treatment with 17-AAG. For example, some cases in our own studies in human colon cancer cell lines showed morphological evidence of mitotic arrest, supported by an accumulation in G_2M phase as measured by flow cytometry; other cell lines had no G_2M block but rather a G_1 arrest (36,37). Similarly, apoptosis was observed in some lines but not others. Differentiation induced by geldanamycins has also been reported in breast cancer-cell lines (34,35). The mechanisms responsible for these differences have not been determined, but they may relate to the interactions between client protein depletion and the cell-cycle checkpoint status of the cancer cell. It has been suggested that G_1 arrest may be RB-dependent in breast cancer-cell lines (34,35), but this simple relationship does not appear to hold true in colon cancer-cell lines (36,37). For a more detailed discussion of possible mechanisms, *see* ref. *17*. Further work is required to elucidate the factors downstream of client-protein depletion that determine how a particular cell will respond to 17-AAG and other HSP90 inhibitors.

3.1.2. GENES INVOLVED IN SENSITIVITY TO 17-AAG

We have used cDNA microarrays to profile the changes in global gene-expression patterns of cancer-cell lines in response to HSP90 inhibition (36). The objective was to gain a better understanding of the molecular mechanism of action of these agents, and also to identify pharmacodynamic markers that could be used in clinical trials. Interestingly, no changes in the mRNA for client proteins were observed. Thus, following depletion of client proteins, there appears to be no feedback loop that results in increased expression of the cognate genes. The most consistent change seen on the gene-expression microarrays was upregulation of the mRNA for HSP70, an effect that has also been consistently observed at the protein level by several groups. Like HSP90, HSP70 is a heat shock protein and molecular chaperone. Its expression is known to be regulated via the transcription factor heat shock factor 1 (HSF1) *(38)*. HSP70 is believed to exert anti-apoptotic effects by blocking both assembly of the apoptosome and initiation of the caspase cascade. Thus, it is interesting to speculate that one of the consequences of HSP70 induction by HSP90 inhibitors may be to protect to some extent against the induction of apoptosis *(17)*.

A particularly fascinating observation seen during our gene-expression profiling studies was the cell line-dependent response of HSP90 itself at the mRNA level following treatment with 17-AAG *(36)*. Thus, HCT116 human colon cancer cells had a significant increase in mRNA levels for HSP90α, the major form expressed in cancer-cell lines. In contrast, the HT29 human colon cancer-cell line did not show an increase in HSP90α mRNA. At the protein level, a similar increase was seen for HSP90 in HCT116 cells, whereas a decrease was actually seen for HT29. On the basis of these results, it is tempting to speculate that the way in which the cell responds in terms of expressing the gene for the HSP90 target may be an important factor in sensitivity to the drug. In support of this, HCT116 cells do appear to recover more rapidly from treatment with 17-AAG, whereas HT29 cells recover less quickly and are more sensitive to the drug. In the microarray study, we also noted that genes that encode keratin 8, keratin 18, and caveolin-1 were deregulated in a cell line-dependent manner in response to 17-AAG *(36)*. The expression of these genes is controlled by the Ras-Raf-MEK-ERK1/2 signaling pathway, so it is possible that the effects of 17-AAG on this pathway may play a role in their deregulation. Notably, the changes in caveolin-1 expression were validated at the protein level.

We observed in a follow-up study in the same panel of human colon cancer-cell lines that one of the lines did not undergo apoptosis in response to 17-AAG *(37)*. This line (KM12), in contrast to the others that were able to undergo apoptosis in response to 17-AAG, expressed high levels of the anti-apoptotic Bag-1 protein and failed to express the pro-apoptotic Bax protein. Levels of Bad were similar across the panel; rather surprisingly, 17-AAG had no effect on the phosphorylation status of Bad. Although these findings highlight interesting areas for future study, it is important to avoid overinterpretation of such correlative findings. Using gene transfection and siRNA to modulate the expression of genes that are suspected of being involved in sensitivity to HSP90 inhibitors, experiments will be carried out to investigate cause-and-effect relationships more rigorously.

Gene-transfer experiments have been in our laboratory to evaluate the mechanistic effects of two genes identified from correlative and other observations as potential factors in sensitivity to HSP90 inhibition. In the first of these, transfection of the gene that encodes quinone reductase NQO1 (DT-diaphorase) was found to have a major sensitizing effect toward 17-AAG (but not toward its principal 17-amino metabolite or to geldanamycin) *(33)*. This observation is being followed up, since human tumors are known to exhibit major differences in DT-diaphorase; there is also a fairly common polymorphism that leads to a loss of enzyme activity *(39)*.

In another set of transfection experiments, the effects of transfer of the gene encoding the client protein ErbB2 into ovarian cancer cells was investigated *(40)*. Overexpression was associated with increased motility, thereby demonstrating the functional activity of the transfected gene product. Interestingly, overexpression of ErbB2, which occurs naturally in some ovarian tumors as well as many other cancers, was associated with a statistically significant fivefold increase in sensitivity to geldanamycin. However, this was not seen with 17-AAG, although there was also an insignificant twofold increase in sensitivity to radicicol. The implications of these findings require further investigation.

Overall, there are likely to be a number of genes that influence the sensitivity of the cell to 17-AAG and other HSP90 inhibitors. Furthermore, changes in gene expression in response to 17-AAG may provide valuable pharmacodynamic markers for use in clinical trials. For instance, we have validated a molecular signature of HSP90 inhibition that appears to be robust and reproducible. This molecular signature represents an increase in levels of HSP70 protein expression and a simultaneous decrease in the expression of the client proteins Raf-1 and CDK *(36)*. This signature appears to be applicable to various cells and tissues *(41)*. In peripheral-blood lymphocytes, a decrease in Src family member LCK, another client protein, is also a useful biomarker of HSP90 inhibition. A decrease in ErbB2 can also provide a sensitive pharmacodynamic readout for tumors that express this particular client protein.

Table 1

Potential Limitations of 17AAG

- Limited stability and complex formulation
- Modest potency against the HSP90 target
- Substrate for P-glycoprotein
- Activated by NQO1/DT-diaphorase
- Metabolism by polymorphic cytochrome P450
- Low oral bioavailability
- Limited therapeutic index

Ongoing gene-expression profiling has revealed more intriguing changes that have yet to be validated. In addition, we have collaborated with Professor Mike Waterfield's group (Ludwig Institute, University College, London) to carry out global proteomic profiling alongside the mRNA analysis. This has yielded valuable, complementary data that are also being followed up.

3.1.3. CLINICAL TRIALS WITH 17-AAG

As mentioned earlier in this chapter, 17-AAG has entered clinical trials as the first-in-class HSP90 inhibitor. Now nearing completion, these Phase I trials have not yet been published as full papers. However, several interim reports have appeared in abstract form (e.g., refs. *42–45*). The drug is given intravenously. Studied schedules include daily dosing for 5 d followed by a 3-wk gap; a weekly dosing schedule is also being investigated at our institution. Encouragingly, we have observed plasma levels above the IC_{50} for growth inhibition in cancer-cell lines. We have also seen changes in the molecular signature used to provide a pharmacodynamic readout in both peripheral-blood lymphocytes and tumor biopsies, and there is evidence of clinical benefit in some patients.

Clearly, the need for tumor biopsies in order to measure changes in biomarkers is a limitation in such studies. Because of this, we are working with our collaborators to identify minimally invasive pharmacodynamic readouts using positron emission tomography (PET; with Professor Pat Price and Dr. Eric Aboagye, Christie Hospital, Manchester and Hammersmith Hospital, London) or magnetic resonance spectroscopy/imaging (MRS/MRI; Professor Martin Leach and colleagues at our own institution/Royal Marsden Hospital and Professor John Griffiths and colleagues at St. George's Hospital Medical School, London, UK). To date, studies are promising. Using MRS in human tumor xenografts, we have observed an interesting and unusual increase in phosphoethanolamine and phosphocholine levels after treatment with 17-AAG *(46)*. These may reflect changes in membrane turnover, or even in lipid signaling. We are also carrying out experiments to pave the way for the use of appropriately labeled choline as a PET tracer *(47)*. The use of molecular and functional imaging has enormous potential for minimally invasive imaging of pharmacodynamics in new drug development *(48,49)*.

3.2. Prospects for New HSP90 Inhibitors

The emerging data suggest that 17-AAG shows promise as the first-in-class HSP90 inhibitor in the clinic. However, it does have some limitations that could be minimized in a follow-up compound. These are summarized in Table 1.

Of particular note, 17-AAG has limited solubility, and the current formulation is rather cumbersome. Ideally, the drug should not be used as a substrate for the P-glycoprotein efflux pump and the attentions of metabolizing enzymes that may introduce significant variability in pharmacokinetics, response, and toxicity. An orally bioavailable drug would provide greater scheduling opportunities, particularly for chronic use, and maximizing the therapeutic window makes good sense.

A number of approaches can be taken to help attain this improved drug profile. Various derivatives of 17AAG or geldanamycin could be evaluated. One of these is 17-dimethylaminoethylamino-17-demethoxygeldanamycin (17-DMAG, NSC 707545) which is more soluble than 17-AAG and has potentially superior antitumor activity *(50)*. The radicicol structure could also be explored further (Fig. 4). Purine-based compounds designed to compete with ATP in the *N*-terminal domain of HSP90 have been described *(51,52)*. For example, PU3 (Fig. 4) has been shown to inhibit HSP90 in cancer cells, and to block cell growth. Another compound, novobiocin, has been reported to inhibit HSP90 *(18)*. A high-throughput screen designed to find inhibitors of the ATPase activity of HSP90 has been reported *(53)*. Use of the so-called TRAP assay (target-related affinity profiling) to identify new HSP90 inhibitors has also been described *(54)*.

3.3. Current Issues with the Development of HSP90 Inhibitors

Clearly, we are still at an early stage with HSP90 inhibitors, but they do show significant promise, par-

Table 2

**Some Current Issues And Challenges
with HSP90 Inhibitors**

- What is the optimal treatment regime?
- How to use the drug as a single agent?
- How to use the drug in combination with cytotoxics
  —e.g., paclitaxel and platinum drugs?
- Will any tumor types be particularly sensitive?
- Are any particular client proteins especially important
  for response in certain tumor settings?
- Will particular genomic abnormalities predispose
  to sensitivity or resistance?

---

ticularly in their potential to provide a unified approach to the issue of combinatorial oncogenesis. A number of questions and challenges remain; some of these are listed in Table 2.

In particular, we need to understand how to use these agents optimally, and to reach a better comprehension of exactly how they work in different settings. As mentioned, one of the most attractive features of HSP90 inhibitors is their potential for single-agent activity. Nevertheless, practical concerns make it likely that even these agents will be evaluated in combination. That may be desirable, or even necessary, either because blockade of certain pathways is incomplete or because of the potential for resistance mechanisms to develop. In addition, since 17-AAG exerts predominantly a cytostatic rather than an overt cytotoxic effect, the addition of cytotoxic chemotherapy could provide the opportunity for cytoreduction and regression, alongside long-term maintenance therapy provided by HSP90 inhibition. Furthermore, there is also the possibility of using HSP90 inhibitors deliberately to potentiate the effects of cytotoxic chemotherapy or to overcome resistance to conventional therapy, an approach that is being evaluated with other signal-transduction inhibitors. Laboratory studies are already underway; certain schedules involving combinations of 17-AAG with paclitaxel have been reported to show promise (35). We have also found combinations of 17-AAG with platinum drugs to be effective in cell-culture studies (55).

3.4. HSP90 Inhibitors in the Chemoprevention Setting

Initial trials with 17-AAG are aimed at patients with advanced disease. It has been proposed that HSP90 inhibitors may be particularly effective when multiple genetic abnormalities are involved in maintaining the malignant state or in driving tumor progression in late-stage disease. However, it seems probable that HSP90 inhibitors could also find utility in the chemoprevention setting.

It is clear that HSP90 is required for maintenance of the transformed phenotype. HSP90 is overexpressed in cancer cells (17). This may be an early response to stress induced by the adverse environment of the cancer cells, or to allow cell survival in the presence of unbalanced signaling associated with mutation or deregulated expression of oncogenes (56). For example, it has been shown that transformation by the H-ras oncogene is reduced in mouse embryo fibroblasts (MEFs) from Hsf-1 knockout mice as compared to MEFs from wild-type littermates (56). In addition, geldanamycin was found to reduce transformation by H-ras in the same system. Furthermore, it was reported many years ago that geldanamycin was able to block transformation of rat embryo cells by the carcinogen 3-methylcholanthrene (57).

Also relevant to the potential use of HSP90 inhibitors in chemoprevention or early-stage disease is the ability of HSP90 to act as a buffer against genetic mutation (20,21). Thus HSP90 may allow both early- and late-stage cancer cells to tolerate the abnormal deregulation of proliferation and survival pathways that would otherwise trigger a lethal effect. Therapeutic intervention at an early stage with HSP90 inhibitors could also block the initial transforming event, as well as the subsequent emergence of multiple oncogenic abnormalities.

Another potential advantage of early treatment with HSP90 inhibitors is that it could prevent development of drug-resistant cells. Interestingly, using the standard approach of continuous exposure to incremental concentrations of 17-AAG, we have found it extremely difficult to induce resistance to 17-AAG itself in cultured cancer cells (A. Maloney and P. Workman, unpublished data). This may be because simultaneous blockade of multiple signal-transduction pathways is able to prevent resistance from arising via activation of alternative survival pathways when the primary oncogenic and antiapoptotic lesion is blocked.

Aside from their uses in a chemoprevention setting, HSP90 inhibitors could also find a role in various non-malignant diseases involving HSP90 client proteins, or situations in which stress responses (e.g., stroke, heart attack) or protein misfolding/aggregation (e.g., scrapie,

Creutzfeldt-Jakob disease, Huntington's chorea, and Alzheimer's disease) are responsible for the condition.

4. CONCLUSION

The field of molecular cancer therapeutics offers remarkable potential for solving the problem of multistep, combinatorial oncogenesis in cancer *(58)*. It has been established that drugs such as Gleevec, Herceptin and Iressa can show clinical benefit. It seems likely that we can do even better by paying greater attention to the particular combination of deregulated genes, proteins, and pathways that drive a given cancer in an individual patient, and then targeting the treatment or prevention strategy accordingly with combinations of individual molecular therapeutic agents as they emerge. In addition, HSP90 inhibitors show early promise for use as single agents with which to attack multistep oncogenesis *(60)*. In addition to their use in advanced malignancy, there is a good rationale and preliminary data to support a role for the use of HSP90 inhibitors in early stage disease, and potentially in a chemoprevention setting.

ACKNOWLEDGMENTS

The work of the author and the Centre for Cancer Therapeutics (http:/www.icr.ac.uk/cctherap/index.html) is funded by a core grant (C309/A2984) from Cancer Research UK (http://www.cancerresearchuk.org). The author is also a Cancer Research UK Life Fellow. I thank the members of the Signal Transduction and Molecular Pharmacology Team and my other colleagues and co-workers in the Centre and elsewhere for their collaboration and stimulating discussions. I also thank Dr. Ted McDonald and colleagues for Fig. 4.

REFERENCES

1. Workman P. Scoring a bull's-eye against genome targets. *Curr Opin Pharmacol* 2001;1:342–352.
2. Workman P. Changing times: developing drugs in genomeland. *Curr Opin Investig Drugs* 2001;2:1128–1135.
3. Reddy A, Kaelin WG. Using cancer genetics to guide the selection of anticancer drug targets. *Curr Opin Pharmacol* 2002;2:366–373.
4. Venter JC, Adams MD, Myers EW, et al. The sequence of the human genome. *Science* 2001;291:1304–1351.
5. International Human Genome Sequencing Consortium. Initial sequencing and analysis of the human genome. *Nature* 2001;409:860–921.
6. Davies H, Bignell GR, Cox C, et al. Mutations of the *BRAF* gene in human cancer. *Nature* 2001;417:949–954.
7. Workman P and Kaye SB (eds.) A Trends Guide to Cancer Therapeutics. *Trends Mol Med* 2002;8:S1–S73.
8. Mills GB, Lu Y, Kohn EC. Linking molecular therapeutics to molecular diagnostics: Inhibition of the FRAP/RAFT/TOR component of the PI3K pathway preferentially blocks PTEN mutant cells *in vitro* and *in vivo*. *Proc Natl Acad Sci USA* 2001;98:10,031–10,033.
9. Ponder BA. Cancer genetics. *Nature* 2002;411:336–341.
10. Volgestein B, Kinzler K. The multiple nature of cancer. *Trends Genet* 1993;9:138–141.
11. Evan GI, Vousden KH. Proliferation, cell cycle and apoptosis in cancer research. *Nature* 2001;411:342–348.
12. Weinstein IB. Addiction to oncogenes. *Science* 2002;297:63–64.
13. Druker BJ. STI571 (Gleevec) as a paradigm for cancer therapy. *Trends Mol Med* 2001;8:4 (Suppl):S14–S18.
14. De Bono J, Rowinsky EK. The ErbB receptor family: a therapeutic target for cancer. *Trends Mol Med* 2001;4 (Suppl): S19–S26.
15. Giaconne G, Johnson DH, Manegold C, et al. A Phase III clinical trial of ZD1839 ('Iressa') in combination with gemacitabine and cisplatin in chemotherapy-naive patients with advanced non-small cell lung cancer (INTACT I). *Ann Oncol* 2002;13 Suppl 5:40.
16. Johnson DH, Herbst R, Giacoone G, et al. ZD1839 (Iressa) in combination with paclitaxel & carboplatin in chemotherapy-naive patients with advanced non-small cell lung cancer (NSCLC): results from a Phase III trial (INTACT 2). *Ann Oncol* 2002;13 Suppl 5: 4680.
17. Maloney A, Workman P. HSP90 as a new therapeutic target for cancer therapy: the story unfolds. *Expert Opin Biol Ther* 2002;2:3–24.
18. Neckers L. Hsp90 inhibitors as novel cancer chemotherapeutic agents. *Trends Mol Med* 2001;8:S55–S61.
19. Hanahan D, Weinberg RA. The hallmarks of cancer. *Cell* 2000;100:57–70.
20. Rutherford LI, Lindquist S. Hsp90 as a capacitator for morphological evolution. *Nature* 1998;396:336–342.
21. Queitshc C, Sangster TA, Linquist S. Hsp90 as a capacitor variation. *Nature* 2002;417:618–624.
22. DeBoer C, Meulman PA, Wnuk RJ, Peterson DH. Geldanamycin, a new antibiotic. *J Antibiot* 1970;23:442–447.
23. Uehara U, Hori M, Takeuchi T, Umezawa H. Phenotypic change from transformed to normal induced by benzoquinoid ansamycins accompanies inactivation of p60src in rat kidney cells infected with Rous sarcoma virus. *Mol Cell Biol* 1986;6:2198–2206.
24. Whitesell L, Mimnaugh EG, Decosta B, et al. Inhibition of heat shock protein HSP90-pp60-src heteroprotein complex formation by benzoquinone ansamycins: essential role for stress proteins in oncogenic transformation. *Proc Natl Acad Sci USA* 1994;91:8324–8328.
25. Prodromou C, Roe SM, O'Brien R, et al. Identification and structural characterization of the ATP/ADP-binding site in the Hsp90 molecular chaperone. *Cell* 1997;90:65–75.

26. Stebbins CE, Russo AA, Schneider C, et al. Crystal structure of an Hsp90-geldanamycin complex: targeting of a protein chaperone by an antitumor agent. *Cell* 1997;89:239–250.

27. Prodromou C, Panaretou B, Chohan S et al. The ATPase cycle of Hsp90 drives a molecular 'clamp' via transient dimerization of the N-terminal domains. *EMBO J* 2000;19:4383–4392.

28. Brunton VG, Steele G, Lewis AD, Workman P. Geldanamycin-induced toxicity in human colon-cancer cell lines: evidence against the involvement of c-Src or DT-diaphorase. *Cancer Chemother Pharmacol* 1998;41:417–422.

29. Supko JG, Hickman RL, Grever MR, Malspeis L. Preclinical pharmacologic evaluation of geldanamycin as an antitumour agent. *Cancer Chemother Pharmacol* 1995;36:305–310.

30. Schnur RC, Corman ML, Gallascun RJ, et al. Inhibition of the oncogene product p185erbB2 in vitro and in vivo by geldanamycin and dihydrogeldanamycin derivatives. *J Med Chem* 1995;38:3806–3812.

31. Schnur RC, Corman ML, Gallascun RJ, et al. ErbB2 oncogene inhibition by geldanamycin derivatives: synthesis, mechanism of action, and structure-activity relationships. *J Med Chem* 1995;38:3813–3820.

32. Schulte TW, Neckers LM. The benzoquinone ansamycin 17-allylamino-17-deemthoxygeldanamcyin binds to HSP90 and shares important biologic activities with geldanamycin. *Cancer Chemother Pharmacol* 1998;42:273–279.

33. Kelland L, Sharp S, Rogers P, et al. DT-diaphorase expression and tumour cell sensitivity to 17-allylamino, 17-demethoxygeldanamycin, and inhibitor of heat shock protein 90. *J Natl Cancer Inst* 1999;91:1940–1949.

34. Strethapakdi M, Liu F, Tavorath R, Rosen N. Inhibition of Hsp90 function by ansamycins causes retinoblastoma gene product-dependent G1 arrest. *Cancer Res* 2000;60:3940–3946.

35. Munster PN, Basso A, Solit D, et al. Modulation of Hsp90 function by ansamycins sensitises breast cancer cells to chemotherapy-induced apoptosis in an RB-and schedule-dependent manner. *Clin Cancer Res* 2001;7:2228–2236.

36. Clarke P, Hostein I, Banerji U, et al. Gene expression profiling of human colon cancer cells following inhibition of signal transduction by 17-allylamno-17demethoxygeldanamycin, an inhibitor of hsp90 molecular chaperone. *Oncogene* 2000;19:4125–4133.

37. Hostein I, Robertson D, Di Stefano F, et al. Inhibition of signal transduction by the Hsp90 inhibitor 17-allylamino-17-demethoxygeldanamycin results in cytostasis and apoptosis. *Cancer Res* 2001;61:4003–4009.

38. Morimoto RI. Regulation of the heat shock transcriptional response: cross talk between a family of heat shock factors, molecular chaperones, and negative regulators. *Genes Dev* 1998;12:3788–3796.

39. Fitzsimmons SA, Workman P, Grever M, et al. Reductase enzyme expression across the National Cancer Institute tumour cell line panel: correlation with sensitivity to mitomycin C and EO9. *J Natl Cancer Inst* 1996;88:259–269.

40. Smith V, Hobbs S, Court W, et al. ErbB2 overexpression in an ovarian cancer cell line confers sensitivity to the HSP90 inhibitor geldanamycin. *Anticancer Res* 2002;22:1993–2000.

41. Banerji U, Walton M, Raynaud F, et al. Validation of pharmacodynamic endpoints for the Hsp90 molecular chaperone inhibitor 17-allylamino 17-demethoxygeldanamycin (17AAG) in a human tumor xenograft model. *Proc Am Assoc Cancer Res* 2001;42:4473.

42. Wilson RH, Takimoto CH, Agnew EB et al. Phase I pharmacologic study of 17-(Allylamino)-17-demethoxygeldanamycin (AAG) in adult patients with advanced solid tumors. *Proc Am Soc Clin Oncol* 2001;20:325.

43. Banerji U, O'Donnell A, Scurr M et al. Phase I trial of the heat shock protein 90 (HSP90) inhibitor 17-allylamino-17-demethoxy-geldanamycin (17AAG). Pharmacokinetic (PK) profile and pharmacodynamic (PD) endpoints. *Proc Am Soc Clin Oncol* 2001;20:326.

44. Munster PN, Tong W, Schwartz L, et al. Phase I trial of 17-(allylamino)-17-demethoxygeldanamycin (17-AAG) in patients (Pts) with advanced solid malignancies. *Proc Am Soc Clin Oncol* 2001;20:327.

45. Erlichman C, Toft D, Reid J, et al. A Phase I trial of 17-allyl-amino-geldanamycin in patients with advanced cancer. *Proc Am Assoc Cancer Res* 2001;42:4474.

46. Chung YL, Troy H, Banerji U, et al. The pharmacodynamic effects of 17-AAG on HT29 xenografts in mice monitored by magnetic resonance spectroscopy. *Proc Am Assoc Cancer Res* 2002;43:73, abstr 371.

47. Lui D, Hutchinson OC, Osman S, et al. Use of radiolabelled choline as a pharmacodynamic marker for the signal transduction inhibitor geldanamycin. *Br J Cancer* 2002;87:783–789.

48. Workman P. Challenges of PK/PD measurements in modern drug development. *Eur J Cancer* 2002;38:2189–2193.

49. Workman P. How much gets there and what does it do? The need for better pharmacokinetic and pharmacodynamic endpoints in contemporary drug discovery and development. *Curr Pharm Des* 2003;9:891–902.

50. Smith V, Sausville EA, Camalier RF, et al. 17-DMAG (NSC 707545), a water soluble geldanamycin analog, has superior *in vitro* and *in vivo* activity compared to the HSP90 inhibitor 17-AAG. *Eur J Cancer* 2002;38:S60, abs. 189.

51. Chiosis G, Timaul MN, Lucas B, et al. A small molecule designed to bind to the adenine nucleotide pocket of HSP90 causes Her2 degradation and the growth arrest and differentiation of breast cancer cells. *Chem Biol* 2001;8:289–299.

52. Chiosis G, Huezo H, Lucas B, Rosen N. Development of a purine-based novel class of Hsp90 binders that inhibit the proliferation of cancer cells and induce the degradation of Her2 tyrosine kinase. *Bioorg Med Chem* 2002;10:3555–3564.

53. Rowlands MG, Newbatt YM, Turlais F, et al. High throughput screening assay for inhibitors of heat-shock protein 90 ATPase activity. *Clin Cancer Res* 2001;7:3749s, abst 475.

54. Beroza P, Meng F, Bears DJ, et al. Efficient discovery of novel small molecule cancer drugs using Telik's target-related affinity profiling (TRAP^(tm)) technology. *Proc Am Assoc Cancer Res* 2002;43:37, abst 191.

55. Banerji U, Walton M, Judson P, Workman P. Combination of the heat shock protein 90 (HSP90) chaperone inhibitor

17-allylamino, 17-demethoxygeldanamycin (17AAG) and conventional cytotoxic agents in an ovarian cancer cell line model. *Eur J Cancer* 2002;38:S52 abst 161.

56. Whitesell L, Bagatell R, Falsey R. The stress response: implications for the clinical development of Hsp90 inhibitors. *Current Drug Targets* 2003;3:349–358.

57. Price PJ, Sk WA, Skeen PC, et al. Geldanamycin inhibition of 3-methylcholantrene-induced rat embryo cell transformation. *Proc Soc Exp Biol Med* 1977;155:461–463.

58. Workman P. The opportunities and challenges of personalized genome-based molecular theropies for cancer: targets, technologies and molecular chaperones. *Cancer Chemother Pharmacol* 2003;52:S45–S60.

59. Workman V. Overview Translating Hsp 90 biology into Hsp 90 drugs. *Curr Canc. Drug Targets* 2003;3:297–300.

23 Therapeutic Strategies Targeting Polyamines

Debora L. Kramer, PhD and Eugene W. Gerner, PhD

CONTENTS

INTRODUCTION
BACKGROUND
TARGETING ODC IN CHEMOPREVENTION
CLINICAL CHEMOPREVENTION STUDIES WITH DFMO
ALTERNATIVE STRATEGIES TO REDUCE CELLULAR POLYAMINE POOLS
CONCLUSION
REFERENCES

1. INTRODUCTION

Although polyamines have been recognized as major biological entities for more than 50 yr, interest flourished when they were positively associated with cell growth. Both pharmacological *(1–3)* and genetic *(3–5)* studies demonstrated that they were essential for cell proliferation, and this attracted broad interest in their potential as a therapeutic target. Polyamines are ubiquitous, abundant, and loosely bound to multiple intracellular sites; therefore, identification of their role in cell proliferation has been an ongoing challenge. The recent definition of regulatory linkages between polyamine biosynthesis and specific oncogenic signaling networks including *c-myc* *(6)*, adenomatous polyposis coli *(APC)* *(7)*, and activated *ras (8)* provides important leads for meeting this challenge. Especially promising is the finding that ornithine decarboxylase (ODC), the key biosynthetic enzyme for polyamines, is transactivated by the proto-oncogene *c-myc (6)*. The additional finding that *c-myc* is upregulated by inactivation of the *APC* tumor suppressor gene *(9)* could, in turn, account for elevations in ODC activity during gastrointestinal (GI) carcinogenesis *(7)*. These linkages may explain why polyamine biosynthesis is typically higher in colorectal tumors than in surrounding normal mucosa *(10–14)*. This example suggests a role for polyamine biosynthesis among tumorigenic events required for dysregulated cell growth.

The association of enhanced polyamine biosynthesis with cell proliferation *(15)* led investigators at the Merrell Dow Research Institute (now Aventis Pharmaceuticals, Inc.) to develop biosynthetic inhibitors *(16–20)*. Of these, the irreversible ODC inhibitor α-diflouromethylornithine (DFMO, clinically known as eflornithine) *(18)* has emerged as an invaluable tool to study the role of polyamines in various cellular processes. DFMO proceeded to clinical trials based on its demonstrated ability to reduce tumor growth in preclinical model systems *(1)*. In these initial trials, the lack of obvious antitumor activity often sidelined DFMO as a chemotherapeutic agent *(1,19,21)*. Nevertheless, because of its low toxicity and preventive efficacy in carcinogenic model systems, DFMO has advanced as a chemopreventive agent. During the past decade, DFMO (licensed by ILEX Oncology) has been evaluated in more than a dozen Phase I and II chemopreventive trials *(see* Table 1) targeting epithelial cancers of the colon, skin, prostate, bladder, breast, and cervix. Although new therapeutic indications for DFMO continue to unfold, including its use as an FDA-approved topical cream to prevent growth of unwanted facial hair (marketed as Vaniqa™), alternate intervention strategies targeting polyamines are being developed *(see* Subheading 5).

2. BACKGROUND

Intracellular polyamines are maintained at millimolar levels in order to support growth *(15,22)*, differentiation *(23)*, and development *(3–5,24)*. They are flexible polycationic organic amines that bind electrostatically

From: Cancer Chemoprevention, Volume 1: Promising Cancer Chemoprevention Agents
Edited by: G. J. Kelloff, E. T. Hawk, and C. C. Sigman © Humana Press Inc., Totowa, NJ

Table 1

Cancer Prevention Trials with DFMO

Phase	Organ Site	DFMO Dose[1]	Duration(mo)	Reference
Pilot	Colon	3.0 g/m²/d	1	Boyle, 1992 (229)
IIA	Colon	De-escalation 0.5–0.075 g/m²/d	1	Meyskens, 1994 (88)
IIB	Colon	Randomized 0.2–0.4 g/m²/d	12	Meyskens, 1998 (89)
IIB	Colon	Randomized, placebo vs 0.5 g + 0.15 g Sulindac/d	36	Meyskens (in progress, http://clinicaltrials.gov/) (3)
II	Colon	Randomized, 0.5 g/m²/d	12	Love, 1998 (166)
II	Colon, FAP[2]	Randomized, Placebo vs 0.5 g/d + 200 mg Celecoxib bid	12	Sinicrope (in progress, http://clinicaltrials.gov/) (3)
I	Skin	Dose escalation 0.125–1.0 g/m²/d	1	Love, 1993 (195)
I	Skin	0.5 g/m²/day + Piroxicam	1	Carbone, 1998 (193)
II	Skin, Actinic Keratosis	Placebo-controlled, randomized, topical (10% cream)	6	Alberts, 2000 (92)
II	Skin, Actinic Keratosis	Placebo-controlled, randomized, topical (10% cream) ± Triamcinolone	6	Alberts (in progress, http://clinicaltrials.gov/) (3)
II	Esophagus	1.5 g/m²/d	3	Gerner, 1994 (170)
II	Prostate	Randomized, Placebo vs 0.5 g/d	12	Meyskens (in progress, http://clinicaltrials.gov/)
II	Prostate	Randomized, Placebo vs 0.5 g/d + 50 µg Casodex/d	1	Urban (in progress, http://clinicaltrials.gov/) (3)
II	Bladder	Randomized, 0.25–1.0 g/m²/d	12	Loprinzi, 1996 (230)
I	Cervix	De-escalation 1.0–0.25 g/m²/d	1	Mitchell, 1998 (93)
II	Breast	Randomized, 0.5 g/m²/d	6	Klemp, 2000 (231)

[1]Oral DFMO doses have been administered as a liquid and prescribed in units of g/m2/d. Note trials that are still in progress are prescribing DFMO in g/d. DFMO is now available in 250 mg tablets (ILEX Oncology, San Antonio, TX). Topical DFMO is prepared in a cream for application (92).

[2]FAP, familial adenomatous polyposis, an autosomal dominant inherited syndrome associated with high risk of colon and other cancers.

[3]Affiliations for trials in progress are as follow, F. Meyskens, UC-Irvine, CA; F. Sinicrope, MD Anderson, Houston, TX; D. Alberts, U. Arizona, Tucson, AZ; D. Urban, U. Alabama, Birmingham, AL.

to negatively charged macromolecules including nucleic acids, acidic proteins, and membranes (25). Examples of polyamine function include their ability to catalyze B- to Z-DNA transition (26,27), to alter triplex formation (28), and to stimulate DNA, RNA, and protein synthesis (3,29). Recently, Igarashi and colleagues (30) used binding constants to predict that 70–80% of the polyamines were complexed with RNA and that <30% remained unbound. This is consistent with our own findings that ~20% of the intracellular polyamine pools regulate their own biosynthesis (31) and transport (32), presumably because they are unbound. It has been difficult to determine the intracellular distribution of polyamines because their labile binding allows for redistribution during cellular disruption. One group used cytochalasin B to rapidly induce enucleation (33) and found that nuclei contained three-fold higher polyamine levels than the cytosol. Two rare examples of polyamines incorporating into macromolecules include the transglutaminase reaction in which they are crosslinked to peptides (34), and synthesis of initiating factor eIF-5A, during which spermidine (Spd) serves as a precursor for a hypusine modification (35).

Intracellular polyamine pools are maintained within a constant range through sensitively regulated homeostatic mechanisms that include polyamine biosynthesis, catabolism, transport, and export (Fig. 1). The various effectors that control each of these processes present

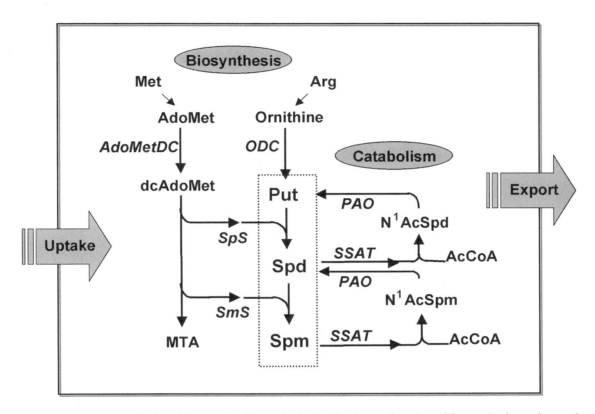

Fig. 1. Levels of intracellular Put, Spd, and Spm pools (shown in dashed box) are a function of four main determinants that include the following: uptake by a polyamine specific transporter (arrow in); biosynthesis by ODC, AdoMetDC, Spd synthase (SpS), and Spm synthase (SmS); catabolism by SSAT and PAO that also liberate H_2O_2 and 3-acetamidopropanal; and export (arrow out) of Put, Spd, Spm, and acetylated products (N[1]-AcSpd and N[1]-AcSpm). A supply of methionine (Met) and arginine (Arg) are required for synthesis of the two initial substrates AdoMet and ornithine, respectively.

opportunities to interfere with pool levels and cell growth. Of the three major mammalian polyamines, putrescine (Put) largely serves as a precursor to the higher polyamines, Spd is best able to support growth-related functions *(21,36–38),* and spermine (Spm) typically displays highest binding potential for most sites *(39)* and maintains viability in the absence of Put and Spd *(40,41).* These functional designations are not absolute because there is a certain level of redundancy among them; therefore, the greatest reduction of cell growth and viability is achieved when all three pools are depleted *(37,38,41).* Structure-activity studies show that structure is quite stringent for Spd and Spm function. For example, derivatives with single carbon increases or decreases in the intra-amine carbon bridges or ethylation of the terminal amines are unable to support cell growth or viability *(42–46).*

In general, the highest polyamine levels are found in highly metabolic (*e.g.*, liver and pancreas) and proliferative (*e.g.*, GI mucosa) tissues *(47).* One novelty

among tissues is that extremely high levels of Spm are produced in the prostate gland for secretion into the seminal fluid *(11,48).* Because of the unique physiology of the prostate gland, polyamine pools may be under the control of novel homeostatic mechanisms that could be selectively exploited in treating or preventing prostate carcinoma *(49–53).* In fact, one early clinical trial found that in patients with chronic prostatitis, DFMO treatment for 1 mo reduced pain and prostate size, and 50% remained disease-free for 3–6 mo *(54).*

2.1. Biosynthesis

Polyamine biosynthesis (Fig. 1) begins with arginine and methionine that are converted into ornithine and *S*-adenosylmethionine (AdoMet), respectively. In a step unique to polyamine biosynthesis, ornithine is decarboxylated by ODC to produce the four-carbon diamine, Put. Put activates AdoMet decarboxylase (AdoMetDC), leading to the synthesis of decarboxylated AdoMet. Both Spd and Spm synthase reactions utilize decarboxylated AdoMet to add an aminopropyl group onto Put to form Spd, and onto Spd to form Spm, respectively. Several comprehensive reviews detail these reactions (2,21,25). Both ODC and AdoMetDC are rate-limiting, and are characterized by short half-lives (t½ = <1 h) and high inducibility. Both proteins are negatively regulated by Spd and/or Spm at the level of translation (55,56), so that when pool sizes are in excess, the decarboxylase activities are low and vice versa. In addition, ODC is regulated by a polyamine-inducible protein known as antizyme that accelerates ODC proteosomal degradation by polyamine excess (57,58). Because polyamines are relatively stable molecules, the biosynthetic activity is low in non-proliferating cells. However, in proliferating cells, cell cycle-dependent increases in ODC and AdoMetDC activities are observed (3,11,23). Specific inhibitors have been developed to target the four biosynthetic enzymes (3,21,38), and the most effective antiproliferative inhibitors target either ODC (19) or AdoMetDC (20,37,59). Typically, ODC inhibitors decrease Put and Spd pools, but do not affect Spm pools (18). AdoMetDC inhibitors decrease Spd and Spm pools while causing high levels of Put accumulation. Thus, the greatest antiproliferative effect is achieved when both enzymes are inhibited to deplete both Spd and Spm pools without accumulating Put (37,41,60). When these inhibitors are used alone, the incomplete pool depletion may be responsible for their cytostatic rather than cytotoxic effects.

2.2. Catabolism

Polyamine biosynthesis is balanced through two key enzymes that compose the catabolic pathway (Fig. 1); (61,62). Spm is first acetylated by spermidine/spermine-N^1acetyltransferase (SSAT) and then oxidized by polyamine oxidase (PAO) to form Spd and stoichiometric amounts of 3-acetamidopropanal and hydrogen peroxide. Spd is similarly acted upon to form Put. With the ability to interconvert polyamines, the pathway has the potential to help normalize pool imbalances. For example, the catabolism of Spm can supply Spd for growth functions. In fact, blocking the oxidation of both acetylated products with a specific inhibitor of PAO (63,64) significantly enhanced the antitumor response to DFMO in animals (65–67). By comparison, PAO is in greater abundance with a longer half-life, while SSAT is short-lived and rate-limiting. SSAT is highly inducible and positively regulated by higher polyamines to increase Spd and Spm acetylation and

oxidation and/or excretion out of the cell (61) during polyamine excess, a potentially toxic condition. Casero's group (68) recently cloned a mammalian PAO and showed that its expression is also inducible. On the other hand, Vujcic et al. (69) found that conditional overexpression of SSAT in cultured breast cancer cells could deplete Spd and Spm pools, and eventually slow cell growth. The findings suggest that induced polyamine catabolism could represent an alternative antiproliferative strategy in addition to the inhibition of biosynthesis (70). Strategies to enhance catabolism by SSAT induction or block recycling by PAO inhibition are further discussed later in this chapter.

2.3. Transport

The mammalian transporter is highly specific for polyamines and polyamine derivatives. In fact, transport recognition requires that polyamine derivatives retain the positively-charged amine groups (42,43,71). Although the bacterial polyamine transporter has been cloned (72,73), the identity of the mammalian protein(s) remains elusive. Similar to both biosynthetic enzymes, polyamine transport is regulated by intracellular polyamine pools. Thus, transport activity is increased during polyamine depletion (74) and decreased by polyamine excess (33,74) via the ODC antizyme protein (57).

It has long been recognized that tumor cell salvaging of exogenous polyamines can compromise the antiproliferative activity of polyamine inhibitors such as DFMO, and this is facilitated by upregulation of the polyamine transporter (75–79). Under in vivo conditions, polyamines can be derived from the surrounding tissues, diet, or from the microbial flora of the gut (62,80,81). This was demonstrated by implanting animals with a tumor that was deficient in polyamine transport, and finding them more responsive to DFMO than animals bearing the wild-type tumor (82). Thus, the approaches used to lower the exogenous polyamine supply include antibiotic sterilization of the gut, polyamine-deficient diets, and a PAO inhibitor to block back-conversion of Spm to Spd and Put (66,67,81,83,84), which in combination with DFMO completely suppressed xenograft tumor growth. To circumvent this potential clinical limitation for DFMO, investigators at MediQuest Therapeutics, Inc. (formerly Oridigm Corporation) are developing an effective polyamine transport inhibitor to be used in combination with biosynthetic inhibitors, such as DFMO. This innovative approach will provide a means to further

Role of Polyamines in Epithelial Cancers

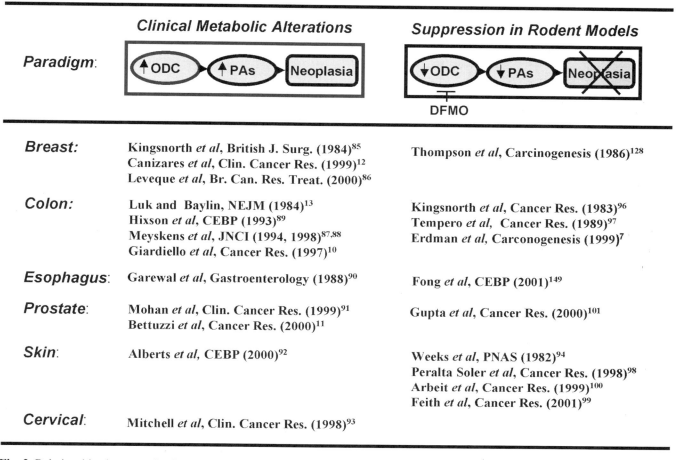

Fig. 2. Relationships between ODC enzyme expression, polyamine contents, and epithelial cancers in humans (left), and the influence of DFMO, an irreversible ODC inhibitor, on polyamine contents and epithelial carcinogenesis in rodent models (right). Representative citations supporting these two paradigms are listed. See text for additional details.

evaluate the functional significance and therapeutic potential of the transporter. Because polyamine transport is an active process and is typically higher in growing vs quiescent cells *(71)*, this process already has therapeutic relevance. In fact, use of the transporter remains a critical feature of most polyamine analog strategies discussed here *(42,43,71)*.

3. TARGETING ODC IN CHEMOPREVENTION

The rationale for targeting polyamine biosynthesis in chemoprevention derives from both preclinical and clinical observations. During the last 20 years, numerous studies found elevated levels of ODC activity and polyamines in tumor tissues taken from patients with breast *(12,85,86)*, colon *(10,13,87–89)*, esophagus *(90)*,

prostate *(11,91)*, skin *(92)*, and cervical *(93)* cancers (Fig. 2). In one breast cancer study *(12)*, carcinoma specimens ($N = 100$) displayed on average fivefold higher ODC activities and two- to threefold higher polyamine levels compared with benign tumors or normal breast tissue. Similarly, analysis of prostate cancer showed threefold higher mean ODC activities in tumor ($N = 31$) vs pair-matched benign tissue *(91)*. Moreover, Bettuzzi et al. *(11)* reported elevations in the transcripts for ODC, ODC antizyme, AdoMetDC, and SSAT in prostate cancer specimens. These findings and others shown in Fig. 2 support the paradigm that polyamine metabolism is elevated in clinical tumor tissues, and provide the rationale for the treatment paradigm that proposes a specific ODC inhibitor will deplete polyamine pools and subsequently alter progression toward neoplasia (Fig. 2).

One of the earliest preclinical indications that ODC activity was involved in tumorigenesis came from the association of ODC induction with tumor promotion by 12-O-tetradecanoylphorbol-13-acetate (TPA) in mouse skin (94). Later, O'Brien's group found that overexpression of ODC in mouse skin was sufficient to promote tumor formation (95). These findings, together with those generated from chemically induced (94,96,97) or genetically engineered (7,98–100) cancers in rodent models clearly established a relationship between polyamine metabolism and tumor formation. Subsequent models have extended these findings. Gupta et al. (101) found in the transgenic adenocarcinoma mouse prostate (TRAMP) model that ODC activity increased four- to fivefold in the dorsolateral prostate prior to detection of prostate tumors, suggesting that ODC is an early event in tumor development.

Molecular changes responsible for increases in polyamines during transformation are being delineated in the multiple intestinal neoplasia (Min) mouse model for intestinal carcinogenesis. Min mice express a mutated APC tumor-suppressor gene similar to the truncated form found in human familial adenomatous polyposis (FAP) (102). APC forms protein complexes to sequester—for instance, the oncogene β-catenin (103), and functions as a gatekeeper to control growth in normal intestinal mucosa (102). In addition to the germline APC mutations seen in FAP, somatic APC mutations are seen in the majority of sporadic colorectal cancers (104,105). Polyamine biosynthetic activity is directly affected by APC status. ODC and polyamine pools were found to be elevated in the flat mucosa of patients with colonic polyposis (13), an association that was further refined by genotyping to include only those presymptomatic FAP patients positive for the APC mutation (10). The correlation between ODC expression and APC mutation was confirmed in the Min mouse, in which ODC transcripts in the small intestine mucosa were found to be elevated compared to wild-type mice and ODC antizyme transcripts were lowered (7). In parallel with an elevation in ODC expression, increases in Put, Spd and Spm pools were also observed (7). The causal linkage between ODC expression and the APC network of transcription factors has recently been elucidated. It is based on the observations by Vogelstein's group that wild-type APC normally suppresses expression of c-myc, and inactivation of APC leads to c-myc activation (9). Thus, combined with the earlier observation by Cleveland and others (6,106) that ODC is transactivated by c-myc, one

could deduce that APC mutation leads to upregulation of the c-Myc protein that, in turn, increases transcription of ODC. Recently, Fultz and Gerner (107) found APC also activates expression of Mad1, a c-myc antagonist that is decreased with APC inactivation.

In addition to the APC gene, the oncogenic Ras network of proteins is also involved in regulation of ODC expression during transformation. For example, certain growth factors selectively induced ODC expression in H-ras transformed mouse fibroblasts but not in normal fibroblasts (108). Furthermore, Holtta and others (8,109) have shown that transformation of NIH-3T3 cells by c-Ha-ras requires ODC activation, and this occurred via c-myc upregulation, an immediate early response to the ras-dependent Raf/MEK/MAP kinase pathway (110). These data raise the possibility that ODC activation via c-myc may be similarly mediated by multiple signaling events during colorectal tumorigenesis (e.g., by mutations that inactivate APC and/or activate K-ras (102). Because the ODC promoter contains responsive sequences (TATA-, GC-, and E-box) to hormones, growth factors, tumor promoters, and oncogenes, ODC transcription can be regulated by multiple signaling pathways. In addition to c-Myc binding the E-box motif, (6), there are response elements for phorbol esters (111), androgens (112), cyclic-adenosine 5' monophosphate (AMP) (113), protein kinase A (113), transcription factors Sp1 (114), c-Fos (115), ZBP-89 (116), and WT1 tumor suppressor (117,118). Together, the upregulation of polyamine biosynthesis by oncogenic signaling pathways, and during malignancy in both rodent models and patient samples, provides a compelling rationale for targeting ODC as a prevention strategy (119).

3.1. Preclinical Studies Validating ODC as a Target in Prevention

Consistent with the evidence indicating that ODC is elevated in epithelial cancers, studies in rodent models indicate that inhibition of ODC by DFMO can suppress tumor development (Fig. 2). The first assessment of DFMO in cancer prevention was performed in the two-stage initiation/promotion model for mouse-skin carcinogenesis (94,120,121). Application of tumor promoters to mouse skin induced ODC transcripts (122) and activity (122–125) and increased Put and Spd pools by 15- and threefold, respectively (94). More recently, similar results were obtained in mice bearing an ODC transgene specifically expressed in follicular keratinocytes *(126)*, a condition that mimicked tumor promotion and increased sensitivity to carcinogen treatment *(95)*. In both models, DFMO treatment was found to block papilloma formation. Similar observations were made in two other transgenic mouse models. In one, skin papillomas induced by a viral protein transgene were prevented with DFMO *(100)*, and in the other, the ODC antizyme *(99)* was used as a transgene to suppress carcinogen-induced ODC activity and inhibit papilloma formation. Similar findings were also observed in mouse models for other epithelial cancers (Fig. 2). For example, treating *Min* mice with 2% DFMO in their drinking water from 7 to 17 wk post-birth suppressed Min-specific increases in Put and reduced tumor formation in the small intestine by 50% *(7)*. Dramatic effects were observed in the TRAMP mouse model following treatment with 1% DFMO from 8–28 wk postbirth. There was a >50% reduction in ODC activity, and the typical increases in prostate gland weight and volume were completely prevented *(101)*. Characterization of the DFMO-fed group showed well-differentiated prostate histology, a significant reduction in two proliferation markers, probasin and proliferating cell nuclear antigen (PCNA) and an elevated apoptotic index. In addition, the treated group showed no evidence of metastasis *(101)*. DFMO was also found to be similarly efficient in suppressing development of carcinogen-driven mammary tumors in rats *(127)*. In this early study, investigators found that ODC activity and polyamine pools in mammary tumors were depleted by DFMO in a dose-dependent manner *(128,129)*, and that cotreatment with Put partially blocked the antitumor response, confirming specificity for polyamine depletion. In addition, reductions in tumor incidence could be achieved with DFMO doses as low as 0.125% *(130)*. In contrast to the carcinogen-based rat mammary tumor model, less dramatic DFMO effects were observed in transgenic mice that spontaneously develop mammary carcinomas, perhaps because DFMO was delivered in the diet rather than by drinking water. Here, the number of preinvasive neoplastic lesions was not affected, but DFMO did reduce tumor multiplicity by 50% and tumor weight by 70% *(131)*.

The mechanism for DFMO inhibition of carcinogenesis is currently unresolved, but several hypotheses are emerging. Inhibition of ODC by DFMO causes polyamine pool depletion and cytostatic growth inhibition in most epithelial and nonepithelial cultured cells *(18,21,37,38)*. Cytostasis by polyamine depletion

has also been associated with accumulation of cells in G_1 phase *(60,132–136)*. Recently, G_1 arrest was optimized in melanoma cells by combining DFMO with the AdoMetDC inhibitor MDL-73811, and G_1 arrest followed marked upregulation of the cyclin-dependent kinase (CDK) inhibitor p21[WAF1/CIP1] *(60)*. Another study found that in colon tumor cells, DFMO decreased c-Myc expression by >90% in addition to its antiproliferative effects *(137)*. Two in vivo studies demonstrated that overexpression of ODC in mouse skin promoted cell proliferation *(138)*, activated protein kinase CK2 *(139)*, and increased cyclin-dependent CDK2 kinase activity *(138)*. It remains an intriguing possibility that prolonged DFMO treatment in vivo may minimize stimulation of certain cycle-related proteins and/or upregulate CDK inhibitors in precancerous lesions. Early studies indicated that DFMO acted to suppress skin carcinogenesis primarily by inhibiting the conversion of benign papillomas to invasive squamous carcinomas *(94)*. The mechanism underlying this effect may involve expression of the matrix metalloproteinases (MMPs) a class of secreted proteases involved in cancer invasion whose expression is polyamine dependent *(140–142)*. Recently, prevention of prostate metastasis in the TRAMP mouse model by DFMO was attributed to its ability to prevent the loss of the cellular adhesion proteins E-cadherin and β-catenin *(101)*. Other studies indicated that DFMO suppression of carcinogenesis depended on specific changes in signaling pathways, such as *ras* activation. When colon tumor-derived Caco-2 cells expressed an activated K-*ras* oncogene, their response to DFMO became cytotoxic *(143)*. In transgenic mice that expressed ODC in the skin, chemically induced skin papilloma formation was decreased by DFMO; however, in double transgenic mice that overexpressed both ODC and an activated H-*ras* oncogene, spontaneously developed papillomas actually regressed with DFMO treatment *(144)*.

Thus, although DFMO may act to suppress transformation through its antiproliferative effects *(101)*, it also has antiangiogenic *(145,146)*, antimetastatic *(101,147,148)*, and apoptotic *(101,145,149)* properties as well as the potential to alter cell adhesion *(140–142,150)* and protein expression *(60,101,137–139)*.

3.2. DFMO as a Cancer-Therapeutic Agent

DFMO, originally developed as a cancer-therapeutic agent *(151,152)*, was well-tolerated in humans except at very high doses (>10 g/m²/d), during which reversible mild thrombocytopenia, anorexia, and bilateral ototoxicity occurred *(153,154)*. In a Phase I trial *(155)*, temporary hearing loss was identified as a major dose-limiting toxicity DLT for orally administered DFMO ranging from 2–12 g/m²/d given over periods from 2–50 wk. Less than 10% of subjects developed hearing loss at cumulative DFMO doses of 150 g/m², and 75% experienced hearing loss at >250 g/m² In Phase II studies, disease stabilization was reported in a few patients *(151,152)*, especially with recurrent neural gliomas *(156)*. However, there were no lasting responses for a specific cancer type. Although DFMO was found to be cytotoxic to small-cell lung carcinoma (SCLC) in preclinical systems *(157,158)*, this was not realized clinically *(159)*. The lack of clinical activity with DFMO is usually attributed to its nontoxic tumoristatic action *(21)*, a property considered desirable for a candidate chemopreventive agent. In further attempts to develop the anticancer potential of DFMO, investigators examined its usefulness in drug combinations *(27)*, and found that it sensitized cultured tumor cells to killing by DNA-damaging drugs *(160)*. Subsequent studies in both in vitro and in vivo systems showed favorable interactions with a variety of known antineoplastic agents *(161)*. Interestingly, DFMO found clinical utility in treatment of African trypanosomiasis, a protozoal parasitic disease *(152,162)*, and pneumonia in acquired immuno deficiency syndrome (AIDS) patients *(163)*.

3.3. Clinical Evaluation of Safety and Efficacy of DFMO

The rationale for use of DFMO in chemoprevention trials includes the finding that ODC, the selective target for DFMO, is upregulated as a consequence of mutation or aberrant expression of several tumor-suppressor proteins and oncogenes. Animal studies indicated that DFMO was able to inhibit ODC activity and decrease one or more of the polyamines in target tissues. These observations provided the basis for an evaluation of tissue polyamine contents of clinical specimens to determine the biochemical efficacy of DFMO in patients. Quantitative measures of polyamines from colonic mucosa of normal human volunteers, obtained for comparison with those who have benign colon polyps and invasive colon cancers, proved to be reliable, reproducible, and sensitive *(87,164)*. Using polyamine levels as a primary endpoint, a Phase IIa *(88)* and a placebo-controlled Phase IIb *(89)* trial in patients with

colon polyps were designed to determine the minimal DFMO dose required to suppress polyamine contents in colorectal tissue. These and other trials concluded that daily oral DFMO doses as low as 0.2 or 0.4 g/m²/d over a 12-mo period could effectively reduce Put levels by 10% or 34%, respectively, in colorectal tissue *(88,89,165,166)*. Decreases in Spd pools and Spd/Spm ratios were significant, but lesser in magnitude. Importantly, there was no detectable hearing loss at doses up to 0.5 g/m²/d *(89)*.

This initial evaluation of DFMO supports the conclusion that a single daily dose of ~0.5 g/m²/d would be safe and effective for future chemoprevention studies. In fact, current studies evaluating DFMO at ≤0.5 g/m²/d did not produce hearing deficits in subjects treated for up to 3 yr (Dr. Frank L. Meyskens, personal communication). Since the average person has a surface area of ~2 m², some trials have converted to dose prescriptions of 0.25 g/d. More extensive safety evaluations are in progress in a placebo-controlled, randomized Phase IIb trial, not yet unblinded, designed to evaluate colon polyp prevention in 40–80-yr-old patients using low doses of oral DFMO (0.5 g/d) combined with the nonsteroidal antiinflammatory drug (NSAID) sulindac (0.15 g/d) for more than 1 yr. Preliminary observations found equivalent toxicities that were minor and manageable in both the placebo and treated groups (Dr. Frank L. Meyskens, personal communication). Thus, low doses of DFMO appear to be biochemically effective—at least in colorectal tissue—and safe, alone or in combination with low-dose sulindac. To facilitate oral delivery in future trials, ILEX Oncology (San Antonio, TX) has completed formulation of DFMO into tablet form.

4. CLINICAL CHEMOPREVENTION STUDIES WITH DFMO

Table 1 presents a summary of previous and current cancer prevention studies using DFMO. As indicated in this table, studies are evaluating this agent in a variety of patient populations and target tissues, including the bladder, breast, colon, esophagus, prostate, and skin. When DFMO was evaluated as a single agent, a uniform finding supports the conclusion that DFMO is well tolerated in reproductively inactive humans from 40–80 yr of age (as discussed previously). The completed clinical chemoprevention studies described in Table 1 were designed to measure effects on surrogate endpoints (e.g., polyamine contents, ODC activity,

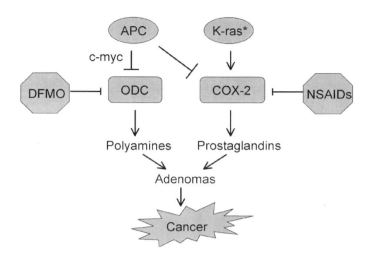

Fig. 3. Rationale for the combination chemoprevention strategy utilizing DFMO and cyclooxygenase inhibitors in colon cancer prevention. Sporadic (not genetic) forms of colon carcinogenesis in humans are associated with high frequencies of mutations in the APC tumor-suppressor gene and the K-*ras* oncogene *(102)*. Both ODC and COX-2 are expressed in cells by *APC*- and K-*ras*-dependent mechanisms *(107,232–234)*, and inhibitors of these enzymes block intestinal tumor formation in rodent models *(179,184)*.

proliferative markers), and not cancer incidence. Several studies, listed as in progress, will evaluate the effects of DFMO on incidence or recurrence of precancerous lesions in the bladder and colon, and should be available within the next 5 yr. The reader should view this modest progress in the context of the field of cancer prevention. Thus far, calcium supplementation is the only intervention that demonstrates even minimally suppressive effects on colon polyp formation *(167)*. Several other recent clinical trials have failed to demonstrate any dietary effects of fiber supplementation *(168)* or fat reduction *(169)* on the recurrence of colorectal adenomas.

Thus far, DFMO has been shown to suppress tissue polyamine contents in a number of sites in the GI tract *(89)*, squamous esophageal mucosa and Barrett's esophageal lesions *(170)*, and the prostate *(171)*. However, DFMO did not suppress proliferation markers (e.g., Ki-67 or BrdU incorporation) in apparently normal colorectal mucosa *(88)*. The following possibilities may explain these results: DFMO may exert its preventive effects by suppressing invasion and/or angiogenesis, or by inducing apoptosis; DFMO selectively prevents ODC induction in the genetically altered cells undergoing transformation that are too few for detection; or DFMO treatment may not reduce the proliferation rate of colonic epithelial cells, but change their distribution, as observed for calcium treatment *(172)*.

4.1. Combination Chemoprevention Trials With DFMO

Among the ongoing trials evaluating DFMO, two of particular interest include the combinations of DFMO and the antiandrogen Casodex for patients who are at risk for prostate cancer, and DFMO and sulindac for patients with colon polyps (discussed here). The rationale for the later arose from the fact that the cyclooxygenase (COX)-2 enzyme, responsible for prostaglandin synthesis, was found to be upregulated in the majority of colonic adenomas *(173,174)*, similar to ODC. Genetic models demonstrate that COX-2 is a downstream effector of *APC (175)* and K-*ras (143)* mutations, and that the *Min* mice that were null for COX-1 and COX-2 expression had reduced colon tumor formation *(176)*. Furthermore, specific inhibitors of COX-2, namely celecoxib, were also able to significantly reduce adenomatous polyposis in both carcinogen-induced *(177,178)* and genetic *(179,180)* rodent models. Finally, FAP patients treated for 6 mo with either sulindac *(181)* or celecoxib *(182)* had fewer adenomas. Together, these data laid the foundation for combining DFMO with the nonselective COX inhibitors piroxicam or sulindac, also known as NSAIDs, which are among the most potent chemopreventive agents studied in rodent models *(183)*. By in vitro analysis, growth inhibition with DFMO and sulindac appear additive in colon tumor cells *(143)*. DFMO

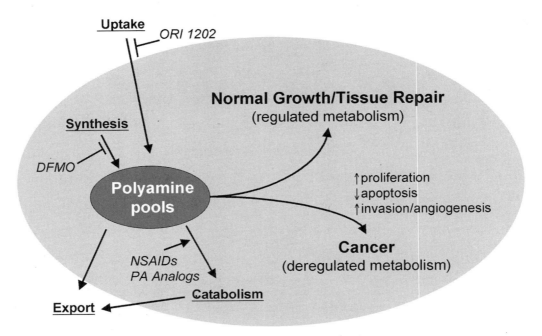

Fig. 4. Intracelullar polyamine pools are influenced by uptake, synthesis, catabolism, and export. These pools participate in a number of cellular processes during normal growth and tissue repair, including proliferation and tissue remodeling. Therefore, during carcinogenesis, upregulation of this metabolic pathway potentially contributes to dysregulated cell proliferation, decreased apoptosis, and invasive properties. The strategies proposed to deplete intracellular polyamine pools include transport inhibition (i.e., ORI-1202) to block uptake from exogenous sources, biosynthetic inhibition (i.e., DFMO) to block new synthesis, or catabolic stimulation (i.e., NSAIDs or polyamine analogs) to reduce intracellular pools and enhance export.

and piroxicam potently inhibited intestinal carcinogenesis in the *Min* mouse model *(184)*. These and other preclinical studies *(185–188)* have led to the recent chemoprevention strategy (Fig. 3) that combines low-dose DFMO (~0.5 g/d) with low-dose sulindac (~0.15 g/d) in FAP patients. Sulindac was the preferred NSAID because of the high levels of GI toxicity associated with piroxicam *(189)*. The preliminary evaluation of toxicities observed with this combination is discussed in the previous section. In addition to the NSAIDs, DFMO has also been shown to be efficacious in rodent models combined with cyclosporin *(190,191)* and selenium *(192)*.

4.2. Surrogate Endpoint Biomarkers (SEBs) for Modulators of Polyamine Metabolism

A number of polyamine parameters have been evaluated as potential SEBs for DFMO in chemoprevention trials. Polyamine contents and Spd/Spm ratios have been validated in the colonic mucosa of normal human volunteers *(87,164)*. Unfortunately, basal ODC activity was too low and variable to be considered a reliable SEB in this tissue *(87)*. Subsequent studies demonstrated that DFMO suppresses Put and Spd pools, and lowers the

Spd/Spm pool ratios in normal mucosa of at-risk individuals *(166)* or those with colon polyps *(88,89,165)*. Changes in Spd/Spm ratios have also been shown to be a reliable SEB in skin *(193,194)* and cervical *(93)* tissues. Several trials *(92,193–195)* have evaluated ODC activity in isolated skin tissue as a possible SEB by measuring both basal and TPA-induced activity. DFMO given at 0.5 g/m2/d suppressed the TPA-induced ODC activity by 50–80%, but the relationship between inhibition of this induced activity and changes in tissue polyamine contents has not been firmly established.

Results from recent trials show that DFMO treatment had no effect on proliferation *(88)* or apoptosis markers in intestinal tissue (Eugene W. Gerner, unpublished results). Consequently, tissue polyamine levels remain the only validated and reliable SEB for DFMO treatment, and ideally, measurements of the target tissue polyamines will be the most informative method to detect changes. However, if biopsies are unattainable, excretion of urinary polyamines could also reliably monitor DFMO action *(196)*. In fact, a Phase I trial noted that a FAP patient with high initial urinary polyamines showed a significant decline in these levels with DFMO treatment, as well as an almost total disappearance of rectal polyps *(196)*.

5. ALTERNATIVE STRATEGIES TO REDUCE CELLULAR POLYAMINE POOLS

Given the success of DFMO as a chemopreventive agent in preclinical models, it is useful to consider alternative strategies for targeting polyamines. These strategies are predicated based on the fact that the intracellular levels polyamines are sensitively maintained by multiple regulatory systems involving metabolism, uptake, and export *(2,21)*, each of which provides an opportunity to disrupt polyamine homeostasis and inhibit cell growth (Fig. 4). The following approaches are discussed: inhibition of polyamine transport; inhibition of AdoMetDC; activation of SSAT to stimulate acetylation and export; inhibition of PAO to block recycling; and more potent ODC inhibition.

5.1. Inhibition of Uptake

Many animal studies (*see* Subheading 2.3.) have demonstrated that exogenously available polyamines from the surrounding normal tissues, diet, and intestinal flora *(62,80,81)* serve to attenuate the antitumor effects of polyamine inhibitors such as DFMO. Although some investigators are exploring dietary control of polyamines *(81,84)*, others are targeting the polyamine transporter. Investigators at MediQuest Therapeutics, Inc., for example, have undertaken a synthetic chemistry program designed to identify compounds that would selectively inhibit polyamine uptake into cells *(197,198)*. Compounds are screened for their ability to potently inhibit Spd uptake and/or to prevent cell growth in the presence of DFMO and 0.5–1 μM Spd—conditions designed to mimic in vivo events. Using these systems, N^1-spermine-L-lysinyl amide (ORI 1202) was selected from a series of Spm/amino acid conjugates *(198)* for its ability to inhibit polyamine uptake in the nanomolar range. In the micromolar range, ORI 1202 enhanced the growth-inhibitory response to DFMO in a large panel of tumor-cell lines and improved depletion of Put and Spd pools. Importantly, ORI 1202 enhanced the antitumor responses to DFMO in the MDA-MB-231 breast *(197)* and PC-3 prostate *(199)* xenografts, thereby validating this novel approach. In support of this strategy, another group reported that the antitumor activity of DFMO was enhanced by blocking proteoglycan assembly, a cell-surface modification found to decrease uptake of exogenous polyamines *(200)*.

5.2. Inhibition of AdoMetDC

It has been demonstrated in vitro that the most effective depletion of polyamine pools and inhibition of cell growth was achieved by inhibiting both ODC and AdoMetDC. AdoMetDC produces dcAdoMet, the rate-limiting substrate for Spd and Spm synthesis. Several product-based nucleoside analogs have been developed as specific inhibitors of AdoMetDC *(20,21,36,37,73)*. Although they have been useful for biosynthetic intervention in cell culture, these particular inhibitors are rapidly degraded in vivo, and have been ineffective as antitumor agents. Investigators at Ciba-Geigy (now Novartis) who are aware of this shortcoming, designed a series of methylglyoxal *bis* (guanylhydrazone) analogs that proved to be metabolically stable and very potent inhibitors of AdoMetDC *(201,202)*. In particular, CGP-48664 (clinically SAM486A) inhibits AdoMetDC in the nanomolar range and effectively inhibits growth of human tumor xenografts *(203)*. A Phase I study *(204)* found that SAM486A was well-tolerated, and that neutropenia was the major toxicity. Although it has been difficult to convincingly validate drug action clinically, analysis of paired melanoma specimens before and after SAM486A treatment showed that Spm and dcAdoMet levels decreased and Put pools increased, consistent with AdoMetDC inhibition. As recent studies indicate *(205,206)*, other sites of action almost certainly contribute to the antiproliferative activity of SAM486A. However, it is possible that specificity for AdoMetDC with SAM486A may be achieved using lower-dose levels appropriate for chemoprevention strategies.

5.3. Stimulation of SSAT

Polyamine analogs were designed to regulate polyamine biosynthetic enzymes as an alternative strategy to inhibiting them *(161,207–210)*. In addition, spermine analogs were found to potently upregulate polyamine catabolism at the level of SSAT activity in certain tumor types *(211–216)*, and consequently to accelerate polyamine pool depletion. These analogs cause rapid cytostatic or cytotoxic responses in certain tumor types *(213,216)*, and often correlate with analog induction of SSAT activity *(46,73,125)*. This latter correlation led investigators to consider that SSAT may be a critical determinant of drug action, and that SSAT induction alone may be sufficient to inhibit tumor-cell growth. The observation that SSAT induction appeared to be higher in tumor than normal tissues suggested that enzyme induction might be a selective means for depleting tumor-cell polyamines. Indeed, an evaluation of diethyl Spm analogs showed that N^1,N^{11}-*bis* (ethyl)norspermine (DENSPM) induced the highest SSAT levels, was the least toxic to mice, and the most effective at inhibiting growth of human tumor xenografts *(217–219)*. DENSPM entered Phase I clinical trials in patients with advanced malignancies *(220,221)*, and represents the first polyamine analog to be clinically evaluated as an anticancer agent. To further support SSAT induction as a antiproliferative strategy, Vujcic et al. *(69)* recently reported that 5–10-fold increases in SSAT activity achieved via conditional expression led to depletion of Spd and Spm pools and a progressive slowing of cell growth. Unrelated to polyamines, monoterpene geraniol *(222)* and certain NSAIDs *(223)* currently being studied as potential chemopreventive agents were also found to stimulate SSAT. Thus, SSAT induction by nontoxic agents may provide a mechanistic rationale for selecting drugs for combinations with DFMO and other polyamine-directed agents.

5.4. Inhibition of PAO

The cellular consequences of PAO inhibition were not apparent until the design and synthesis of the specific enzyme inhibitor MDL-72527. This inhibitor is very effective at blocking endogenous polyamine oxidation in both cell cultures and animals, but it generally does not affect cell growth, and is nontoxic to animals. The cytotoxicity seen in certain cell types is generally attributed to nonspecific effects involving lysosomal swelling *(224)*. Thus far, its most promising application may be in combination with DFMO, where it is used to prevent restoration of Spd pools from Spm via the back-conversion pathway. In this regard, MDL-72527 has been used with DFMO in animal studies to enhance Spd depletion and increase the antitumor response *(66,67)*. These animal data suggest that inhibitors targeting PAO may have usefulness in chemoprevention—an indication that has not yet been studied.

5.5. More Potent ODC Inhibition

Although valuable as a highly specific inhibitor of ODC under both in vitro and in vivo conditions, DFMO has features that have undoubtedly limited its clinical success. It is transported poorly into cells *(225)*, and requires micromolar amounts to effectively compete with ornithine for the active site *(115)*. Other mechanism-based irreversible inhibitors of ODC were

developed in order to improve upon these deficiencies. Methyl ester derivatives of DFMO and putrescine analogs penetrated cells more effectively and had greater affinity for the enzyme *(41,226–228)*. As opposed to the millimolar concentrations of DFMO required to inhibit growth of cultured cells, 2R,5R,-6-methylacetylinic putrescine (RR-MAP) was effective in the mid-micromolar range. Whereas DFMO depleted only Put and Spd, RR-MAP decreased all three polyamines in certain cell types *(227,228)*. Both RR-MAP and ester derivatives of DFMO inhibited ODC at 10-fold lower doses than DFMO and achieved significantly greater antitumor responses in animals with no apparent toxicity *(151,226)*. Although developed more than 25 yr ago, these significantly improved ODC inhibitors have not yet been evaluated clinically.

6. CONCLUSION

There is now convincing evidence to show that new polyamine biosynthesis is induced either directly or indirectly by the genetic changes that lead to dysregulated growth during carcinogenesis. More specifically, ODC and other enzymes in polyamine metabolism are now included among the important downstream mediators of tumor-suppressor genes and oncogenes, and as such, are being considered as potential targets for cancer prevention and treatment. Those signals that alter polyamine metabolism result in higher polyamine contents that may ultimately influence gene expression through nucleic acid associations. Polyamine-dependent increases in expression of certain proteins, such as the matrix metalloproteinases, cell adhesion molecules, and cell cycle-related proteins could also influence cell behaviors. The fact that DFMO, the specific ODC inhibitor, significantly reduced polyamine pools and prevented tumor formation in transgenic rodent models was instrumental in promoting its clinical development. It is encouraging to find that DFMO can be safely administered orally for years, and will effectively deplete polyamine pools at target sites. With efficacy trials still underway, the success of DFMO as a preventive agent will undoubtedly further the development of additional polyamine-directed agents to target biosynthesis, uptake, and catabolism.

REFERENCES

1. Janne J, Alhonen L, Leinonen P. Polyamines: from molecular biology to clinical applications. *Ann Med* 1991;23:241–259.
2. Pegg AE. Recent advances in the biochemistry of polyamines in eukaryotes. *Biochem J* 1986;234:249–262.

3. Tabor CW, Tabor H. Polyamines. *Annu Rev Biochem* 1984;53:749–790.

4. MacRae M, Kramer DL, Coffino P. Developmental effect of polyamine depletion in Caenorhabditis elegans. *Biochem J* 1998;333:309–315.

5. Pendeville H, Carpino N, Marine JC, et al. The ornithine decarboxylase gene is essential for cell survival during early murine development. *Mol Cell Biol* 2001;21:6549–6558.

6. Bello-Fernandez C, Packham G, Cleveland JL. The ornithine decarboxylase gene is a transcriptional target of c-Myc. *Proc Natl Acad Sci USA* 1993;90:7804–7808.

7. Erdman SH, Ignatenko NA, Powell MB, et al. APC-dependent changes in expression of genes influencing polyamine metabolism, and consequences for gastrointestinal carcinogenesis, in the *Min* mouse. *Carcinogenesis* 1999;20:1709–1713.

8. Holtta E, Sistonen L, Alitalo K. The mechanisms of ornithine decarboxylase deregulation in c-Ha-*ras* oncogene-transformed NIH 3T3 cells. *J Biol Chem* 1988;263:4500–4507.

9. He TC, Sparks AB, Rago C, et al. Identification of c-MYC as a target of the APC pathway. *Science* 1998;281:1509–1512.

10. Giardiello FM, Hamilton SR, Hylind LM, et al. Ornithine decarboxylase and polyamines in familial adenomatous polyposis. *Cancer Res* 1997;57:199–201.

11. Bettuzzi S, Davalli P, Astancolle S, et al. Tumor progression is accompanied by significant changes in the levels of expression of polyamine metabolism regulatory genes and clusterin (sulfated glycoprotein 2) in human prostate cancer specimens. *Cancer Res* 2000;60:28–34.

12. Canizares F, Salinas J, de las Heras M, et al. Prognostic value of ornithine decarboxylase and polyamines in human breast cancer: correlation with clinicopathologic parameters. *Clin Cancer Res* 1999;5:2035–2041.

13. Luk GD, Baylin SB. Ornithine decarboxylase as a biologic marker in familial colonic polyposis. *N Engl J Med* 1984;311:80–83.

14. Herrera-Ornelas L, Porter C, Pera P, et al. A comparison of ornithine decarboxylase and *S*-adenosylmethionine decarboxylase activity in human large bowel mucosa, polyps, and colorectal adenocarcinoma. *J Surg Res* 1987;42:56–60.

15. Janne J, Poso H, Raina A. Polyamines in rapid growth and cancer. *Biochim Biophys Acta* 1978;473:241–293.

16. Bey P, Gerhart F, Van Dorsselaer V, Danzin C. α-(Fluoromethyl)dehydroornithine and α-(fluoromethyl)dehydroputrescine analogues as irreversible inhibitors of ornithine decarboxylase. *J Med Chem* 1983;26:1551–1556.

17. Danzin C, Bey P, Schirlin D, Claverie N. α-monofluoromethyl and α-difluoromethyl putrescine as ornithine decarboxylase inhibitors: in vitro and in vivo biochemical properties. *Biochem Pharmacol* 1982;31:3871–3878.

18. Mamont PS, Duchesne MC, Grove J, Bey P. Anti-proliferative properties of DL-α-difluoromethyl ornithine in cultured cells. A consequence of the irreversible inhibition of ornithine decarboxylase. *Biochem Biophys Res Commun* 1978;81:58–66.

19. McCann PP, Pegg AE. Ornithine decarboxylase as an enzyme target for therapy. *Pharmacol Ther* 1992;54:195–215.

20. Pegg AE, McCann PP. S-adenosylmethionine decarboxylase as an enzyme target for therapy. *Pharmacol Ther* 1992;56:359–377.

21. Pegg AE. Polyamine metabolism and its importance in neoplastic growth and as a target for chemotherapy. *Cancer Res* 1988;48:759–774.

22. Luk GD, Marton LJ, Baylin SB. Ornithine decarboxylase is important in intestinal mucosal maturation and recovery from injury in rats. *Science* 1980;210:195–198.

23. Heby O. Role of polyamines in the control of cell proliferation and differentiation. *Differentiation* 1981;19:1–20.

24. Fozard JR, Part ML, Prakash NJ, et al. L-ornithine decarboxylase: an essential role in early mammalian embryogenesis. *Science* 1980;208:505–508.

25. Williams-Ashman HG, Canellakis ZN. Polyamines in mammalian biology and medicine. *Perspect Biol Med* 1979;22:421–453.

26. Shapiro JT, Stannard BS, Felsenfeld G. The binding of small cations to deoxyribonucleic acid. Nucleotide specificity. *Biochemistry* 1969;8:3233–3241.

27. Marton LJ. Effects of treatment with DNA-directed cancer chemotherapeutic agents after polyamine depletion. *Pharmacol Ther* 1987;32:183–190.

28. Thomas T, Thomas TJ. Polyamines in cell growth and cell death: molecular mechanisms and therapeutic applications. *Cell Mol Life Sci* 2001;58:244–258.

29. Cohen S. *A Guide to Polyamines.* Oxford University Press, Oxford, UK, 1998, pp.1–543.

30. Igarashi K, Kashiwagi K. Polyamines: mysterious modulators of cellular functions. *Biochem Biophys Res Commun* 2000;271:559–564.

31. Porter CW, Pegg AE, Ganis B, et al. Combined regulation of ornithine and *S*-adenosylmethionine decarboxylases by spermine and the spermine analogue $N^1 N^{12}$ - bis(ethyl)spermine. *Biochem J* 1990;268:207–212.

32. Kramer DL, Miller JT, Bergeron RJ, et al. Regulation of polyamine transport by polyamines and polyamine analogs. *J Cell Physiol* 1993;155:399–407.

33. McCormick F. Polyamine metabolism in enucleated mouse L-cells. *J Cell Physiol* 1977;93:285–292.

34. Folk JE, Park MH, Chung SI, et al. Polyamines as physiological substrates for transglutaminases. *J Biol Chem* 1980;255:3695–700.

35. Park MH, Folk JE. Biosynthetic labeling of hypusine in mammalian cells. Carbon-hydrogen bond fissions revealed by dual labeling. *J Biol Chem* 1986;261:14,108–14,111.

36. Pegg AE, Jones DB, Secrist JA III. Effect of inhibitors of *S*-adenosylmethionine decarboxylase on polyamine content and growth of L1210 cells. *Biochemistry* 1988;27:1408–1415.

37. Kramer DL, Khomutov RM, Bukin YV, et al. Cellular characterization of a new irreversible inhibitor of *S*-adenosylmethionine decarboxylase and its use in determining the relative abilities of individual polyamines to sustain growth and viability of L1210 cells. *Biochem J* 1989;259:325–331.

38. Kramer DL. Polyamine inhibitors and analogs, in Nishioka K, ed. *Polyamines in Cancer: Basic Mechanisms and Clinical Approaches.* RG Landes, Austin, TX, 1996:151–189.

39. Feuerstein BG, Pattabiraman N, Marton LJ. Molecular mechanics of the interactions of spermine with DNA: DNA bending as a result of ligand binding. *Nucleic Acids Res* 1990;18:1271–1282.

40. Steglich C, Scheffler IE. An ornithine decarboxylase-deficient mutant of Chinese hamster ovary cells. *J Biol Chem* 1982;257:4603–4609.

41. Mamont PS, Danzin C, Kolb M, et al. Marked and prolonged inhibition of mammalian ornithine decarboxylase in vivo by esters of (E)-2-(fluoromethyl)dehydroornithine. *Biochem Pharmacol* 1986;35:159–165.

42. Porter CW, Bergeron RJ. Spermidine requirement for cell proliferation in eukaryotic cells: structural specificity and quantitation. *Science* 1983;219:1083–1085.

43. Porter CW, Cavanaugh PF Jr, Stolowich N, et al. Biological properties of N^4- and N^1,N^8-spermidine derivatives in cultured L1210 leukemia cells. *Cancer Res* 1985;45:2050–2057.

44. Bergeron RJ, McManis JS, Weimar WR, et al. The role of charge in polyamine analogue recognition. *J Med Chem* 1995;38:2278–2285.

45. Shappell NW, Miller JT, Bergeron RJ, Porter CW. Differential effects of the spermine analog, N^1,N^{12}-bis(ethyl)-spemine, on polyamine metabolism and cell growth in human melanoma cell lines and melanocytes. *Anticacer Res* 1992;12:1083–1089.

46. Kramer DL, Fogel-Petrovic M, Diegelman P, et al. Effects of novel spermine analogues on cell cycle progression and apoptosis in MALME-3M human melanoma cells. *Cancer Res* 1997;57:5521–5527.

47. Bachrach U, Heimer YM. *The Physiology of Polyamines.* CRC Press, Inc., Boca Raton, FL:1989:pp.1–106.

48. Williams-Ashman HG, Pegg AE, Lockwood DH. Mechanisms and regulation of polyamine and putrescine biosynthesis in male genital glands and other tissues of mammals. *Adv Enzyme Regul* 1969;7:291–323.

49. Kadmon D. Chemoprevention in prostate cancer: the role of difluoromethylornithine (DFMO). *J Cell Biochem Suppl* 1992;16H:122–127.

50. Heston WD. Prostatic polyamines and polyamine targeting as a new approach to therapy of prostatic cancer. *Cancer Surv* 1991;11:217–238.

51. Nelson PS, Gleason TP, Brawer MK. Chemoprevention for prostatic intraepithelial neoplasia. *Eur Urol* 1996;30:269–278.

52. Smith RC, Litwin MS, Lu Y, Zetter BR. Identification of an endogenous inhibitor of prostatic carcinoma cell growth. *Nat Med* 1995;1:1040–1045.

53. Walczak J, Wood H, Wilding G, et al. Prostate cancer prevention strategies using antiproliferative or differentiating agents. *Urology* 2001;57:81–85.

54. Dunzendorfer U, Knoner M. Therapy with inhibitors of polyamine biosynthesis in refractory prostatic carcinoma. An experimental and clinical study. *Onkologie* 1985;8:196–200.

55. Hayashi S, Murakami Y. Rapid and regulated degradation of ornithine decarboxylase. *Biochem J* 1995;306:1–10.

56. Heby O, Persson L. Molecular genetics of polyamine synthesis in eukaryotic cells. *Trends Biochem Sci* 1990;15:153–158.

57. Hayashi S. Antizyme-dependent degradation of ornithine decarboxylase. *Essays Biochem* 1995;30:37–47.

58. Canellakis ES, Kyriakidis DA, Rinehart CA Jr, et al. Regulation of polyamine biosynthesis by antizyme and some recent developments relating the induction of polyamine biosynthesis to cell growth. Review. *Biosci Rep* 1985;5:189–204.

59. Madhubala R, Secrist JA III,. Pegg AE. Effect of inhibitors of *S*-adenosylmethionine decarboxylase on the contents of ornithine decarboxylase and *S*-adenosylmethionine decarboxylase in L1210 cells. *Biochem J* 1988;254:45–50.

60. Kramer DL, Chang BD, Chen Y, et al. Polyamine depletion in human melanoma cells leads to G1 arrest associated with induction of p21WAF1/CIP1/SDI1, changes in the expression of p21-regulated genes, and a senescence-like phenotype. *Cancer Res* 2001;61:7754–1762.

61. Seiler N. Functions of polyamine acetylation. *Can J Physiol Pharmacol* 1987;65:2024–2035.

62. Seiler N, Bolkenius FN, Rennert OM. Interconversion, catabolism and elimination of the polyamines. *Med Biol* 1981;59:334–346.

63. Bolkenius FN, Bey P, Seiler N. Specific inhibition of polyamine oxidase in vivo is a method for the elucidation of its physiological role. *Biochim Biophys Acta* 1985;838:69–76.

64. Bey P, Bolkenius FN, Seiler N, Casara P. N-2,3-Butadienyl-1,4-butanediamine derivatives: potent irreversible inactivators of mammalian polyamine oxidase. *J Med Chem* 1985;28:1–2.

65. Claverie N, Wagner J, Knodgen B, Seiler N. Inhibition of polyamine oxidase improves the antitumoral effect of ornithine decarboxylase inhibitors. *Anticancer Res* 1987;7:765–772.

66. Moulinoux JP, Darcel F, Quemener V, et al. Inhibition of the growth of U-251 human glioblastoma in nude mice by polyamine deprivation. *Anticancer Res* 1991;11:175–179.

67. Moulinoux JP, Quemener V, Cipolla B, et al. The growth of MAT-LyLu rat prostatic adenocarcinoma can be prevented in vivo by polyamine deprivation. *J Urol* 1991;146:1408–1412.

68. Wang Y, Devereux W, Woster PM, et al. Cloning and characterization of a human polyamine oxidase that is inducible by polyamine analogue exposure. *Cancer Res* 2001;61:5370–5373.

69. Vujcic S, Halmekyto M, Diegelman P, et al. Effects of conditional overexpression of spermidine/spermine N^1-acetyltransferase on polyamine pool dynamics, cell growth, and sensitivity to polyamine analogs. *J Biol Chem* 2000;275:38,319–38,328.

70. Seiler N. Potential roles of polyamine interconversion in the mammalian organism in *Progress in Polyamine Research.* Pegg AE, Zappia V, eds. Plenum Press, New York NY, 1988, pp. 127–145.

71. Seiler N, Dezeure F. Polyamine transport in mammalian cells. *Int J Biochem* 1990;22:211–218.

72. Igarashi K, Kashiwagi K. Polyamine transport in bacteria and yeast. *Biochem J* 1999;344 Pt 3:633–642.

73. Casero RA Jr, Woster PM. Terminally alkylated polyamine analogues as chemotherapeutic agents. *J Med Chem* 2001;44:1–26.

74. Byers TL, Pegg AE. Regulation of polyamine transport in Chinese hamster ovary cells. *J Cell Physiol* 1990;143:460–467.

75. Heston WD, Kadmon D, Covey DF, Fair WR. Differential effect of α-difluoromethylornithine on the in vivo uptake of ^{14}C-labeled polyamines and methylglyoxal *bis* (guanylhydrazone) by a rat prostate-derived tumor. *Cancer Res* 1984;44:1034–1040.

76. Heston WD, Kadmon D, Lazan DW, Fair WR. Copenhagen rat prostatic tumor ornithine decarboxylase activity (ODC)

and the effect of the ODC inhibitor α-difluoromethylornithine. *Prostate* 1982;3:383–389.

77. Kadmon D, Heston WD, Lazan DW, Fair WR. Difluoromethylornithine enhancement of putrescine uptake into the prostate: concise communication. *J Nucl Med* 1982;23:998–1002.

78. Chaney JE, Kobayashi K, Goto R, Digenis GA. Tumor selective enhancement of radioactivity uptake in mice treated with α-difluoromethylornithine prior to administration of 14C-putrescine. *Life Sci* 1983;32:1237–1241.

79. Alhonen-Hongisto L, Seppanen P, Janne J. Intracellular putrescine and spermidine deprivation induces increased uptake of the natural polyamines and methylglyoxal *bis*(guanylhydrazone). *Biochem J* 1980;192:941–945.

80. Sarhan S, Knodgen B, Seiler N. The gastrointestinal tract as polyamine source for tumor growth. *Anticancer Res* 1989;9:215–223.

81. Quemener V, Moulinoux JP, Havouis R, Seiler N. Polyamine deprivation enhances antitumoral efficacy of chemotherapy. *Anticancer Res* 1992;12:1447–1453.

82. Persson L, Holm I, Ask A, Heby O. Curative effect of DL-2-difluoromethylornithine on mice bearing mutant L1210 leukemia cells deficient in polyamine uptake. *Cancer Res* 1988;48:4807–4811.

83. Hessels J, Kingma AW, Muskiet FA, et al. Growth inhibition of two solid tumors in mice, caused by polyamine depletion, is not attended by alterations in cell-cycle phase distribution. *Int J Cancer* 1991;48:697–703.

84. Leveque J, Burtin F, Catros-Quemener V, et al. The gastrointestinal polyamine source depletion enhances DFMO induced polyamine depletion in MCF-7 human breast cancer cells in vivo. *Anticancer Res* 1998;18:2663–2668.

85. Kingsnorth AN, Wallace HM, Bundred NJ, Dixon JM. Polyamines in breast cancer. *Br J Surg* 1984;71:352–356.

86. Leveque J, Foucher F, Bansard JY, et al. Polyamine profiles in tumor, normal tissue of the homologous breast, blood, and urine of breast cancer sufferers. *Breast Cancer Res Treat* 2000;60:99–105.

87. Hixson LJ, Emerson SS, Shassetz LR, Gerner EW. Sources of variability in estimating ornithine decarboxylase activity and polyamine contents in human colorectal mucosa. *Cancer Epidemiol Biomark Prev* 1994;3:317–323.

88. Meyskens FL Jr, Emerson SS, Pelot D, et al. Dose de-escalation chemoprevention trial of α-difluoromethylornithine in patients with colon polyps. *J Natl Cancer Inst* 1994;86:1122–1130.

89. Meyskens FL Jr, Gerner EW, Emerson S, et al. Effect of α-difluoromethylornithine on rectal mucosal levels of polyamines in a randomized, double-blinded trial for colon cancer prevention. *J Natl Cancer Inst* 1998;90:1212–1218.

90. Garewal HS, Sampliner R, Gerner E, et al. Ornithine decarboxylase activity in Barrett's esophagus: a potential marker for dysplasia. *Gastroenterology* 1988;94:819–821.

91. Mohan RR, Challa A, Gupta S, et al. Overexpression of ornithine decarboxylase in prostate cancer and prostatic fluid in humans. *Clin Cancer Res* 1999;5:143–147.

92. Alberts DS, Dorr RT, Einspahr JG, et al. Chemoprevention of human actinic keratoses by topical 2-(difluoromethyl)-dl-ornithine. *Cancer Epidemiol Biomark Prev* 2000;9:1281–1286.

93. Mitchell MF, Tortolero-Luna G, Lee JJ, et al. Phase I dose de-escalation trial of α-difluoromethylornithine in patients with grade 3 cervical intraepithelial neoplasia. *Clin Cancer Res* 1998;4:303–310.

94. Weeks CE, Herrmann AL, Nelson FR, Slaga TJ. α-Difluoromethylornithine, an irreversible inhibitor of ornithine decarboxylase, inhibits tumor promoter-induced polyamine accumulation and carcinogenesis in mouse skin. *Proc Natl Acad Sci USA* 1982;79:6028–6032.

95. O'Brien TG, Megosh LC, Gilliard G, Soler AP. Ornithine decarboxylase overexpression is a sufficient condition for tumor promotion in mouse skin. *Cancer Res* 1997;57:2630–2637.

96. Kingsnorth AN, King WW, Diekema KA, et al. Inhibition of ornithine decarboxylase with 2-difluoromethylornithine: reduced incidence of dimethylhydrazine-induced colon tumors in mice. *Cancer Res* 1983;43:2545–2549.

97. Tempero MA, Nishioka K, Knott K, Zetterman RK. Chemoprevention of mouse colon tumors with difluoromethylornithine during and after carcinogen treatment. *Cancer Res* 1989;49:5793–5797.

98. Peralta Soler A, Gilliard G, Megosh L, et al. Polyamines regulate expression of the neoplastic phenotype in mouse skin. *Cancer Res* 1998;58:1654–1659.

99. Feith DJ, Shantz LM, Pegg AE. Targeted antizyme expression in the skin of transgenic mice reduces tumor promoter induction of ornithine decarboxylase and decreases sensitivity to chemical carcinogenesis. *Cancer Res* 2001;61:6073–6081.

100. Arbeit JM, Riley RR, Huey B, et al. Difluoromethylornithine chemoprevention of epidermal carcinogenesis in K14-HPV16 transgenic mice. *Cancer Res* 1999;59:3610–3620.

101. Gupta S, Ahmad N, Marengo SR, et al. Chemoprevention of prostate carcinogenesis by α-difluoromethylornithine in TRAMP mice. *Cancer Res* 2000;60:5125–5133.

102. Kinzler KW, Vogelstein B. Lessons from hereditary colorectal cancer. *Cell* 1996;87:159–170.

103. Rubinfeld B, Albert I, Porfiri E, et al. Binding of GSK3β to the APC-β-catenin complex and regulation of complex assembly. *Science* 1996;272:1023–1026.

104. Powell SM, Zilz N, Beazer-Barclay Y, et al. APC mutations occur early during colorectal tumorigenesis. *Nature* 1992;359:235–237.

105. Miyoshi Y, Nagase H, Ando H, et al. Somatic mutations of the APC gene in colorectal tumors: mutation cluster region in the APC gene. *Hum Mol Genet* 1992;1:229–233.

106. Pena A, Reddy CD, Wu S, et al. Regulation of human ornithine decarboxylase expression by the c-Myc-Max protein complex. *J Biol Chem* 1993;268:27,277–27,285.

107. Fultz KE, Gerner EW. APC-dependent regulation of ornithine decarboxylase in human colon tumor cells. *Mol Carcinog* 2002;34:10–18.

108. Hurta RA, Huang A, Wright JA. Basic fibroblast growth factor selectively regulates ornithine decarboxylase gene expression in malignant H-*ras* transformed cells. *J Cell Biochem* 1996;60:572–583.

109. Shantz LM, Pegg AE. Ornithine decarboxylase induction in transformation by H-Ras and RhoA. *Cancer Res* 1998;58:2748–2753.

110. Aziz N, Cherwinski H, McMahon M. Complementation of defective colony-stimulating factor 1 receptor signaling and mitogenesis by Raf and v-Src. *Mol Cell Biol* 1999;19:1101–1115.

111. Reddig PJ, Kim YJ, Verma AK. Localization of the 12-O-tetradecanoylphorbol-13-acetate response of the human ornithine decarboxylase promoter to the TATA box. *Mol Carcinog* 1996;17:92–104.

112. Berger FG, Szymanski P, Read E, Watson G. Androgen-regulated ornithine decarboxylase mRNAs of mouse kidney. *J Biol Chem* 1984;259:7941–7946.

113. Abrahamsen MS, Li RS, Dietrich-Goetz W, Morris DR. Multiple DNA elements responsible for transcriptional regulation of the ornithine decarboxylase gene by protein kinase A. *J Biol Chem* 1992;267:18,866–18,873.

114. Kumar AP, Mar PK, Zhao B, et al. Regulation of rat ornithine decarboxylase promoter activity by binding of transcription factor Sp1. *J Biol Chem* 1995;270:4341–4348.

115. Wrighton C, Busslinger M. Direct transcriptional stimulation of the ornithine decarboxylase gene by Fos in PC12 cells but not in fibroblasts. *Mol Cell Biol* 1993;13:4657–4669.

116. Law GL, Itoh H, Law DJ, et al. Transcription factor ZBP-89 regulates the activity of the ornithine decarboxylase promoter. *J Biol Chem* 1998;273:19,955–19,964.

117. Moshier JA, Skunca M, Wu W, et al. Regulation of ornithine decarboxylase gene expression by the Wilms' tumor suppressor WT1. *Nucleic Acids Res* 1996;24:1149–1157.

118. Li RS, Law GL, Seifert RA, et al. Ornithine decarboxylase is a transcriptional target of tumor suppressor WT1. *Exp Cell Res* 1999;247:257–266.

119. Pegg AE, Shantz LM, Coleman CS. Ornithine decarboxylase as a target for chemoprevention. *J Cell Biochem Suppl* 1995;22:132–138.

120. Takigawa M, Verma AK, Simsiman RC, Boutwell RK. Polyamine biosynthesis and skin tumor promotion: inhibition of 12-O-tetradecanoylphorbol-13-acetate-promoted mouse skin tumor formation by the irreversible inhibitor of ornithine decarboxylase α-difluoromethylornithine. *Biochem Biophys Res Commun* 1982;105:969–976.

121. Slaga TJ, Fischer SM, Weeks CE, et al. Specificity and mechanism(s) of promoter inhibitors in multistage promotion. *Carcinog Compr Surv* 1982;7:19–34.

122. Verma AK, Erickson D, Dolnick BJ. Increased mouse epidermal ornithine decarboxylase activity by the tumour promoter 12-O-tetradecanoylphorbol 13-acetate involves increased amounts of both enzyme protein and messenger RNA. *Biochem J* 1986;237:297–300.

123. Gilmour SK, Verma AK, Madara T, O'Brien TG. Regulation of ornithine decarboxylase gene expression in mouse epidermis and epidermal tumors during two-stage tumorigenesis. *Cancer Res* 1987;47:1221–1225.

124. Koza RA, Megosh LC, Palmieri M, O'Brien TG. Constitutively elevated levels of ornithine and polyamines in mouse epidermal papillomas. *Carcinogenesis* 1991;12:1619–1665.

125. O'Brien TG, Simsiman RC, Boutwell RK. Induction of the polyamine-biosynthetic enzymes in mouse epidermis by tumor-promoting agents. *Cancer Res* 1975;35:1662–1670.

126. Megosh L, Gilmour SK, Rosson D, et al. Increased frequency of spontaneous skin tumors in transgenic mice which over-express ornithine decarboxylase. *Cancer Res* 1995;55:4205–4209.

127. Thompson HJ, Herbst EJ, Meeker LD, et al. Effect of D,L-α-difluoromethylornithine on murine mammary carcinogenesis. *Carcinogenesis* 1984;5:1649–1651.

128. Thompson HJ, Ronan AM, Ritacco KA, Meeker LD. Effect of tamoxifen and D,L-2-difluoromethylornithine on the growth, ornithine decarboxylase activity and polyamine content of mammary carcinomas induced by 1-methyl-1-nitrosourea. *Carcinogenesis* 1986;7:837–840.

129. Manni A, Wright C, Pontari M. Polyamines and estrogen control of growth of the NMU-induced rat mammary tumor. *Breast Cancer Res Treat* 1985;5:129–136.

130. Thompson HJ, Meeker LD, Herbst EJ, et al. Effect of concentration of D,L-2-difluoromethylornithine on murine mammary carcinogenesis. *Cancer Res* 1985;45:1170–1173.

131. Green JE, Shibata MA, Shibata E, et al. 2-difluoromethylornithine and dehydroepiandrosterone inhibit mammary tumor progression but not mammary or prostate tumor initiation in C3(1)/SV40 T/t-antigen transgenic mice. *Cancer Res* 2001;61:7449–7455.

132. Heby O, Andersson G, Gray JW. Interference with S and G^2 phase progression by polyamine synthesis inhibitors. *Exp Cell Res* 1978;111:461–464.

133. Seidenfeld J, Block AL, Komar KA, Naujokas MF. Altered cell cycle phase distributions in cultured human carcinoma cells partially depleted of polyamines by treatment with difluoromethylornithine. *Cancer Res* 1986;46:47–53.

134. Muller R, Mumberg D, Lucibello FC. Signals and genes in the control of cell-cycle progression. *Biochim Biophys Acta* 1993;1155:151–179.

135. Koza RA, Herbst EJ. Deficiencies in DNA replication and cell-cycle progression in polyamine-depleted HeLa cells. *Biochem J* 1992;281:87–93.

136. Ray RM, Zimmerman BJ, McCormack SA, et al. Polyamine depletion arrests cell cycle and induces inhibitors p21(Waf1/Cip1), p27(Kip1), and p53 in IEC-6 cells. *Am J Physiol* 1999;276:C684–C691.

137. Celano P, Baylin SB, Giardiello FM, et al. Effect of polyamine depletion on c-*myc* expression in human colon carcinoma cells. *J Biol Chem* 1988;263:5491–5494.

138. Gilmour SK, Birchler M, Smith MK, et al. Effect of elevated levels of ornithine decarboxylase on cell cycle progression in skin. *Cell Growth Differ* 1999;10:739–748.

139. Shore LJ, Soler AP, Gilmour SK. Ornithine decarboxylase expression leads to translocation and activation of protein kinase CK2 in vivo. *J Biol Chem* 1997;272:12536–12543.

140. Smith MK, Goral MA, Wright JH, et al. Ornithine decarboxylase overexpression leads to increased epithelial tumor invasiveness. *Cancer Res* 1997;57:2104–2108.

141. Wallon UM, Shassetz LR, Cress AE, et al. Polyamine-dependent expression of the matrix metalloproteinase matrilysin in a human colon cancer-derived cell line. *Mol Carcinog* 1994;11:138–144.

142. Kubota S, Kiyosawa H, Nomura Y, et al. Ornithine decarboxylase overexpression in mouse 10T1/2 fibroblasts: cellular transformation and invasion. *J Natl Cancer Inst* 1997;89:567–571.

143. Lawson KR, Ignatenko NA, Piazza GA, et al. Influence of K-ras activation on the survival responses of Caco-2 cells to the chemopreventive agents sulindac and difluoromethylornithine. *Cancer Epidemiol Biomark Prev* 2000;9:1155–1162.

144. Smith MK, Trempus CS, Gilmour SK. Co-operation between follicular ornithine decarboxylase and v-Ha-*ras* induces spontaneous papillomas and malignant conversion in transgenic skin. *Carcinogenesis* 1998;19:1409–1415.

145. Takahashi Y, Mai M, Nishioka K. α-difluoromethylornithine induces apoptosis as well as anti-angiogenesis in the inhibition of tumor growth and metastasis in a human gastric cancer model. *Int J Cancer* 2000;85:243–247.

146. Jasnis MA, Klein S, Monte M, et al. Polyamines prevent DFMO-mediated inhibition of angiogenesis. *Cancer Lett* 1994;79:39–43.

147. Kubota S, Ohsawa N, Takaku F. Effects of DL-α-difluoromethylornithine on the growth and metastasis of B16 melanoma in vivo. *Int J Cancer* 1987;39:244–247.

148. Sunkara PS, Rosenberger AL. Antimetastatic activity of DL-α-difluoromethylornithine, an inhibitor of polyamine biosynthesis, in mice. *Cancer Res* 1987;47:933–935.

149. Fong LY, Nguyen VT, Pegg AE, Magee PN. α-Difluoromethylornithine induction of apoptosis: a mechanism which reverses pre-established cell proliferation and cancer initiation in esophageal carcinogenesis in zinc-deficient rats. *Cancer Epidemiol Biomark Prev* 2001;10:191–199.

150. Takigawa M, Nishida Y, Suzuki F, et al. Induction of angiogenesis in chick yolk-sac membrane by polyamines and its inhibition by tissue inhibitors of metalloproteinases (TIMP and TIMP-2). *Biochem Biophys Res Commun* 1990;171:1264–1271.

151. Sjoerdsma A, Schechter PJ. Chemotherapeutic implications of polyamine biosynthesis inhibition. *Clin Pharmacol Ther* 1984; 5:287–300.

152. Schechter PJ, Barlow JLR, Sjoerdsma A. Clinical aspects of inhibition of ornithine decarboxylase with emphasis on therapeutic trials of eflornithine (DFMO) in cancer and protozoan diseases, in *Inhibition of Polyamine Metabolism. Biological Significance and Basis for New Therapies*. McCann PP, Pegg AE, Sjoerdsma A, eds. Academic Press, Inc., Orlando; 1987 pp. 345–364.

153. Abeloff MD, Slavik M, Luk GD, et al. Phase I trial and pharmacokinetic studies of α-difluoromethylornithine—an inhibitor of polyamine biosynthesis. *J Clin Oncol* 1984;2:124–130.

154. Maddox AM, Keating MJ, McCredie KE, et al. Phase I evaluation of intravenous difluoromethylornithine—a polyamine inhibitor. *Investig New Drugs* 1985;3:287–922.

155. Croghan MK, Aickin MG, Meyskens FL. Dose-related α-difluoromethylornithine ototoxicity. *Am J Clin Oncol* 1991;14:331–335.

156. Marton LJ, Pegg AE. Polyamines as targets for therapeutic intervention. *Annu Rev Pharmacol Toxicol* 1995;35:55–91.

157. Luk GD, Goodwin G, Marton LJ, Baylin SB. Polyamines are necessary for the survival of human small-cell lung carcinoma in culture. *Proc Natl Acad Sci USA* 1981;78:2355–2358.

158. Luk GD, Abeloff MD, McCann PP, et al. Long-term maintenance therapy of established human small cell variant lung carcinoma implants in athymic mice with a cyclic regimen of difluoromethylornithine. *Cancer Res* 1986;46:1849–1853.

159. Abeloff MD, Rosen ST, Luk GD, et al. Phase II trials of α-difluoromethylornithine, an inhibitor of polyamine synthesis, in advanced small cell lung cancer and colon cancer. *Cancer Treat Rep* 1986;70:843–845.

160. Marton LJ, Levin VA, Hervatin SJ, et al. Potentiation of the antitumor therapeutic effects of 1,3-*bis*(2-chloroethyl)-1-nitrosourea by α-difluoromethylornithine, an ornithine decarboxylase inhibitor. *Cancer Res* 1981;41:4426–4431.

161. Porter CW, Janne J. Modulation of antineoplastic drug action by inhibitors of polyamine biosynthesis, in *Inhibition of Polyamine Metabolism. Biological Significance and Basis for New Therapies*. Academic Press, Orlando; 1987, pp 203–248.

162. Bacchi CJ, Garofalo J, Mockenhaupt D, et al. In vivo effects of α-DL-difluoromethylornithine on the metabolism and morphology of *Trypanosoma brucei brucei*. *Mol Biochem Parasitol* 1983;7:209–225.

163. Gilman TM, Paulson YJ, Boylen CT, et al. Eflornithine treatment of *Pneumocystis carinii* pneumonia in AIDS. *JAMA* 1986;256:2197–2198.

164. Hixson LJ, Garewal HS, McGee DL, et al. Ornithine decarboxylase and polyamines in colorectal neoplasia and mucosa. *Cancer Epidemiol Biomark Prev* 1993;2:369–374.

165. Meyskens FL Jr, Gerner EW. Development of difluoromethylornithine (DFMO) as a chemoprevention agent. *Clin Cancer Res* 1999;5:945–951.

166. Love RR, Jacoby R, Newton MA, et al. A randomized, placebo-controlled trial of low-dose α-difluoromethylornithine in individuals at risk for colorectal cancer. *Cancer Epidemiol Biomark* Prev 1998;7:989–992.

167. Baron JA, Beach M, Mandel JS, et al. Calcium supplements for the prevention of colorectal adenomas. Calcium Polyp Prevention Study Group. *N Engl J Med* 1999;340:101–107.

168. Alberts DS, Martinez ME, Roe DJ, et al. Lack of effect of a high-fiber cereal supplement on the recurrence of colorectal adenomas. Phoenix Colon Cancer Prevention Physicians' Network. *N Engl J Med* 2000;342:1156–1162.

169. Schatzkin A, Lanza E, Corle D, et al. Lack of effect of a low-fat, high-fiber diet on the recurrence of colorectal adenomas. Polyp Prevention Trial Study Group. *N Engl J Med* 2000;342:1149–1155.

170. Gerner EW, Garewal HS, Emerson SS, Sampliner RE. Gastrointestinal tissue polyamine contents of patients with Barrett's esophagus treated with α-difluoromethylornithine. *Cancer Epidemiol Biomark Prev* 1994;3:325–330.

171. Simoneau AR, Gerner EW, Phung M, et al α-Difluoromethylornithine and polyamine levels in the human prostate: results of a Phase IIa trial. *J Natl Cancer Inst* 2001;93:57–59.

172. Bostick RM, Fosdick L, Wood JR, et al. Calcium and colorectal epithelial cell proliferation in sporadic adenoma patients: a randomized, double-blinded, placebo-controlled clinical trial. *J Natl Cancer Inst* 1995;87:1307–1315.

173. Eberhart CE, Coffey RJ, Radhika A, et al. Up-regulation of cyclooxygenase 2 gene expression in human colorectal adenomas and adenocarcinomas. *Gastroenterology* 1994;107:1183–1188.

174. Dannenberg AJ, Zakim D. Chemoprevention of colorectal cancer through inhibition of cyclooxygenase-2. *Semin Oncol* 1999;26:499–504.

175. Oshima M, Dinchuk JE, Kargman SL, et al. Suppression of intestinal polyposis in Apc delta716 knockout mice by inhibition of cyclooxygenase 2 (COX-2). *Cell* 1996;87:803–809.

176. Chulada PC, Thompson MB, Mahler JF, et al. Genetic disruption of Ptgs-1, as well as Ptgs-2, reduces intestinal tumorigenesis in Min mice. *Cancer Res* 2000;60:4705–4708.

177. Kawamori T, Rao CV, Seibert K, Reddy BS. Chemopreventive activity of celecoxib, a specific cyclooxygenase-2 inhibitor, against colon carcinogenesis. *Cancer Res* 1998;58:409–412.

178. Reddy BS, Hirose Y, Lubet R, et al. Chemoprevention of colon cancer by specific cyclooxygenase-2 inhibitor, celecoxib, administered during different stages of carcinogenesis. *Cancer Res* 2000;60:293–297.

179. Jacoby RF, Seibert K, Cole CE, et al. The cyclooxygenase-2 inhibitor celecoxib is a potent preventive and therapeutic agent in the min mouse model of adenomatous polyposis. *Cancer Res* 2000;60:5040–5044.

180. Oshima M, Murai N, Kargman S, et al. Chemoprevention of intestinal polyposis in the Apc$^{\Delta 716}$ mouse by rofecoxib, a specific cyclooxygenase-2 inhibitor. *Cancer Res* 2001;61:1733–1740.

181. Waddell WR, Loughry RW. Sulindac for polyposis of the colon. *J Surg Oncol* 1983;24:83–87.

182. Steinbach G, Lynch PM, Phillips RK, et al. The effect of celecoxib, a cyclooxygenase-2 inhibitor, in familial adenomatous polyposis. *N Engl J Med* 2000;342:1946–1952.

183. Wargovich MJ, Jimenez A, McKee K, et al. Efficacy of potential chemopreventive agents on rat colon aberrant crypt formation and progression. *Carcinogenesis* 2000;21:1149–1155.

184. Jacoby RF, Cole CE, Tutsch K, et al. Chemopreventive efficacy of combined piroxicam and difluoromethylornithine treatment of Apc mutant *Min* mouse adenomas, and selective toxicity against Apc mutant embryos. *Cancer Res* 2000;60:1864–1870.

185. Li H, Schut HA, Conran P, et al. Prevention by aspirin and its combination with α-difluoromethylornithine of azoxymethane-induced tumors, aberrant crypt foci and prostaglandin E2 levels in rat colon. *Carcinogenesis* 1999;20:425–430.

186. Nigro ND, Bull AW, Boyd ME. Inhibition of intestinal carcinogenesis in rats: effect of difluoromethylornithine with piroxicam or fish oil. *J Natl Cancer Inst* 1986;77:1309–1313.

187. Reddy BS, Nayini J, Tokumo K, et al. Chemoprevention of colon carcinogenesis by concurrent administration of piroxicam, a nonsteroidal antiinflammatory drug with D,L-α-difluoromethylornithine, an ornithine decarboxylase inhibitor, in diet. *Cancer Res* 1990;50:2562–2568.

188. Rao CV, Tokumo K, Rigotty J, et al. Chemoprevention of colon carcinogenesis by dietary administration of piroxicam, α-difluoromethylornithine, 16 α-fluoro-5-androsten-17-one, and ellagic acid individually and in combination. *Cancer Res* 1991;51:4528–4534.

189. Calaluce R, Earnest DL, Heddens D, et al. Effects of piroxicam on prostaglandin E2 levels in rectal mucosa of adenomatous polyp patients: a randomized Phase IIb trial. *Cancer Epidemiol Biomark Prev* 2000;9:1287–1292.

190. Saydjari R, Townsend CM Jr, Barranco SC, Thompson JC. Differential sensitivity of pancreatic and colon cancer to cyclosporine and α-difluoromethylornithine in vivo. *Investig New Drugs* 1988;6:265–272.

191. Saydjari R, Townsend CM Jr, Barranco SC, Thompson JC. Effects of cyclosporine and α-difluoromethylornithine on the growth of mouse colon cancer in vitro. *Life Sci* 1987;40:359–366.

192. McGarrity TJ, Peiffer LP. Selenium and difluoromethylornithine additively inhibit DMH-induced distal colon tumor formation in rats fed a fiber-free diet. *Carcinogenesis* 1993;14:2335–2340.

193. Carbone PP, Douglas JA, Larson PO, et al. Phase I chemoprevention study of piroxicam and α-difluoromethylornithine. *Cancer Epidemiol Biomark Prev* 1998;7:907–912.

194. Carbone PP, Pirsch JD, Thomas JP, et al. Phase I chemoprevention study of difluoromethylornithine in subjects with organ transplants. *Cancer Epidemiol Biomark Prev* 2001;10:657–661.

195. Love RR, Carbone PP, Verma AK, et al. Randomized Phase I chemoprevention dose-seeking study of α-difluoromethylornithine. *J Natl Cancer Inst* 1993;85:732–737.

196. Pendyala L, Creaven PJ, Porter CW. Urinary and erythrocyte polyamines during the evaluation of oral α-difluoromethylornithine in a Phase I chemoprevention clinical trial. *Cancer Epidemiol Biomark Prev* 1993;2:235–241.

197. Weeks RS, Vanderwerf SM, Carlson CL, et al. Novel lysine-spermine conjugate inhibits polyamine transport and inhibits cell growth when given with DFMO. *Exp Cell Res* 2000;261:293–302.

198. Burns MR, Carlson CL, Vanderwerf SM, et al. Amino acid/spermine conjugates: polyamine amides as potent spermidine uptake inhibitors. *J Med Chem* 2001;44:3632–3644.

199. Devens BH, Weeks RS, Burns MR, et al. Polyamine depletion therapy in prostate cancer. *Prostate Cancer Prostatic Dis* 2000;3:275–279.

200. Belting M, Borsig L, Fuster MM, et al. Tumor attenuation by combined heparan sulfate and polyamine depletion. *Proc Natl Acad Sci USA* 2002;99:371–376.

201. Regenass U, Caravatti G, Mett H, et al. New *S*-adenosylmethionine decarboxylase inhibitors with potent antitumor activity. *Cancer Res* 1992;52:4712–4718.

202. Kramer D, Mett H, Evans A, et al. Stable amplification of the *S*-adenosylmethionine decarboxylase gene in Chinese hamster ovary cells. *J Biol Chem* 1995;270:2124–2132.

203. Regenass U, Mett H, Stanek J, et al. CGP 48664, a new *S*-adenosylmethionine decarboxylase inhibitor with broad spectrum antiproliferative and antitumor activity. *Cancer Res* 1994;54:3210–3217.

204. Siu LL, Rowinsky EK, Hammond LA, et al. A Phase I and pharmacokinetic study of SAM486A, a novel polyamine biosynthesis inhibitor, administered on a daily-times five every three-week schedule in patients with advanced solid malignancies. *Clinical Cancer Res* 2002;8:2157–2166.

205. Manni A, Badger B, Wechter R, et al. Biochemical and growth-modulatory effects of the new *S*-adenosylmethionine decarboxylase inhibitor CGP 48664 in malignant and immortalized normal human breast epithelial cells in culture. *Int J Cancer* 1995;62:485–491.

206. Dorhout B, Odink MF, de Hoog E, et al. 4-amidinoindan-1-one 2'-amidinohydrazone (CGP 48664A) exerts in vitro growth inhibitory effects that are not only related to *S*-adenosylmethionine decarboxylase (SAMdc) inhibition. *Biochim Biophys Acta* 1997;1335:144–152.

207. Pegg AE, Erwin BG. Induction of spermidine/spermine N$_1$-acetyltransferase in rat tissues by polyamines. *Biochem J* 1985;231:285–289.

208. Porter CW, Bergeron RJ. Enzyme regulation as an approach to interference with polyamine biosynthesis—an alternative to enzyme inhibition. *Adv Enzyme Regul* 1988;27:57–79.

209. Porter CW, Sufrin JR. Interference with polyamine biosynthesis and/or function by analogs of polyamines or

methionine as a potential anticancer chemotherapeutic strategy. *Anticancer Res* 1986;6:525–542.

210. Bergeron RJ, Feng Y, Weimar WR, et al. A comparison of structure-activity relationships between spermidine and spermine analogue antineoplastics. *J Med Chem* 1997;40:1475–1494.

211. Libby PR, Bergeron RJ, Porter CW. Structure-function correlations of polyamine analog-induced increases in spermidine/spermine acetyltransferase activity. *Biochem Pharmacol* 1989;38:1435–1442.

212. Libby PR, Henderson M, Bergeron RJ, Porter CW. Major increases in spermidine/spermine-N^1-acetyltransferase activity by spermine analogues and their relationship to polyamine depletion and growth inhibition in L1210 cells. *Cancer Res* 1989;49:6226–6231.

213. Casero RA Jr, Celano P, Ervin SJ, et al. Differential induction of spermidine/spermine N^1-acetyltransferase in human lung cancer cells by the *bis*(ethyl)polyamine analogues. *Cancer Res* 1989;49:3829–3833.

214. Fogel-Petrovic M, Shappell NW, Bergeron RJ, Porter CW. Polyamine and polyamine analog regulation of spermidine/spermine N^1-acetyltransferase in MALME-3M human melanoma cells. *J Biol Chem* 1993;268:19, 118–19,125.

215. Fogel-Petrovic M, Kramer DL, Vujcic S, et al. Structural basis for differential induction of spermidine/spermine N^1-acetyltransferase activity by novel spermine analogs. *Mol Pharmacol* 1997;52:69–74.

216. Shappell NW, Fogel-Petrovic MF, Porter CW. Regulation of spermidine/spermine N^1-acetyltransferase by intracellular polyamine pools. Evidence for a functional role in polyamine homeostasis. *FEBS Lett* 1993;321:179–183.

217. Porter CW, Bernacki RJ, Miller J, Bergeron RJ. Antitumor activity of N^1,N^{11}-*bis*(ethyl)norspermine against human melanoma xenografts and possible biochemical correlates of drug action. *Cancer Res* 1993;53:581–58

218. Bernacki RJ, Bergeron RJ, Porter CW. Antitumor activity of N,N^1-*bis*(ethyl)spermine homologues against human MALME-3 melanoma xenografts. *Cancer Res* 1992;52:2424–2430.

219. Bernacki RJ, Oberman EJ, Seweryniak KE, et al. Preclinical antitumor efficacy of the polyamine analogue N^1,N^{11}-diethylnorspermine administered by multiple injection or continuous infusion. *Clin Cancer Res* 1995;1:847–857.

220. Streiff RR, Bender JF. Phase 1 study of N^1,N^{11}-diethyl-norspermine (DENSPM) administered tid for 6 days in patients with advanced malignancies. *Invest New Drugs* 2001;19:29–39.

221. Creaven PJ, Perez R, Pendyala L, et al. Unusual central nervous system toxicity in a Phase I study of N^1,N^{11} diethyl-

norspermine in patients with advanced malignancy. *Invest New Drugs* 1997;15:227–234.

222. Carnesecchi S, Schneider Y, Ceraline J, et al. Geraniol, a component of plant essential oils, inhibits growth and polyamine biosynthesis in human colon cancer cells. *J Pharmacol Exp Ther* 2001;298:197–200.

223. Babbar N, Ignatenko NA, Casero RA Jr, Gerner EW. Cyclooxygenase-independent induction of apoptosis by sulindac sulfone is mediated by polyamines in colon cancer, *J Biol Chem* 2003;278:47,762–47,775.

224. Dai H, Kramer DL, Yang C, et al. The polyamine oxidase inhibitor MDL-72,527 selectively induces apoptosis of transformed hematopoietic cells through lysosomotropic effects. *Cancer Res* 1999;59:4944–4954.

225. Erwin BG, Pegg AE. Uptake of α-difluoromethylornithine by mouse fibroblasts. *Biochem Pharmacol* 1982;31:2820–2823.

226. Bartholeyns J, Mamont P, Casara P. Antitumor properties of (2R,5R)-6-heptyne-2,5-diamine, a new potent enzyme-activated irreversible inhibitor of ornithine decarboxylase, in rodents. *Cancer Res* 1984;44:4972–4977.

227. Mamont PS, Siat M, Joder-Ohlenbusch AM, et al. Effects of (2R, 5R)-6-heptyne-2,5-diamine, a potent inhibitor of L-ornithine decarboxylase, on rat hepatoma cells cultured in vitro. *Eur J Biochem* 1984;142:457–463.

228. Pera PJ, Kramer DL, Sufrin JR, Porter CW. Comparison of the biological effects of four irreversible inhibitors of ornithine decarboxylase in two murine lymphocytic leukemia cell lines. *Cancer Res* 1986;46:1148–1154.

229. Boyle JO, Meyskens FL Jr, Garewal HS, Gerner EW. Polyamine contents in rectal and buccal mucosae in humans treated with oral difluoromethylornithine. *Cancer Epidemiol Biomark Prev* 1992;1:131–135.

230. Loprinzi CL, Messing EM, O'Fallon JR, et al. Toxicity evaluation of difluoromethylornithine: doses for chemoprevention trials. *Cancer Epidemiol Biomark Prev* 1996;5:371–374.

231. Klemp J, Brady D, Frank TS, et al. Incidence of BRCA1/2 germ line alterations in a high risk cohort participating in a Phase II chemoprevention trial. *Eur J Cancer* 2000;36:1209–1214.

232. Sistonen L, Holtta E, Makela TP, et al. The cellular response to induction of the p21 c-Ha-ras oncoprotein includes stimulation of jun gene expression. *EMBO J* 1989;8:815–822.

233. Sheng H, Shao J, Dubois RN. K-*ras*-mediated increase in cyclooxygenase 2 mRNA stability involves activation of the protein kinase B_1 *Cancer Res* 2001;61:2670–2675.

234. Hsi LC, Angerman-Stewart J, Eling TE. Introduction of full-length APC modulates cyclooxygenase-2 expression in HT-29 human colorectal carcinoma cells at the translational level. *Carcinogenesis* 1999;20:2045–2049.

24 The Role of Phytoestrogens as Cancer Prevention Agents

Stephen Barnes, PhD and Coral A. Lamartiniere, PhD

Contents

1. INTRODUCTION

The addition or withdrawal of estrogenic substances from a patient's milieu as part of the prevention or treatment of cancer has been a part of modern medicine for over 100 years. It began in 1896 with surgical resection of the ovaries, the principal site of synthesis of physiologic estrogens, as a treatment for breast cancer by British surgeon Sir George Beatson (1). This method has been recently advanced as a prophylactic treatment for women at very high risk for breast cancer who have BRCA-1 and BRCA-2 germline mutations (2,3).

Two main pharmacological approaches have been used to treat breast cancer: cytotoxic agents, most of which also affect uninvolved tissues; and agents that alter the action of estrogens. The latter were developed because approx two-thirds of all breast tumors contain a receptor for the physiologic estrogen 17β-estradiol. Before the 1970s, synthetic estrogens were used clinically to suppress tumor growth (4). The mechanism for what appears to be a paradoxical effect may lie in estrogen's ability to suppress luteinizing hormone release by the pituitary. Since estrogen-dependent breast tumors require both estrogen and progestin to stimulate growth, reduction in the synthesis of the main pathway of steroid biosynthesis leads to suppression of tumor growth. This biphasic effect of estrogens should be expected to reoccur in other scenarios. Indeed, the size of the estrogen dose produces two separate outcomes for mammary tumors induced by 7,12-dimethylbenz[a]anthracene (DMBA) in rats. Low doses markedly stimulated tumor growth, whereas much larger doses inhibited tumor growth (5).

In the early 1970s, the anti-estrogen tamoxifen was introduced clinically to prevent growth of estrogen-dependent breast tumors. It is distinguished from the cytotoxic agents by being tumoristic and having fewer side effects because of its more selective action (6), leading to its use in chemoprevention of breast cancer on the basis that it would stop a subclinical tumor from emerging and therefore requiring treatment (7).

The use of tamoxifen as a chemopreventive agent arose at a time when epidemiologists were trying to provide answers as to why populations in different areas of the world had marked differences in breast and prostate cancer rates (8). Studies on immigrants to the United States revealed that differences in breast cancer risk could only be sustained for one generation (9). Asian men living in the United States have the same risk of prostate cancer as all American men (10). Only a small part of differences in breast and prostate cancer rates could therefore be accounted for by ethnic differences—e.g., at the genetic level. Instead, environmental factors in various countries must play a large role in risk of these cancers (11). One such factor, deliverable to an otherwise healthy population, is food. Of course, the importance of specific foods with regard to our health has been appreciated for at least 250 years. In the first half of the twentieth century, many food components such as vitamins A–K were isolated and chemically characterized. Each is freely available in supplement mixtures along with other nutritional factors

From: Cancer Chemoprevention, Volume 1: Promising Cancer Chemoprevention Agents
Edited by: G. J. Kelloff, E. T. Hawk, and C. C. Sigman © Humana Press Inc., Totowa, NJ

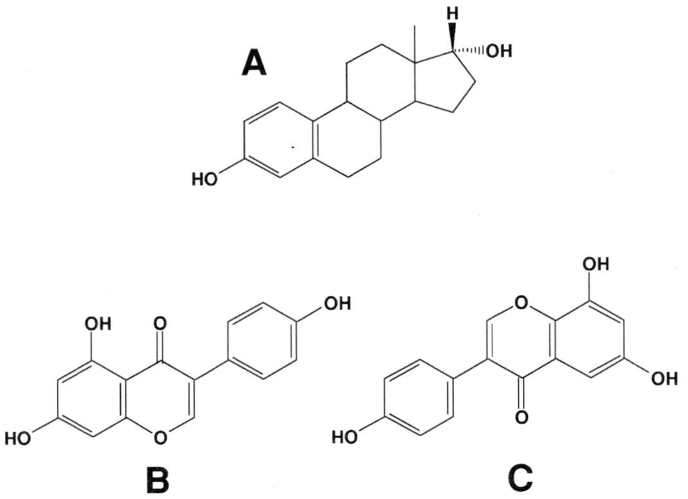

Fig. 1. Revision in the structure of genistein as a phytoestrogen. (**A**) the structure of 17b-estradiol. (**B**) structure of genistein as drawn by the soy community. (**C**) structure of genistein as it is found in the binding pocket of estrogen receptor beta *(19)*.

in most groceries and pharmacies. It is possible that cancer-chemopreventive agents could be delivered in a similar way.

Since the risk of breast cancer is very much lower (although rapidly climbing) in southeast Asia *(12)*, investigators have carefully examined the Asian diet for potential chemopreventive agents. Because the soybean is consumed in greater quantities by southeast Asians than Americans and Western Europeans *(13)*, it became the subject of intensive research *(14–16)*. Soybeans contain several substances with potential anticancer activity. Of these, isoflavones genistein and daidzein and their methylated analogs, biochanin A and formononetin, have received the most attention. They are called phytoestrogens because of their weak activity in stimulating the growth of uteri in ovariectomized rodents *(17)*. Other foods contain several other members of the phytoestrogen family, including plant lignans and their mammalian metabolites, coumestanes, and some fungal products *(18)*. Their estrogenic effects are quite variable, and depend on the species that ingest these foods. Each is a member of the polyphenol family, and characteristically has either a two-carbon or four-carbon bridge between two phenolic rings. Co-crystallization of the ligand-binding domain of estrogen receptor β (ERβ) with genistein *(19)* has forced a change in how the isoflavones are drawn—the B-ring of the genistein should be compared with the A-ring of 17β-estradiol (Fig. 1). Accordingly, several of the phytoestrogens are redrawn to reflect this (Fig. 2).

A major set of reviews on the roles of phytoestrogens in health and disease was published in 1998. It included reviews on the role of phytoestrogens on risk of breast *(18)* and prostate cancer *(20)*, and presented the controversies that existed at that time. Studies conducted in this area since that time represent opinions on preclinical science *(21–27)* and clinical aspects *(28–37)*. In several cases, authors have speculated on the roles of phytoestrogens as selective ER modulators *(38–41)*.

This chapter closely examines the work published on phytoestrogens and cancer since then, and presents the current controversies—which become all the more relevant in light of the National Institutes of Health (NIH) stopping the evaluation of hormone replacement therapy (HRT) in postmenopausal women in the Women's Health Initiative because of an unacceptable increase in cases of breast cancer in the treatment group, as well as other unacceptable risks *(42)*. As a result of this decision, it is anticipated that women will turn to alternative methods to deal with estrogen-dependent issues in the postmenopausal period, often with very little experimental data to support their new choice *(43)*. Since the isoflavones and/or soy allegedly prevent osteoporosis *(44,45)*, postmenopausal symptoms *(46,47)*, neurodegeneration *(48)*, and cardiovascular disease *(49)*, these and other phytoestrogens will be carefully scrutinized by the scientific community. Several investigators have disputed the alleged beneficial effects of isoflavones *(50–52)*.

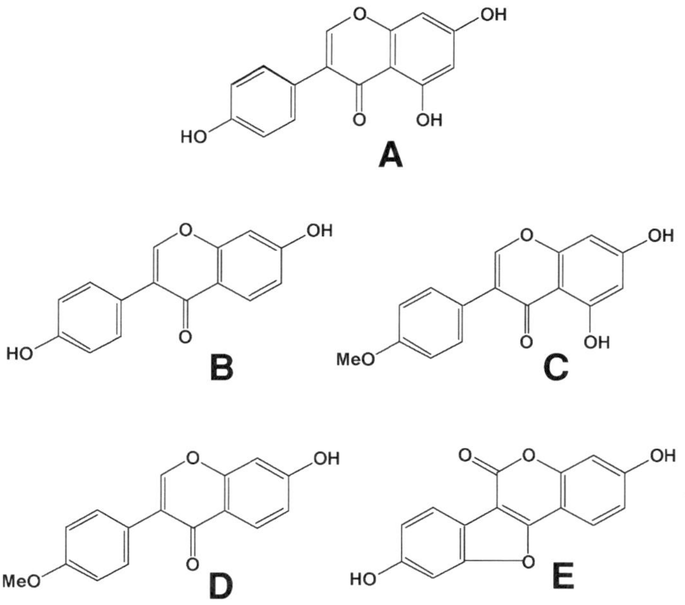

Fig. 2. Revised structure of common phytoestrogens. Structures are as found for genistein in Figure 1C. (**A**) genistein; (**B**) daidzein; (**C**) biochanin A; (**D**) formononetin; (**E**) coumestrol.

2. PHYTOESTROGENS AND BREAST CANCER

In 1998, investigators pondered the paradox of breast cancer chemoprevention by a phytoestrogen (genistein). Genistein had just been shown to be almost as effective an agonist as 17β-estradiol for the newly discovered ERβ *(53)*. Perhaps, in consideration of the effects of high doses of 17β-estradiol in suppressing mammary tumor growth *(4)*, it should not have been so surprising. The mechanism(s) by which it worked was less clear.

Investigators studying phytoestrogens and breast cancer are found in two camps. One group has consistently shown in rodent models that genistein inhibits the appearance of mammary tumors induced by the chemical carcinogens *N*-methyl-*N*-nitrosourea (MNU) and DMBA. *(54)*. This model is a test of cancer chemoprevention. The other group is concerned with a scenario in which already formed human breast cancer cells are induced to grow more rapidly. Much of their work is carried out in the ovariectomized nude mouse model *(55)* implanted with human breast cancer cells. This type of model is more in the category of chemotherapeutics, although the investigators who use it argue that it is also a model of chemoprevention for the emergence of small subclinical cancers.

2.1. Rodent Models of Breast Cancer in Surgically Intact Animals

The National Cancer Institute (NCI) has had a long history of using specific strains of rats and mice to evaluate potential chemoprevention agents. The move in the mid-1980s from using a lab chow diet (containing soy and thus isoflavones) to a defined soy-free diet (AIN-76A) led to a much higher incidence of rats with MNU-induced mammary tumors *(56)*. This prompted studies of the role of soy in prevention of breast cancer *(57,58)* and the emergence of genistein as a potential chemopreventive agent *(59)*. Lamartiniere's group followed up on these early results and rigorously examined the effects of timing exposure of the animals to genistein. They found that genistein given in the diet either in the perinatal *(60)* or prepubertal period *(54)* (but not in later life) was sufficient to prevent DMBA-induced mammary cancer. The early experiments indicated that genistein initially acted like an estrogen by inducing a more rapid proliferation of mammary epithelial cells *(61–63)*. However, it also increased the rate of differentiation *(54,60–63)*, so that by the time of greatest sensitivity to the carcinogen, the mammary gland had become more resistant to chemical carcinogenesis.

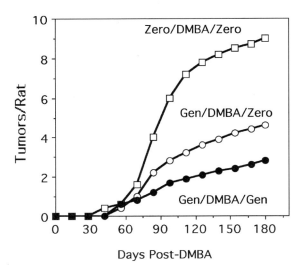

Fig. 3. Adult dietary genistein effect on palpable mammary tumors in rats exposed prepubertally to genistein and as adults to DMBA. Group 1 was fed control AIN-76A diet starting from parturition and continued throughout the study (Zero/DMBA/Zero). Group 2 was fed AIN-76A diet containing 250 mg genistein/kg diet, starting from parturition through d 21 only and then AIN-76A onward (Gen/DMBA/Zero). Group 3 was fed genistein-containing diet from parturition through d 21, AIN-76A only through d 100 postpartum, and genistein-containing diet (Gen/DMBA/Gen) from d 100. All animals received 80 mg DMBA/kg body wt at d 50. Each group consisted of 25 rats. (Adapted from ref.103.)

Table 1
Dietary Genistein, Timing of Exposure, and Mammary Cancer Chemoprevention

Exposure Period	Relative Mammary-Tumor Multiplicity*
No genistein	8.9
Prenatal genistein[a]	8.8
Adult genistein (after tumors)[b]	8.2
Prepubertal genistein[c]	4.3
Prepubertal and adult genistein[b,c]	2.8

Diets contained ± 250 mg genistein/kg AIN-76A.
*All rats were treated with 80 mg DMBA/kg body wt at d 50 postpartum.
[a]Prenatal treatment is throughout gestation;
[b]Adult treatment was initiated at 100 d postpartum;
[c]Prepubertal treatment was from d 1–21 postpartum. (Data adapted from 103).

In 1998, Fritz et al. (60) went further and showed that when genistein was delivered via their mother's milk, young rats were also protected in a dose-dependent manner from DMBA-induced mammary cancer. This important result showed that early postnatal exposure to genistein in the diet was sufficient to prevent breast cancer—in keeping with the epidemiological observation that southeast Asian women who grew up in their home countries and who emigrated to the United States in adult life had a sustained lower rate of breast cancer (64). In contrast, daughters born in the United States who did not eat a diet high in soy had no such protection. This raised a question about women who had not been exposed to substantial levels of isoflavones/soy in their childhood and were now becoming interested in the use of soy or isoflavone supplements. Would the isoflavones behave more like estrogens in promoting breast cancer-cell growth?

One answer to that question is that in surgically intact rodents, genistein does not increase the number of mammary tumors induced by DMBA (54). In fact, it has little effect. Furthermore, Lamartiniere's group has recently shown an important enhancement of the chemopreventive effect of genistein when rats are exposed to it early in life and are also fed genistein for the rest of their lives (Fig. 3; Table 1). This result helps to explain an interesting finding of the NCI-sponsored chemoprevention program. In 1996, NCI chose to go back to using a lab chow diet for its contract studies of chemopreventive agents, because previously well-studied agents failed to have expected effects in experiments that tested interactions between agents using AIN-76A diet. At the same time, because of expressed concerns about possible toxicities of isoflavones, experiments were carried out feeding rats genistein at doses of 200 and 2000 mg/kg diet in the DMBA model of breast cancer. Though genistein had been previously shown to have little or no effect in adult rats, when added to the diet it caused a 44–61% reduction in the number of mammary tumors induced by DMBA (65). Clearly, genistein affects the programming of genes that are expressed in the breast and that may be either turned on or turned off during the period of breast development during puberty.

2.2. Significance of Mouse Models of Breast Cancer

The athymic or nude mouse has been widely used to investigate the effectiveness of therapeutic agents on human breast cancer (66). Specific human breast cancer cells can be added to the mouse as a xenograft without rejection. The mouse can then be treated with the test agent to determine whether the agent can prevent further tumor cell growth or cause apoptosis. When combined with ovariectomy, important assumptions of this model for effects of isoflavones are: their metabolism in mice is similar to that of humans; the immune response, which may affect tumor-cell growth, is independent of the loss of the estrogens; and interactions between these two factors do not occur.

The observation in 1998 that genistein increased the growth of MCF-7 breast cancer-cell xenografts in ovariectomized nude mice caused alarm, since it was contradictory to the direction of chemoprevention research on genistein and other isoflavones at that time (67). However, from 1996 to 1998, several groups had already obtained data from experiments with human breast cancer cells in which all estrogens were carefully removed from the culture medium (in particular from fetal calf serum, but also from the phenol red added to the medium) (68–70). In this estrogen-free system, MCF-7 cells grew very slowly (analogous to the effect of surgically removing ovaries). Under these conditions, addition of genistein increased cell growth, acting as an apparent estrogen, reaching a maximum at doses between 1 and 10 μM. At higher concentrations (>10 μM), genistein inhibited growth (71,72). Genistein at these higher concentrations also inhibited estrogen-induced increases in growth. Thus, genistein has a biphasic action in these estrogen-sensitive cells. In contrast, growth of estrogen-independent breast cancer cells is inhibited at all concentrations of genistein (70,72).

The results in the ovariectomized nude mouse are therefore compatible with those from cell culture experiments. Indeed, Helferich's group has used this model to show that soy protein isolate containing free and conjugated isoflavones (73), as well as conjugated isoflavones alone (74), increase the growth of estrogen-sensitive breast cancer cell xenografts. They also reported that the growth of estrogen-insensitive breast cancer cell xenografts was unresponsive to genistein at dietary levels of 750 ppm (75). They concluded that dietary levels of bioactive genistein do not cause a chemopreventive effect. Instead, they are sufficient to stimulate estrogen-sensitive processes in a dose dependent manner.

What is the significance of these data? Is the ovariectomized athymic nude mouse a suitable model? Interestingly, in another mouse model of breast cancer in which the ovary was left intact, genistein prevented the appearance of mammary tumors (76), or increased the latency period before tumors appeared (77). In this model, spontaneous breast cancer was induced by the mouse mammary tumor virus. Mice fed a plant protein-free but mixed animal protein diet supplemented with biochanin A (4'-methylgenistein) at 200 ppm had a reduction in mammary tumor incidence from 84.6% (for animals fed a control diet) to 35.2% (76). Biochanin A was converted to genistein in these animals, but not in corresponding germ-free animals on the same diets. No chemopreventive effect of biochanin A was observed in the germ-free animals—instead, tumor promotion was observed. Interestingly, daidzein had no chemopreventive effect in either conventional or germ-free mice (76). This confirms the recent findings that daidzein had no effect in the rat DMBA-induced model of breast cancer (78). Since equol levels in both rats and mice were substantially higher than any concentrations observed in humans (76), it is unlikely that equol plays a role in prevention of breast cancer.

In recent study in mice, 4536 murine mammary carcinoma cells were injected into female Balb/c mice to examine the formation of lung metastases (79). Animals were placed on an isoflavone-free AIN-93 diet. Test diets contained 10% or 20% isolated soy protein (ISP). After the tumor had grown to 1 cm, it was resected and the number of lung metastases appearing during the next 3 wk noted. Treatment with ISP decreased tumor incidence (93%, 76%, and 67% incidence—control, 10% ISP and 20% ISP groups, respectively), tumors per animal (5, 2, and 1), cross-sectional area (0.93 mm^2, 0.80 mm^2, and 0.31 mm^2), and volume (0.73 mm^3, 0.56 mm^3, and 0.14 mm^3). In addition, there were fewer microscopically detectable tumors in the ISP group.

A key difference between the ovariectomized athymic nude mouse and other rodent models of breast cancer is the lack of circulating estrogens that result from surgical removal of the ovary. Although widely used, ovariectomy is not an exact model of postmenopausal breast cancer risk. Blood levels of estrogens fall in women after menopause, but not in the catastrophic manner that occurs following removal of the ovaries. Thus, genistein and other phytoestrogens exert their action against a background of estrogens and other steroid hormones. Indeed, ovarian steroid synthesis continues postmenopausally, resulting in androgen biosynthesis and peripheral conversion of androgen to estrogens (80). The ovariectomized, athymic nude mouse model must be modified by adding a steroid hormone background to mimic menopause.

Another difference in the models that has not been addressed or investigated is the role of the immune system. Athymic nude mice have no immune response. This is important because T-cells and B-cells are found on the periphery of most tumors. The absence of an immune response will alter the inflammatory environment around the tumor and may in turn change local metabolism of isoflavones (82). The importance of the latter to tumor cell growth requires further investigation.

2.3. Genistein and Tamoxifen

Since genistein can act as an estrogen, it is of great interest whether genistein reverses the beneficial effects of the clinically effective antiestrogen tamoxifen. Again, controversy reigns. Using the ovariectomized athymic nude mouse model, dietary genistein (1000 ppm) overcame the inhibitory effect of tamoxifen on MCF-7 cell growth (82). A similar result was observed in cell-culture, with genistein reversing the small inhibitory effect of tamoxifen on cell proliferation and G_1 cell-cycle arrest (83).

In contrast, other studies have suggested that genistein and tamoxifen may act synergistically. Gotoh et al. showed in a rat model that a combination of either miso (containing unconjugated isoflavones) or biochanin A with tamoxifen led to a further reduction in MNU-induced mammary tumors than either agent alone (84). Constantinou et al. reported that intact rats treated with tamoxifen and soy protein isolate had fewer DMBA-induced mammary tumors than animals treated with either chemopreventive agent alone (85). Shen et al. showed that tamoxifen and genistein act synergistically to inhibit cell growth in ER-negative human breast cancer cells (86). Tanos et al. (87) found that genistein had a greater inhibitory effect on dysplastic breast epithelial cells than malignant cells. This effect was independent of the presence of ERs, and was additive to the inhibitory effects of tamoxifen.

2.4. Genistein and Prostate Cancer

In 1993, Peterson and Barnes reported that genistein inhibited the growth of human and rat prostate cancer-cell lines (88). Genistein also inhibited epidermal growth factor (EGF)-stimulated growth of LNCAP and DU-145 cells and EGF receptor (EGFR) tyrosine autophosphorylation in DU-145 cells but not in LNCaP cells (88). Soy has been found to have a protective effect against prostatic dysplasia (89) and to inhibit the growth of transplantable human prostate carcinomas and tumor angiogenesis in mice (90,91). Pollard and Luckert (92) have shown that in Lobund-Wistar rats fed high-isoflavone-supplemented soy diet, the incidence of MNU-induced prostate-related cancer was reduced and the disease-free period was prolonged by 27% compared with rats fed the same diet, but low in isoflavones. In 1999, Schleicher et al. demonstrated that genistein directly inhibited growth of transplanted K1 prostate carcinoma cells in Lobund-Wistar rats, albeit at pharmacologic concentrations (93).

Subsequent modifications to the Lobund-Wistar rat model by injection of a chemical carcinogen directly into the dorsal prostate yielded a shorter latency period and more specific origin of cancer. This model provided the opportunity to investigate the potential of chemically synthesized genistein to protect against prostate tumors. In that study, Lobund-Wistar rats were exposed to 0, 25, and 250 mg genistein/kg AIN-76A diet starting at conception and continuing until necropsy at age 11 mo (94). From d 50–66 postpartum, male offspring were given 33 mg flutamide/kg body wt daily by gavage to cause chemical castration. On d 67, 68, and 69, they were injected daily with 25 mg testosterone/kg body wt to stimulate mitosis. On d 70, all rats were anesthetized, and 42 mg MNU/kg body wt was injected into the dorsal prostate for cancer initiation. One week after MNU administration, silastic implants of 25 mg testosterone were administered (and replaced every 12 wk) to stimulate mitosis and promote tumor growth. By 40 wk, palpable prostate tumors were detectable. Animals were necropsied when 48 wk old or when they became moribund. In animals with small tumors, the tumors were confined to the site of MNU injection, demonstrating target organ specificity. Rats fed the control diet, AIN-76A, and subjected to the carcinogenesis protocol developed 86.4% incidence of prostate tumors by age 11 mo (94). Animals exposed to 25 and 250 mg genistein/kg diet had tumor incidences of 77.8% and 63.0%, respectively. The percentage of prostate tumors classified as invasive adenocarcinomas in rats fed 0, 25, and 250 mg genistein/kg diet were 77.3%, 61.1%, and 44.4%, respectively. This significant dose-dependent decrease in prostate adenocarcinoma development demonstrated that lifetime dietary genistein exposure protected against chemically induced prostate cancer development in rats (94).

In 1995, Greenberg et al. (95) described a transgenic mouse model that results in spontaneous development of prostate cancer (TRAMP: TRAnsgenic Mouse Prostate adenocarcinoma). The TRAMP mouse was developed by using the prostate-specific probasin promoter to drive expression of the simian virus (SV40 early gene) in the prostatic epithelium. The SV40 T antigen (Tag) acts as an oncoprotein through interactions with *p53* and retinoblastoma tumor-suppressor gene products. All TRAMP mice develop changes resembling human prostate intraepithelial neoplasia (PIN) and poorly differentiated tumors, ultimately developing prostatic adenocarcinomas that metastasize to distant sites, primarily lymph nodes, bone, and lungs *(96,97)*. About one-half of the transgenic male mice displayed well-differentiated prostatic adenocarcinoma by age 28 wk; the other tumors were divided between moderately differentiated and poorly differentiated adenocarcinomas. To test the potential of genistein to prevent poorly differentiated adenocarcinomas, transgenic males were fed 0, 100, 250, or 500 mg genistein/kg AIN-76A diet starting at age 5–6 wk. Mice remained on the diet until they were age 28–30 wk. The proportion of transgenic males that developed poorly differentiated adenocarcinomas was significantly reduced in a dose-dependent manner by dietary genistein. With the 250 mg genistein/kg diet, there was a 64% decrease in these adenocarcinomas *(98)*. In a recent finding, Lubahn's group has not only confirmed this effect of genistein, but has also found that when the TRAMP mice were crossed with ERα gene-knockout (α ERKO) mice, the chemopreventive effect of genistein was abolished (D. Lubahn, J.D. Day, R. MacDonald, personal communication). This result strongly suggests that genistein exerts its effect by acting as an estrogen.

3. FUTURE DIRECTIONS AND INTERESTING QUESTIONS

The dilemma in 1998 was how a plant estrogen could prevent breast cancer when physiologic estrogens caused breast cancer. Indeed, many physicians and investigators now presume that phytoestrogens cause breast cancer, particularly in high-risk women and those with pre-existing tumors. Although genistein caused orthotopic estrogen-responsive human breast cancer cells to grow in ovariectomized nude mice, genistein-induced increases in mammary tumor formation in surgically intact rats were not observed. A more careful examination of the animal models used to address benefit/risk and lifetime exposure to genistein and other phytoestrogens is sorely needed.

Cotroneo et al. have investigated sex steroid and the EGF signaling pathway in prepubertal rat mammary glands following genistein and estrogen benzoate (EB) treatments in order to elucidate their differential actions *(63)*. Sex-steroid signaling pathways are believed to exert control over proliferation and differentiation of the mammary gland by a complex bidirectional interaction with the EGF signaling pathway. In these studies, female Sprague-Dawley rats were injected with genistein (500 ug/g bw) or EB (500 ng/g bw) on d 16, 18, and 20. Whole-mount analysis of mammary glands from 21-d-old rats showed that both treatments resulted in significantly increased terminal end buds and increased ductal branching, compared to animals that were given the vehicle, DMSO. Both effects were inhibited by blockage of ER function by pretreating with ICI 182,780, a steroidal antiestrogen. Immunoblotting analyis of mammary gland extracts demonstrated increased EGFR and progesterone receptor (PR) expression following treatment with EB or genistein. Tyrosine-phosphorylated EGFR was also increased, but when normalized to total receptors, there was no net effect. The expression and phosphorylation of downstream targets of EGFR, mitogen activating kinase kinase (MEK 1 and 2) and extracellular signal-regulated kinases 1 and 2 (ERK 1 and 2), were not significantly affected. Antiestrogen pretreatment prevented the increase in EGFR, phospho-EGFR, and PR. These data indicate an ER-based mechanism of action for genistein in mammary-gland proliferation and differentiation, which can lead to protection against mammary cancer. However, this does not preclude other growth-factor signaling pathways being differentially regulated by genistein and estrogen and accounting for genistein's health benefits over estrogen's toxic potential. Perhaps a more global approach to understanding differential gene and protein profiles is needed.

Another aspect of the problem is what is meant by an estrogen. This term is very casually used, although this is also true for many other agonists and antagonists. However, in these days of emerging technologies, the effects of estrogens on global gene expression can now be examined. Recent results suggest that in the developing uterus, genistein causes far more changes in gene expression than classical or purely synthetic estrogens *(99)*. In contrast to 17α-ethinyl estradiol, genistein largely downregulates gene expression. Thus, it is wrong to describe genistein as merely an estrogen. Its ability to alter the expression of a much wider range of genes allows it to have many additional properties.

In the prostate, genistein downregulates 11 genes associated with angiogenesis, tumor-cell invasion, and metastasis *(100)*.

Estrogens have important physiological effects at various stages of development and during adult life, and not all of these are related. This can occur because estrogen has both proliferative and differentiation effects. The very high concentrations of estrogens that are present during pregnancy serve to prepare the breast for its use for postnatal care of the infant, and also result in alterations of methylation of specific genes *(101)*. Initial evidence that genistein exposure causes gene methylation has recently been reported *(102)*, and further studies in this area are urgently needed.

In summary, genistein has many physiological actions in the breast and prostate. In the breast, genistein's ability to enhance gland maturation and cell differentiation results in permanent changes to the cellular blueprint that determine how breast tissue responds later in life to hormones and xenobiotics, including carcinogens. We believe that once the initial programming action has taken place through genistein, or some other similar means such as pregnancy or other nutritional differentiating chemical, women can benefit from ingesting soy as adults. For prostate cancer, the action of genistein appears to be direct, whereby the benefits of soy/genistein can be derived in adult life.

ACKNOWLEDGMENTS

The Purdue-UAB Botanicals Center for Age-Related Disease is supported by a grant (P50 AT00477-03) from the National Center for Complementary and Alternative Medicine (SB). The Center for Nutrient-Gene Interaction in Cancer Prevention is supported by a planning grant (P20 CA93753-01) from NCI (SB). CAL receives support from NCI (NIH R01 CA61742), the National Institute of Environmental Health Sciences (NIH RO1-ES-11743), Department of Defense Breast Cancer Program (DOD DAMD 17-00-1-0118, Department of Defense Prostate Cancer Program (DOD DAMD 17-98-1-8582 and DOD DAMD 17-02-1-0662) and a Breast Cancer Predoctoral Training Grant from the Department of Defense (DAMD17-00-1-0119).

REFERENCES

1. Beatson GT. On the treatment of inoperable cases of carcinoma of the mamma: suggestions for a new method of treatment, with illustrative cases. *Lancet* 1896;2:104–107,162–165.
2. Kauff ND, Satagopan JM, Robson ME, et al. Risk-reducing salpingo-oophorectomy in women with a BRCA1 or BRCA2 mutation. *N Engl J Med* 2002;346:1609–1615.
3. Rebbeck TR, Lynch HT, Neuhausen SL, et al. The Prevention and Observation of Surgical End Points Study Group. Prophylactic oophorectomy in carriers of BRCA1 or BRCA2 mutations. *N Engl J Med* 2002;346:1616–1622.
4. Haddow A, Watkinson JM, Patterson E, Koller PC. Influence of synthetic estrogens upon advanced malignant disease. *Br Med J* 1944;2:393–398.
5. Meites J, Cassell E, Clark J. Estrogen inhibition of mammary tumor growth in rats: counteraction by prolactin. *Proc Soc Exp Biol Med* 1971;137:1225–1227.
6. Jordan C. Historical perspective on hormonal therapy of advanced breast cancer. *Clin Ther* 2002;24:A3–A16.
7. Fabian CJ, Kimler BF. Beyond tamoxifen: new endpoints for breast cancer chemoprevention, new drugs for breast cancer prevention. *Ann NY Acad Sci* 2001;952:44–59.
8. Parkin DM, Pisani P, Ferlay J. Estimates of the worldwide incidence of eighteen major cancers in 1985. *Int J Cancer* 54;1993:594–606.
9. Wu AH. Soy and risk of hormone-related and other cancers. *Adv Exp Med Biol* 2001;492:19–28.
10. Shimizu H, Ross RK, Bernstein L, et al. Cancers of the prostate and breast among Japanese and white immigrants in Los Angeles County. *Br J Cancer* 1991;63:963–966.
11. Willett WC. Diet, nutrition, and avoidable cancer. *Environ Health Perspect* 1995;103 (Suppl 8):165–170.
12. Wakai K, Suzuki S, Ohno Y, et al. Epidemiology of breast cancer in Japan. *Int J Epidemiol* 1995;24:285–291.
13. Coward L, Barnes NC, Setchell KDR, Barnes S. The antitumor isoflavones, genistein and daidzein, in soybean foods of American and Asian diets. *J Agric Food Chem* 1993;41:1961–1967.
14. Messina M, Barnes S. Workshop report from the Division of Cancer Etiology, National Cancer Institute, National Institutes of Health. The role of soy products in reducing risks of certain cancers. *J Natl Cancer Inst* 1991;83:541–546.
15. Messina M, Persky V, Setchell KDR, Barnes S. Soy intake and cancer risk: a review of in vitro and in vivo data. *Nutr Cancer* 1994;21:113–131.
16. Messina M, Gardner C, Barnes S. Gaining insight into the health effects of soy but a long way still to go: commentary on the fourth International Symposium on the Role of Soy in Preventing and Treating Chronic Disease. *J Nutr* 2002;132:547S–551S.
17. Degen GH, Janning P, Diel P, Bolt HM. Estrogenic isoflavones in rodent diets. *Toxicol Lett* 2002;128:145–157.
18. Barnes S. Phytoestrogens and breast cancer. *Baillieres Clin Endocrinol Metab* 1998;12:559–579.
19. Pike AC, Brzozowski AM, Hubbard RE, et al. Structure of the ligand-binding domain of oestrogen receptor beta in the presence of a partial agonist and a full antagonist. *EMBO J* 1999;18:4608–4618.
20. Griffiths K, Denis L, Turkes A, Morton MS. Phytoestrogens and diseases of the prostate gland. *Baillieres Clin Endocrinol Metab* 1998;12:625–647.
21. Kim H, Peterson TG, Barnes S. Mechanisms of action of the soy isoflavone genistein: emerging role for its effects via transforming growth factor beta signaling pathways. *Am J Clin Nutr* 1998;68:1418S–1425S.

22. Lamartiniere CA, Zhang JX, Cotroneo MS. Genistein studies in rats: potential for breast cancer prevention and reproductive and developmental toxicity. *Am J Clin Nutr* 1998;68:1400S–1405S.

23. Lamartiniere CA. Protection against breast cancer with genistein: a component of soy. *Am J Clin Nutr* 2000;71:1705S–1707S.

24. Barnes S, Boersma B, Patel R, et al. Isoflavonoids and chronic disease: mechanisms of action. *Biofactors* 2000;12:209–215.

25. Hilakivi-Clarke L, Cho E, deAssis S, et al. Maternal and prepubertal diet, mammary development and breast cancer risk. *J Nutr* 2001;131:154S–157S.

26. Woods CE, Barnes S, Cline JM, in Phytoestrogen action in the breast and uterus. *Phytoestrogens and Health.* Gilani GS, Anderson JJB, eds. AOCS Press, Champaign, IL, 2002, pp.440–469.

27. Sarkar FH, Li YW. Mechanisms of cancer chemoprevention by soy isoflavone genistein. *Cancer Metastasis Rev* 2002;21:265–280.

28. Humfrey CD. Phytoestrogens and human health effects: weighing up the current evidence. *Nat Toxins* 1998;6:51–59.

29. North American Menopause Society. The role of isoflavones in menopausal health: consensus opinion of The North American Menopause Society. *Menopause* 2000;7:215–229.

30. Lawrence JA, Malpas PB, Sigman CC, Kelloff GJ. Clinical development of estrogen modulators for breast cancer chemoprevention in premenopausal vs. postmenopausal women. *J Cell Biochem* 2000;Suppl 34:103–114.

31. Vincent A, Fitzpatrick LA. Soy isoflavones: are they useful in menopause? *Mayo Clin Proc* 2000;75:1174–1184.

32. Wang HK. The therapeutic potential of flavonoids. *Exp Opin Invest Drugs* 2000;9:2103–2119.

33. Wiseman H. The therapeutic potential of phytoestrogens. *Exp Opin Invest Drugs* 2000;9:1829–1840.

34. Wagner JD, Anthony MS, Cline JM. Soy phytoestrogens: research on benefits and risks. *Clin Obstet Gynecol* 2001;44:843–852.

35. Messina MJ, Loprinzi CL. Soy for breast cancer survivors: a critical review of the literature. *J Nutr* 2001:131:3095S–3108S.

36. This B, De La Rochefordiere A, Clough K, et al. The Breast Cancer Group of the Institut Curie. Phytoestrogens after breast cancer. *Endocr Rel Cancer* 2001;8:129–134.

37. Tsourounis C Clinical effects of phytoestrogens. *Clin Obstet Gynecol* 2001;44:836–842.

38. Brzezinski A, Debi A. Phytoestrogens: the "natural" selective estrogen receptor modulators? *Eur J Obstet Gynecol Reprod Biol* 1999;85:47–51.

39. Baker VL, Leitman D, Jaffe RB. Selective estrogen receptor modulators in reproductive medicine and biology. *Obstet Gynecol Surv* 2000;55:S21–S47.

40. Huber J. Phytoestrogens and SERMS, alternatives to classical hormone therapy? *Ther Umsch* 2000; 57: 651–654.

41. Bush TL, Blumenthal R, Lobo R, Clarkson TB. SERMS and cardiovascular disease in women. How do these agents affect risk? *Postgrad Med* 2001;Spec No:17–24.

42. National Heart, Lung, and Blood Institute. NHLBI stops trial of estrogen plus progestin due to increased breast cancer risk, lack of overall benefits. http://www.nhlbi.nih.gov/new/press/02-07-09.htm

43. Kolata G. Race to fill void in menopause-drug market. NY Times, Sep 1, 2002.

44. Barnes, S. Phytoestrogens and osteoporosis—what is a safe dose? *Br J Nutr* 2002 in press.

45. Morabito N, Crisafulli A, Vergara C, et al. Effects of genistein and hormone-replacement therapy on bone loss in early postmenopausal women: a randomized double-blind placebo-controlled study. *J Bone Mineral Res* 2002;17:1904–1912.

46. Albertazzi P, Pansini F, Bottazzi M, et al. Dietary soy supplementation and phytoestrogen levels. *Obstet Gynecol* 1999;94:229–231.

47. Faure ED, Chantre P, Mares P. Effects of a standardized soy extract on hot flushes: a multicenter, double-blind, randomized, placebo-controlled study. *Menopause* 2002; 9;5:329–334.

48. Kim H, Xia H Li L, Gewin J. Attenuation of neurodegeneration-relevant modifications of brain proteins by dietary soy. *Biofactors* 2000;12:243–250.

49. de Kleijn MJ, van der Schouw YT, Wilson PW, et al. Dietary intake of phytoestrogens is associated with a favorable metabolic cardiovascular risk profile in postmenopausal US women: the Framingham study. *J Nutr* 2002;132:276–282.

50. White LR, Petrovitch H, Ross GW, et al. Brain aging and midlife tofu consumption. *J Am Coll Nutr* 2000;19:242–255.

51. Sirtori CR. Risks and benefits of soy phytoestrogens in cardiovascular diseases, cancer, climacteric symptoms and osteoporosis. *Drug Safety* 2001;24:665–682.

52. Van Patten CL, Olivotto IA, Chambers GK, et al. Effect of soy phytoestrogens on hot flashes in postmenopausal women with breast cancer: a randomized, controlled clinical trial. *J Clin Oncol* 2002;20:1449–1455.

53. Kuiper GG, Carlsson B, Grandien K, et al. Comparison of the ligand binding specificity and transcript tissue distribution of estrogen receptors α and β. *Endocrinology* 1997;138:863–870.

54. Lamartiniere CA, Cotroneo MS, Fritz WA, et al. Genistein chemoprevention: timing and mechanisms of action in murine mammary and prostate. *J Nutr* 2002;132:552S–558S.

55. Jordan VC, Gottardis MM, Robinson SP, Friedl A. Immune-deficient animals to study "hormone-dependent" breast and endometrial cancer. *J Steroid Biochem* 1989;34:169–176.

56. Grubbs CJ, Juliana MM, Hill DL, Whitaker LM. Effect of laboratory diets on methylnitrosourea-induced mammary cancers and the efficacy of a chemopreventive agent (retinyl acetate). *Proc Am Assoc Cancer Res* 1986;28:160.

57. Barnes S, Grubbs C, Setchell KDR, Carlson J. Soybeans inhibit mammary tumors in models of breast cancer. *Prog Clin Biol Res* 1990;347:239–253.

58. Hawrylewicz EJ, Zapata J, Blair WH. Soy and experimental cancer: animal studies. *J Nutr* 1995;125:698S–708S.

59. Lamartiniere CA, Moore J, Holland M, Barnes, S. Genistein and chemoprevention of breast cancer. *Proc Soc Exp Biol Med* 1995;208:120–123.

60. Fritz WA, Coward L, Wang J, Lamartiniere CA. Dietary genistein: perinatal mammary cancer prevention, bioavailability and toxicity testing in the rat. *Carcinogenesis* 1998;19:2151–2158.

61. Murrill WB, Brown NM, Zhang J-X, et al. Prepubertal genistein exposure suppresses mammary cancer and enhances gland differentiation in rats. *Carcinogenesis* 1996;17:1451–1457.

62. Brown NM, Lamartiniere CA. Xenoestrogens alter mammary gland differentiation and cell proliferation in the rat. *Environ Health Perspect* 1995;103:708–713.

63. Cotroneo MS, Wang J, Fritz WA, et al. Genistein action in the prepubertal mammary gland in a chemoprevention model. *Carcinogenesis* 2002;23:1467–1474.

64. Wu AH, Wan P, Hankin J, et al. Adolescent and adult soy intake and risk of breast cancer in Asian-Americans. *Carcinogenesis* 2002;23:1491–1496.

65. Lubet RL, Steele VE, Barnes S, et al. Chemopreventive effects of genistein on methylnitrosourea (MNU)-induced mammary tumors. AACR Annual Meeting. *Proc Am Assoc Cancer Res* 2000;41:845, abst 5364.

66. Manzotti C, Audisio RA, Pratesi G. Importance of orthotopic implantation for human tumors as model systems: relevance to metastasis and invasion. *Clin Exp Metastasis* 1993;11:5–14.

67. Hsieh CY, Santell RC, Haslam SZ, Helferich WG. Estrogenic effects of genistein on the growth of estrogen receptor-positive human breast cancer (MCF-7) cells in vitro and in vivo. *Cancer Res* 1998;58:3833–3838.

68. Zava DT, Blen M, Duwe G. Estrogenic activity of natural and synthetic estrogens in human breast cancer cells in culture. *Environ Health Perspect* 1997;105 (Suppl 3):637–645.

69. Willard ST, Frawley LS. Phytoestrogens have agonistic and combinatorial effects on estrogen-responsive gene expression in MCF-7 human breast cancer cells. *Endocrine* 1998;8:117–121.

70. Wang C, Kurzer MS. Effects of phytoestrogens on DNA synthesis in MCF-7 cells in the presence of estradiol or growth factors. *Nutr Cancer* 1998;31:90–100.

71. Peterson TG, Barnes S. Genistein inhibition of the growth of human breast cancer cells: independence from estrogen receptors and the multi-drug resistance gene. *Biochem Biophys Res Commun* 1991;179:661–667.

72. Peterson TG, Barnes S. Genistein inhibits both estrogen and growth factor stimulated proliferation of human breast cancer cells. *Cell Growth Differ* 1996;7:1345–1351.

73. Allred CD, Allred KF, Ju YH, et al. Soy diets containing varying amounts of genistein stimulate growth of estrogen-dependent (MCF-7) tumors in a dose-dependent manner. *Cancer Res* 2001;61:5045–5050.

74. Allred CD, Ju YH, Allred KF, et al. Dietary genistin stimulates growth of estrogen-dependent breast cancer tumors similar to that observed with genistein. *Carcinogenesis* 2001;22:1667–1673.

75. Ju YH, Allred CD, Allred KF, et al. Physiological concentrations of dietary genistein dose-dependently stimulate growth of estrogen-dependent human breast cancer (MCF-7) tumors implanted in athymic nude mice. *J Nutr* 2001;131:2957–2962.

76. Mizunuma H, Kanazawa K, Ogura S, et al. Anticarcinogenic effects of isoflavones may be mediated by genistein in mouse mammary tumor virus-induced breast cancer. *Lab Investig* 2002;62:78–84.

77. Jin ZM, MacDonald RS. Soy isoflavones increase latency of spontaneous mammary tumors in mice. *J Nutr* 2002;132:3186–3190.

78. Lamartiniere CA, Wang J, Smith-Johnson M, Eltoum IE. Daidzein: bioavailability, potential for reproductive toxicity, and breast cancer chemoprevention in female rats. *Toxicol Sci* 2002;65:228–238.

79. Yan L, Li DH, Yee JA. Dietary supplementation with isolated soy protein reduces metastasis of mammary carcinoma cells in mice. *Clin Exp Metastasis* 2002,19;6:535–540.

80. Martin KA. Hormone replacement therapy. http://cme.med.harvard.edu/syl/martin/1.html

81. Ju YH, Doerge DR, Allred KF, et al. Dietary genistein negates the inhibitory effect of tamoxifen on the growth of estrogen-dependent human breast cancer (MCF-7) cells implanted in athymic mice. *Cancer Res* 2002;62:2474–2477.

82. Boersma B, Barnes S, Kirk M, et al. Soy isoflavonoids and cancer—metabolism at the target site. *Mutat Res* 2001;480:121–127.

83. Jones JL. Daley BJ, Enderson BL, et al. Genistein inhibits tamoxifen effects on cell proliferation and cell cycle arrest in T47D breast cancer cells. *Am Surgeon* 2002;68:575–578.

84. Gotoh T, Yamada K, Yin H, et al. Chemoprevention of *N*-nitroso-*N*-methylurea-induced rat mammary carcinogenesis by soy foods or biochanin A. *Jpn J Cancer Res* 1998;89:137–142.

85. Constantinou AI, Xu H, Lucas LM, Lanvit D. Soy enhances tamoxifen's cancer chemopreventive effects in female rats. *J Nutr* 2002;132:576S–577S.

86. Shen F, Xue X, Weber G. Tamoxifen and genistein synergistically down-regulate signal transduction and proliferation in estrogen receptor-negative human breast carcinoma MDA-MB-435 cells. *Anticancer Res* 1999;19:1657–1662.

87. Tanos V, Brzezinski A, Drize O, et al. Synergistic inhibitory effects of genistein and tamoxifen on human dysplastic and malignant epithelial breast cells in vitro. *Eur J Obstet Gynecol Reprod Biol* 2002:102:188–194.

88. Peterson TG, Barnes S. Isoflavones inhibit the growth of human prostate cancer cell lines without inhibiting epidermal growth factor receptor autophosphorylation. *Prostate* 1993; 22:335–345.

89. Sharma OP, Adlercreutz H, Strandberg JD, et al. Soy of dietary source plays a preventive role against the pathogenesis of prostatitis in rats. *J Steroid Biochem Mol Biol* 1992;43:557–564.

90. Aronson WJ, Tymchuk CN, Elashoff RM, et al. Decreased growth of human prostate LNCaP tumors in SCID mice fed a low-fat, soy protein diet with isoflavones. *Nutr Cancer* 1999;35:130–136.

91. Zhou JR, Yu LY, Zhong Y, et al. Inhibition of orthotopic growth and metastasis of androgen-sensitive human prostate tumors in mice by bioactive soybean components. *Prostate* 2002;53:143–153.

92. Pollard M, Wolter W, Sun L. Prevention of induced prostate-related cancer by soy protein isolate/isoflavone-supplemented diet in Lobund-Wistar rats. *In Vivo* 2000;14:389–392.

93. Schleicher RL, Lamartiniere CA, Zheng M, Zhang M. The inhibitory effect of genistein on the growth and metastasis of a transplantable rat accessory sex gland carcinoma. *Cancer Lett* 1999;136:195–201.

94. Wang J, Eltoum I-E, Lamartiniere CA. Dietary genistein suppresses chemically-induced prostate cancer in Lobund-Wistar rats. *Cancer Lett* 2002;186:11–18.

95. Greenberg NM, DeMayo F, Finegold MJ, et al. Prostate cancer in a transgenic mouse. *Proc Natl Acad Sci USA* 1995;92:3439–3443.

96. Gingrich JR, Greenberg NM. A transgenic mouse prostate cancer model. *Toxicol Pathol* 1996;24:502–504.

97. Gingrich JR, Barrios RJ, Kattan MW, et al. Androgen-independent prostate cancer progression in the TRAMP model. *Cancer Res* 1997;57:4687–4691.

98. Mentor-Marcel R, Lamartiniere CA, Eltoum IE, et al. Genistein in the diet reduces the incidence of poorly differentiated prostatic adenocarcinoma in transgenic mice (TRAMP). *Cancer Res* 2001;61:6777–6782.

99. Naciff JM, Jump ML, Torontali SM, et al. Gene expression profile induced by 17α-ethinyl estradiol, bisphenol A, and genistein in the developing female reproductive system of the rat. *Toxicol Sci* 2002;68:184–199.

100. Li YW, Sarkar FH. Down-regulation of invasion and angiogenesis-related genes identified by cDNA microarray analysis of PC3 prostate cancer cells treated with genistein. *Cancer Lett* 2002;186:157–164.

101. McLachlan JA, Burow M, Chiang TC, Li SF. Gene imprinting in developmental toxicology: a possible interface between physiology and pathology. *Toxicol Lett* 2001;120:161–164.

102. Day JK, Bauer AM, DesBordes C, et al. Genistein alters methylation patterns in mice. *J Nutr* 2002;132(8 Suppl):2419S–2423S.

103. Lamartiniere CA, Cotroneo MS, Fritz WA, et al. Genistein chemoprevention: timing and mechanisms of action in murine mammary and prostate. *J Nutr* 2002;132:552S–558S.

25 Cancer Chemopreventive Activity of Monoterpenes and Other Isoprenoids

Pamela L. Crowell, PhD and Michael N. Gould, PhD

CONTENTS

1. INTRODUCTION

d-Limonene and perillyl alcohol—monoterpenes with low toxicity—have cancer-chemopreventive and chemotherapeutic activity against solid cancers and leukemias, which include most of the leading causes of cancer-related death. Monoterpenes are among the numerous and diverse naturally occurring isoprenoids that are synthesized in plants *(1)*. Isoprenoids include monoterpenes (10 carbons), sesquiterpenes (15 carbons), diterpenes (20 carbons), and triterpenes (30 carbons). The monoterpene geraniol and the sesquiterpene farnesol show promise as more potent compounds than *d*-limonene or perillyl alcohol in vivo, and are in development for clinical cancer prevention. Although many reviews have summarized the anticancer activities of isoprenoids *(2–9)*, this chapter focuses on isoprenoid mechanisms of action and clinical applications for *d*-limonene, perillyl alcohol, geraniol, and farnesol (Fig. 1).

2. MECHANISMS OF ACTION

Monoterpenes and other isoprenoids have multiple mechanisms of action in the prevention of cancer during the initiation and the promotion/progression stages of carcinogenesis. Among these are three cellular effects: induction of apoptosis, cell-cycle arrest, and differentiation. The molecular mechanisms responsible for each of these effects are being elucidated, and appear to differ among tissue types in some cases. Unresolved mechanistic questions include the identity of the first molecular interactions between isoprenoids and their targets in various cell types. Emerging technologies such as microarray analysis and proteomics may be valuable in solving these unanswered questions.

2.1. Apoptosis

Apoptosis is a common mechanism for monoterpenes and related isoprenoids in many cancer types. Monoterpene-induced apoptosis of carcinoma cells was first described by Mills et al. *(10)* in a rat liver diethylnitrosamine-induced carcinogenesis model. Rats that consumed a 2% (w/w) perillyl alcohol diet exhibited a 10-fold reduction in liver-tumor mass that was associated with a 10-fold increase in apoptosis and no change in liver-tumor DNA synthesis. Perillyl alcohol-induced apoptosis has also been demonstrated

From: Cancer Chemoprevention, Volume 1: Promising Cancer Chemoprevention Agents
Edited by: G. J. Kelloff, E. T. Hawk, and C. C. Sigman © Humana Press Inc., Totowa, NJ

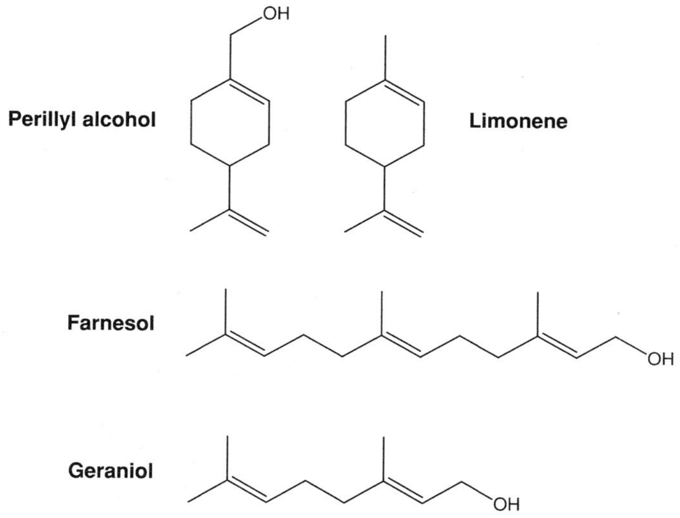

Fig. 1. Isoprenoid structures.

in vivo in colon tumors of that rats that consumed chemopreventive perillyl alcohol diets *(11)* and in chemically induced, regressing rat mammary carcinomas treated with dietary perillyl alcohol *(12)*. Perillyl alcohol also causes apoptosis in cultured pancreatic adenocarcinoma cells *(13)*, *bcr/abl*-transformed myeloid cells *(14)*, and immortalized smooth-muscle cells *(15)*. Other isoprenoids also have apoptotic activity. Farnesol induces apoptosis of acute leukemia *(16)* and Chinese hamster ovary cells *(17)*, and β–ionone induces the apoptosis of cultured melanoma, acute promyelocytic leukemia (APL), and colon adenocarcinoma cells *(18)*. When direct comparisons have been made, isoprenoids consistently induce apoptosis to a much greater extent in cancerous—rather than in noncancerous—normal cells *(10,12–14)*.

The mechanisms responsible for isoprenoid-induced apoptosis include upregulation of the transforming growth factor (TGF)β pathway in perillyl alcohol-treated liver and mammary cancers *(10,12,19,20)*. Perillyl alcohol-treated cancers exhibit upregulation of TGFβ$_1$ as well as the mannose-6 phosphate/insulin-like growth factor (IGF) II receptor, which activates latent TGFβ$_1$, a growth inhibitor, and degrades the growth-stimulating molecule IGF II. TGFβ receptors I and II are upregulated as well. TGFβ is known to stimulate apoptosis, and the in vivo co-localization of TGFβ in perillyl alcohol-treated apoptotic rat mammary carcinoma cells *(12)* strongly implicates this pathway in the anticarcinogenic activity of perillyl alcohol. Other apoptotic mechanisms attributed to perillyl alcohol include increases in AP-1

activity *(21)* and elevated proapoptotic protein (or mRNA) expression. Perillyl alcohol-treated rat mammary tumors have higher levels of Bax and Bad mRNA than untreated tumors *(12)*, and pancreatic adenocarcinoma cells treated with perillyl alcohol exhibit Bak protein induction *(13)*. Thus, although perillyl alcohol induces apoptosis in both mammary and pancreatic cancer cells, the molecular mechanism by which this is accomplished is different among the two cell types.

2.2. Cell-Cycle Regulation

A second mechanism common to a number of isoprenoids in several cancer cell types is inhibition of cell-cycle progression through the G$_1$ phase. Bardon et al. *(22)* first described the accumulation of perillyl alcohol and perillic acid-treated breast cancer cells in the G$_1$ phase of the cell cycle, and demonstrated that a decline in cyclin D$_1$ mRNA level preceded the G$_1$ effect. In addition to the cyclin D$_1$ loss, perillyl alcohol-induced G$_1$ arrest of mammary carcinoma cells has been associated with reduced Rb phosphorylation, increased p21Waf1/Cip1 levels, and reduced cyclin-dependent kinase activity *(12,23)*. Other isoprenoids also cause G$_1$ accumulation in melanoma, acute promyelocytic leukemia, and colon adenocarcinoma cells *(18)*.

2.3. Differentiation

Monoterpenes and related isoprenoids have the ability to induce differentiation and/or tissue remodeling. Haag et al. *(24)* described the remodeling/redifferentiation phenotype of *d*-limonene-treated rat mammary carcinomas undergoing active tumor regression. Shi and Gould *(25)* reported the differentiating effects of perillyl alcohol in cultured neuroblastoma-derived neuro-2A cells. Perillyl alcohol caused neurite outgrowth within 4 h of treatment in a dose-dependent manner. Recent studies by Hanley et al. *(26–28)* have described the particular ability of the sesquiterpene isoprenoid farnesol—and not other isoprenoids—to induce epidermal development in vivo and in cultured human keratinocytes. Furthermore, the transcriptional mechanism responsible for the farnesol-induced differentiation has been partially elucidated *(28)*. Although farnesol has been reported to be a putative ligand for the farnesoid (FXR) nuclear receptor, FXR mRNA was undetectable in the keratinoyces that displayed differentiation in response to farnesol, indicating that the differentiation effects were not likely to involve FXR. Farnesol treatment increased the transcription of differentiation-associated genes, activated peroxisome proliferator-activated receptor (PPAR)α nuclear-receptor activity, and elevated PPARα mRNA levels in the differentiating cells, suggesting a role for PPARα in the farnesol differentiation pathway. Furthermore, farnesol failed to evoke these responses in the epidermis from PPARα-/- knockout mice, indicating that PPARα is required for the differentiation effects of farnesol in the epidermis. It is presently unknown whether farnesol or its metabolite(s) act as direct ligands for PPARα or whether an indirect pathway is responsible for the cell-differentiating effects of farnesol.

2.4. Mevalonate/Cholesterol Pathway

Monoterpenes and other isoprenoids have a number of effects on the mevalonate/cholesterol pathway, the biosynthetic pathway from which all mammalian isoprenoids originate *(30)*. In plants, *d*-limonene is a product of geranylpyrophosphate, an intermediate in the plant plastidic isoprenoid pathway, and it serves as a precursor to all other cyclic monoterpenes, including perillyl alcohol *(1,29)*. In mammalian cells, geraniol and farnesol are produced by dephosphorylation of mevalonate pathway intermediates geranylpyrophosphate and farnesylpyrophosphate, respectively *(6)*. In addition to essential isoprenoids such as cholesterol, ubiquinone, and dolichols, the mammalian mevalonate pathway produces farnesylpyrophosphate and geranylgeranylpyrophosphate, the isoprenoid donors for protein prenylation, the posttranslational modification of proteins by farnesylation or geranylgeranylation, respectively *(30)*. The protein prenylation reactions

are catalyzed by farnesyltransferase and one of two geranylgeranyltransferases. The oncogenic proteins Ras, Rho, and the PRL (PTPCAAX) protein tyrosine phosphatases *(31)* are farnesylated, and farnesylation of Ras, for example, is required for its oncogenic function *(32,33)*. Monoterpenes can inhibit protein prenylation *(34–40)* because of their ability to inhibit farnesyltransferase and geranylgeranyltransferase *(41)*. HMG CoA reductase is the most tightly regulated step in the mevalonate pathway *(30,42)*, and isoprenoids, particularly farnesol, can downregulate HMG CoA reductase *(6,43–45)*. In this way, monoterpenes and farnesol may suppress the farnesylation and thus the oncogenic functions of Ras and perhaps other prenylated proteins. In pancreatic adenocarcinoma cells, perillyl alcohol inhibits Ras farnesylation, but not to the degree necessary to significantly affect the Ras GTP/GDP ratio and signal-transduction activity *(46)*. Thus, mechanisms other than inhibition of Ras farnesylation must account for the antitumor activity of perillyl alcohol toward pancreatic cancer cells. Perillyl alcohol can also inhibit ubiquinone and cholesterol biosynthesis *(47)*, and may thereby inhibit carcinogenesis by limiting ubiquinone availability for electron-transport chain function and suppressing cell division by limiting the cholesterol supply for cell-membrane synthesis.

2.5. Carcinogen Detoxification

Monoterpenes can block cancer initiation by diverting procarcinogen metabolism to less toxic products. The monoterpene *d*-limonene, for example, has chemopreventive activity during the initiation phase of 7,12-dimethylbenz[*a*]anthracene (DMBA) but not *N*-methyl-*N*-nitrosourea (MNU)-induced rat mammary cancer *(48,49)*. DMBA requires metabolic activation, and MNU is a directly acting carcinogen. Limonene blocks DMBA metabolic activation to the ultimate carcinogen principally by inducing phase 2 carcinogen-metabolizing enzymes glutathione-*S*-transferase and uridine diphosphate (UDP)-glucuronyltransferase, and it reduces DMBA-DNA adduct formation and increases DMBA and DMBA metabolite excretion *(50,51)*. Similarly, mice treated with either *d*-limonene or perillyl alcohol show reduced metabolism of 4-(methylnitrosamino)-1-(3-pyridyl)-1-butanone (NNK) by pulmonary and liver microsomes *(52)*, an effect that is consistent with the initiation-phase chemopreventive activity of *d*-limonene in NNK-induced lung carcinogenesis models *(54,58)*.

2.6. Other

Other cancer chemopreventive mechanisms ascribed to monoterpenes and other isoprenoids include the downregulation of Ras oncoprotein levels by perillyl alcohol (55,56), inhibition of polyamine biosynthesis and cell proliferation by limonene (57) and geraniol (58), and inhibition of phosphatidylcholine biosynthesis by farnesol (16,17).

3. PREVIOUS EFFICACY

3.1. Preclinical Studies

Preclinical investigations have revealed the widespread chemopreventive activity of d-limonene, perillyl alcohol, farnesol, and other isoprenoids toward a diverse array of solid cancers and leukemias at every stage of carcinogenesis. Other reviews have also addressed the antitumor activity of isoprenoids (2–4,6–9,55,59).

Limonene, perillyl alcohol, and related compounds, including natural products and synthetic derivatives, have chemopreventive and chemotherapeutic activity in rat mammary cancer models (24,48,49,54,60–65). Gastrointestinal cancer chemoprevention by monoterpenes and other isoprenoids is also well-established. Liver cancer chemoprevention by monoterpenes includes the prevention of chemically induced liver cancer by perillyl alcohol (10) and the suppression of transplanted hepatoma growth by geraniol (66). Colon cancer prevention by monoterpenes has been demonstrated by the chemoprevention of colonic aberrant crypt foci (ACF) formation by limonene (67) and the prevention of chemically induced colon cancer by perillyl alcohol (11). Inhibition of pancreatic cancer growth by perillyl alcohol, geraniol, and farnesol (68,69) has been reported, as has the chemoprevention of chemically induced pancreatic cancer by limonene (70). Similarly, limonene has chemopreventive activity toward N-methyl-N'-nitro-N-nitrosoguanidine-induced gastric cancer (57,71). Both limonene (72) and perillyl alcohol (73) have chemopreventive activity toward NNK-induced lung cancer, and limonene is effective in other lung cancer models as well (53,54). Other examples of the chemopreventive effects of isoprenoids include the prevention of chemically induced skin cancer by limonene (74) and ultraviolet (UV)-induced skin cancer by perillyl alcohol (75), and the suppression of B16 melanoma growth by β-ionone (76). In addition, leukemic-cell growth is markedly impaired by geraniol (77) and perillyl alcohol (14).

3.2. Epidemiological Studies

The principal dietary source for limonene is citrus peel oil (78). Two recent case-control epidemiology studies reported an association between higher citrus peel (but not citrus fruit or citrus juice) consumption and lower incidence of squamous cell carcinoma of the skin (79,80). Furthermore, there was a dose-responsive effect of citrus peel consumption on squamous-cell carcinoma incidence.

3.3. Clinical Studies

Clinical intervention studies have been conducted for the monoterpenes limonene and perillyl alcohol. Vigushin et al. (81) reported initial clinical trial results with oral limonene. One breast cancer patient treated with the maximum tolerated limonene dose of 8 g/m^2 per d had a partial response of 11 mo in duration, and prolonged stable disease occurred in several colorectal cancer (CRC) patients. No responses of this type occurred in a follow-up study. Perillyl alcohol antitumor activity has been evaluated in several Phase I clinical trials. One objective response in a patient with metastatic colorectal cancer (CRC) was reported (82), and a number of prostatic and colon cancer patients had prolonged stable disease with oral perillyl alcohol treatment (82–84). Farnesol and geraniol have been selected for clinical development through the NCI's Rapid Access to Preventive Intervention Development (RAPID) program.

4. SAFETY

Monoterpenes and other isoprenoids have low toxicity in animal and human subjects. The most common side effects reported in high-dose Phase I therapeutic clinical trials with advanced cancer patients are Grade I and Grade II fatigue and gastric reflux (81–84). For example, an individual who had a complete response to CRC following perillyl alcohol showed no toxicity over a 2-yr period while receiving daily divided doses totaling 4.8 g/m^2 per d.

5. PHARMACOLOGY

Limonene (35,37,81,85,86) and perillyl alcohol (64,82–84,87,88) (Fig. 1) are extensively metabolized in vivo, and form the common circulating metabolites perillic acid and dihydroperillic acid.

Higher circulating metabolite plasma concentrations are achieved with oral perillyl alcohol than with higher doses of limonene. The metabolite half-lives are approx 2 h in human subjects, and peak plasma concentrations at the highest tolerated perillyl alcohol doses are >400 μM for perillic acid and >20 μM for dihydroperillic acid *(82–84)*.

6. POPULATIONS THAT BENEFIT FROM INTERVENTION/POTENTIAL CLINICAL STUDIES

6.1. Populations for Intervention

Because monoterpenes and related isoprenoids have chemopreventive activity toward lung, colon, breast, pancreatic, and prostate cancers—all leading causes of cancer deaths—there are innumerable human populations that may benefit from cancer chemoprevention with these agents. Chemoprevention of lung cancer could be tested in smokers, particularly those with documented premalignant lesions. Colon cancer chemoprevention could be tested in individuals with inherited predisposition to the disease, such as those diagnosed with familial adenomatous polyposis (FAP) or in patients with sporadic benign adenomas. Patients at risk for breast cancer who may benefit from monoterpene chemoprevention include those with an inherited *BRCA1* or *BRCA2* mutation, or individuals with premalignant disease. Similarly, subjects with pancreatic K-*ras* oncogene mutation, chronic pancreatitis, or benign pancreatic neoplasms may benefit from chemoprevention with isoprenoids. Furthermore, because pancreatic cancer mortality is extremely high, chemoprevention of pancreatic adenocarcinoma recurrence after surgery or chemoprevention of disease progression to metastatic disease may be feasible. Prostate cancer chemoprevention may be feasible in individuals diagnosed with benign prostatic hyperplasia. In addition, chemoprevention of leukemia progression could be tested in individuals with Philadelphia chromosome positive (e.g., *bcr/abl* oncogene-positive) leukemia.

6.2. Use in Combinations

A second consideration for clinical trials with perillyl alcohol and other isoprenoids is mechanism-related. Because these compounds have mechanisms distinct from those of other chemopreventive agents, combination treatment among agents with different mechanisms may be warranted. For example, perillyl alcohol may be useful in combination with antiestrogens in the prevention of breast cancer in order to target both estrogen receptor (ER) positive and ER-negative cancers.

7. PROMISING ENDPOINTS (BIOMARKERS)

7.1. Measure Biomarkers in Preneoplastic/Malignant Cells

Perillyl alcohol and other isoprenoids are highly selective in vivo for malignant and premalignant lesions over normal tissues. For example, Ariazi et al. *(12)* reported a number of gene-expression changes from perillyl alcohol-treated rat mammary neoplasms that were undetectable in corresponding normal mammary tissues, and Mills et al. *(10)* found similarly selective effects of perillyl alcohol on liver neoplasms vs normal liver. These findings indicate that normal tissue or cell specimens are likely to be unsuitable for surrogate biomarker analysis of isoprenoid function, and thus biomarkers from preneoplastic or malignant tissues are most relevant in the evaluation of isoprenoid chemopreventive activity.

7.2. Surrogate Endpoint Biomarkers

Based on the known mechanisms of action of chemopreventive isoprenoids, a number of surrogate endpoint biomarkers have emerged. Apoptosis is the most widespread mechanism reported for isoprenoids *(10–16,18,58,70)*, and thus measurement of apoptosis itself is a key endpoint for many isoprenoid chemoprevention studies. Apoptosis can be evaluated by cell or nuclear morphology, DNA fragmentation analysis, e.g., by TUNEL or DNA laddering, annexin labeling, or caspase activation. Molecular regulators of apoptosis that are known to be affected by monoterpenes and other isoprenoids include TGFβ, TGFβ receptors, and the mannose-6-phosphate/IGF II receptor *(10,12,19,20)* in liver and mammary tissues, and regulators of the mitochondrial apoptotic pathway, namely Bax *(12)* and Bad in mammary tissue *(12)*, and Bak in the pancreas *(13)*. In a similar vein, G_1 cell-cycle phase accumulation often occurs in response to isoprenoids *(18,22,23)*, and thus general biomarkers of cell proliferation such as BrDU labeling or PCNA staining are appropriate. The specific cell-cycle associated changes reported in monoterpene-treated mammary cells include p21Waf1/Cip1 and cyclin D *(12,22)*. Additional biomarkers of isoprenoid chemopreventive activity may include Ras farnesylation *(34,83)*, Ras protein concentration *(56,83)*, and Phase II carcinogen-metabolizing enzyme concentrations *(50)*.

8. SUMMARY

In summary, diverse monoterpenes and sesquiterpenes show promising cancer chemopreventive activity in preclinical systems, and low toxicity has been observed with some responses in early clinical trials. Many molecular mechanisms of action for these compounds have been described, and future clinical studies will utilize the relevant biomarkers to monitor the effectiveness of the chemopreventive agents.

REFERENCES

1. McGarvey DJ, Croteau R. Terpenoid metabolism. *Plant Cell* 1995;7:1015–1026.
2. Crowell PL. Monoterpenes in breast cancer chemoprevention. *Breast Cancer Res Treat* 1997;46:191–197.
3. Crowell PL. Prevention and therapy of cancer by dietary monoterpenes. *J Nutr* 1999;129:775S–778S.
4. Crowell PL, Elson CE. Isoprenoids, health and disease, in *Handbook of Nutraceuticals and Functional Foods*. Wildman RC, ed. CRC Press, NY, 2001, pp.31–53.
5. Crowell PL, Gould MN. Chemoprevention and therapy of cancer by d-limonene. *Crit Rev Oncog* 1994;5:1–22.
6. Elson CE. Suppression of mevalonate pathway activities by dietary isoprenoids: protective roles in cancer and cardiovascular disease. *J Nutr* 1995;125:1666S-1672S.
7. Elson CE, Yu SG. The chemoprevention of cancer by mevalonate-derived constituents of fruits and vegetables. *J Nutr* 1994;124:607–614.
8. Gould MN. Prevention and therapy of mammary cancer by monoterpenes. *J Cell Biochem Suppl* 1995;22:139–144.
9. Gould MN. Cancer chemoprevention and therapy by monoterpenes. *Environ Health Perspect* 1997;105 Suppl 4:977–979.
10. Mills JJ, Chari RS, Boyer IJ, et al. Induction of apoptosis in liver tumors by the monoterpene perillyl alcohol. *Cancer Res* 1995;55:979–983.
11. Reddy BS, Wang CX, Samaha H, et al. Chemoprevention of colon carcinogenesis by dietary perillyl alcohol. *Cancer Res* 1997;57:420–425.
12. Ariazi EA, Satomi Y, Ellis MJ, et al. Activation of the transforming growth factor beta signaling pathway and induction of cytostasis and apoptosis in mammary carcinomas treated with the anticancer agent perillyl alcohol. *Cancer Res* 1999;59:1917–1928.
13. Stayrook KR, McKinzie JH, Burke YD, et al. Induction of the apoptosis-promoting protein Bak by perillyl alcohol in pancreatic ductal adenocarcinoma relative to untransformed ductal epithelial cells. *Carcinogenesis* 1997;18:1655–1658.
14. Sahin MB, Perman SM, Jenkins G, Clark SS. Perillyl alcohol selectively induces G0/G1 arrest and apoptosis in Bcr/Abl-transformed myeloid cell lines. *Leukemia* 1999;13:1581–1591.
15. Unlu S, Mason CD, Schachter M, Hughes AD. Perillyl alcohol, an inhibitor of geranylgeranyl transferase, induces apoptosis of immortalized human vascular smooth muscle cells in vitro. *J Cardiovasc Pharmacol* 2000;35:341–344.
16. Voziyan PA, Haug JS, Melnykovych G. Mechanism of farnesol cytotoxicity: further evidence for the role of PKC-dependent signal transduction in farnesol-induced apoptotic cell death. *Biochem Biophys Res Commun* 1995;212:479–486.
17. Wright MM, Henneberry AL, Lagace TA, et al. Uncoupling farnesol-induced apoptosis from its inhibition of phosphatidylcholine synthesis. *J Biol Chem* 2001;276:25,254–25,261.
18. Mo H, Elson CE. Apoptosis and cell-cycle arrest in human and murine tumor cells are initiated by isoprenoids. *J Nutr* 1999;129:804–813.
19. Ariazi EA, Gould MN. Identifying differential gene expression in monoterpene-treated mammary carcinomas using subtractive display. *J Biol Chem* 1996;271:29,286–29,294.
20. Jirtle RL, Haag JD, Ariazi EA, Gould MN. Increased mannose 6-phosphate/insulin-like growth factor II receptor and transforming growth factor beta 1 levels during monoterpene-induced regression of mammary tumors. *Cancer Res* 1993;53:3849–3852.
21. Satomi Y, Miyamoto S, Gould MN. Induction of AP-1 activity by perillyl alcohol in breast cancer cells. *Carcinogenesis* 1999;20:1957–1961.
22. Bardon S, Picard K, Martel P. Monoterpenes inhibit cell growth, cell cycle progression, and cyclin D1 gene expression in human breast cancer cell lines. *Nutr Cancer* 1998;32:1–7.
23. Shi W, Gould MN. Induction of cytostasis in mammary carcinoma cells treated with the anticancer agent perillyl alcohol. *Carcinogenesis* 2002;23:131–142.
24. Haag JD, Lindstrom MJ, Gould MN. Limonene-induced regression of mammary carcinomas. *Cancer Res* 1992;52:4021–4026.
25. Shi W, Gould MN. Induction of differentiation in neuro-2A cells by the monoterpene perillyl alcohol. *Cancer Lett* 1995;95:1–6.
26. Hanley K, Jiang Y, Crumrine D, et al. Activators of the nuclear hormone receptors PPARalpha and FXR accelerate the development of the fetal epidermal permeability barrier. *J Clin Invest* 1997;100:705–712.
27. Hanley K, Komuves LG, Bass NM, et al. Fetal epidermal differentiation and barrier development in vivo is accelerated by nuclear hormone receptor activators. *J Investig Dermatol* 1999;113:788–795.
28. Hanley K, Komuves LG, Ng DC, et al. Farnesol stimulates differentiation in epidermal keratinocytes via PPARα *J Biol Chem* 2000;275:11,484–11,491.
29. Lange BM, Croteau R. Isopentenyl diphosphate biosynthesis via a mevalonate-independent pathway: isopentenyl monophosphate kinase catalyzes the terminal enzymatic step. *Proc Natl Acad Sci USA* 1999;96:13,714–13,719.
30. Goldstein JL, Brown MS. Regulation of the mevalonate pathway. *Nature* 1990;343:425–430.
31. Cates CA, Michael RL, Stayrook KR, et al. Prenylation of oncogenic human PTP(CAAX) protein tyrosine phosphatases. *Cancer Lett* 1996;110:49–55.
32. Kato K, Cox AD, Hisaka MM, et al. Isoprenoid addition to Ras protein is the critical modification for its membrane

association and transforming activity. *Proc Natl Acad Sci USA* 1992;89:6403–6407.

33. Kato K, Der CJ, Buss JE. Prenoids and palmitate: lipids that control the biological activity of Ras proteins. *Semin Cancer Biol* 1992;3:179–188.

34. Crowell PL, Chang RR, Ren ZB, et al. Selective inhibition of isoprenylation of 2–6-kDa proteins by the anticarcinogen d-limonene and its metabolites. *J Biol Chem* 1991;266:17,679–17,685.

35. Crowell PL, Lin S, Vedejs E, Gould MN. Identification of metabolites of the antitumor agent d-limonene capable of inhibiting protein isoprenylation and cell growth. *Cancer Chemother Pharmacol* 1992;31:205–212.

36. Crowell PL, Ren Z, Lin S, et al. Structure-activity relationships among monoterpene inhibitors of protein isoprenylation and cell proliferation. *Biochem Pharmacol* 1994;47:1405–1415.

37. Hardcastle IR, Rowlands MG, Barber AM, et al. Inhibition of protein prenylation by metabolites of limonene. *Biochem Pharmacol* 1999;57:801–809.

38. Kawata S, Nagase T, Yamasaki E, et al. Modulation of the mevalonate pathway and cell growth by pravastatin and d-limonene in a human hepatoma cell line (Hep G2). *Br J Cancer* 1994;69:1015–1020.

39. Ren Z, Elson CE, Gould MN. Inhibition of type I and type II geranylgeranyl-protein transferases by the monoterpene perillyl alcohol in NIH3T3 cells. *Biochem Pharmacol* 1997;54:113–120.

40. Schulz S, Buhling F, Ansorge S. Prenylated proteins and lymphocyte proliferation: inhibition by d-limonene related monoterpenes. *Eur J Immunol* 1994;24:301–307.

41. Gelb MH, Tamanoi F, Yokoyama K, et al. The inhibition of protein prenyltransferases by oxygenated metabolites of limonene and perillyl alcohol. *Cancer Lett* 1995;91:169–175.

42. Elson CE, Peffley DM, Hentosh P, Mo H. Isoprenoid-mediated inhibition of mevalonate synthesis: potential application to cancer. *Proc Soc Exp Biol Med* 1999;221:294–311.

43. Clegg RJ, Middleton B, Bell GD, White DA. Inhibition of hepatic cholesterol synthesis and S-3-hydroxy-3-methylglutaryl-CoA reductase by mono and bicyclic monoterpenes administered in vivo. *Biochem Pharmacol* 1980;29:2125–2127.

44. Clegg RJ, Middleton B, Bell GD, White DA. The mechanism of cyclic monoterpene inhibition of hepatic 3-hydroxy-3-methylglutaryl coenzyme A reductase in vivo in the rat. *J Biol Chem* 1982;257:2294–2299.

45. Correll CC, Ng L, Edwards PA. Identification of farnesol as the non-sterol derivative of mevalonic acid required for the accelerated degradation of 3-hydroxy-3-methylglutaryl-coenzyme A reductase. *J Biol Chem* 1994;269:17,390–17,393.

46. Stayrook KR, McKinzie JH, Barbhaiya LH, Crowell PL. Effects of the antitumor agent perillyl alcohol on H-Ras vs K-Ras farnesylation and signal transduction in pancreatic cells. *Anticancer Res* 1998;18:823–828.

47. Ren Z, Gould MN. Inhibition of ubiquinone and cholesterol synthesis by the monoterpene perillyl alcohol. *Cancer Lett* 1994;76:185–190.

48. Elson CE, Maltzman TH, Boston JL, et al. Anti-carcinogenic activity of d-limonene during the initiation and promotion/progression stages of DMBA-induced rat mammary carcinogenesis. *Carcinogenesis* 1988;9:331–332.

49. Maltzman TH, Hurt LM, Elson CE, et al. The prevention of nitrosomethylurea-induced mammary tumors by d-limonene and orange oil. *Carcinogenesis* 1989;10:781–783.

50. Elegbede JA, Maltzman TH, Elson CE, Gould MN. Effects of anticarcinogenic monoterpenes on phase II hepatic metabolizing enzymes. *Carcinogenesis* 1993;14:1221–1223.

51. Maltzman TH, Christou M, Gould MN, Jefcoate CR. Effects of monoterpenoids on in vivo DMBA-DNA adduct formation and on phase I hepatic metabolizing enzymes. *Carcinogenesis* 1991;12:2081–2087.

52. Morse MA, Toburen AL. Inhibition of metabolic activation of 4-(methylnitrosamino)-1-(3- pyridyl)-1-butanone by limonene. *Cancer Lett* 1996;104:211–217.

53. Wattenberg LW, Coccia JB. Inhibition of 4-(methylnitrosamino)-1-(3-pyridyl)-1-butanone carcinogenesis in mice by D-limonene and citrus fruit oils. *Carcinogenesis* 1991;12:115–117.

54. Wattenberg LW, Sparnins VL, Barany G. Inhibition of N-nitrosodiethylamine carcinogenesis in mice by naturally occurring organosulfur compounds and monoterpenes. *Cancer Res* 1989;49:2689–2692.

55. Hohl RJ. Monoterpenes as regulators of malignant cell proliferation. *Adv Exp Med Biol* 1996;401:137–146.

56. Hohl RJ, Lewis K. Differential effects of monoterpenes and lovastatin on RAS processing. *J Biol Chem* 1995;270:17,508–17,512.

57. Yano H, Tatsuta M, Iishi H, et al. Attenuation by d-limonene of sodium chloride-enhanced gastric carcinogenesis induced by N-methyl-N'-nitro-N-nitrosoguanidine in Wistar rats. *Int J Cancer* 1999;82:665–668.

58. Carnesecchi S, Schneider Y, Ceraline J, et al. Geraniol, a component of plant essential oils, inhibits growth and polyamine biosynthesis in human colon cancer cells. *J Pharmacol Exp Ther* 2001;298:197–200.

59. Crowell PL, Siar Ayoubi A, Burke YD. Antitumorigenic effects of limonene and perillyl alcohol against pancreatic and breast cancer. *Adv Exp Med Biol* 1996;401:131–136.

60. Crowell PL, Kennan WS, Haag JD, et al. Chemoprevention of mammary carcinogenesis by hydroxylated derivatives of d-limonene. *Carcinogenesis* 1992; 13:1261–1264.

61. Elegbede JA, Elson CE, Qureshi A, et al. Inhibition of DMBA-induced mammary cancer by the monoterpene d-limonene. *Carcinogenesis* 1984;5:661–664.

62. Elegbede JA, Elson CE, Tanner MA, et al. Regression of rat primary mammary tumors following dietary d-limonene. *J Natl Cancer Inst* 1986;76:323–325.

63. Gould MN, Moore CJ, Zhang R, et al. Limonene chemoprevention of mammary carcinoma induction following direct *in situ* transfer of v-Ha-ras. *Cancer Res* 1994;54:3540–3543.

64. Haag JD, Gould MN. Mammary carcinoma regression induced by perillyl alcohol, a hydroxylated analog of limonene. *Cancer Chemother Pharmacol* 1994;34:477–483.

65. Russin WA, Hoesly JD, Elson CE, et al. Inhibition of rat mammary carcinogenesis by monoterpenoids. *Carcinogenesis* 1989;10:2161–2164.

66. Yu SG, Hildebrandt LA, Elson CE. Geraniol, an inhibitor of mevalonate biosynthesis, suppresses the growth of hepatomas and melanomas transplanted to rats and mice. *J Nutr* 1995;125:2763–2767.

67. Kawamori T, Tanaka T, Hirose Y, et al. Inhibitory effects of d-limonene on the development of colonic aberrant crypt

foci induced by azoxymethane in F344 rats. *Carcinogenesis* 1996;17:369–372.

68. Burke YD, Stark MJ, Roach SL, et al. Inhibition of pancreatic cancer growth by the dietary isoprenoids farnesol and geraniol. *Lipids* 1997;32:151–156.

69. Stark MJ, Burke YD, McKinzie JH, et al. Chemotherapy of pancreatic cancer with the monoterpene perillyl alcohol. *Cancer Lett* 1995;96:15–21.

70. Nakaizumi A, Baba M, Uehara H, et al. d-Limonene inhibits N-nitrosobis(2-oxopropyl)amine induced hamster pancreatic carcinogenesis. *Cancer Lett* 1997;117:99–103.

71. Uedo N, Tatsuta M, Iishi H, et al. Inhibition by D-limonene of gastric carcinogenesis induced by N-methyl- N'-nitro-N-nitrosoguanidine in Wistar rats. *Cancer Lett* 1999;137:131–136.

72. El-Bayoumy K, Upadhyaya P, Desai DH, et al. Effects of 1,4-phenylenebis(methylene)selenocyanate, phenethyl isothiocyanate, indole-3-carbinol, and *d*-limonene individually and in combination on the tumorigenicity of the tobacco-specific nitrosamine 4-(methylnitrosamino)-1-(3-pyridyl)-1-butanone in A/J mouse lung. *Anticancer Res* 1996;16:2709–2712.

73. Lantry LE, Zhang Z, Gao F, et al. Chemopreventive effect of perillyl alcohol on 4-(methylnitrosamino)-1-(3-pyridyl)-1-butanone induced tumorigenesis in (C3H/HeJ X A/J)F1 mouse lung. *J Cell Biochem Suppl* 1997;27:20–25.

74. Elegbede JA, Maltzman TH, Verma AK, et al. Mouse skin tumor promoting activity of orange peel oil and d-limonene: a re-evaluation. *Carcinogenesis* 1986;7:2047–2049.

75. Barthelman M, Chen W, Gensler HL, et al. Inhibitory effects of perillyl alcohol on UVB-induced murine skin cancer and AP-1 transactivation. *Cancer Res* 1998;58:711–716.

76. He L, Mo H, Hadisusilo S, et al. Isoprenoids suppress the growth of murine B16 melanomas in vitro and in vivo. *J Nutr* 1997;127:668–674.

77. Shoff SM, Grummer M, Yatvin MB, Elson CE. Concentration-dependent increase of murine P388 and B16 population doubling time by the acyclic monoterpene geraniol. *Cancer Res* 1991;51:37–42.

78. Duke JA. Handbook of phytochemical constituents of GRAS herbs and other economic plants, CRC Press, Boca Raton, FL, 1992.

79. Hakim IA, Harris RB. Joint effects of citrus peel use and black tea intake on the risk of squamous cell carcinoma of the skin. *BMC Dermatol* 2001;1:3

80. Hakim IA, Harris RB, Ritenbaugh C. Citrus peel use is associated with reduced risk of squamous cell carcinoma of the skin. *Nutr Cancer* 2000;37:161–168.

81. Vigushin DM, Poon GK, Boddy A, et al. Phase I and pharmacokinetic study of D-limonene in patients with advanced cancer. Cancer Research Campaign Phase I/II Clinical Trials Committee. *Cancer Chemother Pharmacol* 1998;42:111–117.

82. Ripple GH, Gould MN, Arzoomanian RZ, et al. Phase I clinical and pharmacokinetic study of perillyl alcohol administered four times a day. *Clin Cancer Res* 2000;6:390–396.

83. Hudes GR, Szarka CE, Adams A, et al. Phase I pharmacokinetic trial of perillyl alcohol (NSC 641066) in patients with refractory solid malignancies. *Clin Cancer Res* 2000;6:3071–3080.

84. Ripple GH, Gould MN, Stewart JA, et al. Phase I clinical trial of perillyl alcohol administered daily. *Clin Cancer Res* 1998;4:1159–1164.

85. Crowell PL, Elson CE, Bailey HH, et al. Human metabolism of the experimental cancer therapeutic agent d-limonene. *Cancer Chemother Pharmacol* 1994;35:31–37.

86. Poon GK, Vigushin D, Griggs LJ, et al. Identification and characterization of limonene metabolites in patients with advanced cancer by liquid chromatography/mass spectrometry. *Drug Metab Dispos* 1996;24:565–571.

87. Phillips LR, Malspeis L, Supko JG. Pharmacokinetics of active drug metabolites after oral administration of perillyl alcohol, an investigational antineoplastic agent, to the dog. *Drug Metab Dispos* 1995;23:676–680.

88. Zhang Z, Chen H, Chan KK, et al. Gas chromatographic-mass spectrometric analysis of perillyl alcohol and metabolismlites in plasma. *J Chromatogr B Biomed Sci Appl* 1999;728:85–95.

26 Development of an Inhibitor of raf Kinase

Frank McCormick, PhD, FRS

CONTENTS

SELECTION OF RAF AS A TARGET
PRODUCTION OF RECOMBINANT RAF
PRECLINICAL TESTING
CLINICAL EXPERIENCE
CONCLUSION
REFERENCES

1. SELECTION OF RAF AS A TARGET

Our efforts to develop raf kinase inhibitors derive from the clear, causal role of Ras proteins in human cancer, and the understanding that raf kinase is a direct downstream effector of Ras action. K-*ras* is activated by mutation in more than 20% of all solid tumors, N-*ras* in 30% of leukemias and lymphomas, and H-*ras* in small numbers of solid and liquid tumors. In addition, normal Ras alleles are frequently amplified in human tumors, and pathways upstream of Ras are amplified (HER2/neu, for example) or activated by gene rearrangement *(bcr-abl)* or mutation such as epidermal growth factor (EGF)-receptor in glioblastoma, for example. For these reasons, Ras has long been considered a promising target for therapeutic intervention (reviewed in *1*).

Strategies for inhibiting Ras directly have been complicated by several factors. First, mutant Ras proteins resemble activated guanosine 5' triphosphate (GTP)-bound forms of their normal counterparts, from the structural perspective, and do not appear to offer opportunities for selective binding of small-molecule drugs. The critical differences lie in their ability to undergo guanosine triphosphatase-activating protein (GAP)-mediated GTP hydrolysis; residues involved in this process are buried within the protein and may not be easily accessible to inhibitor. Development of molecules that block mutant Ras directly and specifically have not seemed feasible. However, antibodies that recognize amino acid substitutions at position 12

of Ras proteins block transformation by the appropriate mutant Ras proteins without affecting normal Ras function *(2)*. These experiments suggest that inner components of the Ras protein become accessible, perhaps as the protein cycles between active and inactive states, and that strategies directed at this accessible, nucleotide-free form of Ras may be worth reconsidering. Likewise, strategies to restore GTPase activity of mutant Ras proteins that would convert the active, GTP-bound form to the inactive state were abandoned after crystal structures suggested that failure of mutant proteins to hydrolyze GTP was the result of steric hindrance by substituting amino acids *(3)*. More recently, it has been suggested that positioning charged residues close to the γ-phosphate of bound GTP could trigger GTP hydrolysis even in mutant Ras proteins, raising the possibility that drugs could be developed to selectively turn off mutant Ras proteins *(4)*. However, these approaches for the inhibition of mutant Ras proteins have not yet been translated into drug candidates, and are not discussed further in this chapter.

The possibility of blocking Ras by preventing post-translational farnesylation has been pursued aggressively by a large number of groups, and farnesyl transferase inhibitors have been in extensive clinical trials. Unfortunately, K-Ras proteins can be modified by geranylgeranyl transferase, restoring their biological function. Farnesyl transferase inhibitors are therefore ineffective at blocking K-Ras function *(5)*.

From: Cancer Chemoprevention, Volume 1: Promising Cancer Chemoprevention Agents
Edited by: G. J. Kelloff, E. T. Hawk, and C. C. Sigman © Humana Press Inc., Totowa, NJ

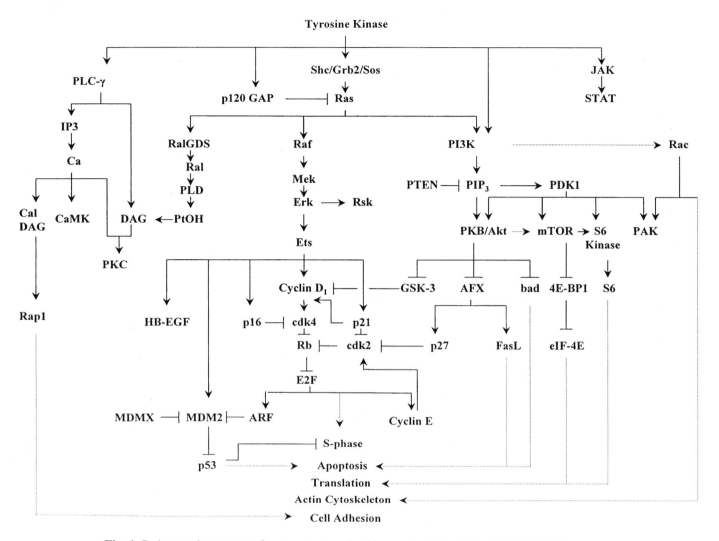

Fig. 1. Pathways downstream for receptor tyrosine kinases that include the Raf/MEK/ERK cascade.

We have taken the approach of targeting pathways directly downstream of Ras, as a surrogate to blocking Ras itself. In 1992, pioneering antibody microinjection experiments from Stacey and colleagues showed that Raf kinase is downstream of Ras and is necessary for Ras function. In 1993, these proteins were found to interact directly *(6)*. Binding Ras to Raf induces kinase activity through a number of steps that are not fully understood. In cells, Ras-binding recruits Raf to the plasma membrane, and a number of kinases and regulatory proteins, participate in the activation process *(7)*. Phosphatase 2a removes inhibitory phosphates, and PAK and Src kinases phosphorylate Raf and contribute to its activation. 14-3-3 binding is determined by these phosphorylation events, playing a key role in regulating Raf kinase activity *(8)*. In vitro, Ras binding to Raf appears to activate the kinase by allosteric mechanisms

that depend on the presence of lipids, but do not depend on autophosphorylation or trans-phosphorylation *(9,10)*.

Raf kinase activated by Ras binds phosphorylates and activates mitogen-activated protein (MAP) kinase kinase (MEK) on two sites, and thus initiates the familiar MAP kinase cascade (Fig. 1). Currently, it is believed that most of Raf kinase's biological activity is mediated by this pathway, but the possibility of MEK-independent functions cannot be dismissed. We therefore conclude that Raf inhibitors are likely to block signal transmission from Ras to MEK and on down the MAP kinase cascade.

Transformation of cells in culture by Ras depends on Raf in most cases. However, other Ras effectors are also necessary, and it seems likely that the full transforming power of Ras depends on complex interactions between multiple Ras effector pathways

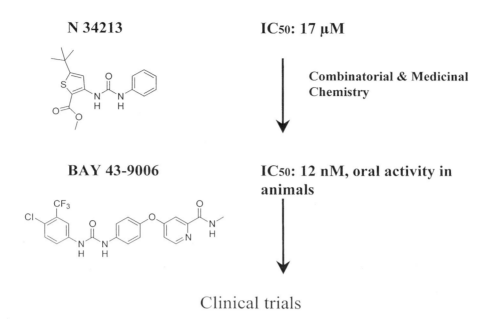

N 34213

IC50: 17 µM

Combinatorial & Medicinal Chemistry

BAY 43-9006

IC50: 12 nM, oral activity in animals

Clinical trials

Fig. 2. Structures of the precursor compound and the final compound BAY 43-9006.

(11). One such interaction involves stable expression of cyclin D$_1$, a key mediator of Ras transformation in vivo *(12)*. Transcription of this gene is mediated by the Raf/MEK/MAP kinase pathway, and cyclin D$_1$ protein is stabilized by another Ras effector pathway initiated by binding to phosphoinositol 3-kinase (PI3K) *(13)*. Similarly, the Raf/MEK/MAP kinase pathway stimulates transcription of murine double mutant 2 (MDM2) *(14)*, whereas the PI3K pathway provokes nuclear accumulation of this p53 regulatory protein *(15)*. The practical importance of these synergistic interactions is that inhibitors of either pathway can profoundly affect Ras activity and thus present potential drug targets.

Until recently, it has been difficult to determine which Ras effector pathway is most critical to the causal role of Ras in development of human cancer. However, the recent discovery that malignant melanomas contain either activated B-Raf or activated N-Ras *(16)* strongly suggests that—at least in this disease—activation of Ras and Raf may be biologically equivalent, although more analysis must be performed on these tumors. For example, phosphatase and tensin homolog (PTEN) is often deleted in melanomas, and a reciprocal relationship has been reported for PTEN loss and Ras activation *(17,18)*. This suggests that both Raf kinase and the PI3K pathway may be upregulated in melanomas that retain wild-type Ras. If so, we would conclude that both effector pathways are necessary for Ras transformation.

In any case, activated B-Raf presents an attractive target for therapy in this disease and others where B-Raf is also activated—colon cancers, breast cancers, and other tumors at lower frequency.

2. PRODUCTION OF RECOMBINANT RAF

Raf kinase exists as a protein complex with 14-3-3 family members—HSP90 and possibly other proteins. Raf itself is modified by phosphorylation on several residues. Purification of active Raf kinase complexes for high-throughput screening has been achieved from Sf9 insect cells using baculovirus vectors expression epitope tagged c-Raf-1 and, in separate vectors, active v-*src* *(19)*. Using this material, we began screening Raf inhibitors in 1992 at ONYX Pharmaceuticals. We identified a weakly active lead compound (N34213, Ki of 17 µM: Fig. 2) from such screens. This compound was subject to extensive medicinal and combinatorial chemistry at Bayer Pharmaceuticals, ultimately identifying a clinical candidate, BAY 43-9006 *(20,21)*.

3. PRECLINICAL TESTING

Effects of blocking the Raf/MEK/MAP kinase have been anticipated by analyzing the effects of MEK inhibitors on cells in culture and in mouse models *(22)*, and effects of expressing dominant-negative forms of MEK that are believed to bind Raf and block MEK activation. Preclinical testing of BAY 43-9006 showed promising activity at levels that were not toxic *(23)*.

4. CLINICAL EXPERIENCE

The orally active Raf kinase inhibitor BAY 43-9006 entered Phase I clinical trials in 2000, and is now in Phase II *(24)*. Initially, it was studied in 46 heavily pretreated patients with refractory solid tumors. Diarrhea was the dose-limiting toxicity (DLT) of this compound, which was observed at doses of 800 mg twice daily. Disease stabilization of greater than 6 mo was observed in seven of the 46 patients. One patient suffering from hepatocellular carcinoma achieved a partial response at 20 wk on a dose schedule of 400 mg twice daily. Expression of activated extracellular signal-regulated kinase (ERK) was measured as a surrogate for Raf kinase inhibition, using cells from peripheral blood. Significant inhibition of ERK phosphorylation was detected, and the most dramatic results are apparent in patients receiving 400 mg twice daily, although significant reductions have also been seen at lower doses in which side effects were minimal.

5. CONCLUSION

BAY 43-9006 is the first orally active Raf kinase inhibitor to enter clinical trials. It was originally developed as part of a strategy to block activated mutant Ras in human cancers, and this may be the clinical situation in which the compound is effective. However, the discovery of mutations in B-*raf* in melanoma and other types of cancer suggests that these may be the more promising diseases to explore the potential of this agent. Obviously, combinations of this drug with others will be tested extensively, since its toxicity is tolerable. Furthermore, the effectiveness of this agent will undoubtedly be compared with that of MAP kinase inhibitors that entered clinical trials a little later. Hopefully, these approaches will prove effective, and will provide clinical benefit to patients who suffer from cancer in the near future.

REFERENCES

1. McCormick F. Small-molecule inhibitors of cell signaling. *Curr Opin Biotechnol* 2000;11:593–597.
2. Feramisco JR, Clark R, Wong G, et al. Transient reversion of ras oncogene-induced cell transformation by antibodies specific for amino acid 12 of ras protein. *Nature* 1985;314:639–642.
3. Wittinghofer A, Franken SM, Scheidig AJ, et al. Three-dimensional structure and properties of wild-type and mutant H-ras-encoded p21. *Ciba Found Symp* 1993;176:6–21.
4. Ahmadian MR, Zor T, Vogt D, et al. Guanosine triphosphatase stimulation of oncogenic Ras mutants. *Proc Natl Acad Sci USA* 1999;96:7065–7070.
5. Prendergast GC, Rane N. Farnesyltransferase inhibitors: mechanism and applications. *Expert Opin Investig Drugs* 2001;10:2105–2116.
6. Van Aelst L, Barr M, Marcus S, et al. Complex formation between RAS and RAF and other protein kinases. *Proc Natl Acad Sci USA* 1993;90:6213–6217.
7. Kolch W. Meaningful relationships: the regulation of the Ras/Raf/MEK/ERK pathway by protein interactions. *Biochem J* 2000;351:289–305.
8. Freed E, Symons M., Macdonald SG, et al. Binding of 14-3-3 proteins to the protein kinase Raf and effects on its activation. *Science* 1994;265:1713–1716.
9. Stokoe D, McCormick F. Activation of c-Raf-1 by Ras and Src through different mechanisms: activation in vivo and in vitro. *EMBO J* 1997;16:2384–2396.
10. Shimizu K, Ohtsuka T, Takai Y. Cell-free assay system for Ras- and Rap1-dependent activation of MAP-kinase cascade. *Methods Mol Biol* 1998;84:173–183.
11. Hamad NM, Elconin JH, Karnoub AE, et al. Distinct requirements for Ras oncogenesis in human versus mouse cells. *Genes Dev* 2002;16:2045–2057.
12. Yu Q, Geng Y, Sicinski P. Specific protection against breast cancers by cyclin D1 ablation. *Nature* 2001;411:1017–1021.
13. Diehl JA, Cheng M, Roussel MF, et al. Glycogen synthase kinase-3β regulates cyclin D1 proteolysis and subcellular localization. *Genes Dev* 1998;12:3499–3511.
14. Ries SJ, Biederer C, Woods D, et al. Opposing effects of Ras on p53: transcriptional activation of mdm2 and induction of p14ARF. *Cell* 2000;103:321–330.
15. Mayo LD, Donner DB. A phosphatidylinositol 3-kinase/Akt pathway promotes translocation of Mdm2 from the cytoplasm to the nucleus. *Proc Natl Acad Sci USA* 2001;98:11,598–11,603.
16. Davies H, Bignell Gr, Cox C, et al. Mutations of the BRAF gene in human cancer. *Nature* 2002;417:949–954.
17. Ikeda T, Yochinaga K, Suzuki A, et al. Anticorresponding mutations of the KRAS and PTEN genes in human endometrial cancer. *Oncol Rep* 2000;7:567–570.
18. Tsao H, Zhang X, Fowlkes K, et al. Relative reciprocity of NRAS and PTEN/MMAC1 alterations in cutaneous melanoma cell lines. *Cancer Res* 2000;60:1800–1804.
19. Macdonald SG, Crews CM, Wu L, et al. Reconstitution of the Raf-1-MEK-ERK signal transduction pathway in vitro. *Mol Cell Biol* 1993;13:6615–6620.
20. Lyons JF, Wilhelm S, Hibner B, et al. Discovery of a novel Raf kinase inhibitor. *Endocr Relat Cancer* 2001;8:219–225.
21. Lowinger TB, Riedl B, Dumas J, et al. Design and discovery of small molecules targeting raf-1 kinase. *Curr Pharm Des* 2002;8:2269–2278.
22. Sebolt-Leopold JS, Dudley DT, Herrera R, et al. Blockade of the MAP kinase pathway suppresses growth of colon tumors in vivo. *Nat Med* 1999;5:810–816.
23. Wilhelm S, Chien DS. BAY 43-9006: preclinical data. *Curr Pharm Des* 2002;8:2255–2257.
24. Hotte SJ, Hirte HW. BAY 43-9006: early clinical data in patients with advanced solid malignancies. *Curr Pharm Des* 2002;8:2249–2253.

27 Abnormalities in Cell Cycle Control in Human Cancer and Their Relevance to Chemoprevention

Alessandro Sgambato, MD, PhD and I. Bernard Weinstein, MD

CONTENTS

1. INTRODUCTION

Carcinogenesis is a multistep process characterized by the progressive acquisition of mutations and epigenetic abnormalities in expression of a variety of cellular genes, which eventually leads to the appearance of a fully malignant cancer. The genes involved in the carcinogenic process have been subdivided into two major categories: oncogenes, dominant-acting genes with increased activity that contributes to tumor development; and tumor-suppressor genes, recessive-acting genes whose functional loss enhances tumor development *(1,2)*. These genes have highly diverse functions, and contribute to cancer formation through multiple mechanisms. Intracellular pathways are involved in signal transduction and gene expression, cell-cycle control, DNA repair and genomic stability, and cell-fate determination—e.g., differentiation, senescence, and apoptosis. Extracellular pathways to cancer formation include tumor invasion, metastasis, and angiogenesis. Within the past decade, it has become apparent that abrogation of normal cell-cycle control is a common event in human tumorigenesis, and that a variety of oncogenes and tumor-suppressor genes act through this mechanism (reviewed in *3–8*). This chapter briefly reviews our knowledge of the mechanisms that control the normal mammalian cell cycle, and major abnormalities that have been discovered in various types of human cancers, and then discusses the current and future relevance of these findings to cancer chemoprevention.

2. MAMMALIAN CELL CYCLE

The cell cycle of proliferating eukaryotic cells is typically subdivided into four distinct phases: G_1, S, G_2, and M. After cell division, daughter cells undergo G_1 phase in which cell size increases and cells prepare for DNA synthesis. The cells then progress into the S phase, during which DNA and histone synthesis occur. They then proceed through the G_2 phase and prepare for mitosis, which occurs in the M phase. Not all cells in normal adult tissues and in many cancers are actively dividing. Many are terminally differentiated, and are unable to reenter the cell cycle. Others may have exited the cell cycle, and are in a non-proliferative or quiescent state known as G_0. In response to specific mitogens, cells in G_0 can re-enter the cell cycle at G_1 and then proceed through the S, G_2, and M phases. The decision between continued proliferation vs differentiation or quiescence is usually made by cells during the G_1

From: Cancer Chemoprevention, Volume 1: Promising Cancer Chemoprevention Agents
Edited by: G. J. Kelloff, E. T. Hawk, and C. C. Sigman © Humana Press Inc., Totowa, NJ

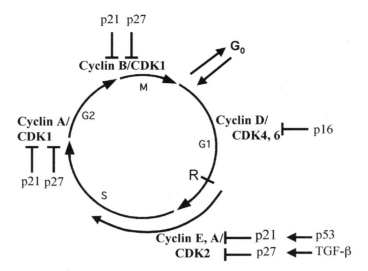

Fig. 1. A schematic diagram of the mammalian cell cycle indicating the major cyclins, cyclin-dependent kinases (CDKs), and CDK inhibitors (p16[Ink4a], p21[Cip1], p27[Kip1]), which regulate transitions through the specific phases of the cell cycle. "R" indicates the restriction point beyond which progression of the cell cycle continues even if mitogenic signals are removed. When hypophosphorylated, the Rb protein inhibits G_1-S transition. For additional details, *see* Fig. 3 and text.

phase of the cell cycle. Progression through G_1 is dependent on stimulation by mitogens (growth factors, cytokines, etc.) until a critical "restriction point" (R) is reached, after which further progression through the cell cycle continues even if mitogenic signals are removed or protein synthesis is inhibited *(9)*.

2.1. Cyclins, Cyclin-Dependent Kinases (CDK), and CDK Inhibitors (CDI)

The orderly progression of dividing mammalian cells through various phases of the cell cycle is governed by a series of proteins known as cyclins *(7,10)*. Cyclins display a remarkable periodicity in changes in abundance during the cell cycle, essentially functioning as positive regulatory subunits of a family of serine/threonine protein kinases called cyclin-dependent kinases (CDKs) *(7,10,11)*. Specific cyclins bind to specific CDKs, activating their kinase activity. Each of these cyclin/CDK complexes is activated at a specific point during the cell cycle and has a specific set of substrates. Sequential activation and subsequent inactivation of these cyclin-CDK complexes govern the progression of eukaryotic cells through the cell cycle. Since CDKs are usually constitutively expressed, and expression of cyclins oscillates with respect to the cell cycle, cyclins control the timing of CDK activation. In mammalian cells, sequential oscillations in levels of cyclins are mainly regulated at the transcriptional level, but also involve other mechanisms, including the

ubiquitin-dependent proteolytic machinery that regulates protein degradation *(7,10)*.

To date, nine different cyclin-dependent kinases (CDK1–9) and at least 15 different cyclins (from cyclin A to T) have been identified in mammalian cells *(7)*. However, only four CDKs (1, 2, 4, and 6) and 8 cyclins (D_1, D_2, D_3, E, A_1, A_2, B_1, B_2) are known to play specific roles in cyclin/CDK control of cell-cycle progression. A schematic representation of the mammalian cell cycle and phases in which major cyclins and CDKs act is shown in Fig. 1. As mentioned previously, quiescent G_0 cells can re-enter the cell cycle in response to external mitogenic stimuli. Cyclins D (1, 2, and 3) are then expressed, bind to and activate CDK4 and/or CDK6 depending on the particular cell type, and thus drive progression through G_1. Cyclin E and cyclin A are then sequentially expressed, bind to CDK2, and allow cells to move into and traverse the S phase. Cyclin A/CDK1 (also called cdc2) then drive the transition from S to G_2 phase. Cyclin B/CDK1 complexes accumulate in the G_2 phase, and are required for progression of cells through the M phase. Following completion of anaphase, cyclin B is degraded by proteolysis, returning cells to a G_1 state from which they can proceed to a new cycle or exit to a quiescent state.

Cyclin accumulation and binding to CDKs is not the only mechanism that regulates CDK activity. Both positive and negative phosphorylation events, as well

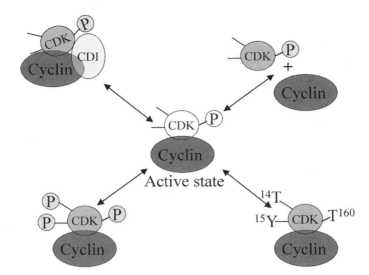

Fig. 2. A simplified scheme of mechanisms that regulate cyclin/CDK activity. CDKs are positively regulated by binding to cyclins and phosphorylation on a specific threonine (Thr 160 in CDK2). They are negatively regulated by phosphorylation on conserved threonine and tyrosine residues near the aminoterminus (Thr 14 and Tyr 15 in mammalian CDK2) and by binding to specific CDIs.

as association with specific inhibitory proteins, are critical in regulating activation of cyclin/CDK complexes during cell-cycle progression (6,7,12). These complexes become activated by phosphorylation at specific sites on CDKs by a CDK-activating kinase (CAK), a multi-subunit enzyme whose catalytic subunit, CDK7, is bound to cyclin H (7). A single CAK can activate all major cyclin/CDK complexes involved in mammalian cell-cycle control. CAK protein levels appear to remain constant during the cell cycle. Changes in CAK activity are mainly dependent on the availability of CDK-Thr[160] for phosphorylation. A still unidentified CDK phosphatase (CAP) is responsible for dephosphorylating these threonine residues, thus inactivating CDK activity. On the other hand, phosphorylation of other conserved threonine and tyrosine residues (Thr 14 and Tyr 15 in mammalian CDK2) located near the aminoterminus negatively regulates CDK activity. The Wee and Myt1 kinases phosphorylate these residues in yeast, but their mammalian counterparts have not yet been definitively identified. The CDC25 (A, B and C) phosphatases remove these inhibitory phosphate groups on CDKs, activating CDK activity. A schematic representation of this complex regulation of cyclin/CDK activity is shown in Fig. 2.

A series of specific CDK inhibitory proteins (CDIs) have been identified in mammalian cells. They are classified into two major categories. The INK4 family includes p16[Inka], p15[Inkb], p18[Inkc], and p19[Inkd], which specifically inhibit CDK4 and CDK6 by binding directly to these CDKs (3,4,7,10,11). The Cip/Kip family includes p21[Cip1] (also known as p21[Waf1]), p27[Kip1], and p57[Kip2] (7,12). These proteins inhibit a broad range of CDKs by binding to various cyclin/CDK complexes, but are most effective in blocking cyclin E/CDK2 and cyclin A/CDK2 complexes. It has been shown that members of the Cip/Kip family are also required to assemble active cyclin D/CDK complexes (6). These complexes retain their catalytic activity when bound to Cip/Kip inhibitors at low stoichiometric ratios, but high concentrations of these CDIs inhibit kinase activities of cyclin/CDK complexes. There is evidence that p27[Kip1] manifests its major inhibitory effect on the cell cycle by binding to and inhibiting the cyclin E/CDK2 complex. A decrease in the cyclin D_1 protein—for example, by withdrawal of growth factors—, can cause a shift of p27[Kip1] from cyclin D_1/CDK4,6 complexes to cyclin E/CDK2 complexes, thus arresting G_1 progression (6).

p21[Cip1] is directly induced when the p53 protein is activated as a result of DNA damage, but it can also be induced by a variety of other conditions via a p53-independent pathway. p57[Kip1] appears to play a role in cell differentiation and apoptosis in various tissues. p27[Kip1] has been implicated in negatively regulating cell proliferation in response to extracellular signals. Induced upon serum deprivation, it is required for the

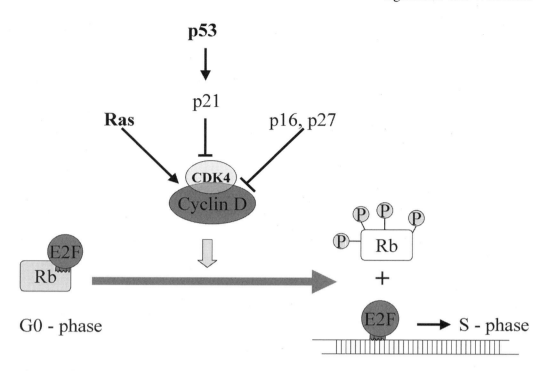

Fig. 3. The retinoblastoma protein (pRb) is the major target of cyclin D/CDK4 kinase activity. Phosphorylation of pRb prevents its binding to and inhibition of transcription factor E2F. When pRb is hyperphosphorylated, free E2F can activate the transcription of genes required for progression through the S phase. CDK activity is inhibited by the CDK inhibitors p21[Cip1], p16[Ink4a], and p27[Kip1]. In response to DNA damage, p53 activates the expression of p21[Cip1], thus causing cell-cycle arrest. Expression of cycin D1 is enhanced by Ras and various growth stimuli.

resulting arrest of cells in G_1. In normal epithelial cells, increased expression of p27[Kip1] also mediates the G_1 arrest induced by transforming growth factor (TGF-β), contact inhibition, or growth in suspension *(7,11,12)*. On the other hand, p27[Kip1] is downregulated when quiescent fibroblasts or epithelial cells are stimulated with growth factors; degradation of p27[Kip1] is essential for progression of T-cells from quiescence to S phase on exposure to interleukin-2 *(4)*. p27[Kip1] expression is mainly regulated at the post-transcriptional level. In fact, while p27[Kip1] mRNA levels are constant during the cell cycle, the p27[Kip1] protein can undergo rapid degradation by the ubiquitin proteasome pathway. This proteolysis is dramatically reduced in resting cells *(13,14)*. p27[Kip1] can act as a substrate of cyclin E/CDK2 kinase activity, and this phosphorylation triggers its ubiquitin-mediated degradation. Once activated, cyclin E/CDK2 promotes p27[Kip1] degradation, accounting in part for the irreversibility of the subsequent entry into S phase *(4)*.

Cyclin/CDK complexes exert their cell cycle-related functions in the nucleus. Thus, it is essential that cyclin/CDK complexes, or the individual subunits, enter the nucleus. The Cip/Kip proteins are necessary

for assembly of cyclin D/CDK complexes, and promote cyclin D/CDK activity by directing them to the nucleus *(15)*. Since only the nuclear component of active cyclin/CDK complexes can regulate the cell cycle, it has been suggested that abnormalities in cytoplasmic vs nuclear localization of cell-cycle regulatory proteins may play a role in perturbing cell-cycle control in cancer cells *(4,16)*.

2.2. CDK Substrates: The Retinoblastoma Protein (pRb)

One of the best-characterized substrates of cyclin/CDK complexes is the protein product of the retinoblastoma *(Rb)* gene *(17)*. The *Rb* gene encodes a nuclear phosphoprotein (pRb) which in early G_1 is hypophosphorylated and acts as a negative regulator of cell cycle progression. The pRb protein becomes progressively more phosphorylated as cells progress through the G_1 phase. Hypophosphorylated pRb binds to a class of transcription factors known as E2F, whose activity is required for entry into S phase, and thus inhibits the ability of E2F to activate S phase genes. The phosphorylation of pRb prevents its binding to

E2F. Thus, when pRb is hyperphosphorylated ("ppRb"), free E2F is released which can then activate transcription of genes required for progression through the S phase (Fig. 3). In vitro and in vivo studies have shown that pRb can be phosphorylated by different cyclin-CDK complexes. In vivo cyclin D- and cyclin E-associated CDK activities contribute sequentially to this process from early-mid to late G_1. Cyclin A and cyclin B-dependent CDK activities maintain pRb in the ppRb form until cells exit mitosis. Then a multimeric complex of protein phosphatase type 1 (PP1) assists in dephosphorylation of ppRb, returning the protein to pRb, its suppressive state. pRb can stimulate the expression of cyclin D_1, and cyclin D_1 expression is repressed in the presence of ppRb, leading to inactivation of CDK4 and CDK6 (6,7). These findings suggest the existence of an autoregulatory loop between pRb and cyclin D_1 that regulates the progression of mammalian cells through the G_1 phase of the cell cycle. This autoregulatory loop also involves CDI p16[Ink4a], since expression of this protein is increased in the presence of pRb, contributing to inactivation of cyclin D_1/CDK4/6 kinase activity. This increase in pRb then sequesters the E2F transcription factors, as described here, resulting in downregulation of p16[Ink4a] expression (18).

Although additional biological substrates of the cyclin D/CDK complexes have thus far not been definitively identified, cyclin E/CDK2 complexes may have a broader range of specificity, since in addition to phosphorylating pRb they can phosphorylate histone H1, p27[Kip1], and probably substrates involved in the initiation of DNA replication. It is essential to identify other substrates for cyclin/CDK complexes, in order to clarify the specific cellular functions regulated by these complexes. Recent studies indicate that in addition to its critical role in controlling the G_1 phase of the cell cycle, cyclin D_1 has several CDK-independent functions. Thus, cyclin D_1 itself can bind directly to the estrogen receptor and stimulate its activity. It can also bind to the androgen receptor and inhibit its activity, and it can bind to and modulate the activities of several transcription factors, including thyroid hormone receptors (19–22).

3. MECHANISTIC STUDIES ON EFFECTS OF DYSREGULATION OF CELL CYCLE CONTROL PROTEINS

3.1. Tumor-Suppressor Genes and Oncogenes

Since precise regulation of the cell cycle is vital to the control of both cell proliferation and cell fate (dif-

Table 1

Cell-Cycle Alterations Associated With Human Cancers

Gene Involved	Type of Abnormality
Cyclin D	Chromosomal translocation causing constitutive high expression
	Gene amplification associated with increased expression
	Increased expression without amplification
Cyclin E	Increased expression and aberrant low mol-wt forms
Cyclin A	Site of integration of hepatitis B virus, yielding increased expression
Cyclin B1	Increased expression
CDK1	Increased expression
CDK2	Amplification and increased expression
CDK4	Amplification and increased expression
	Mutation disrupting p16[INK4a] binding site
CDK6	Amplification and increased expression
CDC25B	Increased expression
p16[Ink4a]	Loss of expression resulting from deletion, mutations, or promoter methylation
p15[Ink4b]	Loss of expression resulting from deletion or promoter methylation
p21[Cip1]	Decreased expression resulting from mutations in the p53 gene
p27[Kip1]	Reduced expression resulting from increased ubiquitin-mediated degradation
pRb	Loss of function caused by gene deletion and/or mutations, or inactivation by viral proteins
p53	Loss of function caused by gene deletion and/or mutations, or inactivation by cellular or viral proteins
Id proteins	Increased expression
hCdc4/Fbw7/Ago	Gene mutation

ferentiation, senescence, and apoptosis), dysregulation of various cell-cycle control proteins would be expected to be critical in carcinogenesis. Indeed, a variety of mutations and/or non-mutational disturbances in expression of cyclins and cyclin-related genes have been found in various types of human cancer (5,7; Table 1). This aspect is discussed later in this chapter. Furthermore, there is an intriguing linkage between cell-cycle machinery and functions of certain classic tumor-suppressor genes and oncogenes. As discussed previously, the Rb gene, the first identified tumor-suppressor gene, is vital in regulating the G_1-to-S transition of the cell cycle. The functions of the p53 tumor-suppressor gene, mutated in about 40–50% of human cancers, are also linked to the cell cycle. The p53 protein, a transcription factor activated in response to DNA damage and a variety of stress signals, is important in a variety of cellular functions, including cell-cycle progression, apoptosis, DNA repair, cell differentiation, and apoptosis (reviewed in 23). Several protein kinases, including CDK1, phosphorylate p53 and modulate its activity. Activation of p53 is frequently associated with induction of the CD1 p21[Cip1]. Cells lacking the p21[Cip1] gene are deficient in the G_1 arrest mediated by p53 (23). As discussed previously, p21[Cip1] blocks the kinase activity of CDKs responsible for phosphorylation of pRb in the G_1 phase. The specificity of p21[Cip1] is quite broad, so it is likely that several CDKs are inhibited simultaneously as a result of wild-type p53 activation (7,10,11). This may in part explain the observation that high inducible expression of p53 can cause cell-cycle arrest in both G_1 and G_2. Because of the numerous ways by which p53 influences cell cycle control and apoptosis (23), it is not surprising that this gene is so frequently mutated in human cancers, and that these mutations alter cell responses to various types of external stresses, including chemotherapeutic and probably chemopreventive agents (23). Several agents can induce p21[Cip1] expression by a p53-independent mechanism, which provides a strategy for antitumor drugs that are effective even in p53 mutant cancer cells or precursor lesions. Activation or overexpression of proteins encoded by several oncogenes or growth-enhancing factors, including TGFα, epidermal growth factor receptor (EGFR), ras, MAP kinases, β-catenin, Stat3, and NFκβ, can activate transcription of the cyclin D_1 gene and thereby enhance cell-cycle progression and proliferation (24–27). Little is known about the effects of these and other oncogenes and growth-enhancing factors on transcription of other cyclins. The c-myc oncogene is also implicated in the control of cell-cycle progression through mechanisms that have not yet been elucidated (28). In addition to the classic oncogenes and tumor-suppressor genes, some cell-cycle regulatory molecules shown in Fig. 1 can also act as oncogenes or tumor-suppressor genes.

3.2. G₁ Cyclins and CDK Inhibitors (CDIs)

Since the major regulatory events leading to cell proliferation and differentiation occur in the G_1 phase, deranged expression of G_1 cyclins and their related partners can play a central role in the loss of normal growth control during tumorigenesis. Experimental in vitro and in vivo data directly implicate cyclin D_1 in the process of neoplastic transformation. Thus, overexpression of cyclin D_1 in fibroblasts caused a decrease in duration of G_1, increased growth, decreased cell size, and enhanced the ability of these cells to form tumors in nude mice (29). Cyclin D_1 also cooperates with other oncogenes to induce in vitro cell transformation. Furthermore, overexpression of cyclin D_1 in transgenic mice was associated with an increase in mammary hyperplasia and mammary carcinomas when driven by a mouse mammary tumor virus (MMTV) promoter, and with dysplasia in the tongue, esophagus, and forestomach when driven by an Epstein-Barr virus (EBV) promoter (5–7). One study found that overexpression of cyclin D_1 in normal human oral squamous epithelial cells enhanced cell proliferation and extended the cells' replicative lifespan. The combination of cyclin D_1 overexpression and p53 inactivation led to immortalization of these cells through a telomerase-independent telomere-lengthening mechanism (30). In contrast, deletion of cyclin D_1 in mice led to hypoplasia of the mammary gland (31). Normal cells have checkpoint controls at the G_1/S and G_2/M transitions that delay further cell-cycle progression to permit repair of damaged DNA. A defect in these cell cycle checkpoints resulting from loss of the p53 tumor-suppressor gene is associated with genomic instability (23). Deregulated expression of cyclin D_1 can also enhance genomic instability. We demonstrated that overexpression of cyclin D_1 in a rat liver epithelial cell line with a normal p53 gene markedly increased the occurrence of gene amplification (32). These results indicate that overexpression of cyclin D_1 has multiple effects on tumorigenesis, including disturbances in growth control, enhancing cell transformation, and accelerating tumor progression by enhancing genomic instability.

As mentioned here, the pRb protein is the major target of the cyclin D1/CDK4 complex; its phosphorylation by cyclin/CDK complexes abolishes its E2F inhibitory activity. An intriguing reciprocal relation-

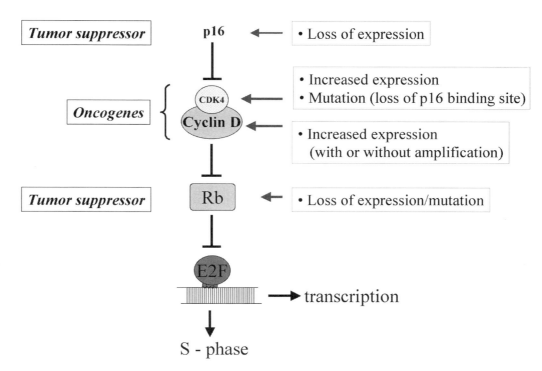

Fig. 4. Multiple mechanisms for disruption of the p16-cyclin D_1-CDK4-pRb pathway in cancer cells. Inactivation of the inhibitory role of pRb on cell-cycle progression can occur through loss of the Rb gene itself or by increased phosphorylation of the pRb protein by CDK4/6. Increased CDK4-associated kinase activity can be caused by increased expression of the protein, an increase in the amount of cyclin D, a decrease in the amount of the negative regulator p16[Ink4a], or a mutation in the p16[Ink4a]-binding site in CDK4. Each of these events enhances the G_1-S transition of the cell cycle and cell proliferation, and have been found in various human cancers.

ship between overexpression of cyclin D_1 and loss of expression of the Rb protein has been reported for several types of cancer (33,34), confirming that both of these alterations target the same pathway of cell transformation. Loss of expression of p16[Ink4a] and, other mechanisms that enhance inactivation of pRb have also been identified in cancer cells (18; Fig. 4).

Accumulation of cyclin E and activation of the cyclin E/CDK2 complex is also a rate-limiting event for the G_1-to-S transition. Indeed, overexpression of cyclin E accelerates the G_1-to-S transition, decreases cell size, and reduces the serum requirement for growth in both human and rat fibroblasts. Overexpression of cyclin E in mammary cells of transgenic mice is associated with an increase in mammary hyperplasia and mammary carcinomas (35). Cyclin E cooperates with cyclin D_1 to phosphorylate the pRb tumor-suppressor protein in mid-late G_1. However, the functions of cyclins D1 and E are not redundant (5–7). The protein hCdc4/Fbw7/Ago binds to cyclin E and targets it for ubiquitin-mediated degradation. This protein acts as a suppressor gene because inactivation of mutations in

tumor cells results in high levels of cyclin E, thus promoting cell proliferation and probably genomic instability (36).

The role of p16[Ink4a] in tumor development has been established by results obtained with knockout mice, since p16[Ink4a]-deficient mice develop spontaneous tumors at an early age and are highly sensitive to tumor induction by chemical carcinogens. Moreover, p16[Ink4a] (also known as MTS1, CDKN2, and CDK1) maps to *9p21*, a region that undergoes frequent genomic deletion in human cancers. Since the p15[Ink4b] (also known as MTS2) gene is adjacent to the p16[Ink4a] locus, the majority of homozygous deletions that inactivate p16[Ink4a] in tumor cells also inactivate p15[Ink4b]. Diverse mechanisms can contribute to the inactivation of this gene at the DNA level. The 5' untranslated region of p16[Ink4a] contains numerous CG dinucleotides (the so-called "CpG island") that are unmethylated in the transcriptionally active gene, but can be aberrantly methylated in many cancer cell lines as well as in many primary tumors, including lung, bladder, prostate, and colon cancers. This event is associated with a tightly compacted chromatin conformation involving the p16^{Ink4a} promoter, resulting in inactivation of gene expression. This is an example of epigenetic inactivation of gene expression, which is potentially reversible with exposure to demethylating agents such as 5-aza-2'-deoxycytidine (5–7).

Recent studies indicate that the p16^{Ink4a} locus plays a central role in tumor development because it is able to generate two distinct products: the p16^{Ink4a} protein and the p19ARF protein. Mice lacking only the alternative reading frame (ARF) sequence are highly tumor-prone, and die of cancer at a young age. The p19ARF protein acts by preventing the inhibitory effects of Mdm2 on p53. Mdm2 binds to p53, blocking its transcriptional activity and targeting it for degradation. The p19ARF protein localizes exclusively in the nucleolus, where it sequesters Mdm2, preventing its nuclear export. Loss of p19ARF is therefore associated with reduced accumulation of p53 in response to genotoxic stress. Introduction of p19ARF into cells causes a p53-dependent cell-cycle arrest, confirming that it acts upstream of p53 (37).

p21^{Cip1}-deficient mice undergo normal development; unlike p53-deficient mice, they do not exhibit early tumorigenesis, although fibroblasts from these mice are defective in G$_1$ arrest in response to DNA damage and nucleotide-pool depletion. p27^{Kip1}-deficient mice also complete an apparently normal prenatal development; their fibroblasts display a normal G$_1$ arrest in response to a variety of extracellular stimuli. However, these mice exhibit multiple organ hyperplasia and retinal dysplasia, and develop pituitary tumors, suggesting that disruption of p27^{Kip1} impairs normal control of cell proliferation. Furthermore, both p27^{Kip1} heterozygous (p27$^{+/-}$) and homozygous (p27$^{-/-}$) deficient mice show an increased predisposition to tumors in multiple tissues when exposed to radiation or a chemical carcinogen. Thus, p27^{Kip1} is haplo-insufficient for tumor suppression in mice since inactivating one allele, which causes only a moderate decrease in p27^{Kip1} protein expression, is sufficient to enhance tumorigenesis (3,6,7). Other experimental data also implicate p27^{Kip1} in the process of neoplastic transformation. The dominantly acting oncogenes *ras* and c-*myc* can inhibit p27^{Kip1} activity and/or expression, and the growth-suppressive activity of the normal phosphatase and tensin homolog (PTEN) tumor-suppressor gene has been related, in part, to its ability to induce cell-cycle arrest by upregulating p27^{Kip1} expression (38). Furthermore, loss of tuberin, a putative tumor-suppressor gene involved in the pathogenesis of tuberosclerosis (TSC), is associated with inhibition of p27^{Kip1} activity through sequestration of the p27^{Kip1} protein in the cytoplasm (39).

3.3. Other Cell Cycle Related Genes

CDKs are activated by both specific cyclins and a series of phosphatases, known as CDC25 A, B, and C, which remove inhibitory phosphate groups from specific tyrosine and threonine residues (*see* Fig. 2). Human CDC25A or CDC25B can cooperate with an activated *ras* oncogene or deleted Rb gene in in vitro transformation of cell lines. Transgenic mice that overexpress CDC25B in the mammary gland display increased sensitivity to mammary tumor induction by 7,12-dimethylbenz[*a*]anthracene DMBA (40). Furthermore, CDC25A and CDC25B are overexpressed in several human cancer cell lines and in human breast, colon, esophageal, non-small-cell lung, and head and neck cancers (3). Another group of proteins recently linked to the cell cycle are the Id proteins (inhibitor of DNA binding/differentiation). These proteins negatively regulate activities of the basic helix-loop-helix (bHLH) family of transcription factors involved in tissue-specific differentiation and other cellular functions. Id proteins are also involved in the control of cell proliferation by regulating expression of CDK inhibitors, and several studies have reported increased expression of Id proteins in primary human tumors and cancer-cell lines (41).

4. ABNORMALITIES IN CELL CYCLE CONTROL PROTEINS IN HUMAN CANCERS

Compelling evidence indicates that abnormalities in the expression of cell-cycle regulatory proteins play a pivotal role in development of several types of human cancer, and that these changes can affect the biological and clinical behavior of these cancers. Table 1 lists major abnormalities found thus far in human cancers.

4.1. Cyclins

The strongest association of cyclin overexpression in human cancer relates to cyclin D$_1$, first identified as the PRAD-1 oncogene, which is frequently rearranged and overexpressed in parathyroid adenomas. Subsequently it was found to be identical to the *bcl*-1 gene, which is translocated and overexpressed in a subset of B-cell neoplasms. Cyclin D$_1$ is normally located on human chromosome 11q13, and is amplified in several types of human tumors. However, human tumors that do not display this amplification also frequently overexpress cyclin D_1 because of increased transcription of this gene *(5,7)*. Increased levels of β-catenin in human colon cancer and other cancers can enhance cyclin D_1 transcription because β-catenin activates the tissue coding factor/leukokinesis-enhancing factor (TCF/LEF) element present in the cyclin D_1 promoter *(42)*. Other transcription factors with activities that are often upregulated in cancer can also enhance the transcriptional activity of the cyclin D_1 promoter *(24–27)*. Cyclin D_1 overexpression, with or without gene amplification, is often seen in head and neck, esophageal, gastric, liver, colon, breast, and other cancers *(5,7)*. Indeed, as one of the most frequent abnormalities seen in human cancers, it is a clinically useful marker of poor prognosis in some human malignancies. Cyclin D_1 overexpression can be an early event in the multistage process of carcinogenesis, since it has been detected in adenomatous polyps of the colon, Barrett's esophagus, preinvasive bronchial lesions, *in situ* carcinomas of the breast, and premalignant lesions of the oropharynx mucosa *(43–46)*. These findings suggest that cyclin D_1 might be a useful biomarker as well as a target for cancer chemoprevention.

The cyclin E gene is only rarely amplified in cancer cells; evidence for a role in oncogenesis is more circumstantial than for cyclin D_1. However, expression of the cyclin E protein is deregulated in several types of human cancers. Overexpression of multiple cyclin E-related proteins has been reported in human cancer cell lines and several types of primary cancers; this has been correlated with an adverse patient prognosis *(5,7)*. A recent large-scale study of breast cancer patients demonstrated that those with high levels of total cyclin E had higher death hazard ratios than those associated with other biological markers examined, including lymph node status *(47)*. If these results are confirmed, assays for cyclin E may provide a valuable prognostic marker in clinical studies, and possibly a useful surrogate marker to evaluate the efficacy of breast cancer chemoprevention or therapy.

Thus far, limited evidence links abnormalities in expression of non-G_1 cyclins to cancer development. In an early study, overexpression of cyclin A was discovered in a human hepatocellular carcinoma and attributed to integration of the hepatitis B virus (HBV) into the cyclin A gene locus. However, this appears to be a rare event in these cancers. Overexpression of cyclin A has been reported in several human primary cancers and cancer-cell lines, but its significance is not known. Deregulated expression of cyclin B and CDK1 have been reported in a variety of primary human cancers and cancer-derived cell lines. In colon cancer cells, increased expression of cyclin B1 has been associated with inactivation of p53 *(48)*. Overexpression of these proteins is frequently associated with loss of cell cycle phase-specificity and abnormalities in their subcellular localization, and can have prognostic significance *(5,7,49)*. The functional significance of these changes is unknown, but they might contribute to genomic (chromosomal) instability, or alter the apoptotic responses of cancer cells *(50)*.

4.2. CDKs and CDK Inhibitors

CDKs are normally expressed at relatively high levels throughout the cell cycle; their activities are mainly dependent on their state of phosphorylation, the availability of cyclins, and the levels of specific CDIs. However, abnormalities leading to overexpression of CDKs can perturb cell-cycle regulation, thus promoting cell proliferation and malignant transformation, since increased expression of CDK4 or CDK6 provides an alternative way to inactivate pRb. Indeed, amplification and increased expression of CDK4 or CDK6 occur at relatively high frequency in soft-tissue sarcomas and in gliomas, but occur only rarely in other types of human cancer. In some human melanomas, a mutated form of CDK4 prevents the binding of p16^{Ink4a}, thus disrupting its negative regulatory activity (Fig. 4). Amplification of CDK2 has been reported in a subset of colon carcinomas. Evidence implicating other CDKs in human tumorigenesis is limited *(5,7)*.

Since CDK inhibitors are potent negative regulators of the cell cycle, they can function as tumor-suppressor genes. Therefore, loss of their expression would be expected to play an important role in the development of human cancers. Indeed, abnormalities in the INK4 locus, including gene mutation, deletion, and/or aberrant methylation, have been seen in a variety of human cancers. As discussed previously, the INK4 locus encodes both the p16^{Ink4} and the p19ARF proteins, so events that affect this locus can result in loss of expression of both proteins, simultaneously impairing both the pRb and the p53 tumor-suppressor pathways. Mutations, homozygous deletion, or hypermethylation of the p16^{Ink4a} locus occur with a relatively high frequency in many human cancer cell lines and also in primary human cancers, including familial melanoma, leukemia, and glioma, as well as carcinomas of the esophagus, pancreas, bladder, prostate, and ovary.

Indeed, the incidence of decreased p16^{Ink4a} expression in human cancers is second only to that of inactivating mutations in the p53 gene. Among the CDIs, only p16^{Ink4a} can be classified as a tumor-suppressor gene by the genetic criterion of loss of heterozygosity (LOH). In some familial melanomas, one defective copy is inherited, and the second is lost during tumor development. Since loss of function of p16^{Ink4a} enhances pRb phosphorylation, it is functionally equivalent to overexpression of cyclin D$_1$, CDK4, or CDK6 (Fig. 4), thus providing an alternative mechanism for inactivating pRb function. In fact, lack of expression of p16^{Ink4a} or pRb occurs in distinct subsets of human cancers of a particular tissue type (3,5,18). A striking recent finding is that decreased expression and/or hypermethylation of the p16^{Ink4a} gene is often found in premalignant lesions of the bronchial epithelium and in bronchial-epithelial cells of former smokers (51). This remarkable finding has implications for chemoprevention.

Initially, the Cip/Kip proteins were not believed to be tumor-suppressor genes, since several independent studies found that alterations in the integrity of human p27^{Kip1} and p21^{Cip1} genes are rare events in primary human cancers and cancer cell lines (5,7). p21^{Cip1} is transcriptionally induced by p53, whose function is missing in a high percentage of human tumors (23). Several studies have demonstrated a decrease in p21^{Cip1} expression in various carcinomas when compared to normal epithelial tissues. Inactivation of p57^{Kip1} has been reported to play a role in the pathogenesis of a subset of cases of Beckwith-Wiedemann syndrome, a cancer-predisposing syndrome, and also in some cases of Wilm's tumors (3,5,18). The p27^{Kip1} gene is located on the short arm of human chromosome 12. It maps to a region (p12–p13.1) which is frequently rearranged and/or deleted in leukemia and mesothelioma. Although the p27^{Kip1} gene is only rarely mutated in cancer cells, reduced expression of the p27^{Kip1} protein has been observed in a variety of human malignancies (3,4,18). Comparisons of immunohistochemical analysis and in situ hybridization showed a discordance between p27^{Kip1} protein and mRNA levels, suggesting that, as in normal cells, p27^{Kip1} is mainly regulated at a posttranscriptional level. Indeed, reduced expression of p27^{Kip1} in human cancers appears to be the result of increased proteasome-dependent degradation of this protein (3,4,18). It is of interest that loss of p27^{Kip1} can be an early event in the multistep process of human tumorigenesis (4). Progressive loss of p27^{Kip1} is

commonly observed during progression from normal to benign and malignant tumors, and decreased expression has been related to the acquisition of a metastatic potential and a poorer prognosis (3,4,18). Since loss of p27^{Kip1} expression may play an important role in tumor progression, agents that increase cellular levels of p27^{Kip1} might be useful in cancer chemoprevention.

Only the nuclear component of the p27^{Kip1} protein can bind to and inhibit cyclin/CDK complexes present in the nucleus. Thus, sequestration in the cytosol can inactivate the inhibitory function of p27^{Kip1}. This mechanism appears to be important in maintaining high cyclin/CDK activity in the nucleus of anchorage-independent transformed cell lines (52). Sequestration in the cytosol might also play a role in the inactivation of this protein during tumor development. Indeed, cytoplasmic localization of p27^{Kip1} has been reported in various types of human cancers (3,4,18,53,54). The nuclear localization signal of p27^{Kip1} contains an AKT consensus site; in breast cancer, phosphorylation by AKT has been demonstrated to impair nuclear import of the p27^{Kip1} protein. Thus, cytoplasmic retention of p27^{Kip1} has been observed in breast cancers in conjunction with AKT activation, and has been correlated with cancer aggressiveness and poor patient prognosis (54). Cytoplasmic sequestration of other CDIs may also limit their inhibitory activities (55).

5. THE CELL CYCLE MACHINERY AS A TARGET FOR CANCER CHEMOPREVENTION

Abnormalities in the expression of several proteins that regulate the cell cycle have been found in a variety of human cancers (Table 1). Increasing evidence shows that these abnormalities can also occur in cancer precursor lesions, including Barrett's esophagus, dysplastic lesions of the oropharynx and bronchus mucosa, adenomatous polyps of the colon, and in situ breast cancer (4,5,7). These abnormalities may provide molecular targets for novel natural products and pharmaceutical agents in cancer chemoprevention and/or treatment (56). Model studies in cell culture systems lend credence to this approach. In early studies, introducing an antisense cyclin D$_1$ cDNA construct into a human esophageal cancer cell line in which the cyclin D$_1$ gene was amplified and overexpressed reduced expression of the cyclin D$_1$ protein, causing a marked inhibition of both anchorage-dependent and -independent growth in vitro and a complete loss of tumorigenicity in nude (athymic) mice *(57)*. Similar results were subsequently obtained by us and other investigators in human colon, lung, and pancreatic cancer cell lines *(58–60)*. A recent study found that cyclin D$_1$ is amplified and overexpressed in a subset of melanoma, and that anti-sense-mediated downregulation of cyclin D$_1$ in a melanoma cell line induced apoptosis in vitro and tumor shrinkage in mouse xenografts *(61)*. These results indicate that overexpression of cyclin D$_1$ in various types of human cancer can be critical in maintaining the malignant phenotype. Therefore, cyclin D$_1$ or related molecules are candidate targets for intervention strategies. Restoration of p16^{Ink4a} in esophageal cancer cells using an adenoviral vector also markedly inhibited cell proliferation and tumorigenicity *(62)*; similar results have been obtained in other types of cancer cells *(63)*. We found that when we introduced a p27^{Kip1}-sense cDNA sequence into the MCF-7 human breast cancer cell line, derivatives that expressed increased levels of the p27^{Kip1} protein displayed growth inhibition and decreased tumorigenicity *(64)*. Results obtained with these gene-transfer studies in cell culture systems provided early support for the hypothesis that drugs targeting the activities of CDKs either directly or indirectly may be useful in cancer chemoprevention and therapy. Thus far, it has not been possible to directly demonstrate similar effects in cell cultures established from cancer precursor lesions because it is difficult to grow these cells in culture—a general limitation of in vitro studies on cancer chemoprevention. Nevertheless, studies with cancer cell lines are likely to be instructive, since cancer precursor lesions often share several abnormalities with their respective types of cancer. For example, advanced lesions of the upper aerodigestive tract frequently display overexpression of cyclin D$_1$ and decreased expression of p16^{Ink4a}. These abnormalities are associated with tumor progression, and appear to influence responses of these lesions to chemoprevention with retinoids *(65)*.

A number of natural products, as well as synthetic nonsteroidal antiinflammatory drugs (NSAIDs) and related agents that have cancer-chemopreventive activity in rodent models of carcinogenesis and in some human cancers, have profound effects on cellular levels and/or activities of several cell cycle control proteins (Table 2). These compounds may achieve their chemopreventive effects, at least in part, by inhibiting cell cycle-related events. Thus, various retinoids (in Dmitrovsky et al., this volume) can increase cells in the

Table 2

Cancer Chemopreventive Agents that Alter the Expression and/or Activity of Proteins Involved in Cell Cycle Control

Agent	Molecular Targets	Ref.
Retinoids	⊥p27^{Kip1}, p21^{Cip1}; ⊕cyclin D1, ppRb	66–68,81
Green tea EGCG	⊥p27^{Kip1}, p21^{Cip1}; ⊕cyclin D1, ppRb	69–71
Selenium	⊕cyclin D1	74–76
Flavonoids	⊕cyclin, CDKS; ⊥CDIs	72
N-acetylcysteine	⊥p16^{Ink4a}, p21^{Cip1}	77
NSAIDs, Sulindac Sulfone	⊕cyclin D1; ⊥p27^{Kip1}, p21^{Cip1}	79
Tamoxifen	⊕cyclins D1, E; ⊥p27^{Kip1}	80
Curcumin	⊕cyclins D1, E	72
Resveratrol	⊥p21^{Cip1}; ⊕cyclins D1,A, and B1	73
Soybean Lunasin	⊕Histone acetylation	98
S-allylmercapto-cysteine (SAMC)	Mitotic spindle	78,78a

⊥: indicates increased expression and/or activity.
⊕: indicates decreased expression and/or activity.

G$_1$ phase of the cell cycle, presumably because they are known to induce decreased cellular levels of cyclin D$_1$ and increased levels of the CDIs p21^{Cip1} and p27^{Kip1}, decreasing levels of ppRb *(66–68)*. The polyphenolic antitumor compound epigallocatechin-3-gallate (EGCG) present in tea (*see* Chapter 30) causes similar effects in cancer cell lines *(69–71)*. Other polyphenolic compounds that display chemopreventive activity, including curcumin, resveratrol, and various flavonoids, have also shown effects on the expression of various cell cycle control proteins *(72,73)*. In some cancer cell lines, resveratrol inhibits progression through the S phase of the cell cycle, which is associated with decreases in levels of expression of cyclins D$_1$, A, and B$_1$ *(73)*. Selenium is believed to be an important cancer chemopreventive agent in the human diet *(74)* (*see* Chapter 35). Selenium compounds can affect the expression of several genes involved in cell cycle control *(75,76)*. Prolongation of the G$_1$ phase of the cell cycle, resulting from increased expression of p16^{Ink4a} and p21^{Cip1}, is induced by *N*-acetylcysteine, an antioxidant with chemopreventive activity *(77)* (*see* Chapter 3). We found that the garlic constituent *S*-allylmercaptocysteine (SAMC) arrests cancer cells in metaphase, apparently because it directly binds to

Table 3

Drugs that Target or Alter the Expression of Cell Cycle Control Proteins That Might be Useful in Cancer Chemoprevention

Mechanism of Action	Specific Agents	Targets/Effects	Ref.
Inhibition of CDK activity	Flavopiridol	CDKs, 1, 2, 4, 6	56,82–84
	UCN-01	CDKs 1, 2, 4	56,85
	Butyrolactone	CDKs 1, 2	56,89
	E7070	CDK 2	86
	Olomoucine and Roscovitine	CDKs 1, 2, 5	87
	Oxindole I, Urea II, NSC 680434, Fascaplysin, PD0183812, CINK4	CDKs 4, 6	88–93
Inhibition of mTOR	Rapamycin	$\oplus$Cyclins D, A; $\perp$p21^{Kip1}	89,94–96
Proteasome inhibition	PS-341, Lactacystin	$\perp$ Cyclins A, B, and p21^{Cip1}	100,101
Inhibition of histone deacetylation	MS-275, Butyrate, Trichostatin A	$\perp$p21^{Cip1}	97–99
Demethylation of DNA	5-Aza-2'-deoxycytidine	$\perp$p16^{Ink4a}	102

$\perp$: indicates increased expression and/or activity.
$\oplus$: indicates decreased expression and/or activity.

tubulin, thereby disrupting the function of the mitotic spindle *(78,78a)*. The NSAID sulindac and the related compound sulindac sulfone (exisulind) inhibit cell-cycle progression in G_1 and cause decreased cellular levels of cyclin D_1 (reviewed in *79*). We should emphasize that most of the results summarized in Table 2 were obtained in cell-culture systems. However, these types of findings are not restricted to in vitro assays; when rats bearing *N*-methyl-*N*-nitrosourea (MNU)-induced mammary tumors were administered tamoxifen, tumors displayed an increase in G_0/G_1 cells and decreased levels of cyclin D_1 and cyclin E proteins and their related mRNAs *(80)*. It has not been determined whether other chemopreventive agents exert specific in vivo effects on cell-cycle-related events in rodent or human tumors.

A limited number of studies examined the precise mechanisms by which agents listed in Table 2 produce the indicated effects. The decrease in cyclin D_1 seen with 9-*cis*-retinoic acid and acyclic retinoid (ACR) is caused by inhibition of cyclin D_1 transcription, but that seen with all-*trans*-retinoic acid (ATRA) is due to posttranslational proteolysis of the cyclin D_1 protein *(81)*. The decrease in cyclin D_1 seen with EGCG and sulindac sulfone is also caused by inhibition of transcription *(71)*. The increase in p21^{Cip1} seen with 9-*cis*-retinoic acid and ACR is remarkable because it occurs rapidly (within 3 h), involves *de novo* transcription, and is p53-independent *(81)*. We should emphasize that the arrest in cell cycle progres-

sion seen in cell-culture systems with several agents listed in Table 2 is often followed by apoptosis. Obviously, the same series of events occurring in vivo would markedly contribute to the chemopreventive effects of these agents.

Table 3 lists several novel agents, currently at various stages of development with respect to cancer treatment, that target cell cycle control proteins. Most of these agents are not yet determined to have cancer chemopreventive activity in preclinical or clinical studies; also unknown is whether potential toxicities might limit their use in long-term cancer chemoprevention studies. Since CDKs are pivotal in regulating cell cycle progression, there is a major effort to develop pharmacological agents that target one or more specific CDKs. Some of these agents are briefly described here.

Of the CDK inhibitors, flavopiridol has been most extensively examined in clinical studies. It is a semi-synthetic flavone derived from rohitukine, an alkaloid isolated from the *Dysoxylum binectarieferum* plant, which is indigenous to India. It inhibits several CDKs (including CDK4 and CDK6), reduces cyclin D_1 expression, and induces cell-cycle arrest and apoptosis in a variety of cancer cells *(82–84)*. UCN-01, originally discovered as a PKC inhibitor, was subsequently found to also inhibit several CDKs and induce cell cycle arrest. This arrest is accompanied by hypophosphorylation of pRb and the accumulation of p21^{Cip1} and p27^{Kip1}. Its action appears to be independent of the p53 and Rb status of cells (85). Both flavopiridol and UCN-01 have been tested in clinical trials, and display promising results (56). The antitumor sulfonamide E7070 causes an accumulation of cells in the G_1 phase of the cell cycle by suppressing cyclin E expression and inhibiting CDK2 activation (86). Olomucine and roscovitine, members of a family of purine-based compounds that inhibit several CDKs and CDK-dependent cellular activities, can induce G_1 and G_2 cell cycle arrest (87). As emphasized here, increased kinase activity of cyclin D_1/CDK4 or cyclin D_1/CDK6 complexes frequently occurs in human cancer and in several premalignant lesions. However, except for flavopiridol, none of the CDK inhibitors mentioned here have a high affinity for CDK4 or CDK6; flavopiridol lacks specificity because it also inhibits other CDKs and has additional cellular targets (82,83). Therefore, several compounds that appear to be specific inhibitors of CDK4 and CDK6 kinase activity are of great interest. The CDK4-specific inhibitors oxindole I and urea II preferentially inhibit proliferation of pRb+ cancer cell lines (88,89). The CDK4 inhibitor 3-amino thioacridone (NSC 680434) and related compounds were identified by their ability to selectively inhibit cancer-cell lines with decreased expression of p16[Ink4a] (90). Fascaplysin is a marine product that specifically inhibits CDK4 by binding to the adenosine 5' triphosphate (ATP) pocket of this kinase and arrests pRb+ cells in G_1 (91). PD 0183812, a [2,3] pyridopyrimidine, is a potent and selective inhibitor of CDK4 and CDK6 kinase activity that also causes G_1 arrest in cancer-cell lines that express pRb (92); CINK4 is a triaminopyrimidine derivative that inhibits tumor-cell growth both in vitro and in vivo (93).

Certain new classes of anticancer agents that display a wide spectrum of biologic activity also have effects on cell cycle-related molecules and cell-cycle progression (89,93) These include rapamycin, histone deacetylase inhibitors, and proteasome inhibitors. Rapamycin is a macrolide fungicide that binds intracellularly to the immunophilin FKBP12. The resultant complex inhibits the activity of a 290-kDa kinase called mTOR. This kinase is activated in response to growth-stimulatory signals acting through the PI3K/Akt pathway (94). Rapamycin causes G_1 cell-cycle arrest by increasing cyclin D1 turnover, upregulating p27[Kip1], and inhibiting cyclin A-dependent kinase activity (95,96). Histone deacetylase inhibitors, including butyrate, trichostatin A, and MS-275, are potent inducers of growth arrest and differentiation

(97), and potentially important chemopreventive agents (98) (see Chapter 43). MS-275 induces p53-independent accumulation of p21[Cip1] and cell cycle arrest (99). It has significant growth-inhibitory effects on several human cancer-cell lines, and is absorbed orally, with good bioavailability.

The ubiquitin-proteasome pathway is active in cell-cycle regulation through precisely programmed degradation of specific cyclins and CDIs. Inhibition of proteasome activity can lead to accumulation of CDIs and cell-cycle arrest. Several proteasome inhibitors have been identified, including lactacystin, peptide aldehydes, and the dipeptide boronate derivatives (e.g., PS-341), some of which are being tested in cancer therapy clinical trials. Proteasome inhibitors can cause accumulation of cyclins A and B and p21[Kip1] and arrest cells in the S and G_2/M phases (100,101). Since they negatively affect the cell cycle machinery and inhibit cell proliferation, they are also potential chemopreventive agents (see Chapter 41). Restoring p16[Ink4a] expression has a dramatic inhibitory effect on growth and tumorigenicity of cancer cells (62,63). The DNA demethylating agent 5-aza-2'-deoxycytidine (DAC) can restore p16[Ink4a] expression and mediate significant growth inhibition in cancer cells that exhibit p16[Ink4a] promoter methylation (102). Of interest, TGF-β, interferon γ, interferon β, cyclic 5' adenine monophosphate (cAMP), and rapamycin can cause an increase in cellular levels of p27[Kip1] (4); increased expression of p27[Kip1] and/or p21[Cip1] have been seen in cells treated with various chemopreventive agents (Table 2).

Further development of agents that inhibit the expression of cyclin D_1 and possibly other cyclins, directly inhibit the activities of specific CDKs, or cause increased cellular levels of CDIs p16[Ink4a], p21[Cip1] or p27[Kip1], may provide useful strategies for cancer chemoprevention. Since the expression or activities of these cell-cycle control proteins is frequently aberrant in premalignant lesions, and several known chemopreventive agents lead to alterations in their expression, these proteins may also provide valuable biomarkers, or surrogate endpoints, in experimental and clinical studies on cancer chemoprevention.

6. CONCLUSIONS AND FUTURE PERSPECTIVES

Abundant evidence has identified perturbation of cell cycle control as a hallmark of the multistage process of carcinogenesis. The resulting abnormalities provide attractive targets for molecular interventions. The most frequently seen abnormalities are in the p16-cyclin D_1-CDK4-pRb pathway. Indeed, abnormalities in one or more components of this pathway occur in a majority of human cancers. The specific abnormality in this pathway can vary with the type of cancer. Although they occur with lesser frequency, abnormalities in other pathways that control the cell cycle (see Table 1) may also provide targets for chemoprevention of specific cancers.

Our own studies have emphasized that subsets of human cancers can display an increase rather than a decrease in expression of cell-cycle inhibitors, including pRb, p27^{Kip1}, p21^{Cip1}, and p16^{Ink4a} (8). A recent study indicates that p21^{Cip1} is frequently overexpressed in both pancreatic intraepithelial neoplastic lesions and in pancreatic cancers (103). In addition, about 65% of gastric cancers overexpress p16^{Ink4a} compared with nonneoplastic gastric mucosa (104). The increased expression of these cell-cycle inhibitors in some types of cancers seems paradoxical. We hypothesize that these events reflect unusual states of homeostasis between positive and negative regulators of the cell cycle that occur during the multistage carcinogenic process and in established cancers. Furthermore, our studies on the effects of an antisense sequence to cyclin D_1 and related studies with other oncogenes suggest that the circuitry of cancer cells may be highly dependent on, even addicted to, specific oncogenes (8). Together, these findings suggest that cancer cells and premalignant lesions might be much more susceptible than normal cells to the inhibitory or cytotoxic effects of agents that alter expression or activity of specific cell cycle control proteins. This is an optimistic scenario with respect to developing chemopreventive agents that have minimal toxicity to the host. The ubiquitous nature of perturbations in cell cycle control proteins in human cancers suggest that they might also be exploited as biomarkers or surrogate endpoints in cancer chemoprevention studies, as some of these abnormalities (for example, increased expression of cyclin D_1 or decreased expression of CDIs) are seen in precursor lesions.

Our understanding of the mechanisms regulating cell cycle progression in mammalian cells and the knowledge that deregulation of cell cycle machinery occurs in the majority of human cancers holds promise for development of novel strategies for cancer chemoprevention. It would not be surprising to see several cell cycle targeting drugs enter the clinic within the next few years for use in both cancer chemoprevention and treatment. Because of the problem of heterogeneity of cell types in cancer-precursor lesions and cancers, it will be important to test these new drugs in combination with agents that target other abnormalities in precursor lesions and cancer cells. Hopefully, these mechanism-based approaches will have a major impact on the reduction of both cancer incidence and mortality.

ACKNOWLEDGMENT

This research was supported by NIH Grant CA63467, AIBS grant DAMRD 17-94-J-4101, and awards from the National Foundation for Cancer Reseach, the T.J. Martell Foundation, and the National Colorectal Cancer Research Association to I.B.W; and by a grant from Compagnia di San Paolo, to A.S. We are grateful to Barbara Castro for valuable assistance in preparing this chapter. We apologize to authors whose work we did not directly cite in the references. For purposes of brevity, we have frequently cited previous review articles or only representative publications.

REFERENCES

1. Fearon ER. Tumor suppressor genes, in *The Genetic Basis of Human Cancer* Vogelstein B, Kinzler KW, eds. McGraw-Hill, New York, NY, 1998, pp.229–236.
2. Park M. Oncogenesis, in *The Genetic Basis of Human Cancer*. Vogelstein B, Kinzler KW, eds. McGraw-Hill, New York, NY, 1998, pp.205–228.
3. Lee MH, Yang HY. Negative regulators of cyclin-dependent kinases and their roles in cancers. *Cell Mol Life Sci* 2001;58:1907–1922.
4. Sgambato A, Cittadini A, Faraglia B, Weinstein IB. Multiple functions of p27Kip1 and its alterations in tumor cells: a review. *J Cell Physiol* 2000;183:18–27.
5. Sgambato A, Flamini G, Cittadini A, Weinstein IB. Abnormalities in cell cycle control in cancer and their clinical implications. *Tumori* 1998;84:421–433.
6. Sherr CJ, Roberts JM. CDK inhibitors: positive and negative regulators of G_1-phase progression. *Genes Dev* 1999;13:1501–1512.
7. Weinstein IB, Zhou P. Defects in cell cycle control genes in human cancern, in *Encyclopedia of Cancer, Vol. 1.* Bertino JR, ed. Academic Press, New York, NY, 1997, pp.256–267.
8. Weinstein IB. Disorders in cell circuitry during multistage carcinogenesis: the role of homeostatis. *Carcinogenesis* 2000;21:857–864.
9. Pardee AB. G_1 events and regulation of cell proliferation. *Science* 1989;246:603–608.
10. Sherr CJ. D-type cyclins. *Trends Biochem Sci* 1995;20:187–190.

11. Draetta GF. Mammalian G_1 cyclins. *Curr Opin Cell Biol* 1994;6:842–846.

12. Sherr CJ, Roberts JM. Inhibitors of mammalian G_1 cyclin-dependent kinases. *Genes Dev* 1995;9:1149–1163.

13. Carrano AC, Eytan E, Hershko A, Pagano, M. SKP2 is required for ubiquitin-mediated degradation of the CDK inhibitor p27Kip1. *Nat Cell Biol* 1999;1:193–199.

14. Hara T, Kamura T, Nakayama K, et al. Degradation of p27Kip1 at the G_0–G_1 transition mediated by a Skp2-independent ubiquination pathway. *J Biol Chem* 2001;276:48,937–48,943.

15. LaBaer J, Garrett MD, Stevenson LF, et al. New functional activities for the p21 family of CDK inhibitors. *Genes Dev* 1997;11:847–862.

16. Davezac N, Baldin V, Gabrielli B, et al. Regulation of CDC25B phosphatases subcellular localization. *Oncogene* 2000;19:2179–2185.

17. Weinberg RA. The retinoblastoma protein and cell cycle control. *Cell* 1995;81:323–330.

18. Nevins JR. The Rb/E2F pathway and cancer. *Hum Mol Genet* 2001;10:699–703.

19. Lin HM, Zhao L, Cheng SY. Cyclin D_1 is a ligand-independent co-repressor for thyroid hormone receptors. *J Biol Chem* 2002;277:28,733–28,741.

20. Reutens AT, Fu M, Wang C, et al. Cyclin D_1 binds the androgen receptor and regulates hormone-dependent signaling in a p300/CBP-associated factor (P/CAF)-dependent manner. *Mol Endocrinol* 2001;15:797–811.

21. Zwijsen RM, Wientjens E, Klompmaker R, et al. CDK-independent activation of estrogen receptor by cyclin D_1. *Cell* 1997;88:405–415.

22. Yao Y, Doki Y, Jiang W, et al. Cloning and characterization of DIP1, a novel protein that is related to the Id family of proteins. *Exp Cell Res* 2000;257:22–32.

23. Ozbun MA, Butel JS. P53 tumor suppressor gene: structure and function, in *Encyclopedia of Cancer, Vol. 2*. Bertino JR, ed. Academic Press, New York, NY, 1997, pp.1240–1257.

24. Aktas H, Cai H, Cooper GM. Ras links growth factor signaling to the cell cycle machinery via regulation of cyclin D_1 and the Cdk inhibitor p27^{Kip1}. *Mol Cell Biol* 1997;17:3850–3857.

25. Joyce, D., Albanese, C., Steer, J., et al. NF-κB and cell-cycle regulation: the cyclin connection. *Cytokine Growth Factor Rev* 2001;12:73–90.

26. Smalley MJ, Dale TC. Wnt signalling in mammalian development and cancer. *Cancer Metastasis Rev* 1999;18:215–230.

27. Turkson J, Jove R. STAT proteins: novel molecular targets for cancer drug discovery. *Oncogene* 2000;19:6613–6626.

28. Grandori C, Cowley SM, James LP, Eisenman RN. The Myc/Max/Mad network and the transcriptional control of cell behavior. *Annu Rev Cell Dev Biol* 2000;16:653–699.

29. Jiang W, Kahn SM, Zhou P, et al. Overexpression of cyclin D1 in rat fibroblasts causes abnormalities in growth control, cell cycle progression and gene expression. *Oncogene* 1993;8:3447–3457.

30. Opitz OG, Suliman Y, Hahn WC, et al. Cyclin D_1 overexpression and p53 inactivation immortalize primary oral keratinocytes by a telomerase-independent mechanism. *J Clin Investig* 2001;108:725–732.

31. Fantl V, Stamp G, Andrews A, et al. Mice lacking cyclin D_1 are small and show defects in eye and mammary gland development. *Genes Dev* 1995;9:2364–2372.

32. Zhou P, Jiang W, Weghorst CM, Weinstein IB. Overexpression of cyclin D_1 enhances gene amplification. *Cancer Res* 1996;56:36–39.

33. Bartkova J, Lukas J, Muller H, et al. Cyclin D_1 protein expression and function in human breast cancer. *Int J Cancer* 1994;57:353–361.

34. Jiang W, Zhang Y-J, Kahn SM, et al. Altered expression of the cyclin D1 and retinoblastoma genes in human esophageal cancer. *Proc Natl Acad Sci USA* 1993;90:9026–9030.

35. Bortner DM, Rosenberg MP. Induction of mammary gland hyperplasia and carcinomas in transgenic mice expressing human cyclin E. *Mol Cell Biol* 1997;17:453–459.

36. Strohmaier H, Spruck CH, Kaiser P, et al. Human F-box protein hCdc4 targets cyclin E for proteolysis and is mutated in a breast cancer cell line. *Nature* 2001;413:316–322.

37. Sherr CJ. Tumor surveillance via the ARF-p53 pathway. *Genes Dev* 1998;12:2984–2991.

38. Mammilapalli R, Gavrilova N, Mihaylova VT, et al. PTEN regulates the ubiquitin-dependent degradation of the cdk inhibitor p27kip1 through the ubiquitin 3 ligase SCF (SKP2). *Curr Biol* 2001;11:263–267.

39. Soucek T, Yeung RS, Hengstschlager M. Inactivation of the cyclin-dependent kinase inhibitor p27 upon loss of the tuberous sclerosis complex gene-2. *Proc Natl Acad Sci USA* 1998;95:15,653–15,658.

40. Yao Y, Slosberg ED, Wang L, et al. Increased susceptibility to carcinogen-induced mammary tumors in MMTV-Cdc25B transgenic mice. *Oncogene* 1999;18:5159–5166.

41. Pagliuca A, Gallo P, De Luca P, Lania L. Class A helix-loop-helix proteins are positive regulators of several cyclin-dependent kinase inhibitors' promoter activity and negatively affect cell growth. *Cancer Res* 2000;60:1376–1382.

42. Tetsu O, McCormick F. Beta-catenin regulates expression of cyclin D1 in colon carcinoma cells. *Nature (London)* 1999;398:422–426.

43. Arber N, Hibshoosh H, Moss SF, et al. Increased expression of cyclin D_1 is an early event in multistage colorectal carcinogenesiss. *Gastroenterology* 1996;110:669–674.

44. Arber N, Lightdale C, Rotterdam H, et al. Increased expression of the cyclin D_1 gene in Barrett's esophagus. *Cancer Epidemiol Biomarkers Prev* 1996;5:457–459.

45. Brambilla E, Gazzeri S, Moro D, et al. Alterations of the Rb pathway (Rb-p16INK4-cyclin D_1) in preinvasive bronchial lesions. *Clin Cancer Res* 1999;5:243–250.

46. Weinstat-Saslow D, Merino MJ, Manrow RE, et al. Overexpression of cyclin D1 mRNA distinguishes invasive and *in situ* breast carcinomas from non-malignant lesions. *Nat Med* 1995;1:1257–1260.

47. Keyomarsi K, Tucker SL, Buchholz TA, et al. Cyclin E and survival in patients with breast cancer. *N Engl J Med* 2002;347:1566–1575

48. Yu M, Zhan Q, Finn OJ. Immune recognition of cyclin B1 as a tumor antigen is a result of its overexpression in human tumors that is caused by non-functional p53. *Mol Immunol* 2001;38:981–987.

49. Soria JC, Jang SJ, Khuri FR, et al. Overexpression of cyclin B1 in early-stage non-small cell lung cancer and its clinical implication. *Cancer Res* 2000;60:4000–4004.

50. Sarafan-Vasseur N, Lamy A, Bourguignon J, et al. Overexpression of B-type cyclins alters chromosomal segregation. *Oncogene* 2002;21:2051–2057.

51. Soria JC, Rodriguez M, Liu DD, et al. Aberrant promoter methylation of multiple genes in bronchial brush samples from former cigarette smokers. *Cancer Res* 2002;62:351–355.

52. Orend G, Hunter T, Ruoslahti E. Cytoplasmic displacement of cyclin E-cdk2 inhibitors p21^{Cip1} and p27^{Kip1} in anchorage-independent cells. *Oncogene* 1998;16:2575–2583.

53. Singh SP, Lipman J, Goldman H, et al. Loss or altered subcellular localization of p27 in Barrett's associated adeno-carcinomas. *Cancer Res* 1998;58:1730–1735.

54. Blain SW, Massaguè J. Breast cancer banishes p27 from the nucleus *Nat Med* 2002;8:1076–1078.

55. Blagosklonny MV. Are p27 and p21 cyctoplasmic oncopro-teins? *Cell Cycle* 2002;1:391–393.

56. Owa T, Yoshino H, Yoshimatsu K, Nagasu T. Cell cycle regulation in the G$_1$ phase: a promising target for the devel-opment of new chemotherapeutic anticancer agents. *Curr Med Chem* 2001;8:1487–1503.

57. Zhou P, Jiang W, Zhang Y, et al. Antisense to cyclin D$_1$ inhibits growth and reverses the transformed phenotype of human esophageal cancer cells. *Oncogene* 1995;11:571–580.

58. Schrump DS, Chen A, Consoli U. Inhibition of lung cancer proliferation by antisense cyclin D. *Cancer Gene Ther* 1996;3:131–135.

59. Arber N, Doki Y, Han EK-H, et al. Antisense to cyclin D$_1$ inhibits the growth and tumorigenicity of human colon cancer cells. *Cancer Res* 1997;57:1569–1574.

60. Sauter ER, Nesbit M, Litwin S, et al. Antisense cyclin D$_1$ induces apoptosis and tumor shrinkage in human squamous carcinomas. *Cancer Res* 1999;59:4876–4881.

61. Sauter ER, Yeo UC, Von Stemm A, et al. Cyclin D$_1$ is a candidate oncogene in cutaneous melanoma. *Cancer Res* 2002;62:3200–3206.

62. Schrump DS, Chen GA, Consuli U, et al. Inhibition of esophageal cancer proliferation by adenovirally mediated delivery of p16INK4. *Cancer Gene Ther* 1996; 3: 357–364.

63. Jin X, Nguyen D, Zhamg WW, Roth JA. Cell cycle arrest and inhibition of tumor cell proliferation by the p16INK gene mediated by an adenovirus vector. *Cancer Res* 1995;55:3250–3253.

64. Sgambato A, Zhang Y-J, Ciaparrone M, et al. Overexpression of p27^{kip1} inhibits the growth of both nor-mal and transformed human mammary epithelial cells. *Cancer Res* 1998;58:3448–3454.

65. Papadimitrakopoulou VA, Izzo J, Mao L, et al. Cyclin D$_1$ and p16 alterations in advanced premalignant lesions of the upper aerodigestive tract: role in response to chemopreven-tion and cancer development. *Clin Cancer Res* 2001;7:3127–3134.

66. Dragnew KH, Freemantle SJ, Spinella MJ, Dmitrovsky E. Cyclin proteolysis as a retinoid cancer prevention mechanism. *Ann NY Acad Sci* 2001;952:13–22.

67. Langenfeld J, Kiyokawa H, Sekula D, et al. Posttranslational regulation of cyclin D$_1$ by retinoic acid: a chemopreventive mechanism. *Proc Natl Acad Sci USA* 1997;94:12070–12074.

68. Masuda M, Toh S, Koike K, et al. The roles of JNK1 and Stat3 in the response of head and neck cancer cell lines to combined treatment with all-*trans*-retinoic acid and 5-FU. *Jpn J Cancer Res* 2002;9:329–339.

69. Lin JK, Liang YC, Lin-Shiau SY. Cancer chemoprevention by tea polyphenols through mitotic signal transduction blockade. *Biochem Pharmacol* 1999;58:911–915.

70. Ahmad N, Adhami VM, Gupta S, et al. Role of the retinoblas-toma (pRb)-E2F/DP pathway in cancer chemopreventive effects of green tea polyphenol epigallocatechin-3-gallate. *Arch Biochem Biophys* 2002;398:125–131.

71. Masuda M, Suzui M, Weinstein IB. Effects of epigal-loctechin-3-gallate (EGCG) on growth, EGFR signaling pathways, gene expression and chemosensitivity in human head and neck squamous cell carcinoma cell lines. *Clin Cancer Res* 2001;7:4220–4229.

72. Casagrande F, Darbon JM. Effects of structurally related flavonoids on cell cycle progression of human melanoma cells: regulation of cyclin-dependent kinases CDK2 and CDK1. *Biochem Pharmacol* 2001;61:1205–1215.

73. Joe AK, Liu H, Suzui M, et al. Resveratrol induces growth inhibition, S-phase arrest, apoptosis, and changes in bio-marker expression in several human cancer cell lines. *Clin Cancer Res* 2002;8:893–903.

74. Ip C. Lessons from basic research in selenium and cancer prevention. *J Nutr* 1998;128:1845–1854.

75. Ip C, Thompson HJ, Ganther HE. Selenium modulation of cell proliferation and cell cycle biomarkers in normal and premalignant cells of the rat mammary gland. *Cancer Epidemiol Biomark Prev* 2000;9:49–54.

76. Rao L, Puschner B, Prolla TA. Gene expression profiling of low selenium status in the mouse intestine: transcriptional activation of genes linked to DNA damage, cell cycle control and oxidative stress. *J Nutr* 2001;131:3175–3181.

77. Liu M, Wikonkal NM, Brash DE. Induction of cyclin-dependent kinase inhibitors and G$_1$ prolongation by the chemopreventive agent *N*-acetylcysteine. *Carcinogenesis* 1999;20:1869–1872.

78. Shirin H, Pinto JT, Kawabata Y, et al. W. Antiproliferative effects of *S*-allylmercaptocysteine on colon cancer cells, when tested alone or in combination with sulindac sulfide. *Cancer Res* 2001;61:725–731.

78a. Xiao D, Pinto JT, Soh JW, et al. Induction of apoptosis by the garlic-derived compound S-allylmercaptocysteine (SAMC) is associated with microtubule depolymerization and c-Jun NH(2)-terminal Kinase 1 activation. *Cancer Res* 2003;63:6825–6837.

79. Soh J-W, Mao Y, Liu L, et al. Protein kinase G activates the JNK1 pathway via phosphorylation of MEKK1. *J Biol Chem* 2001;19:16,404–16,410.

80. Christov K, Ikui A, Shilkaitis A, et al. Cell proliferation, apoptosis and expression of cyclin D1 and cyclin E as poten-tial biomarkers in tamoxifen treated mammary tumors. *Breast Cancer Res* 2003;77:253–264.

81. Suzui M, Masuda M, Lim JTE, et al. Growth inhibition of human hepatoma cells by acylic retinoid is associated with inhibition of expression of cyclin D$_1$. *Cancer Res* 2002;62:3997–4006.

82. Carlson BA, Dunbay MM, Sausville EA, et al. Flavopiridol induces G$_1$ arrest with inhibition of cyclin dependent kinase (CDK) 2 and CDK4 in human breast carcinoma cells. *Cancer Res* 1996;56:2973–2978.

83. Carlson B, Lahusen T, Singh S, et al. Down-regulation of cyclin D$_1$ by transcriptional repression in MCF-7 human breast carcinoma cells induced by flavopiridol. *Cancer Res* 1999;59:4634–4641.

84. Schrump DS, Matthews W, Chen GA, et al. Flavopiridol mediates cell cycle arrest and apoptosis in esophageal cancer cells. *Clin Cancer Res* 1998;4:2885–2890.

85. Akiyama T, Yoshida T, Tsujita T, et al. G_1 phase accumulation induced by UCN-01 is associated with dephosphorylation of Rb and CDK2 proteins as well as induction of CDK inhibitor p21/Cip1/WAF1/Sdi1 in p53-mutated human epidermoid carcinoma A431 cells. *Cancer Res* 1997;57:1495–1501.

86. Owa T, Yoshino H, Okauchi T, et al. Discovery of novel antitumor sulfonamides targeting G1 phase of the cell cycle. *J Med Chem* 1999;42:3789–3799.

87. De Azevedo WF, Leclerc S, Meijer L, et al. Inhibition of cyclin-dependent kinases by purine analogue: crystal structure of human cdk2 complexed with roscovitine. *Eur J Biochem* 1997;243:518–526.

88. Bramson H N, Corona J, Davis ST, et al. Oxindole-based inhibitors of cyclin-dependent kinase 2 (CDK2): design, synthesis, enzymatic activities, and X-ray crystallographic analysis. *J Med Chem* 2001;44:4339–4358.

89. Kent LL, Hull-Campbell NE, Lau T, et al. Characterization of novel inhibitors of cyclin-dependent kinases. *Biochem Biophys Res Commun* 1999;260:768–774.

90. Kubo A, Nakagawa K, Varma RK, et al. The p16 status of tumor cell lines identifies small molecule inhibitors specific for cyclin-dependent kinase 4. *Clin Cancer Res* 1999;5:4279–4286.

91. Soni R, Muller L, Furet P, et al. Inhibition of cyclin-dependent kinase 4 (Cdk4) by fascaplysin, a marine natural product. *Biochem Biophys Res Commun* 2000;275:877–884.

92. Fry DW, Bedford DC, Harvey PH, et al. Cell cycle and biochemical effects of PD 0183812. A potent inhibitor of the cyclin D-dependent kinases CDK4 and CDK6. *J Biol Chem* 2001;276:16,617–16,623.

93. Soni R, O'Reilly T, Furet P, et al. Selective in vivo and in vitro effects of a small molecule inhibitor of cyclin-dependent kinase 4. *J Natl Cancer Inst* 2001;93:436–446.

94. Sekulic A, Hudson CC, Homme JL, et al. A direct linkage between the phosphoinositide 3-kinase-AKT signaling pathway and the mammalian target of rapamycin in mitogen-stimulated and transformed cells. *Cancer Res* 2000;60:3504–3513.

95. Hashemolhosseini S, Nagamine Y, Morley SJ, et al. Rapamycin inhibition of the G_1 to S transition is mediated by effects on cyclin D_1 mRNA and protein stability. *J Biol Chem* 1998;273:14,424–14,429.

96. Kawamata S, Sakaida H, Hori T, et al. The upregulation of p27Kip1 by rapamycin results in G1 arrest in exponentially growing T-cell lines. *Blood* 1998;91:561–569.

97. Marks PA, Richon VM, Breslow R, Rifkind RA. Histone deacetylase inhibitors as new cancer drugs. *Curr Opin Oncol* 2001;13:477–483.

98. Galvez AF, Chen N, Macasieb J, de Lumen BO. Chemopreventive property of a soybean peptide (lunasin) that binds to deacetylated histones and inhibits acetylation. *Cancer Res* 2001;61:7473–7478.

99. Saito A, Yamashita T, Mariko Y, et al. A synthetic inhibitor of histone deacetylase, MS-27-275, with marked in vivo antitumor activity against human tumors. *Proc Natl Acad Sci USA* 1999;96:4592–4597.

100. An WG, Hwang SG, Trepel JB, Blagosklonny MV. Protease inhibitor-induced apoptosis: accumulation of wt p53, p21WAF1/CIP1 and induction of apoptosis are independent markers of proteasome inhibition. *Leukemia* 2000;14:1276–1283.

101. Elliott PJ, Ross JS. The proteasome: a new target for novel drug therapies. *Am J Clin Pathol* 2001;116:637–646.

102. Otterson GA, Khleif SN, Chen W, et al. CDKN2 gene silencing in lung cancer by DNA hypermethylation nad kinetics of p16INK4 protein induction by 5-aza-2' deoxycytidine. *Oncogene* 1995;11:1211–1216.

103. Biankin AV, Kench JG, Morey AL, et al. Overexpression of p21(WAF1/CIP1) is an early event in the development of pancreatic intraepithelial neoplasia. *Cancer Res* 2001;61:8830–8837.

104. Tsujie M, Yamamoto H, Tomita N, et al. Expression of tumor suppressor gene p16[Ink4] products in primary gastric cancer. *Oncology* 2000;58:126–136.

28 Select Cyclic Nucleotide Phosphodiesterase Inhibitors in Colon Tumor Chemoprevention and Chemotherapy

Melissa K. Reeder, PhD, Rifat Pamakcu, MD, PhD,
I. Bernard Weinstein, MD, Kirk Hoffman, PhD,
and W. Joseph Thompson, PhD

CONTENTS

1. INTRODUCTION

Exisulind, and later generation drugs including CP461, are members of a group of new anticancer compounds known as Selective Apoptotic Antineoplastic Drugs (SAANDs). These drugs act by selectively inducing apoptosis in precancerous and cancerous tissues. Exisulind is a metabolite of sulindac, a nonsteroidal antiinflammatory drug (NSAID). Although initially developed to prevent colon cancer, exisulind and CP461 are currently being tested in clinical trials as chemotherapeutics against many types of cancer, including breast, colon, lung, prostate, chronic lymphocytic leukemia, and renal cell carcinoma. SAANDs were screened as cyclic 5' guanosine monophosphate (cGMP) phosphodiesterase (PDE) inhibitors with a preference for the PDE5 gene family. Published data have shown that in a colon cancer model, these drugs increase cGMP levels, activate cGMP-dependent protein kinase G (PKG) to stimulate the Jun kinase (JNK) regulatory cascade, and cause a decrease in accumulated nuclear and cytosolic β-catenin followed by reduced cyclin D$_1$ transcription.

2. SULINDAC METABOLISM: PATH TO EXISULIND

Many NSAIDs have varying degrees of antineoplastic activity, but may also have adverse side effects that include significant gastrointestinal, (GI), renal, and hematological toxicities. The NSAID sulindac, a proven anticancer agent that causes regression of adenomatous colorectal polyps in patients with familial adenomatous polyposis (FAP)*(1–4)*, is a prodrug metabolized primarily into sulfide and sulfone derivatives (Fig. 1) *(5,6)*. The sulfide component inhibits prostaglandin biosynthesis through the inhibition of cyclooxygenases (COX) 1 and 2, responsible for many of the adverse effects of sulindac *(7)*. Studies of the sulfone oxidative metabolite of sulindac led to the discovery of exisulind and a later analog, CP461. Exisulind (sulindac sulfone) designated (Z)-5-fluoro-2-methyl-1-

From: Cancer Chemoprevention, Volume 1: Promising Cancer Chemoprevention Agents
Edited by: G. J. Kelloff, E. T. Hawk, and C. C. Sigman © Humana Press Inc., Totowa, NJ

Fig. (A) Sulindac metabolic pathway. **(B)** Chemical structure of exisulind and CP461.

[(4-[methylsulphonyl]phenyl)methylene]-indene-3-ylacetic acid, does not convert back to sulindac or to the sulfide, and is cleared primarily by the kidneys as the glucuronidated end metabolite. Unlike the sulfide derivative, the sulfone does not inhibit prostaglandin biosynthesis or have significant antiinflammatory properties, because it does not fit in COX active sites *(8)*. Diarylheterocycle COX-2 inhibitors achieve reversible binding in the entry channel of the COX-2 active site, followed by a series of stronger bindings that brings the inhibitors further into the active site, leading to a nearly irreversible and time-dependent inhibition. Sulindac sulfide achieves the reversible initial binding, but this binding cannot lead to the stronger irreversible second-step binding because of the narrow COX-2 entry channel *(9)*, which makes the sulfide more of a COX-1 than a COX-2 inhibitor. Therefore it is not surprising from a molecular point of view that the sulfone, like the sulfide, is very different from the newer COX-2-selective inhibitors. Exisulind was the first of a new class of

Table 1

Summary of Growth Inhibition and Apoptosis Induction for Exisulind and CP461

Cell Line	Tumor	Growth IC_{50} μM		Apoptosis EC_{50} μM	
		Exisulind	CP461	Exisulind	CP4611
3-HTB, HT1376	Bladder	124±27	0.75±0.21	303	1.6±0.85
MDA-MB-231,MDA-MB-435s, UISO-BCA-1, MCF7/S	Breast	106±74	0.77±0.39	454±179	1.73±2.2
MCF-10F,184B5,HBL-100,MDA-MB-436 MDA-MB-453, BT-474, SK-BR-3, BT-20					
HTS	Cervix	200	ND	ND	ND
HT-29, HCT-15, HCT116, Colo205, SW-620, DLD-1, SW480, T84, VACO-2	Colon	218±96	1.3±0.67	515±30	2.33±1.18
RE282	Esophageal (rat)	180	ND	ND	ND
HS746T	gastric	420	ND	ND	ND
U87, U137, U373, A172, GB1, GB2,GB3,GB4	Glioma (human)	162±35	1.14±0.21	ND	ND
9L,C6, F98, D74	Glioma(rat)	145±37	0.98±0.17	ND	ND
k NRK fibroblasts	Kidney	240	ND	ND	ND
K562, CCRF-CEM, MOLT-4, MEG-01, WSU-CLL	Leukemia	287±147	1.1±0.59	432±216	0.98±0.27
A549, HTB-177, A427,NCI-H23, NCI-H322M, NCIH-460, NCI-H82	Lung	277±110	1.8±0.30	494±157	1.55±0.21
UACC375	Melanoma	100	ND	ND	ND
NIH-3T3	Ms.fibro-blast	200	1.5	ND	ND
RPMI-8226	Myeloma	445	1.2	Low response	21
OVCAR-3	Ovary	ND	1.2	ND	ND
PaCa2, BxPc3, CFPAC, PANC-1	Pancreatic	242±132	1.47±0.64	380±178	1.6±0.14
LNCap, DU145, PC-3, BPH	Prostate	180±96	1.4±44	487±80	1.55±0.92
786-0, ACHN, Caki	Renal	185±77	1.1±0.18	565	1.11±0.10
MES-SA, MES-SA/Dx5	Sarcoma	199±62	0.4±0.01	ND	2.13±1.6

Numbers listed are μM concentrations of drug needed to obtain 50% growth inhibition (IC_{50}) or 50% apoptosis induction (EC_{50}). concentrations are average of data for multiple cell lines from one tumor type. ND = concentrations not determined.

antineoplastic drugs that act by selectively inducing apoptosis in precancerous and cancerous tissues.

The antiinflammatory properties of NSAIDs are known to be mediated by COX inhibition (10,11). Their antineoplastic properties have also been suggested to be a result of their ability to reduce prostaglandin levels in the target tissue. (12) Contrary to this, exisulind does not inhibit prostaglandin metabolism. In a mammary carcinogensis study of rats in which tumors were induced with N-methyl-N-nitrosourea (MNU), exisulind and sulindac both increased latency and decreased the numbers of cancers per rat and the overall tumor burden (13). The same study reported that exisulind did not inhibit either COX-1 or COX-2 activity at concentrations much higher than concentrations at which sulindac sulfide inhibited both. In another study in which rat colon carcinogenesis was induced by azoxymethane (AOM), sulindac and exisulind both decreased tumor incidence and multiplicity, and caused a reduction of the colon tumor burden (14). However,

exisulind exhibited no decrease in prostaglandin E$_2$ or inhibition of 5- or 15-lipoxygenase and phospholipase A$_2$. These results clearly show that unlike the sulfide metabolite of sulindac, exisulind exhibits no effect on COX activity. A practical and logical consequence of this property of the drug is that exisulind would not be expected to induce the adverse side effects of NSAIDs.

3. CELLULAR RESPONSE

3.1. Growth Inhibition

Exisulind and the CP461 analog both show consistent growth inhibition in a wide variety of human tumor cell lines (15–18). Cell culture studies have shown that in colon cancer (15) and prostate (19) cell lines, both sulindac sulfide and exisulind exhibit growth-inhibitory properties, but only sulindac sulfide inhibited COX-1 and/or COX-2 activity. Growth inhibition is determined using dye-binding assays (e.g., sulforodamine) to compare growth of cells treated with drug for 6 d to

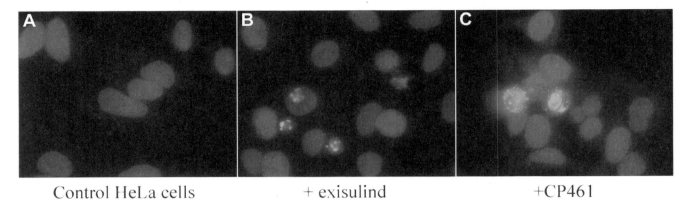

Fig. 2. Induction of apoptosis by exisulind and CP461. HeLa cells untreated (**A**) and treated with 600 μ*M* exisulind (**B**) and 1 μ*M* CP461 (**C**) for 16 h undergo apoptosis as determined by immunofluorescence staining of caspase-cleaved cytokeratin 18 with M30 monoclonal antibody.

growth of untreated cells. Table 1 shows a summary of growth inhibition in response to exisulind and CP461 in cultured human cell lines derived from various tissue origins. The IC_{50} values (concentrations needed to inhibit growth by 50%) show that CP461 is approx 173-fold more potent than exisulind in most tumor cells in culture. These drugs exhibit growth inhibition regardless of the histogenesis of the tumor from which the cell lines were derived, and are also effective in cells derived from precancerous lesions (VACO-235 or BPH-1 cells that were derived from human colonic adenomas or benign prostatic hypertrophy, respectively).

3.2. Apoptosis Induction

Apoptosis or programmed cell death (PCD) is a normal physiologic process used to eliminate unnecessary or aberrant cells without inflammation. This process is in opposition to necrotic cell death, which triggers an inflammatory response. Apoptosis involves a highly regulated and redundant sequence of events arising from the activation of specific proteases (caspases) and endonucleases that produce condensed nuclear and cytoplasmic components while maintaining membrane integrity. PCD comprises intrinsic (mitochondrial) and extrinsic (death receptor) pathways that are both important drug targets.

In vitro and in vivo studies show that apoptosis primarily accounts for growth inhibition by exisulind and lower-affinity SAANDs, and CP461 and higher-affinity analogs have additional antiproliferative effects. Tissue-culture studies have shown that exisulind significantly induces apoptosis, as detected by DNA fragmentation, morphology, and caspase activity *(15,19,20)*. Table 2 lists multiple tumor-

derived cell lines that have tested positive for apoptosis in response to exisulind and/or CP461. Published and unpublished studies in breast- and prostate-cell lines have demonstrated that SAANDs induce apoptosis in tumor cell lines, but not in normal cell-line counterparts *(19)*. Additionally, an in vivo animal study using a human prostate cancer xenograph in nude mice showed that exisulind inhibited tumor growth, and that grafts on the treated mice showed statistically increased apoptosis *(21)*. CP461 was also shown to increase apoptosis and reduce tumor volume in an orthotopically induced human non-small-cell lung cancer (NSCLC) nude rat model *(22,23)*. A study of patients with FAP found that treatment with exisulind resulted in a regression of small polyps *(24)*, resulting from exisulind-induced stimulation of mucus differentiation in cells of the adenomatous glands, along with an increased apoptotic labeling index in the polyps as determined by both morphological changes and TdT-mediated nick-end labeling (TUNEL) assay. Importantly, there was no significant change in the apoptotic index in the normal appearing mucosa. From these and other studies, it is clear that the primary method of growth inhibition by exisulind and CP461 is induction of apoptosis, and an example of this is shown in Fig. 2.

4. MECHANISM OF ACTION

4.1. p53 and Bcl-2 Independent Apoptosis

Early experiments with exisulind revealed that apoptosis induced by SAANDs is independent of p53 and Bcl-2 status *(15,19)*. Many chemotherapeutic drugs induce apoptosis through a p53-dependent path-

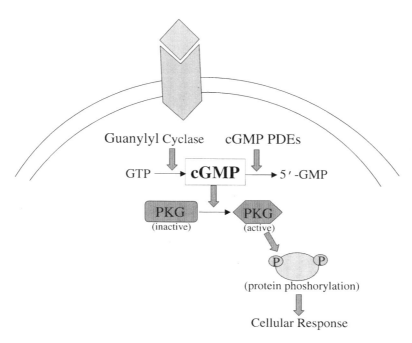

Fig. 3. cGMP Homeostasis. cGMP, guanosine 3',5'-cyclic monophosphate; GTP, guanosine triphosphate; PKG, protein kinase G; PDE, phosphodiesterase.

way; many human tumors contain mutated p53, which may explain the resistance of these neoplastic cells to drugs that utilize this pathway. To study the importance of p53 in an exisulind pathway, HT-29 colon carcinoma cells were treated with exisulind or the chemotherapeutic drugs 5-fluorouracil (5-FU) (50 μM) or etoposide (10 μM). All these treatments induced apoptosis, but only 5-FU and etoposide increased p53 expression (15). Moreover, exisulind was shown to induce apoptosis in Saos-2 cells lacking functional p53. A potential role for the anti-apoptotic protein Bcl-2 in the apoptotic response to exisulind was studied using hormone-dependent and -independent prostate cell lines expressing low, intermediate, or high levels of Bcl-2 (19). Apoptosis was induced with exisulind regardless of the level of Bcl-2 protein expression. Although these two studies revealed that SAANDs molecules use an apoptosis mechanism other than p53 or Bcl-2, a study from our laboratory showed that colon cell lines treated with concentrations of exisulind or CP461 that induce apoptosis respond by altering Bax/Bcl-2 protein ratio levels (25). The amount of Bax protein in these cells increases while the amount of Bcl-2 protein decreases. Thus, it is possible that the intrinsic pathway of apoptosis regulation may play some role in the actions of these drugs in colon tumor-cell lines.

4.2. cGMP PDE Inhibition and PKG Activation

The mechanism of action of exisulind, CP461, and analogs has been studied most extensively in colon tumor cells, primarily because exisulind causes regression and prevents the recurrence of polyps in patients with FAP (24,26,27) and regression of sporadic polyps (28) through an apoptosis mechanism. Numerous colon cancer-cell lines were used to show that exisulind induces apoptosis by inhibiting cGMP PDEs, thereby increasing cGMP levels and PKG activity. This finding has led to the identification and development of more potent exisulind analogs, including CP461, based on screening the drugs for PDE5 inhibition.

Cyclic nucleotide PDEs consist of 11 gene families, and each family contains subtypes—up to 21 subtypes in humans. PDEs hydrolyze the 3'-phosphoester bond of cyclic 5' adenosine monophosphate (cAMP) and cGMP second messengers to their biologically inactive, noncyclic 5'-nucleotides (reviewed in 29,30). These enzymes have a hydrolytic domain that is specific for hydrolyzing cAMP, cGMP or both, and a regulatory domain that keeps the enzymes in a low activity state until activated by various regulatory mechanisms, such as phosphorylation or binding of modulators. PDE4, PDE7, and PDE8 are all relatively specific or selective for cAMP. PDE3 and PDE10 can hydrolyze cGMP, but are generally classified as cAMP PDEs. PDE2 and

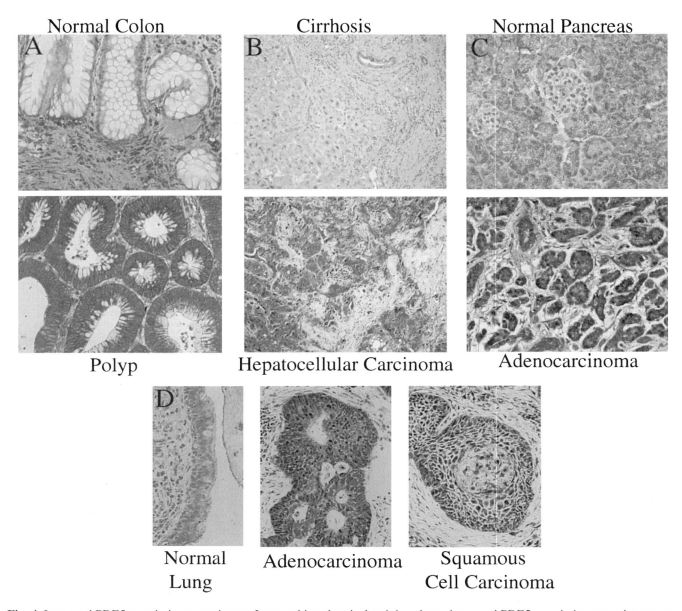

Fig. 4. Increased PDE5 protein in tumor tissues. Immunohistochemical staining shows increased PDE5 protein in tumor tissues corresponding to (**A**) colon, (**B**) liver, (**C**) pancreas, and (**D**) lung normal tissues.

PDE11 have dual activity, but they differ because PDE2 is specifically stimulated by cGMP. PDE6, PDE5, and PDE9 are cGMP-specific; PDE6 is expressed only in retinal rods and cones, where it functions in light capture. PDE1 is stimulated by calcium/calmodulin and has a higher affinity for cGMP than cAMP, although some isoforms do have high affinity for cAMP. The cGMP-specific PDE5 and PDE9 differ, as PDE5 contains a non-active cGMP binding site which triggers a conformational change in PDE5 that allows phosphorylation by PKG.

PDE enzymes have been used for several years to develop new pharmaceuticals that manipulate various cellular processes (*31,32*), but only recently have been investigated for use as anticancer agents (*33,34*). These enzymes contribute to the establishment of cellular cGMP levels. Cyclic GMP levels are determined by a combination of soluble and particulate guanylyl cyclases (GCs) that generate cGMP and cGMP PDEs, cGMP export pumps, and cGMP-binding sites that break down, export, or occupy cGMP, respectively (*30*). Cytosolic cGMP binds to and activates PKG, leading to

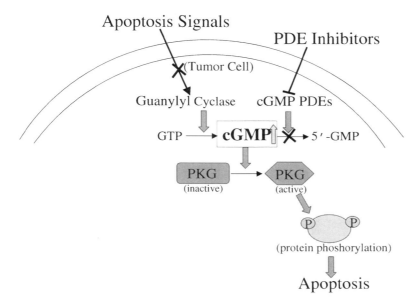

Fig. 5. Mechanism of SAANDs-induced apoptosis through cGMP PDE inhibition. cGMP, guanosine 3',5'-cyclic monophosphate; GTP, guanosine triphosphate; PKG, protein kinase G; PDE, phosphodiesterase.

protein phosphorylation and various cellular responses (Fig. 3). cGMP binding sites also regulate many ion channels. Highly expressed in colon epithelium, GC-C has been used as a diagnostic marker for metastatic colorectal tumors in human extraintestinal tissues *(35)*. PDE5 and PDE2 also have increased expression in colon, lung, pancreatic, breast, and bladder tumor tissues *(36–39)*. Figure 4 shows increased PDE5 protein levels in tumor tissue compared to normal tissue derived from the colon, liver, pancreas, and lung.

Colon cell-line models consisting of SW480, HT29, T84, and HCT116 cells have been used to elucidate the mechanism of SAANDs-induced apoptosis *(40–43)*. Activity of cGMP PDEs in these cells was inhibited by both exisulind and higher-affinity analogs. A similar rank of potency was seen in PDE inhibition as with apoptosis induction and cell-growth inhibition. Compared with exisulind, CP461 is approx 50× more potent in PDE inhibition, 150× more potent in cell growth inhibition, and 200× more potent in apoptosis induction. Exisulind and CP461 also increased cGMP levels at 1, 24, and 72 h after treatment. This cGMP increase is essential to the mechanism; the PDE inhibitors E4021 and zaprinast do not increase cGMP, and also do not induce apoptosis. In addition, the GC activator 3-(5'-hydroxymethyl-2'-furyl)-benzyl(imidazole) (YC-1) and the cGMP analog 8-bromo-cGMP were able to inhibit growth and induce apoptosis. Moreover, exisulind and CP461 significantly increased PKG

activation—presumably through induction of increased cGMP levels.

A fragment of PDE5 used as substrate increased PKG activity as early as 5 min after treatment, and sustained it for 24 h *(43)*. PKG activity increased in a dose-dependent manner both in the absence and presence of added cGMP, indicating that the activity is specific to PKG. PKG protein levels were also increased by drug treatment starting at 8 h and peaking at 48 h of treatment. The drugs did not directly activate PKG in vitro, as cGMP and 8-bromo-cGMP did. Activation was induced by treatment with YC-1 but not forskolin, indicating activation was indeed caused by the increased levels of cGMP. These results have led a model in which SAANDs inhibit PDE, thereby increasing cGMP levels to induce and activate PKG (Fig. 5). This model is strengthened by the previously mentioned overexpression of target cGMP PDEs in the colon, lung, pancreas, breast, prostate, urinary bladder, and renal tumor tissues, all of which respond to SAANDs with growth inhibition/apoptosis (Table 1).

4.3. JNK Pathway Activation

c-Jun NH_2-terminal kinase (JNK1) is a member of the stress-response signaling cascade. JNK1 is involved in apoptotic signaling pathways triggered by various agents, including ultraviolet (UV) and γ irradiation *(44)* and benzyl isothiocyanate *(45)*. Activated JNK1 activates the AP-1 transcription factor, leading

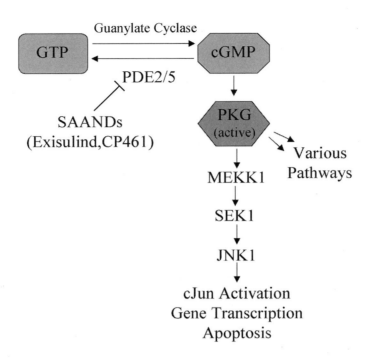

Fig. 6. Model of SAANDs mechanism of JNK activation leading to apoptosis. cGMP, guanosine 3',5'-cyclic monophosphate; GTP, guanosine triphosphate; PKG, protein kinase G; PDE phosphodiesterase; MEKK, mitogen-activated protein kinase kinase kinase; SEK, stress-activated-protein/ERK kinase 1; JNK, c-Jun NH₂-terminal kinase.

to induction of several genes involved in apoptosis *(46)*. In the colon-cell line model in which SAANDs treatment led to increased cGMP and PKG activity, Weinstein et al. *(41)* also detected increased JNK activity. Exisulind and analogs increased JNK activity in SW480 colon cancer cells, as did treatment with cGMP modulators, but not cAMP modulators. SEK1, the kinase directly upstream from JNK1, was also activated by exisulind analogs; increased specific phosphorylation of this protein was detected after 30 min treatment of SW480 cells, peaked at 2 h treatment, and lasted through 12 h treatment. This is an atypical activation of JNK that parallels PKG stimulation. Additionally, cells stably transfected to express a dominant-negative JNK construct markedly inhibited exisulind analog induction of poly(ADP-ribose)polymerase 1 (PARP) cleavage, a marker of apoptosis. These cells were also more resistant to induction of apoptosis by these drugs.

Further extension of this pathway revealed that PKG can directly phosphorylate MEKK1, a mitogen-activated protein (MAP) kinase that activates SEK1 *(42)*. Also, PKG activation of JNK was blocked by transfection of a dominant-negative MEKK1. When wild-type and dominant-negative MEKK were incubated with PKG and

cGMP, the wild-type protein underwent more extensive phosphorylation than the dominant-negative protein. In the same study, transient transfection reporter assays showed that a constitutively activated form of PKG was able to transactivate c-Jun and activate AP-1 transcription in NIH-3T3 mouse fibroblasts. These results lead to a model in which activated PKG activates the stress kinase and prominent proapoptotic pathway by directly phosphorylating MEKK1, leading to a transcriptional response involved in apoptosis induction (Fig. 6).

4.4. β-Catenin and Cyclin D₁ Reduction

Cell-adhesion phosphoprotein β-catenin has an important function in both embryogenesis and oncogenesis through the Wnt signaling pathways, leading to lymphocyte enhancer-binding factor (Lef)/T cell factor (Tcf)-modulated transcription *(47,48)*. In many types of cancer, Tcf factors can be tumor inducers by aberrantly regulating target gene transcription resulting from accumulated β-catenin *(49)*, which is phosphorylated when it forms a complex with adenomatous polposis coli (APC) protein, phosphatase 2A, glycogen synthase kinase β (GSK3β) and other proteins. This phosphorylation leads to its ubiquitination and degradation by proteasomes. Tumor-suppressing protein APC is also phosphorylated,

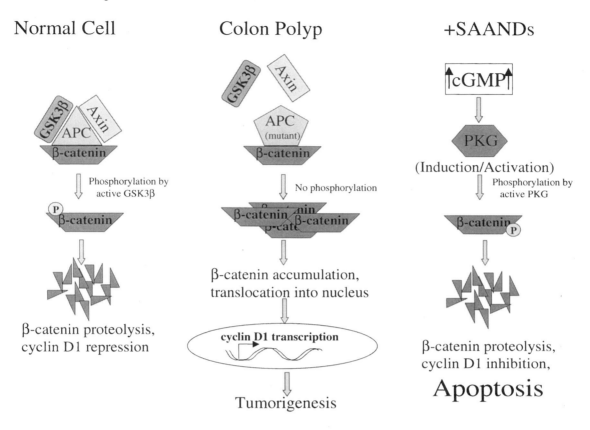

Fig. 7. Model of SAANDs mechanism of β-catenin degradation leading to apoptosis. cGMP, guanosine 3',5'-cyclic monophosphate; PKG, protein kinase G; GSK3β, glycogen synthase kinase 3 beta; APC, adenomatous polyposis coli.

resulting in an increased affinity for β-catenin binding. Mutations in APC or β-catenin occur in sporadic and familial polyps *(50–52)*, presumably causing an accumulation of β-catenin in the nucleus that leads to induction of an oncogenic signal. Treatment of SW480 cells with exisulind and CP461 both reduce β-catenin protein levels, including the nuclear β-catenin *(40)*. PKG has been shown to directly phosphorylate β-catenin in vitro. Treatment of SW480 cells with exisulind or CP461 and CP248 increased β-catenin phosphorylation in intact cells *(43)*. Along with reduced β-catenin levels following SAANDs treatment, reduction of cyclin D_1 protein and mRNA occurs in a time- and dose-dependent manner. Exisulind-induced reduction of β-catenin was not blocked by inhibition of caspase 3 activity; the reduction was detected before early signs of apoptosis *(53)*. Additionally, expression of an *N*-terminal 170-aa fragment of β-catenin decreased exisulind-induced β-catenin degradation, cyclin D_1 reduction, and apoptosis response. Therefore, reduction of accumulated β-catenin by SAANDs occurs before

apoptosis induction. This reduction partially accounts for the proapoptotic effects of these drugs (Fig. 7).

To recapitulate, the mechanism of apoptosis induction by exisulind and CP461 has been demonstrated in colon tumor cells. These drugs inhibit cGMP PDE activity, as evidenced by increased cellular cGMP levels. Both PKG activity and protein levels are increased by these drugs, and although speculative, it is reasonable to propose that increased cellular cGMP causes the initial increase in PKG. PKG activation leads to multiple downstream effects, including activation of the JNK stress-activated signaling pathway, decreased accumulated cytoplasmic and nuclear β-catenin, and the resultant decreased cyclin D_1 mRNA, protein and activity.

The newer generation exisulind derivative CP461 has shown a cellular effect in addition to apoptosis, and initially appears to be independent of PDE inhibition. CP461 blocks tumor cells and normal cells in culture at G_2/M stage of the cell cycle *(22,23,54)*. The mechanism is currently under investigation, but does not involve a direct effect on microtubule binding, as seen with other

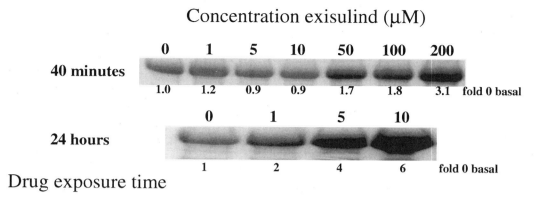

Fig. 8. PKG activation dose requirements for exisulind. Minimum dose requirements for PKG activation in HCT116 colon cancer cells are 50 μM for a 40-min treatment and 1 μM for a 24-h treatment. Activation is represented as increased radiolabeled phosphorylation of PDE5 protein fragment, a PKG-specific substrate.

analogs such as CP248 *(55)*. In normal cells in culture, such as foreskin fibroblasts, CP461 G_2/M block does not induce apoptosis, as in colon and other tumor cells. How the CP461 PDE inhibition as an apoptosis inducer is integrated with the antiproliferative cell cycle block is currently under investigation.

5. THE CONCENTRATION CONTROVERSY

Discussions about the mechanism of action of COX and cyclic nucleotide PDE inhibitors with respect to growth inhibition and apoptosis involve concentrations of drugs used for in vitro assays or cell culture systems. Questions have been raised regarding these biological effects and whether they represent actions or mechanisms that induce clinical activity. Concentrations of exisulind required to achieve effects in intact cells are approx 100 μM for growth inhibition and 400 μM for apoptosis induction, values well within cGMP PDE inhibitory ranges. Studies in rats have shown serum drug concentrations ranging from 200 to 400 μM after oral administration *(14)*, values that are completely consistent with in vitro studies. However, serum concentrations in humans reach only 20–50 μM at clinical doses, calling into question the use of in vitro data for clinical validation. An underlying assumption about serum levels is that they bear an absolute relationship to tissue or tumor concentrations. This is not the case with many drugs; for example, exisulind undergoes enterohepatic circulation and concentration in gastric mucosa. It is important to remember that in vitro assays are optimized and artificial, and may not represent conditions in patient intact cells or tissues, as illustrated for exisulind in Fig. 8 and 9. Depending upon the length of exposure to the drug, colon tumor cells

show several-fold differences in PKG sensitivity (Fig. 8). In addition, when HCT116 cells drug-treated for 5 d instead of optimized shorter time periods are used for apoptosis, the EC_{50} for exisulind-induced apoptosis becomes 5 μM, or well below the serum concentrations of the drug in patients (Fig. 9). CP461, with its much higher affinity, does not show these enhanced sensitivity effects, suggesting that exisulind has some type of concentrating mechanism in epithelial cells.

6. PRECLINICAL STUDIES

6.1. Exisulind

Preclinical studies demonstrate that exisulind inhibits growth and induces apoptosis in various cancer cell lines and xenographs, including the colon, prostate, lung, and breast (Table 1). Exisulind has been shown to be effective in inducing apoptosis and reducing tumor size in such animal models as a colon carcinogenesis rat model, mammary tumor rat model, prostate cancer nude mouse model, bladder cancer rat model, and lung cancer mouse model (reviewed in *56*). Exisulind has also demonstrated additive or synergistic effects in preclinical testing when combined with antineoplastic agents, including docetaxel, paclitaxel, gemcitabine, vinorelbine, irinotecan, trastuzumab, and retinoids in in vitro or in vivo models *(56)*.

The nonclinical safety of exisulind was evaluated in a broad-screen pharmacology screening profile program of 48 different test models. Animal screening was utilized to test exisulind activity on central nervous, GI, cardiovascular, and immunological systems, among others. Additionally, in vivo and in vitro studies using

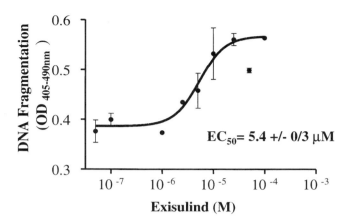

Fig. 9. Apoptosis dose requirements for exisulind. When HCT116 colon cancer cells are treated with exisulind for 5 d, the EC_{50} concentration for apoptosis is decreased to 5 μM.

isolated tissues were used to observe antiinflammatory, metabolic, toxicological, and antagonism effects. These studies demonstrated that exisulind had no activity in any of the screening models, except for some marginal analgesic activity in the phenyl-*p*-quinone writhing assay, and some marginal activity increasing high-density lipoproteins in the metabolic assay when used at high doses. As described previously, exisulind showed minimal or no effect on normal cell apoptosis in cultured cells or in patients, and the mechanism of action is not related to the inhibition of prostaglandin synthesis.

6.2. CP461

CP461 inhibits tumor cell growth and induces apoptosis in vitro in a wide variety of tumor cell types, including breast, prostate, colon, leukemia, and other cancer cell lines (Table 1). Efficacy of CP461 in inducing apoptosis and reducing tumor size has also been demonstrated in vivo in a prostate cancer model in nude mice *(57)*. Synergism of CP461 with docetaxel has been observed in a rodent xenograft model of human lung cancer *(22,23)* and with paclitaxel in human mammary tumor xenographs in nude mice *(8)*.

The nonclinical toxicology program with CP461 indicated that it was well-tolerated for administration to humans in initial Phase I clinical studies. Repeated oral administration to rats and dogs showed no adverse effects at 50 mg/kg/d. At high doses of the drug, increases in liver and thyroid weight were detected, but histopathological changes were limited to hypertophy of these organs in only a small number of animals. Other effects seen at high doses were minimal hepatocellular hypertrophy and increases in liver-specific

alanine aminotransferase (ALT) and liver-nonspecific alkaline phosphatase. The only histological finding noted with the administration of CP461 was hyperplasia of the hepatic biliary canaliculi at doses of 300 mg/kg/d in beagle dogs, which was graded minimal to slight in severity.

7. HUMAN STUDIES

7.1. Pharmacology and Safety

The pharmacokinetics and bioavailibility of exisulind have been evaluated in single-dose studies in healthy volunteers and in multiple-dose studies in patients. Exisulind is rapidly absorbed following single oral doses of 50–400 mg in healthy subjects. Elimination half-life in patients with intact colons ranged from 9 to 14 h; the MRT (mean residence time of unchanged drug in circulation) ranged from 10 to 13 h. The plasma concentration time curve in some patients showed multiple peaks, suggesting enterohepatic recirculation. Exisulind has no effect on the activity of cytochrome P450 enzymes, suggesting that exisulind will not significantly interact with drugs metabolized by these enzymes (Cell Pathways, unpublished results).

A substantial database of over 500 patients (including those with such diseases as sporadic adenomatous polyps, prostate cancer, lung cancer, breast cancer, and Barrett's esophagus) demonstrates the safety of exisulind in humans. Exisulind is generally-well tolerated at doses up to 500 mg/d in patients with intact colons, and 600 mg/d in APC patients with subtotal colectomies. Exisulind has been associated with asymptomatic, dose-related elevations in ALT/aspartate aminotransferase (AST) levels that were rapidly

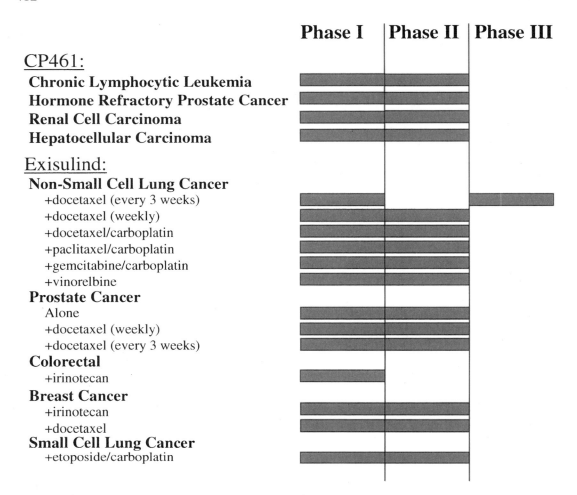

Fig. 10. Completed and current clinical trials for exisulind and CP461.

reversed after discontinuing treatment or reducing the dose. Severe abdominal pain has been reported with exisulind therapy. Some of these cases were associated with biliary events such as acute cholecystitis and obstructive (gallstone) pancreatitis. Exisulind has not been associated with blood dyscrasias, neurologic, or renal events, or any clinically significant changes in vital signs (Cell Pathways, unpublished results).

The pharmacokinetics and safety of CP461 have been evaluated in three Phase I studies, two with healthy volunteers (single dose) and one in patients with solid tumors (repeated dose). Peak plasma concentrations are achieved within 1–2 h after dosing; mean trough levels exceed the in vitro EC_{50} for apoptosis (1 μ*M*) at total daily doses of 400 and 800 mg. CP461 is metabolized in the liver and eliminated completely within 72 h in urine and 144 h in the feces. The half-life of CP461 is 5.4–8.7 h at doses between 100 and 800 mg/d (Cell Pathways, unpublished results).

In safety studies with healthy volunteers, there was no association between the dose of CP461 and the incidence, frequency, or severity of adverse events (AEs). The only AE considered to be possibly related to study medication was a mild arm rash. No clinically significant laboratory changes were reported in vital signs, physical examinations, or electrocardiograms. In the repeated dose study in patients with solid tumors, therapy was generally well-tolerated, and a maximum tolerated dose (MTD) was not reached. Toxicities considered possibly or probably related to drug treatment and National Cancer Institute (NCI) grade 2 or above included asymptomatic AST/ALT elevation, sensory neuropathy in three platinum-pretreated patients, and chest pain (Cell Pathways, unpublished results).

7.2. Human Trials

A summary of current human clinical trials is shown in Fig. 10 for both exisulind and CP461. Results and summaries of Cell Pathways' trials conducted under INDs are as follows.

Exisulind has been evaluated in patients with FAP who had subtotal colectomies. The first Phase I/II study in FAP found that exisulind treatment resulted in statistically significant dose-dependent reductions in colonic adenomatous polyps over time by regressing existing polyps and preventing new polyp formation *(27)*. A randomized, double-blind, placebo-controlled, 12-mo Phase II/III study demonstrated that exisulind (150 mg qid) decreased new polyp formation by 25% compared to placebo (p = ns). The lack of statistical significance may have been caused by the high variability in polyp formation rates between the two groups *(26)*. An open-label, 12-mo extension of this study resulted in an additional 54% decrease (p = 0.004) in polyp formation in patients who continued exisulind, and a 32% decrease (p = 0.001) in polyp formation in patients who crossed over from placebo to exisulind *(58)*. Exisulind was also evaluated in patients who had sporadic adenomatous polyps with intact colons and no familial syndromes. Patients who received exisulind (200 mg bid) had a significantly greater decrease in median polyp size than those who received placebo (p = 0.030). Complete or partial response was significantly higher (54.6%, p = 0.038) and disease progression was significantly less (6.1%, p = 0.017) in the exisulind group compared to placebo *(28)*.

Exisulind at 250 mg bid has been evaluated in men with prostate cancer following radical prostatectomy. In a randomized, double-blind, placebo-controlled, 12-mo study, exisulind suppressed the overall rise in prostate-specific antigen (PSA) levels compared to placebo (p = 0.017, n = 92). The effect was highly significant in men at high risk for metastasis and in those who could not be classified according to risk. In addition, PSA doubling time was lengthened in high-risk patients from 5.6 to 8.8 mo compared to a decrease from 4.9 mo to 2.4 mo in high-risk patients treated with placebo *(59)*. In a 12-mo, open-label extension of this study, the PSA doubling time increased more than twofold for high-risk patients who continued with exisulind *(60)*. Exisulind is currently being evaluated in combination with docetaxel in Phase I/II studies of men with hormone-refractory prostate cancer.

Phase I–III studies evaluating the effect of exisulind in NSCLC are currently being conducted. A Phase I/II study is now determining the activity and tolerable dose regimen of intravenous (iv) docetaxel and oral exisulind administered concurrently. Phase I of the study in patients with advanced cancer is complete, but results have not yet been reported. No unanticipated toxicites or AEs were detected. In the Phase II study, patients with advanced NSCLC who have failed platinum therapy are being treated with exisulind at 250 mg bid plus docetaxel at 36 mg/m^2 iv weekly for 3 of 4 wk until disease progression or toxicity. Efficacy will be evaluated by measuring tumor response and determining time to progression. A randomized, double-blind, placebo-controlled Phase III trial of exisulind at 250 mg bid in combination with docetaxel at 75 mg/m^2 iv every three wk is also being conducted in patients with NSCLC after failure of prior platinum chemotherapy, to determine whether the combination will result in increased overall and 1-yr survival. Tumor responses are examined by chest X-ray or computerized tomography scan to determine the objective rate of response and time to progression. Patients will continue to receive both drugs until disease progression or toxicity.

CP461 has been evaluated in Phase I clinical studies, including single-dose pharmacokinetics and ADME studies in healthy subjects, and a repeated dose study in patients with solid tumors *(61,62)* (Cell Pathways, unpublished results). Additional Phase I–II trials are underway to evaluate the pharmacokinetics, safety, and efficacy of CP461. These studies include a dose response study (400–800 mg/d) in previously untreated patients with chronic lymphocytic leukemia, a pharmacokinetics and dose-escalating (1200–2400 mg/d) study in patients with advanced malignancies, and pilot Phase II studies in chronic lymphocytic leukemia, renal cell carcinoma and hormone-refractory prostate cancer. These studies are in various stages of enrollment.

8. SUMMARY

Exisulind and CP461 are members of a new class of novel compounds known as SAANDs that are intended to prevent and/or treat cancer. These drugs selectively inhibit the growth of a wide variety of tumor cells without affecting normal cell growth. The primary basis for growth inhibition by these drugs is induction of apoptosis in tumor cells. Exisulind is one of very few drugs that has shown apoptosis induction in cell lines, animal xenograph tumors, and adenoma epithelial cells in human patients. The mechanism for apoptosis induction has been eludicated in a colon-tumor model, and involves activation and induction of PKG by the inhibition of cGMP PDEs. PKG is partly activated by the resultant increased cGMP in the cells, but sustained activation of the enzyme suggests other activation mechanisms, such as autophosphorylation, as well as induction of new protein. Apoptosis probably occurs as a result of PKG activation of the JNK stress pathway through MEKK1 phosphorylation and PKG phosphorylation of β-catenin to decrease accumulated β-catenin levels and reverse cyclin D_1 overexpression. In a separate effect, CP461 inhibits the cell cycle at mitosis, which may or may not be related to its PDE inhibition. These drugs have been tested for safety in preclinical and clinical trials, and are well-tolerated in humans, with only mild or moderate AEs. Tested for efficacy in human trials, exisulind has been shown to reduce polyps in patients with FAP and sporadic polyps, and to stabilize or decrease PSA levels and increase PSA doubling times in post-prostatectomy cancer patients. The efficacy of exisulind is being tested in NSCLC patients in combination with docitaxol. CP461 efficacy is currently being tested in chronic lymphocytic leukemia, renal cell carcinoma, and prostate cancer.

It has recently been demonstrated that these drugs cause phosphorylation of vasodilator-stimulated protein (VASP) *(63)*. VASP was originally discovered as a substrate for PKG in human platelets, although it is ubiquitously expressed in most types of cells. This phosphorylation of VASP could prove to be an important biomarker used to determine SAANDs concentration and its effects in the body.

Overall, SAANDs exhibit extraordinary properties that recommend them as promising agents for treatment for a wide variety of cancer disease types. The unique mechanism of action of the lead drugs exisulind and CP461, combined with a broad spectrum of efficacy and low incidence of adverse side effects in humans, make them particularly attractive. It will be exciting to see them at work as instruments of cancer prevention and treatment.

REFERENCES

1. Giardiello FM, Hamilton SR, Krush AJ, et al. Treatment of colonic and rectal adenomas with sulindac in familial adenomatous polyposis. *N Engl J Med* 1993;328:1313–1316.
2. Waddell WR, Ganser GF, Cerise EJ, Loughry RW. Sulindac for polyposis of the colon. *Am J Surg* 1989;157:175–179.
3. Rigau J, Pique JM, Rubio E, et al. Effects of long-term sulindac therapy on colonic polyposis. *Ann Intern Med* 1991;115:952–954.
4. Labayle D, Fischer D, Vielh P, et al. Sulindac causes regression of rectal polyps in familial adenomatous polyposis. *Gastroenterology* 1991;101:635–639.
5. Dobrinska MR, Furst DE, Spiegel T, et al. Biliary secretion of sulindac and metabolites in man. *Biopharm Drug Dispos* 1983;4:347–358.
6. Duggan DE, Hooke KF, Hwang SS. Kinetics of the tissue distributions of sulindac and metabolites. Relevance to sites and rates of bioactivation. *Drug Metab Dispos* 1980;8:241–246.
7. Shen TY, Winter CA. Chemical and biological studies on indomethacin, sulindac and their analogs. *Adv Drug Res* 1977;12:90–245.
8. Haanen C. Sulindac and its derivatives: a novel class of anticancer agents. *Curr Opin Investig Drugs* 2001;2:677–683.
9. Salter EA, Wierzbicki A, Sperl G, Thompson WJ. Molecular modeling study of COX-2 inhibition by diarylheterocycles and sulindac sulfide. *J Mol Struct* 2001;549:111–121.
10. Vane JR, Botting RM. Mechanism of action of anti-inflammatory drugs. *Scand J Rheumatol Suppl* 1996;102:9–21.
11. Vane JR, Botting RM. Mechanism of action of nonsteroidal anti-inflammatory drugs. *Am J Med* 1998;104:2S–8S.
12. Marnett LJ. Aspirin and the potential role of prostaglandins in colon cancer. *Cancer Res* 1992;52:5575–5589.
13. Thompson HJ, Briggs S, Paranka NS, et al. Inhibition of mammary carcinogenesis in rats by sulfone metabolite of sulindac. *J Natl Cancer Inst* 1995;87:1259–1260.
14. Piazza GA, Alberts DS, Hixson LJ, et al. Sulindac sulfone inhibits azoxymethane-induced colon carcinogenesis in rats without reducing prostaglandin levels. *Cancer Res* 1997;57:2909–2915.
15. Piazza GA, Rahm AK, Finn TS, et al. Apoptosis primarily accounts for the growth-inhibitory properties of sulindac metabolites and involves a mechanism that is independent of cyclooxygenase inhibition, cell cycle arrest, and p53 induction. *Cancer Res* 1997;57:2452–2459.
16. Piazza GA, Rahm AL, Krutzsch M, et al. Antineoplastic drugs sulindac sulfide and sulfone inhibit cell growth by inducing apoptosis. *Cancer Res* 1995;55:3110–3116.
17. Hixson LJ, Alberts DS, Krutzsch M, et al. Antiproliferative effect of nonsteroidal antiinflammatory drugs against human colon cancer cells. Cancer *Epidemiol Biomark Prev* 1994;3:433–438.
18. Han EK, Arber N, Yamamoto H, et al. Effects of sulindac and its metabolites on growth and apoptosis in human mammary epithelial and breast carcinoma cell lines. *Breast Cancer Res Treat* 1998;48:195–203.
19. Lim JT, Piazza GA, Han EK, et al. Sulindac derivatives inhibit growth and induce apoptosis in human prostate cancer cell lines. *Biochem Pharmacol* 1999;58:1097–1107.
20. Thompson HJ, Jiang C, Lu J, et al. Sulfone metabolite of sulindac inhibits mammary carcinogenesis. *Cancer Res* 1997;57:267–271.
21. Goluboff ET, Shabsigh A, Saidi JA, et al. Exisulind (sulindac sulfone) suppresses growth of human prostate cancer in a nude mouse xenograft model by increasing apoptosis. *Urology* 1999;53:440–445.
22. Whitehead CM, Earle K, Xu S, et al. CP461 in an orthotopic human NSCLC rat model involves phosphodiesterase targeting, apoptosis induction, G2M block and anti-proliferation. *Proc Am Assoc Cancer Res* 2002;19:924.
23. Whitehead CM, Earle K, Fetter J, et al. CP461 inhibits cGMP PDE activity, induces apoptosis and arrests cell cycle progression in A549 cells in culture and in an orthotopic lung

tumor model. *Apoptosis and Cancer: Basic Mechanisms and Therapeutic Opportunities in the Post-genomic Era.* American Association for Cancer Research Meeting; Waikoloa, Hawaii. February 13–17, 2002.

24. Stoner GD, Budd GT, Ganapathi R, et al. Sulindac sulfone induced regression of rectal polyps in patients with familial adenomatous polyposis. *Adv Exp Med Biol* 1999;470:45–53.

25. Li H, Chen M, David M, et al. CP461, an exisulind analog regulates apoptosis using PKG and Bcl-2 mechanisms. *Apoptosis and Cancer: Basic Mechanisms and Therapeutic Opportunities in the Post-genomic Era.* American Association for Cancer Research Meeting; Waikoloa, Hawaii. February 13–17, 2002.

26. Burke C, van Stolk R, Arber N, et al. Exisulind prevents adenoma formation in familial adenomatous polyposis (FAP). *Gastroenterology* 2000;118:A657, abst. 3604.

27. Burke C. The effect of exisulind on rectal adenomas in adults with familial adenomatous polyposis. *Cancer Investig* 2000;19 (Suppl. 1):26–28.

28. Arber D, Rex D, Sjodahl R, et al. Exisulind induced regression of sporadic adenomatous polyps in a randomized, double-blind, placebo controlled trial. *Gastroenterology* 2002;122 (4 Suppl 1):A70–A71.

29. Dousa TP. Cyclic-3',5'-nucleotide phosphodiesterase isozymes in cell biology and pathophysiology of the kidney. *Kidney Int* 1999;55:29–62.

30. Essayan DM. Cyclic nucleotide phosphodiesterases. *J Allergy Clin Immunol* 2001;108:671–680.

31. Corbin JD, Francis SH. Cyclic GMP phosphodiesterase-5: target of sildenafil. *J Biol Chem* 1999;274:13,729–13,732.

32. Li L, Yee C, Beavo JA. CD3- and CD28-dependent induction of PDE7 required for T cell activation. *Science* 1999;283:848–851.

33. Prasad KN, Becker G, Tripathy K. Differences and similarities btween guanosine 3',5'-cyclic monophosphate phosphodiesterase and adenosine 3',5'-cyclic monophosphate phosphodiesterase activities in neuroblastoma cells in culture. *Proc Soc Exp Biol Med* 1975;149:757–762.

34. Marko D, Pahlke G, Merz KH, Eisenbrand G. Cyclic 3',5'-nucleotide phosphodiesterases: potential targets for anticancer therapy. *Chem Res Toxicol* 2000;13:944–948.

35. Carrithers SL, Barber MT, Biswas S, et al. Guanylyl cyclase C is a selective marker for metastatic colorectal tumors in human extraintestinal tissues. *Proc Natl Acad Sci USA* 1996;93:14,827–14,832. D

36. Piazza GA, Klein-Szanto AJ, Ahnen J, et al. Overexpression of cGMP phosphodiesterase (cG PDE) in colonic neoplasias compared to normal mucosa. *Gastroenterology* 2000;118:590.

37. Piazza GA, Thompson WJ, Pamukcu R, et al. Exisulind, a novel proapoptotic drug, inhibits rat urinary bladder tumorigenesis. *Cancer Res* 2001;61:3961–3968.

38. Piazza GA, Klein-Szanto AJ, Xu A, et al. Phosphodiesterase 5 overexpression in human non-small cell lung tumors compared to normal bronchial epithelium. *Proc Am Assoc Cancer Res* 2001;42,4351.

39. Piazza GA, Sperl G, Whitehead CM, et al. Cyclic GMP phosphodiesterase (cG PDE): overexpression in human pancreatic carcinomas and a target for selective apoptotic antineoplastic drugs. *Gastroenterology* 2001;120 (5 Suppl 1):140.

40. Thompson WJ, Piazza GA, Li H, et al. Exisulind induction of apoptosis involves guanosine 3',5'-cyclic monophosphate

phosphodiesterase inhibition, protein kinase G activation, and attenuated beta-catenin. *Cancer Res* 2000;60:3338–3342.

41. Soh JW, Mao Y, Kim MG, et al. Cyclic GMP mediates apoptosis induced by sulindac derivatives via activation of c-Jun NH2-terminal kinase 1. *Clin Cancer Res* 2000;6:4136–4141.

42. Soh JW, Mao Y, Liu L, et al. Protein kinase G activates the JNK1 pathway via phosphorylation of MEKK1. *J Biol Chem* 2001;276:16,406–16,410.

43. Liu L, Li H, Underwood T, et al. Cyclic GMP-dependent protein kinase activation and induction by exisulind and CP461 in colon tumor cells. *J Pharmacol Exp Ther* 2001;299:583–592.

44. Chen YR, Meyer CF, Tan TH. Persistent activation of c-Jun N-terminal kinase 1 (JNK1) in gamma radiation-induced apoptosis. *J Biol Chem* 1996;271:631–634.

45. Chen YR, Wang W, Kong AN, Tan TH. Molecular mechanisms of c-Jun N-terminal kinase-mediated apoptosis induced by anticarcinogenic isothiocyanates. *J Biol Chem* 1998;273:1769–1775.

46. Basu S, Kolesnick R. Stress signals for apoptosis: ceramide and c-Jun kinase. *Oncogene* 1998;17:3277–3285.

47. Behrens J, von Kries JP, Kuhl M, et al. Functional interaction of beta-catenin with the transcription factor LEF-1. *Nature* 1996;382:638–642.

48. Peifer M, Polakis P. Wnt signaling in oncogenesis and embryogenesis—a look outside the nucleus. *Science* 2000;287:1606–1609.

49. Roose J, Clevers H. TCF transcription factors: molecular switches in carcinogenesis. *Biochim Biophys Acta* 1999;1424:M23–M37.

50. Morin PJ, Sparks AB, Korinek V, et al. Activation of beta-catenin-Tcf signaling in colon cancer by mutations in beta-catenin or APC. *Science* 1997;275:1787–1790.

51. Behrens J. Control of beta-catenin signaling in tumor development. *Ann NY Acad Sci* 2000;910:21–33.

52. Sparks AB, Morin PJ, Vogelstein B, Kinzler KW. Mutational analysis of the APC/beta-catenin/Tcf pathway in colorectal cancer. *Cancer Res* 1998;58:1130–1134.

53. Li H, Liu L, David M, et al. Pro-apoptotic actions of exisulind and CP461 in SW480 colon tumor cells involve β-catenin and cyclin D1 down regulation. *Biochem Pharmacol* 2002;64:1325–1336.

54. Whitehead CM, Fetter J, Xu S, et al. CP461, a pro-apoptotic inhibitor of cGMP phosphodiesterases (PDE), disrupts normal microtubule organization and bipolar spindle formation leading to a prometaphase mitotic block. *Proc Am Assoc Cancer Res* 2002;43:410, abst. 2043.

55. Yoon J-T, Palazzo AF, Xiao D, et al. CP248, a derivative of exisulind, causes growth inhibition, mitotic arrest, and abnormalities in microtubule polymerization in glioma cells. *Mol Cancer Ther* 2002;1:393–404.

56. Goluboff ET. Exisulind, a selective apoptotic antineoplastic drug. *Expert Opin Investig Drugs* 2001;10:1875–1882.

57. Earle K, Piazza G, Lloyd M, et al. Effect of CP-461 on adrogen-independent (PC-3) human prostate cancer xenographs in nude mice. *J Urol* 2000;163 (4 Suppl):38.

58. Phillips RK, Hultcrantz R, Bjork J, et al. Exisulind,a pro-apoptotic drug, prevents new polyp formation in patients with familial adenomatous polyposis. *Gut* 2000;47:A2–A3.

59. Goluboff ET, Prager D, Rukstalis D, et al. Safety and efficacy of exisulind for treatment of recurrent prostate cancer after radical prostatectomy. *J Urol* 2001;166:882–886.

60. Prager D, Goluboff ET, Rukstalis D, et al. Long-term use of exisulind in men with prostate cancer following radical prostatectomy. *Am Soc Clin Oncol* 2002;21:abst. 733.

61. Alila H, Finn TS, Sperl G, et al. A pharmacokinetic and safety study of a selective apoptotic antineoplastic drug (SAAND), CP-461, in healthy volunteers. *Proc Am Soc Clin Oncol* 2000;19:abst 817.

62. Sun W, Stevenson JP, Redlinger M, et al. Phase I clinical and pharmacokinetic (PK) trial of the novel pro-apoptotic compound CP-461 administered orally on a continuous twice-daily schedule to patients with advanced malignancies. *Proc Am Soc Clin Oncol* 2001;20:abst 459.

63. Deguchi A, Soh JW, Li H, et al. Vasodilator-stimulated phosphoprotein (VASP) phosphorylation provides a biomarker for the action of exisulind and related agents that activate protein kinase G. *Mol Cancer Ther* 2002;1:803–809.

V ANTIOXIDANTS, VITAMINS, AND MINERALS

29 Chemoprevention by Fruit Phenolic Compounds

Gary D. Stoner, PhD and Bruce C. Casto, ScD

CONTENTS

INTRODUCTION
PHENOLIC ACIDS
BIOFLAVONOIDS
COMPLEX POLYPHENOLS
SUMMARY
REFERENCES

1. INTRODUCTION

This chapter summarizes available information on the chemopreventive effects of fruit phenolic compounds in various experimental systems. Emphasis is placed on the anticarcinogenic activity of these phenolics and their proposed mechanisms of action.

Epidemiological evidence has suggested a protective effect of polyphenols from fruits and vegetables on human cancer, although some prospective studies have found that definitive evidence is still lacking on their direct involvement. However, experimental studies of the antimutagenic and anticarcinogenic effects of polyphenols have shown that they exhibit antimutagenic activity in vitro; inhibit carcinogen-induced skin, lung, forestomach, oral, esophagus, duodenum, and colon tumors in rodents; and inhibit 12-*O*-tetradecanoylphorbol-13-acetate (TPA)-induced skin tumor promotion in mice. Several mechanisms appear to be responsible for the tumor-inhibitory properties of polyphenols, including modulation of phase 1 and phase 2 enzyme activities, inhibition of chemically induced lipid peroxidation and epidermal ornithine decarboxylase (ODC), reduction in protein kinase C (PKC) and tyrosine protein kinase activities, and reduced cellular proliferation. The phenolics also demonstrate antiinflammatory activity, enhancement of gap-junctional intercellular communication (GJIC), induction of apoptosis, enhancement or prevention of DNA damage, and estrogenic and antiestrogenic activity. These properties, coupled with their many other physiological influences, make them attractive chemopreventive agents that can be used in both the initiation and promotion/progression stages of carcinogenesis.

Compounds from three major categories of fruit phenolics—phenolic acids, bioflavonoids, and complex polyphenols—are discussed here. Polyphenols from roots, stems, and leaves (e.g., tea polyphenols, soy isoflavones) have been presented in other venues, or are discussed in chapters 24 and 30 of this volume. Phenolic compounds from fruit are of great interest, since they possess many properties involved in prevention of cancer and often contain high concentrations of active compounds during fruit maturation. We would like to acknowledge the excellent book, *Fruit Phenolics*, by Drs. Macheix, Fleuriet, and Billot, which provided both the foundation and extremely useful information for this chapter (*1*).

2. PHENOLIC ACIDS

Phenolic acids in fruits are derived from benzoic or cinnamic acids, and differ in the numbers and positions of hydroxylations and methoxylations of the aromatic ring (*1*). Those derived from benzoic acid include gallic, procatechuic, syringic, *p*-hydroxybenzoic, vanillic, and gentisic acids. Those derived from cinnamic acids are caffeic, *p*-coumaric, ferulic, chlorogenic, cinnamic, and sinapic acids. The chemopreventive properties of phenolic acids from these two major groups (hydroxybenzoic and hydroxycinnamic) are presented here to provide further insight into the nature of their chemopreventive activity.

From: Cancer Chemoprevention, Volume 1: Promising Cancer Chemoprevention Agents
Edited by: G. J. Kelloff, E. T. Hawk, and C. C. Sigman © Humana Press Inc., Totowa, NJ

2.1. Hydroxybenzoic Acids and Derivatives

Gallic acid, the most commonly studied hydroxybenzoic acid, is found in fruits in the form of esters with quinic acid (theogallin) and glucose (glucogallin). Free gallic and protocatechuic acids are found in blackberries, raspberries, strawberries, black and red currants, grapes, and the immature fruit of both astringent and nonastringent persimmon (1). Gallic acid is also found during degradation of the hydrolyzable gallotannin. Glucosides of protocatechuic and syringic acids are found in cherries and plums (1).

2.1.1. CHEMOPREVENTION

Lung adenomas in strain A mice, induced by chronic treatment with morpholine and sodium nitrite in drinking water, were greatly inhibited by gallic acid added to the diet (2); gallic acid had a slight inhibitory or no effect on tumorigenesis induced by nitrosomorpholine or mononitrosopiperazine. It was suggested that gallic acid could be useful as a preventive agent when co-administered with drugs that are readily nitrosatable. In a rat hepatocarcinogenesis assay (3), the propyl ester of gallic acid (propyl gallate) at a concentration of 0.25% in the diet significantly but weakly inhibited formation of glutathione-S-transferase (GSH) placental form liver foci induced by diethylnitrosamine. The inhibition of foci was related to the ability to inhibit mutagenesis in the Ames assay, but was unrelated to formation of 8-hydroxy-2'-deoxyguanosine (8-OhdG) adduct levels, suggesting that antioxidant properties of the compounds were not the primary mechanism of foci inhibition.

In a two-stage model of mouse skin carcinogenesis (using 7,12-dimethylbenz[a]anthracene (DMBA) as the initiator and TPA as the promoting agent), gallic acid was the least effective in preventing tumor formation (ED_{50} 5–10 micromoles) of four phenolics found in red wine (4); ellagic acid was the most potent, followed by tannic acid, and n-propyl gallate. The antioxidant and antipromotion activities of gallic acid along with ellagic acid and tannic acid were examined in mouse skin for their ability to inhibit hydroperoxide production and tumor formation induced by TPA (5).

Protocatechuic acid, added to the diet of F344 rats at 500, 1000, or 2000 ppm prior to and during treatment with 4-nitroquinoline 1 oxide (NQO), inhibited the appearance of tongue neoplasms (squamous cell carcinomas and papillomas), hyperplasia, and dysplasia at all concentrations. In addition, when protocatechuic acid was added to the diet 1 wk after NQO treatment, all concentrations effectively and significantly altered the frequency of neoplasms and preneoplastic lesions (6). Oral cancer in the hamster cheek pouch was also inhibited by protocatechuic acid in the diet (200 ppm) approx 2 mo after initiation with DMBA (7). In these reports (6,7), treatment with protocatechuic acid caused a significant decrease in cell proliferation in tongue and cheek pouch epithelium, and decreased polyamine levels in oral mucosa (6).

2.1.2. APOPTOSIS

Human stomach and colon cancer cell lines (KATO III and COLO 205) exposed to gallic acid in vitro showed a concentration- and time-dependent inhibition of growth directly related to induction of apoptosis (8). It was suggested that gallic acid might be an attractive adjunct drug for treating digestive tract cancers that are resistant to chemotherapeutic agents. Similarly, gallic acid was found to induce apoptosis in four human lung cancer cell lines (9) treated in vitro for only 30 min. Effective concentrations (EC_{50}) ranged from 10 to 60 µg/mL; susceptibility to gallic acid induction of apoptosis was not affected in cisplatin-resistant cells. It was again suggested that gallic acid may be effective in drug-resistant cancers.

Differential effects of gallic acid and its alkyl esters (methyl, propyl, octyl, and lauryl gallates) were examined in three different cell lines (10). Three different behaviors were noted, depending on the cell line used for study. Mouse B-cell lymphoma (Wehi 231) cells treated with different gallic acid compounds showed a classic apoptotic DNA ladder fragmentation pattern, whereas the mouse fibroblast line (L929) demonstrated cell shrinkage, chromatin condensation, and the appearance of apoptotic bodies. If peripheral blood lymphocytes were treated with the compounds in a nondividing stage, they were relatively resistant, and required much higher concentrations to demonstrate apoptosis. If the compounds were washed out, the cells divided in a normal manner. However, addition of compounds following mitogen stimulation resulted in an antiproliferative effect. It was emphasized that interest in these compounds stems from the fact that propyl gallate, octyl gallate, and lauryl gallate are currently being used in the European Community as antioxidant food additives (codes E-310, E-311, and E-312, respectively).

Lauryl gallate appears to be more effective in inhibiting tyrosine kinases than either herbimycin or genistein (11). Treatment of mouse B-cell lymphoma cells with lauryl gallate inhibits tyrosine phosphorylation, discharges the mitochondrial membrane potential, and induces mRNA expression of *bcl-2*. Long-term treatment of these cells with lauryl gallate induces several apoptotic biomarkers in addition to the antiapoptotic *bcl-2*, including phosphatidylserine at the cell surface, cytochrome C release, activation of caspases, and a classic fragmentation pattern of DNA.

Esterification of gallic acid with a 3,4-methylenedioxyphenyl group yielded compounds as effective as gallic acid in inducing apoptosis in cancer-cell lines *(12)*, but differential activity was sacrificed, as normal rat hepatocytes and human keratinocytes that are not sensitive to gallic acid were sensitive to cytotoxicity from the esterified compounds. These compounds induced apoptosis by different pathways from those of gallic acid, in that Ca^{2+} chelators, calmodulin inhibitors, and zinc sulfate inhibited apoptotic activity, whereas catalase, *N*-acetylcysteine, and ascorbic acid inhibited apoptosis induced by gallic acid. In a separate report *(13)*, the same investigative group found that apoptosis induced by gallic acid followed different pathways according to the cell line used for bioassay. For example, the human myelogenous leukemic cell line HL-60 included internucleosomal breakdown of chromatin DNA, whereas the rat hepatic cell lines dRLh-84 and PLC/PRF/5 and HeLa cells did not. In addition, prevention of gallic acid-induced apoptosis by antioxidants, calcium chelators, and endonuclease inhibitors was dependent on cell type, implying that the signal pathways were different, but that production of reactive oxygens and elevation of intracellular calcium were similar.

2.1.3. PHARMACOLOGICAL CONSIDERATIONS

The differential activity of gallic acid on tumor cells vs normal cells was explored in cell culture *(14–17)*, where it was found that saliva *(14)* or conditioned medium from normal hepatocytes *(15)* reduced gallic acid-induced apoptosis. Using both sensitive and insensitive cell cultures, it was concluded that catalase content determined the differential effects between cell types, since it was observed that normal cells (e.g., those insensitive to gallic acid-induced apoptosis) produced major amounts of catalase, and sensitive tumor cells produced only small amounts *(16)*.

The ability of galloyl monosaccharides to induce apoptosis was dependent on the number and disposition of phenolic groups *(17)*. For example, tetragalloyl glucose readily induced apoptosis in a human lymphoma (U937) cell line and in human colon and stomach cancer-cell lines, but digalloyl hamamelose and

monogalloyl glucose had only moderate and marginal activity, respectively, in human lymphoma cells.

In addition to their apoptotic-inducing effects, several of the phenolic acids have antiapoptotic and anti-P450 activity. Protocatechuic acid prevents oxidized low-density lipoprotein (LDL)-induced apoptosis in a concentration-dependent manner in cultured endothelial cells. However, the hydroxybenzoic phenolic acid was less effective than the hydroxycinnamic phenolic acids caffeic and ferulic *(18)*. It was theorized that the antiapoptotic effect by protocatechuic acid was the result of its antioxidant activity.

Protocatechuic acid, dodecyl gallate, and propyl gallate were effective inhibitors of cytochrome P450s CYP1A1, CYP1A2, and CYP2B in a murine liver microsome assay *(19)*. Protocatechuic acid was a more effective inhibitor of CYP1A2 and CYP2B activity than dodecyl or propyl gallate, and dodecyl gallate was more selective for CYP2B than propyl gallate; the opposite was true for CYP1A2. The nature of the inhibition was noncompetitive, with no clear structure-activity relationship.

2.2. Hydroxycinnamic Acids and Derivatives

Hydroxycinnamic acids are abundant in fruits and are found in a diversity of species *(1)*. Free hydroxycinnamic acids are rarely found, except under various conditions of extraction, processing, physiological stress, anaerobiosis, or the addition of precursors. In most situations, they are found as two main types of derivatives *(1)*. First are those that involve an ester bond between the carboxyl group of the phenolic acid and an alcohol group of a second compound such as quinic acid or glucose; and second are those that involve a bond with a phenolic group in the compound (e.g., *p*-coumaric acid *O*-glucoside). Caffeic, *p*-coumaric, and ferulic acids (free or bound) are found in essentially every fruit, whereas sinapic acid is found predominantly in lemons, oranges, pineapple, and pumpkin skin, with varied amounts found in tomatoes *(1)*. Other members of this group include chlorogenic and cinnamic acids and coumarins *(1)*.

2.2.1. CHEMOPREVENTION

The phenethyl ester of caffeic acid was evaluated in the C57Bl/6J-Min/+(min/+) mouse model that has a germline mutation in the *APC* gene and is subject to spontaneous intestinal adenomas *(20)*. Caffeic acid ester given in the diet (1500 ppm) reduced tumor formation associated with enterocyte apoptosis by 63%

and decreased expression of β-catenin. Adding ferulic acid (500 ppm) to the diet of NQO-treated male rats significantly reduced the frequency of tongue carcinomas and severe dysplastic lesions, indicating that ferulic acid given post-initiation is an extremely effective agent for oral cancer chemoprevention *(21)*.

An extract containing *p*-coumaric, caffeic, ferulic, sinapic, and methoxycinnamic acids in combination with *p*-coumaric and vanillic acids inhibited viability and the colony-forming capacity of human breast and colon cancer cells in vitro *(22)*. Although caffeic acid was the most effective phenolic acid evaluated as an isolated compound, ferulic and methoxycinnamic acids were also active in both cell viability and clonogenic assays. An extract of *Perilla frutescens* (beefsteak plant) contains several polyphenols found in fruit, including caffeic acid, methyl caffeate, and luteolin. The extract inhibited both DNA synthesis and proliferation of mouse mesanglial cells in culture stimulated by platelet-derived growth factor (PDGF) *(23)*. When components were tested individually, caffeic acid and methyl caffeate were both effective inhibitors of cell proliferation, although luteolin was the most effective *(23)*.

2.2.2. Apoptosis

The caffeic acid phenethyl ester, discussed here as a chemopreventive agent in the Min/+ mouse model *(20)*, causes marked growth inhibition (up to 70%) of the human leukemic HL-60 cell line, mainly because of an apoptotic response *(24)*. Analysis of treated cells revealed a significant decrease in mitochondrial transmembrane potential and depletion of intracellular GSH. Treatment of cells with *N*-acetyl-*l*-cysteine (NAC) reversed GSH depletion and partially inhibited the apoptotic response. The apoptotic event induced by 6 µg/mL of the caffeic acid phenethyl ester is associated with activation of caspase-3, downregulation of *bcl-2*, and upregulation of *Bax* *(25)*—parameters identified with apoptosis in other cell systems.

2.2.3. Pharmacological Considerations

Phenolic acids not only induce apoptosis, but as discussed here for the hydroxybenzoic acids, may also inhibit the induction of apoptosis. Caffeic acid inhibits NFκB-binding activity and apoptosis at low µmol doses; it also inhibits tyrosine kinase activity. Although several other antioxidants have an affect on NFκB activity, they do not inhibit apoptosis (*see* Subheading 2.1.3.), suggesting that the inhibition of apoptosis might be accomplished by antioxidant or nonantioxi-

dant processes *(26)*. Applied to cultures of endothelial cells, caffeic acid was more effective than ferulic, protocatechuic, ellagic, and *p*-coumaric acids in inhibiting apoptosis induced by oxidized LDL *(18)*. Protection against apoptotic induction was suggested to be the result of preventing LDL oxidation and blocking the increase in cytosolic Ca^{2+}.

Epidemiological studies strongly indicate that colorectal cancer (CRC) can be reduced by dietary factors, especially the phenolic compounds. Integrin-mediated cell-matrix contact is responsible for a signaling pathway that regulates cell proliferation, migration, and apoptosis *(27)*. One of the important signaling mediators for this pathway is focal adhesion kinase (FAK). Although not widely explored as a target for chemoprevention, loss of integrin-mediated contact can lead to apoptosis and cell invasion. Applied to colon carcinoma cells in culture, the phenethyl ester of caffeic acid, at doses that did not induce apoptosis, resulted in rearrangement of the actin cytoskeleton and loss of focal adhesion plaques *(27)*. There was also a reduction in tyrosine phosphorylation of FAK (and the associated p130Cas) and cell invasion.

As discussed in Subheading 2.1.3., hydroxybenzoic phenolic acids inhibit cytochrome P450 activity in a murine liver microsome system. Chlorogenic acid was a more effective inhibitor of CYP2B activity than protocatechuic acid or the alkyl esters of gallic acid, but was less effective than protocatechuic acid for the inhibition of CYP1A2 activity *(19)*.

2.3. Ellagic Acid

Ellagic acid is a naturally occurring phenolic constituent of many species from a diversity of fruits. Since its chemopreventive activity and mechanism of action have been discussed in reviews by Stoner and Mukhtar *(28)*, only a brief discussion is given here containing information on its activity published subsequent to the referenced review article. Ellagic acid is usually present in the form of hydrolyzable tannins called ellagitannins—esters of glucose with hexahydroxydiphenic acid—that when hydrolyzed yield ellagic acid, the dilactone of hexahydroxydiphenic acid *(29)*. The highest amounts of ellagic acid in fruits and nuts has been determined to be in blackberries, raspberries, strawberries, cranberries, walnuts, and pecans *(30)*.

2.3.1. Chemoprevention

When administered intraperitoneally or as a dietary admixture, ellagic acid decreased the multiplicity of benzo[*a*]pyrene (B[*a*]P)-induced or NNK-induced lung tumors *(31,32)*; however, significant toxicity was observed following intraperitoneal administration. Topical application of ellagic acid to the skin of Balb/c mice demonstrated a strong protective effect against 3-methylcholanthrene (MCA)-induced skin carcinogenesis *(33)*; however, no inhibitory effect of ellagic acid was found on MCA-induced skin carcinogenesis in CD-1 or Balb/c mice *(34)*. Other organs in which ellagic acid has been shown to exhibit anticarcinogenic effects include the esophagus and liver *(35–37)*.

2.3.2. APOPTOSIS

Ellagic acid was shown to induce cell-cycle arrest, inhibit cell growth, and induce apoptosis in cervical carcinoma cells in vitro *(38)*. Concurrent with these activities was activation of the cyclin dependent kinase (CDK) inhibitory protein (CDI) p21, suggesting that ellagic acid may regulate cell proliferation in tumor cells via this pathway. An extract of *Terminalia chebula*, a *Combretaceae* plant containing ellagic acid as one of its major constituents, was shown to induce apoptosis in human osteosarcoma (HOS-1), breast (MCF-7), and prostate cancer cell lines *(39)*. Ellagic acid was also shown to induce apoptosis in colon cancer cells (SW480) accompanied by downregulation of insulin-like growth factor (IGF-II) and activation of p21 *(40)*.

2.3.3. PHARMACOLOGICAL CONSIDERATIONS

The inhibition of carcinogenesis by ellagic acid may occur through a number of mechanisms in addition to those cited here. Ellagic acid has been shown to inhibit metabolic activation of procarcinogens, promote detoxification by stimulating the activity of various GSH enzyme isoforms, act as a scavenger of reactive carcinogen metabolites, and occupy sites on DNA that might otherwise react with carcinogens or their metabolites *(28)*. With respect to its effects on tumor promotion/progression, ellagic acid inhibits TPA-induced ODC activity, hydroperoxide production, DNA synthesis *(28)*, the activity of PKC isolated from aflatoxin-induced rat liver *(41)*, and all markers of skin-tumor promotion.

Alterations in gene expression induced by ellagic acid were studied in the androgen- sensitive LNCaP human prostate cancer cell line *(42)*. Exposed to ellagic acid for 48 h, a total of 593 genes demonstrated more than twofold differences in expression from untreated cells. Especially intriguing was the demonstration of alterations in p53-responsive genes and in p300, Apaf-1, NFκBp50, and PPAR families of genes involved in signaling pathways leading to growth inhibition.

3. BIOFLAVONOIDS

Extensively reviewed in works by Harborne and colleagues *(43,44)*, flavonoids consist of several classes of compounds, including chalcones, isoflavones, flavones, flavonols, anthocyanins, flavan-3-ols, flavanonols, and flavanones. Except for chalcones, they have a C_1 basic skeleton that varies according to the oxidation level of the central pyran ring *(1)*. Those with reported chemopreventive activity that are discussed here include chalcones (isoliquiritigenin, butein, phloretin, chalconaringenin, and phloridzin), flavones (apigenin, luteolin, nobiletin, robinetin, sinensetin, tangeretin), flavonols (isorhamnetin, kaempferol, myricetin, quercetin, rutin), and flavanones and flavanonols (engeletin, eriocitrin, eriodictyol, hesperidin, naringenin, narginin, and neohesperidin). The remaining classes of flavonoids are discussed in chapters 24 and 30 in this volume or have little published information regarding their chemopreventive action.

3.1. Chalcones

Chalcones play an important role in the biosynthesis of flavonoids, and are characterized by an open 3-C chain in the C_{15} skeleton *(1)*. The isomerization of chalcones into flavanones is a reversible reaction and, this activity may be the reason that chalcones are found in only small amounts in fruits. Some members of this class of flavonoids include: isoliquiritigenin, butein, phloretin, chalconaringenin, and phloridzin. The natural forms are hydroxylated or methoxylated, and many of the chalcones can be extracted from fruits rich in anthocyanins, resulting from the transformation of the anthocyanin flavylium cation into a chalcone *(1)*.

3.1.1. CHEMOPREVENTION

BAP-induced lung tumors of female A/J mice *(45,46)* and mammary tumors of Sprague-Dawley rats were inhibited by chalcones given in the diet 1 wk after final carcinogen treatment, but tumors of the forestomach in A/J mice were not affected. Inhibition of methyl nitrosourea-induced mammary tumors was also demonstrated when chalcones were given 4 wk after carcinogen and alternated at 3-wk intervals thereafter with a control diet *(45)*.

Topical application of isoliquiritigenin inhibited the formation of skin papillomas initiated by DMBA and promoted by TPA or by 7-bromomethylbenz[a]anthracene, a non-TPA type promoter. Isoliquiritigenin also inhibited ODC and PGE_2 induction in intact cells, but did not inhibit 12-lipoxygenase or cyclooxygenase in cellular subfractions (47).

Fifteen (15) natural and synthetic chalcones were evaluated for their ability to inhibit ovarian cancer cell growth in vitro and to interfere with estrogen binding to type II estrogen-binding sites (EBS). Chalcones inhibited cell proliferation and binding of estradiol to type II EBS (48) at concentrations from 0.1 to 10 μM; the relationship between inhibition of cell proliferation and displacement of estrogen bound to EBS were directly related, and were dependent on structural alterations of the chalcone (48). A derivative of chalcone (3'-methyl-3-hydroxy-chalcone, or MeC) inhibited growth of human tumor cell lines from gastric, cervical, and pancreatic cancer, and a neuroblastoma cell line. Inhibition was attributed to a delay at S phase, causing arrest at G_0/G_1. MeC also inhibited the binding of estradiol to EBS and patterns of protein synthesis and phosphorylation of kinases (49).

Inhibition of proliferation of a human colon carcinoma cell line by butein (2 μM) was 4–10× more effective than inhibition induced by a series of hydroxylated chalcones (50). Similarly, isoliquiritigenin and butein were more effective than a series of other flavonoids (e.g., apigenin, luteolin, kaempferol, quercetin, naringenin, and daidzen) in inhibiting cell growth and inducing cell death of B16 mouse melanoma cells in culture (51).

3.1.2. APOPTOSIS

Inhibition of cell growth by isoliquiritigenin and butein in mouse melanoma cells was accompanied by condensation of nuclei, fragmentation of nuclear DNA, elevation of *Bax* expression, and reduced *bcl*-2 expression, characteristic of apoptosis (51). However, it was theorized that the mechanism of apoptosis induction was different for isoliquiritigenin than for butein, since, unlike butein, isoliquiritigenin did not affect *bcl*-2 expression. Also, the addition of extracellular glucose decreased the proportion of cells in apoptosis induced by isoliquiritigenin. These data suggested that isoliquiritigenin induced apoptosis through a glucose transmembrane transport mechanism (51). A group of chalcone analogs was evaluated for growth inhibition in the human breast (MDA-MB 231 and MCF-7) and T-cell leukemic cell lines (52). All the compounds inhibited cell proliferation, and two of the compounds were

more effective than quercetin, the positive control. Two of the most active analogs were further evaluated for their ability to affect the cell cycle, induce apoptosis, affect redox levels, and modulate p-glycoprotein function. With 10 μM, there was a block at G_2/M, induction of apoptosis, and a transient increase of thiol levels, but no effect on p-glycoprotein function (52).

3.1.3. PHARMACOLOGICAL CONSIDERATIONS

Butein was demonstrated to be a specific protein tyrosine kinase inhibitor in the human hepatocellular carcinoma cell line, HepG2 (53). Butein inhibited epidermal growth factor (EGF)-stimulated autophosphotyrosine levels of EGF receptor and its tyrosine-specific protein kinase activities, as well as those of p60c-Src. The inhibition was competitive to adenosine 5' triphosphate (ATP), but not to the phosphate acceptor for EGF receptor tyrosine kinase. Butein also slightly inhibited the activity of serine- and threonine-specific protein kinases such as PKC and cyclic adenosine 5' monophosphate (cAMP)-dependent protein kinase (PKA) (53).

Isoliquiritigenin significantly inhibits the expression of intracellular adhesion molecule-1 (ICAM) and vascular adhesion molecule-1 (VCAM) involved in inflammation and carcinogenesis, in both murine endothelial cells and murine myeloid leukemia cells in vitro (54). The activity of isoliquiritigenin was attributed to the 4-hydroxy group and the coplanar relationship between the phenyl ring and conjugated ketone on the chalcone (54).

Phloretin, a chalcone, demonstrates relatively potent estrogenic activity in a recombinant yeast strain carrying a stably integrated human estrogen receptor (ER) (55). Phloretin also induced cell proliferation in the estrogen-dependent MCF7 breast carcinoma cell line. The feature responsible for activity was the presence of a hydroxyl group on the 4-position of the B-ring of the flavan nucleus.

3.2. Flavones

The flavones have an unsaturated 3-C chain and a double bond between C-2 and C-3, but lack the hydroxyl radical in the 3-position (differentiating them from the flavonols) (1). Although more than 100 different flavones have been described, they are not abundant in fruits, and usually exist as aglycones or glycosides. Examples of the flavones are: apigenin, luteolin, nobiletin, robinetin, sinensetin, and tangeretin. The polymethoxylated flavones are prevalent in the oils from the orange, tangerine, mandarin, and clementine *(1)*. The information presented in this section is primarily focused on apigenin and luteolin, since they have been most extensively studied.

3.2.1. Chemoprevention

Apigenin applied to the skin of SKH-1 mice prior to UVB exposure resulted in ~52% inhibition of skin tumors and an increase in survival of tumor-free animals *(56)*. The reduction in tumors was associated with inhibition of ODC activity in mouse epidermal cells, but neither effect was attributable to absorption of ultraviolet (UV) by apigenin or to a decrease in DNA damage *(56)*.

Both apigenin and robinetin were found to be antimutagenic in the Ames assay when assayed against 2-aminoanthracene or B[a]P. Neither compound was mutagenic by itself and they did not inhibit the mutagenicity of methylnitrosurea or methylnitrosoguanidine *(57)*. When tested for antipromotion properties, both apigenin and robinetin inhibited induction of ODC that was stimulated by TPA after application of the two flavones *(57)*. Applied to the skin of SENCAR mice initiated with DMBA and promoted with TPA, apigenin (5 and 20 µmol) decreased the incidence of papilloma formation from 93.3% to 58% and 39%, and the numbers per mouse from 7.5 to 2.5 and 1.8 *(58)*. The incidence and numbers of carcinomas were also significantly reduced, and the latent period for tumor appearance was delayed by 3 wk. Apigenin also inhibited the conversion of papillomas to carcinomas, although there was no dose-response relationship.

Given by intraperitoneal injection at the time of intramuscular injection of mouse melanoma B16-BL6 cells, apigenin caused a dose-dependent delay of tumor growth and potentiated the inhibition of tumors by a noncytotoxic dose of cisplatin *(59)*. Apigenin also significantly modified the invasion potential of melanoma cells in vitro and decreased the number of colonies in mouse lung in an in vivo metastasis model *(59)*. As part of the invasion and metastasis process, members of the MMP family (MMP-2 and MMP-9) are believed to play an essential role, and are associated with the mitogen-activated protein kinase (MAPK) signaling pathway that is linked to growth and metastasis of breast and renal cell tumors *(60)*. Apigenin inhibits expression of these essential components in breast adenocarcinoma cells, resulting in reduced cell proliferation and invasion through the basement membrane in vitro. In a Wistar rat model of peritoneal metastasis, initiated in the

intestine by azoxymethane (AOM) and potentiated by bombesin, it was found that subcutaneous injections of apigenin on alternate days after carcinogen treatment had no effect on the enhancement of intestinal tumors by bombesin or histologic parameters of the tumors, but did significantly decrease the incidence of metastasis *(61)*. Concurrently, apigenin decreased lymphatic vessel invasion and the bombesin-enhanced phosphorylation of MAPK *(61)*. Related to this inhibition of metastasis, apigenin treatment of the estrogen-insensitive breast cancer-cell line MDA-MB231 resulted in decreased expression of urokinase-plasminogen activator, total inhibition of MMP-9 stimulated by TPA, decreased adhesion to Matrigel, and induction of cell-cycle arrest at G_2/M *(62)*.

Inhibition of growth in vitro has been demonstrated by apigenin and luteolin in a number of human tumor-cell lines. In four human thyroid carcinoma cell lines, apigenin and luteolin at 21 to 32 µmol were the most potent inhibitors of cell proliferation over that effected by other flavonoids such as genistein, chrysin, kaempferol, or biochanin A. The antiproliferative effects were not dependent on estrogen or antiestrogen-binding sites *(63)*. A series of 21 synthetic and natural flavonoids were evaluated for growth inhibition in cell culture in the breast cancer cell line ZR-75-1 (positive for estrogen and other steroid hormones). All compounds inhibited tumor cell growth within a range of concentrations from 2.7 to 34 µg/mL; apigenin was one of the most potent, with an IC_{50} of 3.5 µg/mL *(64)*.

Growth of a murine glomerular mesangial cell line (that forms colonies in soft agar) was inhibited by several extracts of *Perilla frutescens* containing a number of fruit polyphenols, including luteolin 7-*O*-glucuronide-6'-methyl ester. The crude extract inhibited both DNA synthesis and proliferation of PDGF-stimulated mouse mesanglial cells in culture *(23)*. When components were tested individually, luteolin was more effective *(23)* than caffeic acid, methyl caffeate, and rosmarinic acid.

The mechanism of inhibition of human melanoma cell (OCM-1) proliferation by a series of flavonoids, including apigenin and luteolin, was found to be structure-dependent. For example, the presence of a hydroxyl group at the 3' position of the B ring in luteolin was associated with cell-cycle arrest at G_1, whereas its absence in apigenin was associated with arrest at G_2 *(65)*. Arrest at G_1 was correlated with an inhibition of CDK2 activity, possibly by the upregulation of kinase inhibitors p27 and p21, whereas apigenin, which arrested cells in G_2, inhibited the kinase activity of CDK1 presumably linked to phosphorylation of the kinase Tyr15 residue *(65)*. The effect of apigenin on G_2 cell-cycle arrest was also demonstrated in human colon carcinoma cells. Treatment of three cell lines with 0–80 µmol resulted in a time- and dose-dependent reduction in cell number and cell protein. Inhibition was accompanied by a reduction in p34 (cdc2) kinase activity and p34 and cyclin B_1 proteins *(66)*.

In MCF-7 and MDA-MB-468 breast carcinoma cells, it was observed that G_2/M arrest by apigenin was correlated with a significant decrease in cyclins A, D_1, and B_1, and CDK1 and CDK4 protein levels, with a corresponding decrease in cyclin CDK1 kinase activity; expression of cyclin E, CDK2, and CDK6 were unaffected. In MCF-7 cells, apigenin reduced Rb phosphorylation and in MDA-MB-468 cells, it inhibited ERK MAPK phosphorylation *(67)*. Additional information on the mechanism of antiproliferative activity of the flavones apigenin and luteolin was developed using prostate cancer cells, in which both compounds were shown to inhibit proliferation associated with induction of the CDK inhibitor p21. Although both compounds increased p21 levels, apigenin operated through a p53-dependent pathway and luteolin through a p53-independent pathway *(68)*.

In addition to the growth-inhibitory properties of flavonoids discussed here, another way tumor cells can be modified by chemopreventive agents is through induction of differentiation leading to reversion of the transformed phenotype toward a more normal behavior. For example, apigenin has been shown to induce a reversible inhibition of cell growth, and to produce morphological differentiation in rat neuroblastoma cells characterized by elongation and arborization of neurites *(69)*. In a v-H-*ras* transformed NIH-3T3 cell system, apigenin reversed the transformed morphology and ability to clone in soft agar and induced inhibition of cell proliferation. Reversal of the transformed properties was presumably mediated by inhibition of protein tyrosine kinases resulting in alteration of the p21 Ras-mediated signal-transduction pathway *(70)*. In a third system, apigenin and luteolin induced morphological differentiation of the human myeloid leukemia HL-60 cell line into granulocytes, and quercetin and phloretin (a flavonol and a chalcone) induced differentiation into monocytes *(71)*.

3.2.2. Apoptosis

An earlier study *(63)* demonstrated that apigenin and luteolin were the most effective inhibitors of thyroid cancer cell growth among several different classes of flavonoids evaluated. The growth-inhibitory effect of apigenin was evaluated in an anaplastic thyroid carcinoma-cell line, ARO, and the most significant effect observed was a decrease in the level of phosphorylated c-MYC (a substrate for MAPK) subsequently leading to programmed cell death with DNA fragmentation *(72)*.

The selective effect of apigenin was demonstrated in human prostate adenocarcinoma and epidermoid carcinoma cell lines *(73)*. Normal prostate epithelial cells (NHPE), epidermal keratinocytes, and virally transformed prostate epithelial cells (PZ-HPV-7) were only marginally affected by apigenin treatment, whereas cell viability significantly decreased in prostate adenocarcinoma (CA-HPV-10) and human epidermoid carcinoma (A431) cells. Apoptosis was demonstrated in the prostate adenocarcinoma line by DNA ladder, fluorescent microscopy, and TUNEL assays. Apigenin treatment induced cell-cycle arrest at G_2/M in the tumor lines and effected cell death of the normal lines only at high concentrations *(73)*. Apigenin also inhibited growth of the established prostate carcinoma cell line (LNCaP), induced p53-dependent p21, inhibited phosphorylation of Rb protein, and caused induction of apoptosis. This was characterized by DNA fragmentation, poly-(ADP-ribose) polymerase (PARP) cleavage, and a shift in the *Bax:Bcl*-2 ratio toward that found in apoptosis *(74)*.

3.2.3. Pharmacological Considerations

3.2.3.1. Hormonal Activity
Many of the isoflavones isolated from legumes demonstrate estrogenic or antiestrogenic activity, but this class of compounds is rarely found in fruits *(1)*. Other flavonoids found in fruit have received little attention regarding their hormonal activity. The estrogenic, androgenic, and progestational activity of 72 different flavonoids were evaluated in human breast cancer cells (BT-474) at concentrations of 10^{-5} to 10^{-8} M. Among the 72 compounds, 18 demonstrated estrogenic activity, and seven of these had progestational activity. Of this group, luteolin displayed strong estrogenicity, and apigenin induced a robust progestational activity response *(75)*. The estrogenic activity of apigenin and luteolin was further evaluated for their ability to stimulate DNA synthesis in the estrogen-dependent MCF-7 cell line. At low concentrations close to physiological levels of

flavonoids achieved in humans (0.1–10 μmol), apigenin and luteolin induced DNA synthesis in the estrogen-dependent cell line, but at high concentrations (20–90 μmol), DNA synthesis was inhibited. The stimulation of DNA synthesis was selective, and consistent with an estrogenic effect—treatment of the estrogen-independent MDA-MB-231 cells did not trigger DNA synthesis *(76)*. However, variable effects of phytoestrogens are seen in the presence of normal estrogens or growth factors. For example, concentrations of apigenin and luteolin shown to stimulate DNA synthesis in the previously cited work inhibited DNA synthesis when MCF-7 cells were provoked by estradiol. Other flavonoids either inhibited or enhanced DNA synthesis in the presence of estradiol, insulin, or EGF, indicating that the variable effects of phytoestrogens must be taken into consideration when using them as chemopreventive agents *(77)*. The hormonal activity of the phytoestrogens is considerably weaker than that shown by natural or synthetic steroids. As an example, breast cancer-cell lines T-47D and BT-474 stimulated with androgens, progestins, glucocorticoids, and mineralocorticoids respond by producing prostate-specific antigen (PSA). In this system, apigenin exhibited progestational activity at least 10,000-fold weaker than that observed with natural steroid hormones *(78)*. Similarly, the ability of apigenin to stimulate the transcriptional activity of human ER in a recombinant yeast strain was several orders of magnitude below that shown by 17 β-estradiol *(55)*.

The estrogenic and antiestrogenic properties of apigenin were evaluated in the MCF-7 ER-positive cell line using the ER-dependent reporter gene and ER competitive binding assays. Apigenin was found to be unique in that its antiestrogenic activity did not correlate with binding to ER. Therefore, suppression of estrogen-mediated gene transactivation and inhibition of proliferation occurred independently of antagonism at the receptor level *(79)*.

3.2.3.2. Molecular Events (Protein Kinases, Enzyme Induction, Gene Activation)
PKCK2, a serine/threonine kinase, is overexpressed in many human tumors and proliferating tissues. Wnt glycoproteins are secreted factors that are important in embryonic development, but overexpression of Wnts, especially Wnt-1, results in cell transformation and rapid proliferation associated with increased levels of CK2 and Wnt signaling intermediates. Apigenin acts as a selective inhibitor of CK2 and suppresses proliferation of Wnt-1 expressing cells, blocks phosphorylation of beta-catenin, and reduces the level of Wnt signaling intermediates *(80)*.

Apigenin inhibits TPA-mediated promotion of skin tumors in mice accompanied by activation of PKC and several proto-oncogenes *(57,58)*. Apigenin was shown to inhibit TPA-mediated promotion events by competing with ATP to suppress PKC activation, reducing the level of TPA-stimulated phosphorylation of various cellular protein kinases, and inhibiting TPA-induced c-*jun* and c-*fos* expression—activities that lead to inhibition of TPA-induced tumor promotion *(81)*.

Human prostate carcinoma cells contain phosphotyrosine in the oncogenic proline-directed protein kinase factor A (PDPK FA). Treatment of these cells in culture with apigenin strongly induces tyrosine dephosphorylation and inactivates PDPK FA in a concentration-related fashion *(82)*. The data strongly suggest that inhibition of cell proliferation by apigenin may be related to its ability to act as a tyrosine kinase inhibitor (inhibiting PDPK FA-specific tyrosine kinase), inducing tyrosine dephosphorylation and inactivation of the oncogenic PDPK FA oncogenic kinase *(82)*.

Induction of the phase 2 enzyme quinone reductase in murine hepatoma cells is only weakly implemented by apigenin *(83)*, which is less active than kaempferol, quercetin, or myricetin. A 2,3 double bond in the C ring enhanced by a 3-hydroxyl group appears to be essential for induction (kaempferol vs apigenin).

Apigenin may also act as a chemopreventive agent in a manner unrelated to the topics discussed here *(84)*. Apigenin was found to upregulate gap-junction formation in tumors that express some gap junctions, and greatly enhanced gap junctions in cells transfected with the connexin 43 gene. In a tumor cell killing bioassay (10% herpes simplex virus (HSV) thymidine kinase/ganciclovir cells to 90% wild-type tumor cells), apigenin was found to increase the transfer of ganciclovir from HSV thymidine kinase/ganciclovir cells to wild-type tumor cells, resulting in complete remission in 60–70% of mice, as opposed to 30% remission in mice that were not treated with apigenin. These data suggest that the response to antitumor drugs can be significantly improved by manipulation of gap junctions with apigenin *(84)*.

Apigenin may also play a role as an adjunct to radiation therapy. Treatment of cells with apigenin following irradiation of hepatoma cells results in a significant enhancement of radiation-induced cell death attributed to decreased DNA repair *(85)*. Thus, in addition to their other antitumor activities, certain flavonoids may act as radiation enhancers, possibly by affecting the activity of the nuclear enzyme topoisomerase II which is, involved in DNA repair.

3.3. Flavonols

Approximately 200 flavonols, including many that are methylated, have been identified in plants. They are characterized by an unsaturated 3-C chain with a double bond between C-2 and C-3 and a hydroxyl group in the 3-position (3-hydroxyflavone) (1). In addition to the hydroxyl group at 3-, about 90% are also hydroxylated in the 5- and 7-positions. Kaempferol, quercetin, myricetin, and isorhamnetin are glycosides most commonly found in fruits. Quercetin is found in all fleshy fruits, kaempferol in about 80%, and myricetin and isorhamnetin in about 5%. These flavonols are often found in combinations of two or three (quercetin + kaempferol or quercetin + kaempferol + myricetin) (1). Blackberries have the highest amount of flavonols, and raspberries contain about threefold less; quercetin is the most predominant flavonol in elderberries and cranberries (1).

3.3.1. CHEMOPREVENTION

In the Min/+ mouse model, both caffeic acid phenethyl ester and curcumin were found to prevent APC-associated intestinal adenomas (20); however, quercetin and rutin were not effective in prevention at concentrations of up to 2% in the diet (20). However, quercetin significantly inhibited papilloma and squamous cell carcinoma formation when given in the diet, making it extremely effective in the prevention of DMBA-induced oral tumors in the hamster cheek pouch (86).

Both quercetin and kaempferol were found to inhibit cell-cycle progression of human melanoma cells in culture. Quercetin induced cell-cycle arrest at G_1 and kaempferol at G_2/M (65). Quercetin, which induced G_1 block, was found to inhibit CDK2 activity by 40–60%, whereas kaempferol had no effect on this kinase. In contrast, kaempferol inhibited the activity of CDK1 by 50–70%. Quercetin was thought to upregulate CDK inhibitors p21 and p27, leading to inhibition of CDK2 activity. It was believed that inhibition of CDK1 was caused by phosphorylation of the kinase at Tyr15 (65). In the human oral squamous-cell carcinoma cell line (SCC-25), quercetin was compared to cisplatin, genistein, and curcumin for the potential to inhibit cell growth. Cisplatin and curcumin were the most effective

inhibitors of DNA synthesis and cell proliferation, and genistein and quercetin were about 10-fold less potent (87). However, in mouse fibroblast cells, quercetin and myricetin were quite effective in inhibiting TPA-induced transformation, PKC activation, and c-jun expression (88). In a v-H-ras transformed NIH-3T3 cell system described previously for apigenin (70) kaempferol reversed the cell-transformed morphology into a contact-inhibited stage, reduced the ability to clone in soft agar by sixfold, and induced inhibition of cell proliferation in a dose-dependent fashion. Kaempferol also dramatically reduced the phosphotyrosine content of the cells, leading the authors to conclude that reversal of the transformed properties was presumably mediated by alteration of the p21ras-mediated signal-transduction pathway (70).

When quercetin was given to mice by intraperitoneal injection at the same time that mouse melanoma B16-BL6 cells were given by intramuscular injection, quercetin caused a dose-dependent delay of tumor growth and potentiated tumor inhibition by a noncytotoxic dose of cisplatin (59). Quercetin significantly altered the ability of the melanoma cells to colonize in the lungs of mice in a lung metastasis model, and inhibited the invasion of melanoma cells in an in vitro assay (59).

3.3.2. APOPTOSIS

Dietary fruits and vegetables that are rich in flavonoids are preferred over supplemental sources for preventing cancers of the intestinal tract, since intimate contact is maintained with dietary compounds throughout the length of the digestive tract, beginning in the oral cavity. This is especially true for the flavonols, since significant quantities of quercetin, myricetin, and kaempferol are absorbed in the gut with a large fraction remaining in the lumen, exposing the intestine to biologically significant amounts of these flavonols (89). To determine the effect of a series of flavonoids on the growth of colonic tumor cells, compounds ranging from 1 to 100 µmol were added to cells in culture. Growth inhibition and loss of cells was most effective with quercetin, followed by apigenin, fisetin, robinetin, and kaempferol (90), and quercetin was the strongest inducer of apoptosis. Sensitivity to quercetin was correlated with inhibition of EGF receptor kinase. Quercetin, myricetin, and kaempferol induced apoptosis in human HL-60 leukemia cells, with a rapid induction of caspase-3 activity and proteolytic cleavage of PARP. They also induced loss of mitochondrial transmembrane potential and release of cytochrome C, as well as procaspase-9 processing. The potency of apoptotic induction was quercetin>myricetin>kaempferol *(91)*. In breast cancer cells (MBA-MB-468), quercetin inhibited growth more efficiently than kaempferol, and was a more effective inducer of cell-cycle arrest at G_2/M. However, quercetin induced apoptosis, but kaempferol did not *(92)*.

Quercetin induces apoptosis, and will inhibit hydrogen peroxide-induced apoptosis by intervening in the activator protein 1 (AP-1)-mediated apoptotic pathway. In addition, quercetin was shown to block activation of all MAPKs that respond to hydrogen peroxide treatment. It was concluded from several other observations that suppression of the JNK-c-Jun/AP-1 and the ERK-c-Fos/AP-1 pathways is strongly associated with the antiapoptotic effect of quercetin *(93)*.

3.3.3. PHARMACOLOGIC CONSIDERATIONS

3.3.3.1. Hormonal Activity Using a previously described recombinant yeast strain *(55)* that contains a stably integrated human ER, kaempferol was shown to stimulate the transcriptional activity of the ER at a dose several magnitudes higher than that demonstrated by estradiol *(55)*. In estrogen-dependent MCF-7 breast cancer cells, kaempferol induced DNA synthesis at low concentrations (0.1–10 µmol), but at 20–90 µmol, DNA synthesis was dramatically inhibited *(76)*. In experiments designed to define the mechanism of action of estrogenic and antiestrogenic flavonoids, kaempferide did not bind to ER, so it was concluded that the antiestrogenic action of kaempferide occurs independently of direct antagonism of the ER. Based on results seen with other flavonoids, the regulation of breast cancer cell proliferation by ER-binding independent mechanisms is biologically significant *(79)*.

Growth of the androgen-independent prostate tumor cell line (PC-3) was completely inhibited by quercetin and kaempferol, and partially (59%) inhibited by myricetin. Increasing concentrations of these flavonols resulted in a concentration-dependent decrease in cell proliferation, but apoptosis induction by quercetin or kaempferol was not evident in these cells *(94)*.

3.3.3.2. Molecular Events (Phase 2 Enzymes, Protein Kinases, DNA Damage) Kaempferol strongly stimulated the induction of quinone reductase, a phase 2 anticarcinogenic marker enzyme, in murine hepatoma cells, with less activity shown by quercetin

and myricetin *(83)*. A 2,3 double bond in the C ring enhanced by a 3-hydroxyl group (kaempferol) appears to be essential for induction.

Activation of PKC is a driving force in cell proliferation, and suppression of its activity can control proliferation. Modulation of PKC by phenolic compounds revealed that quercetin and kaempferol inhibited enzyme activity in cytosolic, particulate, and nuclear fractions isolated from aflatoxin-induced rat livers *(41)*, whereas ellagic acid and curcumin were effective only on enzymes in the particulate fraction, and curcumin and rutin were only moderately effective against the nuclear enzyme fraction. Furthermore, quercetin and kaempferol significantly induce tyrosine dephosphorylation, and in doing so, inactivate the oncogenic PDPK FA *(82)* in prostate carcinoma cells. Inhibition of tyrosine phosphorylation of this gene represents a novel mechanism for the suppression of cell proliferation *(82)*.

Flavonoids may act as enhancers or inhibitors of DNA damage induced by radiation or peroxides. Quercetin's enhancement of x-irradiation-induced cell death when administered after irradiation, presumably resulting from an adverse effect on DNA repair mechanisms, could potentially be used as an adjunct treatment for tumor radiotherapy *(85)*. In contrast, quercetin prevents DNA single-strand breakage induced by *tert*-butylhydroperoxide via iron-chelating activity *(95)*.

3.4. Flavanones and Flavanonols

These two closely related classes of flavonoids, with a C6-C3-C6 structure where the 3-C chain is saturated and oxygen is in the 4-position, are discussed together in this section. The flavanones correspond to flavones, except that the double bond between carbons 2 and 3 is saturated, and flavanonols have a hydroxyl in the 3-position *(1)*. Among the flavanones are naringenin, nararutin, naringin, hesperidin, and neohesperidin, which are predominantly found in citrus fruits. Flavanonols in fruit are not as well documented, but engeletin and astilbin have been identified and isolated from the skin of white grapes *(1)*.

3.4.1. CHEMOPREVENTION

Hesperidin, given during the initiation and post-initiation phases of oral carcinogenesis in male F344 rats, prevented formation of NQO-induced tongue lesions (neoplasms and preneoplasms). Hesperidin at 1000 ppm in diet prior to and during NQO treatment (20 ppm in drinking water) led to a 75% reduction in tongue carcinoma; when given in the diet 1 wk post-NQO treatment, the frequency of tongue carcinoma was reduced by 62%. Dietary administration of hesperidin significantly decreased polyamine levels and cell proliferation in nonlesional areas of the tongue (96,97). Dietary administration of a powder from the Satsuma mandarin (CHRP), which contains high quantities of β-cryptoxanthine and hesperidin, suppresses AOM-induced aberrant crypt foci through inhibition of cell proliferation and induction of detoxifying enzymes (98). Commercial preparations containing higher amounts of the compounds (MJ, MJ2, MJ5) were evaluated in F344 rats for inhibition of AOM-induced colon tumors (98). Inclusion of the test agents in drinking water beginning 1 wk after the last AOM treatment resulted in 49%, 64%, and 78% reductions in colon carcinomas, respectively. The agents also reduced the level of cyclin D_1 and the number of proliferating cells in tumors, and increased the apoptotic index (98).

3.4.2. Apoptosis

The flavanone from lemon fruit, eriodictyol, causes DNA fragmentation in HL-60 cells in culture that could be suppressed by a caspase inhibitor (99); an apoptotic DNA ladder and chromatin condensation were also observed. Eriodictyol increased cytotoxicity in murine L-929 cells induced by tumor necrosis factor alpha (TNFα), as did naringenin, whereas hesperidin had no protective effect (100). The cytotoxicity induced by TNFα was presumably apoptosis-mediated, since TNFα activates caspase 8 and caspase 3 in mammalian cells, leading to cell death by apoptosis (101,102).

3.4.3. Pharmacological Considerations

Hormonal activity of the flavanone naringenin has been demonstrated in breast cancer-cell lines (55,75,78). In a recombinant yeast strain containing human ER, naringenin was the most potent flavonoid of 23 tested in stimulating transcriptional activity of the integrated ER (55). Similarly, naringenin mimicked natural estrogens and stimulated DNA synthesis in the estrogen-dependent MCF-7-cell line. The estrogenic, androgenic, and progestational activity of 72 flavonoids was evaluated in the BT-474 human breast cancer-cell line at concentrations as low as 10 μmol. In this system, naringenin displayed the strongest estrogenic activity, except for that shown by the soy isoflavones (75). In other work involving the breast cancer-cell lines T-47D and BT-474, naringenin exhibited a weak progestational activity (78).

4. COMPLEX POLYPHENOLS

The tannin complex polyphenols are grouped into two categories: hydrolyzable and nonhydrolyzable. Hydrolyzable tannins are based on gallic acid (gallotannins) or hexahydroxydiphenic acid (ellagitannins) and their derivatives; when degraded, they yield sugars and phenolic acids. Nonhydrolyzable (condensed) tannins include proanthocyanidins and tannins from grape and Japanese persimmon. Certain fruits (primarily berries) contain hydrolyzable tannins with only small amounts of condensed tannins (1). Grapes contain primarily condensed tannins, and other fruits (e.g., strawberries) may contain equal portions of both. A third group of complex polyphenols is the lignans, dimers formed by tail-to-tail linkages of two coniferyl or sinapyl alcohol units (enterodiol, enterolactone, and nordihydroguaiaretic acid, NDGA) (1).

4.1. Chemoprevention

Tannins may act as anti-initiators or antipromoters. An analysis of the effectiveness of tannins as chemopreventive agents has been published (103) in which literature concerning animal models, mechanisms of prevention, and organ sites is reviewed. As an anti-initiator, tannic acid was shown to inhibit the mutagenicity and tumorigenicity of polycyclic aromatic hydrocarbons (PAH). In mouse skin, topical application of tannic acid increased the activity of aryl hydrocarbon hydroxylase by 200%. Application of tannic acid to mouse skin 1 h before B[a]P treatment inhibited binding of the B[a]P-diol-epoxide metabolite to epidermal DNA by 60% (104). Tannic acid and hydrolyzable tannins were examined in a mouse skin-TPA model to determine antioxidant and antipromoting activities in vivo. Pretreatment or posttreatment (36 h after TPA) of mouse skin with tannic acid strongly inhibits the hydroperoxide response to TPA in a dose-dependent manner (105). In addition, hydrolyzable tannins and tannic acid prevented formation of papillomas in mouse skin when given 20 min before each promoter application.

Complex polyphenols and tannins from wine (WCPT) were evaluated for their ability to inhibit colon carcinogenesis in rats (106). WCPT fed in diet (14 or 57 mg/kg/d) before or after AOM had no effect on the number or multiplicity of aberrant crypt foci

(ACF) in the colon. A slight decrease in numbers of cells per crypt was noted, but there was no evidence of increased apoptosis. The high dose of WCPT was equivalent to 10× the dose experienced by a moderate drinker of red wine.

When the antitumor promoting activity of grape seed polyphenols (GSP) was examined in a CD-1 mouse skin model of tumor promotion, pretreatment with GSP resulted in a dose-dependent reduction of TPA-stimulated epidermal ODC activity of up to 70%, and up to 73% inhibition of myeloperoxidase (MPO) activity (107). GSP (5, 10, and 20 mg) added 20 min before TPA application in DMBA-initiated mouse skin resulted in 30%, 40%, and 60% inhibition of skin tumor incidence, respectively. In addition, the number of tumors per mouse decreased by 63%, 51%, and 94% (107).

4.2. Apoptosis

GSP, which are rich in procyanidins, exert a strong growth-inhibitory effect against human prostate carcinoma (DU145) cells in culture. Incubation of 10–100 µg/mL GSP for 2–6 d in cultures of DU145 cells results in significant growth inhibition in a time- and dose-dependent fashion (e.g., 2 d of treatment resulted in 27%, 39%, and 76% growth inhibition at 50, 75, and 100 µg/mL, respectively); up to 98% growth inhibition was observed when cells were treated for 4–6 d with GSP (108). GSP also caused a reduction in ERK-1 and ERK-2 levels, CDK4 and CDK2, and cyclin E, and an increase in p21, resulting in significant growth arrest and apoptotic cell death (108).

GSP produced highly significant growth inhibition in a human breast carcinoma-cell line (MDA-MB-468) when kept in the medium for 1–3 d at concentrations of 25, 50, and 75 µg/mL. Accompanying the growth inhibition was a highly significant inhibition of MAPK and MAPK/p38, a decrease in CDK4, and induction of the CDK inhibitor p21. Cells did not undergo apoptotic cell death, as evidenced by lack of DNA fragmentation, PARP cleavage, and cell morphology. In addition, cells appeared to undergo differentiation, as evidenced by induction of cytokeratin 8 protein levels (109).

Persimmon extract (PS) strongly inhibits the growth of human lymphoid leukemia Molt 4B cells in vitro with only a slight (10–20%) inhibition of ODC activity. Within 3 d after treatment with PS, DNA fragmentation typical of that seen in apoptotic cell death was observed (110).

4.3. Pharmacologic Considerations

Estrogen-dependent MCF-7 cells will undergo DNA synthesis when stimulated by steroids. The lignan enterolactone induces DNA synthesis at low concentrations (0.1–10 µmol) characteristic of an estrogen response, but at higher concentrations inhibits DNA synthesis, indicative of a response that may be independent of the ER (76). In the presence of estradiol, enterolactone enhanced estradiol-induced DNA synthesis (77).

As was shown previously for the phenolic acids, many phenolic compounds have a profound effect on P450 enzyme activity. Among these, tannic acid is the most potent inhibitor of CYP1A1 activity in a murine hepatic microsome in vitro model (19).

In addition to the hormonal activity discussed here, lignans regulate c-fos transcription in human breast cancer cells. Enterodiol and enterolactone have demonstrated a weak inhibition of TPA-induced c-fos mRNA levels, whereas no inhibition was observed with the lignan metabolite (methyl p-hydroxyphenyllactate) and NDGA (111); in contrast, the latter agent actually increased c-fos mRNA levels. None of the compounds inhibited PKC, but NDGA was a potent inhibitor of cell-colony formation (111). In consideration of all parameters, enterodiol, enterolactone, and NDGA would be expected to be less efficacious than other polyphenols as chemopreventive agents.

5. SUMMARY

This chapter clearly demonstrates that fruit contains abundant polyphenolic compounds that exhibit chemopreventive activity both in vitro and in vivo. The data on several of these compounds—e.g., apigenin, quercetin, and ellagic acid—are very extensive, whereas for other compounds, such as the anthocyanins, relatively little information is available. Very few—if any—of these agents have been evaluated for chemopreventive efficacy in human clinical trials. Obviously, much more research is needed with these classes of phenolic compounds before such trials are initiated.

REFERENCES

1. Macheix J-J, Fleuriet A, Billot J. *Fruit Phenolics*, CRC Press, Boca Raton, FL, 1990.
2. Mirvish SS, Cardesa A, Wallcave L, Shubik P. Induction of mouse lung adenomas by amines or ureas plus nitrite and by N-nitroso compounds: effect of ascorbate, gallic acid, thiocyanate, and caffeine. *J Natl Cancer Inst* 1975;55:633–636.
3. Hirose M, Ito T, Takahashi S, et al. Prevention by synthetic phenolic antioxidants of 2-amino-3, 8-dimethylimidazo

[4,5-f] quinoxaline (MeIQx)- or activated MeIQx-induced mutagenesis and MeIQx-induced rat hepatocarcinogenesis, and role of antioxidant activity in the prevention of carcinogenesis. *Eur J Cancer Prev* 1998;7:223–241.

4. Soleas GJ, Grass L, Josephy PD, et al. A comparison of the anticarcinogenic properties of four red wine polyphenols. *Clin Biochem* 2002;35:119–124.

5. Gali HU, Perchellet EM, Klish DS, et al. Hydrolyzable tannins: potent inhibitors of hydroperoxide production and tumor promotion in mouse skin treated with 12-*O*-tetradecanoylphorbol-13-acetate in vivo. *Int J Cancer* 1992;51:425–432.

6. Tanaka T, Kawamori T, Ohnishi M, et al. Chemoprevention of 4-nitroquinoline 1-oxide-induced oral carcinogenesis by dietary protocatechuic acid during initiation and postinitiation phases. *Cancer Res* 1994;54:2359–2365.

7. Ohnishi M, Yoshimi N, Kawamori T, et al. Inhibitory effects of dietary protocatechuic acid and costunolide on 7,12-dimethylbenz[*a*]anthracene-induced hamster cheek pouch carcinogenesis. *Jpn J Cancer Res* 1997;88:111–119.

8. Yoshioka K, Kataoka T, Hayashi T, et al. Induction of apoptosis by gallic acid in human stomach cancer KATO III and colon adenocarcinoma COLO 205 cell lines. *Oncol Rep* 2000;7:1221–1223.

9. Ohno Y, Fukuda K, Takemura G, et al. Induction of apoptosis by gallic acid in lung cancer cells. *Anticancer Drugs* 1999;10:845–851.

10. Serrano A, Palacios C, Roy G, et al. Derivatives of gallic acid induce apoptosis in tumoral cell lines and inhibit lymphocyte proliferation. *Arch Biochem Biophys* 1998;350:49–54.

11. Roy G, Lombardia M, Palacios C, et al. Mechanistic aspects of the induction of apoptosis by lauryl gallate in the murine B-cell lymphoma line Wehi 231. *Arch Biochem Biophys* 2000;383:206–214.

12. Sakaguchi N, Inoue M, Isuzugawa K, et al. Cell death-inducing activity by gallic acid derivatives. *Biol Pharm Bull* 1999;22:471–475.

13. Sakaguchi N, Inoue M, Ogihara Y. Reactive oxygen species and intracellular Ca2+, common signals for apoptosis induced by gallic acid. *Biochem Pharmacol* 1998;55:1973–1981.

14. Aoki K, Ishiwata S, Sakagami H, et al. Modification of apoptosis-inducing activity of gallic acid by saliva. *Anticancer Res* 2001;21:1879–1883.

15. Isuzugawa K, Ogihara Y, Inoue M. Different generation of inhibitors against gallic acid-induced apoptosis produces different sensitivity to gallic acid. *Biol Pharm Bull* 2001;24:249–253.

16. Isuzugawa K, Inoue M, Ogihara Y. Catalase contents in cells determine sensitivity to the apoptosis inducer gallic acid. *Biol Pharm Bull* 2001;24:1022–1026.

17. Saeki K, Hayakawa S, Noro T, et al. Apoptosis-inducing activity of galloyl monosaccharides in human histiocytic lymphoma U937 cells. *Planta Med* 2000;66:124–126.

18. Vieira O, Escargueil-Blanc I, Meilhac O, et al. Effect of dietary phenolic compounds on apoptosis of human cultured endothelial cells induced by oxidized LDL. *Br J Pharmacol* 1998;123:565–573.

19. Baer-Dubowska W, Szaefer H, Krajka-Kuzniak V. Inhibition of murine hepatic cytochrome P450 activities by natural and synthetic phenolic compounds. *Xenobiotica* 1998;28:735–743.

20. Mahmoud NN, Carothers AM, Grunberger D, et al. Plant phenolics decrease intestinal tumors in an animal model of familial adenomatous polyposis. *Carcinogenesis* 2000;21:921–927.

21. Mori H, Kawabata K, Yoshimi N, et al. Chemopreventive effects of ferulic acid on oral and rice germ on large bowel carcinogenesis. *Anticancer Res* 1999;19:3775–3778.

22. Hudson EA, Dinh PA, Kokubun T, et al. Characterization of potentially chemopreventive phenols in extracts of brown rice that inhibit the growth of human breast and colon cancer cells. *Cancer Epidemiol Biomark Prev* 2000;9:1163–1170.

23. Makino T, Ono T, Muso E, Honda G. Inhibitory effect of *Perilla frutescens* and its phenolic constituents on cultured murine mesangial cell proliferation. *Planta Med* 1998;6:541–545.

24. Chen YJ, Shiao MS, Wang SY. The antioxidant caffeic acid phenethyl ester induces apoptosis associated with selective scavenging of hydrogen peroxide in human leukemic HL-60 cells. *Anticancer Drugs* 2001;12:143–149.

25. Chen YJ, Shiao MS, Hsu ML, et al. Effect of caffeic acid phenethyl ester, an antioxidant from propolis, on inducing apoptosis in human leukemic HL-60 cells. *J Agric Food Chem* 2001;49:5615–5619.

26. Nardini M, Leonardi F, Scaccini C, Virgili F. Modulation of ceramide-induced NF-kappaB binding activity and apoptotic response by caffeic acid in U937 cells: comparison with other antioxidants. *Free Radic Biol Med* 2001;30:722–733.

27. Weyant MJ, Carothers AM, Bertagnolli ME, Bertagnolli MM. Colon cancer chemopreventive drugs modulate integrin-mediated signaling pathways. *Clin Cancer Res* 2000;6:949–956.

28. Stoner GD, Mukhtar H. Polyphenols as cancer chemopreventive agents. *J Cell Biochem* Suppl 1995;22:169–180.

29. Bate-Smith EC. Detection and determination of ellagitannins. *Phytochemistry* 1972;11:1153–1156.

30. Daniel EM, Krupnick AS, Heur Y-H, et al. Extraction, stability, and quantitation of ellagic acid in various fruits and nuts. *J Food Compos Anal* 1989;2:338–349.

31. Lesca P. Protective effects of ellagic acid and other plant phenols on benzo(*a*)pyrene-induced neoplasia in mice. *Carcinogenesis* 1983;4:1652–1653.

32. Boukharta M, Jalbert G, Castonguay A. Biodistribution of ellagic acid and dose-related inhibition of lung tumorigenesis in A/J mice. *Nutr Cancer* 1992;18:181–189.

33. Mukhtar H, Das M, Del Tito BJ Jr, Bickers DR. Protection against 3-methylcholanthrene-induced skin tumorigenesis in BALB/c mice by ellagic acid. *Biochem Biophys Res Commun* 1984;119:751–757.

34. Smart RC, Huang MT, Chang RL, et al. Effect of ellagic acid and 3-*O*-decylellagic acid on the formation of benzo(*a*)pyrene-derived DNA adducts *in vivo* and on the tumorigenicity of 3-methylcholanthrene in mice. *Carcinogenesis* 1986;7:1669–1675.

35. Mandal S, Stoner GD. Inhibition of *N*-nitrosobenzylmethylamine-induced esophageal tumorigenesis in rats by ellagic acid. *Carcinogenesis* 1990;11:55–61.

36. Daniel EM, Stoner GD. The effects of ellagic acid and 13-*cis*-retinoic acid on *N*-nitrosobenzylmethylamine-induced esophageal tumorigenesis in rats. *Cancer Lett* 1991;56:117–124.

37. Tanaka T, Iwata H, Niwa K, et al. Inhibitory effect of ellagic acid on *N*-2-fluorenylacetamide-induced liver carcinogenesis in male AC1/N rats. *Jpn J Cancer Res* 1988;79:1297–1303.

38. Narayanan BA, Geoffroy O, Willingham MC, et al. P53/p21(WAF1/CIP1) expression and its possible role in G_1 arrest and apoptosis in ellagic acid treated cancer cells. *Cancer Lett* 1999;136:215–221.

39. Saleem A, Husheem M, Harkonen P, Pihlaja K. Inhibition of cancer cell growth by crude extract and the phenolics of *Terminalia chebula* retz. fruit. *J Ethnopharmacol* 2002;31:327–336.

40. Narayanan BA, Re GG. IGF-II down regulation associated cell cycle arrest in colon cancer cells exposed to phenolic antioxidant ellagic acid. *Anticancer Res* 2001;21:359–364.

41. Mistry KJ, Krishna M, Bhattacharya RK. Modulation of aflatoxin B1 activated protein kinase C by phenolic compounds. *Cancer Lett* 1997;121:99–104.

42. Narayanan BA, Narayanan NK, Stoner GD, Bullock BP. Interactive gene expression pattern in prostate cancer cells exposed to phenolic antioxidants. *Life Sci* 2002;70:1821–1839.

43. Harborne JB, Mabry TJ. *The Flavonoids: Advances in Research.* Chapman and Hall, London/New York, 1982.

44. Harborne JB, Mabry TJ, Mabry H. *The Flavonoids.* Chapman and Hall, London, 1975.

45. Wattenberg LW, Coccia JB, Galbraith AR. Inhibition of carcinogen-induced pulmonary and mammary carcinogenesis by chalcone administered subsequent to carcinogen exposure. *Cancer Lett* 1994;83:165–169.

46. Wattenberg L. Chalcones, myo-inositol and other novel inhibitors of pulmonary carcinogenesis. *J Cell Biochem Suppl* 1995;22:162–168.

47. Yamamoto S, Aizu E, Jiang H, et al. The potent anti-tumor-promoting agent isoliquiritigenin. *Carcinogenesis* 1991;12:317–323.

48. De Vincenzo R, Scambia G, Benedetti Panici P, et al. Effect of synthetic and naturally occurring chalcones on ovarian cancer cell growth: structure-activity relationships. *Anticancer Drug Des* 1995;10:481–490.

49. Satomi Y. Inhibitory effects of 3'-methyl-3-hydroxy-chalcone on proliferation of human malignant tumor cells and on skin carcinogenesis. *Int J Cancer* 1993;55:506–514.

50. Yit CC, Das NP. Cytotoxic effect of butein on human colon adenocarcinoma cell proliferation. *Cancer Lett* 1994;82:65–72.

51. Iwashita K, Kobori M, Yamaki K, Tsushida T. Flavonoids inhibit cell growth and induce apoptosis in B16 melanoma 4A5 cells. *Biosci Biotechnol Biochem* 2000;64:1813–1820.

52. De Vincenzo R, Ferlini C, Distefano M, et al. In vitro evaluation of newly developed chalcone analogues in human cancer cells. *Cancer Chemother Pharmacol* 2000;46:305–312.

53. Yang EB, Zhang K, Cheng LY, Mack P. Butein, a specific protein tyrosine kinase inhibitor. *Biochem Biophy Res Commun* 1998;245:435–438.

54. Tanaka S, Sakata Y, Morimoto K, et al. Influence of natural and synthetic compounds on cell surface expression of cell adhesion molecules, ICAM-1 and VCAM-1. *Planta Med* 2001;67:108–113.

55. Breinholt V, Larsen JC. Detection of weak estrogenic flavonoids using a recombinant yeast strain and a modified MCF7 cell proliferation assay. *Chem Res Toxicol* 1998;11:622–629.

56. Birt DF, Mitchell D, Gold B, et al. Inhibition of ultraviolet light induced skin carcinogenesis in SKH-1 mice by apigenin, a plant flavonoid. *Anticancer Res* 1997;17:85–91.

57. Birt DF, Walker B, Tibbels MG, Bresnick E. Anti-mutagenesis and anti-promotion by apigenin, robinetin and indole-3-carbinol. *Carcinogenesis* 1986;7:959–963.

58. Wei H, Tye L, Bresnick E, Birt DF. Inhibitory effect of apigenin, a plant flavonoid, on epidermal ornithine decarboxylase and skin tumor promotion in mice. *Cancer Res* 1990;50:499–502.

59. Caltagirone S, Rossi C, Poggi A, et al. Flavonoids apigenin and quercetin inhibit melanoma growth and metastatic potential. *Int J Cancer* 2000;87:595–600.

60. Reddy KB, Krueger JS, Kondapaka SB, Diglio CA. Mitogen-activated protein kinase (MAPK) regulates the expression of progelatinase B (MMP-9) in breast epithelial cells. *Int J Cancer* 1999;82:268–273.

61. Tatsuta A, Iishi H, Baba M, et al. Suppression by apigenin of peritoneal metastasis of intestinal adenocarcinomas induced by azoxymethane in Wistar rats. *Clin Exp Metastasis* 2000;18:657–662.

62. Lindenmeyer F, Li H, Menashi S, et al. Apigenin acts on the tumor cell invasion process and regulates protease production. *Nutr Cancer* 2000;39:139–147.

63. Yin F, Giuliano AE, Van Herle AJ. Growth inhibitory effects of flavonoids in human thyroid cancer cell lines. *Thyroid* 1999;9:369–376.

64. Hirano T, Oka K, Akiba M. Antiproliferative effects of synthetic and naturally occurring flavonoids on tumor cells of the human breast carcinoma cell line, ZR-75-1. *Res Commun Chem Pathol Pharmacol* 1989;64:69–78.

65. Casagrande F, Darbon JM. Effects of structurally related flavonoids on cell cycle progression of human melanoma cells: regulation of cyclin-dependent kinases CDK2 and CDK1. *Biochem Pharmacol* 2001;61:1205–1215.

66. Wang W, Heideman L, Chung CS, et al. Cell-cycle arrest at G_2/M and growth inhibition by apigenin in human colon carcinoma cell lines. *Mol Carcinog* 2000;28:102–110.

67. Yin F, Giuliano AE, Law RE, Van Herle AJ. Apigenin inhibits growth and induces G_2/M arrest by modulating cyclin-CDK regulators and ERK MAP kinase activation in breast carcinoma cells. *Anticancer Res* 2001;21:413–420.

68. Kobayashi T, Nakata T, Kuzumaki T. Effect of flavonoids on cell cycle progression in prostate cancer cells. *Cancer Lett* 2002;176:17–23.

69. Sato F, Matsukawa Y, Matsumoto K, et al. Apigenin induces morphological differentiation and G_2-M arrest in rat neuronal cells. *Biochem Biophys Res Commun* 1994;204:578–584.

70. Kuo ML, Lin JK, Huang TS, Yang NC. Reversion of the transformed phenotypes of v-H-ras NIH3T3 cells by flavonoids through attenuating the content of phosphotyrosine. *Cancer Lett* 1994;87:91–97.

71. Takahashi T, Kobori M, Shinmoto H, Tsushida T. Structure-activity relationships of flavonoids and the induction of granulocytic- or monocytic-differentiation in HL60 human myeloid leukemia cells. *Biosci Biotechnol Biochem* 1998;62:2199–2204.

72. Yin F, Giuliano AE, Van Herle AJ. Signal pathways involved in apigenin inhibition of growth and induction of apoptosis

of human anaplastic thyroid cancer cells (ARO). *Anticancer Res* 1999;19:4297–4303.

73. Gupta S, Afaq F, Mukhtar H. Selective growth-inhibitory, cell-cycle deregulatory and apoptotic response of apigenin in normal versus human prostate carcinoma cells. *Biochem Biophys Res Commun* 2001;287:914–920.

74. Gupta S, Afaq F, Mukhtar H. Involvement of nuclear factor-kappa B, Bax and Bcl-2 in induction of cell cycle arrest and apoptosis by apigenin in human prostate carcinoma cells. *Oncogene* 2002;21:3727–3738.

75. Zand RS, Jenkins DJ, Diamandis EP. Steroid hormone activity of flavonoids and related compounds. *Breast Cancer Res Treat* 2000;62:35–49.

76. Wang C, Kurzer MS. Phytoestrogen concentration determines effects on DNA synthesis in human breast cancer cells. *Nutr Cancer* 1997;28:236–247.

77. Wang C, Kurzer MS. Effects of phytoestrogens on DNA synthesis in MCF-7 cells in the presence of estradiol or growth factors. *Nutr Cancer* 1998;31:90–100.

78. Rosenberg RS, Grass L, Jenkins DJ, et al. Modulation of androgen and progesterone receptors by phytochemicals in breast cancer cell lines. *Biochem Biophys Res Commun* 1998;248:935–939.

79. Collins-Burow BM, Burow ME, Duong BN, McLachlan JA. Estrogenic and antiestrogenic activities of flavonoid phytochemicals through estrogen receptor binding-dependent and –independent mechanisms. *Nutr Cancer* 2000;38:229–244.

80. Song DH, Sussman DJ, Seldin DC. Endogenous protein kinase CK2 participates in Wnt signaling in mammary epithelial cells. *J Biol Chem* 2000;275:23,790–23,797.

81. Lin JK, Chen YC, Huang YT, Lin-Shiau SY. Suppression of protein kinase C and nuclear oncogene expression as possible molecular mechanisms of cancer chemoprevention by apigenin and curcumin. *J Cell Biochem Suppl* 1997;28-29:39–48.

82. Lee SC, Kuan CY, Yang CC, Yang SD. Bioflavonoids commonly and potently induce tyrosine dephosphorylation/inactivation of oncogenic proline-directed protein kinase FA in human prostate carcinoma cells. *Anticancer Res* 1998;18:1117–1121.

83. Uda Y, Price KR, Williamson G, Rhodes MJ. Induction of the anticarcinogenic marker enzyme, quinone reductase, in murine hepatoma cells in vitro by flavonoids. *Cancer Lett* 1997;120:213–216.

84. Touraine RL, Vahanian N, Ramsey WJ, Blaese RM. Enhancement of the herpes simplex virus thymidine kinase/ganciclovir bystander effect and its antitumor efficacy in vivo by pharmacologic manipulation of gap junctions. *Hum Gene Ther* 1998;9:2385–2391.

85. van Rijn J, van den Berg J. Flavonoids as enhancers of x-ray-induced cell damage in hepatoma cells. *Clin Cancer Res* 1997;3:1775–1779.

86. Balasubramanian S, Govindasamy S. Inhibitory effect of dietary flavonol quercetin on 7,12-dimethylbenz[a]anthracene-induced hamster buccal pouch carcinogenesis. *Carcinogenesis* 1996;17:887–879.

87. Elattar TM, Virji AS. The inhibitory effect of curcumin, genistein, quercetin and cisplatin on the growth of oral cancer cells in vitro. *Anticancer Res* 2000;20:1733–1738.

88. Lee SF, Lin JK. Inhibitory effects of phytopolyphenols on TPA-induced transformation, PKC activation, and c-jun

expression in mouse fibroblast cells. *Nutr Cancer* 1997;28:177–183.

89. Gee JM, Johnson IT. Polyphenolic compounds: interactions with the gut and implications for human health. *Curr Med Chem* 2001;8:1245–1255.

90. Richter M, Ebermann R, Marian B. Quercetin-induced apoptosis in colorectal tumor cells: possible role of EGF receptor signaling. *Nutr Cancer* 1999;34:88–99.

91. Wang IK, Lin-Shiau SY, Lin JK. Induction of apoptosis by apigenin and related flavonoids through cytochrome c release and activation of caspase-9 and caspase-3 in leukaemia HL-60 cells. *Eur J Cancer* 1999;35:1517–1525.

92. Balabhadrapathruni S, Thomas TJ, Yurkow EJ, et al. Effects of genistein and structurally related phytoestrogens on cell cycle kinetics and apoptosis in MDA-MB-468 human breast cancer cells. *Oncol Rep* 2000;7:3–12.

93. Ishikawa Y, Kitamura M. Anti-apoptotic effect of quercetin: intervention in the JNK- and ERK-mediated apoptotic pathways. *Kidney Int* 2000;58:1078–1087.

94. Knowles LM, Zigrossi DA, Tauber RA, et al. Flavonoids suppress androgen-independent human prostate tumor proliferation. *Nutr Cancer* 2000;38:116–122.

95. Sestili P, Guidarelli A, Dacha M, Cantoni O. Quercetin prevents DNA single strand breakage and cytotoxicity caused by tert-butylhydroperoxide: free radical scavenging versus iron chelating mechanism. *Free Radic Biol Med* 1998;25:196–200.

96. Tanaka T, Makita H, Ohnishi M, et al. Chemoprevention of 4-nitroquinoline 1-oxide-induced oral carcinogenesis in rats by flavonoids diosmin and hesperidin, each alone and in combination. *Cancer Res* 1997;57:246–252.

97. Tanaka T, Makita H, Ohnishi M, et al. Chemoprevention of 4-nitroquinoline 1-oxide-induced oral carcinogenesis by dietary curcumin and hesperidin: comparison with the protective effect of beta-carotene. *Cancer Res* 1994;54:4653–4659.

98. Tanaka T, Kohno H, Murakami M, et al. Suppression of azoxymethane-induced colon carcinogenesis in male F344 rats by mandarin juices rich in beta-cryptoxanthin and hesperidin. *Int J Cancer* 2000;88:146–150.

99. Ogata S, Miyake Y, Yamamoto K, et al. Apoptosis induced by the flavonoid from lemon fruit (Citrus limon BURM.f.) and its metabolites in HL-60 cells. *Biosci Biotechnol Biochem* 2000;64:1075–1078.

100. Habtemariam S. Flavonoids as inhibitors or enhancers of the cytotoxicity of tumor necrosis factor-alpha in L-929 tumor cells. *J Nat Prod* 1997;60:775–778.

101. Goswami R, Kilkus J, Scurlock B, Dawson G. CrmA protects against apoptosis and ceramide formation in PC12 cells. *Neurochem Res* 2002;27:735–741.

102. Liao YC, Liang WG, Chen FW, et al. IL-19 induced production of IL-6 and TNF-alpha and results in cell apoptosis through TNF-alpha. *J Immunol* 2002;169:4288–4297.

103. Nepka C, Asprodini E, Kouretas D. Tannins, xenobiotic metabolism and cancer chemoprevention in experimental animals. *Eur J Drug Metab Pharmacokinet* 1999;24:183–189.

104. Baer-Dubowska W, Gnojkowski J, Fenrych W. Effect of tannic acid on benzo[a]pyrene-DNA adduct formation in mouse epidermis: comparison with synthetic gallic acid esters. *Nutr Cancer* 1997;29:42–47.

105. Gali HU, Perchellet EM, Klish DS, et al. Hydrolyzable tannins: potent inhibitors of hydroperoxide production and tumor promotion in mouse skin treated with 12-*O*-tetrade-canoylphorbol-13-acetate in vivo. *Int J Cancer* 1992;51:425–432.

106. Caderni G, Remy S, Cheynier V, et al. Effect of complex polyphenols on colon carcinogenesis. *Eur J Nutr* 1999;38:126–132.

107. Bomser JA, Singletary KW, Wallig MA, Smith MA. Inhibition of TPA-induced tumor promotion in CD-1 mouse epidermis by a polyphenolic fraction from grape seeds. *Cancer Lett* 1999;135:151–157.

108. Agarwal C, Sharma Y, Agarwal R. Anticarcinogenic effect of a polyphenolic fraction isolated from grape seeds in human prostate carcinoma DU145 cells: modulation of mitogenic signaling and cell-cycle regulators and induc-tion of G_1 arrest and apoptosis. *Mol Carcinog* 2000;28:129–138.

109. Agarwal C, Sharma Y, Zhao J, Agarwal R. A polyphenolic fraction from grape seeds causes irreversible growth inhibi-tion of breast carcinoma MDA-MB468 cells by inhibition mitogen-activated protein kinases activation and inducing G_1 arrest and differentiation. *Clin Cancer Res* 2000;6:2921–2930.

110. Achiwa Y, Hibasami H, Katsuzaki H, et al. Inhibitory effects of persimmon (Diospyros kaki) extract and related polyphe-nol compounds on growth of human lymphoid leukemia cells. *Biosci Biotechnol Biochem* 1997;61:1099–1101.

111. Schultze-Mosgau MH, Dale IL, Gant TW, et al. Regulation of c-fos transcription by chemopreventive isoflavonoids and lignans in MDA-MB-468 breast cancer cells. *Eur J Cancer* 1998;34:1425–1431.

30 Tea Polyphenols as Cancer Chemopreventive Agents

Vaqar M. Adhami, PhD, Farrukh Afaq, PhD, Nihal Ahmad, PhD, Yukihiko Hara, PhD, and Hasan Mukhtar, PhD

Contents

1. INTRODUCTION

In recent years, the concept of chemoprevention has matured to be considered as a practical option to reduce the occurrence of cancer *(1–5)*. Chemoprevention—the use of natural and/or synthetic compounds to intervene in the early precancerous stages of carcinogenesis before the onset of invasive disease—offers a viable approach to define substances, either food components or pharmaceuticals, which can prevent, delay, or completely halt the process of carcinogenesis. Often chemoprevention is referred to as "prevention by delay."

The ultimate aim of chemoprevention is to use the preventive substances in pills or in modified foods as a prevention strategy for people who are at high risk for cancer, much as drugs that reduce cholesterol, blood pressure, and blood clotting benefit people who are at high risk for heart disease and stroke. An ideal chemopreventive agent for human use should have little or no toxicity, high efficacy at multiple sites, capability of oral consumption, a known mechanism of action, low cost, and human acceptance. Of the known chemopreventive agents, greater emphasis is placed on substances that are present in diet and beverages consumed by humans. One reason for this is that, although environmental and natural carcinogens are difficult to control, humans can be motivated to change their dietary habits to consume more chemopreventive substances.

At present, at least 30 different groups of agents that have shown cancer chemopreventive properties in laboratory studies are known. Some of these agents have also shown promise in epidemiological studies *(1–5)*. Polyphenols comprise one such group of agents. Since tea is rich in polyphenols with strong antioxidant potential, we have focused our attention on examining the cancer chemopreventive effects of tea since the late 1980s *(6)*. Tea, the most popular beverage consumed by humans, contains polyphenolic constituents known as catechins *(6–8)*. The anticarcinogenic and antimutagenic activities of polyphenolic agents present in green tea were reported more than a decade ago by this laboratory *(9–10)*. At the present time, more than 900 scientific publications exist on elucidation of tea's

From: Cancer Chemoprevention, Volume 1: Promising Cancer Chemoprevention Agents
Edited by: G. J. Kelloff, E. T. Hawk, and C. C. Sigman © Humana Press Inc., Totowa, NJ

chemopreventive properties. In animal studies, tea consumption has been shown to afford protection against ultraviolet (UV) light-induced skin cancers and chemical carcinogen-induced lung, liver, prostate, colon, stomach, and breast cancers *(6–19)*. All teas are derived from *Camellia sinensis*, an evergreen shrub of the Theaceae family. (A widespread misconception includes herbal teas with products derived from *C. sinensis*. Most herbal infusions should not be mistaken for tea.)

In some parts of the world, consumption of tea has been believed to offer health-promoting potential for many generations *(16–19)*. Epidemiological studies, although inconclusive, suggest that consumption of green tea is associated with a lower cancer risk. This possibility is exciting, because—at least for some populations—tea consumption is hoped to be effective in reducing cancer risk. The challenges are to identify populations that will have potential health benefits, and to discover why tea is ineffective in other populations. The majority of studies that evaluates the use of tea in cancer prevention have been conducted with green tea, although a few studies have also assessed the chemopreventive potential of black tea *(6–19)*. The ratio of studies with green tea alone or its constituents and studies with black tea alone or black tea and green tea is approx 5:1. Based on studies in cell culture, laboratory animals, and epidemiological observations, clinical trials of green tea consumption and cancer risk have been initiated. The major polyphenolic constituents believed to be responsible for the cancer chemopreventive potential of green tea include (–)-epicatechin (EC), (–)-epigallocatechin (EGC), (–)-epicatechin-3-gallate (ECG), and (–)-epigallocatechin-3-gallate (EGCG) (Table 1). Among these, EGCG is believed to be the most active polyphenolic constituent *(8,14,19)*.

2. HISTORY OF TEA CONSUMPTION

The plant *C. sinensis* was originally discovered and grown in Southeast Asia thousands of years ago; according to Chinese mythology, the emperor Shen Nung discovered tea for the first time in 2737 BC *(13)*. Since then, the popularity of this beverage has increased; at present, it is the most popular drink in the world second only to water, with a per capita worldwide consumption of approx 120 mL brewed tea per day. Tea is currently grown and cultivated in at least 30 countries around the world. Many types of tea preparations, originating from *C. sinensis* but

with different processing methods, are consumed today. The three major tea types differing in degree of fermentation include black tea (78%, mainly consumed in western and some Asian countries), green tea (20%, mainly consumed in Asia, and a few countries in North Africa and the Middle East), and oolong tea (2%, consumed in some parts of China and Taiwan) *(5,7,8,14)*.

3. BIOAVAILABILITY OF TEA POLYPHENOLS

The bioavailability of the active polyphenolic constituents after tea consumption in laboratory animals and humans is poorly defined. Yang et al. *(14)* conducted a study of 18 individuals given different amounts of green tea; in which plasma concentrations and urinary excretion of tea catechins were measured as a function of time. After consuming 1.5, 3.0, and 4.5 g of decaffeinated green tea (in 500 mL of water), the maximum plasma concentrations (C_{max}) of EGCG, EGC, and EC were found to be 326 ng/mL, 550 ng/mL, 190 ng/mL respectively, as observed 1.4–2.4 h after ingestion of the tea preparation. When the dose was increased from 1.5–3.0 g, C_{max} values were found to increase by 2.7–3.4-fold, but further increasing the dose to 4.5 g did not increase C_{max} values significantly, suggesting a saturation phenomenon. The half-life of EGCG (5.0–5.5 h) was found to be higher than the half-life of EGC or EC. EGC and EC, but not EGCG, were excreted in urine; 90% of total urinary EGC and EC was demonstrated to be excreted within 8 h. When the tea dosage was increased, the amount of EGC and EC excretion also increased, but a clear dose-response relationship was not observed. This study provided basic pharmacokinetic parameters of green tea polyphenols (GTPs) in humans that may be used to estimate the levels of these compounds after consumption of green tea.

Recently, Saganuma et al. *(18)* studied the distribution of radiolabeled [^{3}H]EGCG in mouse organs following oral administration. Radioactivity was found in many organs, including those in which inhibition of carcinogenesis by EGCG or green tea extract had already been shown. These results suggest that frequent consumption of green tea enables the body to maintain a high level of tea polyphenols. These studies may be useful in designing future strategies intended towards development of green tea as a practical chemopreventive agent.

Table 1
Green Tea Catechins and Their Composition

Constituent	Structure	% by Dry Weight
Catechin		—
Epicatechin		2
Gallocatechin		—
Epigallocatechin		10
Epicatechin gallate		2
Gallocatechin gallate		—
Epigallocatechin gallate		11

Table 2
Laboratory Studies on the Chemoprevention of Various
Cancers by Green Tea

Type of Cancer	Agent Used	System Employed	Reference
Skin	GTP, EGCG, EGC, ECG	Cell culture, mice,	52,84–87
Oral	GTP	Hamsters	54
Stomach	EGCG, GTP	Mice, rats	88–93
Colon	EGCG, GTP	Mice, cell culture	61
Lung	GTP, EGCG	Mice, cell culture	91–94
Liver	EGCG, EGC, ECG, EC	Rats, cell culture	95–98
Pancreas	EGCG	Cell culture	99–102
Prostate	EGCG, GTP	Mice, cell culture	76,79,103, 105
Breast	GTP, EGCG	Rats, mice	106–108

4. TEA AND CANCER CHEMOPREVENTION

Epidemiological studies are often considered to provide reliable information on the preventive effect of certain chemical compounds. In 1989, the International Agency for Research on Cancer Working Group reviewed the results of epidemiological studies relating tea consumption to the occurrence of human cancers (20). The review, based on the available literature, concluded that no association between tea consumption and cancer risk exists. Because of inadequate analysis and inconsistent results, it is usually difficult to draw conclusions on the relationship between tea and human cancer risk. Since epidemiological studies involve various intertwined factors that may yield inexplicable results, experiments with animal and in vitro models were considered necessary to establish the conditions that make the chemopreventive effect clear. Around this time, this laboratory showed that GTPs, tannic acid, and quercetin had potential for protecting against skin tumorigenesis (6). Following this pioneering work, a number of in vivo animal studies in various target organ models, conducted in many laboratories around the world, provided convincing evidence that

the polyphenolic antioxidants present in tea are capable of affording protection against cancer initiation and subsequent development (Table 2); (reviewed in 5,7,8 and references therein). These studies and the data from various epidemiological studies conducted in different populations were considered to be of sufficient merit to embark on clinical trials evaluating the association of green tea consumption with cancer risk (5,7,8,17).

Oral consumption or topical application of green tea and/or its polyphenolic constituents has been shown to afford protection against chemical carcinogen- as well as UV radiation- induced skin carcinogenesis in the mouse model (6,9,19). In many other animal studies, the polyphenolic fraction isolated from green tea, the water extract of green tea, or individual polyphenolic antioxidants present in green tea, have also been shown to afford protection against chemically induced carcinogenesis in the lung, liver, esophagus, forestomach, duodenum, pancreas, colon, and breast (5,7,8 and references therein). It is now believed that many cancer chemopreventive properties of green tea are mediated by EGCG (5,7,8). A single cup of brewed green tea contains up to 400 mg of polyphenolic antioxidants, of which 200 mg is EGCG. Other polyphenolic agents present in green tea also contribute to its cancer chemopreventive efficacy. However, it is unclear whether all the polyphenolic compounds of green tea work through similar biochemical pathways or by different mechanisms. It is also interesting to observe that many consumer products such as beverages, ice cream, health-care products, and cosmetics supplemented with green tea extracts are available in the market.

5. MECHANISM(S) OF THE BIOLOGICAL EFFECTS OF GREEN TEA

A proper understanding of mechanisms of the biological effects of green tea is essential in designing and improving strategies for cancer chemoprevention. Initial mechanistic attempts in this direction were largely focused on evaluating the effect of GTPs on preventing mutagenicity and genotoxicity of chemicals, reducing biochemical markers of tumor initiation and promotion, regulating detoxification enzymes, trapping activated metabolites of carcinogens, and regulating antioxidant and free radical scavenging activity (7,16,21 and references therein). Recent studies have evaluated the molecular mechanisms involved with the biological effects of GTPs, and the studies are discussed in the following sections.

5.1. Green Tea Polyphenols Activate the Mitogen-Activated Protein Kinase (MAPK) Pathway

The protective effects of GTPs have been attributed to inhibition of enzymes such as cytochrome P450, which are involved in the bioactivation of carcinogens (22). Other in vivo studies have also demonstrated the involvement of phase 2 detoxification enzymes during the biological response to green tea. Because the 5' flanking regions of phase 2 enzyme genes contain an antioxidant-responsive element (ARE) believed to mediate induction of phase 2 enzymes by many drugs, the involvement of the MAPK pathway with ARE was studied as a mechanism of biological response to GTPs. This study demonstrated that the activation of the MAPK pathway by GTPs might be a potential signaling pathway involved in regulation of ARE-mediated phase 2 enzyme gene expression (22). It was also demonstrated that GTP treatment of human hepatoma (HepG2) cells transfected with a plasmid construct containing ARE and a minimal glutathione S-transferase Ya promoter linked to the chloramphenicol acetyltransferase (CAT) reporter gene caused induction of CAT activity, suggesting that GTPs stimulate the transcription of phase 2 detoxifying enzymes through ARE. GTPs also resulted in significant activation of MAPK, extracellular signal-regulated kinase 2 (ERK2), and c-Jun N-terminal kinase 1 (JNK1), and increased mRNA levels of early response genes c-*jun* and c-*fos*.

5.2. EGCG Inhibits Urokinase Activity

The anticancer activity of EGCG has been associated with inhibition of urokinase, one of the most frequently expressed enzymes in human cancers (23). Employing computer-based molecular modeling, it was demonstrated that EGCG binds to urokinase, blocking histidine 57 and serine 195 of the urokinase catalytic triad and extending toward arginine 35 from a positively charged loop of urokinase. These calculations were verified by using the spectrophotometric amidolytic assay to evaluate the inhibition of urokinase activity. However, the applicability of these results at achievable dose levels was challenged by Yang (24).

5.3. Green Tea Induces Apoptotic Cell Death and Cell-Cycle Arrest

Because the life-span of both normal and cancer cells within a living system are significantly affected by the rate of apoptosis (25), chemopreventive agents that modulate apoptosis may affect the steady-state cell population. Several cancer chemopreventive agents induce apoptosis; on the other hand, tumor-promoting agents have been found to inhibit apoptosis (26–28). Therefore, it can be assumed that chemopreventive agents with proven effects in animal tumor bioassay systems and/or human epidemiology plus the ability to induce cancer cell apoptosis may have wider implications for cancer management. At present, a limited number of chemopreventive agents are known to cause apoptosis (29,30). In our laboratory, we showed that EGCG induces apoptosis and cell-cycle arrest in human epidermoid carcinoma (A431) cells (31). Importantly, this apoptotic response was specific for cancer cells—EGCG treatment also resulted in induction of apoptosis in human carcinoma keratinocytes HaCaT, human prostate carcinoma cells DU145, and mouse lymphoma cells LY-R, but not in normal human epidermal keratinocytes.

Another study (32) compared the effect of EGCG on the growth of SV40 virally transformed human fibroblasts (WI38VA) with that of normal WI38 cells. In this study, EGCG was found to inhibit the growth of transformed WI38VA cells, but not of their normal counterparts. This study further demonstrated a similar differential growth-inhibitory effect of EGCG between human colorectal cancer (CRC) (Caco-2) cells, breast cancer (Hs578T) cells, and their respective normal counterparts. EGCG treatment also induced apoptosis and enhanced serum-induced expression of c-*fos* and c-*myc* genes in transformed WI38VA cells, but not in the normal WI38 cells. This study suggested that the differential modulation of certain genes, such as c-*fos* and c-*myc*, could be responsible for these differential responses of EGCG.

In another study (33), it was demonstrated that EGCG and other tea polyphenols inhibit the growth of human lung cancer (PC-9) cells with a G_2/M phase arrest of the cell cycle. This study demonstrated that [^{3}H]EGCG administered by oral intubation into the mouse stomach results in small amounts of ^{3}H activity in many organs, such as the skin, stomach, duodenum, colon, liver, lung, and pancreas, where EGCG and green tea extract have been shown to have anticarcinogenic effects. In this study, involvement of the tumor necrosis factor (TNF)-α pathway was suggested as a mechanism of EGCG-mediated biological responses.

In another study by Yang et al. *(34)*, the growth-inhibitory effects of GTPs were investigated using four human cancer-cell lines. Growth inhibition was measured by ^{3}H thymidine incorporation after 48 h of treatment. EGCG and EGC displayed strong growth-inhibitory effects against lung tumor-cell lines H661 and H1299, with estimated IC_{50} values of 22 μ*M*, but were less effective against the lung-cancer cell line H441 and colon-cancer cell line HT-29 with IC_{50} values two- to threefold higher. ECG was found to have lower activities, whereas EC was even less effective. In another set of experiments within this study, exposure of H661 cells to a dose of 30 μM EGCG, EGC, or theaflavins for 24 h resulted in dose-dependent apoptosis. The incubation of H661 cells with EGCG also resulted in dose-dependent formation of H_2O_2. The addition of H_2O_2 to H661 cells was found to result in an apoptotic response similar to EGCG. EGCG-induced apoptosis in H661 cells was found to be completely inhibited by exogenously added catalase (50 U/mL), suggesting that tea polyphenol-mediated H_2O_2 production results in apoptosis of cells, contributing to the growth-inhibitory potential of tea polyphenols in vitro.

5.4. EGCG Inhibits Cellular Proliferation and Fhe Epidermal Growth-Factor Receptor (EGFR) Pathway

Activation of EGFR tyrosine kinase by its ligand is believed to initiate multiple cellular responses associated with cell proliferation, and overexpression of EGFR is shown to produce a neoplastic phenotype. Based on these observations, a recent study *(35)* demonstrated that EGCG significantly inhibits DNA synthesis and protein tyrosine kinase (PTK) activities of EGFR, PDGFR, and FGFR, but not pp60^{v-src}, protein kinase (PK) C and PKA in A431 cells. EGCG was also found to inhibit the auto-phosphorylation of EGFR by EGF and block binding of EGF to its receptor. This study suggests that EGCG might inhibit tumor development by blocking the EGFR pathway.

5.5. EGCG Inhibits Induction of Nitric Oxide Synthase (NOS) via Downregulation in the Transcription Factor Nuclear Factor-κB (NFκB)

Since NO is a bioactive molecule that plays an important role in inflammation and carcinogenesis, in a recent study *(36)*, Lin and Lin evaluated the effects of GTPs on modulation of NOS in thioglycollate-elicited and lipopolysaccharide (LPS)-activated peritoneal macrophages. Gallic acid (GA), EGC, and EGCG were found to inhibit the protein expression of inducible NOS (iNOS) as well as generation of NO. This study further demonstrated that EGCG inhibits activation of the transcrition factor NFκB, an event believed to be associated with the induction of iNOS. As a whole, these data suggested that EGCG may block an early event of NOS induction via inhibiting the binding of transcription factor NFκB to the iNOS promoter, thereby inhibiting induction of iNOS transcription. The involvement of NO in the biological response of EGCG was validated by another study *(37)* where it was demonstrated that EGCG causes inhibition of LPS- and interferon (IFN) γ- activated iNOS mRNA expression in a cell-culture system. EGCG was also found to inhibit enzyme activities of iNOS and neuronal KNOS (nNOS).

Peroxynitrite (OONO) is a highly toxic oxidizing and nitrating species produced in vivo via a reaction between superoxide radical (O_2^-) and NO. In another study, Pannala et al. *(38)* demonstrated the ability of GTPs (catechin, epicatechin, ECG, EGC, and EGCG) to inhibit OONO-mediated tyrosine-nitration and limit surface-charge alteration of low-density lipoprotein (LDL). In this study, all tested compounds were found to be potent OONO scavengers, effective in preventing tyrosine nitration. These polyphenols were also found to protect against OONO-mediated LDL modification.

EGCG was found to differentially regulate expression of NFκB in cancer cells vs normal cells *(39)*. EGCG treatment of human epidermoid carcinoma (A431) cells resulted in dose-dependent lowering of NFκB levels in both the cytoplasm and nucleus, yet inhibition of constitutive and induced expression of NFκB was observed only at higher concentrations in normal human epidermal keratinocytes *(39)*

5.6. EGCG Inhibits Tumor Promoter-Mediated Activator Protein-1 (AP-1) Activation and Cell Transformation

Because many studies have suggested that AP-1 activation plays an important role in tumor promotion, downregulation of this transcription factor is believed to be a general therapeutic strategy against cancer *(40)*. In a study employing an extensively used JB6 mouse epidermal-cell line in vitro model system for tumor-promotion studies, Dong et al. *(41)* investigated the antitumor-promoting effects of EGCG and theaflavins. Both were found to inhibit EGF- or TPA-induced cell transformation, AP-1-dependent transcriptional activity, and DNA-binding activity. This study further showed that inhibition of AP-1 activation occurs via inhibition of a c-Jun NH_2-terminal kinase-dependent pathway.

5.7. EGCG Treatment Results in Cell-Cycle Dysregulation

Disruption of the cell cycle is the hallmark of a cancer cell. EGCG treatment of A431 cells resulted in inhibition of cell growth and arrest of cells in the G_0/G_1 phase of the cell cycle, and induction of apoptosis possibly mediated through inhibition of NFκB *(42)*. In another study, Ahmad et al. *(42)* provided evidence for the involvement of cyclin kinase inhibitor (cki)-cyclin-cyclin-dependent kinase (CDK) machinery during cell-cycle deregulation by EGCG. More recently, we have shown involvement of the retinoblastoma-E2F/DP pathway in the antiproliferative effects of EGCG in A431 cells *(43)*.

5.8. EGC Inhibits PTK Activity, c-jun mRNA Expression, and JNK1 Activation

Lu et al. *(44)* investigated some possible mechanisms involved with the antiproliferative ability of EGC. Employing rat aortic smooth muscle (A7r5) cells, it was demonstrated that EGC inhibited serum-stimulated membranous PTK activity. EGC was also found to reduce phosphorylation at tyrosine of many proteins with different mol wts, indicating that EGC may inhibit PTK activity or stimulate protein phosphatase activity of these proteins. It was further demonstrated that EGC reduces levels of c-*jun* mRNA, phosphorylated JNK1, and JNK1-kinase activity. These data suggest that the antiproliferative effect of EGC—at least in part—is mediated through inhibition of PTK activity, reducing c-*jun* mRNA expression, and inhibiting JNK1 activation.

The involvement of PTK activity and protein phosphorylation was further examined in another study, in which Kennedy et al. *(45)* evaluated the antiproliferative mechanism of GTPs in Ehrlich ascites tumor cells. In this study, EGC and EGCG treatments were found to result in a significant decrease in cell viability. EGC, but not EGCG, stimulated PTK activity. EGC treatment also resulted in tyrosine phosphoryla-tion of 42- and 45-kDa proteins, and ornithine decarboxylase (ODC), a key enzyme in polyamine biosynthesis in cells.

5.9. Green Tea Inhibits Angiogenesis and Tumor Invasion

The ability of cancer cells to move from their original sites and invade surrounding tissue is a phenomenon that makes cancer a deadly or life-threatening disease. Once tumors become aggressive and metastasize to other organs, even systemic chemotherapy may be in vain. Jankun et al. *(46)* showed that the main flavonol of green tea, EGCG, inhibits urokinase, one of the hydrolases implicated in tumor invasion. EGCG was found to inhibit tumor-cell invasion and directly suppress the activity of matrix metalloproteases (MMP) 2 and MMP9, two proteases most frequently overexpressed in cancer and angiogenesis that are essential in cutting through basement membrane barriers *(47)*. Oral feeding of GTPs to animals that spontaneously develop prostate cancer inhibited tumor growth, metastasis, and angiogenesis, as a result of the inhibition of vascular endothelial growth factor (VEGF), a marker of angiogenesis, and also because of suppression of MMP2 and MMP9 activities *(48)*. In vitro studies have also suggested that EGCG treatment of human umbilical-vein endothelial cells results in dose-dependent inhibition of endothelial cells, possibly through inhibition of MMPs *(49)*.

6. GREEN TEA AND SKIN CANCER

Skin is the largest body organ, and serves as a protective barrier against environmental insults such as UV radiation-induced damage. Much of the deleterious effect of solar UV radiation is caused by UVB (290–320 nm). Although the long-term abnormalities of UVB typically become evident in the population age 50 yr and older, epidemiologic studies indicate that much of the critical sunlight exposure responsible for these adverse effects is received at a young age. Recent epidemiological observations suggest that sun-exposed individuals with a history of non-melanoma skin cancer have an increased risk of melanoma and certain non-cutaneous cancers. UVB induces skin cells to produce reactive oxygen species (ROS), eicosanoids, proteinases, and cytokines; the inhibition of these mediators is considered to reduce skin damage. Antioxidants such as ascorbic acid and α-tocopherol have been demonstrated to produce photoprotective effects in some in vitro and in vivo studies (reviewed in *50,51*).

Studies have suggested that GTPs may afford protection against inflammatory responses and the risk of skin cancer. Topical application of GTPs to mouse skin inhibits 12-*O*-tetradecanoylphorbol-13-acetate and other skin tumor promoter caused induction of protein and mRNA expression of the proinflammatory cytokines interleukin (IL)-1α and TNFα. In C3H/HeN mice, skin application of GTPs inhibits UV-radiation-induced local responses, and systemic administration suppresses contact hypersensitivity and edema responses. Many in vitro studies have shown preventive effects of GTPs or crude extracts of green tea in systems that are considered essential to inflammatory and carcinogenic processes *(5,7,8)*.

The relevance of extensive in vitro and in vivo laboratory data to adverse effects caused by solar UVB in human skin is unclear. This information can be based on epidemiological studies in high-risk populations, or based on the use of short-term assays with noninvasive techniques and acceptable protocols in human volunteers. We evaluated the effect of skin-applied GTPs against UV-induced erythema in human volunteers. In this study, a polyphenolic fraction obtained from green tea was applied on the untanned backs of normal volunteers, and 30 min later the sites were exposed to twice the minimal erythemogenic dose (MED) of UV radiation from a solar simulator. Sites pretreated with GTPs exhibited significantly less erythema compared to vehicle-treated sites. The photoprotective effects of GTPs were dependent on the dose of GTPs applied with maximum protection observed with 200 μL of a 5% solution. In time-course studies, a GTP-mediated cutaneous photoprotective effect was evident even when UV irradiation was delayed for many hours. The protective effects lasted for at least 72 h, thus indicating a relatively long-term protection, particularly against chronic low-dose environmental insult. Skin application of GTPs to human volunteers also resulted in significant protection against 2X MED-induced enhancements of sunburn cell formation and depletion of CD1a⁺ Langerhans-cell density *(52)*.

We also investigated whether topical application of EGCG protects against UVB-induced adverse effects in human skin *(53)*. In this study, we evaluated the effect of EGCG treatment on inhibition of UVB-induced infiltration of leukocytes (macrophage/neutrophils), a potential source of generation of ROS and prostaglandin (PG) metabolites, which play critical roles in skin tumor promotion in multistage skin carcinogenesis. Human subjects were exposed to UVB radiation (at 4× MED doses) on sun-protected skin, and skin biopsies or keratomes were obtained 24 or 48 h later. We found that topical application of EGCG (3 mg/2.5 cm²) before UVB exposure to human skin significantly blocked UVB-induced infiltration of leukocytes and reduced myeloperoxidase activity; leukocyte infiltration is considered the major source of ROS generation. In the same set of experiments, we found that topical application of EGCG before UVB exposure decreased UVB-induced erythema. In additional experiments, we found that EGCG treatment before UVB exposure produced significantly lower PG metabolites, particularly PGE₂, in the epidermal microsomal fraction of the skin compared to non-pretreated skin. Histological examination of EGCG-pretreated and UVB-exposed human skin revealed fewer dead cells in the epidermis compared to non-pretreated UVB exposed skin. These data demonstrate that EGCG has the potential to block UVB-induced infiltration of leukocytes and the subsequent generation of ROS in human skin. This may be responsible, at least in part, for the antiinflammatory effects of green tea.

Based on the work described here, it is tempting to suggest that the use of GTP in cosmetic preparations may be a novel approach for preventing adverse effects associated with UV radiation in humans. It is of interest that many low-priced cosmetics marketed by small companies, as well as expensive lines of cosmetics marketed by name-brand companies, are supplementing their products with green tea extracts.

7. GREEN TEA AND CANCER OF THE DIGESTIVE TRACT

Using 7,12-dimethylbenz *[a]* anthracene (DMBA) to induce cancer in the buccal pouch of Syrian hamsters is an animal model of carcinogenesis that closely resembles events involved in the development of precancerous lesions and cancer in the human oral cavity *(54)*. A mixed tea preparation containing 1.5% green tea extract given as the sole source of drinking water before and during DMBA treatment of hamster buccal pouches significantly reduced mean tumor burden and the incidence of dysplasia and oral carcinoma *(55)*. Green tea extracts inhibit *N*-nitrosomethyl-benzylamine (NMBA)-induced esophageal tumorigenesis in rats *(56–58)*. EGCG treatment at a dose of 1 m*M* in drinking water reduces the percentage of tumors in an animal model of N-methyl-N'-nitrosoguanidine (MNNG)-induced stomach cancer (59). The reduction in tumors was attributed to decreased ODC activity and lower polyamine levels, suggesting that EGCG inhibits cellular proliferation of gastric mucosa during the promotion stage of MNNG-induced gastric carcinogenesis. Green tea catechins and EGCG reduce the incidence of large intestinal cancers induced by 1,2-dimethylhydrazine and metastasis of these tumors to lungs in rats (60). Green tea extract given at a dose of 0.01% to 0.1% in the drinking water of rats after treatment with the carcinogen azoxymethane inhibited colon carcinogenesis. EGCG also inhibits proliferation of the human colon carcinoma-cell line SW620, which is resistant to doxorubicin (61).

8. GREEN TEA AND LIVER AND LUNG CANCER

Mice given the carcinogen diethylnitrosamine (DEN) and treated with 1.25% of green tea extract in drinking water show a 50% decrease in the number of lung and liver tumors (62). Tea extracts given in the diet at doses of 0.05% to 0.1% significantly reduce the number of preneoplastic foci in rats treated with DEN and phenobarbital (63). Catechins are effective when administered during or after carcinogenic treatment; they appear to act during both tumor initiation and promotion stages. Green tea extract at doses of 1% to 2% inhibits spontaneous formation of lung tumors in mice (64). Green tea at a dose of 2% and EGCG at 1.2 mM in the drinking water inhibits lung tumorigenesis in mice treated with a potent nitrosoamine found in tobacco smoke (65,66). Green tea or EGCG suppressed increases in the level of 8-OH-dG in mouse lung DNA as a result of nitrosoamine treatment. Since 8-OH-dG is a DNA lesion caused by oxidative damage, EGCG's effect may be partly attributable to its antioxidant activity (65). Oral administration of green tea and EGCG inhibits metastasis of Lewis lung carcinoma LL2 cells in mice (67,68). Since superoxide can enhance the invasiveness of tumor cells (67), EGCG's radical scavenging activity may be related to its inhibition of cancer-cell invasion and metastasis (68). Green tea at a dose of 0.6%, as the sole source of drinking water, reduces tumor multiplicity in transgenic mice treated with 4-(methylnitrosamino)-1-(3-pyridyl)-1-butanone (NNK) (69). Drinking tea for to 4–8 wk reduces NNK-induced expression of mouse lung oncogenes,

such as c-myc, c-raf and c-H-ras, suggesting a possible mechanism of green tea action through modulation of oncogene expression (70).

9. GREEN TEA AND BREAST CANCER

A single dose of DMBA in female SD rats induces mammary gland carcinogenesis (71). Treating these female rats with 1% green tea extract in the diet 1 wk after DMBA administration does not significantly affect the incidence and multiplicity of DMBA-induced mammary tumors. However, starting at 10–18 wk, the average size of palpable mammary tumors is significantly reduced. The survival rate is 94% for the green tea catechins group and 33% for the DMBA-treated group that did not receive the catechins (72). However, when rats are given a diet containing 0.5% of tea extract 13 wk after DMBA treatment, there is no significant effect on tumor incidence and multiplicity (73,74). On the basis of these observations, it appears that green tea catechins are more effective at early post-initiation stages, but not at later stages of tumorigenesis. In another study, green tea catechin extract administered at a dose of 0.5% in drinking water prevented spontaneous mammary tumor incidence and burden in C3H mice and inhibited DMBA-induced mammary tumors in rats (75).

10. GREEN TEA AND PROSTATE CANCER

Green tea and its major constituent EGCG inhibit the growth of a variety of human prostate cancer-cell lines. EGCG treatment of LNCaP (androgen-responsive) and DU145 (androgen-unresponsive) cell lines at a dose of 10–80 µg/mL resulted in dose-dependent inhibition of cell growth, arrest of cell cycle, and induction of apoptosis (76). It appears that cell-cycle arrest produced by EGCG is dependent on p53 status in LNCaP cells, but not in DU145 cells, and is mediated by p21 in both the cell types (76). GTPs also downregulate the androgen receptor in LNCaP cells (77). The transgenic adenocarcinoma mouse prostate (TRAMP) model has recently emerged as an excellent model for prostate cancer (CaP), as it closely mimics progressive forms of human disease from prostatic intraepithelial neoplasia (PIN) to histologic cancer and from histologic to metastasizing prostate carcinoma (78). In TRAMP, the following stages arise sequentially over the 42-wk average lifespan of these mice, which characteristically express the T-antigen oncoprotein by 8 wk of age and develop distinct pathology in the epithelium of the dorsolateral prostate by 10 wk of age. Distant-site metastasis can be detected as early as 12 wk of age, and by 28 wk of age, 100% of animals harbor carcinoma that metastasizes to lymph nodes and lungs (78). In a recent study, the effect of oral GTP at a human-achievable dose on carcinoma development and progression was determined in the TRAMP model. In two independent experiments, oral feeding of 0.1% GTP in the drinking water for 20 wk beginning at 8 wk of age resulted in a substantial reduction in tumor burden, as assessed sequentially during the course of the study by MRI and at termination of the experiment by measuring the size and weight of the dorsolateral prostate and genito-urinary apparatus. Importantly, in GTP-fed mice, significant inhibition in serum insulin growth factor-1 (IGF) and restoration of IGF-binding protein-3 was observed at 7, 14, and 20 wk on test. None of the 20 GTP-fed TRAMP mice exhibited distant-site metastases to lymph nodes and lungs. Further more, these chemopreventive effects of GTP against carcinoma development were confirmed by histopathological examination and proliferating cell nuclear antigen (PCNA) staining in the dorsolateral prostate tissue (79). Further, more GTP treatment of TRAMP mice inhibited metastasis and angiogenesis by inhibiting MMPs and VEGF (48). These data further demonstrate that green tea could be an effective chemopreventive agent against the development of prostate cancer. In a later study by Wang and Mukhtar (80), EGCG treatment of the prostate cancer cell line LNCaP altered expression of genes belonging to the G-protein signaling network. These EGCG-responsive genes may provide key insight that will help to understand mechanisms of action of other polyphenolic compounds in CaP chemoprevention (80).

11. MODULATORY EFFECTS OF GREEN TEA FOR CANCER CHEMOTHERAPY

Green tea can also increase the efficacy of cancer-chemotherapeutic drugs (81). Oral administration of green tea enhanced the tumor-inhibitory effects of doxorubicin on Ehrlich ascites carcinomas implanted in CDF_1 and BDF_1 mice. Green tea treatment resulted in increased availability of doxorubicin to the tumor, but not to normal tissue. If verified in humans, these observations may be relevant to cancer chemotherapy.

12. CONCLUSION AND FUTURE DIRECTIONS

During the last decade, approximately ten million cases of cancer were diagnosed, and four million cancer-related deaths occurred. It is believed that almost one-third of the cancers are caused by dietary and lifestyle-related habits; manipulation of the diet is increasingly being recognized as a potential strategy against cancer (5,7,8,82). The use of tea, especially green tea, as a cancer-chemopreventive agent has only been appreciated in the last 10–12 years. Green tea is a popular beverage, is relatively inexpensive and non-toxic, and has been shown to afford protection against many cancer types. Epidemiological as well as laboratory studies have shown an inverse association of green tea consumption with the development of certain cancer types. Although compelling evidence now indicates green tea's cancer-preventive potential, a clear understanding of the mechanisms associated with its action is far from complete. A complete knowledge of the molecular mechanism(s) involved with the anticarcinogenic efficacy of GTPs may be useful in devising better chemopreventive strategies against cancer.

In view of the available data from laboratory and epidemiological studies, clinical trials are now warranted to evaluate the usefulness of green tea and its polyphenolic antioxidants. Vastag (83) realized that a cup of tea provides an antioxidant boost that may protect against several cancer types, and these tea antioxidants are much more potent than vitamin C and E in their ability to scavenge potentially carcinogenic free radicals. It is important to emphasize here that Phase I clinical trials to evaluate the possible efficacy of formulated green tea in patients with advanced solid tumors are currently underway at the M.D. Anderson Cancer Center and the Memorial Sloan-Kettering Cancer Center.

REFERENCES

1. Kelloff GJ, Hawk ET, Crowell JA, et al. Strategies for identification and clinical evaluation of promising chemopreventive agents. *Oncology* 1996;10:1471–1488.
2. Challa A, Ahmad N, Mukhtar H. Cancer prevention through sensible nutrition (commentary). *Int J Oncol* 1997;11:1387–1392.
3. Pezzuto JM. Plant-derived anticancer agents. *Biochem Pharmacol* 1997;53:121–133.
4. Dragsted LO, Strube M, Larsen JC. Cancer-protective factors in fruits and vegetables: biochemical and biological background. *Pharmacol Toxicol* 1993;72:116–135.
5. Mukhtar H, Ahmad N. Cancer chemoprevention: future holds in multiple agents. *Toxicol Appl Pharmacol* 1999;158:207–210.

6. Khan WA, Wang ZY, Athar M, et al. Inhibition of the skin tumorigenicity of (+/−)-7 beta,8 alpha-dihydroxy-9 alpha,10 alpha-epoxy-7,8,9,10-tetrahydrobenzo[*a*]pyrene by tannic acid, green tea polyphenols and quercetin in Sencar mice. *Cancer Lett* 1988;42:7–12.

7. Katiyar SK, Mukhtar H. Tea in chemoprevention of cancer: epidemiologic and experimental studies. *Int J Oncol* 1996;8:221–238.

8. Ahmad N, Katiyar SK, Mukhtar H. Cancer chemoprevention by tea polyphenols, in *Nutrition and Chemical Toxicity.* Ioannides C, ed.John Wiley & Sons Ltd., West Sussex, England, 1996, pp. 301–343.

9. Wang ZY, Khan WA, Bickers DR, Mukhtar H. Protection against polycyclic aromatic hydrocarbon-induced skin tumor initiation in mice by green tea polyphenols. *Carcinogenesis* 1989;10:411–415.

10. Wang ZY, Cheng SJ, Zhou ZC, et al. Antimutagenic activity of green tea polyphenols. *Mutat Res* 1989;223:273–285.

11. Liao S, Kao YH, Hiipakka RA. Green tea: biochemical and biological basis for health benefits. *Vitam Horm* 2001;62:1–94.

12. Weisburger JH, Rivenson A, Garr K, Aliaga C. Tea, or tea and milk, inhibit mammary gland and colon carcinogenesis in rats. *Cancer Lett* 1997;114:323–327.

13. Harbowy ME, Balentine, DA. Tea chemistry. *Crit Rev Plant Sci* 1997;16:415–480.

14. Yang CS, Wang ZY. Tea and cancer. *J Natl Cancer Inst* 1993;85:1038–1049.

15. Yang CS, Maliakal P, Meng X. Inhibition of carcinogenesis by tea. *Annu Rev Pharmacol Toxicol* 2002;42:25–54.

16. Conney AH, Lu Y, Lou Y, et al. Inhibitory effect of green and black tea on tumor growth. *Proc Soc Exp Biol Med* 1999;220:229–233.

17. Kohlmeier L, Weterings KGC, Steck S, Kok FJ. Tea and cancer prevention: an evaluation of the epidemiologic literature. *Nutr Cancer* 1997;27:1–13.

18. Suganuma M, Okabe S, Oniyama M, et al. Wide distribution of [^{3}H](-)-epigallocatechin-3-gallate, a cancer chemopreventive tea polyphenol, in mouse tissue. *Carcinogenesis* 1998;19:1771–1776.

19. Mukhtar H, Katiyar SK, Agarwal R. Green tea and skin-anticarcinogenic effects. *J Investig Dermatol* 1994;102:3–7.

20. International Agency for Research on Cancer. Coffee, Tea, Mate, Methylxanthines and Methylglyoxal. *IARC Monogr Eval Carcinog Risks Hum* 1991;51:207.

21. Yang CS, Chen L, Lee MJ, et al. Blood and urine levels of tea catechins after ingestion of different amounts of green tea by human volunteers. *Cancer Epidemiol Biomark Prev* 1998;7:351–354.

22. Yu, R, Jiao, JJ, Duh, JL, et al. Activation of mitogen-activated protein kinases by green tea polyphenols: potential signaling pathways in the regulation of antioxidant-responsive element-mediated phase II enzyme gene expression. *Carcinogenesis* 1997;18:451–456.

23. Jankun J, Selman SH, Swiercz R, Skrzypczak-Jankun E. Why drinking green tea could prevent cancer. *Nature* 1997;387:561.

24. Yang CS. Inhibition of carcinogenesis by tea. *Nature* 1997;389:134–135.

25. Fesus L, Szondy Z, Uray I. Probing the molecular program of apoptosis by cancer chemopreventive agents. *J Cell Biochem (Suppl)* 1995;22:151–161.

26. Boolbol SK, Dannenberg AJ, Chadburn A, et al. Cyclooxygenase-2 overexpression and tumor formation are blocked by sulindac in murine model of familial polyposis. *Cancer Res* 1996;56:2556–2560.

27. Mills JJ, Chari RS, Boyer IJ, et al. Induction of apoptosis in liver tumors by the monoterpene perillyl alcohol. *Cancer Res* 1995;55:979–983.

28. Wright SC, Zhong J, Larrick JW. Inhibition of apoptosis as a mechanism of tumor promotion. *FASEB J* 1994;8:654–660.

29. Jiang MC, Yang-Yen HF, Yen JJY, Lin JK. Curcumin induces apoptosis in immortalized NIH 3T3 and malignant cancer cell lines. *Nutr Cancer* 1996;26:111–120.

30. Jee SH, Shen SC, Tseng CR, et al. Curcumin induces p53-dependent apoptosis in human basal cell carcinoma cells. *J Investig Dermatol* 1998;111:656–661.

31. Ahmad N, Feyes DK, Nieminen A-L, et al. Green tea constituent epigallocatechin-3-gallate and induction of apoptosis and cell cycle arrest in human carcinoma cells. *J Natl Cancer Inst* 1997;89:1881–1886.

32. Chen ZP, Schell JB, Ho CT, Chen KY. Green tea epigallocatechin gallate shows a pronounced growth inhibitory effect on cancerous cells but not on their normal counterparts. *Cancer Lett* 1998;129:173–179.

33. Fujiki H, Suganuma M, Okabe S, et al. Cancer inhibition by green tea. *Mutat Res* 1998;402:307–310.

34. Yang GY, Liao J, Kim K, et al. Inhibition of growth and induction of apoptosis in human cancer cell lines by tea polyphenols. *Carcinogenesis* 1998;19:611–616.

35. Liang YC, Lin-shiau SY, Chen CF, Lin JK. Suppression of extracellular signals and cell proliferation through EGF receptor binding by (−)-epigallocatechin gallate in human A431 epidermoid carcinoma cells. *J Cell Biochem* 1997;67:55–65.

36. Lin YL, Lin JK. (−)-Epigallocatechin-3-gallate blocks the induction of nitric oxide synthase by down-regulating lipopolysaccharide-induced activity of transcription factor nuclear factor-kappaB. *Mol Pharmacol* 1997;52:465–472.

37. Chan MM, Fong D, Ho CT, Huang HI. Inhibition of inducible nitric oxide synthase gene expression and enzyme activity by epigallocatechin gallate, a natural product from green tea. *Biochem Pharmacol* 1997;54:1281–1286.

38. Pannala A, Rice-Evans CA, Halliwell B, Singh S. Inhibition of peroxynitrite-mediated tyrosine nitration by catechin polyphenols. *Biochem Biophys Res Commun* 1997;232:164–168.

39. Ahmad N, Gupta S, Mukhtar H. Green tea polyphenol epigallocatechin-3-gallate differentially modulates nuclear factor kappaB in cancer cells versus normal cells. *Arch Biochem Biophys* 2000;376:338–346.

40. McCarty MF. Polyphenol-mediated inhibition of AP-1 transactivating activity may slow cancer growth by impeding angiogenesis and tumor invasiveness. *Med Hypotheses* 1998;50:511–514.

41. Dong Z, Ma W-y, Huang C, Yang CS. Inhibition of tumor promoter-induced activator protein 1 activation and cell transformation by tea polyphenols, (−)-epigallocatechin gallate and theaflavins. *Cancer Res* 1997;57:4414–4419.

42. Ahmad N, Cheng P, Mukhtar H. Cell cycle dysregulation by green tea polyphenol epigallocatechin-3-gallate. *Biochem Biophys Res Commun* 2000;275:328–334.

43. Ahmad N, Adhami VM, Gupta S, et al. Role of retinoblastoma (pRB)-E2F/DP pathway in cancer chemopreventive effects of

green tea polyphenol epigallocatechin-3-gallate. *Arch Biochem Biophys* 2002;398:125–131.

44. Lu, LH, Lee, SS, Huang, HC. Epigallocatechin suppression of proliferation of vascular smooth muscle cells: correlation with c-jun and JNK. *Br J Pharmacol* 1998;124:1227–1237.

45. Kennedy DO, Nishimura S, Hasuma T, et al. Involvement of protein tyrosine phosphorylation in the effect of green tea polyphenols on Ehrlich ascites tumor cells in vitro. *Chem Biol Interact* 1998;110:159–172.

46. Jankun J, Selman SH, Swiercz R, Jankun ES. Why drinking green tea could prevent cancer. *Nature* 1997;387:381.

47. Garbisa S, Biggin S, Cavallarin N, et al. Tumor invasion: molecular shears blunted by green tea. *Nature* 1999;5:1216.

48. Ahmad N, Adhami VM, Gupta S, et al. Involvement of matrix metalloproteinase as a mechanism of inhibition of prostate cancer development and its metastasis by green tea polyphenols in tramp mice. *Proc Am Assoc Cancer Res* 2001;42:141.

49. Singh AK, Seth P, Anthony P, et al. Green tea constituent epigallocatechin-3-gallate inhibits angiogenic differentiation of human endothelial cells. *Arch Biochem Biophys* 2002;401:29–37.

50. Elmets CA, Mukhtar H. Ultraviolet radiation and skin cancer: progress in pathophysiologic mechanisms. *Prog Dermatol* 1996;30:1–16.

51. Mukhtar H, Elmets CA. Photocarcinogenesis: mechanisms, models and human health implications. *Photochem Photobiol* 1996;63:355–447.

52. Mukhtar H, Matsui MS, Maes D, et al. Prevention by green tea polyphenols against ultraviolet-induced erythema in humans. *J Investig Dermatol* 1996;106:846–851.

53. Katiyar SK, Matsui MS, Elmets CA, Mukhtar H. Polyphenolic antioxidant-(–)-epigallocatechin-3-gallate from green tea reduces UVB-induced inflammatory responses and infiltration of leukocytes in human skin. *Photochem Photobiol* 1999;69:148–153.

54. Gimenez-Conti IB, Slaga TJ. The hamster cheek pouch carcinogenesis model. *J Cell Biochem (Suppl)* 1993;17F:83–90.

55. Li N, Han C, Chen J. Tea preparations protect against DMBA-induced oral carcinogenesis in hamsters. *Nutr Cancer* 1999;35:73–79.

56. Chen J. The effects of Chinese tea on the occurrence of esophageal tumors induced by N-nitrosomethylbenzylamine in rats. *Prev Med* 1992;21:385–391.

57. Wang ZY, Wang LD, Lee MJ, et al. Inhibition of N-nitrosomethylbenzylamine-induced esophageal tumorigenesis in rats by green and black tea. *Carcinogenesis* 1995;16:2143–2148.

58. Morse MA, Kresty LA, Steele VE, et al. Effects of theaflavins on N-nitrosomethylbenzylamine-induced esophageal tumorigenesis. *Nutr Cancer* 1997;29:7–12.

59. Yamane T, Takahashi T, Kuwata K, et al. Inhibition of N-methyl-N'-nitro-N-nitrosoguanidine-induced carcinogenesis by (–)-epigallocatechin gallate in the rat glandular stomach. *Cancer Res* 1995;55:2081–2084.

60. Yin P, Zhao J, Cheng S, et al. Experimental studies of the inhibitory effects of green tea catechin on mice large intestinal cancers induced by 1,2-dimethylhydrazine. *Cancer Lett* 1994;79:33–38.

61. Stammler G, Volm M. Green tea catechins (EGCG and EGC) have modulating effects on the activity of doxorubicin in drug-resistant cell lines. *Anticancer Drugs* 1997;8:265–268.

62. Cao J, Xu Y, Chen J, Klaunig JE. Chemopreventive effects of green and black tea on pulmonary and hepatic carcinogenesis. *Fundam Appl Toxicol* 1996;29:244–250.

63. Matsumoto N, Kohri T, Okushio K, Hara Y. Inhibitory effects of tea catechins, black tea extract and oolong tea extract on hepatocarcinogenesis in rat. *Jpn J Cancer Res* 1996;87:1034–1038.

64. Landau JM, Wang ZY, Yang GY, et al. Inhibition of spontaneous formation of lung tumors and rhabdomyosarcomas in A/J mice by black and green tea. *Carcinogenesis* 1998;19:501–507.

65. Xu Y, Ho CT, Amin SG, et al. Inhibition of tobacco-specific nitrosamine-induced lung tumorigenesis in A/J mice by green tea and its major polyphenol as antioxidants. *Cancer Res* 1992;52:3875–3879.

66. Chung FL. The prevention of lung cancer induced by a tobacco-specific carcinogen in rodents by green and black tea. *Proc Soc Exp Biol Med* 1999;220:244–248.

67. Taniguchi S, Fujiki H, Kobayashi H, et al. Effect of (–)-epigallocatechin gallate, the main constituent of green tea, on lung metastasis with mouse B16 melanoma cell lines. *Cancer Lett* 1992;65:51–54.

68. Sazuka M, Murakami S, Isemura M, et al. Inhibitory effects of green tea infusion on in vitro invasion and in vivo metastasis of mouse lung carcinoma cells. *Cancer Lett* 1995;98:27–31.

69. Zhang Z, Liu Q, Lantry LE, et al. A germ-line p53 mutation accelerates pulmonary tumorigenesis: p53-independent efficacy of chemopreventive agents green tea or dexamethasone/myo-inositol and chemotherapeutic agents taxol or adriamycin. *Cancer Res* 2000;60:901–907.

70. Hu G, Han C, Chen J. Inhibition of oncogene expression by green tea and (–)-epigallocatechin gallate in mice. *Nutr Cancer* 1995;24:203–209.

71. Huggins C. Two principles in endocrine therapy of cancers: hormone deprival and hormone interference. *Cancer Res* 1965;25:1163–1167.

72. Hirose M, Mizoguchi Y, Yaono M, et al. Effects of green tea catechins on the progression or late promotion stage of mammary gland carcinogenesis in female Sprague-Dawley rats pretreated with 7,12-dimethylbenz(a)anthracene. *Cancer Lett* 1997;112:141–147.

73. Hirose M, Hoshiya T, Akagi K, et al. Inhibition of mammary gland carcinogenesis by green tea catechins and other naturally occurring antioxidants in female Sprague-Dawley rats pretreated with 7,12-dimethylbenz[a]anthracene. *Cancer Lett* 1994;83:149–156.

74. Tanaka H, Hirose M, Kawabe M, et al. Post-initiation inhibitory effects of green tea catechins on 7,12-dimethylbenz[a]anthracene-induced mammary gland carcinogenesis in female Sprague-Dawley rats. *Cancer Lett* 1997;116:47–52.

75. Bhide SV, Azuine MA, Lahiri M, Telang NT. Chemoprevention of mammary tumor virus-induced and chemical carcinogen-induced rodent mammary tumors by natural plant products. *Breast Cancer Res Treat* 1994;30:233–242.

76. Gupta S, Ahmad N, Nieminen AL, Mukhtar H. Growth inhibition, cell-cycle dysregulation, and induction of apoptosis by green tea constituent (–)-epigallocatechin-3-gallate in androgen-sensitive and androgen-insensitive human

prostate carcinoma cells. *Toxicol Appl Pharmacol* 2000;164:82–90.

77. Ren F, Zhang S, Mitchell SH, et al. Tea polyphenols down-regulate the expression of the androgen receptor in LNCaP prostate cancer cells. *Oncogene* 2000;19:1924–1932.

78. Foster BA, Gingrich JR, Kwon ED, et al. Characterization of prostatic epithelial cell lines derived from transgenic adeno-carcinoma of the mouse prostate. *Cancer Res* 1997;57:3325–3330.

79. Gupta S, Hastak K, Ahmad N, et al. Inhibition of prostate carcinogenesis in TRAMP mice by oral infusion of green tea polyphenols. *Proc Natl Acad Sci USA* 2001;98:10,350–10,355.

80. Wang SI, Mukhtar H. Gene expression profile in human prostate LNCaP cancer cells by (–) epigallocatechin-3-gallate. *Cancer Lett* 2002;182:43–51.

81. Sadzuka Y, Sugiyama T, Hirota S. Modulation of cancer chemotherapy by green tea. *Clin Cancer Res* 1998;4:153–156.

82. Weisburger JH. Tea antioxidants and health, in *Handbook of Antioxidants.* Cadenas E, Packer L, ed. Marcel Dekker, New York, NY, 1996, pp. 469–486.

83. Vastag B. Tea therapy? Out of the cup, into the lab. *J Natl Cancer Inst* 1998;90:1504–1505.

84. Lu YP, Lou YR, Lin Y, et al. Inhibitory effects of orally administered green tea, black tea, and caffeine on skin car-cinogenesis in mice previously treated with ultraviolet B light (high-risk mice): relationship to decreased tissue fat. *Cancer Res* 2001;61:5002–5009.

85. Katiyar SK, Afaq F, Azizuddin K, Mukhtar H. Inhibition of UVB-induced oxidative stress-mediated phosphorylation of mitogen-activated protein kinase signaling pathways in cultured human epidermal keratinocytes by green tea polyphenol (–)-epigallocatechin-3-gallate. *Toxicol Appl Pharmacol* 2001;176:110–117.

86. Katiyar SK, Mukhtar H. Green tea polyphenol (–)-epigal-locatechin-3-gallate treatment to mouse skin prevents UVB-induced infiltration of leukocytes, depletion of anti-gen-presenting cells, and oxidative stress. *J Leukoc Biol* 2001;69:719–726.

87. Nomura M, Kaji A, He Z, et al. Inhibitory mechanisms of tea polyphenols on the ultraviolet B-activated phosphatidylinos-itol 3-kinase-dependent pathway. *J Biol Chem* 2001;276:46,624–46,631.

88. Setiawan VW, Zhang ZF, Yu GP, et al. Protective effect of green tea on the risks of chronic gastritis and stomach cancer. *Int J Cancer* 2001;92:600–604.

89. Hibasami H, Komiya T, Achiwa Y, et al. Induction of apop-tosis in human stomach cancer cells by green tea catechins. *Oncol Rep* 1998;5:527–529.

90. Yamane T, Takahashi T, Kuwata K, et al. Inhibition of *N*-methyl-*N*'-nitro-*N*-nitrosoguanidine-induced carcinogenesis by (–)-epigallocatechin gallate in the rat glandular stomach. *Cancer Res* 1995;55:2081–2084.

91. Katiyar SK, Agarwal R, Mukhtar H. Protective effects of green tea polyphenols administered by oral intubation against chem-ical carcinogen-induced forestomach and pulmonary neoplasia in A/J mice. *Cancer Lett* 1993;73: 167–172.

92. Katiyar SK, Agarwal R, Zaim MT, Mukhtar H. Protection against *N*-nitrosodiethylamine and benzo[a]pyrene-induced forestomach and lung tumorigenesis in A/J mice by green tea. *Carcinogenesis* 1993;14:849–855.

93. Wang ZY, Agarwal R, Khan WA, Mukhtar H. Protection against benzo[a]pyrene- and *N*-nitrosodiethylamine-induced lung and forestomach tumorigenesis in A/J mice by water extracts of green tea and licorice. *Carcinogenesis* 1992;13:1491–1494.

94. Okabe S, Suganuma M, Hayashi M, et al. Mechanisms of growth inhibition of human lung cancer cell line, PC-9, by tea polyphenols. *Jpn J Cancer Res* 1997;88:639–643.

95. Qin G, Ning Y, Lotlikar PD. Chemoprevention of aflatoxin B1-initiated and carbon tetrachloride-promoted hepatocar-cinogenesis in the rat by green tea. *Nutr Cancer* 2000;38:215–222.

96. Uesato S, Kitagawa Y, Kamishimoto M, et al. Inhibition of green tea catechins against the growth of cancerous human colon and hepatic epithelial cells. *Cancer Lett* 2001;170:41–44.

97. Sai K, Kai S, Umemura T, et al. Protective effects of green tea on hepatotoxicity, oxidative DNA damage and cell prolifera-tion in the rat liver induced by repeated oral administration of 2-nitropropane. *Food Chem Toxicol* 1998 36:1043–1051.

98. Cao J, Xu Y, Chen J, Klaunig JE. Chemopreventive effects of green and black tea on pulmonary and hepatic carcinogenesis. *Fundam Appl Toxicol* 1996;29:244–250.

99. Majima T, Tsutsumi M, Nishino H, et al. Inhibitory effects of beta-carotene, palm carotene, and green tea polyphenols on pancreatic carcinogenesis initiated by N-nitrosobis(2-oxopropyl)amine in Syrian golden hamsters. *Pancreas* 1998;16:13–18.

100. Takabayashi F, Harada N, Tahara S, et al. Effect of green tea catechins on the amount of 8-hydroxydeoxyguanosine (8-OHdG) in pancreatic and hepatic DNA after a single administration of *N*-nitrosobis(2-oxopropyl)amine (BOP). *Pancreas* 1997;15:109–112.

101. Takabayashi F, Harada N. Effects of green tea catechins (Polyphenon 100) on cerulein-induced acute pancreatitis in rats. *Pancreas* 1997;14:276–279.

102. Ji BT, Chow WH, Hsing AW, et al. Green tea consumption and the risk of pancreatic and colorectal cancers. *Int J Cancer* 1997;70:255–258.

103. Gupta S, Ahmad N, Mohan RR, et al. Prostate cancer chemoprevention by green tea: in vitro and in vivo inhibition of testosterone-mediated induction of ornithine decarboxy-lase. *Cancer Res* 1999;59:2115–2120.

104. Chung LY, Cheung TC, Kong SK, et al. Induction of apop-tosis by green tea catechins in human prostate cancer DU145 cells. *Life Sci* 2001;68:1207–1214.

105. Paschka AG, Butler R, Young CY. Induction of apoptosis in prostate cancer cell lines by the green tea component, (–)-epigallocatechin-3-gallate. *Cancer Lett* 1998;130:1–7.

106. Pianetti S, Guo S, Kavanagh KT, Sonenshein GE. Green tea polyphenol epigallocatechin-3 gallate inhibits Her-2/neu signaling, proliferation, and transformed phenotype of breast cancer cells. *Cancer Res* 2002;62:652–655.

107. Kavanagh KT, Hafer LJ, Kim DW, et al. Green tea extracts decrease carcinogen-induced mammary tumor burden in rats and rate of breast cancer cell proliferation in culture. *J Cell Biochem* 2001;82:387–398.

108. Liao S, Umekita Y, Guo J, et al. Growth inhibition and regression of human prostate and breast tumors in athymic mice by tea epigallocatechin gallate. *Cancer Lett* 1995;96:239–243.

31 Vitamin E as a Cancer Chemopreventive Agent

Han-Yao Huang, MPH, PhD, Sonja Berndt, PharmD, and Kathy J. Helzlsouer, MD, MHS

CONTENTS

1. INTRODUCTION

Vitamin E, considered the most important lipid-soluble antioxidant in humans, plays a role in cancer chemoprevention that is substantiated by evidence from in vitro studies since the mid-1980s on its antioxidant effects, and more recent studies of effects beyond an antioxidant mechanism, such as antiin-flammation, inhibition of cancer-cell proliferation and growth, apoptosis, and angiogenesis. To date, most studies have focused predominantly on a specific form of vitamin E—e.g., α-tocopherol. In recent years, in vitro studies increasingly suggest that other forms of vitamin E also exert potent cancer-chemopreventive effects.

2. CHEMICAL STRUCTURE(S)

Naturally occurring vitamin E consists of at least eight forms: α-, β-, γ-, δ-tocopherols, and α-, β-, γ-, δ-tocotrienols, which qualitatively possess activities of α-tocopherol. Each of the eight forms consists of a chromanol ring and a side chain (Fig. 1). One form is not convertible to another in humans. The isomers, α-, β-, γ-, and δ-, differ by the number and position of methyl groups on the chromanol ring. Tocotrienols differ from tocopherols in the side chain; the former has an unsaturated isoprenoid side chain, and the latter has a saturated phytyl side chain. For each tocopherol, the positions (R or S) of the methyl groups at positions 2, 4, and 8 along the side chain give rise to eight possible stereoisomers (RRR-, RRS-, RSS-, RSR-, SRS-, SRR-, SSR-, and SSS-tocopherol) *(1)*. Of these, RRR-α-tocopherol is the only stereoisomeric form of α-tocopherol that occurs naturally in food. Natural tocotrienols have 2R and 2S stereoisomers, formed by the chiral center at position 2 on the side chain.

3. OCCURRENCE

Vitamin E exists in a variety of foods, particularly vegetable oil, seeds, nuts, and grains *(2,3)*. Meat contains small amounts of vitamin E (<1 mg total vitamin

From: Cancer Chemoprevention, Volume 1: Promising Cancer Chemoprevention Agents
Edited by: G. J. Kelloff, E. T. Hawk, and C. C. Sigman © Humana Press Inc., Totowa, NJ

Tocopherol

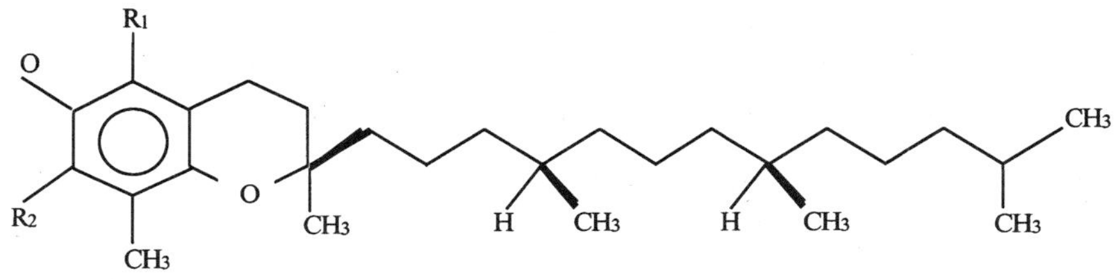

Tocotrienol

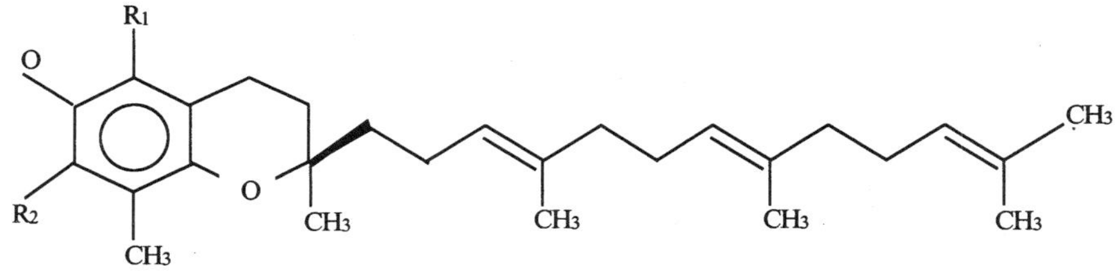

R₁	R₂	Form
CH₃	CH₃	alpha-, α-
CH₃	H	beta-, β-
H	CH₃	gamma-, γ-
H	H	delta-, δ-

Fig. 1. Structures of the tocopherols and tocotrienols.

E/100 g meat) *(3)*. Concentrations of α-tocopherol are higher in wheat germ, almond, sunflower, canola, and safflower oils. γ-Tocopherol is the major form of vitamin E in corn oil and soybean oil. Levels of tocotrienols are high in rice bran, barley, oats, and palm oil.

Because of important biological effects recognized by the scientific community in the past, the major or sole ingredient formulated in vitamin E supplements has been α-tocopherol—either in its free form or as an ester, natural or synthetic. α-Tocopherol esters (e.g., acetate or succinate) have a longer shelf life than α-tocopherol because a masked phenol moiety resists ex vivo oxidation. An α-tocopherol or α-toco-pheryl-ester supplement is either natural (historically and incorrectly labeled as *d*-α-tocopherol, rather than RRR-α-tocopherol) or synthetic (historically and incorrectly labeled as *dl*-α-tocopherol, rather than all-*rac* α-tocopherol). Supplements of RRR-α-toco-pherol that are not naturally occurring, but are derived from methylating γ-tocopherol in vegetable oil, are often commercially labeled as "natural source" vitamin E. Synthetic all-*rac* α-tocopherol represents a mixture of approximately equal amounts

of the eight stereoisomers, RRR-, RRS-, RSS-, RSR-, SRS-, SRR-, SSR-, and SSS-α-tocopherols *(1)*. These stereoisomers do not have the same biological activities. According to resorption-gestation tests in rats, the relative activity of other α-tocopherol acetate stereoisomers as compared to RRR-α-tocopherol acetate was: RRS 90%, RSS 73%, SSS 60%, RSR 57%, SRS 37%, SRR 31%, and SSR 21% *(4)*. Synthetic β-, γ-, or δ-tocopherols have not been made. Synthetic tocotrienols were made via a process that yields a mixture of R- and S-isomers *(5)*. Supplements of combined tocopherols and/or tocotrienols have been made commercially available but little is known about the biological effects of the combination.

4. DIETARY INTAKE

The minimum requirement of vitamin E for optimal body function in humans is uncertain, and may be dependent on the quantity and quality of polyunsaturated fatty acids consumed from food *(6)*, and the propensity for oxidation in the body. In 2000, the Food and Nutrition Board of the US National

Academy of Sciences defined the new recommended dietary allowance (RDA) *(7)* to be 15 mg/d of RRR-α-tocopherol (equivalent to 15 mg/d of 2-R isomeric forms of α-tocopherol or 30 mg/d of synthetic α-tocopherol) for adults, and the tolerable upper intake to be 1000 mg/d of any form of supplemental α-tocopherol. The RDA was determined primarily by induced vitamin E deficiency in humans and the correlation between in vitro hydrogen peroxide-induced erythrocyte hemolysis and plasma α-tocopherol concentrations measured by Horwitt et al. in the 1950s and 1960s *(8,9)*. The Food and Nutrition Board considered only the 2-R stereoisomers of α-tocopherol (e.g., RRR-, RSR-, RRS-, and RSS-α-tocopherol) to be the active components needed to meet vitamin E requirements in humans. The 2-S stereoisomeric forms of α-tocopherol, as well as other tocopherols and tocotrienols, were not included because their concentrations were low in plasma, and thus were considered to have less bioavailability.

According to the Third National Health and Nutrition Examination Survey (NHANES III), the mean dietary intake (excluding supplement use) of vitamin E among US adults from 1988 to 1994 was 10 mg α-tocopherol equivalents (TE) per d in men and 7.57 mg TE per d in women *(10)*. Approximately 20 mg of γ-tocopherol was consumed daily with a typical American diet *(11)*. These intakes were likely to have been underestimated as a result of underreported fat intake and missed vitamin E-fortified food items.

5. ABSORPTION

Vitamin E is lipid-soluble. Following oral ingestion, any esterified form is hydrolyzed to unesterified free form before absorption *(12)*. Both bile salts and pancreatic enzymes are essential for efficient vitamin E absorption *(13–15)*. Unesterified vitamin E is emulsified and incorporated into mixed bile salt micelles that contain hydrolyzed fat and bile salts *(16)*. Mixed micelles then move across the unstirred water layer and, by passive diffusion, are taken up by the brush-border membrane of the intestinal mucosa. Along with apolipoproteins and other lipid-soluble components, vitamin E is reassembled to form chylomicrons. Some vitamin E is delivered to peripheral cells during triglyceride hydrolysis, but most vitamin E-containing chylomicrons are secreted by exocytosis to the lymphatic system, from which chylomicrons reach the blood circulation via the *ductus thoracicus*

(17–20). Chylomicrons are then degraded to remnants by endothelial lipoprotein lipase and exchange apoliproteins with high-density lipoprotein (HDL) before hepatic uptake by apo-E and apo-B receptors *(21,22)*. There appears to be no biodiscrimination among tocopherol isomers, stereoisomers, and esters in the extent of intestinal absorption and delivery to the liver *(23–25)*. However, a 30 K_d α-tocopherol transfer protein (α-TTP) preferentially transfers RRR-α-tocopherol into nascent, very low-density lipoproteins (VLDL) in liver cytoplasm, accounting for higher concentration of RRR-α-tocopherol in plasma lipoproteins than other forms of vitamin E *(25–30)*. Selection by α-TTP is stereospecific and regiospecific because 2-R isomers, and not 2-S isomers, are preferentially incorporated *(31)*. Hence, theoretically, the bioavailability of natural α-tocopherol is approximately twofold that of synthetic α-tocopherol *(32,33)*. Compared to RRR-α-tocopherol, the estimated relative affinity with α-TTP is 38% for β-tocopherol, 9% for γ-tocopherol, 2% for δ-tocopherol, 2% for α-tocopherol acetate, 2% for α-tocopherol quinone, 11% for SRR-α-tocopherol, 12% for α-tocotrienol, and 9% for Trolox *(34)*. These relative affinities also linearly correspond to biological activities as determined by resorption and gestation tests, indicating a significant role for α-TTP in determining the biological activities of vitamin E *(34)*. In addition to the liver, the mRNA for α-TTP has been detected at low levels in the tissues of the brain, spleen, lung, and kidney in rats *(35)*.

The use of α-tocopherol supplements decreases plasma and tissue levels of other forms of vitamin E, possibly as a result of competition for hepatic transport facilitated by α-TTP. Daily supplementation with 800 mg all-*rac*-α-tocopherol for 1 yr decreased γ-tocopherol concentrations in plasma and adipose tissues, and at least 2 yr might be required before a new steady-state α-tocopherol/γ-tocopherol ratio in adipose tissue was achieved *(36)*. Short-term use of all-*rac*-α-tocopherol supplements, 1200 IU/d for 8 wk *(37)* or 800 IU/d for 4 wk *(38)*, also significantly reduced plasma concentrations of β-tocopherol *(37)* and γ-tocopherol *(37,38)*. Adding α-tocopherol to a diet that contained an equal amount of γ-tocopherol increased γ-tocopherol metabolite in bile and urine in vitamin E-deficient rats *(39)*. γ-Tocotrienol was found to have cholesterol-lowering effects by inhibiting the activities of hepatic 3-hydroxy-3-methylglutaryl coenzyme A (HMG-CoA) reductase.

In chickens, this effect was attenuated by α-tocopherol intake, and inhibition of HMG-CoA was observed only when mixed vitamin E was fed with α-tocopherol at less than 10–20% and γ- and δ-tocotrienols greater than 60% *(40)*. In turn, graded dietary levels of RRR-γ-tocopherol increased the concentration of α-tocopherol in serum, heart, liver and muscle of vitamin E-deficient rats that were replete with adequate α-tocopherol *(41)*. It has not been determined whether γ-tocopherol intake enhances circulating and tissue levels of α-tocopherol in humans who are not vitamin E-deficient.

6. DISTRIBUTION

Vitamin E is transported in unesterified forms by plasma lipoproteins to various tissues. Catabolism of triglyceride-rich lipoproteins by lipoprotein lipase, followed by binding to LDL receptor or non-receptor-mediated uptake, are involved in this process *(42,43)*. Plasma concentrations of α-tocopherol linearly increased with doses from 15–150 mg per ingestion *(44)*, and reached a plateau (80–90 μM) after long-term use at high dosages in healthy individuals *(45,46)*. Following a single dose of RRR-α-tocopherol or all *rac*-α-tocopherol, the time to peak concentration in plasma was estimated to be 12–14 h *(47)*, and the elimination half-life was approx 3 d *(48)*. In contrast, time to peak plasma concentration was estimated to be 3–4 h for α-, γ-, and δ-tocotrienol; elimination half-lives were approx 2–4 h *(49)*. The turnover rate of α-tocopherol was estimated to be one pool per d in plasma *(50)*.

Intracellular transport and retention of vitamin E may be modulated by cytosolic tocopherol-associated proteins (46 K_d) discovered in human liver, prostate, brain, heart, and kidney tissue *(51)*. The adult human liver has the highest levels of tocopherol-associated protein; the prostate and brain contain the next two highest levels (39% and 29% of the levels in the liver, respectively) *(51)*. Another tocopherol-binding protein (14.2 K_d) was found in the cytosol of human placenta *(52)*. The exact function of these tocopherol-binding proteins remains unclear.

The rate at which tissue vitamin E levels reach equilibrium varies with the site. In general, equilibrium of vitamin E uptake is achieved most rapidly in the heart, lung, brain, kidney, and liver, less rapidly in muscle and skin, and very slowly in adipose tissues *(53,54)*. A rapid rate does not always reflect the equilibrium concentrations that may depend on tocopherol-binding proteins, tissue lipid content, oxidative stress, and other antioxidants *(54)*. For example, although it is slow to reach equilibrium, adipose tissue contains approx 90% of vitamin E in the body *(55)*. In the hairless mouse, α-tocopherol is generally higher in all tissues except for the skin—where tocotrienol concentrations were found to be higher, followed by γ-tocopherol *(56)*. In contrast, brain tissue contained no detectable levels of tocotrienols, but appeared to have mechanisms for greater α-tocopherol retention and/or uptake than other tissues *(56)*. The various tocopherol and tocotrienol compositions by tissue site imply that mechanisms exist to select specific forms of vitamin E for particular cellular functions.

7. METABOLISM

Unabsorbed vitamin E is excreted into the bile and removed from the body by fecal elimination *(17)*. Oxidation of α-tocopherol results in α-tocopheryl quinone *(57)*, the major metabolite of α-tocopherol in vivo, which can then be reduced to α-tocopherylhydroquinone by NADPH-dependent microsomal and mitochondrial enzymes *(58)*. α-Tocopherylhydroquinone possesses antioxidant properties *(58,59)*. Both tocopherols and tocotrienols can be metabolized to carboxyethyl-hydroxychroman (CEHC) derivatives that are then excreted in urine *(11,60,61)*. For example, 2,5,7,8-tetramethyl-2-(2'-carboxyethyl)-6-hydroxychroman (α-CEHC) is a metabolite of α-tocopherol; 2,7,8-trimethyl-2-(2'-carboxyethyl)-6-hydroxychroman (γ-CEHC) is a metabolite of γ-tocopherol. These metabolites are not oxidative products of the chromanol ring, but of chain-shortening of tocopherols or tocotrienols, presumably via a P450-mediated process *(62)*. Only a small proportion (approx 1%) of ingested α-tocopherol is recovered as α-CEHC metabolite in urine *(63)*, and urinary α-CEHC was detectable only after plasma α-tocopherol concentrations exceeded a threshold (7–9 μmol/g total lipids). Thus, α-CEHC was suggested as an indicator of adequate α-tocopherol intake in humans *(64)*. In contrast, approx 50% of dietary γ-tocopherol was metabolized to γ-CEHC *(11)*. γ-CEHC is reported to have blood pressure-lowering *(65)*, antioxidant *(66)*, and antiinflammatory effects *(67)* in vitro, but its in vivo physiological role is rarely known. Interestingly, from doses of 125 mg/d or 250 mg/d for 1 wk in humans, only 4–6% of ingested γ-tocotrienyl acetate and 1–2% of ingested α-tocotrienyl acetate were recovered as the corresponding CEHC metabolites in urine *(61)*.

8. SAFETY CONSIDERATIONS

Tocopherols are listed as Generally Recognized As Safe (GRAS) by the Food and Drug Administration, Department of Health and Human Services (21CFR582.3890). Most toxicity studies of vitamin E focused on α-tocopherol, suggesting that it is not mutagenic, teratogenic, or carcinogenic (68). The hypothesis of a possible pro-oxidant effect of vitamin E (69,70), has not been extensively tested in vivo. In 1986, the FAO/WHO Expert Committee on Food Additives established the Acceptable Daily Intake for humans to be 0.15–2.0 mg α-tocopherol/kg body wt. From a toxicological point of view, daily doses between 10 and 150 mg were considered "absolutely safe," and daily doses of 100–300 mg were considered harmless (71). A high dose (3200 IU/d) of RRR-α-tocopheryl succinate for 9 wk in 36 patients with angina pectoris caused no major side effects except for gastrointestinal (GI) symptoms reported in isolated cases (72). Supplementation with 800 IU/d of all-rac-α-tocopherol for 4 mo had no adverse effects on a variety of outcome measures, including nutrient status, liver enzyme function, thyroid hormones, renal function, serum nonspecific immunoglobulin concentrations or anti-DNA, and anti-thyroglobulin antibodies, and hematological status, including bleeding time (73). The impact of long-term use of α-tocopherol supplements is uncertain. α-Tocopherol may exacerbate the anticoagulation defect caused by vitamin K deficiency. Thus, persons with vitamin K deficiency or those on antiplatelet therapy should avoid taking high doses of α-tocopherol.

Published data on the safety and toxicity of other forms of tocopherols and tocotrienols is limited. In a pharmacokinetics study, a single dose (1000 mg) of γ-tocopherol reportedly caused no side effects (74). Transient GI symptoms were reported in four of 12 and one of 13 hypercholesterolemic patients who used 250 mg γ-tocotrienol acetate and α-tocotrienol acetate, respectively, for 1 wk. No adverse effects were reported from subjects who used 250 mg δ-tocotrienol acetate/d (75). In one study, 125 mg/d γ-tocotrienyl acetate, 500 mg/d γ-tocotrienyl acetate, 125 mg/d α-tocotrienyl acetate, and 500 mg/d α-tocotrienyl acetate supplements were used sequentially, each for 1 wk, for a total supplementation course of 1 mo (61). In another study, 25 patients with carotid atherosclerosis took an α- and γ-tocotrienol-enriched palm oil fraction (160–240 mg of tocotrienols/d) for 18 mo. Significant atherosclerosis regression was observed in the treatment group compared to the placebo group (76). No adverse effects were reported from these two studies. A 13-wk oral toxicity evaluation of supplements containing α-, β-, γ-, and δ-tocotrienols in rats suggested that the no-observed-adverse-effect level (NOAE) for tocotrienol supplements was 0.19% of diet (120–130 mg/kg/d), based on hematological changes observed in female rats and pathological changes in the liver of male rats at high doses (77).

9. MECHANISMS OF ACTION

9.1. Antioxidant Effects

Antioxidants represent compounds that are capable of undergoing oxidation and preventing or mitigating oxidation of other compounds. All tocopherols and tocotrienols can undergo oxidation via donation of an electron or hydride group from the hydroxyl group on the chromanol ring. α-Tocopherol is considered the most important lipid-soluble antioxidant in vivo, primarily because of its abundance in tissues, erythrocytes, and plasma, which results from favorable α-TTP-facilitated hepatic transport. A potent chain-breaking antioxidant, α-tocopherol intercepts the propagation of lipid peroxidation induced by peroxyl radicals (lipid-OO•) or alkoxyl radicals (lipid-O•), thus protecting lipoproteins and biomembranes from damage by free radicals. Studies in vitro showed that, in lipid peroxidation chain reactions, α-tocopherol may donate a hydrogen atom to become an unusually stable α-tocopheryl radical that couples with another α-tocopheryl radical, or reacts with other antioxidants such as ascorbic acid or glutathione to regenerate α-tocopherol (78). However, in vivo data on the regeneration of α-tocopherol by ascorbic acid is inconsistent (53,79,80). α-Tocopherol may also undergo two-electron redox cycles involving α-tocopherol oxidation to 8a-substituted tocopherones that are subsequently hydrolyzed to α-tocopherylquinone (81).

Both α-tocopherol and γ-tocopherol have been shown to react with nitric oxide (NO)-related compounds such as peroxynitrite (OONO), a strong nitrating and oxidizing electrophile produced from the reaction of NO and superoxide. Because of the unsubstituted carbon at C-5 of the chromanol ring, γ-tocopherol reacts with OONO at this position to form 5-nitroso-γ-tocopherol (82), whereas α-tocopherol is oxidized by OONO to form α-tocopherylquinone

(82,83). In one study, γ-tocopherol was found to be more effective than α-tocopherol in scavenging electrophiles (83). Another study showed that OONO-mediated nitration of γ-tocopherol did not occur unless α-tocopherol was depleted, and suggested that α-tocopherol spares γ-tocopherol from nitration by reacting with transient γ-tocopherol intermediates (84).

In vitro studies suggest that the antioxidant effects of tocotrienols are equivalent to α-tocopherol in homogeneous solutions (85), but are much stronger than α-tocopherol in liposome systems (86–88). For example, α-tocotrienol was found to protect against $(Fe^{2+} + NADPH)$-induced and $(Fe^{2+} + ascorbate)$-induced lipid peroxidation in rat liver microsomes with potency of 40- to 60-fold that of α-tocopherol (88). The isoprenoid side chain of tocotrienol may contribute to its higher antioxidant activity than tocopherol by a higher mobility, a more homogeneous distribution in biomembranes, and a stronger disordering of membrane lipids (88,89).

9.2. Inhibition of Nitrosamine

N-Nitroso compounds, such as nitrosamines, are converted from dietary nitrites in the GI tract, and may contribute to the formation of gastric tumors (90). α-Tocopherol inhibits in vitro (91) and in vivo (92) formation of nitrosamines by reducing nitrous acid to NO. One study showed that serum levels of dimethylnitrosamine were lower in rats after being fed with α-tocopherol (93).

9.3. Antiinflammation

α-Tocopherol, α-tocopheryl succinate, and γ-tocopherol were shown to inhibit activation of nuclear factor κB (NF-κB), a transcription factor involved in inflammatory reactions (94–101). RRR-α-tocopherol inhibited macrophage prostaglandin (PG) E_2 production in mice via inhibition of cyclooxygenase (COX)-2 activities (2). In vitro, γ-tocopherol and its metabolite, γ-CEHC, inhibited COX-2-catalyzed synthesis of PGE_2, and γ-tocopherol reduced nitric oxide synthase (NOS) and nitrite accumulation in macrophages and epithelial cells (67). In activated human monocytes, incubation with α-tocopherol inhibited 5-lipoxygenase and thus inhibited leukotriene B_4 and proinflammatory cytokine interleukin (IL)-1β activity (103). In addition, α-tocopherol inhibited signal transduction involved in the surface expression of adhesion molecules by leukocytes and endothelial cells, suggesting an antiinflammatory effect (104).

9.4. Inhibition of Cell Proliferation and Growth

α-Tocopherol at physiological concentrations inhibits protein kinase C (PKC) (105,106), a family of kinases that are involved in cell growth, proliferation, and death. Inhibition was believed to act through a non-antioxidant mechanism because the antioxidant β-tocopherol did not have such effects (107,108). Furthermore, α-tocopheryl succinate, a non-antioxidant in in vitro settings, inhibited PKC activity at concentrations of 1–25 μM (109). α-Tocopheryl oxybutyric acid, another non-antioxidant vitamin E derivative, inhibited the elevated activity and expression of a rate-limiting enzyme of polyamine biosynthesis, ornithine decarboxylase (ODC), in the promotion phase of lung tumorigenesis in mice (110). The inhibitory effect of α-tocopherol on PKC activity may occur via activation of phospholipase A_2, which is involved in dephosphorylation of PKC-α at the G_0 and G_1 transition (111). α-Tocopoherol may also reduce the generation of membrane-derived diacylglycerol, a lipid that activates PKC translocation and activity (112,113).

α-Tocopheryl succinate inhibits in vitro proliferation and growth of various human cancer cells, including breast cancer (114–116), prostate cancer (117), colorectal carcinoma (118), gastric cancer (119), oral squamous carcinoma (120), leukemia (121), lymphoma (122), and melanoma (123). The antiproliferative effects in breast cancer-cell lines were independent of estrogen-receptor status (114), and independent of androgen sensitivity in prostate cancer-cell lines (117). Inhibition of colorectal cancer (CRC) cell proliferation was found to be p53-independent (118). Studies suggest that both succinyl and α-tocopheryl moieties are necessary to exert maximum inhibitory effects on cell proliferation (124–126). For example, RRR-α-tocopheryl succinate, but not RRR-α-tocopheryl acetate, inhibited MCF7 and MDAMB-435 breast cancer-cell growth (125).

Tocotrienols also exert potent antiproliferative effects on melanoma cells (127,128) and breast cancer cells (129–132), independent of estrogen receptors (129). At similar cellular levels, tocotrienols exert higher antiproliferative and cytotoxic effects than tocopherol on preneoplastic and neoplastic mouse mammary cell lines (132). The IC_{50}s for inhibition of B16 melanoma-cell growth were 10, 20, and 110 μM for δ-, γ-, and α-tocotrienols, respectively, whereas α-tocopoherol at >1600 μM had no inhibitory effect (132). A proposed mechanism of the antiproliferative property of tocotrienol relates to its isoprenoid side chain, which is involved in the production of isoprenoid intermediates from the mevalonate biosynthetic pathway *(133)*. These intermediates are considered to be important in the prenylation of several signal-transduction proteins that are crucial to normal cell growth *(134,135)*. Two new tocotrienols, P-21 desmethyl tocotrienol and P-25 didesmethyltocotrienol, which have no methyl group on the chromanol ring, have been isolated from rice bran *(136)*. These tocotrienols have much greater hypocholesterolemic effects, in vitro antioxidant effects, and suppressive effects on B16 melanoma-cell proliferation than α-tocopherol and α-, γ-, and δ-tocotrienols *(136)*. Although studies of tocotrienols in vitro show promise for cancer-chemopreventive activities, the weak affinity of these agents to α-TTP hinders their circulation with plasma lipoproteins after oral intake. An alternative route of administration is through the skin. Tocotrienols have been found to penetrate murine skin, with a higher accumulation in papillary dermis than α-tocopherol *(137)*. A tocotrienol-rich fraction of palm oil protected murine skin from oxidative stress produced by ultraviolet (UV) light *(138)* and ozone *(139)*.

9.5. Apoptosis

α-Tocopheryl succinate induces apoptosis in human cancer cells in vitro and in vivo through a mechanism that has not been fully elucidated, but may involve tumor necrosis factor (TNF)-related apoptosis-inducing ligand *(140)*, lysosomal instability *(141)*, and signaling pathways of transforming growth factor (TGF)-β *(142,143)*, Fas (CD95/APO-1) *(144,145)*, and c-Jun N-terminal kinase (JNK) mitogen-activated protein kinase (MAPK) *(146–148)*. The intact succinyl ester appears to be required for maximum apoptotic effects *(126)*. α-tocopheryl succinate had stronger apoptotic effects than α-tocopherol and γ-tocopherol in vitro *(132,149,150)* and in vivo *(140)*, possibly because of reduced lipophilicity, faster turnover in plasma, and better tissue accumulation *(140,151)*. Because the succinyl ester is hydrolyzed after oral ingestion, studies have administered α-tocopheryl succinate via injection to investigate its in vivo effects.

A tocotrienol-rich fraction of palm oil (containing α-, γ-, and δ-tocotrienols) induced apoptosis in breast cancer-cell lines *(149)*. Apoptosis occured along with cell-cycle arrest in the G_1 phase, and was shown to be independent of p53 and *ras (149)*.

9.6. Immune Function

The effects of vitamin E on immune function are rarely studied. Supplementation of the diet with RRR-α-tocopherol in vitamin E-depleted rats corrected the increase in plasma IgG, suggesting a role for vitamin E in maintaining the autoimmune system *(152)*. Vitamin E may enhance phagocytic-dependent, cell-mediated immunity *(153)*, such as interferon-γ, IL-2, and tumor necrosis factor (TNF) β that are produced by Th1 lymphocytes. In contrast, vitamin E may attenuate humoral immunity, such as IL-4, IL-5, IL-6, IL-9, IL-10 and IL-13, which are produced by Th2 lymphocytes *(154)*. The mechanism by which vitamin E enhances immune function is uncertain, but may result from antioxidant effects that protect immune cells from oxidative damage.

9.7. Angiogenesis

Tumors undergo angiogenesis—the development of new blood vessels—to facilitate growth and metastasis. Vascular endothelial growth factor (VEGF), also known as vascular permeability factor, is one of the main pro-angiogenic growth factors *(155)*. α-Tocopheryl succinate was found to suppress the gene expression of VEGF in MDA-MD-231 human breast cancer cells *(156)* and in hormone-refractory prostate cancer cells *(157)*.

10. EVIDENCE FROM HUMAN STUDIES

10.1. Epidemiological Observational Studies

Numerous epidemiological observational studies, including retrospective case-control studies and prospective studies, have been conducted to investigate the association between cancer outcomes and vitamin E, measured by dietary intake, supplement use, or serum concentrations. Findings from retrospective case-control studies are inconsistent *(158–207; Table 1)*. Several design limitations in these studies hinder interpretation of the results. For example, dietary or serum levels of vitamin E are assessed at or after cancer diagnoses, and the temporal relationship of vitamin E and cancer outcomes cannot be determined. Moreover, measurements of dietary or supplemental intakes are prone to recall-bias when cancer patients are likely to make more effort in recalling intakes than controls. These limitations may be avoided by prospective study designs in which information about vitamin E is collected prior to the occurrence of cancer.

To date, the majority of prospective nested case-control studies did not find statistically significant

Table 1

Retrospective Case-Control Studies of Dietary or Supplemental Vitamin E Intake,
Serum Vitamin E Concentrations and Cancerous Outcomes

Reference	Time Period	Population	Age (Mean or Median)	Exposure	Cancer Site(s)	Odds Ratio* (95% CI)	P Trend
Sahl et al. (158)	1990–1992	46 cases; 46 clinic controls	65 yr	Dietary vitamin E	Basal-cell skin	No significant difference	
Vena et al. (159)	1979–1985	351 cases; 855 population controls	35–90 yr (range)	Dietary vitamin E	Bladder	No significant association	
Riboli et al. (160)	1983–1986	432 cases; 792 hospital and population controls	<80 yr	Dietary vitamin E	Bladder	0.72 (0.48–1.09)	0.11
Giles et al. (161)	1987–1991	416 cases; 409 population controls	50 yr for males; 49 yr for females	Dietary vitamin E	Brain (glioma)	Male: 1.68 (1.07–2.63) Female: 1.09 (0.62–1.92)	
Hu et al. (162)	1993–1995	129 cases; 258 hospital controls	40–49 yr	Dietary vitamin E	Brain (glioma and meningioma)	0.16 (0.1–0.5)	<0.01
Yeum et al. (163)	Prior to 1998	44 cases; 46 clinic controls with benign breast tumors	44 yr for cases; 38 yr for controls	Serum α-tocopherol	Breast	No significant difference	
				Serum γ-tocopherol		No significant difference	
Gerber et al. (164)	Prior to 1991	48 cases; 50 hospital controls	25–65 yr (range)	Plasma vitamin E	Breast	Higher levels in cases (p<0.01)	
				Plasma vitamin E/cholesterol ratio		No significant difference	
				Leukocyte vitamin E		Higher levels in cases (p<0.01)	
				Erythrocyte vitamin E		No significant difference	
Negri et al. (165)	1991–1994	2,569 cases; 2,588 hospital controls	55–64 yr	Dietary vitamin E	Breast	0.75 (0.6–0.9)	<0.01
Richardson et al. (166)	1983–1987	409 cases; 515 hospital controls	52 yr for cases; 50 yr for controls	Dietary vitamin E	Breast	1.3 (0.9–1.8)	NS
Ronco et al. (167)	1994–1997	400 cases; 405 hospital controls	60–69 yr	Dietary vitamin E	Breast	0.50 (0.30–0.82)	0.009
Yuan et al. (168)	1984–1986	834 cases; 834 community controls	20–69 yr (range)	Dietary vitamin E	Breast	0.7 (0.5–1.1)	
Levi et al. (169)	1993–1999	289 cases; 442 hospital controls	55–64 yr	Dietary vitamin E	Breast	0.37 (0.23–0.59)	<0.001

458

Reference	Years	Cases; controls	Age	Vitamin E measure	Cancer site	Result	p value
Mezzetti et al. (170)	1991–1994	2569 cases; 2588 hospital controls	20–74 yr (range)	Dietary vitamin E	Breast	0.83 (0.69–1.01)	0.1
Ambrosone et al. (171)	1986–1991	633 cases; 711 population controls	40–85 yr (range)	Dietary vitamin E	Breast	FH+: 0.2 (0.1–1.1) FH−: 0.4 (0.3–0.7)	<0.01
Braga et al. (172)	1991–1994	2569 cases; 2,588 hospital controls	20–74 yr (range)	Dietary vitamin E	Breast	Premenopause: 0.80 (0.7–1.0) Postmenopause: 0.75 (0.6–0.9)	<0.05 <0.01
Bohlke et al. (173)	1989–1991	820 cases; 1548 hospital controls	56 yr for cases; 54 yr for controls	Dietary vitamin E	Breast	0.71 (0.48–1.05) Premenopausal: 0.50 (0.25–1.02) Postmenopausal: 0.85 (0.53–1.36)	0.04 0.03 0.25
Männistö et al. (174)	1990–1995	289 cases; 433 community controls	25–75 yr (range)	Dietary + supplemental vitamin E	Breast	No significant difference	
Freudenheim et al. (175)	1986–1991	297 white cases; 311 white population controls	≥40 yr	Dietary vitamin E Vitamin E supplement	Breast (premenopausal)	0.55 (0.34–0.88) 0.95 (0.58–1.55)	0.03 0.99
London et al. (176)	1986–1988	377 stage 1 or 2 breast cancer cases; 403 clinic controls	64 yr for cases; 62 yr for controls	Serum α-tocopherol Dietary vitamin E Dietary + supplemental vitamin E	Breast (postmenopausal)	0.8 (0.5–1.2) 0.4 (0.2–0.9) 0.7 (0.4–1.3)	0.19 0.02 0.07
van 't Veer et al. (177)	1991–1992	347 cases; 347 population controls	62 yr	Adipose tissue α-tocopherol	Breast (postmenopausal)	1.15 (0.75–1.77)	0.42
Potischman et al. (178)	Prior to 1991	387 cases; 670 community and hospital controls		Serum α-tocopherol	Cervical	1.14 (0.6–2.1)	0.63
Peng et al. (179)	1990–1991	27 cases; 27 hospital controls	49 yr	Serum γ-tocopherol Plasma α-tocopherol	Cervical	2.09 (1.1–3.9) Lower levels in cases (p < 0.05)	0.03

(continued)

459

Table 1 (continued)

Reference	Time Period	Population	Age (Mean or Median)	Exposure	Cancer Site(s)	Odds Ratio* (95% CI)	P Trend
				Plasma γ-tocopherol		No significant difference	
				Cervical tissue α-tocopherol		Higher levels in cases (p < 0.05)	
				Cervical tissue γ-tocopherol		Higher levels in cases (p < 0.05)	
Ferraroni et al. (180)	1985–1992	1,326 cases; 2,024 hospital controls	62 yr for cases; 55 yr for controls	Dietary vitamin E	Colorectal	0.60 (0.45–0.80)	<0.05
La Vecchia et al. (181)	1992–1996	1,953 cases; 4,154 hospital controls	62 yr for cases; 58 yr for controls	Dietary vitamin E	Colorectal	0.63 (0.5–0.8)	<0.001
Slattery et al. (182)	1991–1994	1,993 cases; 2,410 population controls	30–79 yr (range)	Dietary α-tocopherol	Colon	Men: 0.99 (0.69-1.42) Women: 1.08 (0.71–1.62)	
				Dietary β-tocopherol		Men: 1.05 (0.77–1.42) Women: 1.14 (0.81–1.62)	
				Dietary γ-tocopherol		Men: 1.11 (0.78–1.57) Women: 1.16 (0.78–1.72)	
				Dietary δ-tocopherol		Men: 1.10 (0.79–1.53) Women: 1.12 (0.77–1.64)	
				Dietary vitamin E (all forms)		Men: 0.97 (0.68–1.40) Women: 0.92 (0.61–1.40)	
				Vitamin E supplement		Men: 0.99 (0.78–1.27) Women: 0.90 (0.69–1.16)	
Ghadirian et al. (183)	1989–1993	402 cases; 668 population controls	35–79 yr (range)	Dietary vitamin E	Colon	0.53 (0.36–0.78)	
				Dietary α-tocopherol		0.63 (0.43–0.94)	
White et al. (184)	1985–1989	444 cases; 427 population controls	30–62 yr (range)	Vitamin E supplement	Colon	0.43 (0.26–0.71)	<0.001
Ferraroni et al. (180)	1985–1992	828 cases; 2,024 hospital controls	62 yr for cases; 55 yr for controls	Dietary vitamin E	Colon	0.58 (0.42–0.81)	<0.05

Reference	Years	Cases; controls	Age	Nutrient	Site	OR (95% CI)	p
La Vecchia et al. (181)	1992–1996	1,225 cases; 4,154 hospital controls	62 yr for cases; 58 yr for controls	Dietary vitamin E	Colon	0.73 (0.6–0.9)	
Ferraroni et al. (180)	1985–1992	498 cases; 2,024 hospital controls	62 yr for cases; 55 yr for controls	Dietary vitamin E	Rectal	0.67 (0.45–0.98)	NS
La Vecchia et al. (181)	1992–1996	728 cases; 4,154 hospital controls	62 yr for cases; 58 yr for controls	Dietary vitamin E	Rectal	1.14 (1.0–1.4)	
Freudenheim et al. (185)	1978–1986	277 male cases; 277 male community controls	64 yr	Dietary vitamin E	Rectal	1.04 (0.64–1.66)	NS
		145 female cases; 145 female community controls	65 yr			0.75 (0.44–1.27)	NS
Charpiot et al. (186)	Prior to 1989	70 cases; 78 hospital or clinic controls	65 yr for cases; 59 yr for controls	Serum α-tocopherol	Digestive (e.g., esophageal, gastric, biliary, colorectal, and pancreatic)	Lower levels in cases (p = 0.002)	
Negri et al. (187)	1988–1994	368 cases; 713 hospital controls	62 yr fo cases; 61 yr for controls	Dietary vitamin E	Endometrial	0.9	0.09
Goodman et al. (188)	1985–1993	332 cases; 511 population controls	59 yr for cases, 57 yr for controls	Dietary vitamin E	Endometrial	0.86 (0.43–1.71)	0.75
Barone et al. (189)	Prior to 1992	133 cases; 264 hospital controls	55–64 yr	Vitamin E supplement	Esophageal	0.4 (0.2–1.0)	
Terry et al. (190)	1995–1997	185 cases; 815 population controls	69 yr for cases; 68 yr for controls	Dietary vitamin E	Esophageal (adenocarcinoma)	0.9 (0.5–1.6)	0.80
		165 cases; 815 population controls	67 yr for cases; 68 yr for controls	Dietary vitamin E	Esophageal (squamous-cell)	0.5 (0.2–1.0)	0.09
Zhang et al. (191)	1992–1994	95 cases; 132 clinic controls		Dietary vitamin E	Esophageal and gastric cardia (adenocarcinoma)	0.7 (0.5–1.1)	0.13
Terry et al. (190)	1995–1997	258 cases; 815 population controls	66 yr for cases; 68 yr for controls	Dietary vitamin E	Gastric (adenocarcinoma)	1.2 (0.8–1.7)	0.38

(continued)

461

Table 1 (*continued*)

Reference	Time Period	Population	Age (Mean or Median)	Exposure	Cancer Site(s)	Odds Ratio* (95% CI)	P trend
Ekström et al. (192)	1989–1995	74 cardia cases; 406 noncardia cases; 1,067 population controls	40–79 yrs (range)	Dietary vitamin E	Gastric	Cardia: 0.6 (0.3–1.2) Noncardia: 0.6 (0.4–0.9)	0.18 0.05
Kumagai et al. (193)	1995	22 cases; 63 hospital controls	58 yr for cases; 55 yr for controls	Serum vitamin E	Gastric	1.8 (0.6–5.0)	NS
Battisti et al. (194)	1994–1996	51 cases; 49 controls	64–72 yr (range)	Serum vitamin E	Gastric	No significant difference	
López-Carrillo et al.(195)	1989–1990	220 cases; 752 population controls	57 yr for cases; 59 yr for controls	Dietary vitamin E	Gastric	0.36 (0.16–0.82)	<0.001
Freudenheim et al. (196)	1975–1985	250 cases; 250 community controls	62 yr	Dietary vitamin E	Laryngeal	0.73 (0.36–1.49)	0.38
LeGardeur et al. (197)	Prior to 1990	59 cases; hospital and community controls	58 yr	Serum vitamin E	Lung	Lower levels in cases (p = 0.04)	
Kumagai et al. (193)	1995	58 cases; 63 hospital controls	57 yr for cases; 55 yr for controls	Serum vitamin E	Lung	0.3 (0.1–0.8)	<0.01
Stefani et al. (198)	1993–1997	541 cases; 540 hospital controls	60–69 yr	Dietary vitamin E	Lung	0.50 (0.34–0.74)	<0.001
Mayne et al. (199)	1982–1985	413 cases; 413 population controls	67 yr for cases; 68 yr for controls	Supplemental vitamin E	Lung	0.55 (0.35–0.85)	
Stryker et al. (200)	1982–1985	204 cases; 248 dermatology clinic patients	48 yr for male cases, 42 yr for female cases, 41 yr for male controls, 38 yr for female controls	Plasma α-tocopherol	Malignant melanoma	1.0	0.4
				Dietary vitamin E (food + supplements)		0.6	0.4

Reference	Study years	Cases; controls	Age	Vitamin E measure	Cancer site	OR (95% CI)	p
Barone et al. (189)	Prior to 1992	290 cases; 576 hospital controls	55–64 yr	Dietary vitamin E (food)	Oral	0.6	0.03
				Vitamin E supplement	Oral	0.5 (0.3–0.9)	
Negri et al. (201)	1992–1997	344 oral cases; 410 pharyngeal cases; 1,775 hospital controls	50–59 yr	Dietary vitamin E	Oral and pharyngeal	0.44 (0.28–0.71)	<0.01
Gridley et al. (202)	1984–1985	190 black cases; 201 black population controls	57 yr	Dietary vitamin E	Oral and pharyngeal	Men: 0.4 Women: NA	0.07 NS
Lu et al. (253)	1993–1995	65 cases; 132 controls recruited from blood bank	60 yr for cases; 42 yr for controls	Plasma α-tocopherol	Prostate	1.02 (0.23–4.62)	0.12
				Plasma γ-tocopherol		0.66 (0.22–1.97)	0.41
				Dietary vitamin E		0.38 (0.09–1.68)	0.59
Deneo-Pellegrini et al. (203)	1994–1997	175 cases; 233 hospital controls	70–79 yr	Dietary vitamin E	Prostate	0.6 (0.3–1.1)	0.03
Ramon et al. (254)	1994–1998	217 cases; 434 hospital and community controls	71–80 yr	Dietary vitamin E	Prostate	1.3 (0.9–2.0)	0.09
Kristal et al. (204)	1993–1996	697 cases; 666 population controls	55–59 yr	Vitamin E supplement	Prostate	0.76 (0.54–1.08)	0.12
Wolk et al. (205)	1989–1991	1185 cases; 1,526 population controls	62 yr for males; 63 yr for females	Dietary vitamin E	Renal-cell	0.90 (0.69–1.16)	
				Dietary + supplemental vitamin E		0.86 (0.62–1.19)	
Horn-Ross et al. (206)	1989–1993	141 cases; 191 population controls	57 yr	Dietary + supplemental vitamin E	Salivary gland	1.2 (0.6–2.3)	0.54
D'Avanzo et al. (207)	1986–1992	399 cases; 617 hospital controls	44 yr for cases, 46 yr for controls	Dietary vitamin E	Thyroid	0.67 (0.4–1.0)	NS

*Odds ratios are expressed as the risk of cancer for highest compared to lowest vitamin E level/intake.

Abbreviations: NS (not significant), FH− (no family history), and FH+ (family history).

associations between pre-diagnostic serum concentrations of α-tocopherol and the risk of developing bladder, breast, cervical, gastric, pancreatic, rectal, basal cell skin, or squamous cell skin cancers (Table 2). The association with colon cancer was not statistically significant in individual studies, but a pooled analysis of five cohorts suggests a protective association [OR = 0.7(0.4–1.1)] *(208)*. With few exceptions *(209,210)*, most studies did not find a protective association of α-tocopherol with the risk of developing lung *(211–215)* and prostate cancer *(211,216–218)*.

In line with findings for serum concentrations, α-tocopherol supplement use was not associated with cancer risk in most prospective cohort studies (Table 3). The few exceptions include the inverse association between the risk of lung cancer and dietary vitamin E and serum α-tocopherol observed in the Alpha-Tocopherol Beta-Carotene (ATBC) trial *(220)*, and the inverse association between the risk of colon cancer and total vitamin E intake observed in the Iowa Women's Health Study *(221)*.

Several reasons may explain the null or weak association of circulating α-tocopherol concentrations or α-tocopherol supplement use with cancer risk. First, the chemopreventive effects of vitamin E may be dose-dependent, and the optimal dose and duration of use is uncertain. Second, the specific forms of vitamin E and routes of administration may be crucial for conferring benefits. Finally, use of α-tocopherol supplements decreases circulating levels of other forms of vitamin E *(37,38)*, and the chemopreventive effects may have been compromised. For example, in a prospective study, prediagnostic plasma γ-tocopherol concentrations were strongly inversely associated with the risk of prostate cancer *(216)*, and a protective association of plasma α-tocopherol was observed only when γ-tocopherol concentrations were above the median *(219)*. In vitamin E-deficient rats, graded levels of dietary γ-tocopherol increased α-tocopherol levels in several tissues *(41)*. These data suggest the possibility that combined use of several forms of vitamin E, rather than α-tocopherol alone, may confer more chemopreventive benefits.

10.2. Clinical Studies of Effects of α-Tocopherol Supplements on Putative Biomarkers of Cancer

Several clinical studies have been conducted to evaluate the effects of α-tocopherol supplement use on biomarkers considered to be important in carcinogenesis, including markers of oxidative damage to DNA, inflammation, and immune function. (Table 4). The majority of the clinical studies are based on small sample sizes, and found no effect of α-tocopherol on biomarkers. Evidence directly linking these biomarkers to cancer risk in humans is limited.

10.2.1. OXIDATIVE DAMAGE TO DNA

Short-term (2–6 mo) or long-term (3 yr) use of RRR-α-tocopherol supplements of 400 IU/d or 200 mg/d had no effect on oxidative damage to DNA, as measured by urinary excretion of 8-hydroxy-2'-deoxyguanosine (8-OHdG) in smokers and nonsmokers *(79,222–224)*. Similarly, several studies *(225–227)* observed no effect on DNA-strand breaks, except one *(228)*. Supplementing a 15% polyunsaturated fatty acid (PUFA) diet with α-tocopherol of 80 mg/d for 4 wk abolished the PUFA-associated pyrimidine oxidation in peripheral-blood lymphocytes from healthy nonsmokers *(229)*. Daily supplementation with all-*rac* α-tocopherol at 15 mg, 60 mg, or 200 mg for 1 mo in 28 individuals caused no change in DNA repair capacity, as measured by ADP ribosyl transferase and unscheduled DNA synthesis in peripheral mononuclear lymphocytes (PBMC)(230). In contrast, α-tocopherol supplement use of 60 mg/d reduced the auto-antibody against 5-hydroxymethyl-2'-deoxyuridine (HMdU) in plasma *(230)*.

10.2.2. INFLAMMATION

Evidence is limited on the effects of vitamin E on inflammatory markers in humans. The use of RRR-α-tocopherol supplements of 1200 mg/d for 3 mo reduced serum levels of C- reactive protein and monocyte interleukin-6 in type II diabetic patients *(231)*, whereas α-tocopherol at 400 IU did not exert antiinflammatory effects, as measured by soluble cell-adhesion molecules and C-reactive protein *(232)*.

10.2.3. IMMUNE FUNCTION

α-Tocopherol supplement use increased cell-mediated immune function in some but not all studies in elderly individuals. Use of 100 mg/d, but not 50 mg/d, for 6 mo was associated with a statistically nonsignificant increase in delayed-type hypersensitivity *(233)*. In another trial of supplementation with placebo or vitamin E at 60 mg/d, 200 mg/d, or 800 mg/d for 235 d, the group that received 200 mg/d vitamin E had the highest

Table 2

Nested Case Control Studies of Dietary or Supplemental Vitamin E Intake, Serum Vitamin E Concentrations, and Cancerous Outcomes

Reference	Time Period	Population	Age (Mean or Median)	Vitamin E Measure	Cancer Site(s)	Odds Ratio* (95% CI)	P Trend
Wald et al. (255)	1975–1985	271 cases; 533 controls	35–64 yr (range)	Serum vitamin E	All cancers	<1 yr from blood collection: 0.52	0.003
						≥1 yr from blood collection: 1.12	NS
Willett et al. (211)	1973–1979	111 cases; 210 controls	57 yr	Serum vitamin E	All cancers (except non-melanoma skin)	1.2	0.87
Stähelin et al. (213)	1971–1980	47 cancer deaths; 136 controls	62 yr	Plasma vitamin E	Cancers other than lung or gastrointestinal	No significant difference	
Breslow et al. (256)	1974–1992	32 cases; 64 controls	65–74 yr	Serum α-tocopherol	Basal-cell skin	2.6 (0.7–9.2)	0.23
Nomura et al. (212)	1971–1981	27 cases; 302 controls	62 yr	Serum vitamin E	Bladder	No significant difference	
Helzlsouer et al. (257)	1974–1986	35 cases; 70 controls	59 yr	Serum α-tocopherol	Bladder	0.57 (0.12–2.70)	0.18
Knekt et al. (258)	1968–1977	15 cases; 29 controls		Serum α-tocopherol	Bladder	1.25	0.57
Knekt et al. (258)	1968–1977	18 cases; 34 controls		Serum α-tocopherol	Brain	0.62	0.33
Willett et al. (211)	1973–1979	14 cases; 31 controls		Serum vitamin E	Breast	No significant difference	
Wald et al. (259)	1968–1982	39 cases; 78 controls	45–50 yr	Plasma vitamin E	Breast	0.50	<0.01
Dorgan et al. (260)	1977–1987	105 cases; 203 controls	58 yr	Serum α-tocopherol	Breast	1.2 (0.5–2.8)	0.72
Hultén et al. (261)	1985–1997	201 cases; 390 controls		Plasma α-tocopherol	Breast	1.3 (0.6–2.7)	0.47
Batieha et al. (262)	1974–1990	50 cases; 99 controls		Serum α-tocopherol / Serum γ-tocopherol	Cervical	1.02 (0.35–2.94) / 0.93 (0.39–2.22)	1.00 / 0.85
Lehtinen et al. (263)	1983–1994	38 cases; 116 controls	33 yr	Serum α-tocopherol	Cervical	1.3 (0.4–3.3)	NS

(continued)

465

Table 2 (continued)

Reference	Time Period	Population	Age (Mean or Median)	Vitamin E Measure	Cancer Site(s)	Odds Ratio* (95% CI)	P Trend
Knekt et al. (264)	1968–1977	58 cases; 58 controls	62 yr	Serum vitamin E	Colorectal	Men: 3.3 Women: 1.3	0.32 0.76
Stähelin et al. (213)	1971–1980	14 cancer deaths; 33 cancer controls	65 yr	Plasma vitamin E	Colorectal	No significant difference	
Longnecker et al. (208)		Pooled analysis of 289 cases and 1,267 controls from 5 cohorts	15–99 yr (range)	Serum α-tocopherol	Colorectal	0.7 (0.4–1.1)	0.15
Schober et al. (265)	1974–1983	72 cases; 143 controls	58 yr	Serum vitamin E	Colon	0.7 (0.2–1.7)	NS
Nomura et al. (212)	1971–1981	81 cases; 302 controls	62 yr	Serum vitamin E	Colon	No significant difference	
Longnecker et al. (208)		Pooled analysis of 206 cases and 938 controls from 5 cohorts	15–99 yr (range)	Serum α-tocopherol	Colon	0.7 (0.4–1.3)	0.26
Comstock et al. (266)	1974–1989	34 cases; 68 controls		Serum vitamin E	Rectal	1.7	0.40
Nomura et al. (212)	1971–1981	32 cases; 302 controls	65 yr	Serum vitamin E	Rectal	No significant difference	
Longnecker et al. (208)		Pooled analysis of 83 cases and 329 controls from 5 cohorts	15–99 yr (range)	Serum α-tocopherol	Rectal	0.6 (0.2–1.5)	0.41
Knekt et al. (258)	1968–1977	9 cases; 16 controls		Serum α-tocopherol	Esophagus	0.39	0.16
Knekt et al. (264)	1968–1977	87 cases; 87 controls	62 yr	Serum vitamin E	Esophagus and stomach	Men: 1.3 Women: 0.6	0.38 0.06
Nomura et al. (212)	1971–1981	70 cases; 302 controls	64 yr	Serum vitamin E	Gastric	No significant difference	
Stähelin et al. (213)	1971–1980	19 cancer deaths; 37 controls	61 yr	Plasma vitamin E	Gastric	No significant difference	
Botterweck et al. (267)	1986–1992	282 cases; 3123 controls	55–69 yr (range)	Dietary vitamin E	Gastric	0.9 (0.6–1.4)	0.83

Reference	Years	Cases; controls	Age	Vitamin E measure	Cancer site	Relative risk	p value
				Supplements with vitamin E		0.7 (0.4-1.5)	
Willett et al. (211)	1973–1979	11 cases; 22 controls		Serum vitamin E	Gastrointestinal	No significant difference	
Knekt et al. (258)	1968–1977	20 cases; 38 controls		Serum α-tocopherol	Kidney	0.86	0.63
Knekt et al. (258)	1968–1977	11 cases; 17 controls		Serum α-tocopherol	Larynx	0.48	0.18
Willett et al. (211)	1973–1979	11 cases; 23 controls		Serum vitamin E	Leukemia and lymphoma	No significant difference	
Knekt et al. (258)	1968–1977	20 cases; 37 controls		Serum α-tocopherol	Lip, oral cavity, and pharynx	1.26	0.54
Knekt et al. (258)	1968–1977	12 cases; 22 controls		Serum α-tocopherol	Liver and gallbladder	2.23	0.09
Willett et al. (211)	1973–1979	17 cases; 28 controls		Serum vitamin E	Lung	No significant difference	
Nomura et al. (212)	1971–1981	74 cases; 302 controls	63 yr	Serum vitamin E	Lung	No significant difference	
Menkes et al. (209)	1974–1983	99 cases; 196 controls	55–64 yr (range)	Serum vitamin E	Lung	0.40	0.04
Stähelin et al. (213)	1971–1980	35 cancer deaths; 102 controls	63 yr	Plasma vitamin E	Lung	No significant difference;	
Comstock et al. (210)	1974–1993	258 cases; 515 controls	45–64 yr (range)	Serum α-tocopherol	Lung	0.77	0.06
Knekt et al. (214)	1968–1991	92 cases; 183 controls	58 yr	Serum α-tocopherol	Lung	0.83 (0.33–2.07)	0.80
Ratnasinghe et al. (215)	1992–1999	108 cases; 216 controls	63 yr	Serum α-tocopherol	Lung	1.1 (0.6–2.3)	0.29
				Serum γ-tocopherol		1.4 (0.7–2.7)	0.62
Voorrips et al. (268)	1986–1992	939 cases; 1525 controls	55–69 yr (range)	Dietary vitamin E	Lung	1.29 (0.88–1.89)	0.24
				Vitamin E supplement		1.16 (0.70–1.93)	0.40
Breslow et al. (256)	1974–1992	30 cases; 60 controls	45–54 yr (range)	Serum α-tocopherol	Malignant melanoma	2.0 (0.5–8.4)	0.35
Knekt et al. (258)	1968–1977	10 cases; 18 controls		Serum α-tocopherol	Malignant melanoma	0.20	<0.01
Zheng et al. (269)	1974–1990	28 cases; 112 controls		Serum total tocopherol	Oral and pharyngeal	0.89	0.75

(continued)

Table 2 (*continued*)

Reference	Time Period	Population	Age (Mean or Median)	Vitamin E Measure	Cancer Site(s)	Odds Ratio* (95% CI)	P Trend
Helzlsouer et al. (270)	1974–1989	35 cases; 67 controls	53 yr	Serum α-tocopherol		0.31	0.07
				Serum γ-tocopherol		4.04	0.05
				Serum α-tocopherol	Ovarian	3.91 (1.1–14.0)	0.04
Burney et al. (271)	1974–1986	22 cases; 44 controls	60–69 yr (range)	Serum γ-tocopherol		1.04 (0.4–2.9)	NS
				Serum α-tocopherol	Pancreatic	1.96	NS
Willett et al. (211)	1973–1979	11 cases; 21 controls		Serum vitamin E	Prostate	No significant difference	
Huang et al. (216)	1974–1996	182 cases; 364 controls	54 yr	Serum α-tocopherol	Prostate	0.58 (0.31–1.06)	0.11
				Serum γ-tocopherol		0.77 (0.42–1.43)	0.30
	1989–1996	142 cases; 284 controls	66 yr	Plasma α-tocopherol		0.78 (0.41–1.50)	0.46
				Plasma γ-tocopherol		0.21 (0.08–0.54)	<0.001
				Serum γ-tocopherol		0.25 (0.09–0.68)	0.01
Nomura et al. (217)	1971–1993	142 cases; 142 controls	62 yr	Serum total tocopherol	Prostate	0.9 (0.5–1.9)	0.64
				Serum α-tocopherol		1.4 (0.7–2.9)	0.71
				Serum δ-tocopherol		1.0 (0.5–2.0)	0.70
				Serum γ-tocopherol		0.7 (0.3–1.5)	0.27
Hsing et al. (218)	1974–1986	103 cases; 103 controls	71 yr	Serum total tocopherol	Prostate	1.00 (0.37–2.68)	0.90
				Serum α-tocopherol		1.00 (0.29–3.45)	
				Serum γ-tocopherol		1.17 (0.39–3.47)	
Gann et al. (218)	1982–1995	578 cases; 1294 controls	61 yr for cases, 62 yr for controls	Serum α-tocopherol	Prostate	1.06 (0.76–1.48)	0.70
				Serum γ-tocopherol		0.98 (0.71–1.35)	0.89
Breslow et al. (256)	1974–1992	37 cases; 74 controls	55–64 yr (range)	Serum α-tocopherol	Squamous-cell skin	1.5 (0.5–4.6)	0.48
Karagas et al. (288)	Prior to 1997	132 cases; 264 controls	35–84 yr (range)	Plasma α-tocopherol	Squamous-cell skin	0.89 (0.43–1.85)	0.72

*Odds ratios are expressed as the risk of cancer for highest compared to lowest vitamin E level/intake.

Abbreviations: NS (not significant).

Table 3
Prospective Cohort Studies of Dietary or Supplemental Vitamin E Intake, Serum Vitamin E Concentrations, and Cancerous Outcomes

Reference	Time Period	Population	Age (Range)	Exposure	Cancer Site(s)	Relative Risk* (95% CI)	P Trend
Eichholzer et al. (272)	1971–1990	290 cancer deaths in a cohort of 2,974 men	20–79 yr	Plasma vitamin E	All cancers (men)	Low vitamin E: 1.19 (0.92–1.54)	NS
van Dam et al. (273)	1986–1994	3190 cases in a cohort of 43,217 men	40–75 yr	Dietary + supplemental vitamin E	Basal-cell skin	0.94 (0.81–1.09)	0.14
Michaud et al. (274)	1986–1998	320 cases in a cohort of 47,909 men	40–75 yr	Dietary + supplemental vitamin E	Bladder	0.64 (0.45–0.92)	0.03
				Dietary + supplemental α-tocopherol only		0.67 (0.46–0.96)	
				Vitamin E supplement		0.68 (0.45–1.03)	0.03
Michels et al. (275)	1987–1997	1271 cases in a cohort of 59,036 women	40–76 yr	Dietary vitamin E	Breast	0.83 (0.60–1.14)	0.38
Verhoeven et al. (276)	1986–1990	650 cases in a cohort of 62,573 women	55–69 yr	Dietary vitamin E	Breast	1.25 (0.85–1.85)	0.37
Hunter et al. (277)	1980–1988	1439 cases in a cohort of 89,494 women	30–55 yr	Dietary + supplemental vitamin E	Breast	0.90 (0.77–1.06)	0.07
	1984–1988	666 cases in a cohort of 71,312 women	30–55 yr	Dietary + supplemental vitamin E	Breast	0.88 (0.69–1.10)	0.24
	1980–1988	1439 cases in a cohort of 89,494 women	30–55 yr	Vitamin E supplement	Breast	1.01 (0.69–1.49)	0.43
Jacobs et al. (278)	1982–1996	4404 cancer deaths in a cohort of 711,891 men and women	30–80 + yr	Vitamin E supplement	Colorectal	For <10 yrs of use: 0.87 (0.73–1.03) For =10 yrs of use: 1.08 (0.85–1.38)	
Sellers et al. (279)	1986–1995	241 cases in a cohort of 35,216 women	55–69 yr	Dietary + supplemental vitamin E	Colon	No FH: 0.7 (0.5–1.0) FH: 0.9 (0.5–1.7)	0.04 0.7
				Dietary vitamin E		No FH: 0.8 (0.5–1.3) FH: 1.2 (0.5–2.6)	0.4 0.7
				Vitamin E supplement		No FH: 0.6 (0.4–0.9) FH: 0.8 (0.4–1.6)	0.03 0.5
Eichholzer et al. (272)	1971–1990	22 cancer deaths in a cohort of 2,974 men	20–79 yr	Plasma vitamin E	Colon	Low vitamin E: 1.03 (0.39–2.67)	NS
Bostick et al. (221)	1986–1990	212 incidence cases in a cohort of 35,215 women	55–69 yr	Dietary + supplemental vitamin E	Colon	0.32 (0.19–0.54)	<0.0001

(continued)

Table 3 (continued)

Reference	Time Period	Population	Age (Range)	Exposure	Cancer Site(s)	Relative Risk* (95% CI)	P Trend
Eichholzer et al. (272)	1971–1990	28 cancer deaths in of 2974 men	20–79 yr	Plasma vitamin E	Gastric	Low vitamin E: 0.54 (0.18–1.63)	NS
Botterweck et al. (267)	1986–1992	282 incident cases in a cohort of 3123 men and women	55–69 yr	Dietary + supplemental Vitamin E	Gastric	0.80 (0.50–1.20)	0.46
Jacobs, et al. (280)	1982–1998	1725 stomach cancer deaths in 1,045,923 US adults	30–80+ yr	Vitamin E supplement	Stomach	1.02 (0.82–1.27)	NS
Woodson et al. (220)	1985–1993	1144 cases in a cohort of 29,133 male smokers (ATBC trial)	50–69 yr	Serum α-tocopherol	Lung	0.81 (0.67–0.97)	0.09
				Dietary vitamin E		0.77 (0.64–0.93)	0.01
				Dietary α-tocopherol		0.80 (0.66–0.97)	0.02
Knekt et al. (281)	1966–1986	117 cases in a cohort of 4,538 men	20–69 yr	Dietary vitamin E	Lung	Nonsmokers (low vs high): 3.06	0.12
						Smokers (low vs high): 0.80	0.58
Fairfield et al. (282)	1976–1996	301 incident cases in a cohort of 80,326 women		Dietary + supplemental vitamin E	Ovarian	0.88 (0.61–1.29)	NS
Eicholzer et al. (272,283)	1971–1990	30 cancer deaths in a cohort of 2,974 men	20–79 yr	Plasma vitamin E	Prostate	Low vitamin E + smokers: 3.26 (1.27–8.35)	<0.05
						Low vitamin E+ non-smokers: 0.76 (0.25–2.36)	NS
Chan et al. (284)	1986–1996	1896 non-stage A1 cases, 522 extraprostatic cases, and 232 metastatic cases in a cohort of 47,780 men	40–75 yr	Vitamin E supplement	Prostate	Non-stage A1: 1.07 (0.95–1.20) Extraprostatic: 1.22 (0.95–1.52) Metastatic/fatal: 1.14 (0.82–1.59)	
Hartman et al. (285)	1985–1993	317 cases in a cohort of 29,133 male smokers (ATBC trial)	50–69 yr	Serum α-tocopherol	Prostate	No AT supplement: 0.98 (0.60–1.60)	0.80
						AT supplement: 0.76 (0.42–1.37)	0.37
				Dietary α-tocopherol		No AT supplement:	0.28

	1.30 (0.82–2.07)	0.29
Dietary β-tocopherol	AT supplement: 0.70 (0.44–1.31)	0.13
	No AT supplement: 1.42 (0.90–2.25)	0.41
Dietary γ-tocopherol	AT supplement: 0.81 (0.46–1.44)	0.12
	No AT supplement: 1.33 (0.88–1.99)	0.08
Dietary δ-tocopherol	AT supplement: 0.56 (0.32–0.98)	0.02
	No AT supplement: 1.48 (0.99–2.22)	0.36
Dietary α-tocotrienol	AT supplement: 0.70 (0.38–1.26)	0.66
	No AT supplement: 0.93 (0.57–1.52)	0.86
Dietary β-tocotrienol	AT supplement: 1.04 (0.56–1.95)	0.58
	No AT supplement: 1.08 (0.64–1.80)	0.87
Dietary γ-tocotrienol	AT supplement: 1.04 (0.55–1.97)	0.43
	No AT supplement: 1.17 (0.77–1.77)	0.50
Dietary δ-tocotrienol	AT supplement: 0.74 (0.42–1.29)	0.63
	No AT supplement: 1.17 (0.78–1.77)	0.39
	AT supplement: (0.72 (0.40–1.21)	

*Unless otherwise indicated, relative risks are expressed as the risk of cancer for highest compared to lowest vitamin E level/intake.

Abbreviations: NS (not significant), FH (family history of colon cancer), and AT (alpha-tocopherol).

471

Table 4
Clinical Studies of the Effects of α-Tocopherol Supplementation on Biomarkers of Oxidative DNA Damage, Inflammation, and Immunity

Study	Subjects	Dose	Duration	Outcome	Assay	Result
Huang et al. (79)	184 nonsmokers Mean (SD) age = 58(14) yr	400 IU/d RRR-α-tocopheryl acetate vs placebo	2 mo	24-hr urinary 8-OHdG	ELISA	No effect
Jacobson et al. (222)	121 heavy smokers Mean (SD) age =42 (9) yr	400 IU/d α-tocopherol + 500 mg/d vitamin C + 12 mg/d β-carotene vs placebo	6 mo	PAH-DNA adducts in mononuclear and oral cells, 8-oxo-or 8-OHdG in mononuclear and oral cells	ELISA and Imm-uoperoxidase staining	No effect on the four outcome measures
Porkkala-Sar ataho et al. (223)	48 men with hyper-cholesterolemia (smokers and non smokers)	182 mg/d RRR-α-tocopheryl acetate	36 mo	Serum 7β-hydroxyl cholesterol, 24-hr urinary 8-oxodG	Mass spectrometry HPLC/ED	↓ in 7β-hydroxyl cholesterol, no effect on 8-oxodG
Priemé et al. (224)	20 male smokers 20 controls, age 35–65 yr	200 mg/d RRR-α-tocopheryl acetate vs placebo	2 mo	24-hr urinary 8-oxo-dG	HPLC-ED	No effect
Astley et al. (225)	N = 42 IDDM men and women 31 contr-ols age	400 IU/d	8 wk	Single strand break in lymphocyte DNA (H₂O₂-induced)	Comet assay	No effect
Sampson et al. (226)	N = 40 NIDDM 30 controls	400 IU/d α-tocopherol	8 wk	DNA single-strand break in lymphocytes		No effect
Duthie et al. (227)	N = 50 male smokers, 50 male nonsmok-ers, age 50–59 yr	280 mg/d α-tocopherol + 100 mg/d vitamin C + 25 mg/d β-carotene	20 wk	DNA-strand breaks in lymphocytes, oxidized pyrimidine bases in lymphocytes	Alkaline comet assay	No effect on DNA-strand breaks ↓ oxidized pyrimi-dine bases
Sardas et al. (228)	15 IDDM and 48 NIDDM patients Mean (SD) age = 45(14.5) yr	900 mg/d α-tocopherol vs placebo	12 wk	DNA-strand break	Alkaline comet assay	↓ in the numbers of DNA-damaged cells
Jenkinson et al. (229)	21 healthy male non-smokers mean (SD) age = 29 (1) yr	80 mg/d RRR-α-tocopheryl acetate + 5% (or 15%) PUFA diet vs 5%-(or 15%) PUFA diet	4 wk for each diet; 10 wk of washout	Oxidized-pyrimidine (200 µM H₂O₂- induced), DNA strand break in lymphocyte	Alkaline comet assay	α-tocopherol supple-mentation abolish-ed the damaging effects of PUFA (15% of total energy in diet)
Hu et al. (230)	28 healthy smokers and nonsmokers Mean age = 35 yr	15 mg/d, 60 mg/d, and 200 mg/d all-rac α-tocopherol	4 wk	Anti-HMdU Ab in plasma	ELISA	No effect for 15 mg/d, ↓ oxidative DNA damage at 4

Study	Subjects	Treatment	Duration	Outcome	Method	Results
						wk for 60 mg/d and 200 mg/d
						No effect
Goodman et al. (286)	N = 22 adult non-smokers	800 IU/d α-tocopherol + 30 mg/d β-carotene	6 wk	Bleomycin-induced chromosomal breaks in blood lymphocytes		No effect on spontaneous rate of genetic damage in lymphocyte
Fenech et al. (287)	N = 60 male non-smokers, age 50–70 yr	50 mg/d RRR-α-tocopheryl acetate (phase A), 335 mg/d for each phase RRR-α-tocopheryl acetate (phase B) vs placebo	8 wk	Spontaneous genetic damage rate in peripheral-blood lymphocytes	Cytokinesis-block micronucleus assay	
Devaraj et al (231)	47 type II diabetic patients, 25 healthy controls	1200 mg/d RRR-α-tocopherol	3 mo	Serum levels of C-reactive protein monocyte interleukin (IL)-6	High sensitive microparticle enzyme immunoassay ELISA	↓ serum C-reactive protein, ↓ monocyte IL-6
Kaul et al. (232)	26 healthy subjects	400 IU all-rac α-tocopherol	6–8 wk	Plasma-soluble cell adhesion molecule and C-reactive protein	ELISAI immunonephelometry	No effects
Pallast et al. (233)	161 healthy subjects age 65–80 yr	50 mg/d and 100 mg/d vitamin E	6 mo	Delayed-type hypersensitivity (DTH) IL-2, IL4, and IFN-γ	DTH skin tests In vitro production of IL2, IL4, and IFN-γ by PBMC stimulated by phytohemagglutinin	Borderline effects on DTH No effects on IL-2, IL-4, and IFN-γ
Meydani et al. (234)	88 healthy subjects age ≥65 yr	60 mg/d, 200 mg/d, and 800 mg/d vitamin E	235 d	DTH	DTH skin tests	↑ T-cell-mediated immune by vitamin E use of 200 mg/d
Meydani et al. (153)	32 individuals	800 mg/d all-rac α-tocopheryl acetate	30 d	DTH, IL2, PGE2, lipid peroxides		↑DTH and IL2, ↓ PGE2 and lipid peroxides
De Waart et al. (235)	52 elderly subjects 74 elderly subjects	100 mg all-rac α-tocopheryl acetate	3 mo	Cellular immune Humoral immune	Response of PBMC to mitogens IgG, IgG4,IgAab	No effects
Girodon et al. (236)	725 institutional subjects, age ≥ 65 yr	Vitamin E 15 mg/d + Vitamin C 120 mg/d + β-carotene 15 mg/d	2 yr	Cellular immune Humoral immune Survivorship	DTH test Antibody to influenza vaccine Infectious morbidity and mortality	No effects

Abbreviations: Vit C (vitamin C), anti-HMdU Ab (auto-antibody against 5-hydroxymethyl-2'-deoxyuridine), 8-OHdG (8-hydroxy-2'-deoxyguanosine), PAH (polycyclic aromatic hydrocarbon), DTH (delayed-type hypersensitivity); PBMC (peripheral-blood mononuclear cells).

473

Table 5
Effects of α-Tocopherol Supplement Use on Intermediate Endpoints

Reference	Population	Vitamin E Supplements	Time Period	Intermediate Endpoint	Results
Greenberg (237)	864 patients with history of colorectal adenoma	Vitamin E 400 mg/d + vitamin C1000 mg/d or vitamin E 400 mg/d+vitamin C 1000 mg/d + β-carotene 25 mg/d	4 yr	Incidence of recurrence of colorectal adenoma	No effects
McKeown-Eyssen (238)	137 polyp patients previously had surgery for polyp removal	Vitamin E 400 mg/d + vitamin C 400 mg/d	2 yr	Recurrence of polyps	No effects
Hofstad et al. (239)	116 polyp-bearing patients	Vitamin E 75 mg/d+β-carotene 15 mg/d + + vitamin C150 mg/d+ selenium 101 μg/d+calcium 1.6 g/d	3 yr	Polyp growth	No effects
Cahill et al. (240)	40 polyp patients, 20 controls	Vitamin E 160 mg/d	1 mo	Colonic crypt-cell proliferation	No effects
Malila et al. (241)	146 heavy smokers	Vitamin E 50 mg/d	Average 6.3 yr	Incidence of colorectal adenoma	Increase in risk of colorectal adenoma
Zaridze et al. (242)	532 patients of oral leukoplakia and/or chronic esophagitis	(1) Riboflavin 80 mg/wk (2) retinol 100,000 IU/wk + vitamin E 80 mg/wk + β-carotene 40 mg/d (3) Both of the above (4) Placebo	20 mo	Prevalence of oral leukoplakia	Decrease in the prevalence in the (2) group
Liede et al. (243)	409 male smokers in the ATBC trial	(1) α-tocopherol 5 mg/d (2) β-carotene 20 mg/d (3) Both of the above (4) Placebo	5–7 yr	Clinical exam of oral mucosa, Histological exam of lesions showing leukoplakia, Cytological exam of buccal epithelium	No effects

increase in T-cell-mediated immune function *(234)*, as compared to placebo. Use of 800 mg/d all-*rac* α-tocopheryl acetate for 1 mo increased delayed-type hypersensitivity skin response, mitogen-stimulated lymphocyte proliferation, IL-2, and decreased PGE_2 and plasma lipid peroxides *(153)*. However, no effects were observed on humoral immune (IgG, IgG4, and IgA) and in vitro responses of PBMCs to mitogens in a study in which all-*rac* α-tocopheryl acetate of 100 mg/d was used for 3 mo *(235)*. In addition, combined use of vitamin E (15 mg), vitamin C (120 mg), and β-carotene (15 mg) for 2 yr had no significant effects on delayed-type hypersensitivity skin response, antibody after influenza vaccine, urogenital or respiratory infections, and survival in 725 institutionalized elderly persons *(236)*.

10.3. Studies with Intermediate Endpoints

In the Polyp Prevention Study of 864 patients with a history of colorectal adenomas, concomitant use of vitamin E (400 mg/d) and vitamin C (1000 mg/d) or both vitamins with β-carotene (25 mg/d) for 4 yr did not reduce the risk for incidence of new colorectal adenoma *(237;* Table 5*)*. Another study of 137 patients with previous surgery for polyp removal found that vitamin E (400 mg/d) and vitamin C (400 mg/d) for 2 yr *(238)* had no significant effect on polyp recurrences. Daily use of a mixture of β-carotene (15 mg), vitamin C (150 mg), vitamin E (75 mg), selenium (101 μg), and calcium carbonate (1.6 g) for 3 yr in patients with polyps did not suppress polyp growth *(239)*. Vitamin E at 160 mg/d for 1 mo did not reduce colonic crypt-cell proliferation in 40 patients with polyps, as compared to 20 controls *(240)*. An ancillary study of the ATBC trial reported an increased relative risk of polyps in the active vitamin E supplement group, and issues were raised about whether vitamin E at 50 mg/d might have increased rectal bleeding, leading to diagnoses of polyp incidence that would have otherwise been missed *(241)*.

One study suggests that vitamin E alone or in combination with β-carotene and retinol or vitamin C exert inhibitory effects on oral leukoplakia *(242)*. However, an ancillary study of the ATBC trial observed no effects on oral mucosal lesions in heavy smokers *(243)*.

10.4. Large-Scale Intervention Trials

Two large-scale trials have been completed, and one trial is ongoing to test the efficacy of α-tocopherol sup-

plement use in cancer prevention. The completed trials focused on selective populations—e.g., male heavy smokers or the malnourished.

The ATBC trial evaluated the efficacy of α-tocopherol (50 mg/d) and β-carotene (20 mg/d) in prevention of lung cancer in 29,133 Finnish men who smoked five or more cigarettes per d. After a follow-up period of 5–8 yr, no significant α-tocopherol-associated changes were observed on total mortality, lung cancer mortality, or incidence of lung cancer (RR = 0.98; 0.86, 1.12) *(244)*, urothelial cancer (RR = 1.1; 0.8, 1.5) *(245)*, renal cell cancer (RR = 1.1; 0.7, 1.6) *(245)*, colorectal cancer (CRC) (RR = 0.78; 0.55, 1.09) *(246)*, stomach cancer (RR = 0.98; 0.57, 1.69) *(247)*, pancreatic cancer *(248)*, and all cancer sites. Intriguingly, a 32% (95% CI = 12–47%) reduction in prostate cancer risk and a 41% (95% CI= 1%–65%) reduction in prostate cancer mortality were observed in the active supplement group as compared to the placebo group *(249)*.

The Nutrition Intervention Trial, now completed, was designed to determine whether dietary supplementation with specific vitamins and minerals would lower cancer mortality or incidence as well as mortality from other diseases in Linxian, China, where incidence of esophageal/gastric cancer mortality is high. A total of 29,584 individuals were randomized into one of four supplementation groups: retinol and zinc; riboflavin and niacin; vitamin C and molybdenum; and β-carotene, vitamin E, and selenium. After the 5.25-yr intervention period (1986–1991), significant reductions in total mortality (9%), cancer mortality (13% reduction), and stomach cancer mortality (21% reduction) occurred in the group that received beta-carotene (15 mg/d), vitamin E (30 mg/d) and selenium (50 μg/d); no statistically significant reductions in the prevalence of esophageal or gastric dysplasia or cancer were observed *(250,251)*. The individual effect of α-tocopherol in this trial cannot be determined.

Prompted by secondary analysis of the ATBC trial that reported a risk reduction in prostate cancer, the Selenium and Vitamin E Cancer Prevention Trial (SELECT) was launched in 2001 to evaluate the efficacy of supplementation with vitamin E (all-*rac* α-tocopherol, 400 mg/d), alone or in combination with selenium (200 μg/d), in prostate cancer prevention *(252)*. The trial provides optional multivitamins that contain no vitamin E and selenium. The target study population is 32,400 healthy North American men age 55 years or older (age 50 or older for African Americans) and the total study period is 12 yr (5 yr of recruitment and at least 7 yr of follow-up). Results from this trial will provide evidence on the efficacy of α-tocopherol supplement use in primary prostate cancer prevention.

11. SUMMARY

Research has just begun to expand testing the efficacy of α-tocopherol in Phase III trials, and to elucidate effects of other tocopherols, tocotrienols, and α-tocopherol derivatives in in vitro and animal studies. Results from some observational epidemiological studies and a large-scale intervention trial suggest that α-tocopherol may be important in preventing prostate, colorectal, and lung cancers. However, optimal use of vitamin E in regard to dosage, duration, and composition remains uncertain. Because the use of α-tocopherol supplements decreases serum concentrations of γ-tocopherol, and presumably other tocopherols and tocotrienols, concomitant use of all forms of vitamin E may confer more chemopreventive benefits than α-tocopherol alone.

ACKNOWLEDGMENT

This work was supported in part by research grants IUOIAG 18033 and IUOI CA86308–01 from the National Cancer Institute.

REFERENCES

1. Weiser H, Vecchi M. Stereoisomers of alpha-tocopheryl acetate—characterization of the samples by physico-chemical methods and determination of biological activities in the rat resorption-gestation test. *Int J Vitam Nutr Res* 1981;51:100–113.
2. McLaughlin PJ, Weihrauch JL. Vitamin E content of foods. *J Am Diet Assoc* 1979:75:647–665.
3. Lehmann J, Martin HL, Lashley EL, et al. Vitamin E in foods from high and low linoleic acid diets. *J Am Diet Assoc* 1986;86:1208–1216.
4. Weiser H, Vecchi M. Stereoisomers of alpha-tocopheryl acetate. II. Biopotencies of all eight stereoisomers, individually or in mixtures, as determined by rat resorption-gestation tests. *Int J Vitam Nutr Res* 1982;52:351–370.
5. Pearce BC, Parker RA, Deason ME, et al. Hypocholesterolemic activity of synthetic and natural tocotrienols. *J Med Chem* 1992;35:3595–3606.
6. Muggli R. Physiological requirements of vitamin E as a function of the amount and type of polyunsaturated fatty acid. *World Rev Nutr Diet* 1994;75:166–168.
7. Institute of Medicine. Panel on Dietary Antioxidants and Related Compounds. Dietary reference intakes for vitamin C, vitamin E, selenium, and carotenoids. National Academy Press, Washington DC, 2000.
8. Horwitt MK, Harvey CC, Duncan GD, Wilson WC. Effects of limited tocopherol intake in man with relationships to erythrocyte hemolysis and lipid peroxidations. *Am J Clin Nutr* 1956;4:408–419.
9. Horwitt MK, Century B, Zeman AA. Erythrocytes survival time and reticulocyte levels after tocopherol depletion in man. *Am J Clin Nutr* 1963;12: 99–106.
10. Alaimo K, McDowell MA, Briefel RR, et al. Dietary intake of vitamins, minerals, and fiber of persons ages 2 months and over in the United States: Third National Health and Nutrition Examination Survey, Phase 1, 1988–91. Advance Data from Vital and Health Statistics No. 258. Hyattsville, MD: *National Center for Health Statistics*, 1994.
11. Swanson JE, Ben RN, Burton GW, Parker RS. Urinary excretion of 2,7, 8-trimethyl-2-(beta-carboxyethyl)-6-hydroxychroman is a major route of elimination of gamma-tocopherol in humans. *J Lipid Res* 1999;40:665–671.
12. Muller DP, Manning JA, Mathias PM, Harries JT. Studies on the intestinal hydrolysis of tocopheryl esters. *Int J Vitam Nutr Res* 1976;46:207–210.
13. Gallo-Torres HE. Obligatory role of bile for the intestinal absorption of vitamin E. *Lipids* 1970;5:379–384.
14. Harries JT, Muller DP. Absorption of vitamin E in children with biliary obstruction. *Gut* 1971;12:579–584.
15. Sokol RJ, Heubi JE, Iannaccone S, et al. Mechanism causing vitamin E deficiency during chronic childhood cholestasis. *Gastroenterology* 1983;85:1172–1182.
16. Cohn W, Gross P, Grun H, et al. Tocopherol transport and absorption. *Proc Nutr Soc* 1992 ;51:179–188.
17. Drevon CA. Absorption, transport and metabolism of vitamin E. *Free Radic Res Commun* 1991;14:229–246.
18. Losowsky MS, Kelleher J, Walker BE, et al. Intake and absorption of tocopherol. *Ann NY Acad Sci* 1972;203:212–222.
19. Kelleher J, Losowsky MS. The absorption of alpha-tocopherol in man. *Br J Nutr* 1970;24:1033–1047.
20. Pearson CK, Barnes MM. The absorption and distribution of the naturally occurring tocochromanols in the rat. *Br J Nutr* 1970;24:581–587.
21. Fragoso YD, Brown AJ. In vivo metabolism of alpha-tocopherol in lipoproteins and liver: studies on rabbits in response to acute cholesterol loading. *Rev Paul Med* 1998;116:1753–1759.
22. Thellman CA, Shireman RB. In vitro uptake of [3H]alpha-tocopherol from low density lipoprotein by cultured human fibroblasts. *J Nutr* 1985;115:1673–1679.
23. Mathias PM, Harries JT, Peters TJ, Muller DP. Studies on the in vivo absorption of micellar solutions of tocopherol and tocopheryl acetate in the rat: demonstration and partial characterization of a mucosal esterase localized to the endoplasmic reticulum of the enterocyte. *J Lipid Res* 1981;22:829–837.
24. Kiyose C, Muramatsu R, Fujiyama-Fujiwara Y, et al. Biodiscrimination of alpha-tocopherol stereoisomers during intestinal absorption. *Lipids* 1995;30:1015–1018.
25. Traber MG, Burton GW, Hughes L, et al. Discrimination between forms of vitamin E by humans with and without genetic abnormalities of lipoprotein metabolism. *J Lipid Res* 1992;33:1171–1182.
26. Catignani GL. An alpha-tocopherol binding protein in rat liver cytoplasm. *Biochem Biophys Res Commun* 1975;67:66–72.
27. Yoshida H, Yusin M, Ren I, et al. Identification, purification, and immunochemical characterization of a tocopherol-

binding protein in rat liver cytosol. *J Lipid Res* 1992;33:343–350.

28. Kuhlenkamp J, Ronk M, Yusin M, et al. Identification and purification of a human liver cytosolic tocopherol binding protein. *Protein Expr Purif* 1993;4:382–389.

29. Kayden HJ, Traber MG. Absorption, lipoprotein transport, and regulation of plasma concentrations of vitamin E in humans. *J Lipid Res* 1993;34:343–358.

30. Traber MG, Arai H. Molecular mechanisms of vitamin E transport. *Annu Rev Nutr* 1999;19:343–355.

31. Ingold KU, Burton GW, Foster DO, et al. Biokinetics of and discrimination between dietary RRR- and SRR-α- tocopherols in the male rat. *Lipids* 1987;22:163–172.

32. Acuff RV, Thedford SS, Hidiroglou NN, et al. Relative bioavailability of RRR- and all-rac-α-tocopheryl acetate in humans: studies using deuterated compounds. *Am J Clin Nutr* 1994;60:397–402.

33. Burton GW, Traber MG, Acuff RV, et al. Human plasma and tissue α-tocopherol concentrations in response to supplementation with deuterated natural and synthetic vitamin E. *Am J Clin Nutr*1998;67:669–684.

34. Hosomi A, Arita M, Sato Y, et al. Affinity for α-tocopherol transfer protein as a determinant of the biological activities of vitamin E analogs. *FEBS Lett* 1997;409:105–108.

35. Hosomi A, Goto K, Kondo H, et al. Localization of α-tocopherol transfer protein in rat brain. *Neurosci Lett* 1998;256:159–162.

36. Handelman GJ, Epstein WL, Peerson J, et al. Human adipose α-tocopherol and gamma-tocopherol kinetics during and after 1 y of α-tocopherol supplementation. *Am J Clin Nutr* 1994;59:1025–1032.

37. Handelman GJ, Machlin LJ, Fitch K, et al. Oral α-tocopherol supplements decrease plasma γ-tocopherol levels in humans. *J Nutr* 1985;115:807–813.

38. Baker H, Handelman GJ, Short S, et al. Comparison of plasma α and γ tocopherol levels following chronic oral administration of either all-*rac*-α-tocopheryl acetate or RRR-α-tocopheryl acetate in normal adult male subjects. *Am J Clin Nutr* 1986;43:382–387.

39. Kiyose C, Saito H, Kaneko K, et al. α-Tocopherol affects the urinary and biliary excretion of 2,7,8- trimethyl-2 (2'-carboxyethyl)-6-hydroxychroman, γ-tocopherol metabolite, in rats. *Lipids* 2001;36:467–472.

40. Qureshi AA, Pearce BC, Nor RM, et al. Dietary α-tocopherol attenuates the impact of gamma-tocotrienol on hepatic 3-hydroxy-3-methylglutaryl coenzyme A reductase activity in chickens. *J Nutr* 1996;126:389–394.

41. Clement M, Bourre JM. Graded dietary levels of RRR-γ-tocopherol induce a marked increase in the concentrations of α- and γ-tocopherol in nervous tissues, heart, liver and muscle of vitamin-E-deficient rats. *Biochim Biophys Acta* 1997;1334:173–181.

42. Cohn W, Goss-Sampson MA, Grun H, Muller DP. Plasma clearance and net uptake of α-tocopherol and low-density lipoprotein by tissues in WHHL and control rabbits. *Biochem J* 1992;287 (Pt 1):247–254.

43. Traber MG, Kayden HJ. Vitamin E is delivered to cells via the high affinity receptor for low-density lipoprotein. *Am J Clin Nutr* 1984;40:747–751.

44. Traber MG, Rader D, Acuff RV, et al. Vitamin E dose-response studies in humans with use of deuterated RRR- α-tocopherol. *Am J Clin Nutr* 1998;68:847–853.

45. Dimitrov NV, Meyer C, Gilliland D, et al. Plasma tocopherol concentrations in response to supplemental vitamin E. *Am J Clin Nutr* 1991;53:723–729.

46. Jialal I, Fuller CJ, Huet BA. The effect of α-tocopherol supplementation on LDL oxidation. A dose-response study. *Arterioscler Thromb Vasc Biol* 1995;15:190–198.

47. Cheeseman KH, Holley AE, Kelly FJ, et al. Biokinetics in humans of RRR-α-tocopherol: the free phenol, acetate ester, and succinate ester forms of vitamin E. *Free Radic Biol Med* 1995;19:591–598.

48. Ferslew KE, Acuff RV, Daigneault EA, et al. Pharmacokinetics and bioavailability of the RRR and all racemic stereoisomers of α-tocopherol in humans after single oral administration. *J Clin Pharmacol* 1993;33:84–88.

49. Yap SP, Yuen KH, Wong JW. Pharmacokinetics and bioavailability of α-, γ- and Δ-tocotrienols under different food status. *J Pharm Pharmacol* 2001;53:67–71.

50. Traber MG, Ramakrishnan R, Kayden HJ. Human plasma vitamin E kinetics demonstrate rapid recycling of plasma RRR-α-tocopherol. *Proc Natl Acad Sci USA* 1994;91:10,005–10,008.

51. Zimmer S, Stocker A, Sarbolouki MN, et al. A novel human tocopherol-associated protein: cloning, in vitro expression, and characterization. *J Biol Chem* 2000;275:25,672–25,680.

52. Gordon MJ, Campbell FM, Dutta-Roy AK. α-Tocopherol-binding protein in the cytosol of the human placenta. *Biochem Soc Trans* 1996;24:202S.

53. Burton GW, Wronska U, Stone L, et al. Biokinetics of dietary RRR-α-tocopherol in the male guinea pig at three dietary levels of vitamin C and two levels of vitamin E. Evidence that vitamin C does not "spare" vitamin E in vivo. *Lipids* 1990;25:199–210.

54. Blatt DH, Leonard SW, Traber MG. Vitamin E kinetics and the function of tocopherol regulatory proteins. *Nutrition* 2001;17:799–805.

55. Machlin LJ, ed. Handbook of Vitamins, 2nd ed, Marcel Dekker, New York, *NY*,1991.

56. Podda M, Weber C, Traber MG, Packer L. Simultaneous determination of tissue tocopherols, tocotrienols, ubiquinols, and ubiquinones. *J Lipid Res* 1996;37:893–901.

57. Csallany AS, Draper HH, Shah SN. Conversion of α-tocopherol-C14 to tocopheryl-p-quinone in vivo. *Arch Biochem Biophys* 1962;98,142–145.

58. Hayashi T, Kanetoshi A, Nakamura M, et al. Reduction of α-tocopherolquinone to α-tocopherolhydroquinone in rat hepatocytes. *Biochem Pharmacol* 1992;44:489–493.

59. Bindoli A, Valente M, Cavallini L. Inhibition of lipid peroxidation by α-tocopherolquinone and α-tocopherolhydroquinone. *Biochem Int* 1985;10:753–761.

60. Chiku S, Hamamura K, Nakamura T. Novel urinary metabolite of d-Δ-tocopherol in rats. J *Lipid Res* 1984;25:40–48.

61. Lodge JK, Ridlington J, Leonard S, et al. G. α- and γ-Tocotrienols are metabolized to carboxyethyl-hydroxychroman derivatives and excreted in human urine. *Lipids* 2001;36:43–48.

62. Parker RS, Sontag TJ, Swanson, JE. Cytochrome P4503A-dependent metabolism of tocopherols and inhibition by sesamin. *Biochem Biophys Res Commun* 2000;277:531–534.

63. Traber MG, Elsner A, Brigelius-Flohe R. Synthetic as compared with natural vitamin E is preferentially excreted as

α-CEHC in human urine: studies using deuterated α-tocopheryl acetates. *FEBS Lett* 1998:437:145–148.

64. Schultz M, Leist M, Petrzika M, et al. Novel urinary metabolite of α-tocopherol, 2,5,7,8-tetramethyl-2(2'-carboxyethyl)-6-hydroxychroman, as an indicator of an adequate vitamin E supply? *Am J Clin Nutr* 1995;62:15,27S–15,34S.

65. Wechter WJ, Kantoci D, Murray ED Jr, et al. A new endogenous natriuretic factor: LLU-α. *Proc Natl Acad Sci USA* 1996;93:6002–6007.

66. Appenroth D, Karge E, Kiessling G, et al. LLU-α, an endogenous metabolite of γ-tocopherol, is more effective against metal nephrotoxicity in rats than γ-tocopherol. *Toxicol Lett* 2001;122:255–265.

67. Jiang Q, Elson-Schwab I, Courtemanche C, Ames BN. γ-tocopherol and its major metabolite, in contrast to α- tocopherol, inhibit cyclooxygenase activity in macrophages and epithelial cells. *Proc Natl Acad Sci USA* 2000;97:11,494–11,499.

68. Bendich A, Machlin LJ. Safety of oral intake of vitamin E. *Am J Clin Nutr* 1988;48:612–619.

69. Bowry VW, Ingold KU, Stocker R. Vitamin E in human low-density lipoprotein. When and how this antioxidant becomes a pro-oxidant. *Biochem J* 1992;288 (Pt 2):341–344.

70. Ingold KU, Bowry VW, Stocker R, Walling C. Autoxidation of lipids and antioxidation by α-tocopherol and ubiquinol in homogeneous solution and in aqueous dispersions of lipids: unrecognized consequences of lipid particle size as exemplified by oxidation of human low density lipoprotein. *Proc Natl Acad Sci USA* 1993;90:45–49.

71. Kappus H, Diplock AT. Tolerance and safety of vitamin E: a toxicological position report. *Free Radic Biol Med* 1992;13:55–74.

72. Anderson TW, Reid DB. A double-blind trial of vitamin E in angina pectoris. *Am J Clin Nutr* 1974;27:1174–1178.

73. Meydani SN, Meydani M, Blumberg JB, et al. Assessment of the safety of supplementation with different amounts of vitamin E in healthy older adults. *Am J Clin Nutr* 1998;68:311–318.

74. Traber MG, Kayden HJ. Preferential incorporation of α-tocopherol vs γ-tocopherol in human lipoproteins. *Am J Clin Nutr* 1989;49:517–526.

75. O'Byrne D, Grundy S, Packer L, et al. Studies of LDL oxidation following α-, γ-, or Δ-tocotrienyl acetate supplementation of hypercholesterolemic humans. *Free Radic Biol Med* 2000;29:834–845.

76. Tomeo AC, Geller M, Watkins TR, et al. Antioxidant effects of tocotrienols in patients with hyperlipidemia and carotid stenosis. *Lipids* 1995;30:1179–1183.

77. Nakamura H, Furukawa F, Nishikawa A, et al. Oral toxicity of a tocotrienol preparation in rats. *Food Chem Toxicol* 2001;39:799–805.

78. McCay PB. Vitamin E: interactions with free radicals and ascorbate. *Annu Rev Nutr* 1985;5:323–340.

79. Huang HY, Helzlsouer KJ, Appel LJ. The effects of vitamin C and vitamin E on oxidative DNA damage: results from a randomized controlled trial. *Cancer Epidemiol Biomark Prev* 2000;9:647–652.

80. Bendich A, D'Apolito P, Gabriel E, Machlin LJ. Interaction of dietary vitamin C and vitamin E on guinea pig immune responses to mitogens. *J Nutr* 1984;114:1588–1593.

81. Yamauchi R, Yagi Y, Kato K. Oxidation of α-tocopherol during the peroxidation of dilinoleoylphosphatidylcholine in liposomes. *Biosci Biotechnol Biochem* 1996;60:616–620.

82. Cooney RV, Ross PD, Bartolini GL. N-nitrosation and N-nitration of morpholine by nitrogen dioxide: inhibition by ascorbate, glutathione and α-tocopherol. *Cancer Lett* 1986;32:83–90.

83. Cooney RV, Franke AA, Harwood PJ, et al. γ-Tocopherol detoxification of nitrogen dioxide: superiority to α-tocopherol. *Proc Natl Acad Sci USA* 1993;90:1771–1775.

84. Goss SP, Hogg N, Kalyanaraman B. The effect of α-tocopherol on the nitration of γ-tocopherol by peroxynitrite. *Arch Biochem Biophys* 1999;363:333–340.

85. Weber C, Podda M, Rallis M, et al. Efficacy of topically applied tocopherols and tocotrienols in protection of murine skin from oxidative damage induced by UV- irradiation. *Free Radic Biol Med* 1997;22:761–769.

86. Kamat JP, Devasagayam TP. Tocotrienols from palm oil as potent inhibitors of lipid peroxidation and protein oxidation in rat brain mitochondria. *Neurosci Lett* 1995;195:179–182.

87. Kamat JP, Sarma HD, Devasagayam TP, et al. Tocotrienols from palm oil as effective inhibitors of protein oxidation and lipid peroxidation in rat liver microsomes. *Mol Cell Biochem* 1997;170:131–137.

88. Serbinova E, Kagan V, Han D, Packer L. Free radical recycling and intramembrane mobility in the antioxidant properties of α-tocopherol and α-tocotrienol. *Free Radic Biol Med* 1991;10:263–275.

89. Suzuki YJ, Tsuchiya M, Wassall SR, et al. Structural and dynamic membrane properties of α-tocopherol and α-tocotrienol: implication to the molecular mechanism of their antioxidant potency. *Biochemistry* 1993;32:10,692–10,699.

90. Mirvish SS. The etiology of gastric cancer. Intragastric nitrosamide formation and other theories. *J Natl Cancer Inst* 1983;71:629–647.

91. Fiddler W, Pensabene JW, Piotrowski EG, et al. Inhibition of formation of volatile nitrosamines in fried bacon by the use of cure-solubilized α-tocopherol. *J Agric Food Chem* 1978;26:653–656.

92. Mirvish SS. Effects of vitamins C and E on N-nitroso compound formation, carcinogenesis, and cancer. *Cancer* 1986;58:1842–1850.

93. Kamm JJ, Dashman T, Newmark H, Mergens WJ. Inhibition of amine-nitrite hepatotoxicity by α-tocopherol. *Toxicol Appl Pharmacol* 1977;41:575–583.

94. Li Y, Glauert HP, Spear BT. Activation of nuclear factor-κB by the peroxisome proliferator ciprofibrate in H4IIEC3 rat hepatoma cells and its inhibition by the antioxidants N-acetylcysteine and vitamin E. *Biochem Pharmacol* 2000;59:427–434.

95. Maziere C, Conte MA, Degonville J, et al. C. Cellular enrichment with polyunsaturated fatty acids induces an oxidative stress and activates the transcription factors AP1 and NFκB. *Biochem Biophys Res Commun* 1999;265:116–122.

96. Li D, Saldeen T, Mehta JL. γ-Tocopherol decreases ox-LDL-mediated activation of nuclear factor-κB and apoptosis in human coronary artery endothelial cells. *Biochem Biophys Res Commun* 1999;259:157–161.

97. Islam KN, Devaraj S, Jialal I. α-Tocopherol enrichment of monocytes decreases agonist-induced adhesion to human endothelial cells. *Circulation* 1998;98:2255–2261.

98. Nakamura T, Goto M, Matsumoto A, Tanaka I. Inhibition of NF-κ B transcriptional activity by α-tocopheryl succinate. *Biofactors* 1998;7:21–30.

99. Erl W, Weber C, Wardemann C, Weber PC. α-Tocopheryl succinate inhibits monocytic cell adhesion to endothelial cells by suppressing NF-κB mobilization. *Am J Physiol* 1997;273:H634–H640.

100. Maziere C, Auclair M, Djavaheri-Mergny M, et al. Oxidized low density lipoprotein induces activation of the transcription factor NFκB in fibroblasts, endothelial and smooth muscle cells. *Biochem Mol Biol Int* 1996;39:1201–1207.

101. Suzuki YJ, Packer L. Inhibition of NF-κB DNA binding activity by α-tocopheryl succinate. *Biochem Mol Biol Int* 1993;31:693–700.

102. Wu D, Hayek MG, Meydani S. Vitamin E and macrophage cyclooxygenase regulation in the aged. *J Nutr* 2001;131:382S–388S.

103. Devaraj S, Jialal I. α-Tocopherol decreases interleukin-1 beta release from activated human monocytes by inhibition of 5-lipoxygenase. *Arterioscler Thromb Vasc Biol* 1999;19:1125–1133.

104. Yoshikawa T, Yoshida N, Manabe H, et al. α-tocopherol protects against expression of adhesion molecules on neutrophils and endothelial cells. *Biofactors* 1998;7:15–19.

105. Tasinato A, Boscoboinik D, Bartoli GM, et al. d-α-tocopherol inhibition of vascular smooth muscle cell proliferation occurs at physiological concentrations, correlates with protein kinase C inhibition, and is independent of its antioxidant properties. *Proc Natl Acad Sci USA* 1995;92:12,190–12,194.

106. Ozer NK, Palozza P, Boscoboinik D, Azzi A. d-α-Tocopherol inhibits low density lipoprotein induced proliferation and protein kinase C activity in vascular smooth muscle cells. *FEBS Lett* 1993;322:307–310.

107. Fazzio A, Marilley D, Azzi A. The effect of α-Tocopherol and β-tocopherol on proliferation, protein kinase C activity and gene expression in different cell lines. *Biochem Mol Biol Int* 1997;41:93–101.

108. Martin-Nizard F, Boullier A, Fruchart JC, Duriez P. α-Tocopherol but not β-tocopherol inhibits thrombin-induced PKC activation and endothelin secretion in endothelial cells. *J Cardiovasc Risk* 1998;5:339–345.

109. Gopalakrishna R, Jaken S. Protein kinase C signaling and oxidative stress. *Free Radic Biol Med* 2000;28:1349–1361.

110. Yano T, Yano Y, Yajima S, et al. The suppression of ornithine decarboxylase expression and cell proliferation at the promotion stage of lung tumorigenesis in mice by α-tocopheryloxybutyric acid. *Biochem Pharmacol* 2001;61:1177–1181.

111. Ricciarelli R, Tasinato A, Clement S., et al. α-tocopherol specifically inactivates cellular protein kinase Cα by changing its phosphorylation state. *Biochem J* 1998;334 (Pt 1):243–249.

112. Lee IK, Koya D, Ishi H, et al. d-α-Tocopherol prevents the hyperglycemia induced activation of diacylglycerol (DAG)-protein kinase C (PKC) pathway in vascular smooth muscle cell by an increase of DAG kinase activity. *Diabetes Res Clin Pract* 1999;45:183–190.

113. Tran K, Proulx PR, Chan AC. Vitamin E suppresses diacylglycerol (DAG) level in thrombin-stimulated endothelial cells through an increase of DAG kinase activity. *Biochim Biophys Acta* 1994;1212:193–202.

114. Heisler T, Towfigh S, Simon N, McFadden DW. Peptide YY and vitamin E inhibit hormone-sensitive and -insensitive breast cancer cells. *J Surg Res* 2000;91:9–14.

115. Malafa MP, Neitzel LT. Vitamin E succinate promotes breast cancer tumor dormancy. *J Surg Res* 2000;93:163–170.

116. Charpentier A, Groves S, Simmons-Menchaca M, et al. RRR-α-tocopheryl succinate inhibits proliferation and enhances secretion of transforming growth factor-β (TGF-β) by human breast cancer cells. *Nutr Cancer* 1993;19:225–239.

117. Israel K, Sanders BG, Kline K. RRR-α-tocopheryl succinate inhibits the proliferation of human prostatic tumor cells with defective cell cycle/differentiation pathways. *Nutr Cancer* 1995;24:161–169.

118. Nargi JL, Ratan RR, Griffin DE. p53-independent inhibition of proliferation and p21(WAF1/Cip1)-modulated induction of cell death by the antioxidants *N*-acetylcysteine and vitamin E. *Neoplasia* 1999;1:544–556.

119. Rose AT, McFadden DW. α-Tocopherol succinate inhibits growth of gastric cancer cells in vitro. *J Surg Res* 2001;95:19–22.

120. Elattar TM, Lin HS. Inhibition of human oral squamous carcinoma cell (SCC-25) proliferation by prostaglandin E2 and vitamin E succinate. *J Oral Pathol Med* 1993;22:425–427.

121. Turley JM, Sanders BG, Kline K. RRR-α-tocopheryl succinate modulation of human promyelocytic leukemia (HL-60) cell proliferation and differentiation. *Nutr Cancer* 1992;18:201–213.

122. Turley JM, Funakoshi S, Ruscetti FW, et al. Growth inhibition and apoptosis of RL human B lymphoma cells by vitamin E succinate and retinoic acid: role for transforming growth factor β. *Cell Growth Differ* 1995;6:655–663.

123. Schwartz J, Shklar G. The selective cytotoxic effect of carotenoids and α-tocopherol on human cancer cell lines in vitro. *J Oral Maxillofac Surg* 1992;50:367–373.

124. Slack R, Proulx P. Studies on the effects of vitamin E on neuroblastoma N1E 115. *Nutr Cancer* 1989;12:75–82.

125. Kline K, Cochran GS, Sanders BG. Growth-inhibitory effects of vitamin E succinate on retrovirus-transformed tumor cells in vitro. *Nutr Cancer* 1990;14:27–41.

126 Fariss MW, Fortuna MB, Everett CK, et al. The selective antiproliferative effects of α-tocopheryl hemisuccinate and cholesteryl hemisuccinate on murine leukemia cells result from the action of the intact compounds. *Cancer Res* 1994;54:3346–3351.

127. Mo H, Elson CE. Apoptosis and cell-cycle arrest in human and murine tumor cells are initiated by isoprenoids. *J Nutr* 1999;129:804–813.

128. He L, Mo H, Hadisusilo S, et al. Isoprenoids suppress the growth of murine B16 melanomas in vitro and in vivo. *J Nutr* 1997;127:668–674.

129. Guthrie N, Gapor A, Chambers AF, Carroll KK. Inhibition of proliferation of estrogen receptor-negative MDA-MB-435 and -positive MCF-7 human breast cancer cells by palm oil tocotrienols and tamoxifen, alone and in combination. *J Nutr* 1997;127:544S–548S.

130. Nesaretnam K, Guthrie N, Chambers AF, Carroll KK. Effect of tocotrienols on the growth of a human breast cancer cell line in culture. *Lipids* 1995;30:1139–1143.

131. Nesaretnam K, Stephen R, Dils R, Darbre P. Tocotrienols inhibit the growth of human breast cancer cells irrespective of estrogen receptor status. *Lipids* 1998;33:461–469.

132. McIntyre BS, Briski KP, Gapor A, Sylvester PW. Antiproliferative and apoptotic effects of tocopherols and tocotrienols on preneoplastic and neoplastic mouse mammary epithelial cells. *Proc Soc Exp Biol Med* 2000;224:292–301.

133. Theriault A, Chao JT, Wang Q, et al. Tocotrienol: a review of its therapeutic potential. *Clin Biochem* 1999;32:309–319.

134. Dricu A, Wang M, Hjertman M, et al. Mevalonate-regulated mechanisms in cell growth control: role of dolichyl phosphate in expression of the insulin-like growth factor-1 receptor (IGF-1R) in comparison to Ras prenylation and expression of c-*myc*. *Glycobiology* 1997;7:625–633.

135. Zhang FL, Casey PJ. Protein prenylation: molecular mechanisms and functional consequences. *Annu Rev Biochem* 1996;65:241–269.

136. Qureshi AA, Mo H, Packer L, Peterson DM. Isolation and identification of novel tocotrienols from rice bran with hypocholesterolemic, antioxidant, and antitumor properties. *J Agric Food Chem* 2000;48:3130–3140.

137. Traber MG, Rallis M, Podda M, et al. Penetration and distribution of α-tocopherol, α- or γ- tocotrienols applied individually onto murine skin. *Lipids* 1998;33:87–91.

138. Weber C, Podda M, Rallis M, et al. Efficacy of topically applied tocopherols and tocotrienols in protection of murine skin from oxidative damage induced by UV- irradiation. *Free Radic Biol Med* 1997;22:761–769.

139. Thiele JJ, Traber MG, Podda M, et al. Ozone depletes tocopherols and tocotrienols topically applied to murine skin. *FEBS Lett* 1997;401:167–170.

140. Weber T, Lu M, Andera L, et al. Vitamin E succinate is a potent novel antineoplastic agent with high selectivity and cooperativity with tumor necrosis factor-related apoptosis-inducing ligand (Apo2 ligand) in vivo. *Clin Cancer Res* 2002;8:863–869.

141. Neuzil, J., Zhao, M., Ostermann, G., et al. α-Tocopheryl succinate, an agent with in vivo anti-tumour activity, induces apoptosis by causing lysosomal instability. *Biochem J* 2002;362:709–715.

142. Charpentier A, Simmons-Menchaca M, Yu W, et al. RRR-α-tocopheryl succinate enhances TGF-β 1, -β 2, and -β 3 and TGF-β R-II expression by human MDA-MB-435 breast cancer cells. *Nutr Cancer* 1996;26:237–250.

143. Yu W, Heim K, Qian M, et al. Evidence for role of transforming growth factor-β in RRR-α- tocopheryl succinate-induced apoptosis of human MDA-MB-435 breast cancer cells. *Nutr Cancer* 1997;27:267–278.

144. Israel K, Yu W, Sanders BG, Kline K. Vitamin E succinate induces apoptosis in human prostate cancer cells: role for Fas in vitamin E succinate-triggered apoptosis. *Nutr Cancer* 2000;36:90–100.

145. Yu W, Israel K, Liao QY, et al. Vitamin E succinate (VES) induces Fas sensitivity in human breast cancer cells: role for Mr 43,000 Fas in VES-triggered apoptosis. *Cancer Res* 1999;59:953–961.

146. Yu W, Simmons-Menchaca M, You H, et al. RRR-α-tocopheryl succinate induction of prolonged activation of c-*jun* amino-terminal kinase and c-*jun* during induction of apoptosis in human MDA-MB-435 breast cancer cells. *Mol Carcinog* 1998;22:247–257.

147. Yu W, Liao QY, Hantash FM, et al. Activation of extracellular signal-regulated kinase and c-Jun-NH(2)-terminal kinase

148. but not p38 mitogen-activated protein kinases is required for RRR-α-tocopheryl succinate-induced apoptosis of human breast cancer cells. *Cancer Res* 2001;61:6569–6576.

148. Kline K, Yu W, Sanders BG. Vitamin E: mechanisms of action as tumor cell growth inhibitors. *J Nutr* 2001;131:161S–163S.

149. Yu W, Simmons-Menchaca M, Gapor A, et al. Induction of apoptosis in human breast cancer cells by tocopherols and tocotrienols. *Nutr Cancer* 1999;33:26–32.

150. McIntyre BS, Briski KP, Tirmenstein MA, et al. Antiproliferative and apoptotic effects of tocopherols and tocotrienols on normal mouse mammary epithelial cells. *Lipids* 2000;35:171–180.

151. Tirmenstein MA, Leraas TL, Fariss MW. α-tocopheryl hemisuccinate administration increases rat liver subcellular α-tocopherol levels and protects against carbon tetrachloride-induced hepatotoxicity. *Toxicol Lett* 1997;92:67–77.

152. Weimann BJ, Weiser H. Functions of vitamin E in reproduction and in prostacyclin and immunoglobulin synthesis in rats. *Am J Clin Nutr* 1991;53:1056S–1060S.

153. Meydani SN, Barklund MP, Liu S, et al. Vitamin E supplementation enhances cell-mediated immunity in healthy elderly subjects. *Am J Clin Nutr* 1990;52:557–563.

154. Long KZ, Santos JI. Vitamins and the regulation of the immune response. *Pediatr Infect Dis J* 1999;18:283–290.

155. Shklar G, Schwartz JL. Vitamin E inhibits experimental carcinogenesis and tumour angiogenesis. *Eur J Cancer B Oral Oncol* 1996;32B:114–119.

156. El Salahy EM, Ahmed MI, El Gharieb A, Tawfik H. New scope in angiogenesis: role of vascular endothelial growth factor (VEGF), NO, lipid peroxidation, and vitamin E in the pathophysiology of pre-eclampsia among Egyptian females. *Clin Biochem* 2001;34:323–329.

157. Yu A, Somasundar P, Balsubramaniam A, et al. Vitamin E and the Y4 agonist BA-129 decrease prostate cancer growth and production of vascular endothelial growth factor. *J Surg Res* 2002;105:65–68.

158. Sahl WJ, Glore S, Garrison P, et al. Basal cell carcinoma and lifestyle characteristics. *Int J Dermatol* 1995;34:398–402.

159. Vena JE, Graham S, Freudenheim J, et al. Diet in the epidemiology of bladder cancer in western New York. *Nutr Cancer* 1992;18:255–264.

160. Riboli E, Gonzalez CA, Lopez-Abente G, et al. Diet and bladder cancer in Spain: a multi-centre case-control study. *Int J Cancer* 1991;49:214–219.

161. Giles GG, McNeil JJ, Donnan G, et al. Dietary factors and the risk of glioma in adults: results of a case-control study in Melbourne, Australia. *Int J Cancer* 1994;59:357–362.

162. Hu J, La Vecchia C, Negri E, et al. Diet and brain cancer in adults: a case-control study in northeast China. *Int J Cancer* 1999;81:20–23.

163. Yeum KJ, Ahn SH, Rupp de Paiva SA, et al. Correlation between carotenoid concentrations in serum and normal breast adipose tissue of women with benign breast tumor or breast cancer. *J Nutr* 1998;128:1920–1926.

164. Gerber M, Richardson S, Salkeld R, Chappuis P. Antioxidants in female breast cancer patients. *Cancer Investig* 1991;9:421–428.

165. Negri E, La Vecchia C, Franceschi S, et al. Intake of selected micronutrients and the risk of breast cancer. *Int J Cancer* 1996;65:140–144.

166. Richardson S, Gerber M, Cenee S. The role of fat, animal protein and some vitamin consumption in breast cancer: a

case control study in southern France. *Int J Cancer* 1991;48:1–9.

167. Ronco A, De Stefani E, Boffetta P, et al. Vegetables, fruits, and related nutrients and risk of breast cancer: a case-control study in Uruguay. *Nutr Cancer* 1999;35:111–119.

168. Yuan JM, Wang QS, Ross RK, et al. Diet and breast cancer in Shanghai and Tianjin, China. *Br J Cancer* 1995;71:1353–1358.

169. Levi F, Pasche C, Lucchini F, La Vecchia C. Dietary intake of selected micronutrients and breast-cancer risk. *Int J Cancer* 2001;91:260–263.

170. Mezzetti M, La Vecchia C, Decarli A, et al. Population attributable risk for breast cancer: diet, nutrition, and physical exercise. *J Natl Cancer Inst* 1998;90:389–394.

171. Ambrosone CB, Marshall JR, Vena JE, et al. Interaction of family history of breast cancer and dietary antioxidants with breast cancer risk (New York, United States). *Cancer Causes Control* 1995;6:407–415.

172. Braga C, La Vecchia C, Negri E, et al. Intake of selected foods and nutrients and breast cancer risk: an age- and menopause-specific analysis. *Nutr Cancer* 1997;28:258–263.

173. Bohlke K, Spiegelman D, Trichopoulou A, et al. Vitamins A, C and E and the risk of breast cancer: results from a case-control study in Greece. *Br J Cancer* 1999;79:23–29.

174. Mannisto S, Alfthan G, Virtanen M, et al. Toenail selenium and breast cancer—a case-control study in Finland. *Eur J Clin Nutr* 2000;54:98–103.

175. Freudenheim JL, Marshall JR, Vena JE, et al. Premenopausal breast cancer risk and intake of vegetables, fruits, and related nutrients. *J Natl Cancer Inst* 1996;88:340–348.

176. London SJ, Stein EA, Henderson IC, et al. Carotenoids, retinol, and vitamin E and risk of proliferative benign breast disease and breast cancer. *Cancer Causes Control* 1992;3:503–512.

177. van't Veer P, Strain JJ, Fernandez-Crehuet J, et al. Tissue antioxidants and postmenopausal breast cancer: the European Community Multicentre Study on Antioxidants, Myocardial Infarction, and Cancer of the Breast (EURAMIC). *Cancer Epidemiol Biomark Prev* 1996;5:441–447.

178. Potischman N, Herrero R, Brinton LA, et al. A case-control study of nutrient status and invasive cervical cancer. II. Serologic indicators. *Am J Epidemiol* 1991;134:1347–1355.

179. Peng YM, Peng YS, Childers JM, et al. Concentrations of carotenoids, tocopherols, and retinol in paired plasma and cervical tissue of patients with cervical cancer, precancer, and noncancerous diseases. *Cancer Epidemiol Biomarkers Prev* 1998;7:347–350.

180. Ferraroni M, La Vecchia C, D'Avanzo B, et al. Selected micronutrient intake and the risk of colorectal cancer. *Br J Cancer* 1994;70:1150–1155.

181. La Vecchia C, Braga C, Negri E. Intake of selected micronutrients and risk of colorectal cancer. *Int J Cancer* 1997;73(4), 525–530.

182. Slattery ML, Edwards SL, Anderson K, Caan B. Vitamin E and colon cancer: is there an association? *Nutr Cancer* 1998;30:201–206.

183. Ghadirian P, Lacroix A, Maisonneuve P, et al. Nutritional factors and colon carcinoma: a case-control study involving French Canadians in Montreal, Quebec, Canada. *Cancer* 1997;80:858–864.

184. White E, Shannon JS, Patterson RE. Relationship between vitamin and calcium supplement use and colon cancer. *Cancer Epidemiol Biomark Prev* 1997;6:769–774.

185. Freudenheim JL, Graham S, Marshall JR, et al. A case-control study of diet and rectal cancer in western New York. *Am J Epidemiol* 1990;131:612–624.

186. Charpiot P, Calaf R, Di Costanzo J, et al. Vitamin A, vitamin E, retinol binding protein (RBP), and prealbumin in digestive cancers. *Int J Vitam Nutr Res* 1989;59:323–328.

187. Negri E, La Vecchia C, Franceschi S, et al. Intake of selected micronutrients and the risk of endometrial carcinoma. *Cancer* 1996;77:917–923.

188. Goodman MT, Wilkens LR, Hankin JH, et al. Association of soy and fiber consumption with the risk of endometrial cancer. *Am J Epidemiol* 1997;146:294–306.

189. Barone J, Taioli E, Hebert JR, Wynder EL. Vitamin supplement use and risk for oral and esophageal cancer. *Nutr Cancer* 1992;18:31–41.

190. Terry P, Lagergren J, Ye W, et al. Antioxidants and cancers of the esophagus and gastric cardia. *Int J Cancer* 2000;87:750–754.

191. Zhang ZF, Kurtz RC, Yu GP, et al. Adenocarcinomas of the esophagus and gastric cardia: the role of diet. *Nutr Cancer* 1997;27:298–309.

192. Ekstrom AM, Serafini M, Nyren O, et al. Dietary antioxidant intake and the risk of cardia cancer and noncardia cancer of the intestinal and diffuse types: a population-based case-control study in Sweden. *Int J Cancer* 2000;87:133–140.

193. Kumagai Y, Pi JB, Lee S, et al. Serum antioxidant vitamins and risk of lung and stomach cancers in Shenyang, China. *Cancer Lett* 1998;129:145–149.

194. Battisti C, Formichi P, Tripodi SA, et al. Vitamin E serum levels and gastric cancer: results from a cohort of patients in Tuscany, Italy. *Cancer Lett* 2000;151:15–18.

195. Lopez-Carrillo L, Lopez-Cervantes M, Ward MH, et al. Nutrient intake and gastric cancer in Mexico. *Int J Cancer* 1999;83:601–605.

196. Freudenheim JL, Graham S, Byers TE, et al. Diet, smoking, and alcohol in cancer of the larynx: a case-control study. *Nutr Cancer* 1992;17:33–45.

197. LeGardeur BY, Lopez A, Johnson WD. A case-control study of serum vitamins A, E, and C in lung cancer patients. *Nutr Cancer* 1990;14:133–140.

198. Stefani ED, Boffetta P, Deneo-Pellegrini H, et al. Dietary antioxidants and lung cancer risk: a case-control study in Uruguay. *Nutr Cancer* 1999;34:100–110.

199. Mayne ST, Janerich DT, Greenwald P, et al. Dietary β carotene and lung cancer risk in U.S. nonsmokers. *J Natl Cancer Inst* 1994;86:33–38.

200. Stryker WS, Stampfer MJ, Stein EA, et al. Diet, plasma levels of β-carotene and α-tocopherol, and risk of malignant melanoma. *Am J Epidemiol* 1990;131:597–611.

201. Negri E, Franceschi S, Bosetti C, et al. Selected micronutrients and oral and pharyngeal cancer. *Int J Cancer* 2000;86:122–127.

202. Gridley G, McLaughlin JK, Block G, et al. Diet and oral and pharyngeal cancer among blacks. *Nutr Cancer* 1990;14:219–225.

203. Deneo-Pellegrini H, De Stefani E, Ronco A, Mendilaharsu M. Foods, nutrients and prostate cancer: a case-control study in Uruguay. *Br J Cancer* 1999;80:591–597.

204. Kristal AR, Stanford JL, Cohen JH, et al. Vitamin and mineral supplement use is associated with reduced risk of prostate cancer. *Cancer Epidemiol Biomark Prev* 1999;8:887–892.

205. Wolk A, Gridley G, Niwa S, et al. International renal cell cancer study. VII. Role of diet. *Int J Cancer* 1996;65:67–73.

206. Horn-Ross PL, Morrow M, Ljung BM. Diet and the risk of salivary gland cancer. *Am J Epidemiol* 1997;146:171–176.

207. D'Avanzo B, Ron E, La Vecchia C, et al. Selected micronutrient intake and thyroid carcinoma risk. *Cancer* 1997;79:2186–2192.

208. Longnecker MP, Martin-Moreno JM, Knekt P, et al. Serum α-tocopherol concentration in relation to subsequent colorectal cancer: pooled data from five cohorts. *J Natl Cancer Inst* 1992;84:430–435.

209. Menkes MS, Comstock GW, Vuilleumier JP, et al. Serum β-carotene, vitamins A and E, selenium, and the risk of lung cancer. *N Engl J Med* 1986;315:1250–1254.

210. Comstock GW, Alberg AJ, Huang HY, et al. The risk of developing lung cancer associated with antioxidants in the blood: ascorbic acid, carotenoids, α-tocopherol, selenium, and total peroxyl radical absorbing capacity. *Cancer Epidemiol Biomark Prev* 1997;6:907–916.

211. Willett WC, Polk BF, Underwood BA, et al. Relation of serum vitamins A and E and carotenoids to the risk of cancer. *N Engl J Med* 1984;310:430–434.

212. Nomura AM, Stemmermann GN, Heilbrun LK, et al. Serum vitamin levels and the risk of cancer of specific sites in men of Japanese ancestry in Hawaii. *Cancer Res* 1985;45:2369–2372.

213. Stahelin HB, Rosel F, Buess E, Brubacher G. Cancer, vitamins, and plasma lipids: prospective Basel study. *J Natl Cancer Inst* 1984;73:1463–1468.

214. Knekt P, Marniemi J, Teppo L, et al. Is low selenium status a risk factor for lung cancer? *Am J Epidemiol* 1998;148:975–982.

215. Ratnasinghe D, Tangrea JA, Forman MR, et al. Serum tocopherols, selenium and lung cancer risk among tin miners in China. *Cancer Causes Control* 2000;11:129–135.

216. Huang HY, Alberg AJ, Norkus EP, et al. prospective study of antioxidant micronutrients in the blood and the risk of developing prostate cancer, *Am J Epidemiol* 2003;157:335–344.

217. Nomura AM, Stemmermann GN, Lee J, Craft NE. Serum micronutrients and prostate cancer in Japanese Americans in Hawaii. *Cancer Epidemiol Biomark Prev* 1997;6:487–491.

218. Gann PH, Ma J, Giovannucci E, et al. Lower prostate cancer risk in men with elevated plasma lycopene levels: results of a prospective analysis. *Cancer Res* 1999;59:1225–1230.

219 Helzlsouer KJ, Huang HY, Alberg AJ, et al. Association between α-tocopherol, γ-tocopherol, selenium, and subsequent prostate cancer. *J Natl Cancer Inst* 2000;92:2018–2023.

220. Woodson K, Tangrea JA, Barrett MJ, et al. Serum α-tocopherol and subsequent risk of lung cancer among male smokers. *J Natl Cancer Inst* 1999;91:1738–1743.

221. Bostick RM, Potter JD, McKenzie DR, et al. Reduced risk of colon cancer with high intake of vitamin E: The Iowa Women's Health Study. *Cancer Res* 1993;53:4230–4237.

222. Jacobson JS, Begg MD, Wang LW, et al. Effects of a 6-month vitamin intervention on DNA damage in heavy smokers. *Cancer Epidemiol Biomark Prev* 2000;9:1303–1311.

223. Porkkala-Sarataho E, Salonen JT, Nyyssonen K, et al. Long-term effects of vitamin E, vitamin C, and combined supplementation on urinary 7-hydro-8-oxo-2'-deoxyguanosine, serum cholesterol oxidation products, and oxidation resistance of lipids in nondepleted men. *Arterioscler Thromb Vasc Biol* 2000;20:2087–2093.

224. Prieme H, Loft S, Nyyssonen K, et al. No effect of supplementation with vitamin E, ascorbic acid, or coenzyme Q10 on oxidative DNA damage estimated by 8-oxo-7,8-dihydro-2'-deoxyguanosine excretion in smokers. *Am J Clin Nutr* 1997;65:503–507.

225. Astley S, Langrish-Smith A, Southon S, Sampson M. Vitamin E supplementation and oxidative damage to DNA and plasma LDL in type 1 diabetes. *Diabetes Care* 1999;22:1626–1631.

226. Sampson MJ, Astley S, Richardson T, et al. Increased DNA oxidative susceptibility without increased plasma LDL oxidizability in Type II diabetes: effects of α-tocopherol supplementation. *Clin Sci (Lond)* 2001;101:235–241.

227. Duthie SJ, Ma A, Ross MA, Collins AR. Antioxidant supplementation decreases oxidative DNA damage in human lymphocytes. *Cancer Res* 1996;56:1291–1295.

228. Sardas S, Yilmaz M, Oztok U, et al. Assessment of DNA strand breakage by comet assay in diabetic patients and the role of antioxidant supplementation. *Mutat Res* 2001;490:123–129.

229. Jenkinson AM, Collins AR, Duthie SJ, et al. The effect of increased intakes of polyunsaturated fatty acids and vitamin E on DNA damage in human lymphocytes. *FASEB J* 1999;13:2138–2142.

230. Hu JJ, Chi CX, Frenkel K, et al. α-Tocopherol dietary supplement decreases titers of antibody against 5-hydroxymethyl-2'-deoxyuridine (HMdU). *Cancer Epidemiol Biomark Prev* 1999;8:693–698.

231. Devaraj S, Jialal I. α Tocopherol supplementation decreases serum C-reactive protein and monocyte interleukin-6 levels in normal volunteers and type 2 diabetic patients. *Free Radic Biol Med* 2000;29:790–792.

232. Kaul N, Devaraj S, Grundy SM, Jialal I. Failure to demonstrate a major anti-inflammatory effect with alpha tocopherol supplementation (400 IU/day) in normal subjects. *Am J Cardiol* 2001;87:1320–1323.

233. Pallast EG, Schouten EG, de Waart FG, et al. Effect of 50- and 100-mg vitamin E supplements on cellular immune function in noninstitutionalized elderly persons. *Am J Clin Nutr* 1999;69:1273–1281.

234. Meydani SN, Meydani M, Blumberg JB, et al. Vitamin E supplementation and in vivo immune response in healthy elderly subjects. A randomized controlled trial. *JAMA* 1997;277:1380–1386.

235. de Waart FG, Portengen L, Doekes G, et al. Effect of 3 months vitamin E supplementation on indices of the cellular and humoral immune response in elderly subjects. *Br J Nutr* 1997;78:761–774.

236. Girodon F, Galan P, Monget AL, et al. Impact of trace elements and vitamin supplementation on immunity and infections in institutionalized elderly patients: a randomized controlled trial. MIN. VIT. AOX. Geriatric Network. *Arch Intern Med* 1999;159:748–754.

237. Greenberg ER, Baron JA, Tosteson TD, et al. A clinical trial of antioxidant vitamins to prevent colorectal adenoma. Polyp Prevention Study Group. *N Engl J Med* 1994;331:141–147.

238. McKeown-Eyssen G, Holloway C, Jazmaji V, et al. A randomized trial of vitamins C and E in the prevention of recurrence of colorectal polyps. *Cancer Res* 1988;48:4701–4705.

239. Hofstad B, Almendingen K, Vatn M, et al. Growth and recurrence of colorectal polyps: a double-blind 3-year intervention with calcium and antioxidants. *Digestion* 1998;59:148–156.

240. Cahill RJ, O'Sullivan KR, Mathias PM, et al. Effects of vitamin antioxidant supplementation on cell kinetics of patients with adenomatous polyps. *Gut* 1993;34:963–967.

241. Malila N, Virtamo J, Virtanen M, et al. The effect of α-tocopherol and β-carotene supplementation on colorectal adenomas in middle-aged male smokers. *Cancer Epidemiol Biomark Prev* 1999;8:489–493.

242. Zaridze D, Evstifeeva T, Boyle P. Chemoprevention of oral leukoplakia and chronic esophagitis in an area of high incidence of oral and esophageal cancer. *Ann Epidemiol* 1993;3:225–234.

243. Liede K, Hietanen J, Saxen L, et al. Long-term supplementation with α-tocopherol and β-carotene and prevalence of oral mucosal lesions in smokers. *Oral Dis* 1998;4:78–83.

244. The effect of vitamin E and β carotene on the incidence of lung cancer and other cancers in male smokers. The Alpha-Tocopherol, Beta Carotene Cancer Prevention Study Group. *N Engl J Med* 1994;330:1029–1035.

245. Virtamo J, Edwards BK, Virtanen M, et al. Effects of supplemental α-tocopherol and β-carotene on urinary tract cancer: incidence and mortality in a controlled trial (Finland). *Cancer Causes Control* 2000;11:933–939.

246. Albanes D, Malila N, Taylor PR, et al. Effects of supplemental α-tocopherol and β-carotene on colorectal cancer: results from a controlled trial (Finland). *Cancer Causes Control* 2000;11:197–205.

247. Varis K, Taylor PR, Sipponen P, et al. Gastric cancer and premalignant lesions in atrophic gastritis: a controlled trial on the effect of supplementation with α-tocopherol and β-carotene. The Helsinki Gastritis Study Group. *Scand J Gastroenterol* 1998;33:294–300.

248. Rautalahti MT, Virtamo JR, Taylor PR, et al. The effects of supplementation with α-tocopherol and β-carotene on the incidence and mortality of carcinoma of the pancreas in a randomized, controlled trial. *Cancer* 1999;86:37–42.

249. Heinonen OP, Albanes D, Virtamo J, et al. Prostate cancer and supplementation with α-tocopherol and β-carotene: incidence and mortality in a controlled trial. *J Natl Cancer Inst* 1998;90:440–446.

250. Blot WJ, Li JY, Taylor PR, et al. Nutrition intervention trials in Linxian, China: supplementation with specific vitamin/mineral combinations, cancer incidence, and disease-specific mortality in the general population. *J Natl Cancer Inst* 1993;85:1483–1492.

251. Wang GQ, Dawsey SM, Li JY, et al. Effects of vitamin/mineral supplementation on the prevalence of histological dysplasia and early cancer of the esophagus and stomach: results from the General Population Trial in Linxian, China. *Cancer Epidemiol Biomark Prev* 1994;3:161–166.

252. Klein EA, Thompson IM, Lippman SM, et al. SELECT: the next prostate cancer prevention trial. Selenum and Vitamin E Cancer Prevention Trial. *J Urol* 2001;166:1311–1315.

253. Lu QY, Hung JC, Heber D, et al. Inverse associations between plasma lycopene and other carotenoids and prostate cancer. *Cancer Epidemiol Biomark Prev* 2002;10(7):749–756.

254. Ramon JM, Bou R, Romea S, et al. Dietary fat intake and prostate cancer risk: a case-control study in Spain. *Cancer Causes Control* 2000;11:679–685.

255. Wald NJ, Thompson SG, Densem JW, et al. Serum vitamin E and subsequent risk of cancer. *Br J Cancer* 1987;56:69–72.

256. Breslow RA, Alberg AJ, Helzlsouer KJ, et al. Serological precursors of cancer: malignant melanoma, basal and squamous cell skin cancer, and prediagnostic levels of retinol, β-carotene, lycopene, α-tocopherol, and selenium. *Cancer Epidemiol Biomark Prev* 1995;4:837–842.

257. Helzlsouer KJ, Comstock GW, Morris JS. Selenium, lycopene, α-tocopherol, β-carotene, retinol, and subsequent bladder cancer. *Cancer Res* 1989;49:6144–6148.

258. Knekt P, Aromaa A, Maatela J, et al. Serum micronutrients and risk of cancers of low incidence in Finland. *Am J Epidemiol* 1991;134:356–361.

259. Wald NJ, Boreham J, Hayward JL, Bulbrook RD. Plasma retinol, β-carotene and vitamin E levels in relation to the future risk of breast cancer. *Br J Cancer* 1984;49:321–324.

260. Dorgan JF, Sowell A, Swanson CA, et al. Relationships of serum carotenoids, retinol, α-tocopherol, and selenium with breast cancer risk: results from a prospective study in Columbia, Missouri (United States). *Cancer Causes Control* 1998;9:89–97.

261. Hulten K, van Kappel AL, Winkvist A, et al. Carotenoids, α-tocopherols, and retinol in plasma and breast cancer risk in northern Sweden. *Cancer Causes Control* 2001;12:529–537.

262. Batieha AM, Armenian HK, Norkus EP, et al. Serum micronutrients and the subsequent risk of cervical cancer in a population-based nested case-control study. *Cancer Epidemiol Biomark Prev* 1993;2:335–339.

263. Lehtinen M, Luostarinen T, Youngman LD, et al. Low levels of serum vitamins A and E in blood and subsequent risk for cervical cancer: interaction with HPV seropositivity. *Nutr Cancer* 1999;34:229–234.

264. Knekt P, Aromaa A, Maatela J, et al. Serum vitamin E, serum selenium and the risk of gastrointestinal cancer. *Int J Cancer* 1988;42:846–850.

265. Schober SE, Comstock GW, Helsing KJ, et al. Serologic precursors of cancer. I. Prediagnostic serum nutrients and colon cancer risk. *Am J Epidemiol* 1987;126:1033–1041.

266. Comstock GW, Helzlsouer KJ, Bush TL. Prediagnostic serum levels of carotenoids and vitamin E as related to subsequent cancer in Washington County, Maryland. *Am J Clin Nutr* 1991;53:260S–264S.

267. Botterweck AA, van den Brandt PA, Goldbohm RA. Vitamins, carotenoids, dietary fiber, and the risk of gastric carcinoma: results from a prospective study after 6.3 years of follow- up. *Cancer* 2000;88:737–748.

268. Voorrips LE, Goldbohm RA, Brants HA, et al. A prospective cohort study on antioxidant and folate intake and male lung cancer risk. *Cancer Epidemiol Biomark Prev* 2000;9:357–365.

269. Zheng W, Blot WJ, Diamond EL, et al. W. Serum micronutrients and the subsequent risk of oral and pharyngeal cancer. *Cancer Res* 1993;53:795–798.

270. Helzlsouer KJ, Alberg AJ, Norkus EP, et al. Prospective study of serum micronutrients and ovarian cancer. *J Natl Cancer Inst* 1996;88:32–37.

271. Burney PG, Comstock GW, Morris JS. Serologic precursors of cancer: serum micronutrients and the subsequent risk of pancreatic cancer. *Am J Clin Nutr* 1989;49:895–900.

272. Eichholzer M, Stahelin HB, Gey KF, et al. Prediction of male cancer mortality by plasma levels of interacting vitamins: 17-year follow-up of the prospective Basel study. *Int J Cancer* 1996;66:145–150.

273. van Dam RM, Huang Z, Giovannucci E, et al. Diet and basal cell carcinoma of the skin in a prospective cohort of men. *Am J Clin Nutr* 2000;71:135–141.

274. Michaud DS, Spiegelman D, Clinton SK, et al. Prospective study of dietary supplements, macronutrients, micronutrients, and risk of bladder cancer in US men. *Am J Epidemiol* 2000;152:1145–1153.

275. Michels KB, Holmberg L, Bergkvist L, et al. Dietary antioxidant vitamins, retinol, and breast cancer incidence in a cohort of Swedish women. *Int J Cancer* 2001;91:563–567.

276. Verhoeven DT, Assen N, Goldbohm RA, et al. Vitamins C and E, retinol, β-carotene and dietary fibre in relation to breast cancer risk: a prospective cohort study. *Br J Cancer* 1997;75:149–155.

277. Hunter DJ, Manson JE, Colditz GA, et al. A prospective study of the intake of vitamins C, E, and A and the risk of breast cancer. *N Engl J Med* 1993;329:234–240.

278. Jacobs EJ, Connell CJ, Patel AV, et al. Vitamin C and vitamin E supplement use and colorectal cancer mortality in a large American Cancer Society cohort. *Cancer Epidemiol Biomark Prev* 2001;10:17–23.

279. Sellers TA, Bazyk AE, Bostick RM, et al. Diet and risk of colon cancer in a large prospective study of older women: an analysis stratified on family history (Iowa, United States). *Cancer Causes Control* 1998;9:357–367.

280. Jacobs EJ, Connell CJ, McCullough ML, et al. Vitamin C, vitamin E, and multivitamin supplement use and stomach cancer mortality in the Cancer Prevention Study II cohort. *Cancer Epidemiol Biomark Prev* 2002;11:35–41.

281. Knekt P, Jarvinen R, Seppanen R, et al. Dietary antioxidants and the risk of lung cancer. *Am J Epidemiol* 1991;134:471–479.

282. Fairfield KM, Hankinson SE, Rosner BA, et al. Risk of ovarian carcinoma and consumption of vitamins A, C, and E and specific carotenoids: a prospective analysis. *Cancer* 2001;92:2318–2326.

283. Eichholzer M, Stahelin HB, Ludin E, Bernasconi F. Smoking, plasma vitamins C, E, retinol, and carotene, and fatal prostate cancer: seventeen-year follow-up of the prospective Basel study. *Prostate* 1999;38:189–198.

284. Chan JM, Stampfer MJ, Ma J, et al. Supplemental vitamin E intake and prostate cancer risk in a large cohort of men in the United States. *Cancer Epidemiol Biomarkers Prev* 1999;8:893–899.

285. Hartman TJ, Albanes D, Pietinen P, et al. The association between baseline vitamin E, selenium, and prostate cancer in the α-tocopherol, β-carotene cancer prevention study. Cancer Epidemiol *Biomark Prev* 1998;7: 335–340.

286. Goodman MT, Hernandez B, Wilkens LR, et al. Effects of β-carotene and α-tocopherol on bleomycin-induced chromosomal damage. *Cancer Epidemiol Biomark Prev* 1998;7:13–117.

287. Fenech M, Dreosti I, Aitken C. Vitamin-E supplements and their effect on vitamin-E status in blood and genetic damage rate in peripheral blood lymphocytes. *Carcinogenesis* 1997;18:359–364.

288. Karagas MR, Greenberg ER, Nierenberg D, et al. Risk of squamous cell carcinoma of the skin in relation to plasma selenium, α-tocopherol, β-carotene, and retinol: a nested case-control study. *Cancer Epidemiol Biomark Prev* 1997;6:25–29.

32 Vitamin C as a Cancer Chemopreventive Agent

Jane Higdon, PhD and Balz Frei, PhD

CONTENT

1. INTRODUCTION

The writings of Linus Pauling and others have stimulated a great deal of public interest in the use of vitamin C to prevent and treat cancer. Although vitamin C is known to be essential for normal physiologic function, its role in preventing cancer is less clear. Unlike most mammals, humans and other primates have lost the ability to synthesize vitamin C from glucose as a result of a mutation in the gene that encodes L-gulonolactone oxidase, the last enzyme in the biosynthetic pathway of vitamin C *(1)*. Thus, humans must obtain vitamin C through their diets. Severe vitamin C deficiency results in potentially fatal scurvy. To prevent scurvy, an adult must consume about 10 mg/d of vitamin C, easily obtained from as little as one serving/d of most fruits and vegetables. The current recommended dietary allowance (RDA) for vitamin C is 90 mg/d for men and 75 mg/d for women *(2)*, based on the vitamin C intake required for 80% neutrophil saturation with little urinary loss in healthy men. When the recommendation was made, similar data was not available for women, and the RDA was extrapolated on the basis of body wt. At this time, the results of a similar study in women have been published; the authors recommended that the RDA for vitamin C also be raised to 90 mg/d for women *(3)*.

1.1. Physiologic Functions of Vitamin C

The physiologic functions of vitamin C are related to its efficacy as a reducing agent or electron donor. Vitamin C is known to be a specific electron donor for eight human enzymes *(1)*. Three of those enzymes participate in the posttranslational hydroxylation of collagen, which is essential in the formation of stable collagen helices *(4)*. Vitamin C is necessary for the maximal activity of two dioxygenase enzymes required for carnitine biosynthesis; carnitine is required for long-chain fatty acid transport into the mitochondria. Vitamin C is also a cofactor for dopamine-β-monooxygenase, the enzyme that catalyzes the conversion of dopamine to norepinephrine, and two other enzymes required for peptide amidation and tyrosine metabolism. Vitamin C may also play a role in the metabolism of cholesterol to bile acids and in steroid metabolism as a cofactor of enzyme 7α-monooxygenase *(5)*. Hydroxylation of xenobiotics and carcinogens by the cytochrome P450 family of enzymes is also enhanced by reducing agents such as vitamin C *(6)*. Vitamin C has been found to enhance the activity of endothelial nitric oxide synthase (NOS) by maintaining its cofactor tetrahydrobiopterin in the reduced, and thus active, form *(7)*.

1.2. Antioxidant Functions of Vitamin C

Two properties make vitamin C an ideal antioxidant. First, low one-electron reduction potentials of ascorbate and its one electron oxidation product, the ascorbyl radical, enable these compounds to react with and reduce virtually all physiologically relevant reactive oxygen species (ROS) and reactive nitrogen species (RNS), including superoxide, hydroperoxyl radicals,

From: Cancer Chemoprevention, Volume 1: Promising Cancer Chemoprevention Agents
Edited by: G. J. Kelloff, E. T. Hawk, and C. C. Sigman © Humana Press Inc., Totowa, NJ

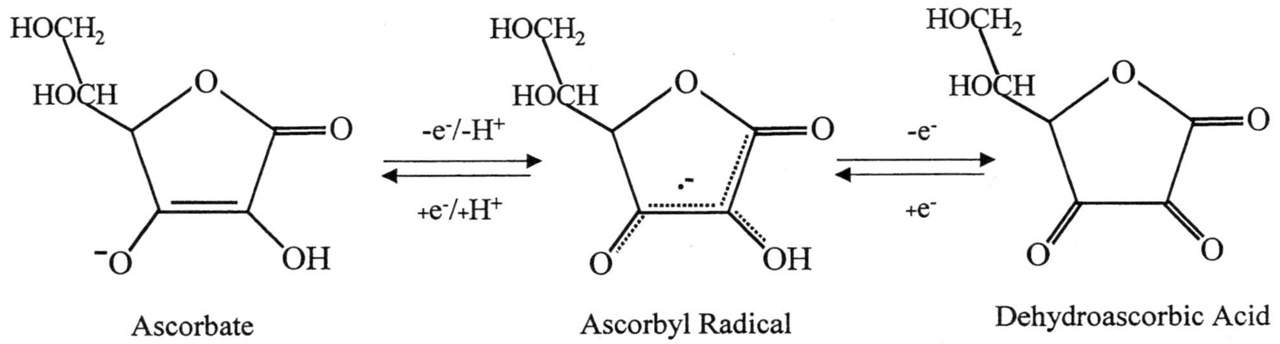

Fig. 1. Oxidation of ascorbate by two successive one-electron oxidation steps to give the ascorbyl radical and dehydroascorbic acid, respectively.

aqueous peroxyl radicals, singlet oxygen, ozone, peroxynitrite (OONO), nitrogen dioxide, nitroxide radicals, and hypochlorous acid. Hydroxyl radicals, which are so reactive that they combine indiscriminately with any substrate at a diffusion-limited rate, also react rapidly with vitamin C (8). Vitamin C acts as a co-antioxidant by regenerating α-tocopherol from the α-tocopheroxyl radical. This may be an important function, because in vitro experiments have shown that α-tocopherol can act as a pro-oxidant in the absence of co-antioxidants such as vitamin C (9).

The second property that makes vitamin C an ideal antioxidant is the low reactivity of the ascorbyl radical formed when ascorbate scavenges ROS or RNS. The ascorbyl radical scavenges another radical, or rapidly dismutates to form ascorbate and dehydroascorbic acid (Fig. 1), or is reduced back to ascorbate by NADH-dependent semidehydroascorbate reductase or the NADPH-dependent selenoenzyme thioredoxin reductase. Dehydroascorbic acid, the two-electron oxidation product of ascorbate, can be reduced back to ascorbate by the glutathione (GSH)-dependent enzyme glutaredoxin, or thioredoxin reductase. Alternatively, dehydroascorbic acid can be irreversibly hydrolyzed to diketogulonic acid (DKG), which does not function as an antioxidant (10).

2. POTENTIAL MECHANISMS OF CANCER CHEMOPREVENTION BY VITAMIN C

2.1. Prevention of Oxidative Damage to DNA

ROS and RNS have been implicated in the initiation and promotion of carcinogenesis. Some carcinogens generate free radicals during their metabolism, which may damage cells and predispose them to malignant changes. Inflammatory cells also generate

ROS and RNS, and chronic inflammation has been associated with cancer development in a number of tissues (11). DNA contains reactive groups in its bases that are highly susceptible to attack by ROS and RNS. It has been proposed that oxidative damage to DNA occurs in vivo at a rate of 10^4 oxidative hits per cell per d (12). Most oxidative lesions are repaired—e.g., by specific DNA glycosylases—but repair is not 100% efficient, and oxidative lesions on DNA accumulate with age (13). If not repaired, oxidative DNA damage may lead to mutations. Such mutations increase the risk of cancer if they occur in critical genes, such as those that encode tumor-suppressor proteins or growth factors. A direct link between cancer and oxidative DNA damage is still lacking (14). However, increased levels of oxidized DNA bases have been observed at sites of chronic inflammation and in preneoplastic lesions (15), and cellular and urinary levels of the oxidized DNA base 8-oxo-guanine are elevated in smokers (16,17). Vitamin C may prevent oxidative DNA damage in vivo by scavenging ROS and RNS, regenerating or sparing other cellular antioxidants, such as α-tocopherol or GSH, or by affecting the expression or activity of DNA repair or antioxidant enzymes (18).

2.2. Chemoprotection Against Mutagenic Compounds

N-Nitroso compounds have been implicated in the etiology of cancers of the nasopharynx, esophagus, stomach, colon, urinary bladder, and lung (19,20). Epidemiologic studies have shown an inverse association between vitamin C intake, mainly from fruits and vegetables, and cancers at these sites (21). Vitamin C may provide protection from these cancers by inhibiting the formation of mutagenic N-nitroso compounds such as

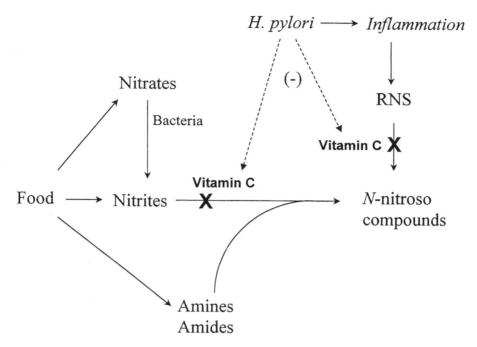

Fig. 2. Inhibition of *N*-nitroso compound formation in the stomach by vitamin C. Food may contain nitrites, nitrates, amines, and amides. Dietary nitrate may be converted to nitrite by oral bacteria. In the acidic environment of the stomach, nitrite interacts with dietary amines or amides to form carcinogenic *N*-nitroso compounds. Vitamin C prevents nitrosation by nitrite and by RNS produced by inflammatory cells. However, *H. pylori* infection is known to decrease the vitamin C content of gastric juice. Adapted from Schorah *(137)*.

nitrosamines *(22)*—which are formed by reactions of amides and amines with nitrite, common in cured foods and cigarette smoke (Fig. 2) *(20)*. Nitrosating compounds can also be formed from nitric oxide (NO) generated by inflammatory cells that express inducible nitric oxide synthase (iNOS) *(23,24)*. Increased vitamin C intake has been shown to decrease nitrosation in humans *(25,26)*.

2.3. Immune System Stimulation

Dysregulation of apoptotic and proliferative functions of the immune system may increase the risk of developing cancer *(27)*. Normally, lymphocyte apoptosis serves immune-regulatory functions, such as immune-response termination and tolerance acquisition. However, some tumors appear able to exploit lymphocyte apoptosis, escaping immune-mediated killing *(28,29)*. A potential chemopreventive property of vitamin C is prevention of immune dysfunction. Phagocytes and lymphocytes take up vitamin C, resulting in intracellular concentrations 100-fold higher than in plasma *(30)*. In vitro, vitamin C has been found to stimulate several indices of phagocytic function in macrophages *(31)* and to inhibit T-cell

apoptosis *(32)*. In humans, studies of the effect of vitamin C on immune function have been somewhat contradictory. Vitamin C depletion reduced the delayed-type hypersensitivity response in otherwise healthy men, but had no effect on lymphocyte proliferation *(33)*. However, two other studies found that vitamin C supplementation of at least 1000 mg/d increased ex vivo measures of lymphocyte proliferation *(34,35)*. Vitamin C supplementation decreased leukocyte apoptosis at doses of 500 and 1000 mg/d for 2 wk, and supplementation of at least 1000 mg/d increased natural killer (NK) cell activity in healthy individuals *(36)* and individuals exposed to immunosuppressing toxic chemicals *(37)*. Chronic inflammation is an important risk factor for a number of cancers *(8)*, even those with no established infectious cause *(38)*. Induction of inflammatory cytokines may suppress cell-mediated immune responses and increase production of oxidants and metabolites, potentially increasing DNA damage and mutations. By scavenging ROS and RNS, vitamin C may also protect tissues and immune cells from oxidative damage by the oxidants produced by phagocytic cells, particularly hypochlorous acid and other chlorinated oxidants *(39)*.

2.4. Cell Cycle Regulation and Apoptosis

Cell cycle arrest and apoptosis are important mechanisms for limiting the adverse effects of DNA damage in living organisms. Following DNA damage, cells can be transiently arrested at the G_1/S, S, or G_2/M damage checkpoints where DNA is repaired or the cell undergoes apoptosis. Inhibition of normal apoptosis pathways in healthy tissue contributes to carcinogenesis by promoting genetic instability and accumulation of mutations. Cancer cells often have mutations that make them resistant to apoptosis and facilitate proliferation *(40)*.

Pretreatment of hamster ovary cells with physiological concentrations of vitamin C (50 μM) enhanced cell-cycle arrest at the G_2/M checkpoint when oxidative stress was induced by a radical generating system *(41)*. In the absence of oxidative stress, vitamin C did not affect cell cycle progression. The p53 tumor-suppressor protein is known to play a critical role in inducing cell cycle arrest at the G_1/S DNA damage checkpoint, and mutations of the p53 gene have been associated with a number of cancers *(8)*. Cervical cells infected with cancer-producing strains of human papillomavirus (HPV) synthesize oncoproteins that target p53 for destruction. The addition of vitamin C to HPV-18-positive HeLa cells resulted in stabilization of p53 and increased sensitivity to apoptosis induced by chemotherapeutic agents *(42)*.

The redox environment of a cell appears to have complex and multifaceted effects on the induction of apoptosis. Although ROS may trigger apoptosis by inducing activation of caspases (a cascade of apoptosis-inducing proteins), sustained oxidative stress can inhibit apoptosis by modification of a critical thiol residue in a caspase catalytic site *(43)*. Sustained exposure to chloramines—chlorinated oxidants generated by myeloperoxidase from inflammatory cells—has been found to block apoptosis in cultured human endothelial cells. Incubation with 1 mM vitamin C, resulting in intracellular concentrations of 1–2 mM, protected cells from this oxidative stress and allowed apoptosis to proceed *(44)*. Overall, the effects of vitamin C on tumor-cell apoptosis in cell culture experiments have been contradictory. Several studies have found that vitamin C inhibits tumor cell death induced by oxidative stress *(45–47)*, and other studies have reported that vitamin C is cytotoxic to tumor cells *(48–50)*. Vitamin C has been shown to interact with different types of cell culture media to produce H_2O_2 at different rates. This effect appears to be related to the availability of free metal ions in the media, and could partly account for conflicting results from cell culture experiments *(51)*. Such findings limit the utility of cell culture results to predict the actions of vitamin C in vivo. In humans, vitamin C doses ranging from 500 mg to 5000 mg have been found to have no effect or a slight inhibitory effect on the apoptosis of leukocytes *(36,52)*.

3. EVIDENCE THAT VITAMIN C PREVENTS DNA DAMAGE

3.1. Biomarkers of Oxidative and Non-Oxidative DNA Damage

More than 20 different oxidative lesions of DNA have been identified, of which 8-oxo-2'-deoxyguanosine (8-oxo-dG) is one of the most frequent and best studied (Fig. 3) *(53,54)*. Attack of guanine in the C-8 position by a hydroxyl radical, OONO, or singlet oxygen results in the formation of 8-oxo-guanine (8-oxo-gua), a mutagenic base damage product. Guanine (G) normally forms a basepair with cytosine (C), but 8-oxo-gua may also pair with adenine (A). After replication, what was formally a G:C basepair is replaced by a T:A basepair, resulting in a transversion mutation. Urinary measurements of damaged DNA bases represent the number of repaired bases from the sum of all organs and cells of the body over a given period—e.g., the net rate of damage. In tissues such as lymphocytes, the measurement is a concentration specific to that tissue, representing the balance between damage and repair at the time of sampling *(55)*. The derivatization required for GC/MS assays of 8-oxo-gua increases the likelihood of artifactual oxidation compared to HPLC-EC methods *(54)*, explaining the higher values reported with GC/MS.

Single-cell alkaline gel electrophoresis (the Comet assay) is a sensitive assay of DNA single-strand breaks. The Comet assay may be adapted to measure oxidative damage to DNA bases by measuring strand breaks induced by treating DNA with relevant repair enzymes—e.g., FapyGua glycosylase (Fpg) for oxidized purine lesions and endonuclease III (EndoIII) for oxidized pyrimidine lesions *(54)*. ^{32}P-postlabeling assays may also be used to identify oxidative DNA damage. However, gamma radiation from the ^{32}P-phosphate can also oxidize guanine, and may explain the high values sometimes recorded with this method.

Micronuclei, chromatin-containing bodies that usually represent chromosomal fragments not incor-

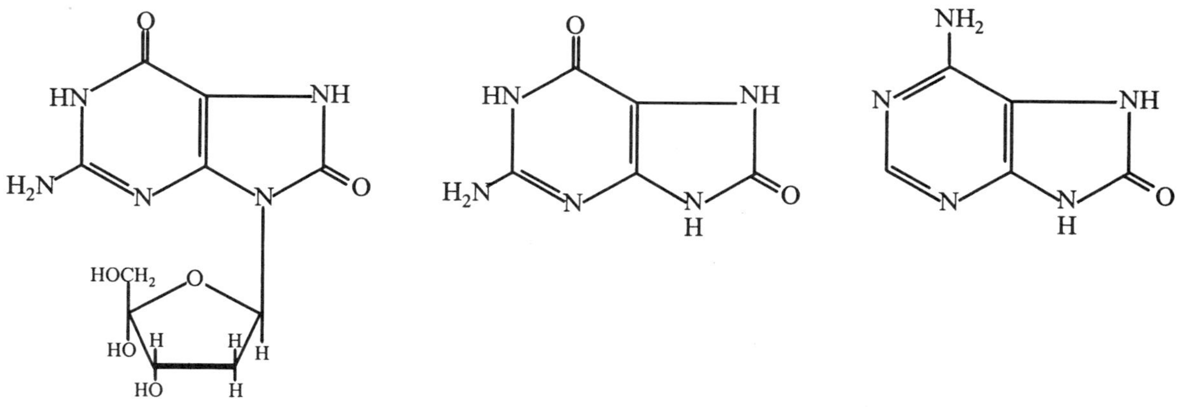

Fig. 3. Some oxidation products of DNA: 8-oxo-2'-deoxyguanosine, 8-oxo-guanine, 8-oxo-adenine.

porated into a nucleus during mitosis, are used as simple indicators of chromosomal damage. Micronuclei in cells may be counted and used as an index of DNA damage in vivo. In the sister chromatid exchange (SCE) assay, an indirect measure of genetic damage that is not well understood, cells are examined to determine whether two sister chromatids exchanged material during mitosis *(56)*.

3.2. Vitamin C and DNA Damage in Animal Models

In most but not all studies using animal models, vitamin C treatment has been found to inhibit DNA damage induced by mutagens. Vitamin C treatment of rats inhibited increases in liver and kidney 8-oxo-dG levels induced by ethinyl estradiol and potassium bromate exposure, respectively *(57,58)*. However, vitamin C did not significantly inhibit pentachlorophenol-induced increases in liver 8-oxo-dG in mice *(59)*. Vitamin C treatment prior to smoke exposure in mice also prevented cigarette smoke-induced single strand breaks in lung, stomach, and liver DNA *(60)*. Unlike mice and rats, guinea pigs cannot synthesize vitamin C, but must obtain it from their diet. However, liver 8-oxo-dG levels did not differ significantly in guinea pigs fed diets that contained widely varying levels of vitamin C (33, 660, and 13,200 mg/kg diet) for 5 wk *(61)*. A vitamin C-deficient diet in guinea pigs resulted in increased DNA damage of lens epithelium after UV-B radiation exposure, and vitamin C inhibited DNA damage in

lens epithelium of rats exposed to UV-B radiation, as determined by the Comet assay *(62)*.

3.3. Vitamin C and DNA Damage in Humans
3.3.1. OBSERVATIONAL STUDIES

A number of observational studies have examined the relationship between measures of vitamin C intake and DNA damage in humans (Table 1). In a study of 194 men, 156 of whom were smokers, plasma vitamin C was 8% lower in smokers than nonsmokers, and SCE increased in the lymphocytes of smokers *(63)*. However, lymphocyte SCE and sputum-cell micronuclei were not correlated with plasma vitamin C concentrations. Vitamin C and vitamin E concentrations were observed to be lower in the seminal fluid of smokers than nonsmokers, and 8-oxo-dG levels in sperm DNA were significantly higher in smokers *(64)*. Increased damage to sperm DNA could result in increased frequencies of heritable mutations. A study of 30 pregnant women, including 11 smokers, also found plasma vitamin C to be lower in smokers, although there was no difference in placental 8-oxo-dG at birth between smokers and nonsmokers *(65)*. Although a study of 53 men and women, including 30 smokers, found smokers to have 50% higher excretion levels of 8-oxo-dG in 24-hr urine samples than nonsmokers, vitamin C intake was not correlated with urine 8-oxo-dG *(66)*. Plasma vitamin C concentrations were not measured in this study; thus, it is unclear whether the smokers also had lower plasma vitamin C levels. Although smoking appears to

Table 1
Vitamin C and DNA Damage in Humans

Reference	Subjects	Treatment/Design	Δ in Vitamin C Concentration	Biomarker of DNA Damage	Results
Observational studies					
Loft et al., 1992 (66)	31 men 53 women	Observational study	Vitamin C intake by diet record	Urine 8-oxodG (HPLC-EC)	No correlation with vitamin C intake
van Poppel et al., 1993 (63)	156 male smokers 38 male nonsmokers	Observational study	Plasma: 8% lower in smokers vs nonsmokers, $p < 0.05$	Lymphocyte SCE Sputum cell micronuclei	Smokers had ↑ SCE. Micronuclei and SCE were not correlated with plasma vitamin C
Fraga et al., 1996 (64)	51 men (22 smokers)	Observational study	Seminal fluid Vitamin C: 17% ↓ in smokers, NS Vitamin E: 32% ↓ in smokers, $p < 0.05$	Sperm 8-oxodG (HPLC-EC)	52% ↑ in smokers vs nonsmokers, $p < 0.01$
Daube et al., 1997 (65)	30 pregnant women (11 smokers, 19 nonsmokers)	Observational study	Plasma vitamin C: 10% ↓ insmokers vs nonsmokers, NS	At term: Placental 8-oxodG (HPLC-EC)	Placental 8-oxodG: no difference between smokers and nonsmokers. No correlation between plasma vitamin C and placental 8-oxodG
Lenton et al., 1999 (67),	105 nonsmokers (37 men 68 women)	Observational study	Lymphocyte vitamin C	Lymphocyte 8-oxodG and 5-OHdC (HPLC-EC)	Inverse correlations between lymphocyte intracellular ascorbate 8-oxodG, $p < 0.01$ 5-OHdC, $p < 0.01$
Huang et al., 2000 (68)	184 nonsmokers	Observational study	Serum vitamin C	Urine 8-oxodG (ELISA kit)	Serum ascorbate inversely associated with 8-oxodG, $p < 0.02$
Supplementation studies: Ex vivo DNA damage					
Pohl & Reidy, 1989 (69)	$n = 8$ in vitamin C group $n = 2$ in control	Parallel design 1) Vitamin C 100 mg/d × 14 days, 1,000 mg/d 14 d 2) Control	Serum: After 100 mg/d: 1.2-fold ↑ After 1,000 mg/d: 2-fold ↑	Chromosomal breaks and exchanges in whole blood after ex vivo bleomycin exposure	% abnormal cells ↓ 25% after 1,000 mg/d $p < 0.01$ Average breaks/cell ↓ 36% after 1,000 mg/d, $p < 0.05$

490

Reference	Subjects	Treatment	Vitamin C status	Assay	Results
Green et al., 1994 (71)	6 men and women	Single dose vitamin C: 500 mg (~35 mg/kg)	ND	Lymphocyte DNA damage with and without ex vivo exposure to ionizing radiation (Comet assay)	↓, $p < 0.001$ with and without ex vivo exposure to ionizing radiation
Anderson et al., 1997 (70)	48 nonsmokers (24 men, 24 women)	Crossover design Vitamin C: 1) 60 mg/d × 14 d 2) 6,000 mg/d × 14 d 3) placebo × 14 d	Plasma: 1) 1.2-fold ↑ 2) 1.8-fold ↑ 3) ↔	Lymphocyte DNA damage with and without ex vivo H_2O_2 exposure (Comet assay) Chromosomal aberrations in whole blood with and without ex vivo bleomycin (Bleomycin assay)	Lymphocyte DNA damage: no difference for either vitamin C treatment vs placebo with or without ex vivo H_2O_2 exposure ↑ in chromosomal aberrations after both vitamin C treatments with ex vivo bleomycin exposure, $p < 0.01$
Panayiotidis & Collins, 1997 (72)	6 smokers 6 nonsmokers	Single dose vitamin C: 1,000 mg	ND	Lymphocyte DNA damage after ex vivo exposure to H_2O_2 (Comet assay)	20% ↓ 2 h after single dose vitamin C in smokers and nonsmokers, $p < 0.05$
Crott & Fenech, 1999 (52)	11 nonsmoking men	Cross-over design Baseline: Antioxidant-poor diet 1) vitamin C: 2 g single dose 2) Placebo	Plasma: 2 h after vitamin C 1.16-fold ↑ 4 h after vitamin C 1.25-fold ↑	0, 2, 4 h after treatment: Lymphocyte micronuclei with and without ex vivo H_2O_2 exposure (cytokinesis block method)	No significant change in micronuclei at 2 h or 4 h with or without ex vivo H_2O_2 exposure
Brennan et al., 2000 (167)	7 nonsmoking men and women	Vitamin C: 1,000 mg/d × 42 d	Plasma: 1.5-fold ↑ Lymphocyte: 1.9-fold ↑	Lymphocyte DNA damage with and without ex vivo H_2O_2 exposure (Comet assay)	Without ex vivo H_2O_2: no effect vs baseline With ex vivo H_2O_2: ↓ vs baseline, $p <0.05$

Supplementation studies: In vivo DNA damage

Reference	Subjects	Treatment	Vitamin C status	Assay	Results
Fraga et al., 1991 (79) Jacobson et al., 1991 (33)	10 men	Depletion-repletion study Vitamin C: 1) 5mg/d × 32 d 2) 10–20 mg/d × 28 d 3) 60–250 mg/d × 28 d	Seminal fluid and plasma: 1) 50% ↓ vs baseline 2) ≥ 50% ↓ persists 3) Return to baseline	Sperm, lymphocyte, and 24 h urine 8-oxodG (HPLC-EC)	Sperm 8 oxodG: 1) ↑ vs baseline, $p < 0.01$ 2) ↑vs baseline, $p < 0.01$ 3) ↓ vs phase 2, $p < 0.01$ No change in lymphocyte and 24 h urine 8-oxodG

(continued)

491

Table 1 (*continued*)

Reference	Subjects	Treatment/Design	Δ in Vitamin C Concentration	Biomarker of DNA Damage	Results
Dyke et al., 1994 (80)	49 GI patients; 41 had atrophic gastritis on endoscopy	Vitamin C: 1,000 mg/d × 28 d	Plasma: ↑ in 43/49, p < 0.001 Gastric mucosa: ↑ in normal mucosa No change in atrophic gastritis	Gastric mucosal DNA damage by ³²P-postlabeling assay	↓ after treatment in 28/43 patients, p < 0.01
Prieme et al., 1997 (78)	Male smokers 1) n = 21 2) n = 21 3) n = 20	Parallel design Vitamin C: 1) 500 mg/d × 60 d 2) 500 mg/d slow-release × 60 d 3) placebo × 60 d	ND	Urine 8-oxodG (HPLC-EC)	No significant difference between vitamin C treatments and placebo
Lee et al., 1998 (73)	Male smokers 1) n = 3 2) n = 3	Parallel design: 1) Vitamin C 500 mg/d × 4 wk 2) Placebo	Plasma 1) 1.8-fold ↑ 2) ↔	Lymphocyte 8-oxodG (HPLC-EC)	No significant change
Podmore et al., 1998 (75) Cooke et al., 1998 (74)	30 nonsmokers (14 men, 16 women)	Sequential design Wk 1–6: calcium carbonate 500 mg/d Wk 7–12 Vitamin C 500 mg/d Wk 13–25: Washout	Wk 12 Plasma: 1.6-fold ↑	Lymphocyte 8-oxoade, 8-oxogua (GC-MS) 8-oxogua, 8-oxodG (HPLC-EC) Serum 8-oxodG, urine 8-oxodG (ELISA)	Vitamin C vs calcium: lymphocyte 8-oxoade ↑ 8-oxogua ↓ 8-oxodG ↑ Serum 8-oxodG ↑, p <0.05 Washout vs calcium: urine 8-oxodG ↑, p < 0.05
Rehman et al., 1998 (76)	10 w/ high plasma C (72 μM) + 9 low plasma C (50 μM) in each treatment group	Parallel design 1) 60 mg/d + 14 mg Fe/d × 12 wk 2) 260 mg/d + 14 mg Fe/d × 12 wk	Plasma: 1) high plasma C: 1.1-fold ↑ low plasma C: ↑ 1.4-fold 2) high plasma C: 1.1-fold ↑ low plasma C: 1.8-fold ↑	At 0, 6, and 12 wk: leukocytes 8-oxogua, 8-oxoade, 5-Me-hydantoin, 5-OH-hydantoin, 5-OH-uracil, 5-Cl-uracil, thymine glycol, 5-OH-cytosine, 5-Me-uracil, FAPY ade, FAPY gua (GC-MS)	High plasma C: ↑ total base damage vs baseline at 6 wk, p < 0.05; no change in total base damage at 12 wks for both treatments Low plasma C: no change in total base damage vs baseline at 6 and 12 wk for both treatments
Proteggente et al 2000 (77)	20 nonsmokers (9 men, 11 women)	Crossover trial 1) 260 mg/d × 6 wk 2) 260 mg/d + 14 mg/d Fe × 6 wk 3) placebo × 6 wk	Plasma: 1) 1.2-fold ↑ 2) 1.2-fold ↑ 3) ↔	At 0 and 6 wk: Leukocyte DNA base damage (GC/MS) (*see* Rehman et al.)	1) No difference vs placebo in individual or total base damage 2) No difference vs placebo in individual or total base damage

492

Reference	Subjects	Design/Treatment	Biomarker (method)	Antioxidant status	DNA damage result
Vojdani et al., 2000 (36)	20 healthy volunteers n = 5 in each treatment group	Parallel design Vitamin C: 1) 500 mg/d × 14 d 2) 1,000 mg/d × 14 d 3) 5,000 mg/d × 14 d 4) placebo	Leukocyte 8-oxodG (HPLC-EC)	Leukocyte: 1) 1.6-fold ↑ 2) 1.5-fold ↑ 3) 1.4-fold ↑	1) 500 mg/d × 14 d: 30% ↓, $p = 0.05$ No change after 1000 mg/d and 5,000 mg/d × 14 d
Huang et al., 2000 (68)	Nonsmokers 1) n = 46 2) n = 47	Parallel design Vitamin C: 1) 500 mg/d × 2 mo 2) placebo × 2 mo	Urine 8-oxodG (ELISA kit)	Serum: 1) 1.2-fold ↑ 2) ↔	No difference vs placebo or baseline
Schneider et al., 2001 (168)	6 smokers + 6 nonsmokers in each group	1) Vitamin C 1,000 mg/d × 7 d, then vitamin C 1,000 mg/d + RRR-α–tocopherol 335 mg/d × 7 d 2) control	Lymphocyte DNA damage: Micronuclei (cytokinesis block method) SCE frequency	Plasma ascorbate: 2.2-fold ↑ in smokers 1.3-fold ↑ in nonsmokers Plasma ascorbyl radical (EPR): 1.1-fold ↑ in smokers, $p < 0.05$ NS in nonsmokers	Micronuclei: 7d (vitamin C): no change in smokers or nonsmokers. 14d (C+E): ↓ micronuclei in smokers, $p < 0.05$; no change in nonsmokers SCE: no change for smokers or nonsmokers at 7d or 14d

increase oxidation of ascorbate and therefore the requirement for it (2), these observational studies did not determine whether increases in DNA damage in smokers are a result of vitamin C depletion or mutagens in cigarette smoke. In nonsmokers, lymphocyte vitamin C concentrations were inversely associated with lymphocyte 8-oxo-dG levels (67), and serum vitamin C concentrations were inversely associated with urine 8-oxo-dG concentrations (68).

3.3.2. VITAMIN C SUPPLEMENTATION AND EX VIVO DNA DAMAGE

Vitamin C supplementation studies have assessed DNA damage in vivo and ex vivo after exposure to mutagens such as ionizing radiation, bleomycin, and H_2O_2 (Table 1). A small study of eight individuals found that a sequential regimen of 100 mg/d of vitamin C for 14 d followed by 1000 mg/d for another 14 d resulted in a 36% decrease in lymphocyte chromosomal aberrations after ex vivo exposure to bleomycin (69). However, a larger crossover trial of 48 men and women found that lymphocyte chromosomal aberrations after ex vivo bleomycin exposure increased following 14-d treatments with 60 mg/d or 6,000 mg/d of vitamin C (70). The increase in chromosomal aberrations caused by ex vivo bleomycin exposure after vitamin C supplementation may be related to the presence of contaminating metal ions in the assay (see Subheading 5). In the same study, lymphocyte DNA damage determined by the Comet assay did not differ from placebo for either vitamin C regimen in the presence or absence of ex vivo H_2O_2 exposure. In contrast, a study of seven men and women who took 1,000 mg/d of vitamin C for 42 d found that lymphocyte DNA damage measured by the Comet assay decreased in the presence of ex vivo exposure to H_2O_2. Two other studies employing the Comet assay found that a single 1000 mg dose of vitamin C resulted in a 20% decrease in lymphocyte DNA damage after ex vivo exposure to H_2O_2 (71), and that a single 500 mg dose of vitamin C decreased lymphocyte DNA damage before and after ex vivo exposure to ionizing radiation (72). A single 2000 mg dose of vitamin C did not result in significant changes in lymphocyte micronuclei with or without ex vivo exposure to H_2O_2 (52).

3.3.3. VITAMIN C SUPPLEMENTATION AND IN VIVO DNA DAMAGE

A number of intervention studies have examined the effect of vitamin C supplementation on lymphocyte 8-oxo-dG concentrations (Table 1). A small study of male smokers found no difference in lymphocyte 8-oxo-dG levels after supplementation with 500 mg/d vitamin C for 4 wk compared to placebo (73), and another small study found that 500 mg/d vitamin C for 2 wk significantly decreased leukocyte 8-oxo-dG by 30% compared to placebo (36). In the same study, leukocyte 8-oxo-dG levels were not different from placebo after vitamin C doses of 1,000 mg/d and 5,000 mg/d for 2 wk. In another supplementation trial, 500 mg/d vitamin C for 6 wk decreased lymphocyte 8-oxo-dG levels measured by high-performance liquid chromatography (HPLC), and decreased lymphocyte 8-oxo-gua levels measured by GC-MS (74,75). However, levels of another oxidized DNA base measured by GC-MS, 8-oxo-adenine (8-oxo-ade), increased. The significance of this study's findings is discussed further in Subheading 5. Two other supplementation trials evaluated changes in 13 oxidized DNA bases measured by GC-MS, including 8-oxo-gua and 8-oxo-ade, after co-supplementation with vitamin C and iron. In those with relatively high plasma vitamin C levels at the start of the study, some oxidized bases decreased after co-supplementation, including 8-oxo-ade, while others increased (76). Lack of a placebo control made this study's result difficult to interpret. In a subsequent placebo-controlled crossover trial conducted by the same laboratory, 6 wk of supplementation with either 260 mg/d vitamin C or 260 mg/d vitamin C + 14 mg/d of iron resulted in lymphocyte 8-oxo-ade and 8-oxo-gua levels that did not significantly differ from placebo (77). Two separate studies examining the effect of 500 mg/d vitamin C for 2 mo on urine 8-oxo-dG in smokers (78) and nonsmokers (68) also found no significant differences from placebo.

Few studies have examined the effect of vitamin C status on DNA damage in human tissues other than leukocytes. Although vitamin C depletion over a period of 2 mo did not affect 8-oxo-dG levels in lymphocytes or urine, 8-oxo-dG levels in sperm DNA significantly increased (33,79). Administration of 1000 mg/d vitamin C to patients with gastrointestinal disease for 28 d resulted in decreased DNA damage assessed by ^{32}P-postlabeling in 28 of 43 patients (80). Although vitamin C has been found to prevent oxidative DNA damage in vitro and to some extent ex vivo, evidence that vitamin C supplementation decreases DNA damage in vivo is inconsistent and obscured by the possibility of artifactual oxidation during measurement.

4. EVIDENCE THAT VITAMIN C PREVENTS CANCER IN HUMANS

4.1. Evidence from Prospective Cohort Studies

4.1.1. ALL CANCERS

Five of nine prospective cohort studies observed a significant inverse relationship between some measure of vitamin C intake and mortality from all cancers (Table 2). In a 7-yr study of more than 11,000 men and women in the United States, the risk of death from cancer was 24% lower in women with a dietary vitamin C intake of more than 225 mg/d, compared to women whose dietary intake was less than 155 mg/d (81). No significant relationship between vitamin C intake and cancer mortality was observed in men. A study of 1556 men followed for 24 yr found that those with dietary vitamin C intake higher than 113 mg/d had a 39% lower risk of death from cancer than those whose dietary vitamin C intake was less than 82 mg/d (82). Of four studies that directly evaluated supplement use, none found a significant association between the use of vitamin C supplements and overall cancer mortality (81,83–85). Serum or plasma vitamin C reflects total (dietary and supplemental) vitamin C intake. Three of four prospective studies that evaluated serum or plasma vitamin C found it to be inversely associated with overall cancer mortality. In a study of 2974 Swiss men followed for 17 yr, plasma vitamin C levels consistent with a vitamin C intake of greater than 55 mg/d were associated with a 25% lower risk of death from cancer than plasma levels reflecting vitamin C intake of less than 55 mg/d (86). A study in the United States followed more than 7000 men and women for 12–16 yr and found that men with serum levels of vitamin C in the highest quartile were 62% less likely to die of cancer than men with plasma levels in the lowest quartile, consistent with intakes of less than 60 mg/d (87). No significant association between the serum vitamin C level and cancer mortality was observed in women. In a study of more than 19,000 men and women followed for 4 yr, men in the highest quintile of plasma vitamin C, corresponding to a mean intake of 109 mg/d, were 53% less likely to die of cancer than men in the lowest plasma vitamin C quintile, corresponding to a mean intake of 51 mg/d (88). Again, no significant association between plasma vitamin C and cancer mortality was observed in women.

4.1.2. LUNG CANCER

Five of 11 prospective cohort studies (89–93) (Table 2) have observed significant inverse associations between vitamin C intake and the risk of lung cancer. In a cohort of 872 Dutch men followed over a perid of 25 yr, dietary vitamin C intakes greater than 100 mg/d were associated with a 50–60% lower risk than intakes of less than 60–80 mg/d (89,94). A much larger cohort of 58,279 Dutch men followed over a period of 6 yr found dietary vitamin C intakes of more than 138 mg/d associated with a 23% lower risk of lung cancer than dietary intakes of less than 82 mg/d (93). In a cohort of 4538 Finnish men, dietary intake of vitamin C was inversely related to the risk of lung cancer only in nonsmokers (90). In a cohort of more than 10,000 United States men and women followed over a period of 19 yr, those with dietary vitamin C intakes greater than 113 mg/d had a 34% decrease in the risk of lung cancer compared to those with dietary intakes less than 23 mg/d (91); a larger study of more than 47,000 United States men and women found total vitamin C intake (diet and supplements) to be inversely related to the risk of lung cancer in men, but not women (92).

Although smoking remains the most significant risk factor for lung cancer, prospective studies suggest that dietary vitamin C intakes of greater than 100 mg/d are associated with a decreased risk of lung cancer in men compared to dietary intakes of less than 60 mg/d. At present, there is little evidence that vitamin C supplementation significantly affects the risk of lung cancer. Although this effect is likely to hold true for women, fewer prospective studies have examined the relationship between vitamin C intake and lung cancer in women, despite the fact that it is the most common cause of cancer mortality in women.

4.1.3. ESOPHAGEAL CANCER

Most epidemiologic research that has evaluated the relationship between vitamin C intake and the risk of esophageal cancer has examined squamous cell carcinoma of the esophagus (95). Two prospective cohort studies found no significant association between dietary vitamin C and the incidence of esophageal cancer, although cases of esophageal cancer were combined with other cancers of the upper digestive tract in each study because so few cases occurred during follow-up (83,96). Evidence from case-control studies indicates that increased dietary vitamin C, rather than vitamin C supplements, may decrease the risk of squamous cell carcinoma of the esophagus (97–104), leaving open the possibility that vitamin C may only be a marker of increased fruit and vegetable consumption.

Table 2

Vitamin C Intake and Cancer Risk: Prospective Cohort Studies

Reference (country)	Population (duration)	Cancer Site (events)	Association	Risk and Associated Vitamin C Intake
Enstrom et al., 1986 (173) (US)	3119 men and women (10 y)	All cancers (68 deaths)	Nonsignificant	≥ 250 mg/d vs < 250 mg/d: NS (crude estimate of vitamin C intake)
Enstrom et al., 1992 (83) (US)	4479 men 6869 women (10 y)	All cancers (228 deaths in men, 169 deaths in women)	Men: nonsignificant Women: nonsignificant	Men: > 50 mg/d + regular supplement vs < 50 mg/d: NS Women: >50 mg/d + regular supplement vs <50 mg/d: NS
Shibata et al., 1992 (81)(US)	4277 men 7300 women (8 y)	All cancers (645 cases in men, 690 cases in women)	Men: nonsignificant Women: inverse	Men: > 210 mg/d vs < 145 mg/d: NS Women: 155–225 mg/d vs < 155 mg/d: ↓ risk by 19% >225 mg/d vs < 155 mg/d: ↓ risk by 24% 500 mg/d supplement vs no supplement: Men and Women: NS
Pandey et al., 1995 (82) (US)	1556 men (24 y)	All cancers (155 deaths)	Inverse	>113mg/d vs < 82 mg/d: ↓ risk by 39% Smokers: ↓ risk by 48% Non-smokers: NS
Losconczy et al., 1996 (84) (US)	11,178 elderly men and women (6 y)	All cancers (761 deaths)	Nonsignificant	Regular supplement use vs no supplement: NS
Sahyoun et al., 1996 (85) (US)	725 elderly men and women (10 y)	All cancers (57 deaths)	Nonsignificant for plasma vitamin C	Vitamin C intake: > 388 mg/d (diet + supplement) vs < 90 mg/d: NS Plasma vitamin C: >88.6 μM vs < 51.7 μM: NS
Eichholzer et al., 1996 (86) (Switzerland)	2974 men (17 y)	All cancers (290 deaths)	Inverse for plasma vitamin C	>22.7 μM1 vs < 22.7 μM: ↓ risk by 25%
Loria et al., 2000 (87) (US)	3347 men 3724 women (12–16 y)	All cancers (228 deaths in men, 155 deaths in women)	Men: inverse for serum vitamin C Women: nonsignificant	Serum vitamin C Men:≥73.8 mM vs < 28.4 mM: ↓ risk by 62% Women:≥85.2 μM vs < 39.7 μM: NS Approximate dietary intakes: Men and Women: 400 mg/d vs < 60 mg/d2,3
Khaw et al., 2001 (88) (UK)	8860 men 10,636 women (4 y)	All cancers (116 deaths in men, 84 deaths in women)	Men: inverse for plasma vitamin C Women: nonsignificant	Plasma vitamin C Men: >72.6 μM vs < 20.8 μM: ↓ risk by 53% Women: > 85.1 μM vs < 30.3 μM: NS Corresponding dietary intakes Men: 109 mg/d vs 51 mg/d Women: 113 mg/d vs 57 mg/d
Shekelle et al., 1981 (174) (US)	1954 men (19 y)	Lung (33 cases)	Nonsignificant	101 mg/d in non cases vs 92 mg/d in cases: NS

496

Study	Population	Cancer site	Result	Details
Kvale et al., 1983 (175) (Norway)	13,785 men (11 y)	Lung (72 cases)	Nonsignificant	Vitamin C index: highest vs lowest quartile: NS
Kromhout, 1987 (89) (Netherlands)	872 men (25 y)	Lung (63 deaths)	Inverse	83–103 mg/d vs < 63 mg/d: ↓ risk by 60% > 103 mg/d vs < 63 mg/d: ↓ risk by 64%
Knekt et al., 1991 (90) (Finland)	4538 men (20 y)	Lung (117 cases)	Nonsmokers: inverse Smokers: nonsignificant	Non-cases: 83 mg/d vs cases: 81 mg/d: NS Highest tertile of intake vs lowest: Nonsmokers: threefold ↓ risk Smokers: NS
Shibata et al., 1992 (81) (US)	4277 men 7300 women (8 y)	Lung (94 cases in men, 70 cases in women)	Men: nonsignificant Women: nonsignificant	Men: > 210 mg/d vs < 145 mg/d: NS Women: > 225 mg/d vs < 155 mg/d: NS 500 mg/d supplement vs no supplement: Men: NS Women: NS
Chow et al., 1992 (176) (US)	17,818 men (20 y)	Lung (219 deaths)	Nonsignificant	Highest quintile (diet) vs lowest: NS
Steinmetz et al., 1993 (177) (US)	41,837 post-menopausal women (4 y)	Lung (138 cases, 2,814 in cancer-free subcohort)	Nonsignificant	≥189 mg/d vs ≤ 99 mg/d (diet):NS ≥ 330 mg/d vs ≤ 123 mg/d (diet + supplements): NS
Ocke et al., 1995 (178) (7 countries study)	>12,000 men (Ecologic/ cohort; 25 y)	Lung (424 deaths)	Nonsignificant	No significant association between vitamin C intake and lung cancer mortality
Eichholzer et al., 1996 (86) (Switzerland)	2974 men (17 y)	Lung (87 deaths)	Nonsignificant for plasma vitamin C	Plasma vitamin C >22.7 μM^1 vs < 22.7 μM: NS
Ocke et al., 1997 (94) (Netherlands)	561 men (20 y)	Lung (54 cases)	Inverse	>102 mg/d vs < 80 mg/d: ↓ risk by 54%
Yong et al., 1997 (91) (US)	3968 men 6100 women (19 y)	Lung (248 cases)	Inverse	Men and women 54–113 mg/d vs < 23 mg/d: ↓ risk by 33% > 113 mg/d vs < 23 mg/d: ↓ risk by 34%
Bandera et al., 1997 (92) (US)	27,544 men 20,456 women (7 y)	Lung (395 cases in men, 130 cases in women)	Men: Inverse Women: nonsignificant	Total vitamin C (diet + supplement) Men: Highest tertile vs lowest: ↓ risk by 37% Women: Highest tertile vs lowest: NS
Voorrips et al., 2000 (93) (Netherlands)	58,279 men (6 y)	Lung (939 cases, 1525 in cancer-free subcohort)	Inverse	>82 mg/d vs < 51 mg/d:↓ risk by 21% > 138 mg/d vs < 51 mg/d: ↓ risk by 23% Supplement use vs no supplement use: NS
Zheng et al., 1995 (96) (US)	34,691 post-menopausal women (7 y)	Mouth, pharynx, esophagus (33 cases)	Nonsignificant	>201 mg/d vs < 91 mg/d (diet): NS
Enstrom et al., 1992 (83) (US)	4479 men 6869 women (10 y)	Esophagus and stomach 18 deaths in men, 5 deaths in women	Men: nonsignificant Women: nonsignificant	Men: > 50 mg/d + regular supplement vs 0–49 mg/d: NS Women: > 50 mg/d + regular supplement vs 0–49 mg/d: NS

(continued)

Table 2 (*continued*)

Reference (country)	Population (duration)	Cancer Site (events)	Association	Risk and Associated Vitamin C Intake
Chyou et al., 1990 (*118*) (US/Hawaii)	8006 men of Japanese ancestry (18 y)	Stomach (111 cases, 361 in cancer-free subcohort)	Nonsignificant	Cases: 101 mg/d vs non-cases: 114 mg/d NS
Ocke et al., 1995 (*178*) (7 countries study)	>12,000 men (Ecologic/ cohort; 25 y)	Stomach (267 deaths)	Inverse	10 mg/d increase in vitamin C intake was associated with a 0.28% lower 25-yr stomach cancer mortality: $p = 0.0003$
Zheng et al., 1995 (*96*) (US)	34,691 post-menopausal women (7 y)	Stomach (26 cases)	Nonsignificant	> 201 mg/d vs <91 mg/d (diet): NS
Eichholzer et al., 1996 (*86*) (Switzerland)	2974 men (17 y)	Stomach (28 deaths)	Nonsignificant for plasma vitamin C	Plasma vitamin C >22.7 μmol/L[1] vs < 22.7 μM: NS
Botterweck et al., 2000 (*117*) (Netherlands)	120,852 men and women (6 y)	Stomach (282 cases, 3,123 in cancer-free subcohort)	Dietary intake: inverse (borderline) Supplement use: nonsignificant	>135 mg/d vs < 55 mg/d:↓ risk by 30%, $p = 0.06$ Supplement use vs no supplement use: NS
Jacobs et al., 2002 (*119*) (US)	1,045,923 men and women (16 y)	Stomach (1,725 cases)	Supplement use < 10 y: inverse	Vitamin C supplement use at enrollment: < 10 y vs nonusers: ↓ risk by 32% ≥ 10 y vs nonusers: NS
Heilbrun et al., 1989 (*121*) (US)	8006 men of Japanese ancestry (16 y)	Colon (102 cases) Rectum (60 cases 361 in cancer free subcohort)	Colon: inverse Rectum: nonsignificant	Colon cancer > 160 mg/d vs < 37 mg/d: ↓ risk by 46% Rectal cancer > 160 mg/d vs < 37 mg/d: NS
Shibata et al., 1992 (*81*) (US)	4277 men 7300 women (8 y)	Colon (97 cases in men, 105 cases in women)	Men: nonsignificant for diet and supplements Women: inverse for diet and supplements	Men: > 210 mg/d vs <145 mg/d: NS Women: > 225 mg/d vs <155 mg/d: ↓ risk by 39% 500 mg/d supplement vs no supplement: Men:NS Women: ↓ risk by 33%
Bostick et al., 1993 (*179*) (US)	35.215 women (5y)	Colon (212 cases)	Nonsignificant for diet and supplements	>201 mg/d vs <91 mg/d (diet): NS >392 mg/d vs <112 mg/d (diet + supplements): NS >Regular supplement vs no supplement: NS
Ocke et al., 1995 (*178*) (7 countries study)	>12,000 men (Ecologic/ cohort; 25 y)	Colon/rectum (130 deaths)	Nonsignificant	No significant association between vitamin C intake and colorectal cancer mortality
Eichholzer et al. 1996 (*86*) (Switzerland)	2974 men (17 y)	Colon (22 deaths)	Nonsignificant for plasma vitamin C	Plasma vitamin C >22.7 μmol/L[1] vs < 22.7 μmol/L[1]: NS

498

Reference	Population	Cancer site (cases)	Result	Details
Jacobs et al., 2001 (123) (US)	711,891 men and women (14 y)	Colon/rectum (4,404 deaths)	Rectal CA: inverse colon CA: nonsignificant	≥10 y of supplement use compared to no supplement use: NS for colorectal CA and colon CA, ↓ risk by 60% for rectal CA
Shibata et al., 1992 (81) (US)	4277 men (8 y)	Bladder (69 cases)	Diet: nonsignificant Supplements: inverse	>210 mg/d vs < 145 mg/d: NS 500 mg/d supplement vs no supplement: ↓ risk by 42%
Zeegers et al., 2001 (125) (Netherlands)	120,852 men and women (6 y)	Bladder (569 cases, 3,123 in cancer-free subcohort)	Nonsignificant	>135 mg/d (diet) vs <55 mg/d: NS
Michaud et al.2001 (124) (US)	51,529 men (12 y)	Bladder (320 cases)	Nonsignificant (inversetrend for supplement use)	>1,159 mg/d vs < 95 mg/d (diet + supplement): NS ≥10 y of supplement use vs no supplement use: ↓ risk by 27% p = 0.08
Shibata et al., 1992 (81) (US)	4277 men (8 y)	Prostate (208 cases)	Nonsignificant	>210 mg/d vs <145 mg/d: NS 500 mg/d supplement vs no supplement: NS
Eichholzer et al., 1996 (86) (Switzerland)	2974 men (17 y)	Prostate (30 deaths)	Nonsignificant for plasma vitamin C	Plasma vitamin C >22.7 μmol/L[1] vs < 22.7 μmol/L: NS
Daviglus et al., 1996 (126) (US)	1899 men (30 y)	Prostate (130 cases)	Nonsignificant	>121 mg/d vs < 74 mg/d: NS
Graham et al., 1992 (129) (US)	18,586 women (7 y)	Breast (344 cases)	Nonsignificant	>79 mg/d vs < 34 mg/d: NS
Shibata et al., 1992 (81) (US)	7300 women (8 y)	Breast (219 cases)	Nonsignificant	>225 mg/d vs < 155 mg/d: NS 500 mg/d supplement vs no supplement: NS
Rohan et al., 1993 (132) (Canada)	56,837 women (5 y)	Breast (519 cases, 1182 in cancer-free subcohort)	Diet: nonsignificant Supplements: positive	>220 mg/d vs < 101 mg/d: NS >250 mg/d (supplement) vs no supplement:↑ risk by 46%
Kushi et al. 1996 (130) (US)	34,387 women (5 y)	Breast (879 cases)	Nonsignificant	>201 mg/d vs < 91 mg/d (diet): NS >392 mg/d vs < 112 mg/d (diet + supplements): NS >Regular supplement vs no supplement: NS
Verhoeven, et al., 1997 (133) (Netherlands)	62,573 women (4 y)	Breast (650 cases)	Nonsignificant (borderline inverse for diet)	>165 mg/d vs < 59 mg/d: NS (23% ↓ in risk, p = 0.08 for trend) Supplement use vs no supplement use: NS
Zhang et al., 1999 (134) (US)	83,234 women (14 y)	Breast (2697 cases)	All women: nonsignificant Family hx of breast CA: inverse	>205 mg/d vs 70 mg/d (diet): NS >710 mg/d vs <83 mg/d (diet + supplement):NS Premenopausal + family hx of breast CA: > 205 mg/d vs < 70 mg/d (diet): ↓ risk by 63%

(continued)

Table 2 (continued)

Reference (country)	Population (duration)	Cancer Site (events)	Association	Risk and Associated Vitamin C Intake
Wu et al., 2000 (135) (US)	14,625 women (5 y)	Breast (119 cases, 119 in cancer-free subcohort)	Nonsignificant	Plasma vitamin C 105—204 µM vs 13–56 µM: NS Estimated vitamin C intake:[3] > 400 mg/d vs 35–100 mg/d
Michels et al., 2001 (131) (Sweden)	59,036 women (8 y)	Breast (1,271 cases)	All women: nonsignificant BMI > 25: inverse	All women: > 110 mg/d vs < 31 mg/d: NS Overweight women (BMI > 25): > 110 mg/d vs < 31 mg/d: ↓ risk by 39%
Fairfield et al.,2001 (180) (US)	80,326 women (16 y)	Ovary (301 cases)	Nonsignificant	>219 mg/d vs < 67 mg/d (diet): NS >762 mg/d vs < 79 mg/d (diet + supplement):NS
Jain et al.,2000 (181) (Canada)	56,837 women (8–13 y)	Endometrium (221 cases, 3,718 in cancer-free subcohort)	Nonsignificant	>196 mg/d (diet) vs < 110 mg/d: NS >205 mg/d (diet + supplements) vs <112 mg/d: NS
Hunter et al., 1992 (182) (US)	73,366 women (4 y)	Skin (basal cell) (771 cases)	Nonsignificant	>200 mg/d (diet) vs < 58 mg/d: NS >679 mg/d (diet + supplements) vs < 67 mg/d: NS
van Dam et al., 2000 (183) (US)	43,217 men (8 y)	Skin (basal cell) (3,190 cases)	Total intake: positive Nonsignificant when adjusted for physical exam frequency	>1,164 mg/d vs < 95 mg/d (diet + supplements):↑ risk by 12%
Zhang et al., 2001 (184) (US)	47,336 men (10 y) 88,410 women (16 y)	Non-Hodgkins lymphoma (111 cases in men, 261 cases in women)	Nonsignificant	Vitamin C supplement use Men: ≥ 700 mg/d vs never used: NS Women: ≥ 700 mg/d vs never used: NS
Zhang et al., 2001 (185) (US)	508,351 men 676,306 women (14 y)	Non-Hodgkins lymphoma (1,571 deaths in men, 1,398 deaths in women)	Nonsignificant	Vitamin C supplement use Men: ≥10 yr of use vs never used: NS Women: ≥ 10 yr of use vs never used: NS

[1]22.7 µM is consistent with vitamin C intake of approximately 55 mg/d.
[2]Based on data from Levine et al. (30).
[3]Based on data from Levine et al. (3).

4.1.4. STOMACH CANCER

Consumption of fruits and vegetables as a source of dietary vitamin C is consistently and strongly inversely related to the risk of gastric cancer in case-control studies (105–116). However, only one of three prospective studies that specifically reported the risk of stomach cancer (96,117,118) observed an inverse association with dietary vitamin C intake. After 6 yr of following up more than 120,000 Dutch men and women, the risk of stomach cancer in those who consumed less than 55 mg/d dietary vitamin C was 30% higher than that of the two-thirds who consumed more than 55 mg/d, $p = 0.06$ (117). A very large prospective study found that the risk of stomach cancer was 32% lower for those who had used vitamin C supplements for less than 10 yr at enrollment than for those who had not used vitamin C supplements (119). However, the risk of stomach cancer in those who had used vitamin C supplements for 10 yr or longer was no different than the risk for nonusers. A prospective study of 2974 Swiss men found that low plasma vitamin C levels consistent with intakes of less than 55 mg/d were associated with increased stomach cancer mortality after 12 yr of follow-up (120), but the inverse relationship was not significant at 17 yr of follow-up (86). The relationship between vitamin C intake and the risk of gastric cancer may be complicated by *Helicobacter pylori* infection, a known risk factor for gastric cancer that may decrease the vitamin C content of gastric juice (see Subheading 4.2.1.).

4.1.5. COLORECTAL CANCER (CRC)

Of three prospective studies that examined the relationship between dietary vitamin C intake and CRC (81,121,122), two found a significant inverse relationship. A nested case-control study in men of Japanese ancestry found a 46% lower risk of colon cancer in men with dietary vitamin C intakes of more than 160 mg/d compared to men with vitamin C intakes averaging less than 37 mg/d (121). In a prospective cohort study that followed 4277 elderly men and 7300 elderly women over a period of 8 yr, women who consumed more than 225 mg/d vitamin C had a 39% lower risk of colon cancer than women who consumed less than 155 mg/d, but no association between vitamin C intake and the risk of colon cancer was observed for men (81). A similar decrease in the risk of colon cancer was observed in women who took vitamin C supplements. A recent study of colon cancer mortality in more than 700,000 United States men and women found vitamin C supplementation for at least

10 yr to be associated with a 60% reduction in the risk of rectal cancer, but not significantly associated with the risk of colon cancer (123). After 17 yr of follow-up, plasma levels of vitamin C at baseline were not associated with the risk of colon cancer in a cohort of 2974 Swiss men (86). Although fruit, and more consistently, vegetable intake is inversely associated with CRC (122), epidemiologic evidence for vitamin C as a specific protective factor is less consistent.

4.1.6. BLADDER CANCER

Dietary vitamin C intake was not significantly associated with bladder cancer in three prospective studies (81,124,125). However, vitamin C supplement use was significantly associated with reduction in the risk of bladder cancer in a cohort of elderly men followed for 8 yr (81), and a trend toward a reduction in risk ($p = 0.08$) was observed for at least 10 yr of vitamin C supplement use in a large cohort of male health professionals (124). Overall, the evidence for a protective effect of dietary vitamin C on bladder cancer is weak, although there is some evidence for a protective effect of supplemental vitamin C, which is more likely to increase urinary vitamin C concentrations.

4.1.7. PROSTATE CANCER

Only two prospective studies have examined the relationship between vitamin C intake and the risk of prostate cancer. Plasma levels of vitamin C were not associated with the risk of prostate cancer over a 17-yr follow-up period in a cohort of 2974 Swiss men (86), and dietary vitamin C was not associated with the risk of prostate cancer in a cohort of 1899 men followed for 30 yr (126). A review of prostate cancer risk and fruits, vegetables, and associated micronutrients concluded that high intakes of vitamin C were unlikely to affect the risk of prostate cancer (127).

4.1.8. BREAST CANCER

Although the etiology of breast cancer is multifactorial and primarily hormone related, increased oxidative stress may also contribute to the risk of breast cancer in susceptible individuals (128). However, the seven prospective studies that evaluated dietary vitamin C intake (81,129–134) and the single prospective study that measured plasma vitamin C levels (135) found no significant association between vitamin C status and the risk of breast cancer in women. Two recent prospective studies found dietary vitamin C intake to be inversely associated with the risk of breast cancer in subgroups. In the Nurses' Health Study, premenopausal women with a family history of breast cancer who consumed an average of 205 mg/d of vitamin C from foods had a 63% lower risk of breast cancer than those who consumed an average of 70 mg/d *(134)*. In the Swedish Mammography Cohort, women with a BMI greater than 25 kg/m² who consumed an average of 110 mg/d vitamin C had a 39% lower risk of breast cancer compared to those who consumed an average of 31 mg/d *(131)*. None of the five prospective studies that evaluated vitamin C supplement use observed significant reductions in the risk of breast cancer *(81,130,132–134)*. Thus, vitamin C intake from fruits and vegetables may decrease the risk of breast cancer, especially in certain high-risk subgroups, but the contribution of vitamin C vis-à-vis fruit and vegetable intake itself has not been fully elucidated.

4.1.9. SUMMARY OF EVIDENCE FROM PROSPECTIVE COHORT STUDIES

In studies that demonstrated inverse associations between vitamin C intake and total cancer risk, less than 82 mg/d of dietary vitamin C were generally associated with increased cancer risk compared to intakes greater than 110 mg/d. Similarly, when inverse associations between plasma vitamin C levels and cancer risk were observed, plasma levels above 50 μ*M* (consistent with dietary vitamin C intakes of at least 100 mg/d) were protective *(136)*. These intake levels are consistent with the amount (100 mg/d) found to result in tissue saturation in healthy young men *(30)*. Findings of a protective effect for vitamin C in women were somewhat less consistent, and two prospective studies found protective effects for women only at intake levels greater than 200 mg/d *(81,134)*. Recent data indicate that tissue saturation in healthy young women requires at least 200 mg/d of vitamin C *(3)*, which may partially explain the less consistent findings of benefit in women. In most cases, fruits and vegetables, rather than vitamin C supplements, were the source of protective effects on total cancer risk. Thus, it cannot be determined from these studies whether vitamin C is itself protective or is simply a marker for consumption of fruit and vegetables, which contain a plethora of (micro)nutrients and phytochemicals that play a role in cancer chemoprevention.

4.2. Human Intervention Trials: Precancerous Lesions and Cancers

4.2.1. *H. PYLORI*, PRECANCEROUS LESIONS, AND GASTRIC CANCER

By scavenging RNS, vitamin C can prevent the formation of potentially carcinogenic *N*-nitroso com-

pounds in the stomach. Chronic infection with *H. pylori* is associated with an increased risk of gastric cancer, and appears to inhibit secretion of vitamin C into the gastric juice. Thus, less vitamin C is available to scavenge RNS and prevent formation of potentially carcinogenic *N*-nitroso compounds *(137)*. In general, first eradicating *H. pylori* makes attempts to increase vitamin C levels in gastric juice through supplementation more successful *(138,139)*. *H. pylori* infection and low serum levels of vitamin C have been associated with increased risk that precancerous conditions of the gastric mucosa, such as atrophic gastritis, intestinal metaplasia, and dysplasia, will progress to gastric cancer in high-risk populations *(140,141)*. The course of gastric atrophy and intestinal metaplasia was followed by gastric biopsy in a randomized controlled trial of standard anti-*H. pylori* therapy compared to β-carotene supplementation (30 mg/d) or vitamin C supplementation (2 g/d) for 6 yr in individuals at very high risk of gastric cancer *(142)*. Each treatment resulted in significantly increased rates of regression. Vitamin C supplementation was associated with a fivefold increase in the rate of gastric atrophy regression and a 3.3-fold increase in the rate of intestinal metaplasia regression. Successful eradication of *H. pylori* resulted in 8.7-fold and 5.4-fold increases in the rates of regression of gastric atrophy and intestinal metaplasia, respectively. A randomized controlled trial of 500 mg/d vitamin C after *H. pylori* eradication therapy in patients with intestinal metaplasia resulted in complete resolution of intestinal metaplasia in nine of 29 patients who took vitamin C for 6 mo compared to one of 29 who took placebo *(143)*. Two additional randomized trials of anti-*H. pylori* therapy and vitamin C supplementation on the course of precancerous gastric lesions are ongoing *(144)*.

A 6-yr randomized controlled trial of four different vitamin/mineral combinations in 29,584 Chinese men and women at very high risk of esophageal and stomach cancer found no difference in the incidence of stomach cancer or mortality after treatment for more than 5 yr with 120 mg/d vitamin C combined with 30 μg/d molybdenum *(145)*. Unfortunately, no attempt was made to eradicate *H. pylori*, which was likely to limit increases in gastric juice vitamin C levels. A randomized trial to evaluate the efficacy of *H. pylori* treatment and/or antioxidant supplementation in reducing the prevalence of gastric dysplasia and gastric cancer in a high-risk area of China is currently underway *(146)*.

4.2.2. ESOPHAGEAL DYSPLASIA AND CANCER

A daily multivitamin/mineral supplement containing 180 mg of vitamin C, given for a period of 6 yr to 3318 Chinese men and women diagnosed with esophageal dysplasia, did not affect the short-term incidence of esophageal or stomach cancer in a very high-risk population *(147)*. A larger population trial of 29,584 men and women from the same high-risk area of China found that daily supplementation with a combination of 120 mg vitamin C and 30 μg molybdenum did not significantly reduce the incidence of esophageal cancer and did not affect the prevalence of esophageal dysplasia or early cancer in 1.3% of participants who underwent endoscopy at the end of the trial *(148)*. Although there is evidence that vitamin C may prevent cancer initiation by inhibiting the formation of *N*-nitroso compounds, intervention trials in this high-risk population suggest that vitamin C may not be effective once initiation has occurred *(19)*.

4.2.3. COLORECTAL ADENOMAS AND COLORECTAL EPITHELIAL CELL PROLIFERATION

Several intervention trials have examined the effect of vitamin C supplementation on colorectal adenomas (precancerous polyps) and biomarkers of CRC. Although four of five familial adenomatous polyposis (FAP) patients who took 3 g/d vitamin C for 4 mo experienced regression of rectal adenomas *(149)*, a placebo-controlled trial of 3 g/d vitamin C for 18 mo in 36 FAP patients found no significant difference between vitamin C and placebo treatment in regression of rectal adenomas *(150)*. Other intervention trials on colorectal adenomas have employed combinations of antioxidant supplements. Although one preliminary trial suggested marked beneficial effects for a combination of vitamins C, E, and A given for 18 mo *(151)*, a large-scale randomized controlled trial in sporadic adenoma patients did not find a combination of 1000 mg/d vitamin C, 400 mg/d of α-tocopherol, and 25 mg/d of β-carotene to reduce adenoma recurrence over a 4-yr period *(152)*.

Several small intervention trials have used indices of colorectal epithelial cell proliferation as intermediate endpoints. Familial polyposis patients who took 3 g/d vitamin C for up to 21 mo showed a significant decrease in the rectal epithelial cell proliferation rate compared to those who took placebo *(150)*. A small trial in adenoma patients given a combination of antioxidants, including 1000 mg vitamin C, 70 mg α-tocopherol, and 30,000 IU vitamin A daily for 6 mo,

found that this antioxidant combination significantly reduced rectal epithelial cell proliferation rates compared to placebo *(153)*. In another trial, adenoma patients given 750 mg/d vitamin C for 1 mo showed a 54% decrease in colonic epithelial cell proliferation rates, yet proliferation rates in those taking a placebo did not change *(154)*. However, a study of colon cancer patients randomized to receive 1 g/d vitamin C plus vitamin E, vitamin A, and calcium or placebo for 6 mo found that colonic epithelial cell proliferation rates decreased in both groups, but did not differ significantly between treatment and placebo groups *(155)*. Although short-term vitamin C therapy has not been found to affect regression or the recurrence of colorectal adenomas in controlled trials, results of placebo-controlled trials using colonic epithelial cell proliferation as a biomarker are encouraging enough to warrant further investigation of vitamin C therapy and precursors for colon cancer *(122)*.

5. DOES VITAMIN C PROMOTE DNA DAMAGE IN VIVO?

Adding vitamin C to purified DNA or isolated nuclei in the presence of redox-active transition metal ions—e.g., iron or copper—results in single strand breaks and oxidative-base modifications such as 8-oxo-dG *(156–158)*. This effect is believed to result from binding of metal ions to DNA, which results in site-specific hydroxyl radical production and oxidative damage *(156)*. However, in the absence of metal ions, vitamin C inhibits the formation of 8-oxo-dG in purified DNA exposed to OONO or ultraviolet (UV) light *(158–160)*. Adding vitamin C to cells in culture has both inhibited *(161–163)* and increased *(70,71,164)* oxidative DNA damage. However, the pro-oxidant effect of vitamin C is likely the result of the presence of metal ions in the media.

Five animal studies measured 8-oxo-dG levels after vitamin C supplementation; two found vitamin C supplementation inhibited carcinogen-induced increases in 8-oxo-dG *(57,58)*, two found no difference in tissue 8-oxodG levels *(59,61)*, and one found no difference in urine 8-oxo-dG levels *(165)*. Four animal studies measured single strand breaks using the Comet assay after vitamin C supplementation, and three found decreases in single strand breaks. The fourth study examined the effect of vitamin C supplementation on radiation-induced single strand breaks in immature erythrocyte DNA from mouse bone marrow *(166)*. Treating mice for 5 d with 50 or 100 mg/kg vitamin C prior to gamma radiation exposure decreased single strand breaks, yet 200 mg/kg had no significant effect and 400 mg/kg increased single strand breaks. However, vitamin C supplementation with 400 mg/kg immediately after radiation exposure decreased single strand breaks.

Of 14 studies that examined the effect of vitamin C supplementation on in vivo DNA damage in humans, four found decreased DNA damage (36,71,79,80), and eight found no significant change (52,68, 70,73,77,78,167,168). Supplemental vitamin C doses in these studies ranged from 250 mg to 6000 mg over periods ranging from 1–60 d. Only two supplementation studies found significant increases in measures of DNA damage (74–76), but they also found significant decreases in other measures of DNA damage.

In 1998, Podmore and colleagues published a highly controversial paper entitled, "Vitamin C exhibits pro-oxidant properties" (75). Thirty (30) healthy volunteers were supplemented with a "placebo" of 500 mg/d calcium carbonate for 6 wk and then switched to a vitamin C supplement of 500 mg/d for 6 wk. Levels of two oxidized bases from DNA of isolated lymphocytes were measured using GC-MS. After vitamin C supplementation, baseline 8-oxo-gua levels significantly decreased relative to baseline or placebo, and levels of 8-oxo-ade significantly increased. Serious issues have been raised in regard to this study. First, GC-MS is prone to artifactual ex vivo oxidation. The levels of 8-oxo-gua reported in this study are 10- to 100-fold higher than those reported by other investigators for human lymphocytes (169). Second, 8-oxo-ade is believed to be at least 10 × less mutagenic than 8-oxo-gua (170). Third, lymphocyte vitamin C levels were not determined, even though this was the tissue in which oxidative damage was evaluated. Baseline plasma levels, which averaged 51 μM, were already saturating with respect to intracellular lymphocyte vitamin C levels. Therefore, supplementation with 500 mg/d vitamin C was not likely to affect lymphocyte levels. Finally, the study design is questionable because it lacked a proper placebo group throughout the study duration (171).

Another study examined the effect of iron and vitamin C co-supplementation on oxidative damage to DNA; healthy volunteers took 14 mg/d iron sulfate and either 60 or 260 mg/d vitamin C (76). Levels of 13 different oxidized DNA bases from white blood cells were measured using GC-MS. One group's baseline plasma levels of vitamin C averaged 72 μM, which did not

change significantly during supplementation. In this group, levels of some oxidized DNA bases—e.g., thymine glycol and 5-hydroxycytosine—were increased after 12 wk of supplementation, and others, including 8-oxo-gua and 8-oxo-ade, were decreased. Another group of volunteers had lower plasma vitamin C levels at baseline, averaging 50 μM, which increased significantly during supplementation. Although levels of oxidized bases were somewhat higher at baseline in this group, they did not change significantly at the end of 12 wk of supplementation. As in the previous study, baseline levels of 8-oxo-gua and 8-oxo-ade were quite high, presumably because of artifactual oxidation during GC-MS analysis. DNA was isolated from white blood cells rather than isolated lymphocytes, so phagocyte activation during sample preparation may also have contributed to artifactual DNA oxidation. Moreover, the study lacked a placebo control group, as well as control groups given either iron or vitamin C alone. A later study published by the same research group addressed the issue of control groups (77). In this crossover study, 20 healthy volunteers sequentially took 260 mg/d vitamin C, 260 mg/d vitamin C + 14 mg/d iron sulfate, and a placebo, each for 6 wk. Although two of 12 oxidized bases increased significantly from baseline during the vitamin C + iron treatment, none increased significantly compared to placebo. The authors concluded that there was no compelling evidence for a pro-oxidant effect of vitamin C supplementation on DNA base damage in the presence or absence of iron supplementation.

The great majority of studies examining the effect of vitamin C supplementation on in vivo DNA damage have not found that vitamin C promotes DNA damage. The single animal study and two human studies that found increases in some measures of DNA damage also found decreases in other measures of DNA damage. At present, little credible evidence supports the idea that vitamin C acts as a pro-oxidant and promotes DNA damage in vivo.

6. CONCLUSIONS

Vitamin C has the potential to inhibit carcinogenesis in a number of ways. It may protect DNA from potentially mutagenic oxidative damage by scavenging ROS and RNS, and regenerating or sparing other antioxidants such as α-tocopherol or GSH (18). When consumed with meals, vitamin C decreases the formation of carcinogenic N-nitroso compounds in the digestive tract, which may explain the protective effect of fruit and vegetable consumption on digestive tract cancers *(19)*. Vitamin C may also play a role in preserving immune function and preventing oxidative damage caused by chronic inflammation. Recent in vitro findings that vitamin C may help preserve cellular apoptotic function in the presence of oxidative stress warrant further investigation *(41,44)*. Controlled trials demonstrating that vitamin C supplementation may decrease colonic epithelial cell proliferation and enhance regression of precancerous gastric lesions after *H. pylori* eradication are also encouraging *(142,143,154)*.

A number of well-designed epidemiologic studies have suggested a protective role for dietary vitamin C, especially with respect to cancers of the lung and digestive tract. For the most part, vitamin C intake from fruits and vegetables, rather than from supplements, appeared to be the source of protective effects. Recently, a study of men who were not taking supplements found that plasma vitamin C was more strongly correlated with fruit and vegetable intake than plasma α-tocopherol, γ-tocopherol, β-carotene, and β-cryptoxanthin *(172)*. Thus, it could be argued that vitamin C plays an important role in the well-established protective effect of fruit and vegetable intake, but its exact relationship to the myriad of other cancer-chemopreventive compounds in fruits and vegetables, such as fiber, folic acid, and other nutrients and phytochemicals, remains unclear. At present, there is little evidence that vitamin C supplementation at doses of 500 mg/d or higher prevents DNA damage or cancer in individuals who already consume adequate dietary vitamin C. On the other hand, there is no convincing evidence that taking vitamin C supplements at doses as high as 5,000 mg/d increases DNA damage or cancer risk. A diet including five or more servings of fruits and vegetables, as recommended by the National Cancer Institute, will generally provide at least 200 mg/d vitamin C *(1)*, a level of intake associated with decreased cancer risk in numerous epidemiologic studies.

REFERENCES

1. Levine M, Rumsey SC, Daruwala R, et al. Criteria and recommendations for vitamin C intake. *JAMA* 1999;281:1415–1423.
2. Food and Nutrition Board, Institute of Medicine. Vitamin C, in *Dietary Reference Intakes for Vitamin C, Vitamin E, Selenium, and Carotenoids.* National Academy Press, Washington, DC, 2000, pp.95–185.
3. Levine M, Wang Y, Padayatty SJ, Morrow J. A new recommended dietary allowance of vitamin C for healthy young women. *Proc Natl Acad Sci USA* 2001;98:9842–9846.
4. Phillips CL, Yeowell HN. Vitamin C, collagen biosynthesis and aging, in, *Vitamin C in Health and Disease.* Packer L, Fuchs J, eds. Marcel Dekker Inc., New York, NY, 1997, pp.205–230.
5. Burri BJ, Jacob RA. Human metabolism and the requirement for vitamin C, in *Vitamin C in Health and Disease.* Packer L, Fuchs J, eds. Marcel Dekker Inc., New York, NY, 1997, pp. 341–366.
6. Tsao CS. An overview of ascorbic acid chemistry and biochemistry, in *Vitamin C in Health and Disease.* Packer L, Fuchs J, eds. Marcel Dekker Inc., New York, NY, 1997, pp.25–58.
7. Huang A, Vita JA, Venema RC, Keaney JF Jr. Ascorbic acid enhances endothelial nitric-oxide synthase activity by increasing intracellular tetrahydrobiopterin. *J Biol Chem* 2000;275:17,399–17,406.
8. Halliwell B, Gutteridge JMC. *Free Radicals in Biology and Medicine, 3rd ed.* Oxford University Press, New York, NY, 1999.
9. Upston JM, Terentis AC, Stocker R. Tocopherol-mediated peroxidation of lipoproteins: implications for vitamin E as a potential antiatherogenic supplement. *FASEB J* 1999;13:977–994.
10. Carr AC, Frei B. Toward a new recommended dietary allowance for vitamin C based on antioxidant and health effects in humans. *Am J Clin Nutr* 1999;69:1086–1107.
11. Wiseman H, Halliwell B. Damage to DNA by reactive oxygen and nitrogen species: role in inflammatory disease and progression to cancer. *Biochem J* 1996;313:17–29.
12. Woodall AA, Ames BN. Diet and oxidative damage to DNA: the importance of ascorbate as an antioxidant, in *Vitamin C in Health and Disease.* Packer L, Fuchs J, eds. Marcel Dekker Inc., New York, NY, 1997, pp.193–204.
13. Ames BN, Shigenaga MK, Hagen TM. Oxidants, antioxidants, and the degenerative diseases of aging. *Proc Natl Acad Sci USA* 1993;90:7915–7922.
14. Collins AR. Oxidative DNA damage, antioxidants, and cancer. *Bioessays* 1999;21:238–246.
15. Halliwell B. Vitamin C and genomic stability. *Mutat Res* 2001;475:29–35.
16. Asami S, Manabe H, Miyake J, et al. Cigarette smoking induces an increase in oxidative DNA damage, 8-hydroxy-deoxyguanosine, in a central site of the human lung. *Carcinogenesis* 1997;18:1763–1766.
17. Poulsen HE, Loft S, Prieme H, et al. Oxidative DNA damage in vivo: relationship to age, plasma antioxidants, drug metabolism, glutathione-*S*-transferase activity and urinary creatinine excretion. *Free Radic Res* 1998;29:565–571.
18. Poulsen HE, Jensen BR, Weimann A, et al. Antioxidants, DNA damage and gene expression. *Free Radic Res* 2000;33:S33–S39.
19. Mirvish SS. Role of *N*-nitroso compounds (NOC) and *N*-nitrosation in etiology of gastric, esophageal, nasopharyngeal and bladder cancer and contribution to cancer of known exposures to NOC. *Cancer Lett* 1995;93:17–48.
20. Hecht SS. Approaches to cancer prevention based on an understanding of *N*-nitrosamine carcinogenesis. *Proc Soc Exp Biol Med* 1997;216:181–191.

21. World Cancer Research Fund. *Food, Nutrition, and the Prevention of Cancer: A Global Perspective.* American Institute for Cancer Research, Washington, DC, 1997.

22. Tannenbaum SR, Wishnok JS, Leaf CD. Inhibition of nitrosamine formation by ascorbic acid. *Am J Clin Nutr* 1991;53:247S–250S.

23. Mannick EE, Bravo LE, Zarama G, et al. Inducible nitric oxide synthase, nitrotyrosine, and apoptosis in *Helicobacter pylori* gastritis: effect of antibiotics and antioxidants. *Cancer Res* 1996;56:3238–3243.

24. Satarug S, Haswell-Elkins MR, Tsuda M, et al. Thiocyanate-independent nitrosation in humans with carcinogenic parasite infection. *Carcinogenesis* 1996;17:1075–1081.

25. Leaf CD, Vecchio AJ, Roe DA, Hotchkiss JH. Influence of ascorbic acid dose on *N*-nitrosoproline formation in humans. *Carcinogenesis* 1987;8:791–795.

26. Mirvish SS, Grandjean AC, Reimers KJ, et al. Effect of ascorbic acid dose taken with a meal on nitrosoproline excretion in subjects ingesting nitrate and proline. *Nutr Cancer* 1998;31:106–110.

27. Ginaldi L, De Martinis M, D'Ostilio A, et al. Cell proliferation and apoptosis in the immune system in the elderly. *Immunol Res* 2000;21:31–38.

28. Radoja S, Frey AB. Cancer-induced defective cytotoxic T lymphocyte effector function: another mechanism how antigenic tumors escape immune-mediated killing. *Mol Med* 2000;6:465–479.

29. O'Connell J, Bennett MW, Nally K, et al. Altered mechanisms of apoptosis in colon cancer: Fas resistance and counterattack in the tumor-immune conflict. *Ann NY Acad Sci* 2000;910:178–192.

30. Levine M, Conry-Cantilena C, Wang Y, et al. Vitamin C pharmacokinetics in healthy volunteers: evidence for a recommended dietary allowance. *Proc Natl Acad Sci USA* 1996;93:3704–3709.

31. Del Rio M, Ruedas G, Medina S, et al. Improvement by several antioxidants of macrophage function in vitro. *Life Sci* 1998;63:871–881.

32. Campbell JD, Cole M, Bunditrutavorn B, Vella AT. Ascorbic acid is a potent inhibitor of various forms of T cell apoptosis. *Cell Immunol* 1999;194:1–5.

33. Jacob RA, Kelley DS, Pianalto FS, et al. Immunocompetence and oxidant defense during ascorbate depletion of healthy men. *Am J Clin Nutr* 1991;54:1302S–1309S.

34. Anderson R, Oosthuizen R, Maritz R, et al. The effects of increasing weekly doses of ascorbate on certain cellular and humoral immune functions in normal volunteers. *Am J Clin Nutr* 1980;33:71–76.

35. Panush RS, Delafuente JC, Katz P, Johnson J. Modulation of certain immunologic responses by vitamin C. III. Potentiation of in vitro and in vivo lymphocyte responses. *Int J Vitam Nutr Res Suppl* 1982;23:35–47.

36. Vojdani A, Bazargan M, Vojdani E, Wright J. New evidence for antioxidant properties of vitamin C. *Cancer Detect Prev* 2000;24:508–523.

37. Heuser G, Vojdani A. Enhancement of natural killer cell activity and T and B cell function by buffered vitamin C in patients exposed to toxic chemicals: the role of protein kinase-C. *Immunopharmacol Immunotoxicol* 1997;19:291–312.

38. O'Byrne KJ, Dalgleish AG. Chronic immune activation and inflammation as the cause of malignancy. *Br J Cancer* 2001;85:473–483.

39. Hughes DA. Effects of dietary antioxidants on the immune function of middle-aged adults. *Proc Nutr Soc* 1999;58:79–84.

40. Reed JC. Dysregulation of apoptosis in cancer. *J Clin Oncol* 1999;17:2941–2953.

41. Bijur GN, Briggs B, Hitchcock CL, Williams MV. Ascorbic acid-dehydroascorbate induces cell-cycle arrest at G_2/M DNA damage checkpoint during oxidative stress. *Environ Mol Mutagen* 1999;33:144–152.

42. Reddy VG, Khanna N, Singh N. Vitamin C augments chemotherapeutic response of cervical carcinoma HeLa cells by stabilizing P53. *Biochem Biophys Res Commun* 2001;282:409–415.

43. Hampton MB, Orrenius S. Modulation of cell death by oxidants and antioxidants, in *Vitamin C: The State of the Art in Disease Prevention Sixty Years After the Nobel Prize.* Paoletti R, Sies H, Bug J, et al., eds. Springer-Verlag, Milan, 1998, pp.13–20.

44. Vissers MC, Lee WG, Hampton MB. Regulation of apoptosis by vitamin C. Specific protection of the apoptotic machinery against exposure to chlorinated oxidants. *J Biol Chem* 2001;276:46,835–46,840.

45. Savini I, D'Angelo I, Ranalli M, et al. Ascorbic acid maintenance in HaCaT cells prevents radical formation and apoptosis by UV-B. *Free Radic Biol Med* 1999;26:1172–1180.

46. Witenberg B, Kalir HH, Raviv Z, et al. Inhibition by ascorbic acid of apoptosis induced by oxidative stress in HL-60 myeloid leukemia cells. *Biochem Pharmacol* 1999;57:823–832.

47. Yallampalli S, Micci MA, Taglialatela G. Ascorbic acid prevents beta-amyloid-induced intracellular calcium increase and cell death in PC12 cells. *Neurosci Lett* 1998;251:105–108.

48. Sakagami H, Satoh K, Fukuchi K, et al. Effect of an iron-chelator on ascorbate-induced cytotoxicity. *Free Radic Biol Med* 1997;23:260–270.

49. Sakagami H, Satoh K, Hakeda Y, Kumegawa M. Apoptosis-inducing activity of vitamin C and vitamin K. *Cell Mol Biol* 2000;46:129–143.

50. Satoh K, Ida Y, Hosaka M, et al. Induction of apoptosis by cooperative action of vitamins C and E. *Anticancer Res* 1998;18:4371–4375.

51. Clement MV, Ramalingam J, Long LH, Halliwell B. The in vitro cytotoxicity of ascorbate depends on the culture medium used to perform the assay and involves hydrogen peroxide. *Antioxid Redox Signal* 2001;3:157–163.

52. Crott JW, Fenech M. Effect of vitamin C supplementation on chromosome damage, apoptosis and necrosis ex vivo. *Carcinogenesis* 1999;20:1035–1041.

53. Halliwell B. Can oxidative DNA damage be used as a biomarker of cancer risk in humans? Problems, resolutions and preliminary results from nutritional supplementation studies. *Free Radic Res* 1998;29:469–486.

54. Loft S, Poulsen HE. Antioxidant intervention studies related to DNA damage, DNA repair and gene expression. *Free Radic Res* 2000;33:S67–S83.

55. Loft S, Deng XS, Tuo J, et al. Experimental study of oxidative DNA damage. *Free Radic Res* 1998;29:525–539.

56. Hoffman GR. Genetic toxicology, in *Toxicology: The Basic Science of Poisons, 5th ed.* Klassen CD, ed. McGraw-Hill, New York, NY, 1996, pp.269–300.

57. Sai K, Umemura T, Takagi A, et al. The protective role of glutathione, cysteine and vitamin C against oxidative DNA damage induced in rat kidney by potassium bromate. *Jpn J Cancer Res* 1992;83:45–51.

58. Ogawa T, Higashi S, Kawarada Y, Mizumoto R. Role of reactive oxygen in synthetic estrogen induction of hepatocellular carcinomas in rats and preventive effect of vitamins. *Carcinogenesis* 1995;16:831–836.

59. Sai-Kato K, Umemura T, Takagi A, et al. Pentachlorophenol-induced oxidative DNA damage in mouse liver and protective effect of antioxidants. *Food Chem Toxicol* 1995;33:877–882.

60. Tsuda S, Matsusaka N, Ueno S, et al. The influence of antioxidants on cigarette smoke-induced DNA single-strand breaks in mouse organs: a preliminary study with the alkaline single cell gel electrophoresis assay. *Toxicol Sci* 2000;54:104–109.

61. Cadenas S, Barja G, Poulsen HE, Loft S. Oxidative DNA damage estimated by oxo8dG in the liver of guinea-pigs supplemented with graded dietary doses of ascorbic acid and alpha-tocopherol. *Carcinogenesis* 1997;18:2373–2377.

62. Reddy VN, Giblin FJ, Lin LR, Chakrapani B. The effect of aqueous humor ascorbate on ultraviolet-B-induced DNA damage in lens epithelium. *Invest Ophthalmol Vis Sci* 1998;39:344–350.

63. van Poppel G, Verhagen H, van 't Veer P, van Bladeren PJ. Markers for cytogenetic damage in smokers: associations with plasma antioxidants and glutathione S-transferase mu. *Cancer Epidemiol Biomark Prev* 1993;2:441–447.

64. Fraga CG, Motchnik PA, Wyrobek AJ, et al. Smoking and low antioxidant levels increase oxidative damage to sperm DNA. *Mutat Res* 1996;351:199–203.

65. Daube H, Scherer G, Riedel K, et al. DNA adducts in human placenta in relation to tobacco smoke exposure and plasma antioxidant status. *J Cancer Res Clin Oncol* 1997;123:141–151.

66. Loft S, Vistisen K, Ewertz M, et al. Oxidative DNA damage estimated by 8-hydroxydeoxyguanosine excretion in humans: influence of smoking, gender and body mass index. *Carcinogenesis* 1992;13:2241–2247.

67. Lenton KJ, Therriault H, Fulop T, et al. Glutathione and ascorbate are negatively correlated with oxidative DNA damage in human lymphocytes. *Carcinogenesis* 1999;20:607–613.

68. Huang HY, Helzlsouer KJ, Appel LJ. The effects of vitamin C and vitamin E on oxidative DNA damage: results from a randomized controlled trial. *Cancer Epidemiol Biomark Prev* 2000;9:647–652.

69. Pohl H, Reidy JA. Vitamin C intake influences the bleomycin-induced chromosome damage assay: implications for detection of cancer susceptibility and chromosome breakage syndromes. *Mutat Res* 1989;224:247–252.

70. Anderson D, Phillips BJ, Yu TW, et al. The effects of vitamin C supplementation on biomarkers of oxygen radical generated damage in human volunteers with "low" or "high" cholesterol levels. *Environ Mol Mutagen* 1997;30:161–174.

71. Green MH, Lowe JE, Waugh AP, et al. Effect of diet and vitamin C on DNA strand breakage in freshly-isolated human white blood cells. *Mutat Res* 1994;316:91–102.

72. Panayiotidis M, Collins AR. Ex vivo assessment of lymphocyte antioxidant status using the comet assay. *Free Radic Res* 1997;27:533–537.

73. Lee BM, Lee SK, Kim HS. Inhibition of oxidative DNA damage, 8-OHdG, and carbonyl contents in smokers treated with antioxidants (vitamin E, vitamin C, β-carotene and red ginseng). *Cancer Lett* 1998;132:219–227.

74. Cooke MS, Evans MD, Podmore ID, et al. Novel repair action of vitamin C upon in vivo oxidative DNA damage. *FEBS Lett* 1998;439:363–367.

75. Podmore ID, Griffiths HR, Herbert KE, et al. Vitamin C exhibits pro-oxidant properties. *Nature* 1998;392:559.

76. Rehman A, Collis CS, Yang M, et al. The effects of iron and vitamin C co-supplementation on oxidative damage to DNA in healthy volunteers. *Biochem Biophys Res Commun* 1998;246:293–298.

77. Proteggente AR, Rehman A, Halliwell B, Rice-Evans CA. Potential problems of ascorbate and iron supplementation: pro-oxidant effect in vivo? *Biochem Biophys Res Commun* 2000;277:535–540.

78. Prieme H, Loft S, Nyyssonen K, et al. No effect of supplementation with vitamin E, ascorbic acid, or coenzyme Q10 on oxidative DNA damage estimated by 8-oxo-7,8-dihydro-2'-deoxyguanosine excretion in smokers. *Am J Clin Nutr* 1997;65:503–507.

79. Fraga CG, Motchnik PA, Shigenaga MK, et al. Ascorbic acid protects against endogenous oxidative DNA damage in human sperm. *Proc Natl Acad Sci USA* 1991;88:11,003–11,006.

80. Dyke GW, Craven JL, Hall R, Garner RC. Effect of vitamin C supplementation on gastric mucosal DNA damage. *Carcinogenesis* 1994;15:291–295.

81. Shibata A, Paganini-Hill A, Ross RK, Henderson BE. Intake of vegetables, fruits, β-carotene, vitamin C and vitamin supplements and cancer incidence among the elderly: a prospective study. *Br J Cancer* 1992;66:673–679.

82. Pandey DK, Shekelle R, Selwyn BJ, et al. Dietary vitamin C and beta-carotene and risk of death in middle-aged men. The Western Electric Study. *Am J Epidemiol* 1995;142:1269–1278.

83. Enstrom JE, Kanim LE, Klein MA. Vitamin C intake and mortality among a sample of the United States population. *Epidemiology* 1992;3:194–202.

84. Losonczy KG, Harris TB, Havlik RJ. Vitamin E and vitamin C supplement use and risk of all-cause and coronary heart disease mortality in older persons: the Established Populations for Epidemiologic Studies of the Elderly. *Am J Clin Nutr* 1996;64:190–196.

85. Sahyoun NR, Jacques PF, Russell RM. Carotenoids, vitamins C and E, and mortality in an elderly population. *Am J Epidemiol* 1996;144:501–511.

86. Eichholzer M, Stahelin HB, Gey KF, et al. Prediction of male cancer mortality by plasma levels of interacting vitamins: 17-yr follow-up of the prospective Basel study. *Int J Cancer* 1996;66:145–150.

87. Loria CM, Klag MJ, Caulfield LE, Whelton PK. Vitamin C status and mortality in US adults. *Am J Clin Nutr* 2000;72:139–145.

88. Khaw KT, Bingham S, Welch A, et al. Relation between plasma ascorbic acid and mortality in men and women in EPIC-Norfolk prospective study: a prospective population study. European Prospective Investigation into Cancer and Nutrition. *Lancet* 2001;357:657–663.

89. Kromhout D. Essential micronutrients in relation to carcinogenesis. *Am J Clin Nutr* 1987;45:1361–1367.

90. Knekt P, Jarvinen R, Seppanen R, et al. Dietary antioxidants and the risk of lung cancer. *Am J Epidemiol* 1991;134:471–479.

91. Yong LC, Brown CC, Schatzkin A, et al. Intake of vitamins E, C, and A and risk of lung cancer. The NHANES I epidemiologic followup study. First National Health and Nutrition Examination Survey. *Am J Epidemiol* 1997;146:231–243.

92. Bandera EV, Freudenheim JL, Marshall JR, et al. Diet and alcohol consumption and lung cancer risk in the New York State Cohort (United States). *Cancer Causes Control* 1997;8:828–840.

93. Voorrips LE, Goldbohm RA, Brants HA, et al. A prospective cohort study on antioxidant and folate intake and male lung cancer risk. *Cancer Epidemiol Biomark Prev* 2000;9:357–365.

94. Ocke MC, Bueno-de-Mesquita HB, Feskens EJ, et al. Repeated measurements of vegetables, fruits, β-carotene, and vitamins C and E in relation to lung cancer. The Zutphen Study. *Am J Epidemiol* 1997;145:358–365.

95. Fontham E. Prevention of upper gastrointestinal tract cancers, in *Preventive Nutrition: The Comprehensive Guide for Health Professionals, 2nd ed.* Bendich A, Deckelbaum RJ, eds. Humana Press, Totowa, NJ, 2001, pp.21–45.

96. Zheng W, Sellers TA, Doyle TJ, et al. Retinol, antioxidant vitamins, and cancers of the upper digestive tract in a prospective cohort study of postmenopausal women. *Am J Epidemiol* 1995;142:955–960.

97. Ziegler RG, Morris LE, Blot WJ, et al. Esophageal cancer among black men in Washington, D.C. II. Role of nutrition. *J Natl Cancer Inst* 1981;67:1199–1206.

98. Mettlin C, Graham S, Priore R, et al. Diet and cancer of the esophagus. *Nutr Cancer* 1981;2:143–147.

99. Tuyns AJ. Protective effect of citrus fruit on esophageal cancer. *Nutr Cancer* 1983;5:195–200.

100. Brown LM, Blot WJ, Schuman SH, et al. Environmental factors and high risk of esophageal cancer among men in coastal South Carolina. *J Natl Cancer Inst* 1988;80:1620–1625.

101. De Stefani E, Ronco A, Mendilaharsu M, Deneo-Pellegrini H. Diet and risk of cancer of the upper aerodigestive tract—II. Nutrients. *Oral Oncol* 1999;35:22–26.

102. Franceschi S, Bidoli E, Negri E, et al. Role of macronutrients, vitamins and minerals in the aetiology of squamous-cell carcinoma of the oesophagus. *Int J Cancer* 2000;86:626–631.

103. Launoy G, Milan C, Day NE, et al. Diet and squamous-cell cancer of the oesophagus: a French multicentre case-control study. *Int J Cancer* 1998;76:7–12.

104. Mayne ST, Risch HA, Dubrow R, et al. Nutrient intake and risk of subtypes of esophageal and gastric cancer. *Cancer Epidemiol Biomark Prev* 2001;10:1055–1062.

105. Boeing H, Frentzel-Beyme R, Berger M, et al. Case-control study on stomach cancer in Germany. *Int J Cancer* 1991;47:858–864.

106. Correa P, Fontham E, Pickle LW, et al. Dietary determinants of gastric cancer in south Louisiana inhabitants. *J Natl Cancer Inst* 1985;75:645–654.

107. Ekstrom AM, Serafini M, Nyren O, et al. Dietary antioxidant intake and the risk of cardia cancer and noncardia cancer of the intestinal and diffuse types: a population-based case-control study in Sweden. *Int J Cancer* 2000;87:133–140.

108. Graham S, Haughey B, Marshall J, et al. Diet in the epidemiology of gastric cancer. *Nutr Cancer* 1990;13:19–34.

109. Hansson LE, Nyren O, Bergstrom R, et al. Nutrients and gastric cancer risk. A population-based case-control study in Sweden. *Int J Cancer* 1994;57:638–644.

110. Gonzalez CA, Riboli E, Badosa J, et al. Nutritional factors and gastric cancer in Spain. *Am J Epidemiol* 1994;139:466–473.

111. Kaaks R, Tuyns AJ, Haelterman M, Riboli E. Nutrient intake patterns and gastric cancer risk: a case-control study in Belgium. *Int J Cancer* 1998;78:415–420.

112. La Vecchia C, Ferraroni M, D'Avanzo B, et al. Selected micronutrient intake and the risk of gastric cancer. *Cancer Epidemiol Biomark Prev* 1994;3:393–398.

113. Palli D, Russo A, Decarli A. Dietary patterns, nutrient intake and gastric cancer in a high-risk area of Italy. *Cancer Causes Control* 2001;12:163–172.

114. Ramon JM, Serra-Majem L, Cerdo C, Oromi J. Nutrient intake and gastric cancer risk: a case-control study in Spain. *Int J Epidemiol* 1993;22:983–988.

115. Risch HA, Jain M, Choi NW, et al. Dietary factors and the incidence of cancer of the stomach. *Am J Epidemiol* 1985;122:947–959.

116. You WC, Blot WJ, Chang YS, et al. Diet and high risk of stomach cancer in Shandong, China. *Cancer Res* 1988;48:3518–3523.

117. Botterweck AA, van den Brandt PA, Goldbohm RA. Vitamins, carotenoids, dietary fiber, and the risk of gastric carcinoma: results from a prospective study after 6.3 yr of follow-up. *Cancer* 2000;88:737–748.

118. Chyou PH, Nomura AM, Hankin JH, Stemmermann GN. A case-cohort study of diet and stomach cancer. *Cancer Res* 1990;50:7501–7504.

119. Jacobs EJ, Connell CJ, McCullough ML, et al. Vitamin C, vitamin E, and multivitamin supplement use and stomach cancer mortality in the Cancer Prevention Study II cohort. *Cancer Epidemiol Biomark Prev* 2002;11:35–41.

120. Stahelin HB, Gey KF, Eichholzer M, et al. Plasma antioxidant vitamins and subsequent cancer mortality in the 12-yr follow-up of the prospective Basel Study. *Am J Epidemiol* 1991;133:766–775.

121. Heilbrun LK, Nomura A, Hankin JH, Stemmermann GN. Diet and colorectal cancer with special reference to fiber intake. *Int J Cancer* 1989;44:1–6.

122. Bostick RM. Diet and colon cancer, in *Preventive Nutrition: the Comprehensive Guide for Health Professionals, 2nd ed.* Bendich A, Deckelbaum RJ, eds. Humana Press, Totowa, NJ, 2001, pp.47–96.

123. Jacobs EJ, Connell CJ, Patel AV, et al. Vitamin C and vitamin E supplement use and colorectal cancer mortality in a large American Cancer Society cohort. *Cancer Epidemiol Biomark Prev* 2001;10:17–23.

124. Michaud DS, Spiegelman D, Clinton SK, et al. Prospective study of dietary supplements, macronutrients, micronutrients, and risk of bladder cancer in US men. *Am J Epidemiol* 2000;152:1145–1153.

125. Zeegers MP, Goldbohm RA, Brandt PA. Are retinol, vitamin C, vitamin E, folate and carotenoid intake associated with bladder cancer risk? Results from the Netherlands Cohort Study. *Br J Cancer* 2001;85:977–983.

126. Daviglus ML, Dyer AR, Persky V, et al. Dietary beta-carotene, vitamin C, and risk of prostate cancer: results

from the Western Electric Study. *Epidemiology* 1996;7:472–477.

127. Chan JM, Giovannucci EL. Vegetables, fruits, associated micronutrients, and risk of prostate cancer. *Epidemiol Rev* 2001;23:82–86.

128. Ambrosone CB. Oxidants and antioxidants in breast cancer. *Antioxid Redox Signal* 2000;2:903–917.

129. Graham S, Zielezny M, Marshall J, et al. Diet in the epidemiology of postmenopausal breast cancer in the New York State Cohort. *Am J Epidemiol* 1992;136:1327–1337.

130. Kushi LH, Fee RM, Sellers TA, et al. Intake of vitamins A, C, and E and postmenopausal breast cancer. The Iowa Women's Health Study. *Am J Epidemiol* 1996;144:165–174.

131. Michels KB, Holmberg L, Bergkvist L, et al. Dietary antioxidant vitamins, retinol, and breast cancer incidence in a cohort of Swedish women. *Int J Cancer* 2001;91:563–567.

132. Rohan TE, Howe GR, Friedenreich CM, et al. Dietary fiber, vitamins A, C, and E, and risk of breast cancer: a cohort study. *Cancer Causes Control* 1993;4:29–37.

133. Verhoeven DT, Assen N, Goldbohm RA, et al. Vitamins C and E, retinol, beta-carotene and dietary fibre in relation to breast cancer risk: a prospective cohort study. *Br J Cancer* 1997;75:149–155.

134. Zhang S, Hunter DJ, Forman MR, et al. Dietary carotenoids and vitamins A, C, and E and risk of breast cancer. *J Natl Cancer Inst* 1999;91:547–556.

135. Wu K, Helzlsouer KJ, Alberg AJ, et al. A prospective study of plasma ascorbic acid concentrations and breast cancer (United States). *Cancer Causes Control* 2000;11:279–283.

136. Gey KF. Vitamins E plus C and interacting conutrients required for optimal health. A critical and constructive review of epidemiology and supplementation data regarding cardiovascular disease and cancer. *Biofactors* 1998;7:113–174.

137. Schorah CJ. Vitamin C and gastric cancer prevention, in *Vitamin C: The State of the Art in Disease Prevention Sixty Years After the Nobel Prize*. Paoletti R, Sies H, Bug J, et al., eds. Springer-Verlag, Milan, 1998, pp.41–49.

138. Jarosz M, Dzieniszewski J, Dabrowska-Ufniarz E, et al. Effects of high dose vitamin C treatment on *Helicobacter pylori* infection and total vitamin C concentration in gastric juice. *Eur J Cancer Prev* 1998;7:449–454.

139. de Sanjose S, Munoz N, Sobala G, et al. Antioxidants, *Helicobacter pylori* and stomach cancer in Venezuela. *Eur J Cancer Prev* 1996;5:57–62.

140. Zhang L, Blot WJ, You WC, et al. Serum micronutrients in relation to pre-cancerous gastric lesions. *Int J Cancer* 1994;56:650–654.

141. You WC, Zhang L, Gail MH, et al. Gastric dysplasia and gastric cancer: *Helicobacter pylori*, serum vitamin C, and other risk factors. *J Natl Cancer Inst* 2000;92:1607–1612.

142. Correa P, Fontham ET, Bravo JC, et al. Chemoprevention of gastric dysplasia: randomized trial of antioxidant supplements and anti-helicobacter pylori therapy. *J Natl Cancer Inst* 2000;92:1881–1888.

143. Zullo A, Rinaldi V, Hassan C, et al. Ascorbic acid and intestinal metaplasia in the stomach: a prospective, randomized study. *Aliment Pharmacol Ther* 2000;14:1303–1309.

144. Reed PI. Vitamin C, *Helicobacter pylori* infection and gastric carcinogenesis. *Int J Vitam Nutr Res* 1999;69:220–227.

145. Blot WJ, Li JY, Taylor PR, et al. Nutrition intervention trials in Linxian, China: supplementation with specific vita-min/mineral combinations, cancer incidence, and disease-specific mortality in the general population. *J Natl Cancer Inst* 1993;85:1483–1492.

146. Gail MH, You WC, Chang YS, et al. Factorial trial of three interventions to reduce the progression of precancerous gastric lesions in Shandong, China: design issues and initial data. *Control Clin Trials* 1998;19:352–369.

147. Li JY, Taylor PR, Li B, et al. Nutrition intervention trials in Linxian, China: multiple vitamin/mineral supplementation, cancer incidence, and disease-specific mortality among adults with esophageal dysplasia. *J Natl Cancer Inst* 1993;85:1492–1498.

148. Taylor PR, Li B, Dawsey SM, et al. Prevention of esophageal cancer: the nutrition intervention trials in Linxian, China. Linxian Nutrition Intervention Trials Study Group. *Cancer Res* 1994;54:2029s–2031s.

149. DeCosse JJ, Adams MB, Kuzma JF, et al. Effect of ascorbic acid on rectal polyps of patients with familial polyposis. *Surgery* 1975;78:608–612.

150. Bussey HJ, DeCosse JJ, Deschner EE, et al. A randomized trial of ascorbic acid in polyposis coli. *Cancer* 1982;50:1434–1439.

151. Roncucci L, Di Donato P, Carati L, et al. Antioxidant vitamins or lactulose for the prevention of the recurrence of colorectal adenomas. Colorectal Cancer Study Group of the University of Modena and the Health Care District 16. *Dis Colon Rectum* 1993;36:227–234.

152. Greenberg ER, Baron JA, Tosteson TD, et al. A clinical trial of antioxidant vitamins to prevent colorectal adenoma. Polyp Prevention Study Group. *N Engl J Med* 1994;331:141–147.

153. Paganelli GM, Biasco G, Brandi G, et al. Effect of vitamin A, C, and E supplementation on rectal cell proliferation in patients with colorectal adenomas. *J Natl Cancer Inst* 1992;84:47–51.

154. Cahill RJ, O'Sullivan KR, Mathias PM, et al. Effects of vitamin antioxidant supplementation on cell kinetics of patients with adenomatous polyps. *Gut* 1993;34:963–967.

155. Cascinu S, Ligi M, Del Ferro E, et al. Effects of calcium and vitamin supplementation on colon cell proliferation in colorectal cancer. *Cancer Invest* 2000;18:411–416.

156. Drouin R, Rodriguez H, Gao SW, et al. Cupric ion/ascorbate/hydrogen peroxide-induced DNA damage: DNA-bound copper ion primarily induces base modifications. *Free Radic Biol Med* 1996;21:261–273.

157. Hu ML, Shih MK. Ascorbic acid inhibits lipid peroxidation but enhances DNA damage in rat liver nuclei incubated with iron ions. *Free Radic Res* 1997;26:585–592.

158. Fischer-Nielsen A, Poulsen HE, Loft S. 8-hydroxy-deoxyguanosine in vitro: effects of glutathione, ascorbate, and 5-aminosalicylic acid. *Free Radic Biol Med* 1992;13:121–126.

159. Wei H, Cai Q, Tian L, Lebwohl M. Tamoxifen reduces endogenous and UV light-induced oxidative damage to DNA, lipid and protein in vitro and in vivo. *Carcinogenesis* 1998;19:1013–1018.

160. Fiala ES, Sodum RS, Bhattacharya M, Li H. (-)-Epigallocatechin gallate, a polyphenolic tea antioxidant, inhibits peroxynitrite-mediated formation of 8-oxodeoxyguanosine and 3-nitrotyrosine. *Experientia* 1996;52:922–926.

161. Noroozi M, Angerson WJ, Lean ME. Effects of flavonoids and vitamin C on oxidative DNA damage to human lymphocytes. *Am J Clin Nutr* 1998;67:1210–1218.

162. Pflaum M, Kielbassa C, Garmyn M, Epe B. Oxidative DNA damage induced by visible light in mammalian cells: extent, inhibition by antioxidants and genotoxic effects. *Mutat Res* 1998;408:137–146.

163. Fischer-Nielsen A, Loft S, Jensen KG. Effect of ascorbate and 5-aminosalicylic acid on light-induced 8-hydroxy-deoxyguanosine formation in V79 Chinese hamster cells. *Carcinogenesis* 1993;14:2431–2433.

164. Singh NP. Sodium ascorbate induces DNA single-strand breaks in human cells in vitro. *Mutat Res* 1997;375:195–203.

165. De Martinis BS, Bianchi MD. Effect of vitamin C supplementation against cisplatin-induced toxicity and oxidative DNA damage in rats. *Pharmacol Res* 2001;44:317–320.

166. Konopacka M, Widel M, Rzeszowska-Wolny J. Modifying effect of vitamins C, E and β-carotene against gamma-ray-induced DNA damage in mouse cells. *Mutat Res* 1998;417:85–94.

167. Brennan LA, Morris GM, Wasson GR, et al. The effect of vitamin C or vitamin E supplementation on basal and H_2O_2-induced DNA damage in human lymphocytes. *Br J Nutr* 2000;84:195–202.

168. Schneider M, Diemer K, Engelhart K, et al. Protective effects of vitamins C and E on the number of micronuclei in lymphocytes in smokers and their role in ascorbate free radical formation in plasma. *Free Radic Res* 2001;34:209–219.

169. Collins A, Cadet J, Epe B, Gedik C. Problems in the measurement of 8-oxoguanine in human DNA. Report of a workshop, DNA oxidation, held in Aberdeen, UK, 19–21 January, 1997. *Carcinogenesis* 1997;18:1833–1836.

170. Wood ML, Esteve A, Morningstar ML, et al. Genetic effects of oxidative DNA damage: comparative mutagenesis of 7,8-dihydro-8-oxoguanine and 7,8-dihydro-8-oxoadenine in *Escherichia coli*. *Nucleic Acids Res* 1992;20:6023–6032.

171. Carr A, Frei B. Does vitamin C act as a pro-oxidant under physiological conditions? *FASEB J* 1999;13:1007–1024.

172. Block G, Norkus E, Hudes M, et al. Which plasma antioxidants are most related to fruit and vegetable consumption? *Am J Epidemiol* 2001;154:1113–1118.

173. Enstrom JE, Kanim LE, Breslow L. The relationship between vitamin C intake, general health practices, and mortality in Alameda County, California. *Am J Public Health* 1986;76:1124–1130.

174. Shekelle RB, Lepper M, Liu S, et al. Dietary vitamin A and risk of cancer in the Western Electric study. *Lancet* 1981;2:1185–1190.

175. Kvale G, Bjelke E, Gart JJ. Dietary habits and lung cancer risk. *Int J Cancer* 1983;31:397–405.

176. Chow WH, Schuman LM, McLaughlin JK, et al. A cohort study of tobacco use, diet, occupation, and lung cancer mortality. *Cancer Causes Control* 1992;3:247–254.

177. Steinmetz KA, Potter JD, Folsom AR. Vegetables, fruit, and lung cancer in the Iowa Women's Health Study. *Cancer Res* 1993;53:536–543.

178. Ocke MC, Kromhout D, Menotti A, et al. Average intake of anti-oxidant (pro)vitamins and subsequent cancer mortality in the 16 cohorts of the Seven Countries Study. *Int J Cancer* 1995;61:480–484.

179. Bostick RM, Potter JD, McKenzie DR, et al. Reduced risk of colon cancer with high intake of vitamin E: the Iowa Women's Health Study. *Cancer Res* 1993;53:4230–4237.

180. Fairfield KM, Hankinson SE, Rosner BA, et al. Risk of ovarian carcinoma and consumption of vitamins A, C, and E and specific carotenoids. *Cancer* 2001;92:2318–2326.

181. Jain MG, Rohan TE, Howe GR, Miller AB. A cohort study of nutritional factors and endometrial cancer. *Eur J Epidemiol* 2000;16:899–905.

182. Hunter D, Colditz G, Stampfer M, et al. Diet and risk of basal cell carcinoma of the skin in a prospective cohort of women. *Ann Epidemiol* 1992;2:231–239.

183. van Dam RM, Huang Z, Giovannucci E, et al. Diet and basal cell carcinoma of the skin in a prospective cohort of men. *Am J Clin Nutr* 2000;71:135–141.

184. Zhang SM, Giovannucci EL, Hunter DJ, et al. Vitamin supplement use and the risk of non-Hodgkin's lymphoma among women and men. *Am J Epidemiol* 2001;153:1056–1063.

185. Zhang SM, Calle EE, Petrelli JM, et al. Vitamin supplement use and fatal non-Hodgkin's lymphoma among US men and women. *Am J Epidemiol* 2001;153:1064–1070.

33 Carotenoids

Susan T. Mayne, PhD and Brenda Cartmel, PhD

CONTENTS

1. INTRODUCTION

Carotenoids—plant pigments that are generally found in fruits and vegetables—are widespread in plants and in photosynthetic bacteria, where they serve two essential functions: as accessory pigments in photosynthesis and in photoprotection. These two functions are a result of the conjugated polyene structure of carotenoids (Fig. 1), which allows the molecule to absorb light and quench, or inactivate, singlet oxygen and free radicals. Although several hundred different carotenoids are found in nature, humans generally ingest and absorb significant quantities of relatively few carotenoids, particularly lycopene, β- and α-carotene, lutein, zeaxanthin, and β-cryptoxanthin. The carotenoid profile of an individual's blood is a reflection of the carotenoid composition of that individual's diet. Normative intake data and plasma concentrations from the Third National Health and Nutrition Examination Survey in the United States (NHANES III) have been made available for these carotenoids (1,2), as shown in Table 1. Lycopene, a red pigment derived almost exclusively from tomatoes/tomato products, is the predominant carotenoid in the United States population as a whole. Persons in the United States generally consume substantial quantities of foods containing tomato products, such as pastas with tomato sauce, pizza, and lasagna. In countries where tomatoes are not widely consumed, lycopene concentrations in blood can be low relative to other carotenoids.

The carotenoids mentioned here comprise the vast majority (more than 90%) of those that humans ingest and absorb systemically, so they will be the focus of this chapter. Lycopene is covered in chapter 34 in this volume, and thus is not discussed in detail here.

2. MECHANISMS OF ACTION

Carotenoids are reported to have numerous biological effects that could be consistent with possible antitumor activity. This literature has been extensively reviewed by the International Agency for Research on Cancer (IARC) (3), and is only briefly reviewed here.

As described by Krinsky (4), carotenoids have biological functions and biological actions. They function as accessory pigments in photosynthesis via singlet excited carotenoid; offer protection against photosensitization via triplet excited carotenoid; and some carotenoids serve as provitamin A compounds via central and excentric (see Fig. 2) cleavage. Mechanisms for these functions are reasonably well characterized.

With regard to provitamin A activity, some carotenoids are known to be metabolized into retinol by the enzyme 15,15'-dioxygenase (so-called central cleavage). These are known as provitamin A carotenoids

From: Cancer Chemoprevention, Volume 1: Promising Cancer Chemoprevention Agents
Edited by: G. J. Kelloff, E. T. Hawk, and C. C. Sigman © Humana Press Inc., Totowa, NJ

MAJOR HUMAN SERUM CAROTENOIDS

PROVITAMIN A CAROTENOIDS   **NON-PROVITAMIN A CAROTENOIDS**

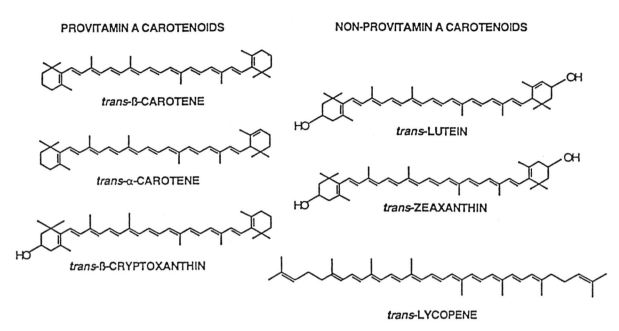

Fig. 1. Structures of the major provitamin A and non-provitamin A carotenoids present in human blood (adapted from *51* with permission).

Table 1
Median Intakes and Serum Carotenoid Concentrations of Persons 4 yr and Older, United States, NHANES III, 1988–1994

	Median Intake mg/d	Median Plasma Concentration ug/dL
Lycopene	8.06	22.4
β-Carotene	1.66	14.7
Lutein + zeaxanthin	1.46	18.9
β-Cryptoxanthin	0.09	8.0
α-Carotene	0.04	3.4

Data taken from Institute of Medicine *(1,2)*.

and include the following: β-carotene, α-carotene, and β-cryptoxanthin. Lycopene and lutein/zeaxanthin do not possess an unsubstituted β-ionone ring, and therefore cannot be converted into retinol. In addition to central cleavage, there is evidence that carotenoids undergo excentric cleavage to produce primarily a series of carotenoic acids. These carotenoic acids can ultimately be converted into retinoic acid. Therefore, when evaluating possible mechanisms of action, retinoid-like effects of carotenoids must be considered, given the possibility that they are metabolized into retinoids, including retinoic acid.

In addition to vitamin A activity in humans and antioxidant activity in plants and photosynthetic bacteria, carotenoids are also reported to have a number of biological actions in humans, including antioxidant activity, immunoenhancement, inhibition of mutagenesis and transformation, and regression of premalignant lesions. In contrast to the carotenoid functions, mechanisms of carotenoid action are far from clear. Some actions of carotenoids, such as regression of premalignant lesions, are shared by the retinoids, with the potential for a similar mechanism of action. However, carotenoids and retinoids also have distinct differences in action, most notably antioxidant activity.

Many carotenoids, including β-carotene, have the ability to quench singlet oxygen, a highly reactive form of oxygen, in a physical reaction in which the energy of the excited oxygen is transferred to the carotenoid, forming an excited-state molecule *(4)*. Quenching of singlet oxygen is the basis for β-carotene's well-known therapeutic efficacy in erythropoietic protoporphyria, a photosensitivity disorder *(5)*. In addition to singlet oxygen, carotenoids are also believed to quench oxygen radicals, and perhaps nitrogen radicals as well. However, the ability of β-carotene and other carotenoids to quench reactive oxygen radicals may be limited, because the carotenoid itself can be oxidized during the process (autoxidation). Burton and

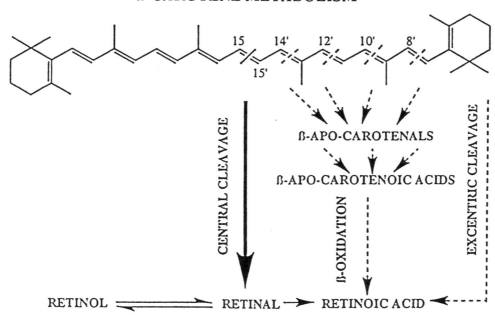

Fig. 2. Metabolism of β-carotene to retinal via central cleavage and to retinoic acid via excentric cleavage (adapted from *51* with permission).

Ingold et al. *(6)* have shown that β-carotene autoxidation in vitro is dose-dependent, and is dependent upon oxygen concentrations.

Since a relatively large body of literature has linked oxygen free radicals with carcinogenesis *(7)*, there is considerable interest in antioxidant compounds and antioxidant activity as a mechanism for cancer prevention. Despite the focus on antioxidants and cancer, and clear evidence of β-carotene's chemopreventive efficacy in some animal carcinogenesis models *(3)*, antioxidant activity has not been proven to be responsible for the chemoprotective effects observed in the animal studies. For example, β-carotene-induced immunological enhancement could play a significant role in tumor inhibition by increasing natural killer (NK) cells and activating immunoregulatory lymphocytes that are important in host defense *(8)*. Various carotenoids have been reported to affect gap-junctional communication, which is related to their ability to upregulate the expression of the connexin43 gene *(9)*; this activity was not related to antioxidant activities of the various carotenoids. Supplementary β-carotene also has been reported to increase the expression of transforming growth factor (TGF) β-1 in cervical biopsy specimens *(10)*. These and other potential mechanisms reviewed elsewhere *(3)* suggest that it is biologically plausible that carotenoids may have chemopreventive activity.

Considering the interest in antioxidant activity as a potential mechanism for chemopreventive efficacy, it is not surprising that other dietary antioxidants have been studied along with β-carotene for such efficacy in humans, particularly vitamins E and C and selenium. These agents are often evaluated in combination, as discussed in Subheading 3.3.

3. PREVIOUS EFFICACY

3.1. Preclinical

β-Carotene, in particular, has been studied extensively in animal carcinogenesis models; other carotenoids have been studied to a lesser extent. The literature on carotenoids in animal models of carcinogenesis was comprehensively reviewed by the IARC in their Chemoprevention handbook series *(3)*, and the reader is referred to that volume for details of animal studies of carotenoids. The following briefly summarizes carotenoid efficacy in animal carcinogenesis models.

3.1.1. β-CAROTENE

The IARC *(3)* concluded that:

"There is sufficient evidence for cancer-preventive activity of β-carotene in experimental animals. This evaluation is based on models of skin carcinogenesis

in mice and buccal pouch carcinogenesis in hamsters. Findings in models of liver carcinogenesis in rats and pancreatic carcinogenesis in rats and hamsters provide further support to this conclusion."

More specifically, the IARC report noted that β-carotene had been evaluated in more than 20 studies of skin carcinogenesis in mice; it was effective against skin carcinogenesis in nearly all of these. Similarly, nearly 20 studies of β-carotene in the hamster buccal pouch model of oral carcinogenesis have suggested its efficacy. Tumor-site specificity in β-carotene efficacy in animal models was noted. For example, β-carotene was not consistently effective in models of respiratory tract carcinogenesis. Thus, animal models of carcinogenesis clearly indicate that β-carotene as a single agent has efficacy in selected models of carcinogenesis, most notably in models of skin and buccal pouch carcinogenesis, but that efficacy was not universal in all tumor sites examined.

3.1.2. α-CAROTENE, LYCOPENE, LUTEIN

Carotenoids other than β-carotene have received more limited attention in animal carcinogenesis studies. The IARC report *(3)* also reviewed animal studies of these and other carotenoids, and concluded the following:

"There is limited evidence that α-carotene has cancer-preventive activity from single studies of models of liver, lung, skin and colon carcinogenesis. There is limited evidence that lycopene has cancer-preventive activity from models of colon, liver, mammary gland and lung carcinogenesis. There is limited evidence that lutein has cancer-preventive activity from experimental models of colon and skin carcinogenesis."

Therefore, although selected studies indicate efficacy for these other carotenoids, the number of studies examining carotenoids other than β-carotene was rather limited.

3.2. Observational Epidemiology

Two different approaches have been used to evaluate carotenoid exposure in epidemiological studies of carotenoids and cancer risk. One approach relies on an estimation of the usual intake of specific carotenoids in the diet, and a second approach relies on biochemical assessment of specific carotenoids and/or total carotenoids in blood samples. The two approaches are both considered valid methods for evaluating carotenoid exposure, since blood levels are correlated with dietary intake. The evaluation of blood carotenoids and risk of cancer is most commonly used in prospective cohort studies, in which blood samples can be obtained from subjects prior to the development of cancer. Many studies use biochemical measures of exposure to carotenoids and their association with risk of various cancers; these are comprehensively reviewed and discussed in the IARC report *(3)*. The IARC noted that:

"the results for lung cancer were remarkably consistent, almost all studies showing an inverse association between blood β-carotene or total carotene status and lung cancer risk... The results of the few studies on cervical and oral and pharyngeal cancer are also consistent. For other sties, the aggregate results are less compelling, and the evidence for an inverse association is less strong."

These biochemical epidemiologic studies thus strongly support the notion that those who consume a carotenoid-rich diet resulting in higher blood carotenoid concentrations have a lower risk of developing certain cancers.

Hundreds of studies that estimate carotenoid intake and risk of various cancers are now available and reviewed elsewhere. More than 20 case-control studies on lung cancer and carotene intake are reviewed in the IARC monograph *(3)*, which concluded that nearly all the studies found a lower risk of lung cancer among people with a high dietary intake of carotenoids. However, a majority of the studies found stronger inverse trends with vegetable and fruit intake than with estimated carotenoid intake. After an exhaustive review of the literature on carotenoids and cancer risk by tumor site, the IARC report noted significant inverse associations for laryngeal and esophageal cancer, and consistent risk reduction with increasing consumption of carotene containing foods with regard to gastric cancer. In contrast to these cancer sites, the IARC report found no consistent inverse association between carotene intake and the risk of colorectal, breast, and prostate cancers.

In all observational studies, it is not possible to determine whether or not observed associations are causal, because of the potential for uncontrolled confounding. Individuals who consume greater amounts of carotenoids in the diet may have other health behaviors associated with a lower risk of cancer, such as less exposure to tobacco. Also, it is difficult to sort out whether protective effects result from other protective factors in fruits and vegetables, or from the carotenoids themselves; the evidence thus far most strongly supports

Table 2
Randomized Trials of β-Carotene: Premalignant Endpoints as Outcome

Reference	Population	Intervention	N	Endpoint	Result	p Value
Stich (1984) (32)	Philippines—betel quid users	β-carotene (180 mg/wk) Placebo	25 18	Oral micronuclei	↓ 66% ↓ 1%	p < 0.001
Stich (1985) (33)	Inuits—smokeless tobacco users	β-carotene (180 mg/wk) Placebo	23 31	Oral micronuclei	↓ 60% ↓ 0.5%	p < 0.001
Stich (1988) (34)	India—betel nut chewers	β-carotene (180 mg/wk) β-carotene & retinol (100,000 IU/wk) Placebo	31 51 30	Oral micronuclei	↓ 71%/↓ 75%[a] ↓ 71%/↓ 71% ↑ 8%/↓ 7%	p < 0.001 p < 0.001
Stich (1988) (34)	India—betel nut chewers	β-carotene (180 mg/wk) β-carotene & retinol (100,000 IU/wk) Placebo	27 51 33	Oral leukoplakia (complete remission)	14.8% 27.5% 3%	p = NS p < 0.05
Sankaranarayanan (1997) (35)	India	Vitamin A (300.000 IU/wk) β-carotene (360 mg/wk) Placebo	50 55 55	Complete regression Oral Leukoplakia	52% 33% 10%	p < 0.0001
Zaridze (1993) (36)	Uzbekistan—oral leukoplakia,	β-carotene (40 mg/d) + retinol (100,000 IU/wk) + vitamin E (80 mg/wk) vs placebo	384	Leukoplakia prevalence	OR = 0.62 (0.39–0.98)	p < 0.05
	Esophagitis		291	Progression/stable vs regression	OR = 0.66 (0.37–1.16)	p = NS
McLarty (1995) (30)	US—male asbestos workers	Retinol (25,000 Q.O.D.) + β-carotene (50 mg/d) vs placebo	755 total	Sputum atypia	OR = 1.24 (0.78–1.96)	p = NS
Van Poppel (1992) (37)	Netherlands—male smokers	β-carotene (20 mg/d) vs placebo	114 total	Sputum micronuclei	↓ 27% (9–41%)	p < 0.05
deVet (1991) (38)	Netherlands—cervical dysplasia	β-carotene(10 mg/d) vs placebo	278 total	Regression	OR = 0.68[b] (0.28–1.60)	p = NS
Romney (1997) (39)	US—cervical dysplasia	β-carotene (30 mg/d) vs placebo	69 total	Persistent CIN	OR = 1.53	p = NS
Mackerras (1999) (40)	Australia—cervical atypia or dysplasia	β-carotene (30 mg/d) +/- vitamin C (500 mg/d) vs placebo	141 total	Regression	HR = 1.58 (0.86–2.93)	p = NS
Keefe (2001) (41)	US—cervical dysplasia	β-carotene (30 mg/d) vs placebo	103 total	Regression	25% 38%	p = NS
Greenberg (1994) (42)	US—resected adenoma	β-carotene (25 mg/d) +/- vitamin C (1 g/d) + vitamin E (400 mg/d) vs placebo	751 total	Recurrent adenoma	β-carotene: RR = 1.01 (0.85–1.20)	p = NS
Kikendall (1991) (43)	US—resected adenoma	β-carotene (15 mg/d) vs placebo	132[c] 125	Recurrent polyps	29% 24%	p = NS

(continued)

Table 2 (continued)

Reference	Population	Intervention	N	Endpoint	Result	p Value
MacLennan (1995) (44)	Australia—resected adenoma	β-carotene (20 mg/d) +/− wheat bran +/− low-fat diet vs placebo	390 total	Recurrent adenoma	OR = 1.4 (0.8–2.3)	p = NS
Hofstad (1998) (45)	Norway—adenoma patients	β-carotene (15 mg/d) + vitamin C, vitamin E, selenium, calcium vs placebo	116 total	Recurrent adenoma/ adenoma growth	Overall no difference between intervention and Control	p = NS
Correa (2000) (11)	Columbia—gastric dysplasia	β-carotene (30 mg/d) +/− vitamin C, triple therapy vs placebo	852 total 631[d]	Regression: subjects with atrophy	RR = 5.1 (1.7–15.0)	p < 0.05
				Regression: subjects with intestinal metaplasia	RR = 3.4 (1.1–9.8)	p < 0.05

[a]change in leukoplakia and normal mucosa, respectively.
[b]based upon broad definition of regression (major and minor).
[c]number completing 36 mo.
[d]number completing trial.
HR, hazard ratio; OR, odds ratio; RR, relative risk; Se, selenium.

516

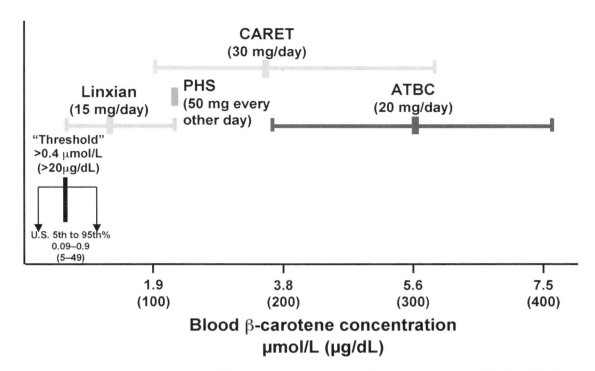

Fig. 3. Median, 25th and 75th percentiles of blood β-carotene concentrations achieved in the ATBC and CARET trials, during which β-carotene apparently increased the risk of lung cancer in heavy smokers, and in the Linxian, China, Cancer Prevention Study, during which persons who received β-carotene had favorable outcomes. An approximate threshold associated with a reduced risk of cancer and all-cause mortality is indicated. (Median and interquartile ranges were provided by the investigators of the trials, except PHS; the U.S. normative data are published in ref *1*.) (Adapted. from *52* with permission.)

a generalized fruit and vegetable effect rather than a specific carotenoid effect. Thus, observational epidemiologic studies generally support a cancer preventive effect of a carotenoid-rich diet in humans, at least for certain common tumor sites, but it is unclear whether observed associations reflect carotenoid effects *per se*.

3.3. Clinical Intervention Studies

β-Carotene (supplemental) has been one of the most widely studied agents in clinical intervention studies aimed at the prevention of precancerous lesions or invasive malignancies. Table 2 summarizes the results of randomized intervention trials of β-carotene that use precancerous lesions as the primary outcome, and Table 3 summarizes the results of randomized intervention trials of β-carotene that use invasive cancers as the primary outcome. Carotenoids other than β-carotene (and excluding lycopene, which is discussed in Chapter 34) have not been evaluated in clinical intervention studies aimed at cancer prevention.

3.3.1. CLINICAL INTERVENTION STUDIES: PRECANCEROUS ENDPOINTS

Supplemental β-carotene has been evaluated as a single agent, and in combination with related nutrients for chemopreventive efficacy in the setting of oral precancerous lesions, gastric precancerous lesions, bronchial preneoplasia (atypical cells in sputum), cervical dysplasia, and adenomatous polyps. As is evident from Table 2, these trials provide strong evidence that short-term supplementation with β-carotene lacks efficacy in preventing or regressing bronchial neoplasia, cervical precancerous lesions, and adenomatous polyps. One randomized trial of supplemental β-carotene in patients with gastric precancerous lesions suggested efficacy *(11)*, but this observation requires confirmation, particularly because of the relatively small number of subjects in the placebo group for this trial (*n* = 100 of 852 total randomized). Efficacy of supplemental β-carotene is currently most convincing for oral precancerous lesions, as reviewed elsewhere *(12)*; a total of nine trials have investigated the effects of supplemental

Table 3
Randomized Trials of β-Carotene: Invasive Cancer as Endpoint

Reference	Population	Intervention	N	Endpoint	Result	p Value
Hennekens et al. (1996) (25)	US—male physicians	β-carotene (50 mg/qod) vs placebo	22,071 total	Total cancer	RR = 0.98 (0.91–1.06)	p = NS
Lee et al. (1999) (46)	US—female health professionals	β-carotene (50 mg/qod) vs placebo	19,939 19,937	All cancers	RR = 1.03 * (0.89–1.18)	p = NS
Heart Protection Study Group (2002) (47)	UK—adults at risk for CHD	β-carotene (20 mg/d) + vitamin E (600 mg/d) + vitamin C (250 mg/d) vs placebo	20,536 total	Total cancer (except non-melanoma skin cancer)	Intervention: 7.8% Placebo: 8.0%	p = NS
ATBC (1994) (16)	Finland—male smokers	β-carotene (20 mg/d) +/– vitamin E (50 mg/d) vs placebo	29,133 total	Lung cancer	BC:RR = 1.18 (1.03–1.36)	p < 0.05
Omenn et al. (1996) (17)	US—smokers and asbestos workers	β-carotene (30 mg/d) + retinol (25,000 IU/d) vs placebo	18,314 total	Lung cancer	RR = 1.28 (1.04–1.57)	p < 0.05
Greenberg et al. (1990) (48)	US—prior skin cancer	β-carotene (50 mg/d) vs placebo	1805 total	Second skin cancer	RR = 1.05 (0.91–1.22)	p = NS
Green et al. (1999) (49)	Australia	β-carotene (30 mg/d) vs placebo	1383 total	Incident squamous cell skin cancer	RR = 1.35 (0.84–2.19)	p = NS
				Incident basal cell skin cancer	RR = 1.04 (0.73–1.27)	p = NS
Blot et al. (1993) (14)	Linxian county, China—general population	β-carotene (15 mg/d) + vitamin E (30 mg/d) + selenium (50 ug/d) vs placebo	29,584 total	Stomach cancer death	RR = 0.79 (0.64–0.99)	p < .05
				Esophageal cancer death	RR = 0.96 (0.78–1.18)	p = NS
Li et al. (1993) (50)	Linxian county, China—esophageal dysplasia	Multivite/multimineral + β-carotene (15 mg/d) vs placebo	3,318 total	Stomach cancer death	RR = 1.18 (0.76–1.85)	p = NS
				Esophageal cancer death	RR = 0.84 (0.54–1.29)	p = NS
Mayne et al. (2001) (15)	US—prior early stage mouth/throat cancer	β-carotene (50 mg/d) vs placebo	135 129	Second mouth/throat cancer	RR = 0.69 (0.39–1.25)	p = NS
				Lung cancer	RR = 1.44 (0.62–3.39)	p = NS

*Results for β-carotene only (trial continuing for vitamin E and aspirin).
OR, odds ratio; RR, relative risk.

518

β-carotene, alone or in combination with other agents, on regression of oral leukoplakia. Six non-randomized studies reported response rates ranging from 44–97%. However, the response rates from these uncontrolled studies must be interpreted cautiously for three reasons: leukoplakias can regress spontaneously; varying response criteria were used; and there was no apparent dose-response relationship. Three placebo-controlled trials of β-carotene and oral leukoplakia are available, all suggesting chemopreventive efficacy (Table 2). Although these trials of supplemental β-carotene in oral premalignancy have some limitations, it is notable that consistent efficacy of retinoids—structural analogs of β-carotene—has been reported in the setting of oral precancerous lesions, as reviewed elsewhere (13).

3.3.2. CLINICAL INTERVENTION STUDIES: INVASIVE CANCER AS PRIMARY ENDPOINTS

Supplemental β-carotene has been evaluated as a single agent or in combination with related nutrients for chemopreventive efficacy in the primary prevention of total cancers, lung cancers, esophageal/gastric cancers, and in the secondary prevention of non-melanoma skin cancers and oral/pharynx/larynx cancers. As seen in Table 3, these trials provide strong evidence of supplemental β-carotene's lack of efficacy in preventing total cancers, primary or secondary lung cancers, and secondary non-melanoma skin cancers. With regard to lung cancer, evidence supports either no effect or a possible adverse effect of supplemental β-carotene, particularly in current smokers. This finding is discussed in greater depth in Subheading 7.

To date, only one clinical intervention trial involving supplemental β-carotene to prevent invasive cancers, the Linxian County trial in China, reported statistically significant evidence of chemopreventive efficacy (14). In this trial, the combination of supplemental β-carotene, selenium, and vitamin E significantly reduced gastric but not esophageal cancer mortality. Another trial of supplemental β-carotene observed a nonsignificant decrease in the incidence of second cancers of the oral cavity, pharynx, and larynx, but also observed a nonsignificant increase in the incidence of lung cancer (15). It is possible that efficacy observed in the Linxian trial could result from selenium or vitamin E given along with β-carotene, and the suggestion of possible benefit against secondary head and neck cancers is consistent with chance, given the wide confidence intervals. However, it is notable that significant

chemopreventive efficacy has been observed in these two sites (gastric and oral) in trials involving precancerous lesions, and efficacy for one of these sites is consistent with the results of animal carcinogenesis studies (buccal pouch model).

In summary, evidence from clinical intervention trials indicates that supplemental β-carotene has potential efficacy against gastric cancers/precancerous lesions, and possibly oral cancers/oral precancerous lesions. In contrast, there is strong evidence of a lack of efficacy against total cancers, lung cancers, non-melanoma skin cancers, cervical dysplasia, and adenomatous polyps, and evidence of harm in certain subgroups of the population (see Subheading 7).

4. SAFETY

The safety of carotenoids has been reviewed carefully as part of the Dietary Reference Intake (DRI) evaluation undertaken by the Institute of Medicine in 2000 (1). The DRI process includes a formal hazard identification review, in order to derive tolerable upper intake levels (ULs) for each nutrient. This evaluation considered the safety of carotenoids obtained from foods, and also from supplemental sources.

It has long been known that those who consume high-carotenoid diets can develop a condition known as carotenodermia—yellow pigmentation in the skin caused by carotene accumulation. If the condition results from high lycopene intake, it is generally referred to as lycopenodermia. Both conditions are harmless and reversible, and are not considered a safety concern. No other side effects have been linked conclusively to a high consumption of carotenoids from foods.

However, as described in the previous section on clinical intervention studies, high-dose supplemental β-carotene has been shown to increase the incidence of lung cancer in smokers in two clinical trials. One trial, the α-Tocopherol β-Carotene Trial, or ATBC (16), evaluated 20 mg β-carotene per d, and the Carotene and Retinol Efficacy Trial, or CARET, evaluated 30 mg β-carotene per d given in combination with retinol (25,000 IU/d) (17). Although the lowest β-carotene dose associated with adverse effects (20 mg/d) is only threefold higher than high intakes of β-carotene obtained from foods (99th percentile of β-carotene intake in all subjects was 6.6 mg/d in NHANES III) (2), the bioavailability of supplemental β-carotene vastly exceeds that of β-carotene from foods. If risk is characterized as a function of plasma β-carotene concentrations (see Fig. 3), it is apparent that the concentrations associated with possible adverse effects on lung cancer are well beyond the concentrations achieved from consumption of carotenoids in foods, pertaining only to high-dose β-carotene supplements. Carotenoids other than β-carotene have not yet been studied in large clinical intervention studies, so there is very little data on the safety of other carotenoid supplements.

5. PHARMACODYNAMICS

The pharmacodynamics of carotenoids, both from diet and from supplements, have been widely studied (18). Carotenoids are lipid-soluble compounds whose absorption is influenced by many factors, including dietary fat. Micellar solubilization is necessary for carotenoid absorption. Carotenoids can either be absorbed intact or metabolized in the enterocyte. Provitamin A carotenoids can be converted into retinal via the enzyme 15-15'-dioxygenase, which has now been cloned. If carotenoids are not metabolized but are absorbed intact, they are carried in the circulation first by chylomicrons, which carry them to the liver, a major storage depot for carotenoids. The liver repackages them into very low-density lipoproteins (VLDLs), which are subsequently converted into low-density lipoproteins (LDL). LDL is the primary carrier of carotenoids in human blood, although they are also found in lesser concentrations in other lipoprotein fractions.

The lipoproteins distribute carotenoids to various tissues throughout the body; they are found in the highest concentrations (per g tissue weight) in tissues including the adrenals, testes, and corpus luteum (3). Because these tissues are relatively minor in weight, they serve as only minor storage sites for carotenoids. More important storage tissues for carotenoids are fat, liver, skin, and plasma, given their larger tissue weights (3). Tissue-selective effects on carotenoid absorption have been suggested. For example, the human macula concentrates lutein and zeaxanthin, but not the other major dietary carotenoids (19). The mechanisms for tissue-specific effects on absorption or retention of specific carotenoids are unknown at this time.

Carotenoid depletion and repletion studies have been carried out in humans in order to estimate half-lives in plasma. When low-carotenoid diets were fed to healthy men, plasma carotenoids depleted relatively rapidly, with estimated mean depletion half-lives of < 12 d for β-carotene, α-carotene, and cryptoxanthin, between 12 and 33 d for lycopene, and between 33 and 61 d for lutein/zeaxanthin (20). These values are consistent with techniques using octadeuterated β-carotene in humans, in which β-carotene was estimated to have

a mean residence time (MRT) of 9–13 d in plasma and 51 d in the entire system (21,22). Carotenoids are known to accumulate in adipose tissue; however, the pharmacokinetics of carotenoid depletion and repletion have not been well characterized in tissues other than plasma.

6. PHARMACEUTICAL SCIENCE

β-Carotene is the most widely studied carotenoid supplement in the prevention of cancer or other chronic diseases. Clinical intervention trials nearly always use synthetic β-carotene, which generally comes in the all-trans configuration (>90–95%). Since β-carotene is an extremely hydrophobic compound, manufacturers have developed various formulations to increase water-solubility and bioavailability. One such formulation widely studied in animal models is β-carotene beadlets, wherein the β-carotene is encapsulated in a gelatin and starch matrix (10% β-carotene by weight) with various stabilizers added. These and other supplemental forms of β-carotene have dramatically better bioavailability than β-carotene as generally encountered in a food matrix. For example, the absorption of β-carotene in supplements solubilized with emulsifiers and protected by antioxidants can be 70 % or more (1). In contrast, less than 5% bioavailability of carotenes has been reported from raw foods such as carrots (1).

Although most cancer prevention trials have used single nutrient supplements of β-carotene, some of these formulations appear to also contain small amounts of α-carotene. For example, β-carotene concentrations in plasma increased approx 10-fold, and plasma α-carotene concentrations nearly doubled in one multi-year cancer prevention clinical trial involving supplemental β-carotene (23).

Although synthetic supplements have been the supplement of choice for large-scale intervention trials to date, natural source supplements of carotenoids including β-carotene have been used in human intervention research. One commercial mixed carotenoid supplement (β-tene, Cognis Corporation, LaGrange, IL,) is derived from the algae *Dunaliella salina* and contains a mixture of the following carotenoids: β-carotene (54% all-trans, 37% 9-cis, 9% 13-cis, and other isomers), α-carotene, zeaxanthin, cryptoxanthin, and lutein (24). Considering the different composition of natural source carotenoid supplements as compared to synthetic supplements, it is evident that efficacy comparisons from one class of supplements are not readily generalizable to the other.

7. POPULATIONS THAT BENEFIT OR ARE HARMED BY INTERVENTION

In contrast to most other chemopreventive agents in this volume, clinical trials of supplemental β-carotene to prevent human cancer have advanced to the point where it is now reasonably clear which populations are most likely to benefit or be harmed, at least with regard to high-dose supplementation. As described in Subheading 3.3 there is some evidence that supplemental β-carotene may have benefit in reducing the progression of gastric precancerous lesions and in reducing gastric cancer incidence/mortality. Trials supporting these possible benefits were conducted in countries in which micronutrient intake may be suboptimal (especially in Linxian County, China), suggesting that the populations most likely to benefit may be those at higher risk of gastric cancer and with suboptimal micronutrient intake. Also, as described in Subheading 3.3., supplemental β-carotene has documented efficacy in regressing oral precancerous lesions, and possible efficacy in preventing cancers of the oral cavity, pharynx, and larynx. Risk factors for oral precancerous lesions and oropharyngeal cancers are similar: chronic use of tobacco and alcohol, and relatively low consumption of fruits and vegetables. Inadequate micronutrient status is common in patients with head and neck cancers, again suggesting that populations with relatively poor micronutrient intake/status may be most likely to benefit from supplementation. However, widespread use of tobacco in this patient population probably precludes the use of β-carotene as a high-dose supplement, because the evidence—although not entirely consistent *(25)*—indicates that concurrent use of high-dose supplemental β-carotene in current smokers may increase the incidence of lung cancer.

More specifically, in the ATBC study population, which included only men who were current smokers at the time of randomization, supplemental β-carotene was found to increase the risk of lung cancer. Additional analyses of ATBC data indicated that this apparent adverse effect of β-carotene supplementation was only noted in those who smoked more heavily: the RR for lung cancer in the supplemental β-carotene group as compared to placebo was 0.97 for men who smoked 5–19 cigarettes per d, 1.25 for men who smoked 20–29 cigarettes per d, and 1.28 in men who smoked >29 cigarettes per d *(26)*. CARET included both current and former smokers; supplemental β-carotene plus retinol increased the risk of lung cancer in current (RR = 1.42) but not former (RR = 0.80) smokers *(17)*. In contrast, 12 yr of intervention with supplemental β-carotene did not increase the risk of lung cancer in current or former smokers in the Physicians' Health Study, as compared to placebo *(25)*.

The finding that high-dose supplemental β-carotene may interact with concurrent tobacco exposure to promote rather than inhibit lung carcinogenesis is receiving considerable attention in mechanistic research studies; for example, squamous metaplasia has been produced in the lungs of ferrets exposed to both cigarette smoke and high-dose β-carotene *(27)*. Clarification of the mechanism of this unexpected adverse finding with β-carotene should be a high priority, as it may have implications for other carotenoids being considered for intervention studies (e.g., lycopene for prostate cancer prevention).

8. POTENTIAL CLINICAL STUDIES

Clinical studies of β-carotene for cancer prevention are limited at this time, pending results of mechanistic studies aimed at understanding the promotional effects observed in lungs of current smokers taking high-dose supplements of β-carotene. Lycopene is the only other carotenoid currently being evaluated in human cancer prevention/intermediate endpoint studies, as discussed elsewhere in this volume. Clinical studies of β-carotene-rich/carotenoid-rich foods for cancer prevention are underway *(28)*. These studies are more difficult to implement, requiring a major dietary behavioral change, rather than taking a daily supplement. However, these trials are a more direct test of the hypothesis that has emerged from observational epidemiological studies—that dietary β-carotene (in the form of fruits and vegetables) is associated with a lower risk of various cancers. Two very interesting clinical questions regarding supplemental β-carotene remain unanswered at this time. The first is whether or not lower doses of supplemental β-carotene (e.g., 6 mg/d) might have favorable effects with regard to lung or other cancers, as recent animal experiments have suggested *(29)*. The second unresolved question is whether or not former or non-smokers might benefit from supplemental β-carotene, particularly in populations with suboptimal micronutrient status. These hypotheses are not currently being tested because of safety concerns regarding the use of supplemental β-carotene in long-term clinical trials.

9. PROMISING ENDPOINTS (BIOMARKERS)

To date, cancer prevention trials involving β-carotene have failed to support its efficacy in humans. One contribution these trials may make to the larger field of chemoprevention research is that β-carotene has been studied in trials of intermediate endpoints and of invasive cancer at the same tumor site (albeit in different trials), allowing an examination of the predictive value of intermediate endpoints. Sputum cytology, one such intermediate endpoint, is used for lung cancer. β-Carotene in combination with retinol was found to have no effect; if anything, it increased atypia in sputum cells *(30)*. The CARET study, which used the same combination intervention, reported that it had no benefit and instead increased the risk of lung cancer when compared to placebo. Similarly, retinoids have been shown to have no effect on bronchial metaplasia *(13)*, another intermediate endpoint for lung cancer, and also had no overall benefit with regard to second primary prevention of lung cancer *(31)*. Collectively, these trials support the possible value of intermediate endpoints for lung cancer as promising biomarkers of chemopreventive efficacy (or lack of efficacy) in lung cancer.

Oral precancerous lesions have also been used as an intermediate endpoint to screen compounds for possible chemopreventive efficacy in oral cancers, and as reviewed earlier, β-carotene has been shown to reverse/regress oral precancerous lesions. The largest trial of supplemental β-carotene for oropharyngeal and laryngeal cancer prevention *(15)* suggested possible chemopreventive efficacy for supplemental β-carotene in oropharyngeal/laryngeal tumor sites (RR = 0.69); however, the result was not statistically significant, since this trial closed recruitment prematurely as a result of the CARET trial findings. A larger trial of 13-*cis*-retinoic acid in secondary prevention of oropharyngeal and laryngeal cancer is underway; (Preliminary results of the trial are now available [Khuri F, Lee JJ, Lippman SM, et al. Isotretinoin effects on head and neck cancer recurrence and second primary tumors. *Proc Am Soc Clin Oncol* 2003;22:90 (abstr 359)]) if that trial observes chemopreventive efficacy for both carotenoids and retinoids as is seen in oral precancerous lesions *(12,13)*, the weight of evidence will support the value of using site-specific intermediate endpoints to evaluate the potential efficacy of agents for prevention of lung and oral cancers.

REFERENCES

1. Institute of Medicine, National Academy of Sciences, Food and Nutrition Board, Panel on Dietary Antioxidants and Related Compounds. *Dietary Reference Intakes for Vitamin C, Vitamin E, Selenium, and Carotenoids.* National Academy Press, Washington, DC, 2000.
2. Institute of Medicine, National Academy of Sciences, Food and Nutrition Board, Panel on Micronutrients. *Dietary Reference Intakes for Vitamin A, Vitamin K, Arsenic, Boron,*
Chromium, Copper, Iodine, Iron, Manganese, Molybdenum, Nickel, Silicon, Vanadium, and Zinc. National Academy Press, Washington, DC, 2001.
3. IARC Working Group on the Evaluation of Cancer Preventive Agents. *IARC* International Agency for Research on Cancer, World Health Organization, *Handbooks of Cancer Prevention, Volume 2, Carotenoids.* Oxford University Press, Carey, NC, 1998.
4. Krinsky NI. Actions of carotenoids in biological systems. *Annu Rev Nutr* 1993;13:561–587.
5. Mathews-Roth MM. Carotenoids in erythropoietic protoporphyria and other photosensitivity diseases. *AnnNY Acad Sci* 1993;691:127–138.
6. Burton GW, Ingold KU.β-carotene: an unusual type of lipid antioxidant. *Science* 1984;224:569–573.
7. Floyd RA. Role of free radicals in carcinogenesis and brain ischemia. *FASEB J* 1990;4:2587–2597.
8. Watson RR, Rybski J. Immunomodulation by retinoids and carotenoids, in *Nutrition and Immunology*. Chandra RK, ed. Alan R. Liss, New York, NY 1988, pp. 87–99.
9. Zhang LX, Cooney RV, Bertram JS. Carotenoids enhance gap junctional communication and inhibit lipid peroxidation in C3H/10T1/2 cells: relationship to their cancer chemopreventive action. *Carcinogenesis* 1991;12:2109–2114.
10. Comerci JT Jr, Runowicz CD, Fields AL, et al. Induction of transforming growth factor β-1 in cervical intraepithelial neoplasia in vivo after treatment with β-carotene. *Clin Cancer Res* 1997;3:157–160.
11. Correa P, Fontham ETH, Bravo JC, et al. Chemoprevention of gastric dysplasia: randomized trial of antioxidant supplements and anti-*Helicobacter pylori* therapy. *J Natl Cancer Inst* 2000;92:1881–1888.
12. Mayne ST, Cartmel B, Morse DE. Chemoprevention of oral premalignant lesions, in *Head and Neck Cancer*. Ensley JF, Gutkind JS, Jacobs JR, Lippman SM, eds. Elsevier Science, New York, NY, 2003, pp. 261–269.
13. Mayne ST, Lippman SM. Cancer prevention: diet and chemopreventive agents.Retinoids, carotenoids, and micronutrients, in Principles and Practice of Oncology, 6th ed. DeVita VT Jr, Hellman S, Rosenberg SA, eds. Lippincott Williams & Wilkins, Philadelphia, PA, 2001, pp.575–590.
14. Blot WJ, Li J-Y, Taylor PR, et al. Nutrition intervention trials in Linxian, China: supplementation with specific vitamin/mineral combinations, cancer incidence, and disease-specific mortality in the general population. *J Natl Cancer Inst* 1993;85:1483–1492.
15. Mayne ST, Cartmel B, Baum M, et al. Randomized trial of supplemental β-carotene to prevent second head and neck cancer. *Cancer Res* 2001;61:1457–1463.
16. The Alpha-Tocopherol, Beta Carotene Cancer Prevention Study Group.The effect of vitamin E and β carotene on the incidence of lung cancer and other cancers in male smokers. *N Engl J Med.* 1994;330:1029–1035.
17. Omenn GS, Goodman GE, Thornquist MD, et al. Effects of a combination of β carotene and vitamin A on lung cancer and cardiovascular disease. *N Engl J Med.* 1996;334:1150–1155.
18. Boileau TW, Moore AC, Erdman JW Jr. Carotenoids and vitamin A, in *Antioxidant Status, Diet, Nutrition, and Health.* Papas AM, ed. CRC Press, Boca Raton, FL, 1999, pp.133–158.
19. Schalch W, Dayhaw-Barker P, Barker FM II. The carotenoids of the human retina, in *Nutritional and*

Environmental Influences on the Eye. Taylor A, ed. CRC Press, Boca Raton, FL, 1992, pp.215–250.

20. Rock CL, Swendseid ME, Jacob R, McKee RW. Plasma carotenoid levels in human subjects fed a low carotenoid diet. *J Nutr* 1992;122:96–100.

21. Novotny JA, Dueker SR, Zech LA, Clifford AJ. Compartmental analysis of the dynamics of β-carotene metabolism in an adult volunteer. *J Lipid Res* 1995;36:1825–1838.

22. Novotny JA, Zech LA, Furr HC, et al. Mathematical modeling in nutrition:constructing a physiologic compartmental model of the dynamics of β-carotene metabolism. *Adv Food Nutr Res* 1996;40:25–54.

23. Mayne ST, Cartmel B, Silva F, et al. Effect of supplemental β-carotene on plasma concentrations of carotenoids, retinol and α-tocopherol in humans. *Am J Clin Nutr* 1998;68:642–647.

24. Stahl W, Schwarz W, von Laar J, Sies H. All-*trans* β-carotene preferentially accumulates in human chylomicrons and very low density lipoproteins compared with the 9-*cis* geometrical isomer. *J Nutr* 1995;125:2128–2133.

25. Hennekens CH, Buring JE, Manson JE, et al. Lack of effect of long-term supplementation with β carotene on the incidence of malignant neoplasms and cardiovascular disease. *N Engl J Med* 1996;334:1145–1149.

26. Albanes D, Heinonen OP, Taylor PR, et al. α-Tocopherol and β-carotene supplements and lung cancer incidence in the Alpha-Tocopherol, Beta-Carotene Cancer Prevention Study: effects of baseline characteristics and study compliance. *J Natl Cancer Inst* 1996;88:1560–1570.

27. Wang XD, Liu C, Bronson RT, et al. Retinoid signaling and activator protein-1 expression in ferrets given β-carotene supplements and exposed to tobacco smoke. *J Natl Cancer Inst* 1999;91:60–66.

28. McEligot AJ, Rock CL, Flatt SW, et al. Plasma carotenoids are biomarkers of long-term high vegetable intake in women with breast cancer. *J Nutr* 1999;129:2258–2263.

29. Liu C, Wang X-D, Bronson RT, et al. Effects of physiological *versus* pharmacological β-carotene supplementation on cell proliferation and histopathological changes in the lungs of cigarette smoke-exposed ferrets. *Carcinogenesis* 2000;21:2245–2253.

30. McLarty JW, Holiday DB, Girard WM, et al. β-Carotene, vitamin A and lung cancer chemoprevention: results of an intermediate endpoint study. *Am J Clin Nutr* 1995;62:1431S–1438S.

31. Lippman SM, Lee JJ, Karp DD, et al. Randomized Phase III intergroup trial of isotretinoin to prevent second primary tumors in stage I non-small-cell lung cancer. *J Natl Cancer Inst* 2001;93:605–618.

32. Stich HF, Rosin MP, Vallejera MO.Reduction with vitamin A and β-carotene administration of proportion of micronucleated buccal mucosal cells in Asian betel nut and tobacco chewers. *Lancet* 1984;1:1204–1206.

33. Stich HF, Hornby P, Dunn BP.A pilot β-carotene intervention trial with Inuits using smokeless tobacco. *Int J Cancer* 1985;36:321–327.

34. Stich HF, Rosin MP, Hornby AP, et al. Remission of oral leukoplakias and micronuclei in tobacco/betel quid chewers treated with β-carotene and with β-carotene plus vitamin A. *Int J Cancer* 1988;42:195–199.

35. Sankaranarayanan R, Mathew B, Varghese C, et al. Chemoprevention of oral leukoplakia with vitamin A and β carotene: an assessment. *Oral Oncol* 1997;33:231–236.

36. Zaridze D, Evstifeeva T, Boyle P. Chemoprevention of oral leukoplakia and chronic esophagitis in an area of high incidence of oral and esophageal cancer. *Ann Epidemiol* 1993;3:225–234.

37. van Poppel G, Kok FJ, Hermus RJJ. β-Carotene supplementation in smokers reduces the frequency of micronuclei in sputum. *Br J Cancer* 1992;66:1164–1168.

38. de Vet HC, Knipschild PG, Willebrand D, et al. The effect of β-carotene on the regression and progression of cervical dysplasia: a clinical experiment. *J Clin Epidemiol* 1991;44:273–283.

39. Romney SL, Ho GY, Palan PR, et al. Effects of β-carotene and other factors on outcome of cervical dysplasia and human papillomavirus infection. *Gynecol Oncol* 1997;65:483–492.

40. Mackerras D, Irwig L, Simpson JM, et al. Randomized double-blind trial of β-carotene and vitamin C in women with minor cervical abnormalities. *Br J Cancer* 1999;79:1448–1453.

41. Keefe KA, Schell MJ, Brewer C, et al. A randomized, double blind, Phase III trial using oral β-carotene supplementation for women with high-grade cervical intraepithelial neoplasia. *Cancer Epidemiol Biomark Prev* 2001;10:1029–1035.

42. Greenberg ER, Baron JA, Tosteson TD, et al. A clinical trial of antioxidant vitamins to prevent colorectal adenoma. *N Engl J Med* 1994;331:141–147.

43. Kikendall JW, Mobarhan S, Nelson R, et al. Oral β carotene does not reduce the recurrence of colorectal adenomas. *Am J Gastroenterol* 1991;36:1356 (abstr).

44. MacLennan R, Macrae F, Bain C, et al. Randomized trial of intake of fat, fiber, and β carotene to prevent colorectal adenomas. *J Natl Cancer Inst* 1995;87:1760–1766.

45. Hofstad B, Almendingen K, Vatn M, et al. Growth and recurrence of colorectal polyps: a double-blind 3-year intervention with calcium and antioxidants. *Digestion* 1998;59:148–156.

46. Lee IM, Cook NR, Manson JE, et al. β-Carotene supplementation and incidence of cancer and cardiovascular disease: The Women's Health Study. *J Natl Cancer Inst* 1999;91:2102–2106.

47. Heart Protection Study Collaborative Group. MRC/BHF Heart Protection Study of antioxidant vitamin supplementation in 20,536 high-risk individuals: a randomized placebo-controlled trial. *Lancet* 2002;360:23–33.

48. Greenberg ER, Baron JA, Stukell TA, et al. A clinical trial of β carotene to prevent basal-cell and squamous-cell cancers of the skin. *N Engl J Med* 1990;323:789–795.

49. Green A, Williams G, Neale R, et al. Daily sunscreen application and β-carotene supplementation in prevention of basal-cell and squamous-cell carcinomas of the skin:a randomized controlled trial. *Lancet* 1999;354:723–729.

50. Li J-Y, Taylor PR, Li B, et al. Nutrition intervention trials in Linxian, China: multiple vitamin/mineral supplementation, cancer incidence, and disease-specific mortality among adults with esophageal dysplasia. *J Natl Cancer Inst* 1993;85:1492–1498.

51. Krinsky NI, Mayne ST. Current views on carotenoids: biology, epidemiology and trials, in *Vitamin A and Retinoids: An Update of Biological Aspects and Clinical Applications.* Livrea MA, ed. Birkhauser Verlag, Basel, 2000, pp.45–57.

52. Mayne ST. β-Carotene, carotenoids, and cancer prevention. *Principles Pract Oncol Updates* 1998;12:1–15.

34

Lycopene, a Dietary Cancer Chemopreventive Agent

Andreas I. Constantinou, PhD and Richard B. van Breemen, PhD

CONTENTS

INTRODUCTION
CLINICAL STUDIES OF LYCOPENE
ANIMAL MODELS AND STUDIES OF LYCOPENE CANCER PREVENTION
CELL-BASED STUDIES OF LYCOPENE
SUMMARY AND CONCLUSIONS
ACKNOWLEDGMENTS
REFERENCES

1. INTRODUCTION

Lycopene (Fig. 1), β-carotene, and lutein are the three most abundant carotenoids in the human diet *(1)*. Of more than 600 natural carotenoids, lycopene is the most efficient singlet oxygen quencher, and is therefore a potent antioxidant *(2,3)*. Although twice as efficient as β-carotene at quenching singlet oxygen *(3,4)*, lycopene has no provitamin A activity, so its potential pharmacological effects cannot be associated with vitamin A. Lycopene is found in food primarily as the all-*trans* isomer, the form that is biosynthesized by plants and found in tomatoes, watermelon, and pink grapefruit *(5)*. However, when exposed to heat and light during cooking or food processing, lycopene will produce a variable mixture of all-*trans*-lycopene and *cis* isomers.

Reviews by Gerster *(6)* and van Poppel *(7)* examined the findings of more than 77 retrospective dietary studies and 55 prospective dietary or blood-level studies investigating the anticarcinogenic effects of carotenoids. These data overwhelmingly support the hypothesis that a diet rich in fresh fruits and vegetables reduces the incidence of cancer at certain sites. The overriding question posed by these reviews is, "What are the active anticancer agents in these diets?" Hydrocarbon carotenes and oxygenated xanthophylls comprise the highly conjugated class of pigments known as carotenoids *(8)*.

Many key biological roles are ascribed to various carotenoids in both the plant *(9)* and animal kingdoms *(10)*. In addition, a growing body of evidence acquired over the past decade suggests that carotenoids may function to prevent and/or attenuate certain deleterious human health conditions *(11)*. In most dietary carotenoid studies to date, β-carotene intake and/or blood levels were measured and correlated with cancer prevention. However, few epidemiological studies have included measurements of the blood or tissue levels of other carotenoids. Furthermore, because of analytical limitations, the amounts of *cis*- vs all-*trans* carotenoid isomers could not be examined until most recently. For example, the separation of all-*trans*-lycopene from various *cis* isomers using current high-pressure liquid chromatography (HPLC) technology and on-line mass spectrometric detection is shown in Fig. 2. Synthetic β-carotene used for dietary supplementation is all-*trans*. Fresh root vegetables such as carrots and sweet potatoes contain exclusively all-*trans* carotenoids *(12)*. Green leaves, vegetables exposed to sunlight, and cooked vegetables including cooked carrots and sweet potatoes have significant levels of *cis* carotenoids *(12)*.

Since lycopene is such a potent antioxidant, its anticancer activity might be the result of chemoprotection from oxidative stress that results from an imbalance in the prooxidant/antioxidant ratio in favor of the oxidants *(13,14)*. The most important oxidants responsible for oxidative stress are free radicals and other reactive oxygen species (ROS), which can be formed as a result of exposure to toxic agents such as chemotherapeutic drugs or cigarette smoke (oxidants or prooxidants) or by inadequate dietary supplies of antioxidants *(15)*.

From: Cancer Chemoprevention, Volume 1: Promising Cancer Chemoprevention Agents
Edited by: G. J. Kelloff, E. T. Hawk, and C. C. Sigman © Humana Press Inc., Totowa, NJ

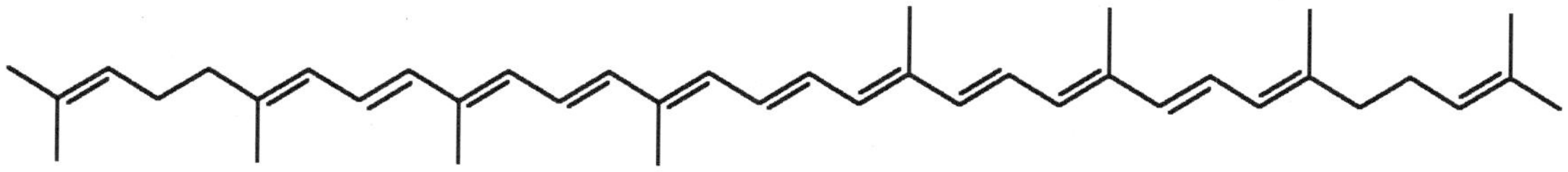

Fig. 1. All-*trans*-lycopene.

Oxidative stress might contribute to aging, arteriosclerosis, rheumatoid arthritis, and cancer *(15)*. Several reviewers have presented strong evidence that ROS play an important role in the development of cancer *(15,16)*.

A great deal of evidence supports the link between oxidative stress and cancer. Clinical trials using antioxidants (i.e., the Linxian, China studies *(17)* and numerous case-control investigations) demonstrated that cancer prevention was associated with higher levels of plasma nutrient antioxidants *(18,19)*. More than 200 cancer studies with animal models demonstrated a protective effect (at the levels of both initiation and promotion) of nutrient antioxidants and a large variety of nonnutritive antioxidants *(20–22)*. An increased risk of cancer has been found in conditions that produce ROS, such as chronic inflammation *(23)*. Free radicals are known to mediate the activation of carcinogens, which can be prevented by the addition of antioxidants *(24)*. Cellular prooxidative states that result in increases in ROS, such as exposure to organic peroxides and the hydroxy radical, can promote initiated cells to neoplastic growth *(25)*. And finally, many tumor promoters are prooxidants, or produce prooxidative states *(26)*.

This chapter summarizes the increasing clinical and preclinical evidence suggesting that lycopene might serve as a chemopreventive agent in certain forms of cancer.

2. CLINICAL STUDIES OF LYCOPENE

Numerous epidemiological studies have investigated which components of dietary fruits and vegetables are most responsible for their cancer preventive effects. Overall, these studies suggest that dietary intake of carotenoids is inversely correlated with the incidence of many forms of cancers, and lycopene in particular is indicated for prevention of certain types of cancer *(27–31)*. For example, Cramer et al. *(32)* carried out a dietary questionnaire-based study of 549 women with ovarian cancer and 516 control subjects. They found that the consumption of lycopene, especially in the form of tomato sauce, was significantly and inversely associated with the risk of ovarian cancer in premenopausal women. In contrast, α-carotene and carrot consumption were more significant for reducing the risk of ovarian cancer in postmenopausal women. To date, no reports of prospective epidemiological studies or lycopene intervention trials have confirmed these findings regarding ovarian cancer chemoprevention by lycopene.

In a study by Helzlsouer and colleagues *(33)*, lycopene was suggested to reduce the risk of bladder cancer. The objective of the study was to examine the association between serum nutrients and the development of bladder cancer. Lycopene, selenium, α-tocopherol, β-carotene, and retinol were measured in serum collected from more than 25,000 persons and kept frozen for 12 yr. During that period, 35 cases of bladder cancer developed among participants. Nutrient serum levels among the cancer cases were compared to those of two matched controls for each case. It was found that lycopene and selenium were lower among the cancer cases, suggesting that these two compounds might provide protection against bladder cancer. In a related prospective study of this same study population by Sato et al. *(34)*, 295 cases of breast cancer and 295 matched controls were evaluated, and dietary lycopene was among the carotenoids associated with a reduced risk of breast cancer.

In a pilot study of 32 women, Kanetsky *(35)* used dietary recall interviews and noted that women in the upper levels of lycopene intake were one-fourth as likely to suffer from cervical dysplasia as women in the lower intake groups. Cervical dysplasia is a risk factor for developing cervical carcinoma. In a similar study, Goodman et al. *(36)* reported on 238 women, 147 with dysplasia and 191 controls, and found that mean levels of lycopene were significantly lower among women with cervical dysplasia than in control subjects. Furthermore, inverse dose-response trends were observed for the carotenoids lycopene and α-cryptoxanthin and the antioxidants vitamin C and α-tocopherol. To the best of our knowledge, no clinical intervention studies have evaluated the chemopreventive activity of lycopene in digestive cancer, bladder cancer, cervical dysplasia, and cancer of the cervix.

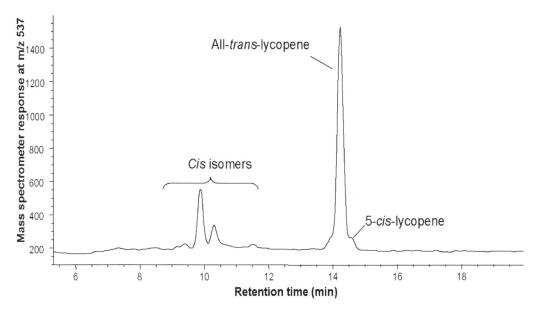

Fig. 2. LC-MS analysis of all-*trans*-lycopene and various *cis*-lycopene isomers using a commercially available C_{30} reversed-phase HPLC column engineered for carotenoid isomer analysis interfaced to a mass spectrometer equipped for positive ion atmospheric pressure chemical ionization. For more information, *see* van Breemen et al. *(45)*.

By far the most compelling evidence so far in support of lycopene as a cancer chemoprevention agent has been in studies of men with prostate cancer, the second leading cause of cancer death among American men over age 65. In 1995, Giovannucci et al. *(37)* reported the results of a single dietary assessment with follow-up of 51,529 male health professionals; 773 of these developed prostate cancer over a 6-yr period. Higher intake of lycopene and tomato products was found to be associated with lower risk of prostate cancer. Giovannucci *(38)* reaffirmed these results in a review of the epidemiological evidence available from multiple sources. Recently, Gann et al. *(39)* and Giovannucci et al. *(40)* reported results for a prospective study of this same cohort of men with multiple dietary assessments during a period of 12 yr. During this extended period of time, 2481 cases of prostate cancer occurred in the study group. These prospective epidemiological analyses confirmed the inverse correlation between prostate cancer and the consumption of tomato products.

Coincident with the epidemiological studies of lycopene and prostate cancer reported by Giovannucci and colleagues, Clinton et al. *(41)* measured lycopene in a variety of human tissues, finding that lycopene and particularly its *cis* isomers, are selectively concentrated in the human prostate. These results suggest that lycopene might be an active component of the tomato

that serves as a prostate cancer chemopreventive agent. In support of this hypothesis, prospective and retrospective epidemiological studies reported by Giovannucci et al. showed a significantly lower risk of prostate cancer in men who consumed tomato products that were rich in lycopene. These statistically significant findings all suggest that lycopene shows promise as a cancer chemopreventive agent in the human prostate.

In addition to these epidemiological studies, a four-arm Phase II clinical trial in progress, under the direction of van Breemen, is investigating the efficacy of lycopene as a prostate cancer chemopreventive agent. In this study, lycopene is administered as a tomato oleoresin at 30 mg/d and measured in the serum of men before and after a 21-d intervention period. Lycopene is also being measured in prostate tissue biopsy specimens. DNA oxidation products, including 8-oxo-deoxyguanosine (8-oxo-dG), 5-hydroxymethyluridine, and 8-oxo-deoxyadenosine (8-oxo-dA) are being measured in peripheral-blood leukocytes before and after lycopene intervention. These DNA modifications are also measured in prostate tissue taken from biopsy specimens and are evaluated as intermediate endpoints for preventing DNA oxidation by lycopene. In addition, prostate-specific antigen (PSA) is measured in blood before and after the intervention period.

Intervention with tomato sauce was evaluated in a completed unblinded fifth arm of this study *(42)*.

Table 1
Results of Tomato Sauce-Based Lycopene Intervention in Men With Prostate Cancer Who Consumed 30 mg Lycopene/d
in Tomato Sauce for 21 Days[1]

Measurement	Change From Baseline Value or Untreated Controls	p Value
Serum lycopene	1.97-fold increase[2]	<0.001
Prostate lycopene	2.93-fold increase[2]	<0.001
Serum PSA	17.5% decrease[2]	=0.002
Leukocyte 8-oxo-dG	21.3% decrease[2]	=0.005
Prostate 8-oxo-dG	28.3% lower[3]	=0.03

[1]Sample Size (N): 32 men with prostate adenocarcinoma
[2]Compared to baseline value
[3]Compared to 8-oxo-dG in resected prostate tissue from untreated men (N=7) with prostate adenocarcinoma

Among the 32 men who completed this preliminary dietary study, 75% were African-American, an ethnic group at particularly high risk for prostate cancer. Each patient served as his own control, since blood and prostate tissue biopsies were obtained at the start of the intervention period and blood and prostate tissue (from prostatectomy) were obtained after the 21-d dietary intervention period. Serum and prostate lycopene levels increased two- and threefold, respectively, following administration of 30 mg/d of dietary, tomato-based lycopene. The results of these assays are summarized in Table 1. Although these results indicate that an imperfect correlation exists between serum lycopene and prostate levels, they confirm studies by other groups showing that oral administration of lycopene or food rich in lycopene results in elevated serum levels (43,44). These data also confirm the observations of other groups who have found a trend between serum and prostate levels of lycopene in men who are undergoing prostate surgery (45). However, the bioavailability of lycopene and the amount of an oral dose that reaches the prostate could not be determined from these studies; other studies should be designed to elicit this information.

In addition to measuring total lycopene levels in prostate tissue and serum from these men who consumed dietary, tomato-based lycopene, van Breemen and colleagues (46) used liquid chromatography-mass spectrometry (LC-MS) with C$_{30}$ reversed-phase chromatography and atmospheric pressure chemical ionization (APCI) to measure the ratio of cis/trans-lycopene in these serum and prostate tissue extracts (see example in Fig. 2). This analytical method facilitated the detection of all-trans-lycopene and up to 14 cis-isomer peaks in a single LC-MS chromatogram with a limit of detection of 0.93 pmol. They found that serum contained approx 28.9% all-trans-lycopene before dietary intervention and 31.7% all-trans-lycopene after intervention, despite the fact that the administered form of lycopene was 83% all-trans. This percentage of all-trans-lycopene is essentially identical to the 30.6% value measured in a solution containing a thermodynamic mixture of lycopene isomers, suggesting that lycopene rapidly isomerizes in serum just as it does in solution. In contrast, the percentage of all-trans-lycopene in human prostate tissue (lower than that in human serum) increased from 12.4–22.7% as a result of dietary intervention with tomato sauce.

A comparable observation was reported earlier by Clinton et al,. who found that in the human prostate, all-trans-lycopene constituted 12–21% of the total (41). These studies showed that cis-lycopene accumulates preferentially in the human prostate and the proportion of cis-lycopene in human prostate tissue is greater than that in human serum. The mechanism for this accumulation and the reasons for different ratios of cis and all-trans isomers in prostate compared to serum remain unknown. Our data are consistent with the hypothesis that all-trans-lycopene is taken up preferentially by the prostate and then isomerized to cis forms. Other explanations are possible, including selective absorption of cis-lycopene isomers by the prostate, selective stabilization of cis isomers, and selective degradation of all-trans-lycopene in the prostate. The correct explanation for these results requires additional investigation.

Finally, total PSA levels were measured in blood samples at baseline, and again at completion of the tomato sauce intervention period in order to evaluate lycopene's possible effect on PSA levels (results shown in Table 1). This dietary intervention study found that levels of PSA decreased by a statistically significant 17.5%. These results were confirmed in a pilot study reported by Kucuk et al. *(28)* in which 15 men with prostate cancer received 30 mg lycopene/d for 21 d following the same design as that of the van Breemen study. However, the study by Kucuk lacked sufficient power to be statistically significant.

PSA is produced by the epithelial cells of the prostate and secreted into the seminal fluid *(47)*. Compared to the concentration of PSA in seminal fluid, the concentration of PSA in blood is small. Increased levels of PSA in blood are not the result of greater production of PSA by cells, but of abnormalities in the prostate gland architecture, which can be caused by trauma or disease *(48)*. Because of its relative tissue specificity, serum PSA is used in combination with the digital rectal examination to screen men for prostate cancer. Currently, biopsy is recommended in men with PSA levels that exceed 4 ng/mL. Cancer is detected in approx 25% of men with PSA values between 4 and 10 ng/mL; more than one-half of men with PSA values exceeding 10 ng/mL have advanced cancer *(49)*. PSA is also used to monitor the success of radiotherapy, chemotherapy, and surgery for the treatment of prostate cancer *(50)*. Given the association of high serum PSA levels with prostate cancer, it is a significant finding that administration of 30 mg/d of lycopene for just 21 d reduced serum PSA levels in men with prostate cancer. Whether this indicates that lycopene might have value as a chemotherapeutic agent for prostate cancer, in addition to efficacy as a chemopreventive agent, has not yet been determined.

3. ANIMAL MODELS AND STUDIES OF LYCOPENE CANCER PREVENTION

Although the consumption of lycopene-containing tomatoes has been clearly associated with a reduced risk of prostate cancer, these epidemiological results have not been reproduced in animal models of prostate cancer. In male F344 rats, ventral prostate cancer was induced with 3,2'-dimethyl-4-aminobiphenol (DMAB) and 2-amino-1-methylimidazo[4,5-*b*]pyridine (PhIP). Dietary lycopene of up to 45 mg/kg failed to prevent DMAB-induced ventral prostate carcinomas *(51)*. In the prostate of lacZ mice, both benzo*[a]*pyrene (B*[a]*P)-induced and spontaneous mutagenesis were only slightly inhibited by oleoresin *(52)*. The uptake and tissue distribution of lycopene in F344 rats fed a diet supplemented with 10 mg/kg of lycopene for 2 mo was compared to that of humans. In rats, lycopene concentration was determined to be highest in the spleen (21.2 nmol/g) and liver (20.3 nmol/g), followed by the prostate (0.3 nmol/g) and lung (0.1 nmol/g) *(30)*. Interestingly, the human prostate accumulates higher lycopene levels (0.8 nmol/g) than the rat prostate *(30)*. It is unlikely that the difference in tissue levels is solely responsible for the failure of lycopene to prevent tumors in the rat prostate. There are several possible explanations for the failure of animal prostate cancer models to reproduce human epidemiological data. Animal models of prostate cancer may be flawed because they use large doses of carcinogens that do not mimic the human situation. Lycopene is metabolized differently in the animal prostate because of anatomical differences between human and rat or mouse prostate. Lycopene does not reach effective concentrations in the rat prostate. And, finally, animal studies that use purified lycopene (or the tomato extract oleoresin) do not derive the benefit of synergism between different food components.

Animal models of breast cancer have revealed mixed results. Young female Sprague-Dawley rats treated with 7,12-dimethylbenz*[a]*anthracene (DMBA) or *N*-methyl-*N*-nitrosourea (MNU) develop mammary tumors. DMBA requires metabolic activation, whereas MNU is a direct-acting carcinogen. Intraperitoneal administration of lycopene-enriched tomato oleoresin suppressed DMBA-induced mammary tumor development in rats *(53)*. In this study, rats were injected with oleoresin (10 mg/kg, twice per wk) for 2 wk prior to tumor induction by DMBA and for an additional 16 wk after carcinogen administration. Oleoresin-treated rats developed significantly fewer tumors, and tumor volume was smaller than that of the unsupplemented rats. In contrast, β-carotene was found to be ineffective *(53)*.

Dietary oleoresin and pure lycopene were evaluated in the MNU-induced mammary tumorigenesis model in female Sprague-Dawley rats *(54)*. Rats were fed diets supplemented with 250 and 500 mg/kg lycopene, or oleoresin providing equivalent amounts of lycopene. The rats began eating the experimental or control diets 1 wk before initiation with MNU and continued for an additional 18 wk. Pure lycopene and oleoresin did not exert an inhibitory effect on tumor incidence, latency, multiplicity, volume, or total tumors per group compared with unsupplemented controls. In this study, total lycopene concentration of about 0.16 μM was measured in the serum of rats fed the high dose of oleoresin. Administration of lycopene to female rats at doses ranging from 0.001–0.1 g/kg bw per d for 2 wk resulted in lycopene plasma concentration ranging from 0.016 μM at the low dose to 0.067 μM at the high dose (55). According to Stahl and Sies (56), lycopene concentrations in rats are much lower than those reported in human populations, where the plasma concentration of lycopene ranges from 0.22 to 1.06 μM or from 0.07 to1.790 μM, according to Breinholt and colleagues (55). For example, men who consumed a tomato-rich diet had a mean serum lycopene concentration of 1.3 μM (46). Elderly women who consume diets rich in fruits and vegetables had a plasma mean concentration of total lycopene of 0.43 μM (the concentration of lycopene in younger women or younger or older men was higher) (57). Conflicting results in the two models of chemoprevention might be the result of differences in the two carcinogens, one being a direct-acting carcinogen (MNU) and the other (DMBA) requiring activation by the host. Differences in the route of lycopene administration further complicate comparisons between the two studies. In the Cohen et al. study (54), lycopene or oleoresin incorporated into the diet mimicked the human situation. In contrast, the intraperitoneal administration of lycopene in the study of Sharoni et al. (53) circumvented the process of digestion and absorption into lymphatic chylomicrons.

Through its action on cytochrome P450, lycopene may diminish the effects of carcinogens requiring metabolic activation such as DMBA. Breinholt et al. (55) determined the drug metabolizing capacity and antioxidant status of female rats exposed to lycopene diets. They found that the activities of the liver cytochrome P450-dependent enzymes, benzyloxyresorufin O-dealkylase and ethoxyresorufin O-dealkylase, were significantly induced by lycopene administration. Also, the phase II detoxification enzymes, glutathione S-transferase (GST) and quinone reductase, were induced by lycopene in the liver. Superoxide dismutase (SOD), glutathione reductase, and glutathione peroxidase in the blood were also induced by the administration of lycopene. These studies suggest that modulation of antioxidant and drug metabolizing enzymes might indeed be stronger in humans whose plasma lycopene levels are several-fold higher than those reported in rats (55).

An investigation by Kim et al. evaluated the chemopreventive potential of lycopene during the post-initiation stage in a multi-organ carcinogenesis model (58). B6C3F$_1$ mice of both sexes were subjected to treatment with a combination of three carcinogens, diethylnitrosamine (DEN), MNU, and 1,2-dimethyl-hydrazine (DMH), for up to 9 wk after birth. Lycopene at 25 and 50 mg/kg diet was given after wk 11. Aberrant crypt foci (ACF) and tumors in the colon, kidney, liver, and lung were determined. The incidence and multiplicity of lung adenomas plus carcinomas were significantly reduced only in the group of male mice that received 50 mg/kg-diet lycopene. No such effect was observed for females. Although the effect of lycopene on hepatocellular carcinomas was inconclusive, the carotenoid was ineffective in preventing colon and kidney tumors in this study. The results suggest that lycopene exerts a chemopreventive effect limited to male lung carcinogenesis when given in the post-initiation stage to B6C3F$_1$ mice. In A/J mice, oleoresin (up to 8.3 g/kg diet) was ineffective against B[a]P plus 4-(methyl-nitrosamino)-1-(3-pyridyl)-1-butanone (NNK)-induced lung tumorigenesis (59).

Inhibition of colon carcinogenesis by lycopene and tomato juice was investigated in young female F344 rats (60). Rats received MNU, and had free access to plain drinking water containing lycopene, or water containing diluted tomato juice. The incidence of colon cancer was significantly lower in the group that received tomato juice but not the group that received lycopene (60). These results show that tomato juice furnishes protection against colon carcinogenesis, and suggest that lycopene and other components of oleoresin might act synergistically. In a related study, the effects of oleoresin on long-term (spontaneous) carcinogenesis were compared to B[a]P-induced short-term effects in lacZ mice (52). Oleoresin inhibited spontaneous but not B[a]P-induced mutagenesis in the prostate and the colon. This study suggests that the antioxidant action of oleoresin might neutralize low levels of pro-oxidants that occur during normal metabolism, but not high levels that are introduced by carcinogens in short time intervals.

Based on the observation that patients with hepatitis and cirrhosis have low plasma lycopene levels (61), the effects of lycopene on occurrence of hepatic neoplasia were evaluated in rats. Lycopene-containing oleoresin was added to the diet at 5 g/kg. It offered no protection against spontaneous hepatocarcinogenesis or enhanced survival in rats (62). Although oxygen radicals play an important role in the development of hepatitis and subsequent liver cancer, it appears that the antioxidative activities of lycopene might be insufficient to prevent hepatocarcinogenesis in the rat. However, hepatic fibrogenesis was suppressed in a strain of rats that consumed lycopene in their diet *(63)*. The mechanism of this preventive effect was through inhibition of stellate-cell activity. Dietary lycopene has been shown to decrease the initiation of liver carcinomas in male C3H/He mice after combined treatment with 4-nitroquinoline-1-oxide and glycerol *(64)*. In rats, oxidative stress introduced by ferric nitrilotriacetate (Fe-NTA) was determined to cause increased 8-oxo-dG levels in the liver accompanied by histopathological changes *(65)*. Lycopene (10 mg/kg body wt) almost completely prevented this oxidative damage and protected the liver against observed histological alterations.

Tomato juice exerts an inhibitory effect on development of urinary bladder carcinoma induced by N-butyl-N-(4-hydroxybutyl)nitrosamine (BBN) in rats *(66)*. The carcinogen was administered in the drinking water of male F344 rats for 8 wk followed by diluted tomato juice for 12 wk. In the group that was given tomato juice, the numbers—but not the incidence of—urinary bladder transitional cell carcinomas were decreased. Nodullopapillary hyperplasias, invasion, or differentiation of transitional cell carcinomas were not affected by this treatment *(66)*. In the same animal model, piroxicam—a nonsteroidal antiinflammatory drug (NSAID)—in combination with lycopene significantly decreased the incidence and number of transitional cell carcinomas *(67)*.

Recently, Boileau et al. *(68)* reported that *cis* isomers of lycopene were more bioavailable than all-*trans*-lycopene in the ferret. This information, in combination with measurements showing that *cis*-lycopene isomers often constitute more than 50% of total lycopene in human blood and tissues *(41,69)*, has prompted speculation that *cis*-lycopenes might be more readily absorbed by humans. However, data on the human bioavailability of lycopene and its isomers are scarce. Since human tissue specimens are often limited to biopsies less than 10 mg, a reliable and sensitive method is needed to simultaneously measure *cis*- and *trans*-lycopene in these samples. Recently, van Breemen et al. *(46)* developed a highly sensitive and specific LC-MS method to address this problem and applied it to the analysis of lycopene isomers in human serum and prostate tissue of men with prostate cancer before and after lycopene intervention. An example of this analysis is presented in Fig. 2. This new analytical capability might allow scientists to determine if *cis*-lycopene isomers are more bioavailable than *trans*-lycopene.

4. CELL-BASED STUDIES OF LYCOPENE

Lycopene has been found to inhibit the proliferation of several types of cancer cells, including those of prostate, breast, endometrium, leukemia, and lung *(70–76)*. Although the precise mode of action is not fully understood, several molecular pathways have been proposed.

Lycopene, as well as other acyclic carotenoids such as phytofluene and ζ-carotene, present in the tomato, significantly reduced the viability of PC-3, DU-145 and LNCaP human prostate cancer cell lines *(70)*. However, lycopene tended to reduce cell viability at a lower concentration than did the other acyclic carotenoids. Generally, 5 μM lycopene reduced cell viability to about the same magnitude as 20 μM of phytofluene and ζ-carotene. In a previous study, Pastori et al. reported that lycopene at 1.8 μM inhibited the proliferation of PC-3 and DU-145 cells when given in combination with 50 μM α-tocopherol *(71)*. These concentrations, considered physiologically relevant, inhibited by almost 90% the growth of both types of prostate cancer cells. The synergism between lycopene and α-tocopherol was not shared by β-tocopherol, ascorbic acid, and probucol *(71)*.

Karas et al. *(72)* have shown that, in MCF-7 breast cancer cells, growth stimulation by insulin-like growth factor I (IGF-I) was reduced by physiological concentrations of lycopene. IGF-I acts as a mitogen, and is considered a risk factor in breast and prostate cancer. The inhibitory effect of lycopene on IGF signaling was associated with suppression of cell cycle progression without being associated with apoptotic or necrotic cell death. A delay in the progression of MCF-7 cells from G_1 to S was also observed in response to lycopene or acycloretinoic acid treatments *(73)*. Since the concentrations of acycloretinoic acid and lycopene required for inducing cell growth inhibition were similar, it was concluded that acycloretinoic acid is unlikely to be the active metabolite of lycopene. Based on the low affinity of lycopene for retinoic acid receptor (RAR) and a low efficacy in activating the receptor, it was also determined that RAR does not mediate the growth-inhibitory effect of the agent. Since lycopene inhibited growth of both the estrogen receptor (ER)-positive MCF-7 and ER-negative MDA-MB-231 cells, it was concluded that ER is not involved in the inhibition of breast cancer cells (74).

Nahum et al. dissected the mechanism by which lycopene (2–3 μM) delays cell cycle in synchronized human breast (MCF-7, T47D) and endometrial (ECU-1) cancer cells (75). In these cells, inhibition of growth and block in cell cycle progression at the G_1 phase was associated with reduced cyclin-dependent kinase (CDK)4 and CDK2 activities. A decrease was also evident in cyclin D_1 and cyclin D_3 levels that was not accompanied by reduced cyclin E levels. Cyclin D_1 is a known oncogene, and its overexpression is associated with malignancy. Based on alterations in the levels of CDK inhibitors p21(Cip1/Waf1) and p27(Kip1) in lycopene-treated (cell cycle-arrested) or serum-stimulated cells, the following chain of events was proposed to explain the inhibitory effect of lycopene on cell cycle progression. Retention of p27 in the cyclin E-CDK2 complex causes a decrease in cyclin D, which leads to reduction in CDK4 kinase activity and subsequent decrease in pRb phosphorylation, resulting in inhibition of G_1/S transition (75).

In human fetal skin fibroblasts (HFFF2 cells), lycopene at a concentration of 0.1 μM was found to be an effective inducer of gap-junctional communication. This was determined by microinjecting fluorescent Lucifer Yellow CH dye into selected HFFF2 cells in a confluent culture that had been treated or not with lycopene, and then measuring the transfer of fluorescence to adjacent cells 5 min later (77). The lycopene oxidation product acycloretinoic acid also increased gap-junctional communication but required a 10-fold higher concentration for the same effect. Induction of gap-junctional communication, unlike that of retinoic acid and other carotenoids, was not mediated by stabilizing the mRNA of connexin43 (78). Induction of gap-junctional communication in the lycopene-treated cells was suggested to be related to cancer prevention (79).

In the HL-60 promyelocytic leukemia cell line, a concentration-dependent reduction in HL-60 cell growth was shown to be accompanied by cell differentiation and delay in the G_0/G_1 phase of the cell cycle (76). More importantly, lycopene was shown to act synergistically with 1,25-dihydroxyvitamin D_3 in both inhibiting HL-60-cell proliferation and inducing the differentiation of these cancer cells (76). These results may suggest that dietary carotenoids may act as chemopreventive agents only in conjunction with other dietary components, providing a possible explanation for the failure of human

intervention studies in which β-carotene was used only in conjunction with either α-tocopherol (80,81) or with retinyl palmitate (82).

Matos et al. (83) investigated the antioxidant effects of lycopene against iron-induced oxidative stress, using Fe-NTA, known to induce lipid peroxidation, DNA damage, and renal carcinomas in rats. The effect of lycopene on lipid peroxidation and on formation of 8-oxo-dG was determined in green monkey kidney fibroblasts (CV1-P) exposed to Fe-NTA plus ascorbate. Lycopene produced an 86% reduction in Fe-NTA/ascorbate-induced lipid peroxidation, which was associated with a substantial decrease in 8-oxo-dG levels. These results indicate that lycopene, by protecting mammalian cells against membrane and DNA damage, might prevent tumor promotion associated with oxidative stress.

In an interesting study, lycopene was entrapped in human albumin and its effect against oxidative $^1O_2$ attack was determined by detecting 8-oxo-dG and 4-hydroxy-8-oxo-dG. The lycopene/albumin complex reduced oxidative DNA damage by 50–70% compared to the control. This experiment suggested that lycopene entrapped in albumin can be an efficient quencher of $^1O_2$ and in this manner may provide protection against the deleterious effect of this ROS (84). Furthermore, lycopene has been shown to exhibit much more potent antiproliferative effects than either α- or β-carotene against endometrial (Ishikawa), mammary (MCF-7), and lung (NCI-H226) human cancer cells, with half-maximal inhibitory concentrations of 1–2 μM (85). In comparison, α- or β-carotene required from four- to 10-fold higher concentrations to exert the same antiproliferative effect as lycopene.

5. SUMMARY AND CONCLUSIONS

A large number of prospective and retrospective epidemiological studies suggest an inverse relationship between prostate cancer and the consumption of tomato products. In men, the consumption of tomato products is associated with increased levels of lycopene in serum and especially in the prostate gland. The results of the first human intervention studies with tomato sauce show a marked increase in lycopene levels in the prostate 3 wk after the intervention, accompanied by a decrease in PSA levels and a decrease in oxidative DNA damage (42). The tissue concentration of lycopene as well as the chemical form might be important for chemopreventive efficacy; emerging studies suggest that the *cis* isomer found in prostate and liver, especially after castration, might be the effective form *(68,86)*. Consumption of tomato products has also been linked to a reduced risk for ovarian cancer, urinary bladder cancer, breast cancer, cancer of the digestive system, and cancer of the cervix. However, the evidence that tomato products or lycopene might be beneficial for organs other than the prostate is slim, based mainly on dietary recall interview studies and cell culture studies.

Studies in rat models of prostate cancer chemoprevention have generally failed to show the expected outcome. This might be caused by either the high doses of carcinogens that are routinely used in these models or the bioavailability and tissue distribution of lycopene in the rat prostate, which seems to be different from that of the human prostate. Most animal studies have also shown that lycopene and oleoresin are generally ineffective in preventing chemically induced colon, lung, and liver cancer. Lycopene seems to provide better protection against spontaneous tumors that (unlike induced tumors) do not require exposure to high doses of carcinogens—a quality consistent with its ability to quench free radicals. Studies in cultured cells showed clearly that lycopene can prevent certain types of oxidative DNA damage at physiologically relevant concentrations, but also revealed other possible mechanisms of action. These include an antiproliferative effect caused by cell cycle arrest, induction of differentiation, and stimulation of gap-junctional communication *(73,75,76)*. Studies in cultured cells also revealed that lycopene might be more effective as an antitumor agent when given in combination with other agents (e.g., vitamin D_3 or α-tocopherol) *(71,76)*. This latter observation provides a possible explanation of why animal studies generally show that lycopene is ineffective, and human studies suggest the opposite. In humans that eat a variety of foods, synergism between lycopene and other dietary components is possible, yet animals fed purified lycopene or oleoresin have little chance for synergism unless the experiment is designed to evaluate that question.

In conclusion, efficacy of lycopene may depend on its tissue distribution, bioavailability, and the presence of other dietary components that may work together in a synergistic manner. The mechanisms of lycopene action involve protection against oxidative DNA damage and membrane damage either directly through chemical quenching or indirectly through the activation of phase II detoxification enzymes. Further studies are needed in all levels (in vitro, cell culture, animal models of cancer, and clinical intervention) to elucidate the precise mechanism of action and to determine the chemopreventive efficacy of this promising carotenoid. Particular emphasis should be given to a possible synergism between *cis*-lycopene isomers and other food components, especially other antioxidants.

ACKNOWLEDGMENTS

We are grateful to Kevin Grandfield for editorial assistance.

REFERENCES

1. Scott K, Hart D. The carotenoid composition of vegetables and fruits commonly consumed in the UK. Norwich: Institute for Food Research, 1994.
2. Woodall A, Britton G, Jackson M. Antioxidant activity of carotenoids in phosphatidylcholine vesicles: chemical and structural considerations. *Biochem Soc Trans* 1995;23:133S.
3. Di Mascio P, Kaiser S, Sies H. Lycopene as the most efficient biological carotenoid singlet oxygen quencher. *Arch Biochem Biophys* 1989;274:532–538.
4. Conn P, Schalach W, Truscott T. The singlet oxygen and carotenoid interaction. *J Photochem Photobiol B* 1991;11:41–47.
5. Shi J, Le Maguer M. Lycopene in tomatoes: chemical and physical properties affected by food processing. *Crit Rev Food Sci Nutr* 2000;40:1–42.
6. Gerster H. Anticarcinogenic effect of common carotenoids. *Internat J Vit Nutr Res* 1993;63:93–121.
7. van Poppel G. Carotenoids and cancer: an update with emphasis on human intervention studies. *Eur J Cancer* 1993;29A:1335–1344.
8. Isler O. *Carotenoids*. Birkhauser Verlag, Basel, 1971.
9. Goodwin TW. Function of carotenoids, in *The Biochemistry of the Carotenoids, 2nd ed., vol. 1*. Chapman and Hall, New York, NY, 1980, pp.77–95.
10. Goodwin TW. *Mammals, in The Biochemistry of Carotenoids, 2nd ed., vol. 2*. Chapman and Hall, New York, NY, 1980,pp.173–195.
11. Olson J. Carotenoids and vitamin A: An overview, in *Lipid-Soluble Antioxidants: Biochemistry and Clinical Applications*. Ong SH, Packer L, eds. Birkhauser Verlag, Basel, 1992, pp.178–192.
12. Chandler L, Schwartz S. HPLC separation of *cis-trans* carotene iosmers in fresh and processed fruits and vegetables. *J Food Sci* 1987;52:669–672.
13. Sies H. Oxidative stress: introduction, in *Oxidative Stress: Oxidants and Antioxidants*. Sies H. ed. Academic Press, New York, NY 1991, pp.xv–xxii.
14. Halliwell B, Cross C. Oxygen-derived species— their relation to human disease and environmental stress. *Environ Health Perspec* 1994;102:5–12.
15. Guyton K, Kensler T. Oxidative mechanisms in carcinogenesis. *Br Med Bull* 1993;49:523–544.
16. Frenkel K. Carcinogen-mediated oxidant information and oxidative DNA damage. *Pharmacol Ther* 1992;53:127–166.

17. Blot W, Li J, Taylor P, et al. Nutrition intervention trials in Linxian, China: supplementation with specific vitamin/mineral combinations, cancer incidence, and disease-specific mortality in the general population. *J Natl Cancer Inst* 1993;85:1483–1492.

18. Garland M, Willett W, Manson J, Hunter D. Antioxidant micronutrients and breast cancer. *J Am Coll Nutr* 1992;12:400–411.

19. Byers T, Perry G. Dietary carotenes, vitamin C, and vitamin E as protective antioxidants in human cancers. *Annu Rev Nutr* 1992;12:139–159.

20. Krinsky N. Actions of carotenoids in biological systems. *Annu Rev Nutr* 1991;13:561–587.

21. Kahl R. Protective and adverse biological actions of phenolic antioxidants, in *Oxidative Stress: Oxidants and Antioxidants*. Sies H, ed. Academic Press, New York, NY, 1991, pp.245–273.

22. Statland B. Nutrition and cancer. *Clin Chem* 1992;38:1587–1594.

23. Calabresi P, Chabner B. Antineoplasitc agents, in *Goodman and Gilman's The Pharmacological Basis of Therapeutics, 8th ed.* Gilman A, Rall T, Niew A, Taylor P, eds. Pergamon Press, New York, NY, 1990, pp.1209–1262.

24. Trush M, Kensler T. Role of free radicals in carcinogen activation, in *Oxidative Stress: Oxidants and Antioxidants*. Sies H, ed. Academic Press, New York, NY, 1991, pp.277–318.

25. Cerutti P. Prooxidation states and tumor promotion. *Science* 1985;227:375–381.

26. Cerutti P. Tumor promotions by oxidants, in *Theories of Carcinogenesis*. Iverson O, ed. Hemisphere Publishing, Washington DC, 1988, pp.221–230.

27. Lu Q, Hung J, Heber D, et al. Inverse associations between plasma lycopene and other carotenoids and prostate cancer. *Cancer Epidemiol Biomark Prev* 2001;10:749–756.

28. Kucuk O, Sarkar F, Sakr W, et al. Phase II randomized clinical trial of lycopene supplementation before radical prostatectomy. *Cancer Epidemiol Biomark Prev* 2001;10:861–868.

29. Clinton S. The dietary antioxidant network and prostate carcinoma. *Cancer* 1999;86:1629–1631.

30. Agarwal S, Rao AV. Tomato lycopene and its role in human health and chronic diseases. *Can Med Assoc J* 2000;163:739–744.

31. Rao AV, Agarwal S. Role of antioxidant lycopene in cancer and heart disease. *J Am Coll Nutr* 2000;19:563–569.

32. Cramer D, Kuper H, Harlow B, Titus-Ernstoff L. Carotenoids, antioxidants and ovarian cancer risk in pre- and postmenopausal women. *Int J Cancer* 2001;94:128–134.

33. Helzlsouer KJ, Comstock GW, Morris JS. Selenium, lycopene, alpha-tocopherol, beta-carotene, retinol, and subsequent bladder cancer. *Cancer Res* 1989;49:6144–6148.

34. Sato R, Helzlsouer KJ, Alberg AJ, et al. Prospective study of carotenoids, tocopherols, and retinoid concentrations and the risk of breast cancer. *Cancer Epidemiol Biomark Prev* 2002;11:451–457.

35 Kanetsky P, Gammon M, Mandelblatt J, et al. Dietary intake and blood levels of lycopene: association with cervical dysplasia among non-Hispanic, black women. *Nutr Cancer* 1998;31:31–40.

36. Goodman M, Kiviat N, McDuffie K, et al. The association of plasma micronutrients with the risk of cervical dysplasia in Hawaii. *Cancer Epidemiol Biomark Prev* 1998;7:537–544.

37. Giovannucci E, Ascherio A, Rimm E, et al. Intake of carotenoids and retinol in relation to risk of prostate cancer. *J Natl Cancer Inst* 1995;87:1767–1776.

38. Giovannucci E. Tomatoes, tomato-based products, lycopene, and cancer: review of the epidemiological literature. *J Natl Cancer Inst* 1999;91:317–331.

39. Gann P, Ma J, Giovannucci E, et al. Lower prostate cancer risk in men with elevated plasma lycopene levels: results of a prospective analysis. *Cancer Res* 1999;59:1225–1230.

40. Giovannucci E, Rimm E, Liu Y, et al. A prospective study of tomato products, lycopene, and prostate cancer risk. *J Natl Cancer Inst* 2002;94:391–398.

41. Clinton SK, Emenhiser C, Schwartz SJ, et al. *cis-trans* lycopene isomers, carotenoids, and retinol in the human prostate. *Cancer Epidemiol Biomark Prev* 1996;5:823–833.

42. Chen L, Stacewicz-Sapuntzakis M, Duncan C, et al. Tomato sauce consumption decreases serum PSA and oxidative damage in prostate cancer patients. *J Natl Cancer Inst* 2001;93:1872–1879.

43. Paerau I, Khachik F, Brown E, et al. Chronic ingestion of lycopene-rich tomato juice or lycopene supplements significantly increases concentrations of lycopene and related carotenoids in human. *Am J Clin Nutr* 1998;68:1187–1195.

44. Sutherland W, Walker R, De Jong S, Upritchard J. Supplementation with tomato juice increases plasma lycopene but does not alter susceptibility to oxidation of low-density lipoproteins from renal transplant recipients. *Clin Nephrol* 1999;52:30–36.

45. Freeman V, Meydani M, Yong S, et al. Prostatic levels of tocopherols, carotenoids, and retinol in relation to plasma levels and self-reported usual dietary intake. *Am J Epidemiol* 2000;151:109–118.

46. van Breemen R, Xu X, Viana M, et al. Liquid chromatography-mass spectrometry of *cis-* and all-*trans*-lycopene in human serum and prostate tissue after dietary supplementation with tomato sauce. *J Agric Food Chem* 2002;50:2214–2219.

47. Noldus J, Chen Z, Stamey T. Isolation and characterization of free form prostate specific antigen (f-PSA) in sera of men with prostate cancer. *J Urol* 1997;158:1606–1609.

48. Christensson A, Laurell C-B, Lilja H. Enzymatic activity of prostate specific antigen and its reactions with extracellular serine proteinase inhibitors. *Eur J Biochem* 1990;194:755–763.

49. Catalona W, Colberg J, Smith D, et al. Measurement of percent-free PSA improves specificity for lower PSA cutoffs in prostate cancer screening. *J Urol* 1996;155:422A.

50. Oesterling J. Prostate specific antigen: a critical assessment of the most useful tumor marker for adenocarcinoma of the prostate. *J Urol* 1991;145:907–923.

51. Imaida K, Tamaon S, Kato K, et al. Lack of chemopreventive effects of lycopene and curcumin on experimental rat prostate carcinogenesis. *Carcinogenesis* 2001;22:467–472.

52. Guttenplan JB, Chen M, Kosinska W, et al. Effects of a lycopene-rich diet on spontaneous and benzo*[a]*pyrene-induced mutagenesis in prostate, colon and lungs of the lacZ mouse. *Cancer Lett* 2001;164:1–6.

53. Sharoni Y, Giron E, Rise M, Levy J. Effects of lycopene-enriched tomato oleoresin on 7,12-dimethylbenz*[a]*anthracene-induced rat mammary tumors. *Cancer Detect Prev* 1997;21:118–123.

54. Cohen LA, Zhao Z, Pittman B, Khachik F. Effect of dietary lycopene on *N*-methylnitrosourea-induced mammary tumorigenesis. *Nutr Cancer* 1999;34:153–159.

55. Breinholt V, Lauridsen ST, Daneshvar B, Jakobsen J. Dose-response effects of lycopene on selected drug-metabolizing and antioxidant enzymes in the rat. *Cancer Lett* 2000;154:201–210..

56. Stahl W, Sies H. Lycopene: a biologically important carotenoid for humans? *Arch Biochem Biophys* 1996;336:1–9.

57. Yeum KJ, Booth SL, Sadowski JA, et al. Human plasma carotenoid response to the ingestion of controlled diets high in fruits and vegetables. *Am J Clin Nutr* 1996;64:594–602.

58. Kim DJ, Takasuka N, Kim JM, et al. Chemoprevention by lycopene of mouse lung neoplasia after combined initiation treatment with DEN, MNU and DMH. *Cancer Lett* 1997;120:15–22.

59. Hecht SS, Kenney PM, Wang M, et al. Evaluation of buty-lated hydroxyanisole, myo-inositol, curcumin, esculetin, resveratrol and lycopene as inhibitors of benzo[*a*]pyrene plus 4-(methylnitrosamino)-1-(3-pyridyl)-1-butanone-induced lung tumorigenesis in A/J mice. *Cancer Lett* 1999;137:123–130.

60. Narisawa T, Fukaura Y, Hasebe M, et al. Prevention of *N*-methylnitrosourea-induced colon carcinogenesis in F344 rats by lycopene and tomato juice rich in lycopene, *Jpn J Cancer Res* 1998;89:1003–1008.

61. Yamamoto Y, Yamashita S, Fujisawa A, et al. Oxidative stress in patients with hepatitis, cirrhosis, and hepatoma evaluated by plasma antioxidants. *Biochem Biophys Res Commun* 1998;247:166–170.

62. Watanabe S, Kitade Y, Masaki T, et al. Effects of lycopene and Sho-saiko-to on hepatocarcinogenesis in a rat model of spontaneous liver cancer. *Nutr Cancer* 2001;39:96–101.

63. Kitade Y, Watanabe S, Masaki T, et al. Inhibition of liver fibrosis in LEC rats by a carotenoid, lycopene, or a herbal medicine, Sho-saiko-to. *Hepatol Res* 2002;22:196–205.

64. Nishino H. Cancer prevention by natural carotenoids. *J Cell Biochem Suppl* 1997;27:86–91.

65. Matos HR, Capelozzi VL, Gomes OF, et al. Lycopene inhibits DNA damage and liver necrosis in rats treated with ferric nitrilotriacetate. *Arch Biochem Biophys* 2001;396:171–177.

66. Okajima E, Tsutsumi M, Ozono S, et al. Inhibitory effect of tomato juice on rat urinary bladder carcinogenesis after *N*-butyl-*N*-(4-hydroxybutyl)nitrosamine initiation. *Jpn J Cancer Res* 1993;89:22–26.

67. Okajima E, Ozono S, Endo T, et al. Chemopreventive efficacy of piroxicam administered alone or in combination with lycopene and beta-carotene on the development of rat urinary bladder carcinoma after *N*-butyl-*N*-(4-hydroxy-butyl)nitrosamine treatment. *Jpn J Cancer Res* 1997;88:543–552.

68. Boileau AC, Merchen NR, Wasson K, et al. *cis*-Lycopene is more bioavailable than *trans*-lycopene in vitro and in vivo in lymph-cannulated ferrets. *J Nutr* 1999;129:1176–1181.

69. Stahl W, Sies H. Uptake of lycopene and its geometrical isomers is greater from heat-processed than from unprocessed tomato juice in humans. *J Nutr* 1992;122:2162–2166.

70. Kotake-Nara E, Kushiro M, Zhang H, et al. Carotenoids affect proliferation of human prostate cancer cells. *J Nutr* 2001;131:3303–3306.

71. Pastori M, Pfander H, Boscoboinik D, Azzi A. Lycopene in association with alpha-tocopherol inhibits at physiological concentrations proliferation of prostate carcinoma cells. *Biochem Biophys Res Commun* 1998;250:582–585.

72. Karas M, Amir H, Fishman D, et al. Lycopene interferes with cell cycle progression and insulin-like growth factor I signaling in mammary cancer cells. *Nutr Cancer* 2000;36:101–111.

73. Ben-Dor A, Nahum A, Danilenko M, et al. Effects of acyclo-retinoic acid and lycopene on activation of the retinoic acid receptor and proliferation of mammary cancer cells. *Arch Biochem Biophys* 2001;391:295–302.

74. Prakash P, Russell RM, Krinsky NI. In vitro inhibition of proliferation of estrogen-dependent and estrogen-independent human breast cancer cells treated with carotenoids or retinoids. *J Nutr* 2001;131:1574–1580.

75. Nahum A, Hirsch K, Danilenko M, et al. Lycopene inhibition of cell cycle progression in breast and endometrial cancer cells is associated with reduction in cyclin D levels and retention of p27(Kip1) in the cyclin E-cdk2 complexes. *Oncogene* 2001;20:3428–3436.

76. Amir H, Karas M, Giat J, et al. Lycopene and 1,25-dihy-droxyvitamin D_3 cooperate in the inhibition of cell cycle progression and induction of differentiation in HL-60 leukemic cells. *Nutr Cancer* 1999;33:105–112.

77. Stewart WW. Functional connections between cells as revealed by dye-coupling with a highly fluorescent naphthalimide tracer. *Cell* 1978;14:741–759.

78. Zhang LX, Cooney RV, Bertram JS. Carotenoids up-regulate connexin43 gene expression independent of their provitamin A or antioxidant properties. *Cancer Res* 1992;52:5707–5712.

79. Zhang LX, Cooney RV, Bertram JS. Carotenoids enhance gap junctional communication and inhibit lipid peroxidation in C3H/10T1/2 cells: relationship to their cancer chemopreventive action. *Carcinogenesis* 1991;12:2109–2114.

80. Albanes D, Heinonen OP, Taylor PR, et al. Alpha-tocopherol and beta-carotene supplements and lung cancer incidence in the alpha-tocopherol, beta-carotene cancer prevention study: effects of base-line characteristics and study compliance. *J Natl Cancer Inst* 1996;88:1560–1570.

81. Albanes D, Heinonen OP, Huttunen JK, et al. Effects of alpha-tocopherol and beta-carotene supplements on cancer incidence in the Alpha-Tocopherol Beta-Carotene Cancer Prevention Study. *Am J Clin Nutr* 1995;62:1427S–1430S.

82. Omenn GS, Goodman G, Thornquist M, et al. The beta-carotene and retinol efficacy trial (CARET) for chemoprevention of lung cancer in high risk populations: smokers and asbestos-exposed workers. *Cancer Res* 1994;54:2038s–2043s.

83. Matos HR, Di Mascio P, Medeiros MH. Protective effect of lycopene on lipid peroxidation and oxidative DNA damage in cell culture. *Arch Biochem Biophys* 2000;383:56–59.

84. Yamaguchi LF, Martinez GR, Catalani LH, et al. Lycopene entrapped in human albumin protects 2'-deoxyguanosine against singlet oxygen damage. *Arch Latinoam Nutr* 1999;49:12S–20S.

85. Levy J, Bosin E, Feldman B, et al. Lycopene is a more potent inhibitor of human cancer cell proliferation than either alpha-carotene or beta-carotene. *Nutr Cancer* 1995;24:257–266.

86. Boileau TW, Clinton SK, Erdman JW Jr. Tissue lycopene concentrations and isomer patterns are affected by androgen status and dietary lycopene concentration in male F344 rats. *J Nutr* 2000;130:1613–1618.

35 Not All Chemopreventive Selenium Compounds are Created Equal

Karam El-Bayoumy, PhD

CONTENTS

1. INTRODUCTION

In the United States (US), nearly two-thirds of cancer deaths can be linked to tobacco use and diet (reviewed in *1*). The effective control and prevention of tobacco consumption, and reduction of exposure to known environmental carcinogens remain major goals for cancer prevention. To reduce the epidemic proportions of tobacco-related cancers, especially lung cancer, chemoprevention (although still in a phase of extensive development) offers an attractive and plausible approach. However, chemoprevention should never be viewed as a substitute for primary prevention efforts. To fully elucidate how dietary constituents can be effectively harnessed for cancer control, a stepwise approach must be taken. Thus, we are searching for optimal diets and for naturally occurring agents in routinely consumed foods that may inhibit cancer development. Structural modification of established, naturally occurring chemopreventive agents has led to synthetic agents with greater efficacy and lower toxicity.

In previous investigations of several animal model systems that utilize numerous synthetic carcinogens present in tobacco and food contaminants, a significant reduction of cancer incidence and/or multiplicity of tumors has been demonstrated for a wide variety of chemopreventive agents including selenium compounds. However, at present, the overall effectiveness of these agents leaves much to be desired. One would hope to completely eliminate tumor formation—that is, to achieve zero incidence at low levels of toxicity in assays with more potent and relevant carcinogens. Therefore, efforts are being continued to develop novel chemopreventive agents that are more effective and less toxic than those already in use. Moreover, there is a great need for chemopreventive agents effective when given after the carcinogenic insult, in the post-initiation period of carcinogenesis; a limited number of agents (e.g., selenium compounds) have been shown to have this property.

A special issue [Larry C. Clark Memorial Issue, Vol. 40 (1) 2001] of *Nutrition and Cancer*, an international journal, is devoted to a single topic, selenium and cancer. This issue contains several reports that cover the entire spectrum, ranging from the role of selenium as a nutrient; its cancer-chemopreventive effects in laboratory animals; cellular and molecular mechanisms in vitro and in vivo that may account for its chemopreventive as well as antiangiogenic activity; and the utilization of this

From: Cancer Chemoprevention, Volume 1: Promising Cancer Chemoprevention Agents
Edited by: G. J. Kelloff, E. T. Hawk, and C. C. Sigman © Humana Press Inc., Totowa, NJ

micronutrient in several clinical intervention trials. Readers are encouraged to refer to this issue for detailed information on the role of selenium in cancer prevention.

In this chapter, the author analyzes the available knowledge and briefly provides readers with a current understanding of the role of selenium in cancer prevention. This chapter is not meant to provide a comprehensive review of the subject, but to provide basic information on the role of dose and form (structure) of selenium compounds in cancer chemoprevention, metabolism leading to active selenium intermediates, and suggested mechanism(s) for cancer prevention. Potential new avenues for future research studies are proposed.

2. EPIDEMIOLOGIC STUDIES

More than 30 years ago, Shamberger and Frost observed a protective role of selenium against cancer development (2); this suggestion was based on the inverse relationship between geographical distribution of selenium in American forage crops and local cancer mortality rates. Epidemiological studies have suggested that an increased risk for certain human diseases, including cancer, is related to insufficient intake of selenium; however, some inconsistencies remain (3). It is not intended to review all published studies on the role of selenium in cancer prevention in this section, but to mention a few, especially on the role of selenium in prevention of the cancers (lung, prostate, breast, and colon) most commonly observed in Western countries. In a meta-analysis from a number of studies comparing the significance of serum selenium, retinol, β-carotene and vitamin E, selenium emerged as the factor with the most protective effect (4). Low selenium status and the risk of lung cancer has been reported (5,6). In a cohort study, men in the highest quintile of selenium intake had only one-half the odds ratio of prostate cancer compared to men in the lowest quintile (7). The selenoenzyme known as iodothyronine deiodinase is responsible for the synthesis of triiodothryonine (T_3). In a study of postmenopausal breast cancer patients, a strong inverse relationship was observed between T_3 levels and breast cancer between the highest and lowest tertiles of intake (8); levels of selenium in toenails were positively associated with T_3 levels in both cases and controls. In a study of selenium intake and colorectal cancer (CRC) that adjusted for possible confounders, individuals in the lowest quartile of plasma selenium had 4× the risk of colorectal adenomas compared to those in the highest quartile (9).

3. PRECLINICAL INVESTIGATIONS

Although the suggestion made in 1969 by Shamberger and Frost stimulated extensive experimental studies in laboratory animals (2), more than 50 yr ago, Clayton and Baumann had already demonstrated the protective role of selenium against chemically induced cancer in rats (10).

In general, preclinical studies conducted in our laboratories and elsewhere showed that at doses well above the physiological requirement, selenium is a proven chemopreventive agent in several animal models for tumorigenesis. Supplementing the diet or drinking water with inorganic selenium protects laboratory animals against cancer of the mammary gland, colon, lung, oral cavity, pancreas, liver, and skin (11,12). Both inorganic selenium compounds and naturally occurring selenium-containing amino acids such as selenomethionine (SM) were equally effective chemopreventive agents, and had comparable toxicity (11). Yet this toxicity inhibited further research until we introduced novel synthetic organoselenium compounds; the rationale for synthesizing these agents is clearly stated in our previous report (13). In our laboratories, achieving optimal chemopreventive potency with the lowest toxicity continues to be a primary goal in the development of organoselenium compounds that can be employed in clinical trials. Nevertheless, it is of paramount importance to emphasize that studies have shown that chemically induced cancer in rodents, especially those cancers commonly observed in humans in Western countries (lung, breast, colon), can be inhibited by various forms of selenium compounds, particularly at levels higher than nutritionally required (11). It is of interest to note that although the naturally occurring SM protects rats from carcinogen-induced mammary cancer (reviewed in 14), it lacks efficacy in other animal model systems (15–17). Clearly, SM lacks a protective effect against the development of prostate, colon, and lung cancers in animal models (15–17). Furthermore, although 1,4-phenylenebis(methylene)selenocyanate (p-XSC) is an effective chemopreventive agent against the development of lung tumors induced by the tobacco-specific carcinogen 4-(methylnitrosamino)-1-(3-pyridyl)-1-butanone (NNK), the naturally occurring SM and Se-methylselenocysteine (SMC) showed no protective effect (18). The synthetic organoselenium compounds developed in our laboratories—especially p-XSC—are superior to inorganic selenite, SM, and SMC in the lung, colon, mammary, and oral can-

Table 1
Clinical Trials That Showed Inhibition After Intervention With Selenium Alone
or in Combination With Other Minerals and Vitamins

Country, Type of Cancer	Patient Population	Level of Selenium	Form of Selenium	References
China, liver cancer	Hepatitis surface antigen carriers; no quality control	200 µg Se/d	Se-enriched yeast	21,22
China, liver cancer	Hepatitis surface antigen carriers; no quality control	15 mg/kg Se	Selenite	21,22
China, stomach cancer	General population; Double-blind, placebo-controlled	50 µg Se/d	Se-enriched yeast with β-carotene and vitamin E	23
India, Oral lesions	Reverse smokers	100 µg Se/d 6 mo; 50 µg Se/d–6 mo	Sodium selenite with Vitamin A, riboflavin, and zinc	25
US, Lung, colon, prostate	Randomized; double-blind placebo-controlled	200 µg Se/d	Se-enriched yeast	19,20

cer models (12,15–18). Consequently, there is an urgent need to determine the efficacy of p-XSC in a prostate cancer model.

Since the etiology of most human cancers remains unknown, the selection of chemopreventive selenium compounds should be based on demonstrated efficacy in several animal models against tumors induced by various chemical carcinogens, and should not be limited to naturally occurring compounds. However, the structure of synthetic organoselenium compounds should be tailored to enhance efficacy and minimize toxic side effects. A promising candidate that fulfills the previously mentioned requirements is p-XSC.

4. CLINICAL INTERVENTION STUDIES

The use of selenium in human clinical trials is thus far limited (19–25). Successful clinical trials after intervention with selenium alone or in combination with other minerals and vitamins are presented in Table 1. These trials have been conducted in China, India, and the US with selenium in the form of selenite, selenate, and selenium-enriched yeast. In certain trials, it was difficult to tease out the form of selenium that was given. In some trials, selenium was given as a cocktail including other minerals and vitamins. Populations with various risk factors were recruited for these trials. Linxian (China) cancer prevention tri-

als have shown that giving a combination of selenium, β-carotene, and α-tocopherol resulted in significantly fewer cases and lower mortality from stomach cancer than observed in the placebo groups (23). When selenium was given in combination with 25 other vitamins and minerals, it had no effect on the development of esophageal cancer (24). However, some of the studies performed in China suffered from methodologic problems, such as lack of quality controls (21,22). In a study conducted in India, selenium was given in combination with vitamins A, C, and E, as well as zinc (25); here the results clearly showed a protective effect of this cocktail against the development of oral lesions in subjects who practice reverse smoking. One of the most exciting clinical trials in the US, conducted by Clark et al., supported a protective effect of selenium-enriched yeast against cancer of the prostate, colon, and lung (19,20). The outcome of this trial instigated two new clinical trials: PRECISE in three European countries and SELECT in the US (26–28). A clinical pilot study conducted by our group was designed to evaluate the influence of selenium-enriched yeast supplementation on biomarkers of oxidative damage and hormone status in healthy adult males (29). The results clearly showed that selenium-enriched yeast can enhance the levels of plasma glutathione (GSH) but inhibit prostate-specific antigen (PSA), yet it has no effect on androgen metabolism (29).

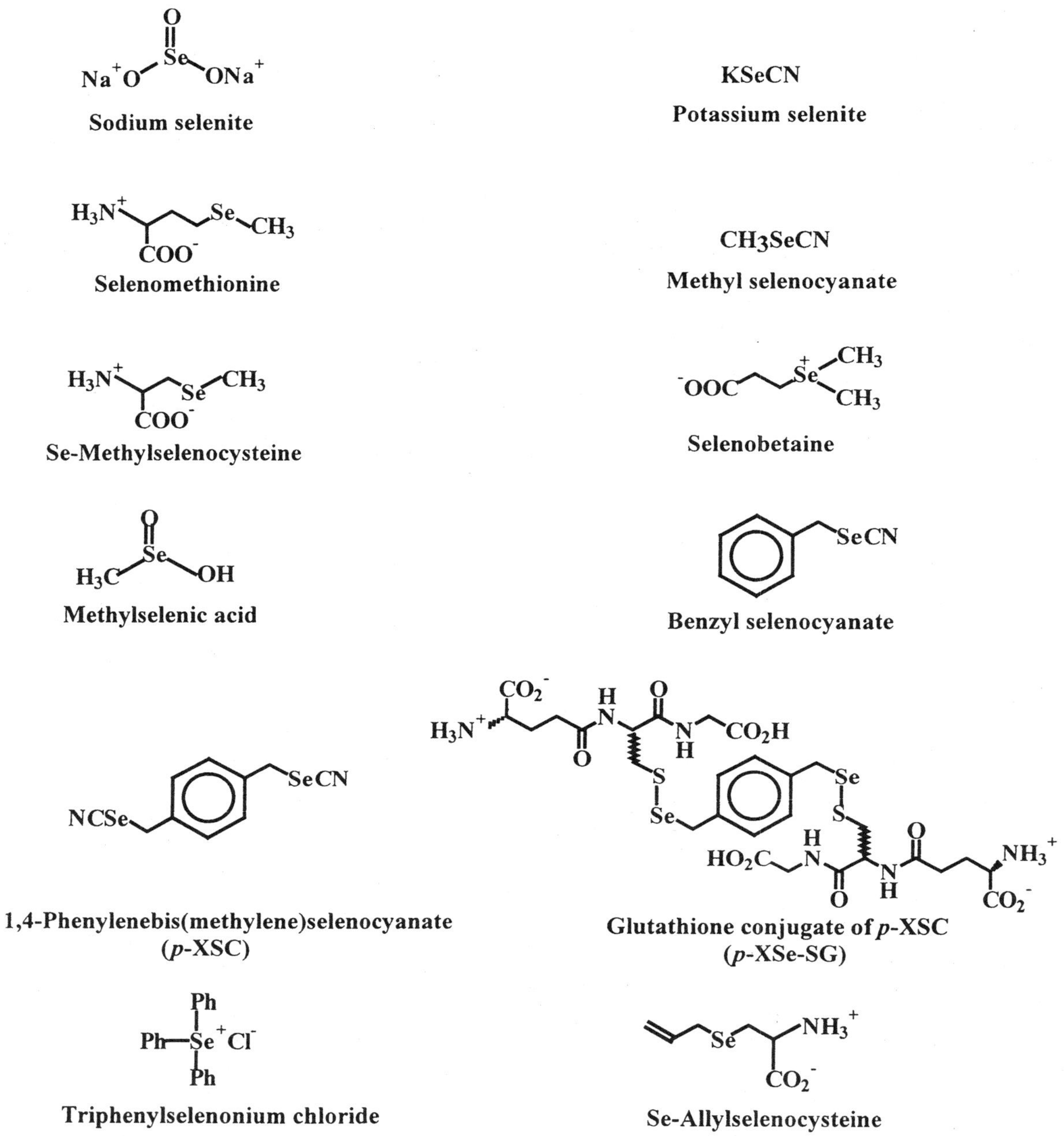

Fig. 1. Chemical structures of various selenium compounds listed in Table 2.

5. ROLE OF DOSE AND FORMULATION (STRUCTURE) OF SELENIUM IN CHEMOPREVENTION

Understanding the metabolism of selenium compounds is an essential step in determining whether the parent compound and/or its metabolites are responsible for chemoprevention. Our results, supported by those described in the literature, indicate that the chemopreventive efficacy of selenium as an anticarcinogen depends on the chemical form in which it is administered, indicating that metabolism is a key step in cancer prevention *(30)*. It is now well established that the antitumor properties of the inorganic form (selenite) are strongly influenced by its metabolism. After absorption, selenite is reduced by thiols (GSH) and NADPH-dependent reductase through selenodiglutathione (GSSeSG) to the highly toxic hydrogen selenide (H_2Se), which can be incorporated as selenocysteine into selenoproteins such as GSH peroxidase, type I

Table 2
Chemopreventive Efficacy of Various Selenium Compounds
in the DMBA-Induced Mammary Tumor Model[a]

Compound[b]	ED_{50}[c] (ppm Se)	MTD[d] (ppm Se)	Chemo-preventive Index[e]
Sodium selenite	3	4	1.3
Potassium selenocyanate	3	4	1.3
Selenomethionine	4–5	5–6	1–1.5
Methyl selenocyanate	2	4	2.0
Se-methylselenocysteine	2	5	2.5
Selenobetaine	2	5	2.5
Methylseleninic acid	2	5	2.5
Benzyl selenocyanate	2	5	2.5
1,4-phenylenebis(methylene) selenocyanate (p-XSC)	5	20	4.0
Triphenylselenonium chloride	10–20	>200	>10
p-XSe-SG	>5–6	ND	ND
Se-allylselenocysteine	≤1	ND	ND

[a]Data obtained from *(14,35,61)*.

[b]Each compound was administered before DMBA and continued until the end of the experiment; all selenium compounds were added to the diet. Selenomethionine and Se-methylselenocysteine are naturally occurring compounds, all others are synthetic.

[c]ED_{50} is defined as the effective dose that produces 50% inhibition in total tumor yield.

[d]MTD is the maximum tolerable dose; ND, not determined in this model.

[e]Chemopreventive index = MTD/ED_{50}.

iodothyronine deiodinase, the 57-kDa plasma protein, and selenoprotein. H_2Se is methylated to mono-, di- and trimethylated derivatives before excretion. Published studies have indicated that the chemopreventive action of selenium compounds is likely caused by intermediates such as methyl selenol (CH_3SeH) *(14,30,31)*. It is of particular interest that certain potent chemopreventive agents such as *p*-XSC and its GSH conjugate and triphenyl selenonium chloride do not release selenium in a form that can be incorporated into Se-containing enzymes *(31–34)*. These results support the notion that the contribution of selenium-containing enzymes to the chemopreventive activity is still questionable, since the activity of these enzymes (e.g., GSH peroxidase) is already maximum at normal nutritional

levels of selenium—e.g., achieving nutritional requirements is insufficient for chemoprevention.

As described here, studies in our laboratories have focused on the design of synthetic organoselenium compounds with improved chemopreventive efficacy and lower toxicity than those reported historically. Their efficacy and toxicity largely depend on the dose and form in which they are administered. In this report, we selected a rat model using 7,12-dimethyl-benz[*a*]anthracene (DMBA)-induced mammary adenocarcinoma to compare several synthetic, naturally occurring selenium compounds, as well as inorganic selenium compounds (Fig. 1; Table 2), for the efficacy and tolerability of these agents.

In a mammary-cancer chemoprevention study, the term "chemopreventive index" *(35)* was introduced. As a simple approach for comparison, it is defined as the ratio of the maximum tolerated dose (MTD) of a given selenium compound divided by the dose which results in a 50% inhibition of cancer (ED_{50}).

In addition to CH_3SeH, intermediates such as aromatic selenols are likely to play a critical role in cancer prevention by synthetic organoselenium compounds, as shown in Table 2. In the early 1990s, we proposed that because selenols are strong nucleophiles (pKa-value ≅ 5), they have the capacity to form adducts with thiol bond (–SH) functionality of enzymes via the formation of Se-S bond *(36)*. Following metabolism, the stability of released selenol intermediates undoubtedly will determine the reactivity and selectivity of the reaction with proteins. In addition to covalent binding of active selenium intermediates to proteins in plasma, Combs' laboratory reported on the detection of noncovalently bound selenium in human plasma *(31)*. Therefore, it is essential to determine which structural requirements govern and which provide optimal biological activity of selenium compounds. Moreover, the development of sensitive analytical methods to biomonitor protein adducts with various selenols would be highly useful in intervention trials.

6. MECHANISM(S) OF CHEMOPREVENTION BY SELENIUM COMPOUNDS

The bulk of our knowledge on the mechanisms of cancer prevention by selenium is based on animal data and studies conducted in in vitro systems. The mechanisms by which selenium compounds inhibit tumor formation during the initiation phase of carcinogenesis

Table 3
Molecular Targets Modulated by Selenium

Targets	References
Phase 1, 2 enzymes	44–46
Selenoenzymes	
(-Se-S-protein adducts, redox enzymes)	37,38
Protein kinase C	37,39–42
Specific kinase (Jun N-kinase)	49
NF-κB	47
AP-1	52
Sp1, Sp3	48
gadd activation	50
Tumor-suppressor gene p53	51
DNA cytosine methyltransferase	53
Eicosanoid biosynthesis	54

have been explored in vitro and in well-defined animal models (12). Oxidative damage has been implicated in the development of cancer during the initiation phase, but more so during the promotion phase of carcinogenesis. Yet, the mechanisms that can actually account for chemoprevention by selenium during the promotion/progression phase of carcinogenesis must be fully explored. Medina et al. (14) and the author of this chapter (12) reviewed the effects of various forms of selenium compounds on multiple molecular and cellular targets of the multi-step carcinogenesis process (Table 3). Briefly, molecular targets that can be modulated by selenium include selenoenzymes and selenium-binding protein adducts (e.g., redox enzymes), (30,37,38) protein kinase C (PKC) (39–42), protein phosphorylation (40,43), phase 1 and 2 enzyme activities (41,42,44–46), nuclear factor κB activity (47), Sp1 and Sp3 (48) specific kinases (49), gadd activation (50), tumor-suppressor gene p53 (51), activator protein-1 (AP-1) binding to DNA (52), DNA cytosine methyltransferase (53), and eicosanoid biosynthesis (54).

Of particular interest is that inorganic selenium compounds in cell culture systems at levels of 5–10 μM can induce single strand breaks in DNA and cell death by necrosis. However, certain organoselenium compounds, even at higher levels of selenium (10–50 μM), can cause cell death by apoptosis with no evidence of DNA single strand breaks (14). Although various selenium compounds with diverse chemical structures are known to inhibit cell proliferation in vitro, little is known regarding selenium intake and its effect

on cell proliferation in vivo in normal growing cells or in neoplastic cells of the same organ following carcinogen treatment. However, in an in vivo study, it was reported that the effect of selenium on cell proliferation and cell cycle biomarkers varies depending on its form, and whether cells are normal or transformed (55); the findings of this study suggest that early transformed cells are sensitive to selenium intervention, whereas normal cells are not. Moreover, an in vivo study conducted by Rao et al. showed that p-XSC inhibits PKC activities in the colonic mucosa and in tumors of rats treated with azoxymethane (56). As discussed here, there are numerous plausible biomarkers that can be selected as targets in the design of future clinical chemoprevention intervention strategies. The feasibility of utilizing a cDNA microarray approach in elucidating cellular and molecular targets for selenium intervention trials should be explored. To this end, limited studies in rodents have been reported (57–60). However, the author of this report strongly believes that extensive pilot studies are required to test and validate the most appropriate biomarkers that will be highly useful in the area of cancer prevention trials, not only in cancer patients or populations at high risk for a given cancer, but more importantly in healthy people, as those intended in the SELECT study (26,27). The author of this report conducted a preliminary clinical pilot study (cf. section on Clinical Intervention Studies) aimed at determining the influence of selenium-enriched yeast supplementation on biomarkers of oxidative damage and hormone status in healthy African and White Americans (29).

7. SUGGESTED RECOMMENDATION OF SELENIUM INTAKE

The average selenium intake of a US resident is about 70–100 μg per d. At this level, standard criteria for nutritional requirements are satisfied, but they are insufficient for cancer prevention. Selenium intake in most parts of Europe is considered to be lower than in the US; the mean plasma selenium level in US residents is 100 ± 30 S.D. $\mu g/g$ (12).

Intake of 200 μg selenium per d has been proven safe in the clinic (19,20); 400 $\mu g/d$ is considered the upper limit (reviewed in 12). In Clark's trial (19,20), persons with plasma selenium levels <106 ng/mL at the beginning of the trial achieved the greatest benefit from selenium supplementation. Because human clinical trials are limited, Combs, Jr. suggested (31)—based on

Clark's data *(19,20)*—that for cancer prevention, it is necessary to raise human plasma levels to >120 ng/mL.

8. SUMMARY AND FUTURE DIRECTIONS

Today, our knowledge of the mechanism(s) of action responsible for cancer prevention by selenium compounds, including those developed in our laboratories, is based primarily on studies conducted in preclinical animal models and in in vitro systems. The form and dose of selenium and not the element *per se* are the determining factors in cancer chemoprevention. It is essential to determine which types of selenium compounds provide optimal protection against genetic damage (specific molecular and/or cellular targets) with the least toxicity. We have clearly demonstrated that structural modification of synthetic organoselenium compounds achieves greater chemopreventive efficacy with minimal toxic side effects. Evidence thus far supports the role of selenium metabolites containing a selenol moiety (−SeH) in cancer prevention. Selenols could be derived from aliphatic and aromatic selenium compounds. Such intermediates, because of their strong nucleophilic character, are likely to form covalent adducts with thiol (−SH)-containing proteins that are involved in numerous biological functions. Thus, it is essential to develop sensitive analytical methods to monitor specific molecular targets (e.g., selenol-binding proteins) that may be critical in cancer prevention; these types of studies should be conducted initially in animal models and later in clinical pilot studies. Upon close examination of chemopreventive indices in the rat mammary-tumor model system (*cf.* Table 2), it can be suggested that selection of selenium compounds in future clinical intervention trials should not be limited to those found naturally. There is an urgent need for extensive pilot studies in humans aimed at determining the role of the most promising agents, such as *p*-XSC, on cellular and molecular targets critical in the multistep carcinogenesis process. To provide better strategies for the design of cancer chemoprevention trials and possibly the discovery of diagnostic markers in clinical intervention trials, the use of cDNA microarray for global gene-expression analysis, especially when combined with proteomics technologies, will be highly valuable.

ACKNOWLEDGMENTS

The work performed in the author's laboratory and described in this chapter was supported by the US Department of Health and Human Services, National Cancer Institute Grants CA-70972 and CA-46589 and Grant DE-13222 from the National Institutes of Dental and Craniofacial Research. Facilities were supported by an NCI Cancer Center Support Grant CA-17613. The author thanks Ms. Elizabeth Appel for preparing and editing the manuscript.

REFERENCES

1. El-Bayoumy K, Hoffmann D. Nutrition and tobacco-related cancer, in *Nutritional Oncology*. Heber D, Blackburn GL, Go VLW, eds. Academic Press, New York, 1999, pp.299–324.
2. Shamberger RJ, Frost DV. Possible protective effect of selenium against human cancer. *Can Med Assoc J* 1969;100:682.
3. Combs GF Jr, Gray WP. Chemopreventive agents: selenium. *Pharmacol Ther* 1998;79:179–192.
4. Comstock GW, Bush TL, Helzlsouer K. Serum retinol, β-carotene, vitamin E, and selenium as related to subsequent cancer of specific sites. *Am J Epidemiol* 1992;135:115–121.
5. Knekt P, Marniemi J, Teppo L, et al. Is low selenium status a risk factor for lung cancer? *Am J Epidemiol* 1998;148:975–982.
6. van den Brandt PA, Goldbohm RA, van't Veer P, et al. A prospective cohort study on selenium status and the risk of lung cancer. *Cancer Res* 1993;53:4860–4865.
7. Yoshizawa K, Willett WC, Morris SJ, et al. Study of prediagnostic selenium level in toenails and the risk of advanced prostate cancer. *J Natl Cancer Inst* 1998;90:1219–1224.
8. Strain JJ, Bokje E, van't Veer P, et al. Thyroid hormones and selenium status in breast cancer. *Nutr Cancer* 1997;27:48–52.
9. Russo MW, Murray SC, Wurzelmann JI, et al. Plasma selenium levels and the risk of colorectal adenomas. *Nutr Cancer* 1997;28:125–129.
10. Clayton CC, Baumann CA. Diet and azo dye tumors: effect of diet during periods when the dye is not fed. *Cancer Res* 1949;9:575–592.
11. El-Bayoumy K. The role of selenium in cancer prevention, in *Cancer Prevention*. DeVita VT, Hellman S, Rosenberg SA, eds. JB Lippincott Company, Philadelphia, PA, 1991, pp.1–15.
12. El-Bayoumy K. The protective role of selenium on genetic damage and on cancer. *Mutat Res* 2001;475:123–139.
13. El-Bayoumy K, Upadhyaya P, Chae Y-H, et al. Chemoprevention of cancer by organoselenium compounds. *J Cell Biochem Suppl* 1995;22:92–100.
14. Medina D, Thompson H, Ganther H, et al. Se-methylselenocysteine: a new compound for chemoprevention of breast cancer. *Nutr Cancer* 2001;40:12–17.
15. McCormick D, Rao K, Lubet R, et al. Differential activity of 9-*cis*-retinoic acid, α-tocopherol, and selenomethionine as chemopreventive agents in the rat prostate. *Proc Am Assoc Cancer Res* 1997;38:261.
16. Reddy BS, Hirose Y, Lubet RA, et al. Lack of chemopreventive efficacy of DL-selenomethionine in colon carcinogenesis. *Int J Mol Med* 2000;5:327–330.
17. Prokopczyk B, Cox JE, Upadhyaya P, et al. Effects of dietary 1,4-phenylenebis(methylene)selenocyanate on 4-(methylni-

trosamino)-1-(3-pyridyl)-1-butanone-induced DNA adduct formation in lung and liver of A/J mice and F344 rats. *Carcinogenesis* 1996;17:749–753.

18. Das A, Desai D, Pittman B, et al. Comparison of the chemopreventive efficacies of 1,4-phenylenebis(methylene)selenocyanate (p-XSC), selenium-enriched yeast, and Se-methylselenocysteine (MSC) on 4-(methylnitrosamino)-1-(3-pyridyl)-1-butanone (NNK)-induced tumorigenesis in A/J mouse lung. *Proc Am Assoc Cancer Res* 2002;43: abst. no. 1531.

19. Clark LC, Combs GF Jr, Turnbull BW, et al. Effects of selenium supplementation for cancer prevention in patients with carcinoma of the skin. A randomized controlled trial. Nutritional Prevention of Cancer Study Group. *JAMA* 1996;276:1957–1963.

20. Clark LC, Dalkin B, Krongrad A, et al. Decreased incidence of prostate cancer with selenium supplementation: results of a double-blind cancer prevention trial. *Br J Urol* 1998;81:730–734.

21. Yu SY, Zhu YJ, Li WG, et al. A preliminary report on the intervention trials of primary liver cancer in high-risk populations with nutritional supplementation of selenium in China. *Biol Trace Elem Res* 1991;29:289–294.

22. Yu SY, Zhu YJ, Li WG. Protective role of selenium against hepatitis B virus and primary liver cancer in Qidong. *Biol Trace Elem Res* 1997;56:117–124.

23. Blot WJ, Li JY, Taylor PR, et al. Nutrition intervention trials in Linxian, China: supplementation with specific vitamin/mineral combinations, cancer incidence, and disease-specific mortality in the general population. *J Natl Cancer Inst* 1993;85:1483–1492.

24. Li JY, Taylor PR, Li B, et al. Nutrition intervention trials in Linxian, China: multiple vitamin/mineral supplementation, cancer incidence, and disease-specific mortality among adults with esophageal dysplasia. *J Natl Cancer Inst* 1993;85:1492–1498.

25. Prasad MPR, Mukundan MA, Krishnaswamy K. Micronuclei and carcinogen DNA adducts as intermediate end points in nutrient intervention trial of precancerous lesions in the oral cavity. *Eur J Cancer B Oral Oncol* 1995;31B:155–159.

26. Klein EA, Thompson IM, Lippman SM, et al. SELECT: the next prostate cancer prevention trial. Selenium and Vitamin E Cancer Prevention Trial. *J Urol* 2001;166:1311–1315.

27. Hoque A, Albanes D, Lippman SM, et al. Molecular epidemiologic studies within the Selenium and Vitamin E Cancer Prevention Trial (SELECT). *Cancer Causes Control* 2001;12:627–633.

28. Rayman MP. The importance of selenium to human health. *Lancet* 2000;356:233–241.

29. El-Bayoumy K, Richie JP Jr, Boyiri T, et al. Influence of selenium-enriched yeast supplementation on biomarkers of oxidative damage and hormone status in healthy adult males: a clinical pilot study. *Cancer Epidemiol Biomark Prev* 2002;11:1459–1465.

30. Ganther HE. Selenium metabolism, selenoproteins and mechanisms of cancer prevention: complexities with thioredoxin reductase. *Carcinogenesis* 1999;20:1657–1666.

31. Combs GF Jr. Considering the mechanisms of cancer prevention by selenium, in *Nutrition and Cancer Prevention*. Kluwer Academic/Plenum Publishers, New York, NY, 2000, pp.107–117.

32. El-Bayoumy K, Upadhyaya P, Sohn OS, et al. Synthesis and excretion profile of 1,4-[^{14}C]phenylenebis(methylene)selenocyanate in the rat. *Carcinogenesis* 1998;19:1603–1607.

33. Ip C, Lisk DJ. Triphenylselenonium and diphenylselenide in cancer chemoprevention: comparative studies of anticarcinogenic efficacy, tissue selenium levels and excretion profile. *Anticancer Res* 1997;17:3195–3199.

34. Ip C, Thompson HJ, Ganther HE. Cytostasis and cancer chemoprevention: investigating the action of triphenylselenonium chloride in in vivo models of mammary carcinogenesis. *Anticancer Res* 1998;18:9–12.

35. Ip C, El-Bayoumy K, Upadhyaya P, et al. Comparative effect of inorganic and organic selenocyanate derivatives in mammary cancer chemoprevention. *Carcinogenesis* 1994;15:187–192.

36. El-Bayoumy K, Upadhyaya P, Date V, et al. Metabolism of [^{14}C]benzyl selenocyanate in the F344 rat. *Chem Res Toxicol* 1991;4:560–565.

37. Allan CB, Lacourciere GM, Stadtman TC. Responsiveness of selenoproteins to dietary selenium. *Annu Rev Nutr* 1999;19:1–16.

38. Mustacich D, Powis G. Thioredoxin reductase [Review]. *Biochem J* 2000;346:1–8.

39. Foiles PG, Fujiki H, Suganuma M, et al. Inhibition of PKC and PKA by chemopreventive organoselenium compounds. *Int J Oncol* 1995;7:685–690.

40. Sinha R, Kiley SC, Lu J, et al. Effects of methylselenocysteine on PKC activity, cdk2 phosphorylation and gadd gene expression in synchronized mouse mammary epithelial tumor cells. *Cancer Lett* 1999;146:135–145.

41. Gopalakrishna R, Gundimeda U, Chen Z-H. Cancer-preventive selenocompounds induce a specific redox modification of cysteine-rich regions in Ca(2+)-dependent isoenzymes of protein kinase C. *Arch Biochem Biophys* 1997;348:25–36.

42. Gopalakrishna R, Chen Z-H, Gundimeda U. Selenocompounds induce a redox modulation of protein kinase C in the cell, compartmentally independent from cytosolic glutathione: its role in inhibition of tumor promotion. *Arch Biochem Biophys* 1997;348:37–48.

43. Stapleton SR, Garlock GL, Foellmi-Adams L, Kletzien RF. Selenium: potent stimulator of tyrosyl phosphorylation and activator of MAP kinase. *Biochim Biophys Acta* 1997;1355:259–269.

44. Fiala ES, Joseph C, Sohn OS, et al. Mechanism of benzylselenocyanate inhibition of azoxymethane-induced colon carcinogenesis in F344 rats. *Cancer Res* 1991;51:2826–2830.

45. Sohn OS, Fiala ES, Upadhyaya P, et al. Comparative effects of phenylenebis(methylene)selenocyanate isomers on xenobiotic metabolizing enzymes in organs of female CD rats. *Carcinogenesis* 1999;20:615–621.

46. Tanaka T, Makita H, Kawabata K, et al. 1,4-Phenylenebis(methylene)selenocyanate exerts exceptional chemopreventive activity in rat tongue carcinogenesis. *Cancer Res* 1997;57:3644–3648.

47. Makropoulos V, Brüning T, Schulze-Osthoff K. Selenium-mediated inhibition of transcription factor NF-kappa B and HIV-1 LTR promoter activity. *Arch Toxicol* 1996;70:277–283.

48. Youn BW, Fiala ES, Sohn OS. Mechanisms of organoselenium compounds in chemoprevention: effects of transcription factor-DNA binding. *Nutr Cancer* 2001;40:28–33.

49. Adler V, Pincus MR, Posner S, et al. Effects of chemopreventive selenium compounds on Jun N-kinase activities. *Carcinogenesis* 1996;19:1849–1854.

50. Kaeck M, Lu J, Strange R, et al. Differential induction of growth arrest inducible genes by selenium compounds. *Biochem Pharmacol* 1997;53:921–926.

51. Lanfear J, Fleming J, Wu L, et al. The selenium metabolite selenodiglutathione induces p53 and apoptosis: relevance to the chemopreventive effects of selenium? *Carcinogenesis* 1994;15:1387–1392.

52. Spyrou G, Bjornstedt M, Kumar S, Holmgren A. AP-1 DNA-binding activity is inhibited by selenite and selenodiglutathione. *FEBS Lett* 1995;368:59–63.

53. Fiala ES, Staretz ME, Pandya GA, et al. Inhibition of DNA cytosine methyltransferase by chemopreventive selenium compounds, determined by an improved assay for DNA cytosine methyltransferase and DNA cytosine methylation. *Carcinogenesis* 1998;19:597–604.

54. Cao YZ, Reddy CC, Sordillo LM. Altered eicosanoid biosynthesis in selenium-deficient endothelial cells. *Free Radic Biol Med* 2000;28:381–389.

55. Ip C, Thompson HJ, Ganther HE. Selenium modulation of cell proliferation and cell cycle biomarkers in normal and premalignant cells of the rat mammary gland. *Cancer Epidemiol Biomark Prev* 2000;9:49–54.

56. Rao CV, Simi B, Hirose Y, et al. Mechanisms in the chemoprevention of colon cancer: modulation of protein kinase C, tyrosine protein kinase and diacylglycerol kinase activities by 1,4-phenylenebis(methylene)selenocyanate and impact of low-fat diet. *Int J Oncol* 2000;16:519–527.

57. Dong Y, Lisk D, Block E, Ip C. Characterization of the biological activity of γ-glutamyl-Se-methylselenocysteine: a novel, naturally occurring anticancer agent from garlic. *Cancer Res* 2001;61:2923–2928.

58. Dong Y, Ganther HE, Stewart C, Ip C. Identification of molecular targets associated with selenium-induced growth inhibition in human breast cells Using cDNA microarrays. *Cancer Res* 2002;62:708–714.

59. Zhu Z, Jiang W, Ganther HE, Thompson HJ. Mechanisms of cell cycle arrest by methylseleninic acid. *Cancer Res* 2002;62:156–164.

60. Narayanan BA, Desai D, Narayanan NK, et al. Comparison of the chemopreventive efficacies of 1,4-phenylenebis(methylene)selenocyanate (*p*-XSC) and its glutathione conjugate *p*-XSeSG on 7,12-dimethyl benz[*a*]anthracene (DMBA)-induced mammary carcinogenesis in the rat: molecular mechanisms using microarray analysis. *Proc Am Assoc Cancer Res* 2002; abst. no. 4088.

61. Ip C, Lisk DJ, Ganther HE. Activities of structurally-related lipophilic selenium compounds as cancer chemopreventive agents. *Anticancer Res* 18:4019–4025.

36 Calcium

John A. Baron, MD, MS, MSc

CONTENTS

1. INTRODUCTION

Calcium is an essential human nutrient, probably best known for its role in bone metabolism *(1)*. Calcium also takes part in several basic cellular processes, functioning as an intracellular second messenger—e.g., in receptor-mediated signaling pathways that transmit outside molecular signals into the cell *(2)*. However, Newmark and colleagues' first proposal that high calcium intake might have antineoplastic effects did not derive from either of these functions. Rather, they hypothesized that calcium would indirectly affect the neoplastic process through a relatively simple chemical reaction with fats and bile acids *(3)*.

As this hypothesis related to colorectal neoplasia, the antineoplastic potential of calcium has been most extensively investigated regarding that malignancy. This chapter summarizes calcium's possible chemopreventive effects, begins with large bowel neoplasia, and subsequently considers possible effects on other cancers. Unfortunately, the effect of calcium intake on carcinogenesis outside the colon and rectum has received much less epidemiological and experimental investigation.

2. CALCIUM AND EXPERIMENTAL CARCINOGENESIS IN THE LARGE BOWEL

The hypothesis set out by Newmark and colleagues derives from the cancer promoting effect that neutral fats and bile acids are believed to exert on colorectal mucosa. In the lumen of the bowel, calcium can form insoluble chemical complexes with these bile acids and fats, precipitate them out of the water phase of the stool, and thus separate them from effective contact with the mucosa *(3)*. Calcium would thus exert an antineoplastic effect by shielding the mucosa from carcinogen contact. In fact, high calcium intake has been found to protect against experimental bowel carcinogenesis in most animal models *(4–12)*, although a few experimental studies have reported increases in tumor numbers *(13,14)*.

The cancer-sparing effect of high calcium intake may vary in ways that shed light on the underlying mechanisms. In some investigations, a protective effect has been more pronounced in rats fed a high-fat diet than in those fed lower-fat diets *(5,6)*. Some studies suggest a greater effect of calcium on carcinomas than on adenomas *(6,15)*, or a reduction in the number of invasive cancers with an increase in numbers of adenomas *(16)*. These latter findings might suggest that calcium

From: Cancer Chemoprevention, Volume 1: Promising Cancer Chemoprevention Agents
Edited by: G. J. Kelloff, E. T. Hawk, and C. C. Sigman © Humana Press Inc., Totowa, NJ

preferentially alters the later stages of carcinogenesis, but effects on aberrant crypt foci (ACF) indicate an impact on earlier stages as well *(17,18)*.

Data support the relevance of the originally proposed mechanistic pathways. High calcium intake can indeed cause loss of fats and bile acids in the stool *(19–24)*. Precipitated fat "soaps" have been observed in the stool after calcium supplementation, and dietary calcium can ameliorate the hyperproliferative effect of carcinogens, bile acids, or small bowel resection on bowel mucosa *(25–30)*. Recent studies have also indicated that higher calcium intake can increase apoptosis in normal mucosa of the large bowel *(18,31)*, particularly in the distal bowel *(31)*.

Despite these findings, it cannot be assumed that the fat-precipitation mechanism definitely explains calcium's effects. For example, one study found that a reduction in proliferation associated with calcium supplementation did not track well with a reduction in tumor occurrence *(12)*. In addition, other mechanisms have been proposed. In particular, extracellular calcium may itself be a first messenger that influences intracellular events related to carcinogenesis through a calcium-sensing receptor *(32–35)*. In cell lines, higher extracellular calcium can suppress proliferation in colon cancer cell lines *(33,36)*.

Although these animal studies clearly provide a mechanistic context for investigating the relationship between calcium intake and human carcinogenesis, several important limitations remain. Correspondence between experimental rodent carcinogenesis and human cancer is far from perfect: the time-course of cancer development, the particular carcinogens involved, and perhaps the genetic background of carcinogenesis may differ in important regards. Also, differences between ameliorating calcium deficiency and supplementing beyond adequate intake may be an issue in the translation from animals to humans.

3. CALCIUM INTAKE AND HUMAN COLORECTAL NEOPLASIA: OBSERVATIONAL DATA

3.1. Dietary Calcium and Colorectal Cancer (CRC)

In part because of promising animal data, a large number of epidemiological studies have investigated the association between calcium intake and the risk of colorectal neoplasia. Some early studies reported an inverse relationship between dietary calcium intake

and CRC risk *(37,38)*. However, epidemiological studies regarding dietary calcium intake and CRC cancer have generally yielded mixed findings *(39,40)*. One cohort study of men reported an age- and energy-adjusted relative risk of 0.61 (95% CI 0.40–0.91) for subjects in the highest quintile of dietary calcium vs those in the lowest. This rose to 0.81 (95% CI 0.52–1.28) after adjustment for other covariates *(41)*. Other follow-up studies found suggestions of an inverse association of dietary or total calcium intake with CRC risk *(42–45)*, but some cohort data have been frankly negative *(46–49)*.

Case-control studies have reported similarly inconsistent results *(39,40)*. Some of these studies have found marked inverse associations of dietary calcium with risk *(37,50–53)*, but others have reported no association, or even suggestions of increased risk *(54–58)*.

Available data do not indicate any particular dose-response pattern. In some studies that observed an inverse association, maximal calcium benefit was apparent at low intakes *(38,44,51,53,59,60)*, suggesting that any cancer-sparing effect might involve a reversal of deficiency. However, other studies suggested that the cancer-sparing effect emerged at higher intakes, or was a continuous, graded one *(37,42,61)*.

There seem to be no important subgroup effects. Studies that report data for both genders have generally reported similar relative risks for both *(37,38,47,48,50–52,54–57,62,63)*. However, some case-control studies have reported suggestions that an inverse association of calcium intake with CRC risk is more pronounced in women than in men *(60,64)*. When found, the protective effects of calcium have been similar in the colon and rectum, and in subsites within the colon *(41,43,50–52,57,59,62,65–69)*. No findings have consistently suggested that the effect of calcium is greater among subjects with a high fat intake *(41,50,51,57,68)*.

3.2. Dietary Calcium and Colorectal Adenomas

Epidemiological studies of dietary calcium and the risk of colorectal adenoma have generally not found strong associations. Two related large cohort studies in women and men found that high calcium intake conferred slight (nonsignificant) increases in risk *(70)*; similar findings were reported in a case-control study from France *(71)*. On the other hand, two case-control studies *(43,72)* and a cohort analysis of incident adenomas *(73)* suggested an inverse relationship. Other studies reported either no association or ambiguous findings *(56,74–77)*. In contrast to the findings for

CRC, an inverse association of calcium with adenoma risk may be greater among individuals with a high fat intake *(70,78)*.

3.3. Calcium Supplements

Observational data regarding the association between calcium supplement use and the risk of CRC or adenomas are as conflicting as the dietary data. One cohort study of women reported that supplements conferred a reduced risk of colon and rectal cancer *(42,45)*. This effect was not seen in another cohort *(47)*, and a case-control study of colon cancer reported only inconsistent suggestions of an inverse association *(63)*. Two adenoma case-control studies *(79,80)* have been negative, but one follow-up study reported decreased adenoma risks associated with the use of calcium supplements *(81)*.

Interpretation of these epidemiological data is difficult. Nutritional assessment necessarily involves considerable measurement error, which, if non-differential, would introduce a conservative bias in both case-control and cohort studies. The possibility of confounding between calcium intake and other dietary constituents further complicates research on this topic. In particular, at least in the United States, dietary calcium and vitamin D are both largely obtained from dairy products *(51,62,82,83)*, a pattern that creates the potential for confounding between these two nutrients.

4. CALCIUM AND COLORECTAL NEOPLASIA: CLINICAL TRIAL DATA

4.1. Biochemical and Cellular Endpoints in Clinical Trials

Cell proliferation seems to play an important role in carcinogenesis generally *(84)*, and hyperproliferation may be a feature of bowel epithelium prone to neoplasia *(85)*. Several studies have investigated the effects of supplemental calcium on mucosal proliferation in the large bowel, and results have been inconsistent. Some of these investigations reported no beneficial effect *(86–90)*, a few reported suggestions of increased proliferation *(87,88,91–93)*, and others reported a reduction in proliferation *(94–100)*. Interpretation of some results is limited by small sample size, lack of controls, and apparently unblinded laboratory measurements.

In some investigations, other anticarcinogenic effects were observed: reduced cytotoxicity of fecal water *(89,101,102)*, reduced proportion of secondary

bile acids in the bile acid pool *(89,102,103)*, and lowered bile acid concentration in fecal water *(103)*. However, no beneficial effects on these parameters were reported in other studies that suggested either no change *(86,101)*, or an increase *(88,91,104)* in bile acid concentrations in the water phase of the stool. In one study, calcium supplementation had no effect on ornithine decarboxylase (ODC) activity in normal colonic mucosa of healthy subjects with a family history of CRC *(105)*.

4.2. Clinical Endpoints in Trials

Several clinical trials of colorectal neoplasia and calcium supplementation have been published. The Polyp Prevention Study Group found that supplementation with elemental calcium (1200 mg daily) reduced recurrent adenoma risk by 18% and recurrent adenoma numbers by 26% *(106)*. Risk reduction did not vary materially with baseline dietary fat intake. Most adenomas found after randomization in this study were small, early lesions without substantial malignant potential. However, calcium's protective effect was more pronounced for adenomas with a more advanced histology. Risk reduction in the calcium group was 12% for tubular adenomas (adjusted risk ratio 0.88; 95% CI 0.69–1.01), but was 36% for more advanced lesions such as tubulovillous or villous adenomas or cancer (adjusted risk ratio 0.64; 95% CI 0.45–0.91) *(107)*.

Broadly similar findings were reported from a smaller European adenoma prevention trial *(108)*. Calcium supplementation (2.0 gm/d) conferred a 34% risk reduction (95% CI 17–62%). The calcium effect was somewhat more pronounced among subjects with baseline calcium intake below the median, but there were no suggestions that the calcium effect was greater among those who had a high fat intake.

Two other clinical trials reported data consistent with a chemopreventive effect of calcium supplementation. In Norway, patients with adenomas were randomized to placebo or a mixture of β-carotene (15 mg), vitamin C (150 mg), vitamin E (75 mg), selenium (101 μg), and calcium (4 g; 1.6 g elemental calcium). The intervention had no effect on the growth of polyps left in place, but reduced the risk of new adenomas (odds ratio 0.31; 95% CI 0.11–0.84) *(109)*. Another small trial, conducted among subjects with familial adenomatous polyposis (FAP) randomized subjects to placebo or calcium carbonate (1500 mg elemental calcium). After 6 mo, polyp counts increased by 64% in the placebo group, and by 47% in the calcium group. Although the increase was smaller in the calcium group, the two rates were not statistically significantly different (110).

4.3. Colorectal Cancer, Calcium, and K-ras

K-ras gene mutations are common early events in colorectal tumorigenesis (111), occurring in 40–60% of CRC. The vast majority of these are in codons 12 and 13 of K-ras (112). K-ras mutations are also found in colorectal adenomas, again predominantly in codons 12 and 13. Reported prevalence in adenomas has varied widely (15–75%), often (but not consistently) higher in larger or more advanced adenomas (reviewed in 113,114).

Little is known about the cause of K-ras somatic mutations in colorectal tumors. One case-control study of CRC from Majorca reported that dietary calcium was associated with a reduced risk of tumors containing mutated K-ras and with a nonsignificant increase in risk of tumors with wild-type K-ras (115). (In this study, dietary calcium was associated with a nonsignificant increase in the overall risk of CRC.) Other studies have not reported these striking findings, although their results are consistent with the idea that at least some ras mutations are less common in patients with a higher calcium intake (116–118).

One investigation of dietary calcium's effects on experimental bowel cancer has reported findings regarding K-ras mutations. In rats fed a moderate fat diet and given dimethylhydrazine (DMH), calcium did not affect the number of animals with tumors, but did reduce the number of tumors per tumor-bearing rat. Cancers in the calcium-supplemented rats had no K-ras mutations, in contrast to 33% of cancers in the unsupplemented rats (119). Thus, calcium intake may specifically protect against K-ras mutations, perhaps through changes in bile acid levels or composition.

5. CALCIUM INTAKE AND OTHER CANCERS OF THE GASTROINTESTINAL TRACT

Because bile acids can potentially contact the mucosa of the entire gastrointestinal (GI) lumen, and may reflux into the pancreatic duct, hypothesized mechanisms of anticarcinogenesis for the colorectum could conceivably be operative in other parts of the GI tract. Indeed, alkaline (bile) reflux into the esophagus seems to be involved in the etiology of adenocarcino-

ma of the distal esophagus and Barrett's esophagus, a premalignant condition related to this malignancy (120). Bile acids have been implicated in some animal models of pancreatic carcinogenesis (121,122).

Epidemiological data regarding the association between calcium intake and upper aerodigestive tract cancers are conflicting. In several studies, a high calcium intake was unrelated to risk of squamous carcinoma of the esophagus or adenocarcinoma of the esophagus/gastric cardia (123–126). One case-control study even an reported an increased risk of oral cavity cancers among subjects with a high calcium intake (127).

In contrast, some studies reported that a high dietary calcium intake was associated with nonsignificantly reduced risks of cancers of the oral cavity, larynx, esophagus (128), or oral cavity and pharynx (129). Similar findings were reported from a cohort study of upper aerodigestive tract cancer from Japan; in this study, the trend of decreasing risk with increasing intake was statistically significant (130). A randomized double-blind trial of calcium supplementation (600 mg/d) in patients with precancerous esophageal lesions found an improvement in esophageal dysplasia and reduction in mucosal proliferation (131). (This study is reported in Chinese with an English abstract.)

A high calcium intake appears to have no substantial protective effect on the risk of stomach cancer. A hospital-based case-control study from Italy reported increased risks in those with high calcium intake (132); there were nonsignificant suggestions of an increased risk in a Spanish case-control study (133). On the other hand, an investigation from China reported protective effects of high dietary calcium (134). Several other studies reported no association (135–139).

Some data suggest a reduced risk of pancreatic cancer with high calcium intake. A population-based case-control study from western Washington reported an odds ratio of 0.5 (95% CI 0.2–1.0) for subjects in the highest quartile of calorie-adjusted calcium intake in comparison to those in the lowest quartile (140). Two other case-control studies reported data consistent with this effect, although the point estimates were much more modest (141) or not statistically significant (142). One population-based case-control study found no association (143). A cohort study conducted among male smokers reported nonsignificant, modestly reduced risks of pancreatic cancer among subjects in the highest two quintiles of calcium intake (144).

6. CANCERS OUTSIDE THE GI TRACT

The bile acid hypothesis set out for CRC seems unlikely to be relevant to carcinogenesis in organs outside the GI tract. However, the antiproliferative effect of extracellular calcium could possibly have an effect at such sites *(145,146)*. Also, changes in bile acid and cholesterol metabolism that have been described in association with high calcium intake could conceivably affect hormonal status. However, such a mechanism has not been investigated, and this possibility remains highly speculative.

6.1. Cancers of the Breast, Ovary, Uterus, and Prostate

The relatively little data that exist regarding the relationship between calcium intake and risk of cancers of the ovary, endometrium, and cervix, suggest that high intake is not associated with a decreased risk of these malignancies *(147–149)*. Indeed, increased risk of endometrial cancer was reported among women with high calcium intake in one study *(150)*.

However, some preclinical data suggest that calcium is protective against mammary tumors in rats *(151,152)*. Some animal studies have found evidence that a calcium-fortified diet can reduce proliferation of the mammary epithelium *(153)*. Increases in extracellular calcium can promote differentiation of breast epithelial cells in culture *(145)*.

Few data are available regarding an association of dietary calcium intake with the risk of human breast cancer. In one cohort study, high calcium intake was associated with a markedly reduced risk *(154)*. Another cohort study *(155)* and several case-control studies have also reported reductions in risk with high intake *(156–160)*, but other studies have not reported similar findings *(58,161–163)*. One investigation reported that high calcium intake was associated with a reduced risk of proliferative benign breast disease *(164)*.

Some investigators have proposed that calcium intake may increase the risk of prostate cancer, presumably by decreasing levels of 1,25-dihydroxyvitamin D_3, a hormone believed to exert antineoplastic effects *(165,166)*. A few cohort analyses have reported such an increased risk in association with a high calcium intake *(167,168)*, as have some case-control studies *(169,170)*. However, other cohort *(171,172)* and case-control studies *(173–176)* have found no association, or have reported protective effects *(177)*. A small clinical trial of calcium supplementation suggested a lower risk of prostate cancer in the supplemented group *(106)*.

6.2. Other Cancers

Bladder cancer does not appear to be associated with dietary calcium intake *(178,179)*. In one case-control study, high dietary intake conferred an increased risk, but this was attenuated after control for saturated fat intake *(179)*. In contrast, a cohort study reported nonsignificantly reduced risks of renal carcinoma in postmenopausal women with a high calcium intake; the use of calcium supplements was significantly inversely related to risk (relative risk 0.52; 95% CI 0.52–0.89) *(180)*.

One cohort study suggested that a high calcium intake was associated with an increased risk of lung cancer *(181)*, but a case-control study from China reported that a high calcium intake was associated with a reduced risk, particularly of adenocarcinoma and large-cell carcinoma *(182)*. Another case-control study from China reported no association *(183)*.

Two studies suggest that a high calcium intake may decrease the risk of gliomas *(184,185)*. Other studies suggest that maternal use of calcium supplements decreases a child's risk of gliomas and neuroectodermal tumors *(186,187)*.

7. OTHER EFFECTS OF HIGH CALCIUM INTAKE

As might be expected from its importance for bone, a high calcium intake has a modest beneficial effect on bone density and may reduce fracture risk *(1,2,188)*. Calcium supplementation also may also have small beneficial effects on blood pressure *(189–192)*, total cholesterol levels *(191)*, and body wt *(193–196)*. A high calcium intake may also decrease platelet aggregation *(197–200)*. These findings suggest that a high calcium intake could reduce the risk of coronary artery disease. Indeed, ecological data are consistent with this hypothesis *(201)*, and some animal experimental findings also support the concept *(197)*. Epidemiological data regarding calcium intake and the risk of myocardial infarction and stroke are limited but consistent with a modest inverse association *(202–205)*.

8. SAFETY OF CALCIUM CHEMOPREVENTION

Calcium supplementation is widely used, and is generally free from acute toxicity. The recommended calcium intake is 1000 mg/d for adults 19–50 yr of age, and 1,200 mg/d for adults 51–70 yr of age *(1)*. Intake up to 2,500 mg in adults is considered safe *(1)*. However, high- dose calcium supplementation can have predictable metabolic toxicity—mainly hypercalcemia, which can lead to renal insufficiency and alkalosis, the "milk-alkali syndrome" *(1,206)*. This syndrome is rare in healthy people, and has not been observed in trials of calcium and vitamin D supplementation using doses of around 1000 mg calcium per day. Although high dietary calcium does not exacerbate a tendency to form kidney stones, calcium supplementation probably does *(207,208)*; therefore, a history of urinary stones is a relative contraindication for calcium supplements. Some natural calcium supplements contain small amounts of lead *(209)*, although the clinical significance of these amounts appears to be limited *(210)*.

In addition to these toxicological issues, the relationship of calcium intake to the risk of prostate cancer is also clearly relevant to safety of calcium supplementation. As noted previously, the data regarding this issue are conflicting, and the matter remains unresolved.

9. SUMMARY

Calcium supplementation clearly reduces the risk of colorectal neoplasia. This effect can be discerned in available, yet somewhat conflicting epidemiological data, but clinical trial confirmation has been required to establish the effect and estimate its magnitude. The mechanisms underlying the anticarcinogenic effects of calcium are unclear, but may involve protection of the colorectal mucosa from bile acid-induced damage.

The association between calcium intake and other malignancies has generally not been extensively investigated; available data are largely derived from studies of dietary calcium intake. These investigations involve considerable measurement error—which would tend to obscure some associations—and also necessarily focus on lower ranges of intake than would be available from supplements. Therefore, a current understanding of calcium's potential to exert chemopreventive effects outside the large bowel must be regarded as tentative.

Although carcinogenesis in the distal esophagus—as in the colorectum—may be promoted by bile acids, there is little evidence of a protective effect of calcium intake on adenocarcinoma of the distal esophagus. An inverse association of calcium intake and risk of pancreatic cancer has been seen in some studies, but data regarding this association are relatively weak, and require further confirmation. Observational data also suggest a benefit of high calcium intake on the risk of breast cancer. Further observational investigation regarding these relationships is needed before more definititive conclusions can be drawn. Clinical trial data regarding the effect of calcium supplementation on the breast would also be very valuable, although this is likely to be difficult. High calcium intake appears to have no substantial effects on risk of other cancers, although available data are very sparse.

Considering these data, it is clear that calcium is an excellent candidate to be a useful chemopreventive agent in the large bowel. The issue of prostate cancer aside, calcium supplements are generally safe and cheap, and probably have a modest beneficial effect on bone. However, the ultimate benefit of calcium supplementation for chemoprevention of CRC must be seen in the context of current clinical practice. For example, it is unclear what the marginal benefit of calcium would be in addition to endoscopic screening.

Despite these uncertainties, the impact of calcium intake on colorectal neoplasia risk provides several relevant insights. Most importantly, effective colorectal chemoprevention is clearly possible. Moreover, this nutrient offers an appealing model for chemopreventive agent development: mechanistic, experimental studies led to epidemiological studies, human biomarker investigations, and ultimately, clinical trials. This agent is available in food and is commonly taken as a supplement, which has made epidemiological studies possible and facilitated progress in understanding its potential. Hopefully, a similar interplay between preclinical studies, epidemiology, human biomarker investigations, and chemoprevention trials will lead to a better understanding of calcium's role in the prevention of neoplasia in other organs.

REFERENCES

1 Standing Committee on the Scientific Evaluation of Dietary Reference Intakes Food and Nutrition Board Institute of Medicine. *Dietary Reference Intakes for Calcium, Phosphorus, Magnesium, Vitamin D and Fluoride.* National Academy Press, Washington, DC, 1997.

2 Weaver CM, Heaney RP. Calcium. in, *Modern Nutrition in Health and Disease, 9th ed.* Shils ME, Olson JA, Shike M, Ross AC, eds. Lippincott Williams & Wilkins, Baltimore, MD, 1999, pp.141–155.

3 Newmark HL, Wargovich MJ, Bruce WR. Colon cancer and dietary fat, phosphate, and calcium: a hypothesis. *J Natl Cancer Inst* 1984;72:1323–1325.

4 Appleton GV, Davies PW, Bristol JB, Williamson RC. Inhibition of intestinal carcinogenesis by dietary supplementation with calcium. *Br J Surg* 1987;74:523–525.

5　Pence BC, Buddingh F. Inhibition of dietary fat-promoted colon carcinogenesis in rats by supplemental calcium or vitamin D$_3$. *Carcinogenesis* 1988;9:187–190.

6　Wargovich M, Allnutt D, Palmer C, et al. Inhibition of the promotional phase of azoxymethane-induced colon carcinogenesis in the rat by calcium lactate: effect of simulating two human nutrient density levels. *Cancer Lett* 1990;53:17–25.

7　Sitrin M, Halline A, Abrahams C, Brasitus T. Dietary calcium and vitamin D modulate 1,2-dimethylhydrazine-induced colonic carcinogenesis in the rat. *Cancer Res* 1991;51:5608–5613.

8　Pence BC, Dunn DM, Zhao C, et al. Chemopreventive effects of calcium but not aspirin supplementation in cholic acid-promoted colon carcinogenesis: correlation with intermediate endpoints. *Carcinogenesis* 1995;16:757–765.

9　Ranhotra GS, Gelroth JA, Glaser BK, et al. Cellulose and calcium lower the incidence of chemically-induced colon tumors in rats. *Plant Foods Hum Nutr* 1999;54:295–303.

10　Belbraouet S, Felden F, Pelletier X, et al. Dietary calcium salts as protective agents and laminin P1 as a biochemical marker in chemically induced colon carcinogenesis in rats. *Cancer Detect Prev* 1996;20:294–299.

11　Adell-Carceller R, Segarra-Soria M, Gibert-Jerez J, et al. Inhibitory effect of calcium on carcinogenesis at the site of colonic anastomosis: an experimental study. *Dis Colon Rectum* 1997;40:1376–1381.

12　Barsoum GH, Thompson H, Neoptolemos JP, Keighley MR. Dietary calcium does not reduce experimental colorectal carcinogenesis after small bowel resection despite reducing cellular proliferation. *Gut* 1992;33:1515–1520.

13　Behling AR, Kaup SM, Choquette LL, Greger JL. Lipid absorption and intestinal tumour incidence in rats fed on varying levels of calcium and butterfat. *Br J Nutr* 1990;64:505–513.

14　Weber T, Connors R, Tracy T Jr, et al. Mucosal proliferation characteristics in ureterosigmoidostomy: effect of calcium supplement. *J Pediatr Surg* 1990;25:130–132.

15　McSherry C, Cohen B, Bokkenheuser V, et al. Effects of calcium and bile acid feeding on colon tumors in the rat. *Cancer Res* 1989;49:6039–6043.

16　Vinas-Salas J, Biendicho-Palau P, Pinol-Felis C, et al. Calcium inhibits colon carcinogenesis in an experimental model in the rat. *Eur J Cancer* 1998;34:1941–1945.

17　Weisburger JH, Braley J, Reinhardt J, et al. The role of fat and calcium in the production of foci of aberrant crypts in the colon of rats fed 2-amino-1-methyl-6-phenylimidazo[4,5-b]-pyridine. *Environ Health Perspect* 1994;102(Suppl 6):53–55.

18　Liu Z, Tomotake H, Wan G, et al. Combined effect of dietary calcium and iron on colonic aberrant crypt foci, cell proliferation and apoptosis, and fecal bile acids in 1,2-dimethylhydrazine-treated rats. *Oncol Rep* 2001;8:893–897.

19　Drenick EJ. The influence of ingestion of calcium and other soap-forming substances on fecal fat. *Gastroenterology* 1961;41:242–244.

20　Fleischman AI, Yacowitz H, Hayton T, Bierenbaum ML. Effects of dietary calcium upon lipid metabolism in mature male rats fed beef tallow. *J Nutr* 1966;88:255–260.

21　Nazir DJ, Mishkel MA. The effect of calcium on plasma lipids and bile acid and fecal fat excretion in normolipidemic subjects. *Clin Chim Acta* 1975;62:117–123.

22　Lutwak L, Laster L, Gitelman HJ, et al. Effects of high dietary calcium and phosphorus on calcium, phosphorus, nitrogen and fat metabolism in children. *Am J Clin Nutr* 1964;14:76–82.

23　Yacowitz H, Fleischman AI, Bierenbaum ML. Effects of oral calcium upon serum lipids in man. *Br Med J* 1965;1:1352–1354.

24　Yacowitz H, Fleischman AI, Amsden RT, Bierenbaum ML. Effects of dietary calcium upon lipid metabolism in rats fed saturated or unsaturated fat. *J Nutr* 1967;92:389–392.

25　Reshef R, Rozen P, Fireman Z, et al. Effect of a calcium-enriched diet on the colonic epithelial hyperproliferation induced by N-methyl-N'-nitro-N-nitrosoguanidine in rats on a low calcium and fat diet. *Cancer Res* 1990;50:1764–1767.

26　Nobre-Leitao C, Chaves P, Fidalgo P, et al. Calcium regulation of colonic crypt cell kinetics: evidence for a direct effect in mice. *Gastroenterology* 1995;109:498–504.

27　Wargovich MJ, Eng VW, Newmark HL, Bruce WR. Calcium ameliorates the toxic effect of deoxycholic acid on colonic epithelium. *Carcinogenesis* 1983;4:1205–1207.

28　Bird RP, Schneider R, Stamp D, Bruce WR. Effect of dietary calcium and cholic acid on the proliferative indices of murine colonic epithelium. *Carcinogenesis* 1986;7:1657–1661.

29　Appleton GV, Bristol JB, Williamson RC. Increased dietary calcium and small bowel resection have opposite effects on colonic cell turnover. *Br J Surg* 1986;73:1018–1021.

30　Van der Meer R, Lapre JA, Govers MJ, Kleibeuker JH. Mechanisms of the intestinal effects of dietary fats and milk products on colon carcinogenesis. *Cancer Lett* 1997;114:75–83.

31　Penman ID, Liang QL, Bode J, et al. Dietary calcium supplementation increases apoptosis in the distal murine colonic epithelium. *J Clin Pathol* 2000;53:302–307.

32　Kallay E, Bajna E, Wrba F, et al. Dietary calcium and growth modulation of human colon cancer cells: role of the extracellular calcium-sensing receptor. *Cancer Detect Prev* 2000;24:127–136.

33　Kallay E, Kifor O, Chattopadhyay N, et al. Calcium-dependent c-myc proto-oncogene expression and proliferation of Caco-2 cells: a role for a luminal extracellular calcium-sensing receptor. *Biochem Biophys Res Commun* 1997;232:80–83.

34　Riccardi D. Calcium ions as extracellular, first messengers. *Z Kardiol* 2000;89(Suppl 2):9–14.

35　Chattopadhyay N, Brown EM. Cellular "sensing" of extracellular calcium (Ca(2+)(o)): emerging roles in regulating diverse physiological functions. *Cell Signal* 2000;12:361–366.

36　Cross HS, Hulla W, Tong WM, Peterlik M. Growth regulation of human colon adenocarcinoma-derived cells by calcium, vitamin D and epidermal growth factor. *J Nutr* 1995;125:2004S–2008S.

37　Slattery ML, Sorenson AW, Ford MH. Dietary calcium intake as a mitigating factor in colon cancer. *Am J Epidemiol* 1988;128:504–514.

38　Macquart-Moulin G, Riboli E, Cornee J, et al. Case-control study on colorectal cancer and diet in Marseilles. *Int J Cancer* 1986;38:183–191.

39　Bergsma-Kadijk JA, van 't Veer P, Kampman E, Burema J. Calcium does not protect against colorectal neoplasia. *Epidemiology* 1996;7:590–597.

40 Martinez ME, Willett WC. Calcium, vitamin D, and colorectal cancer: a review of the epidemiologic evidence. *Cancer Epidemiol Biomark Prev* 1998;7:163–168.

41 Kearney J, Giovannucci E, Rimm EB, et al. Calcium, vitamin D, and dairy foods and the occurrence of colon cancer in men. *Am J Epidemiol* 1996;143:907–917.

42 Bostick RM, Potter JD, Sellers TA, et al. Relation of calcium, vitamin D, and dairy food intake to incidence of colon cancer among older women. The Iowa Women's Health Study. *Am J Epidemiol* 1993;137:1302–1317.

43 Martinez M, Giovannucci E, Colditz G, et al. Calcium, vitamin D, and the occurrence of colorectal cancer among women. *J Natl Cancer Inst* 1996;88:1375–1382.

44 Pietinen P, Malila N, Virtanen M, et al. Diet and risk of colorectal cancer in a cohort of Finnish men. *Cancer Causes Control* 1999;10:387–396.

45 Zheng W, Anderson KE, Kushi LH, et al. A prospective cohort study of intake of calcium, vitamin D, and other micronutrients in relation to incidence of rectal cancer among postmenopausal women. *Cancer Epidemiol Biomark Prev* 1998;7:221–225.

46 Heilbrun L, Hankin J, Nomura A, Stemmermann G. Colon cancer and dietary fat; phosphorus; and calcium in Hawaiian-Japanese men. *Am J Clin Nutr* 1986;1986:306–309.

47 Kampman E, Goldbohm R, Van Den Brandt P, Van't Veer P. Fermented dairy products, calcium, and colorectal cancer in the Netherlands cohort study. *Cancer Res* 1994;54:3186–3190.

48 Wu AH, Paganini-Hill A, Ross RK, Henderson BE. Alcohol, physical activity and other risk factors for colorectal cancer: a prospective study. *Br J Cancer* 1987;55:687–694.

49 Jarvinen R, Knekt P, Hakulinen T, Aromaa A. Prospective study on milk products, calcium and cancers of the colon and rectum. *Eur J Clin Nutr* 2000;55:1000–1007.

50 Kampman E, Slattery ML, Caan B, Potter JD. Calcium, vitamin D, sunshine exposure, dairy products and colon cancer risk (United States). *Cancer Causes Control* 2000;11:459–466.

51 De Stefani E, Mendilaharsu M, Deneo-Pellegrini H, Ronco A. Influence of dietary levels of fat, cholesterol, and calcium on colorectal cancer. *Nutr Cancer* 1997;29:83–89.

52 Whittemore AS, Wu-Williams AH, Lee M, et al. Diet, physical activity, and colorectal cancer among Chinese in North America and China. *J Natl Cancer Inst* 1990;82:915–926.

53 Zaridze D, Filipchenko V, Kustov V, et al. Diet and colorectal cancer: results of two case- control studies in Russia. *Eur J Cancer* 1992;29A:112–115.

54 Kampman E, van 't Veer P, Hiddink GJ, et al. Fermented dairy products, dietary calcium and colon cancer: a case-control study in The Netherlands. *Int J Cancer* 1994;59:170–176.

55 Freudenheim JL, Graham S, Marshall JR, et al. A case-control study of diet and rectal cancer in western New York. *Am J Epidemiol* 1990;131:612–624.

56 Boutron MC, Faivre J, Marteau P, et al. Calcium, phosphorus, vitamin D, dairy products and colorectal carcinogenesis: a French case-control study. *Br J Cancer* 1996;74:145–151.

57 Pritchard RS, Baron JA, Gerhardsson de Verdier M. Dietary calcium, vitamin D, and the risk of colorectal cancer in Stockholm, Sweden. *Cancer Epidemiol Biomark Prev* 1996;5:897–900.

58 Graham S, Marshall J, Haughey B, et al. Dietary epidemiology of cancer of the colon in western New York. *Am J Epidemiol* 1988;128:490–503.

59 Marcus PM, Newcomb PA. The association of calcium and vitamin D, and colon and rectal cancer in Wisconsin women. *Int J Epidemiol* 1998;27:788–793.

60 Ghadirian P, Lacroix A, Maisonneuve P, et al. Nutritional factors and colon carcinoma: a case-control study involving French Canadians in Montreal, Quebec, Canada. *Cancer* 1997;80:858–864.

61 Kato I, Akhmedkhanov A, Koenig K, et al. Prospective study of diet and female colorectal cancer: the New York University Women's Health Study. *Nutr Cancer* 1997;28:276–281.

62 Peters RK, Pike MC, Garabrant D, Mack TM. Diet and colon cancer in Los Angeles County, California. *Cancer Causes Control* 1992;3:457–473.

63 White E, Shannon JS, Patterson RE. Relationship between vitamin and calcium supplement use and colon cancer. *Cancer Epidemiol Biomark Prev* 1997;6:769–774.

64 Meyer F, White E. Alcohol and nutrients in relation to colon cancer in middle-aged adults. *Am J Epidemiol* 1993;138:225–236.

65 Ferraroni M, La Vecchia C, D'Avanzo B, et al. Selected micronutrient intake and the risk of colorectal cancer. *Br J Cancer* 1994;70:1150–1155.

66 Tuyns AJ, Haelterman M, Kaaks R. Colorectal cancer and the intake of nutrients: oligosaccharides are a risk factor, fats are not. A case-control study in Belgium. *Nutr Cancer* 1987;10:181–196.

67 Lee HP, Gourley L, Duffy SW, et al. Colorectal cancer and diet in an Asian population—a case-control study among Singapore Chinese. *Int J Cancer* 1989;43:1007–1016.

68 Stemmermann GN, Nomura A, Chyou PH. The influence of dairy and nondairy calcium on subsite large-bowel cancer risk. *Dis Colon Rectum* 1990;33:190–194.

69 Arbman G, Axelson O, Ericsson-Begodzki AB, et al. Cereal fiber, calcium, and colorectal cancer. *Cancer* 1992;69:2042–2048.

70 Kampman E, Giovannucci E, van 't Veer P, et al. Calcium, vitamin D, dairy foods, and the occurrence of colorectal adenomas among men and women in two prospective studies. *Am J Epidemiol* 1994b;139:16–29.

71 Macquart-Moulin G, Riboli E, Cornee J, et al. Colorectal polyps and diet: a case-control study in Marseilles. *Int J Cancer* 1987;40:179–188.

72 Almendingen K, Trygg K, Larsen S, et al. Dietary factors and colorectal polyps: a case- control study. *Eur J Cancer Prev* 1995;4:239–246.

73 Hyman J, Baron J, Dain B, et al. Dietary and supplemental calcium and the recurrence of colorectal adenomas. *Cancer Epidemiol Biomark Prev* 1998;7:291-295.

74 Little J, Logan RF, Hawtin PG, et al. Colorectal adenomas and diet: a case-control study of subjects participating in the Nottingham faecal occult blood screening programme. *Br J Cancer* 1993;67:177–184.

75 Benito E, Cabeza E, Moreno V, et al. Diet and colorectal adenomas: a case-control study in Majorca. *Int J Cancer* 1993;55:213–219.

76 Tseng M, Murray SC, Kupper LL, Sandler RS. Micronutrients and the risk of colorectal adenomas. *Am J Epidemiol* 1996;144:1005–1014.

77 Lubin F, Rozen P, Arieli B, et al. Nutritional and lifestyle habits and water-fiber interaction in colorectal adenoma etiology. *Cancer Epidemiol Biomark Prev* 1997;6:79–85.

78 Martinez ME, McPherson RS, Annegers JF, Levin B. Association of diet and colorectal adenomatous polyps: dietary fiber, calcium, and total fat. *Epidemiology* 1996;7:264–268.

79 Neugut A, Horvath K, Whelan R, et al. The effect of calcium and vitamin supplements on the incidence and recurrence of colorectal adenomatous polyps. *Cancer* 1996;78:723–728.

80 Peleg I, Lubin M, Cotsonis G, et al. Long-term use of non-steroidal antiinflammatory drugs and other chemopreventors and risk of subsequent colorectal neoplasia. *Dig Dis Sci* 1996;41:1319–1326.

81 Whelan RL, Horvath KD, Gleason NR, et al. Vitamin and calcium supplement use is associated with decreased adenoma recurrence in patients with a previous history of neoplasia. *Dis Colon Rectum* 1999;42:212–217.

82 Peters U, McGlynn KA, Chatterjee N, et al. Vitamin D, calcium, and vitamin D receptor polymorphism in colorectal adenomas. *Cancer Epidemiol Biomark Prev* 2001;10:1267–1274.

83 Levine AJ, Harper JM, Ervin CM, et al. Serum 25-hydroxyvitamin D, dietary calcium intake, and distal colorectal adenoma risk. *Nutr Cancer* 2001;39:35–41.

84 Preston-Martin S, Pike MC, Ross RK, et al. Increased cell division as a cause of human cancer. *Cancer Res* 1990;50:7415–7421.

85 Lipkin M. Biomarkers of increased susceptibility to gastrointestinal cancer: new application to studies of cancer prevention in human subjects. *Cancer Res* 1988;48:235–245.

86 Stern HS, Gregoire RC, Kashtan H, et al. Long-term effects of dietary calcium on risk markers for colon cancer in patients with familial polyposis. *Surgery* 1990;108:528–533.

87 Bostick RM, Potter JD, Fosdick L, et al. Calcium and colorectal epithelial cell proliferation: a preliminary randomized, double-blinded, placebo-controlled clinical trial. *J Natl Cancer Inst* 1993;85:132–141.

88 Kleibeuker JH, Welberg JW, Mulder NH, et al. Epithelial cell proliferation in the sigmoid colon of patients with adenomatous polyps increases during oral calcium supplementation. *Br J Cancer* 1993;67:500–503.

89 Cats A, Kleibeuker JH, van der Meer R, et al. Randomized, double-blinded, placebo-controlled intervention study with supplemental calcium in families with hereditary nonpolyposis colorectal cancer. *J Natl Cancer Inst* 1995;87:598–603.

90 Armitage NC, Rooney PS, Gifford KA, et al. The effect of calcium supplements on rectal mucosal proliferation. *Br J Cancer* 1995;71:186–190.

91 Gregoire RC, Stern HS, Yeung KS, et al. Effect of calcium supplementation on mucosal cell proliferation in high risk patients for colon cancer. *Gut* 1989;30:376–382.

92 Baron JA, Tosteson TD, Wargovich MJ, et al. Calcium supplementation and rectal mucosal proliferation: a randomized controlled trial. *J Natl Cancer Inst* 1995;87:1303–1307.

93 Weisgerber UM, Boeing H, Owen RW, et al. Effect of longterm placebo controlled calcium supplementation on sigmoidal cell proliferation in patients with sporadic adenomatous polyps. *Gut* 1996;38:396–402.

94 Lipkin M, Newmark H. Effect of added dietary calcium on colonic epithelial-cell proliferation in subjects at high risk for familial colonic cancer. *N Engl J Med* 1985;313:1381–1384.

95 Lipkin M, Friedman E, Winawer SJ, Newmark H. Colonic epithelial cell proliferation in responders and nonresponders to supplemental dietary calcium. *Cancer Res* 1989;49:248–254.

96 Rozen P, Fireman Z, Fine N, et al. Oral calcium suppresses increased rectal epithelial proliferation of persons at risk of colorectal cancer. *Gut* 1989;30:650–655.

97 Barsoum GH, Hendrickse C, Winslet MC, et al. Reduction of mucosal crypt cell proliferation in patients with colorectal adenomatous polyps by dietary calcium supplementation. *Br J Surg* 1992;79:581–583.

98 Wargovich MJ, Isbell G, Shabot M, et al. Calcium supplementation decreases rectal epithelial cell proliferation in subjects with sporadic adenoma. *Gastroenterology* 1992;103:92–97.

99 Bostick RM, Fosdick L, Wood JR, et al. Calcium and colorectal epithelial cell proliferation in sporadic adenoma patients: a randomized, double-blinded, placebo-controlled clinical trial. *J Natl Cancer Inst* 1995;87:1307–1315.

100 Rozen P, Lubin F, Papo N, et al. Calcium supplements interact significantly with long-term diet while suppressing rectal epithelial proliferation of adenoma patients. *Cancer* 2001;91:833–840.

101 Lapre JA, De Vries HT, Termont DS, et al. Mechanism of the protective effect of supplemental dietary calcium on cytolytic activity of fecal water. *Cancer Res* 1993;53:248–253.

102 Welberg JW, Kleibeuker JH, Van der Meer R, et al. Effects of oral calcium supplementation on intestinal bile acids and cytolytic activity of fecal water in patients with adenomatous polyps of the colon. *Eur J Clin Invest* 1993;23:63–68.

103 Lupton JR, Steinbach G, Chang WC, et al. Calcium supplementation modifies the relative amounts of bile acids in bile and affects key aspects of human colon physiology. *J Nutr* 1996;126:1421–1428.

104. Alder RJ, McKeown-Eyssen G, Bright-See E. Randomized trial of the effect of calcium supplementation on fecal risk factors for colorectal cancer. *Am J Epidemiol* 1993;138:804–814.

105. Love RR, Verma AK, Surawicz TS, Morrissey JF. Absence of effect of supplemental oral calcium on ornithine decarboxylase (ODC) activity in colonic mucosae of healthy individuals with a family history of colorectal cancer. *J Surg Oncol* 1990;43:79–82.

106. Baron J, Beach M, Mandel J, et al. Calcium supplements for the prevention of colorectal adenomas. *N Engl J Med* 1999;340:101–107.

107. Wallace K, Baron JA, Cole BF, et al. Calcium carbonate chemoprevention in the large bowel: effects on hyperplastic polyps, tubular adenomas, and more advanced lesions. *Proc Am Assoc Cancer Res* 2002;43:163–164, abst. no. 816.

108. Bonithon-Kopp C, Kronborg O, Giacosa A, et al. Calcium and fibre supplementation in prevention of colorectal adenoma recurrence: a randomised intervention trial. European Cancer Prevention Organisation Study Group. *Lancet* 2000;356:1300–1306.

109. Hofstad B, Almendingen K, Vatn M, et al. Growth and recurrence of colorectal polyps: a double-blind 3-year intervention with calcium and antioxidants. *Digestion* 1998;59:148–156.

110. Thomas MG, Tebbutt S, Williamson RC. Vitamin D and its metabolites inhibit cell proliferation in human rectal mucosa and a colon cancer cell line. *Gut* 1992;33:1660–1663.

111. Fearon ER. Molecular genetics of colorectal cancer. *Ann NY Acad Sci* 1995;768:101–110.

112. Vogelstein B, Fearon ER, Hamilton SR, et al. Genetic alterations during colorectal-tumor development. *N Engl J Med* 1988;319:525–532.

113. McLellan EA, Owen RA, Stepniewska KA, et al. High frequency of K-ras mutations in sporadic colorectal adenomas. *Gut* 1993;34:392–396.

114. Jen J, Powell SM, Papadopoulos N, et al. Molecular determinants of dysplasia in colorectal lesions. *Cancer Res* 1994;54:5523–5526.

115. Bautista D, Obrador A, Moreno V, et al. Ki-ras mutation modifies the protective effect of dietary monounsaturated fat and calcium on sporadic colorectal cancer. *Cancer Epidemiol Biomark Prev* 1997;6:57–61.

116. Slattery ML, Curtin K, Anderson K, et al. Associations between dietary intake and Ki-ras mutations in colon tumors: a population-based study. *Cancer Res* 2000;60:6935–6941.

117. Kampman E, Voskuil DW, van Kraats AA, et al. Animal products and K-ras codon 12 and 13 mutations in colon carcinomas. *Carcinogenesis* 2000;21:307–309.

118. Martinez ME, Maltzman T, Marshall JR, et al. Risk factors for Ki-ras protooncogene mutation in sporadic colorectal adenomas. *Cancer Res* 1999;59:5181–5185.

119. Llor X, Jacoby RF, Teng BB, et al. K-ras mutations in 1,2-dimethylhydrazine-induced colonic tumors: effects of supplemental dietary calcium and vitamin D deficiency. *Cancer Res* 1991;51:4305–4309.

120. Triadafilopoulos G. Acid and bile reflux in Barrett's esophagus: a tale of two evils. *Gastroenterology* 2001;121:1502–1506.

121. Ura H, Makino T, Ito S, et al. Combined effects of cholecystectomy and lithocholic acid on pancreatic carcinogenesis of N-nitrosobis(2-hydroxypropyl)amine in Syrian golden hamsters. *Cancer Res* 1986;46:4782–4786.

122. Ikematsu Y, Tomioka T, Kitajima T, et al. Tauroursodeoxycholate and cholestyramine enhance biliary carcinogenesis in hamsters. *World J Surg* 2000;24:22–26.

123. Graham S, Marshall J, Haughey B, et al. Nutritional epidemiology of cancer of the esophagus. *Am J Epidemiol* 1990;131:454–467.

124. Brown LM, Swanson CA, Gridley G, et al. Dietary factors and the risk of squamous cell esophageal cancer among black and white men in the United States. *Cancer Causes Control* 1998;9:467–474.

125. Franceschi S, Bidoli E, Negri E, et al. Role of macronutrients, vitamins and minerals in the aetiology of squamous-cell carcinoma of the oesophagus. *Int J Cancer* 2000;86:626–631.

126. Zhang ZF, Kurtz RC, Yu GP, et al. Adenocarcinomas of the esophagus and gastric cardia: the role of diet. *Nutr Cancer* 1997;27:298–309.

127. Marshall JR, Graham S, Haughey BP, et al. Smoking, alcohol, dentition and diet in the epidemiology of oral cancer. *Eur J Cancer B Oral Oncol* 1992;28B:9–15.

128. Rogers MA, Thomas DB, Davis S, et al. A case-control study of element levels and cancer of the upper aerodigestive tract. *Cancer Epidemiol Biomark Prev* 1993;2:305–312.

129. Negri E, Franceschi S, Bosetti C, et al. Selected micronutrients and oral and pharyngeal cancer. *Int J Cancer* 2000;86:122–127.

130. Chyou PH, Nomura AM, Stemmermann GN. Diet, alcohol, smoking and cancer of the upper aerodigestive tract: a prospective study among Hawaii Japanese men. *Int J Cancer* 1995;60:616–621.

131. Wang LD. Effect of added dietary calcium on human esophageal precancerous lesion in the high risk area for esophageal cancer—a randomized double blind intervention trial. *Chung-Hua Chung Liu Tsa Chih (Chin J Oncol)* 1990;12:332–335.

132. La Vecchia C, Ferraroni M, D'Avanzo B, et al. Selected micronutrient intake and the risk of gastric cancer. *Cancer Epidemiol Biomark Prev* 1994;3:393–398.

133. Ramon JM, Serra-Majem L, Cerdo C, Oromi J. Nutrient intake and gastric cancer risk: a case-control study in Spain. *Int J Epidemiol* 1993;22:983–988.

134. You WC, Blot WJ, Chang YS, et al. Diet and high risk of stomach cancer in Shandong, China. *Cancer Res* 1988;48:3518–3523.

135. Gonzalez CA, Riboli E, Badosa J, et al. Nutritional factors and gastric cancer in Spain. *Am J Epidemiol* 1994;139:466–473.

136. Chyou PH, Nomura AM, Hankin JH, Stemmermann GN. A case-cohort study of diet and stomach cancer. *Cancer Res* 1990;50:7501–7504.

137. Buiatti E, Palli D, Decarli A, et al. A case-control study of gastric cancer and diet in Italy: II. Association with nutrients. *Int J Cancer* 1990;45:896–901.

138. Harrison LE, Zhang ZF, Karpeh MS, et al. The role of dietary factors in the intestinal and diffuse histologic subtypes of gastric adenocarcinoma: a case-control study in the U.S. *Cancer* 1997;80:1021–1028.

139. Palli D, Russo A, Decarli A. Dietary patterns, nutrient intake and gastric cancer in a high-risk area of Italy. *Cancer Causes Control* 2001;12:163–172.

140. Farrow DC, Davis S. Diet and the risk of pancreatic cancer in men. *Am J Epidemiol* 1990;132:423–431.

141. Silverman DT, Swanson CA, Gridley G, et al. Dietary and nutritional factors and pancreatic cancer: a case-control study based on direct interviews. *J Natl Cancer Inst* 1998;90:1710–1719.

142. Baghurst PA, McMichael AJ, Slavotinek AH, et al. A case-control study of diet and cancer of the pancreas. *Am J Epidemiol* 1991;134:167–179.

143. Olsen GW, Mandel JS, Gibson RW, et al. Nutrients and pancreatic cancer: a population-based case-control study. *Cancer Causes Control* 1991;2:291–297.

144. Stolzenberg-Solomon RZ, Pietinen P, Taylor PR, et al. Prospective study of diet and pancreatic cancer in male smokers. *Am J Epidemiol* 2002;155:783–792.

145. Brown EM. G protein-coupled, extracellular Ca2+ (Ca2+(o))-sensing receptor enables Ca2+ (o) to function as a versatile extracellular first messenger. *Cell Biochem Biophys* 2000;33:63–95.

146. Hennings H, Holbrook KA, Yuspa SH. Factors influencing calcium-induced terminal differentiation in cultured mouse epidermal cells. *J Cell Physiol* 1983;116:265–281.

147. Kushi LH, Mink PJ, Folsom AR, et al. Prospective study of diet and ovarian cancer. *Am J Epidemiol* 1999;149:21–31.

148. Barbone F, Austin H, Partridge EE. Diet and endometrial cancer: a case-control study. *Am J Epidemiol* 1993;137:393–403.

149. Liu T, Soong SJ, Wilson NP, et al. A case control study of nutritional factors and cervical dysplasia. *Cancer Epidemiol Biomark Prev* 1993;2:525–530.

150. Negri E, La Vecchia C, Franceschi S, et al. Intake of selected micronutrients and the risk of endometrial carcinoma. *Cancer* 1996;77:917–923.

151. Jacobson EA, James KA, Newmark HL, Carroll KK. Effects of dietary fat, calcium, and vitamin D on growth and mammary tumorigenesis induced by 7,12-dimethyl-benz(*a*)anthracene in female Sprague-Dawley rats. *Cancer Res* 1989;49:6300–6303.

152. Carroll KK, Jacobson EA, Eckel LA, Newmark HL. Calcium and carcinogenesis of the mammary gland. *Am J Clin Nutr* 1991;54:206S–208S.

153. Zhang L, Bird RP, Bruce WR. Proliferative activity of murine mammary epithelium as affected by dietary fat and calcium. *Cancer Res* 1987;47:4905–4908.

154. Knekt P, Jarvinen R, Seppanen R, et al. Intake of dairy products and the risk of breast cancer. *Br J Cancer* 1996;73:687–691.

155. Friedenreich CM, Howe GR, Miller AB. Recall bias in the association of micronutrient intake and breast cancer. *J Clin Epidemiol* 1993;46:1009–1017.

156. Negri E, La Vecchia C, Franceschi S, et al. Intake of selected micronutrients and the risk of breast cancer. *Int J Cancer* 1996;65:140–144.

157. Favero A, Parpinel M, Franceschi S. Diet and risk of breast cancer: major findings from an Italian case-control study. *Biomed Pharmacother* 1998;52:109–115.

158. Landa MC, Frago N, Tres A. Diet and the risk of breast cancer in Spain. *Eur J Cancer Prev* 1994;3:313–320.

159. Katsouyanni K, Trichopoulos D, Boyle P, et al. Diet and breast cancer: a case-control study in Greece. *Int J Cancer* 1986;38:815–820.

160. Zaridze D, Lifanova Y, Maximovitch D, et al. Diet, alcohol consumption and reproductive factors in a case-control study of breast cancer in Moscow. *Int J Cancer* 1991;48:493–501.

161. Witte JS, Ursin G, Siemiatycki J, et al. Diet and pre-menopausal bilateral breast cancer: a case-control study. *Breast Cancer Res Treat* 1997;42:243–251.

162. Potischman N, Swanson CA, Coates RJ, et al. Intake of food groups and associated micronutrients in relation to risk of early-stage breast cancer. *Int J Cancer* 1999;82:315–321.

163. Levi F, Pasche C, Lucchini F, La Vecchia C. Dietary intake of selected micronutrients and breast-cancer risk. *Int J Cancer* 2001;91:260–263.

164. Rohan TE, Jain M, Miller AB. A case-cohort study of diet and risk of benign proliferative epithelial disorders of the breast (Canada). *Cancer Causes Control* 1998;9:19–27.

165. Giovannucci E. Dietary influences of 1,25(OH)2 vitamin D in relation to prostate cancer: a hypothesis. *Cancer Causes Control* 1998;9:567–582.

166. Feldman D, Skowronski RJ, Peehl DM. Vitamin D and prostate cancer. *Adv Exp Med Biol* 1995;375:53–63.

167. Chan JM, Stampfer MJ, Ma J, et al. Dairy products, calcium, and prostate cancer risk in the Physicians' Health Study. *Am J Clin Nutr* 2001;74:549–554.

168. Giovannucci E, Rimm EB, Wolk A, et al. Calcium and fructose intake in relation to risk of prostate cancer. *Cancer Res* 1998;58:442–447.

169. Tzonou A, Signorello LB, Lagiou P, et al. Diet and cancer of the prostate: a case-control study in Greece. *Int J Cancer* 1999;80:704–708.

170. Chan JM, Giovannucci E, Andersson SO, et al. Dairy products, calcium, phosphorous, vitamin D, and risk of prostate cancer (Sweden). *Cancer Causes Control* 1998;9:559–566.

171. Schuurman AG, van den Brandt PA, Dorant E, Goldbohm RA. Animal products, calcium and protein and prostate cancer risk in The Netherlands Cohort Study. *Br J Cancer* 1999;80:1107–1113.

172. Chan JM, Pietinen P, Virtanen M, et al. Diet and prostate cancer risk in a cohort of smokers, with a specific focus on calcium and phosphorus (Finland). *Cancer Causes Control* 2000;11:859–867.

173. Tavani A, Gallus S, Franceschi S, La Vecchia C. Calcium, dairy products, and the risk of prostate cancer. *Prostate* 2001;48:118–121.

174. Kristal AR, Stanford JL, Cohen JH, et al. Vitamin and mineral supplement use is associated with reduced risk of prostate cancer. *Cancer Epidemiol Biomark Prev* 1999;8:887–892.

175. Hayes RB, Ziegler RG, Gridley G, et al. Dietary factors and risks for prostate cancer among blacks and whites in the United States. *Cancer Epidemiol, Biomark Prev* 1999;8:25–34.

176 Ohno Y, Yoshida O, Oishi K, et al. Dietary beta-carotene and cancer of the prostate: a case-control study in Kyoto, Japan. *Cancer Res* 1988;48:1331–1336.

177 Vlajinac HD, Marinkovic JM, Ilic MD, Kocev NI. Diet and prostate cancer: a case-control study. *Eur J Cancer* 1997;33:101–107.

178 Michaud DS, Spiegelman D, Clinton SK, et al. Prospective study of dietary supplements, macronutrients, micronutrients, and risk of bladder cancer in US men. *Am J Epidemiol* 2000;152:1145–1153.

179 Riboli E, Gonzalez CA, Lopez-Abente G, et al. Diet and bladder cancer in Spain: a multicentre case-control study. *Int J Cancer* 1991;49:214–219.

180 Prineas RJ, Folsom AR, Zhang ZM, et al. Nutrition and other risk factors for renal cell carcinoma in postmenopausal women. *Epidemiology* 1997;8:31–36.

181 Shekelle RB, Lepper M, Liu S, et al. Dietary vitamin A and risk of cancer in the Western Electric study. *Lancet* 1981;2:1185–1190.

182 Koo LC. Dietary habits and lung cancer risk among Chinese females in Hong Kong who never smoked. *Nutr Cancer* 1988;11:155–172.

183 Hu J, Johnson KC, Mao Y, et al. A case-control study of diet and lung cancer in northeast China. *Int J Cancer* 1997;71:924–931.

184 Tedeschi-Blok N, Schwartzbaum J, Lee M, et al. Dietary calcium consumption and astrocytic glioma: the San Francisco Bay Area Adult Glioma Study, 1991–1995. *Nutr Cancer* 2001;39:196–203.

185 Hu J, La Vecchia C, Negri E, et al. Diet and brain cancer in adults: a case-control study in northeast China. *Int J Cancer* 1999;81:20–23.

186 Bunin GR, Kuijten RR, Boesel CP, et al. Maternal diet and risk of astrocytic glioma in children: a report from the Childrens Cancer Group (United States and Canada). *Cancer Causes Control* 1994;5:177–187.

187 Bunin GR, Kuijten RR, Buckley JD, et al. Relation between maternal diet and subsequent primitive neuroectodermal brain tumors in young children. *N Engl J Med* 1993;329:536–541.

188 Eastell R. Treatment of postmenopausal osteoporosis. *N Engl J Med* 1998;338:736–746.

189 Allender PS, Cutler JA, Follmann D, et al. Dietary calcium and blood pressure: a meta-analysis of randomized clinical trials. *Ann Int Med* 1996;124:825–831.

190 Bucher HC, Cook RJ, Guyatt GH, et al. Effects of dietary calcium supplementation on blood pressure. A meta-analysis of randomized controlled trials. *JAMA* 1996;275:1016–1022.

191 Bostick RM, Fosdick L, Grandits GA, et al. Effect of calcium supplementation on serum cholesterol and blood pressure. A randomized, double-blind, placebo-controlled, clinical trial. *Arch Fam Med* 2000;9:31–38.

192 Ascherio A, Hennekens C, Willett WC, et al. Prospective study of nutritional factors, blood pressure, and hypertension among US women. *Hypertension* 1996;27:1065–1072.

193 Carruth BR, Skinner JD. The role of dietary calcium and other nutrients in moderating body fat in preschool children. *Int J Obes Relat Metab Disord* 2001;25:559–566.

194. Lin YC, Lyle RM, McCabe LD, et al. Dairy calcium is related to changes in body composition during a two-year exercise intervention in young women. *J Am Coll Nutr* 2000;19:754–760.

195 Zemel MB, Shi H, Greer B, et al. Regulation of adiposity by dietary calcium. *FASEB J* 2000;14:1132–1138.

196 Davies KM, Heaney RP, Recker RR, et al. Calcium intake and body weight. *J Clin Endocrinol Metab* 2000;85:4635–4638.

197 Renaud S, Ciavatti M, Thevenon C, Ripoll JP. Protective effects of dietary calcium and magnesium on platelet function and atherosclerosis in rabbits fed saturated fat. *Atherosclerosis* 1983;47:187–198.

198 Renaud S, Morazain R, Godsey F, et al. Nutrients, platelet function and composition in nine groups of French and British farmers. *Atherosclerosis* 1986;60:37–48.

199 Kang JS, Cregor MD, Smith JB. Effect of calcium on blood pressure, platelet aggregation and erythrocyte sodium transport in Dahl salt-sensitive rats. *J Hypertens* 1990;8:245–250.

200 Otsuka K, Watanabe M, Yue Q, et al. Dietary calcium attenuates platelet aggregation and intracellular Ca^{2+} mobilization in spontaneously hypertensive rats. *Am J Hyperten* 1997;10:1165–1170.

201 Knox EG. Ischaemic-heart-disease mortality and dietary intake of calcium. *Lancet* 1973;1:1465–1467.

202 Bostick RM, Kushi LH, Wu Y, et al. Relation of calcium, vitamin D, and dairy food intake to ischemic heart disease mortality among postmenopausal women. *Am J Epidemiol* 1999;149:151–161.

203 Van der Vijver LP, van der Waal MA, Weterings KG, et al. Calcium intake and 28-year cardiovascular and coronary heart disease mortality in Dutch civil servants. *Int J Epidemiol* 1992;21:36–39.

204 Iso H, Stampfer MJ, Manson JE, et al. Prospective study of calcium, potassium, and magnesium intake and risk of stroke in women. *Stroke* 1999;30:1772–1779.

205 Abbott RD, Curb JD, Rodriguez BL, et al. Effect of dietary calcium and milk consumption on risk of thromboembolic stroke in older middle-aged men. The Honolulu Heart Program. *Stroke* 1996;27:813–818.

206 Whiting SJ, Wood RJ. Adverse effects of high-calcium diets in humans. *Nutr Rev* 1997;55:1–9.

207 Curhan GC, Willett WC, Speizer FE, et al. Comparison of dietary calcium with supplemental calcium and other nutrients as factors affecting the risk for kidney stones in women. *Ann Int Med* 1997;126:497–504.

208 Curhan GC, Willett WC, Rimm EB, Stampfer MJ. A prospective study of dietary calcium and other nutrients and the risk of symptomatic kidney stones. *N Engl J Med* 1993;328:833–838.

209 Ross EA, Szabo NJ, Tebbett IR. Lead content of calcium supplements. *JAMA* 2000;284:1425–1429.

210 Heaney RP. Lead in calcium supplements: cause for alarm or celebration? *JAMA* 2000;284:1432–1433.

37 Folate and Cancer Chemoprevention

Shumin M. Zhang, MD, ScD and Walter C. Willett, MD, DrPH

CONTENTS

1. INTRODUCTION

Folate, a water-soluble B vitamin, is found in a wide variety of foods, particularly vegetables, fruits, and liver. Folic acid, the synthetic form of folate used in vitamin supplements and fortified foods, consists of the base pteridine attached to one molecule of *p*-aminobenzoic acid and one molecule of glutamic acid (glutamate) *(1)*. The most common clinical manifestation of folate deficiency is megaloblastic anemia, which responds rapidly to folic acid *(2)*. Low folate intake during early pregnancy increases the risk of neural-tube defects in the fetus, and the occurrence and recurrence of these defects are significantly reduced by folic acid supplementation *(3,4)*. This is the first clear example of a major adverse health effect of suboptimal vitamin intake in the absence of clinical manifestation of deficiency. Recent evidence suggests that adequate folate intake may also help prevent cancer of the colon, breast, and other organs *(5)*.

2. POTENTIAL MECHANISMS OF ACTION

2.1. Folate Absorption and Transport

Folate in foods is found primarily in the reduced form of 5-methyltetrahydrofolate polyglutamate, which must be deconjugated in the jejunum to the monoglutamate form by folate conjugases for intestinal absorption *(6)*. Most intestinal absorption of folate appears to be carrier-mediated on the brush border membrane, which is saturable and increases with decreasing pH *(7,8)*. Another mechanism of absorption is through a pH-sensitive passive diffusion process *(9)*. Once inside the mucosal enterocyte, folate is reduced to tetrahydrofolate by the enzyme folate reductase *(1,10)*. Serine reversibly transfers a methylene group to tetrahydrofolate to form glycine and 5,10-methylenetetrahydrofolate, which is irreversibly reduced to 5-methyltetrahydrofolate by the enzyme 5,10-methylenetetrahydrofolate reductase (MTHFR) (Fig. 1;*1*)

Folate circulates as 5-methyltetrahydrofolate either freely dissolved or bound to blood proteins. Although some of the folate is nonspecifically bound to a variety of proteins with a low affinity such as albumin and hemoglobin, most of the folate is specifically bound to soluble folate-binding proteins with a higher affinity, which are found both in extracellular fluids (blood, cerebrospinal fluid, and urine) and in cell cytoplasm *(11)*. The uptake of folate by tissues is mediated by three pathways: the reduced folate carrier, membrane-associated folate-binding proteins (receptors), and passive diffusion *(12)*. In the kidney, folate transport across proximal tubular cells is mediated primarily by the folate-binding proteins in the brush border membrane to accumulate and reabsorb folate *(13,14)*. In the liver, folate is either converted to the polyglutamate forms for storage or released into bile to the small

From: Cancer Chemoprevention, Volume 1: Promising Cancer Chemoprevention Agents
Edited by: G. J. Kelloff, E. T. Hawk, and C. C. Sigman © Humana Press Inc., Totowa, NJ

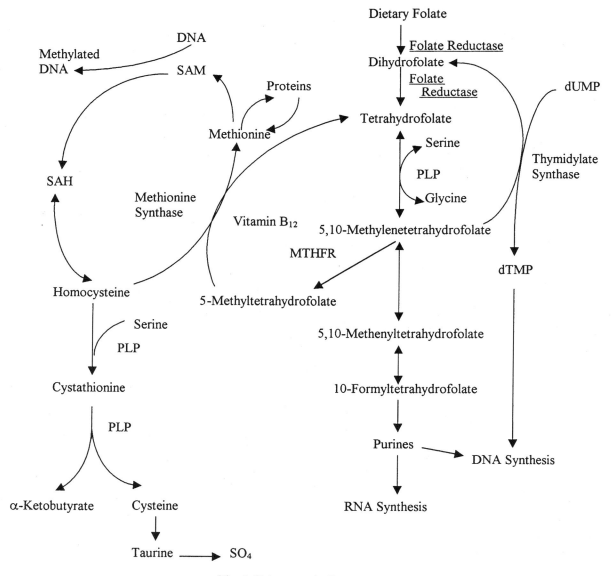

Fig. 1. Folate metabolism pathways.

intestine for reabsorption and subsequent distribution to tissues *(15)*.

2.2. Folate Metabolism

The pathways of folate metabolism are presented in simplified form in Fig 1; *(1,16)*. Within cells, 5-methyltetrahydrofolate donates a methyl group to homocysteine to form methionine and tetrahydrofolate. This methylation reaction is catalyzed by the enzyme methionine synthase, a vitamin B_{12}-dependent methyltransferase. Methionine is the precursor of *S*-adenosylmethionine (SAM), the universal methyl donor for many acceptors including guanidinoacetate, DNA, RNA, proteins, phospholipids, neurotransmitters,

and hormones. *S*-adenosylhomocysteine (SAH), a byproduct of these methylation reactions, is subsequently hydrolyzed to regenerate homocysteine, which then becomes available to start a new cycle of methyl-group transfer. Tetrahydrofolate can be converted to 5,10-methylenetetrahydrofolate, which transfers a methyl group to deoxyuridylate (dUMP) to generate deoxythymidylate (dTMP) by the enzyme thymidylate synthase. Thymidylate is a necessary precursor of DNA synthesis and erythrocyte formation. 5,10-methylenetetrahydrofolate can be oxidized to 10-formyltetrahydrofolate for *de novo* purine synthesis.

Homocysteine can also condense with serine to form cystathionine in an irreversible reaction catalyzed by the pyridoxal-5'-phosphate (PLP)-dependent enzyme, cystathionine β-synthase. Cystathionine is hydrolyzed by a second PLP-dependent enzyme, γ-cystathionase, to form cysteine and α-ketobutyrate. Excess cysteine is oxidized to taurine or inorganic sulfates and excreted in the urine. This transsulfuration pathway effectively catabolizes excess homocysteine that is not required for methyl transfer. Homocysteine is thus at the intersection of two metabolic pathways, remethylation and transsulfuration. The two pathways are modulated by SAM, which can serve as an inhibitor of MTHFR and as an activator of cystathionine β-synthase (1). When intracellular SAM concentration is high, homocysteine is diverted through the transsulfuration pathway because the synthesis of 5-methyltetrahydrofolate is inhibited and cystathionine β-synthase is activated. Conversely, when intracellular SAM concentration is low, homocysteine is diverted through the remethylation pathway.

Methionine can be consumed directly from the diet or formed endogenously via a reaction requiring folate in the form of 5-methyltetrahydrofolate. Methionine thus may have a sparing effect on the folate that otherwise would be used in methionine synthesis. Methionine itself is also likely to be important in carcinogenesis because of its involvement in DNA methylation.

2.3. Effect of Alcohol on Folate Metabolism

It has been known for decades that alcohol consumption suppresses the hematopoietic responses to folic acid therapy in folate-deficient patients with megaloblastic anemia, and that alcohol cessation or larger doses of folic acid can overcome this suppression (17). Alcohol also accelerates the induction of megaloblastic anemia in individuals on a low-folate diet (18). In normal individuals on a low-folate diet, an abrupt fall in serum folate levels follows acute alcohol consumption, returning rapidly to normal when alcohol is stopped (19). Chronic alcohol intake was also associated with lower blood folate levels among nonalcoholic elderly subjects (20).

The mechanism for the detrimental effects of alcohol on folate metabolism remains uncertain, but may be related to reduced intestinal absorption and increased renal excretion (16). Also, oxidation of alcohol generates acetaldehyde, which may directly destroy folate through cleavage of 5-methyltetrahydrofolate at the C^9-N^{10} bond (21) or condensation with tetrahydrofolate (22,23). Alcohol also may impair folate metabolism through the inhibition of methionine synthase in the

liver, which may trap folate as 5-methyltetrahydrofolate, leading to a shortage of tetrahydrofolate and a conditional folate deficiency (23,24). Human colonic bacteria are capable of producing considerable acetaldehyde from alcohol (25–28), which may break down folate in the colon and cause local folate deficiency in colonic mucosa (28). Alcohol thus could increase the requirement for folate intake and modify the association between folate and cancer risk. High alcohol intake may increase the risk of colon adenoma (29,30), colon cancer (31), breast cancer (32,33), and lung cancer (34).

2.4. Folate and DNA Synthesis and Repair

Folate in the form of 5,10-methylenetetrahydrofolate is essential for the de novo biosynthesis of thymidylate and purines (Fig. 1; 1). Folate deficiency may result in misincorporation of uracil into DNA during DNA synthesis (35,36). Wickramasinghe and Fida (35) noted markedly increased misincorporation of uracil into the DNA of bone-marrow cells among patients with megaloblastic anemia caused by folate or vitamin B_{12} deficiency. Blount et al. (36) showed that folate deficiency was associated with massive incorporation of uracil into human DNA and chromosome breaks, and that folic acid supplementation reversed high levels of uracil in DNA and micronucleus frequency (a measure of chromosome breaks) (36). Uracil in DNA is excised by a repair glycosylase, with the formation of a transient single strand break in the DNA; however, two opposing single strand breaks cause a double strand chromosome break, which is difficult to repair (36).

Diets deficient in folate have been associated with impairment of DNA excision repair (37) and induction of DNA strand breaks in lymphocytes (38) and within a highly conserved region (exons 5–8) of the p53 tumor-suppressor gene (39–41), which may cause functional inactivation of p53. Folate supplementation significantly reduced the extent of p53 strand breaks in exons 5–8 (41). The p53 tumor-suppressor gene is often mutated in tumors of the lung, colon, and breast (42–45). p53 serves as a critical brake on tumor development by shutting down multiplication of damaged or stressed cells to inhibit their progress through the cell cycle and by inducing programmed death (apoptosis) of the cells (45,46).

A randomized, double-blind, placebo-controlled trial among 20 patients with colon adenomas after polypectomy showed that daily supplementation with 5 mg folate for 1 yr significantly decreased the extent of p53 strand breaks in exons 5–8 (47). A similar trial conducted in 24 patients with chronic ulcerative colitis demonstrated that daily treatment with 15 mg folic acid for 3 mo significantly reduced cell proliferation in the upper section of the crypts (48). A third randomized, double-blind, placebo-controlled trial in young Australian adults also showed that treatment with a combination of 700 µg of folic acid and 7 µg of vitamin B_{12} for 12 wk followed by 2000 µg of folic acid and 20 µg of vitamin B_{12} for another 12 wk significantly reduced the frequency of micronucleated cells in individuals with a high baseline frequency of micronucleated cells (49). These two trials provide evidence that folic acid supplementation may reduce DNA damage (48,49).

2.5. Folate and DNA Methylation

Folate is an important mediator in the transfer of methyl groups for DNA methylation through the synthesis of SAM, a universal methyl donor for more than 100 biochemical reactions (1). DNA methylation is a heritable state without alteration of nucleotide sequences responsible for encoding the genome (50,51). Gene expression can be modulated by alterations in DNA methylation patterns, which are frequently seen in tumor cells, with wide areas of global hypomethylation along the genome accompanied by localized areas of hypermethylation at certain specific sites, such as the CpG islands (50–53). CpG island methylation of DNA of normal cells is rare (50,52,53), but is related to X-chromosome inactivation in females and genomic imprinting (50–53).

Aberrant CpG island hypermethylation, like mutations and deletions, can silence transcription of associated tumor-suppressor genes, serving as one of the "hits" in the Knudsen two-hit hypothesis for tumor generation (51–53). This epigenetic process disrupts tumor-suppressor gene function, and can predispose to genetic alterations by inactivating DNA-repair genes (50). DNA methylation may thus represent an early event in transformation of the normal cell to a malignant cell and an alternative pathway to cancer (51,52). Almost one-half of tumor suppressor genes that cause familial cancers through germline mutations can be inactivated through promoter CpG island hypermethylation in sporadic cancers; such genes include VHL (angiogenesis), $p16^{INK4a}$ (cyclin-dependent kinase inhibitor), E-cadherin (homotypic epithelial cell-cell adhesion), hMLH1 (DNA mismatch repair), BRCA1 (DNA damage repair), and LKB1 (serine, threonine kinase) (50). Promoter CpG island hypermethylation

has been associated with inactivation of other important genes related to tumor progression, including $p15^{INK4a}$ (cyclin-dependent kinase inhibitor), ER (estrogen receptor), O^6-MGMT (repair of DNA guanosine methyl adducts), GSTPI (prevention of oxidative DNA damage), TIMP3 (metastasis inhibitor), DAPK1 (kinase mediator of interferon-induced apoptosis), and p73 (a p53-like gene) (50). These genes have been implicated in cancers of the colon, breast, ovary, kidney, stomach, endometrium, pancreas, lung, prostate, brain, and thyroid, as well as in leukemia and lymphomas, and other cancers (50,51).

In colon cancer, $p16^{INK4a}$ inactivation is observed only in association with promoter CpG island hypermethylation (54). The majority of colorectal tumors with microsatellite instability have promoter CpG island hypermethylation of the hMLH1 (55–57). Treatment of cell lines from these tumors with the DNA methyltransferase inhibitor 5-aza-2'-deoxycytidine (5-azad-C) causes demethylation of the hMLH1 promoter, reaccumulation of the hMLH1 protein, and restoration of considerable mismatch repair capacity (55). This provides direct evidence that promoter CpG island hypermethylation is associated with loss of function of the tumor-suppressor gene hMLH1. CpG island methylator genotype (CIMP) has recently been described as a distinct pathway of colorectal carcinogenesis characterized by simultaneous methylation of multiple CpG islands, including genes such as $p16^{INK4a}$, hMLH1, and THBS1 (angiogenesis inhibitor) (58). CIMP accounts for the majority of sporadic colon cancer characterized by microsatellite instability related to hMLH1 methylation (58), and has also been observed in colon adenomas (59).

Hypermethylation within the gene itself may induce mutational events. Approximately 51% of the point mutations in p53 are guanine (G):cytosine (C)→adenine (A):thymine (T), and 59% of them are located at a CpG dinucleotide (45). DNA methylation in mammals occurs at the C residue. All 42 CpG dinucleotides, along with exons 5–8 of p53, were found completely methylated regardless of the tissue involved (45,60). Spontaneous deamination of C leading to formation of a uracil (U):G mismatch can be efficiently repaired by a UDNA glycosylase (45). 5-methylcytosine derived from C of CpG dinucleotides on DNA by an enzymatic reaction has a high propensity, as compared with C, to undergo spontaneous deamination to form T (61), resulting in a C→T point mutation (45,51). The DNA repair mechanism may not correctly recognize this mutation because T is a normal nucleotide of human DNA. The complementary strand G may be replaced by A to form the normal T→A opposition, resulting in a G→A point mutation *(51)*.

Indirect evidence for a role of DNA hypermethylation in carcinogenesis derives from the research in mice that are heterozygous for the multiple intestinal neoplasia *(Min)* mutation of the adenomatous polyposis coli *(Apc)* gene. *Min* mice develop multiple intestinal polyps, a condition that resembles human familial adenomatous polyposis (FAP) coli. A decrease in DNA methyltransferase activity was found to drastically suppress the formation of *Apc^min*-induced intestinal polyps *(62)*.

A significant loss of methyl groups in DNA has been observed in human colorectal adenomas and adenocarcinomas *(63–66)*, in the rectal mucosa of patients with chronic ulcerative colitis *(67)*, and in normal rectal mucosa of patients with colorectal adenomas and adenocarcinomas *(66)*. This finding suggests that DNA hypomethylation occurs early in colorectal carcinogenesis. Global DNA hypomethylation has also been observed in cancers of the lung *(63)*, stomach *(68)*, uterine cervix *(69)*, and breast *(70)*. Loss of DNA methylation induced by the hypomethylating agent 5-azacytidene causes undercondensation of human chromosomes and might lead to mitotic nondisjunction *(71)*, resulting in loss or gain of chromosomes and genomic instability *(43)*. Decreased levels of methylation in the cellular oncogenes c-Ha-*ras* and c-Ki-*ras* in human colon and lung tumors *(72)* and c-*myc* in human colorectal adenomas and adenocarcinomas *(73)* have also been reported. However, it is still unclear whether hypomethylation causes overexpression of these protooncogenes, and is not merely a secondary characteristic of cancer cells *(51)*.

Direct links between folate, DNA methylation, and carcinogenesis have been seen in rodents. Dietary deficiency in methyl group donors (methionine, choline, folate, and vitamin B_{12}) appears to lower the threshold for chemical carcinogenesis in the liver and other tissues of rats *(74)*. This is the only nutrient deficiency known to be carcinogenic in itself *(74)*. Prolonged methyl-deficient diets in rats, even without administration of carcinogens, can cause liver tumors *(75,76)*. DNA hypomethylation was detected in the liver after 1 wk *(39,77–79)* with concomitant increases in the mRNA levels of c-myc and c-fos and a smaller increase in c-Ha-*ras* protooncogenes *(78,79)*. After 1 mo of methyl-deficient diets, restoration of methyl-adequate diets gradually reversed the changes in DNA methylation

and gene expression *(79,80)*. Abnormalities of DNA methylation induced by methyl donor-deficient diets precede the development of tumors in rodents, which resemble human colorectal cancer (CRC).

Daily supplementation with 5–10 mg folic acid for 3–12 mo reversed genomic DNA hypomethylation in patients with colon adenomas or adenocarcinomas in three small randomized, double-blind, placebo-controlled studies *(47,66,81)*. However, daily supplementation with 5 mg folic acid for 6 mo had little effect in a trial conducted in patients with chronic ulcerative colitis (UC) *(5)*. In a trial conducted in young Australian adults, a combination of 700 µg of folic acid and 7 µg of vitamin B_{12} for 12 wk followed by 2000 µg of folic acid and 20 µg of vitamin B_{12} for another 12 wk produced no effect on DNA methylation *(49)*.

3. FOLATE DEFICIENCY AND CRC IN THE 1,2-DIMETHYLHYDRAZINE MODEL

The 1,2-dimethylhydrazine (DMH) rodent CRC model has been used extensively to examine the effects of nutritional factors on colon carcinogenesis *(82)*. DMH-induced adenocarcinomas of the colon are similar histologically to human colon tumors *(82,83)*, and their pathologic features include the entire sequence seen in the human colon, from tubular adenomas through polypoid and sessile carcinomas to mucinous adenocarcinomas *(83)*. Genomic events commonly observed in human colon carcinogenesis, such as amplification and overexpression of c-*myc* and activation of ki-*ras*, also are seen in the DMH-induced rodent colon tumors *(84,85)*. In this animal model, folate deficiency has enhanced the action of DMH on the development of colonic neoplasia in rats *(86,87)*; folate-depleted rats had a greater incidence of microscopic colonic dysplasia and carcinoma than folate-repleted rats *(86)*. Also, the incidence and average number of macroscopic tumors per rat decreased progressively in a dose-responsive manner with increasing levels of dietary folate *(87)*.

4. EPIDEMIOLOGIC STUDIES OF FOLATE AND CANCER

4.1. Folate and Colorectal Adenoma and Cancer

4.1.1. FOLATE AND COLORECTAL ADENOMA

Most cancers of the colon and rectum develop from adenomatous polyps *(88,89)*. Studies of these clinical

Table 1
Epidemiologic Studies of Folate and Colorectal Adenoma

Study (Reference), Year	Location	Cases	Exposure	Comparison	Relative Risk (95% CI)
Prospective study					
Giovannucci et al. (29), 1993	United States (US)	564 (F)	Total folate	Highest vs lowest quintile	0.66 (0.46–0.95)
		331 (M)			0.63 (0.41–0.98)
Baron et al. (30), 1998	US	260	Total folate	Highest vs lowest quartile	1.11 (0.69–1.78)
		259	Dietary folate		0.94 (0.53–1.67)
Case-control studies					
Benito et al. (90), 1993	Majorca, Spain	101	Dietary folate	Highest vs lowest quartile	0.27*
Bird et al. (91), 1995	California	152 (F)	Total folate	Highest vs lowest quartile	1.47 (0.73–2.95)
		180 (M)			0.70 (0.36–1.34)
		152 (F)	RBC folate	Highest vs lowest quartile	1.26 (0.65–2.43)
		180 (M)			0.47 (0.24–0.90)
		F†	Plasma folate	Highest vs lowest quartile	0.95 (0.69–1.30)
		M†			0.65 (0.45–0.95)
Tseng et al. (92), 1996	North Carolina	131 (F)	Total folate	Highest vs lowest quartile	0.39 (0.15–1.03)
		105 (M)			0.84 (0.29–2.43)
Boutron-Ruault et al. (93), 1996	Burgundy, France	Small 154	Dietary folate	Highest vs lowest quintile	0.5 (0.3–1.0)
		Large 208	Dietary folate	Highest vs lowest quintile	0.5 (0.3–1.0)
Neugut et al. (95), 1996	New York, NY	Incidence 122 (F)	Multivitamins	≥14 yr vs nonusers	0.8 (0.4–1.6)
		175 (M)		≥16 yr vs nonusers	0.6 (0.3–1.6)
		Recurrence 59 (F)	Multivitamins	≥11 yr vs nonusers	0.8 (0.3–2.4)
		139 (M)		≥12 yr vs nonusers	0.9 (0.4–1.9)
Whelan et al. (94), 1999	New York, NY	Recurrence 183	Multivitamins	Users vs nonusers	0.47 (0.31–0.72)

* 95% CI was not given.

†Exact number of cases was not given for plasma folate.

precursors of invasive cancer can provide information on the earlier stages of the adenoma-carcinoma sequence.

4.1.1.1. Cohort and Case-Control Studies Low folate intake has been related to an increased occurrence of colorectal adenoma in two large prospective cohorts, the Nurses' Health Study and the Health Professionals Follow-up Study in the US (29; Table 1). The highest quintile intake of folate was significantly associated with a decreased risk of colorectal adenoma compared with the lowest quintile of folate intake in women (relative risk = 0.66; 95% CI = 0.46–0.95) and in men (relative risk = 0.63; 95% CI

= 0.41–0.98) (29). Combinations of low folate and high alcohol or low folate and low methionine were associated with an approximately twofold increase in risk of colorectal adenoma (29). Folate supplements and dietary folate were not significantly associated with the overall risk of recurrence of colorectal adenoma in an adenoma prevention trial among patients with at least one recent large-bowel adenoma who were followed by colonoscopy for 1 yr (30). However, in this study, patients with a low-folate, high-alcohol diet had a higher risk than those with intermediate intake of folate and alcohol (relative risk = 1.85; 95% CI = 1.15–2.97), but patients with a high-folate, low-alcohol diet did not have a lower risk (relative risk = 0.99; 95% CI = 0.65–1.49) *(30)*.

Most retrospective case-control studies suggest a protective effect of folate intake or multivitamin use on the occurrence of colorectal adenomas *(90–94;* Table 1). A case-control study conducted in Majorca, Spain of men and women that included colorectal adenoma patients diagnosed by endoscopy and general population control subjects found a relative risk of 0.27 between the highest and lowest quartile intake of folate *(90)*. Among patients who underwent screening by flexible sigmoidoscopy at two southern California Kaiser Permanente medical centers, total folate intake was nonsignificantly associated with a 30% lower risk of colorectal adenomas in men but not in women *(91)*. In an analysis of colonoscopy patients in the University of North Carolina hospitals, total folate intake was inversely associated with colorectal adenoma in women (relative risk = 0.39; 95% CI = 0.15–1.03) but not in men (relative risk = 0.84; 95% CI = 0.29–2.43) *(92)*. A French case-control study found a significant association between high folate intake and 50% lower risk of small or large colorectal adenomas *(93)*. A colonoscopy-based case-control investigation in New York City observed a significant 53% reduction in the recurrence of colon adenomas associated with regular use of multivitamin supplements *(94)*. However, another analysis of patients at three colonoscopy practices in New York City found long-term use of multivitamins only weakly inversely associated with the occurrence or recurrence of colorectal adenomas in men and women *(95)*.

Red blood cell (RBC) and serum levels of folate and colonic mucosa have been shown to respond to folate supplements in clinical trials *(47,96,97)*, and reflect folate concentrations in colonic mucosa *(47,98,99)*. Limited data from three case-control studies that have examined folate blood levels in relation to colon adenomas also support an inverse association (Table 1). The same endoscopy-based case-control study at two southern California Kaiser Permanente medical centers described here also found a significant reduction in risk of colorectal adenomas associated with high levels of RBC folate (relative risk = 0.47; 95% CI = 0.24–0.90) and plasma folate (relative risk = 0.65; 95% CI = 0.45–0.95) only in men; the comparable relative risks in women were 1.26 (95% CI = 0.65–2.43) for RBC folate and 0.95 (95% CI = 0.69–1.30) for plasma folate *(91)*. In a case-control study in Greece, the mean levels of RBC and serum folate of 62 patients whose colonoscopic and histologic evaluation revealed colon adenomas were also found to be significantly lower than those of 50 control patients whose colonoscopic evaluation revealed no abnormality *(100)*. Furthermore, patients with adenomatous polyps had significantly lower folate concentrations in the normal rectosigmoid mucosa than patients with hyperplastic polyps *(98)*.

4.1.1.2. Randomized Trials Only one published double-blind, randomized, placebo-controlled clinical trial has examined daily supplementation with 1 mg folic acid on the recurrence of colon adenomas among 60 men and women who had incident colonic adenomas removed by endoscopic polypectomy. Frequencies of adenoma recurrence detected by colonoscopy were 23% in the folate group and 38% in the placebo group after 12 mo of intervention; frequencies were 13% in the folate group and 28% in the placebo group after 24 mo of intervention, but these differences did not reach statistical significance *(101)*. At least two ongoing randomized, double-blind, placebo-controlled trials with large sample sizes in the US are examining the effect of daily supplementation with 1 mg of folic acid on the recurrence of colon adenoma *(5)*.

4.1.2. FOLATE AND COLORECTAL CANCER CRC

Five prospective cohort studies examining folate and CRC risk strongly support an inverse association between folate intake and CRC, particularly among individuals with a high-alcohol, low-methionine diet *(31,102–105;* Table 2). In the Health Professionals Follow-up Study, although total folate intake was only weakly associated with the risk of colon cancer, a high-alcohol, low-folate, low-methionine diet had a strong positive association with risk of total colon cancer (relative risk = 3.30; 95% CI = 1.58–6.88) and distal colon cancer (relative risk = 7.44; 95% CI = 1.72–32.1) among men *(31)*. In the Nurses' Health Study, women with folate intake >400 µg/d were found to have a significantly lower (31%) risk of colon cancer than women with intake ≤200 µg/d *(103)*. Furthermore, women who took folic acid-containing multivitamins for at least 15 yr were 75% less likely to develop colon cancer than women who did not take multivitamins *(103)*. In a nested case-control study within the Alpha-Tocopherol Beta-Carotene (ATBC) Study cohort among male smokers, total folate intake was inversely associated with the risk of colon cancer (relative risk = 0.51; 95% CI = 0.20–1.31; for top vs bottom quartile) *(102)*. Furthermore, men with a high-alcohol, low-folate,

Table 2
Epidemiologic Studies of Folate and CRC

Study (Reference), Year	Location	Cases	Exposure	Comparison	Relative Risk (95% CI)
Prospective study					
Giovannucci et al. *(31)*, 1995	US	Colon			
		205 (M)	Total folate	Highest vs lowest quintile	0.86 (0.54–1.36)
			Multivitamins	≥10 yr vs nonusers	0.74 (0.47–1.17)
Glynn et al. *(102)*, 1996	Finland	Colon			
		86 (M)	Total folate	Highest vs lowest quartile	0.51 (0.20–1.31)
			Serum folate	Highest vs lowest quartile	0.96 (0.40–2.30)
		Rectum			
		50 (M)	Total folate	Highest vs lowest quartile	2.12 (0.43–10.5)
			Serum folate	Highest vs lowest quartile	2.94 (0.84–10.3)
Ma et al. *(107)*, 1997	US	Colorectal			
		202 (M)	Plasma folate	<3.0 vs ≥3.0 ng/mL	1.78 (0.93–3.42)
Giovannucci et al. *(103)*, 1998	US	Colon			
		442 (F)	Total folate	>400 vs ≤200 µg/d	0.69 (0.52–0.93)
			Multivitamins	≥15 yr vs nonusers	0.25 (0.13–0.51)
Kato et al. *(104)*, 1999	US	Colorectal			
		105 (F)	Total folate	Highest vs lowest quartile	0.88 (0.46–1.69)
			Serum folate	Highest vs lowest quartile	0.52 (0.27–0.97)
Su et al. *(105)*, 2001	US	Colon			
		120 (F)	Dietary folate	Highest vs lowest quartile	0.74 (0.36–1.51)
		99 (M)			0.40 (0.18–0.88)
Kim et al. *(106)*, 2001	North America, Europe	4829	Total folate	Highest vs lowest quintile	0.80 (0.71–0.90)
Case-control studies					
Benito et al. *(108)*, 1991	Majorca, Spain	Colon			
		144	Dietary folate	Highest vs lowest quartile	0.62*
		Rectum			
		130	Dietary folate	Highest vs lowest quartile	0.54*
Freudenheim et al. *(109)*, 1991	Western New York	Colon			
		223 (F)	Dietary folate	Highest vs lowest quartile	0.69 (0.36–1.30)
		205 (M)			1.03 (0.56–1.89)
		Rectum			
		151 (F)	Dietary folate	Highest vs lowest tertile	0.50 (0.24–1.03)
		293 (M)		Highest vs lowest quartile	0.31 (0.16–0.59)
Ferraroni et al. *(110)*, 1994	Italy	Colon			
		828	Dietary folate	Highest vs lowest quintile	0.55 (0.41–0.75)
		Rectum			
		498	Dietary folate	Highest vs lowest quintile	0.49 (0.33–0.71)

(continued)

Table 2 (*continued*)

Study (Reference), Year	Location	Cases	Exposure	Comparison	Relative risk (95% CI)
		Colorectal			
		615 (F)	Dietary folate	Highest vs lowest quintile	0.37 (0.24–0.57)
		711 (M)			0.63 (0.44–0.91)
Meyer et al. *(111)*, 1993	Washington State	Colon			
		186 (F)	Dietary folate	Highest vs lowest quartile	0.54*
		238 (M)			1.24*
Boutron-Ruault et al. *(93)*, 1996	Burgundy, France	Right colon			
		43	Dietary folate	Highest vs lowest quintile	0.8 (0.3–2.4)
		Left colon			
		63	Dietary folate	Highest vs lowest quintile	0.4 (0.1–1.1)
		Rectum			
		65	Dietary folate	Highest vs lowest quintile	3.9 (1.1–13.5)
White et al. *(112)*, 1997	Washington State	Colon			
		193 (F)	Folate supplements	≥400 µg/d vs nonusers	0.44 (0.24–0.80)
		251 (M)			0.59 (0.34–1.01)
			Multivitamins	1 pill/d vs never-users	0.43 (0.26–0.71)
					0.55 (0.34–0.88)
Slattery et al. *(113)*, 1997	California	Colon			
		894 (F)	Dietary folate	Highest vs lowest quintile	0.8 (0.6–1.1)
		1099 (M)			Not given

*95% CI was not given.

low-protein diet were at much higher risk for colon cancer than those with a low-alcohol, high-folate, high-protein diet (relative risk = 4.79; 95% CI = 1.36–16.9) *(102)*. In the National Health and Nutrition Examination Survey (NHANES) I Epidemiologic Follow-up Study, a national probability sample of the US non-institutionalized population, the highest quartile intake of dietary folate was related to a significant 60% lower risk of colon cancer than the lowest quartile intake in men, and women had a nonsignificant 26% lower risk *(105)*. Moreover, compared with a non-alcohol, high-folate, high-methionine diet, a high-alcohol, low-folate, low-methionine diet was related to a significant increase in risk of colon cancer in men (RR = 2.22; 95% CI = 1.03–4.77) but not in women (RR = 1.20; 95% CI = 0.61–2.36) *(105)*. In a nested case-control study within the New York University Women's Health Study, total folate intake was weakly associated with risk of CRC; relative risk was 0.88 (95% CI = 0.46–1.69) among women in the highest quartile compared with

those in the lowest quartile *(104)*. A recent pooled analysis of data from nine ongoing prospective cohorts in North America and Europe reported a significant 11% (95% CI = 2–19%) reduction in risk of CRC for every 400 µg/d increase in total folate intake *(106)*.

Two *(104,107)* of three *(102,104,107)* prospective studies have also suggested that high folate blood levels reduce CRC risk (Table 2). In a nested case-control study within the Physician's Health Study, men with deficient levels of plasma folate (<3 ng/mL) had a greater risk of CRC than did those with adequate levels *(107)*. A nested case-control study within the New York University Women's Health Study also observed a significant 48% lower risk of CRC in the highest compared with the lowest quartile of serum folate *(104)*. In addition, the risk of CRC was double in women with below-median serum folate and above-median alcohol relative to those with above-median serum folate and below-median alcohol (relative risk = 1.99; 95% CI = 0.92–4.29) *(104)*. However, a nested case-control study within the ATBC Study among male smokers described previously found no association between serum folate levels and CRC risk *(102)*.

Several case-control studies have reported on folate intake and CRC risk *(93,108–113)*; most have found a lower risk of CRC among those with the highest folate intake *(108–112;* Table 2). A case-control study in Majorca, Spain associated higher folate intake with a 44% lower risk of CRC among men and women; this inverse association was similar for colon and rectal cancer *(108)*. In the western New York study, higher folate intake was associated with a lower risk of rectal cancer in women (relative risk = 0.50; 95% CI = 0.24–1.03) and men (relative risk = 0.31; 95% CI = 0.16–0.59) and colon cancer in women (relative risk = 0.69; 95% CI = 0.36–1.30) but not in men (relative risk = 1.03; 95% CI = 0.56–1.89) *(109)*. Moreover, the association between folate intake and rectal cancer differed according to alcohol intake; the highest risk for rectal cancer was among men who consumed a high-alcohol, low-folate diet (relative risk = 5.07; 95% CI = 2.17–11.9) relative to those who consumed a low-alcohol, high-folate diet *(109)*. An Italian study related higher intake of folate to a lower risk of colon cancer (relative risk = 0.55; 95% CI = 0.41–0.75) and rectal cancer (relative risk = 0.49; 95% CI = 0.33–0.71); these inverse associations existed among both men and women, but disappeared when the studies also controlled for vitamins C and E and β-carotene *(110)*. In a case-control study conducted in western Washington State, high folate intake was associated with a lower risk of colon cancer among women (relative risk = 0.54), although the association was attenuated after further adjustment for dietary fiber (relative risk = 0.73); no association was seen in men *(111)*. In the same study population, use of folic acid supplements and multivitamins were both associated with a lower risk of colon cancer. The relative risks for individuals consuming ≥400 µg/d of folic acid supplements compared with nonusers were 0.44 (95% CI = 0.24–0.80) in women and 0.59 (95% CI = 0.34–1.01) in men *(112)*. Similarly, the relative risks for individuals who used multivitamins daily for 10 years were 0.43 (95% CI = 0.26–0.71) in women and 0.55 (95% CI = 0.34–0.88) in men compared with nonusers *(112)*. In a French case-control study, high folate intake was associated with a nonsignificant lower risk for colon cancer but a significant higher risk for rectum cancer *(93)*. A large case-control study conducted among men and women enrolled in the Kaiser Permanente Medical Care Program found a weak inverse association between folate intake and colon cancer, but the risk did not differ according to alcohol consumption *(113)*.

4.1.3. FOLATE AND ULCERATIVE COLITIS-RELATED COLON CANCER

Ulcerative colitis (UC) is a relapsing and remitting disease characterized by acute noninfectious inflammation of the colorectal mucosa *(114)*. Patients with chronic UC are at increased risk of developing colonic dysplasia and cancer *(115,116)*. Three small studies have shown that taking folic acid supplements or having high RBC folate levels is associated with lower risk of dysplasia or colon cancer in patients with UC *(117–119)*. In a case-control study with 35 patients with dysplasia or cancer and 64 control patients, folate supplementation was associated with a nonsignificant 62% lower risk of dysplasia or cancer *(117)*. Another study involving six patients with dysplasia or cancer and 61 control patients noted a significant 18% reduction in risk with each 10 ng/mL increase in RBC folate levels *(118)*. In a retrospective cohort of 98 patients with UC, the risk of dysplasia or cancer was 46% lower in patients taking 1 mg/d folic acid supplements for at least 6 mo compared with patients who did not take supplements *(119)*, but the benefit was less for those who took 0.4 mg/d folic acid in a multivitamin (relative risk = 0.76; 95% CI = 0.36–1.61) (119).

4.1.4. FOLATE-METABOLIC GENES AND COLORECTAL ADENOMA AND CANCER

4.1.4.1. Methylenetetrahydrofolate Reductase Genetic differences in folate metabolism could influence the risk of CRC. MTHFR is a key enzyme in folate metabolism, and irreversibly catalyzes the reduction of 5,10-methylenetetrahydrofolate to 5-methyltetrahydrofolate, the predominant circulating form of folate and the cofactor for methylation of homocysteine into methionine (Fig. 1; *120*). As described previously, 5,10-methylenetetrahydrofolate also donates a methyl group in the conversion of deoxyuridylate into the thymidylate necessary for DNA synthesis *(1)*.

A common 677C→T polymorphism of the MTHFR gene has been identified that alters a highly conserved amino acid, alanine, to a valine residue *(120)*. The heterozygous (677CT) or homozygous (677TT) polymorphisms of the MTHFR gene correlate with reduced enzyme activity and increased thermolability *(120,121)*. Individuals homozygous for the mutation (677TT) have significantly elevated levels

Table 3
Epidemiologic Studies of the MTHFR 677C→T and Methionine Synthase 2756A→G Polymorphisms
and Colorectal Adenoma and Cancer

Study (Reference), Year	Location	Cases	Endpoints	Gene	Genotypes	Relative Risk (95%CI)
Prospective studies						
Chen et al. (126), 1996	US	144 (M)	Colorectal cancer	MTHFR	TT vs CT/CC	0.57 (0.30–1.06)
Ma et al. (107), 1997	US	202 (M)	Colorectal cancer	MTHFR	TT vs CC	0.45 (0.24–0.86)
					CT vs CC	0.98 (0.67–1.45)
Ma et al. (138), 1999	US	356 (M)	Colorectal cancer	Methionine synthase	GG vs AA	0.59 (0.27–1.27)
					AG vs AA	0.92 (0.67–1.25)
Chen et al. (129), 1998	US	257 (F)	Colorectal adenoma	MTHFR	TT vs CT/CC	1.35 (0.84–2.17)
				Methionine synthase	GG vs AG/AA	0.66 (0.26–1.70)
Case-control studies						
Park et al. (127), 1999	Korea	200	Colorectal cancer	MTHFR	TT vs CT/CC	0.87*
Slattery et al. (128), 1999	US	643 (F)	Colon Cancer	MTHFR	TT vs CC	0.9 (0.6–1.2)
					CT vs CC	1.0 (0.8–1.3)
		824 (M)		MTHFR	TT vs CC	0.8 (0.6–1.1)
					CT vs CC	1.0 (0.9–1.3)
Ulrich et al. (130), 1999	US	200 (F)	Colorectal adenoma	MTHFR	TT vs CC	1.0 (0.6–1.9)
					CT vs CC	0.7 (0.5–1.1)
		327 (M)		MTHFR	TT vs CC	0.7 (0.4–1.3)
					CT vs CC	1.0 (0.7–1.5)
Levine et al. (131), 2000	Los Angeles	471	Colorectal adenoma	MTHFR	TT vs CC	1.11 (0.71–1.71)
					CT vs CC	0.85 (0.65–1.13)
Marugame et al. (132), 2000	Japan	205 (M)	Colorectal adenoma	MTHFR	TT vs CC	1.17 (0.61–2.23)
					CT vs CC	0.87 (0.56–1.34)
Cross-sectional study						
Ulvik et al. (133), 2001	Norway	47	Colorectal adenoma	MTHFR	TT vs CC	2.41 (0.82–7.06)
					CT vs CC	1.51 (0.76–2.99)

*95% CI was not given.

of plasma homocysteine (120,121), which may increase arteriosclerosis (122,123) and coronary vascular disease (121). The MTHFR 677TT genotype frequencies vary greatly in different ethnic groups, with the highest frequency in Hispanics (21–25%), intermediate frequency in other whites (8–18%) and the lowest frequency in Africans (0%) and African-Americans (1–2%) (124). Adequate folate intake is required to reduce the elevated levels of plasma homocysteine associated with the homozygous mutant genotype (677TT) (121,125).

In two large cohorts of male health professionals in the US, men with the MTHFR 677TT genotype had approximately one-half the CRC risk of those with the homozygous wild-type (677CC) or heterozygous (677CT) genotypes (107,126; Table 3). An adequate dietary methyl supply appears to be important for individuals with the 677TT genotype, and the apparent protection associated with this mutation was absent or weak in men who had lower intakes of methionine or folate (126) or who were folate-deficient (107), and was abolished by alcohol consumption (107,126).

When the dietary methyl supply is high, the MTHFR 677TT genotype may be related to reduced risk of CRC because of the increased availability of 5,10-methylenetetrahydrofolate in the DNA synthesis pathway, which reduces misincorporation of U into DNA that might otherwise result in double strand breaks during the U excision processes (107,126). In contrast, when methionine or 5-methyltetrahydrofolate is low because of a deficiency or alcohol consumption, individuals with the 677TT genotype may be less able to develop an adequate methyl supply, resulting in potentially abnormal DNA methylation with subsequent oncogenic alterations (107,126). However, the MTHFR 677TT genotype was not significantly associated with an overall decreased risk of CRC in two case-control studies (127,128). In the latter study, the inverse association was seen only among individuals with a diet high in folate, vitamin B_6, and vitamin B_{12}, and did not differ according to alcohol consumption or methionine intake (128).

The MTHFR 677TT genotype was not significantly associated with a risk of colon adenomas and did not significantly interact with the consumption of folate, methionine, or alcohol in the Nurses' Health Study (129). Three large endoscopy-based case-control studies in the US (130,131) and Japan (132) also found no overall association between the MTHFR 677C→T polymorphism and the risk of colon adenoma. A small cross-sectional investigation in Norway noted a nonsignificant positive association between the MTHFR 677C→T polymorphism and the risk of colon adenomas (133). Low dietary intake of folate, vitamin B_6, vitamin B_{12}, and methionine (130) or low blood levels of folate (131) was associated with an increased risk of colon adenomas only among those with the TT genotype. Similarly, the TT genotype was significantly associated with an increased risk only among individuals with lower RBC folate levels (133). These findings suggest that the MTHFR 677C→T polymorphism is unlikely to play a major role in the earlier stages of colorectal carcinogenesis.

A second common 1298A→C polymorphism in the MTHFR gene with the allele frequency of 33% changes a glutamate into an alanine residue and results in decreased MTHFR activity (134). This recently identified mutation appears to have a synergistic effect with the 677C8→T polymorphism on plasma levels of homocysteine and folate (134), but the relationship to the risk of colon cancer has not yet been determined.

4.1.4.2. Methionine Synthase Methionine synthase, another gene in folate metabolism, has been cloned (135–137), and a common 2756A→G polymorphism that results in substitution of an aspartic acid (D919) by a glycine residue has been identified (136,137). Methionine synthase, a vitamin B_{12}-dependent enzyme, catalyzes the remethylation of homocysteine to methionine using a methyl group donated by 5-methyltetrahydrofolate (Fig. 1; 1). Compared with the MTHFR 677TT genotype, the methionine synthase 2756GG genotype has relatively low frequency ranging from 3–5% among healthy controls from three large prospective cohorts (129,138). In two large cohorts among US male health professionals, the methionine synthase 2756GG genotype was associated with a nonsignificant 41% lower risk of colon cancer relative to the 2756AA genotype (138). There was also a similar interaction with alcohol consumption described here for the MTHFR polymorphism, in which the protective effect of this methionine synthase polymorphism on the risk of colon cancer was absent in men with low plasma folate or high alcohol consumption (138). In the Nurses' Health Study, the polymorphism of methionine synthase was also associated with a nonsignificant lower risk of colorectal adenomas (129).

4.2. Folate and Breast Cancer

Several epidemiologic investigations, including three large prospective cohorts, found that adequate folate intake appeared to be important in breast cancer prevention (139–147), particularly among women who regularly consume alcohol (139–142,146; Table 4).

In the Nurses' Health Study, higher total folate intake was associated with a lower risk among women who consumed >15 g/d of alcohol (relative risk = 0.55; 95% CI = 0.39–0.76; >600 µg/d vs 150–299 µg/d) and among women with a lower methionine intake (139). In this study, current use of multivitamin supplements was also associated with a lower risk among women who consumed >15 g/d of alcohol (relative risk = 0.74; 95% CI = 0.59–0.93; current vs never-users) (139). In the Canadian National Breast Screening Study, the highest quintile intake of dietary folate was associated with a significantly reduced risk of breast cancer relative to the lowest quintile among women who consumed >14 g/d of alcohol (relative risk = 0.34; 95% CI = 0.18–0.61) (140). In the Iowa Women's Health Study, low dietary folate intake was associated with a significantly increased risk of breast cancer among postmenopausal women who consumed >4 g/d of alco-

Table 4
Epidemiologic Studies of Folate and Breast Cancer

Study (Reference), Year	Location	Cases	Exposure	Comparison	Relative Risk (95% CI)
Prospective studies					
Zhang et al. *(139)*, 1999	US	3483	Total folate	>600 vs 150–299 µg/d	0.91 (0.82–1.01)
				By alcohol: <15 g/d	0.98 (0.88–1.10)
				≥15 g/d	0.55 (0.39–0.76)
			Multivitamins	Current vs nonusers	
				By alcohol: <15 g/d	1.01 (0.90–1.14)
				≥15 g/d	0.74 (0.59–0.93)
Rohan et al. *(140)*, 2000	Canada	1469	Dietary folate	Highest vs lowest quintile	0.99(0.79–1.25)
				By alcohol: ≤14 g/d	1.22 (0.94–1.58)
				>14 g/d	0.34 (0.18–0.61)
Sellers et al.*(141)*, 2001	Iowa	1586	Dietary folate	≤172 vs >294 µg/d	1.21 (0.91–1.61)
				By alcohol: 0 g/d	1.08 (0.78–1.49)
				≤4 g/d	1.33 (0.86–2.05)
				>4 g/d	1.59 (1.05–2.41)
Wu et al. *(148)*, 1999	Maryland	1974 cohort:			
		133	Plasma folate	Lowest vs highest quintile	1.08 (0.50–2.37)
		1989 cohort:			
		110	Plasma folate	Lowest vs highest quintile	0.79 (0.33–1.90)
Case-control studies					
Negri et al. *(142)*, 2000	Italy	2569	Dietary folate	Highest vs lowest quintile	0.73 (0.60–0.88)
				By alcohol: <1 g/d	0.79 (0.60–1.06)
				1-25 g/d	0.77 (0.54–1.09)
				≥25 g/d	0.49 (0.32–0.74)
Levi et al. *(146)*, 2001	Vaud, Switzerland	289	Dietary folate	Highest vs lowest tertile	0.45 (0.27–0.74)
				By alcohol: None	0.67 (0.40–1.12)[‡]
				Drinkers	0.55 (0.33–0.92)[‡]
Graham et al.* *(145)*, 1991	Western New York	439	Dietary folate	Highest vs lowest quartile	0.70 (0.48–1.02)
Freudenheim et al.[†] *(144)*, 1996	Western New York	297	Dietary folate	Highest vs lowest quartile	0.50 (0.31–0.82)
			Folate supplements	≥400 g/d vs nonusers	0.97 (0.67–1.42)
Ronco et al. *(143)*, 1999	Uruguay	400	Dietary folate	Highest vs lowest quartile	0.70 (0.46–1.07)
Potischman et al. *(149)*, 1999	US	568	Dietary folate	Highest vs lowest quartile	0.89 (0.7–1.2)
			Total folate		1.11 (0.8–1.5)
Shrubsole et al. *(147)*, 2001	Shanghai, China	1321	Dietary folate	Highest vs lowest quintile	0.71 (0.56–0.92)

[*]Postmenopausal women only
[†]Premenopausal women only
[‡]For a difference in intake between the median of the 3rd tertile and the median of the 1st tertile

hol (relative risk = 1.59; 95% CI = 1.05–2.41) *(141)*. However, in the only published study using prospectively collected blood, plasma levels of folate and homocysteine were not significantly related to the risk of breast cancer *(148)*.

Two large case-control studies in Italy and Switzerland also found the inverse association of folate intake with the risk of breast cancer was modified by alcohol intake *(142,146)*. In the Italian study, the relative risk for folate intake was strongest among women who consumed ≥25 g/d of alcohol (relative risk = 0.49; 95% CI = 0.32–0.74; top vs bottom quintiles) *(142)*. In the Swiss study, the relative risks were 0.67 (95% CI = 0.40–1.12) among nondrinkers and 0.55 (95% CI = 0.33–0.92) among drinkers *(146)*. Several case-control studies reported findings for folate intake and the risk of breast cancer, but did not consider alcohol intake. Two case-control studies in western New York reported that women in the highest quartile of dietary folate had a significant 50% lower risk of premenopausal breast cancer *(144)* and a nonsignificant 30% lower risk of postmenopausal breast cancer *(145)*. In a case-control study in Uruguay, women with the highest intake of folate had a nonsignificant 30% lower risk of breast cancer than those with the lowest intake *(143)*. A large case-control study in Shanghai, China found higher dietary folate intake was associated with a lower risk of breast cancer (relative risk = 0.62; 95% CI = 0.46–0.82; top vs bottom quintiles) *(147)*. However, a case-control investigation in the US observed no association between folate intake and the risk of breast cancer *(149)*.

4.3. Folate and Cervical Dysplasia (Cervical Intraepithelial Neoplasia) and Cancer

In an early report, cytological changes observed in the cervical squamous epithelium of patients with folic acid deficiency were remarkably similar to those observed in patients following radiation therapy, and folic acid supplementation reversed the former changes *(150)*. In another early report on eight patients, daily treatment with 10 mg folic acid for 3 wk reversed the megaloblastic features in cervical smears associated with oral contraceptive use *(151)*. In a small double-blind trial with 47 patients with mild or moderate dysplasia of the uterine cervix, daily supplementation with 10 mg folic acid for 3 mo decreased manifestations of dysplasia and megaloblastosis of the cervix *(152)*. However, in a randomized, double-blind, placebo-controlled trial involving 235 patients with grade 1 or 2 cervical dysplasia, no changes were seen in patients'

dysplasia status, biopsy results, or prevalence of human papillomavirus (HPV) 16 infection after daily supplementation with 10 mg folic acid for 6 mo *(153)*, suggesting that folic acid supplementation may not alter the progress of cervical dysplasia. Another randomized, double-blind, placebo-controlled clinical trial involving 331 patients also showed little reduction in dysplasia grade after daily supplementation with 5 mg folic acid for 6 mo *(154)*.

Epidemiologic studies attempting to relate folate to cervical dysplasia risk have yielded mixed findings (Table 5). In the only published prospective study, higher folate intake was not significantly associated with the risk of cervical dysplasia in either HPV DNA-positive or HPV DNA-negative women *(155)*. In a hospital-based case-control study, high levels of folate in RBCs, serum, and diet were strongly associated with a decreased risk of cervical dysplasia *(156)*. A small study among Native American women in New Mexico reported a strong inverse association between folate intake and the risk of cervical dysplasia *(157)*, but a large investigation conducted later in the same population observed no association between RBC folate levels and risk *(158)*. Two large case-control studies in Alabama found a weak inverse association between blood folate levels *(159)* or dietary folate intake *(160)* and the risk of cervical dysplasia. A small study in New York City noted an inverse association of cervical dysplasia with dietary folate intake, but not with RBC or serum folate levels *(161)*. In a case-control study in Hawaii, higher levels of plasma folate were not associated with a risk of cervical dysplasia *(162)*, whereas higher intakes of dietary folate were strongly inversely associated with risk *(163)*. Two case-control studies that have examined the MTHFR 677C→T polymorphism and the risk of cervical dysplasia showed an increased risk among women with the heterozygous CT genotype or the homozygous TT genotype *(163, 164)*.

In a case-control study in Alabama, Butterworth et al. *(159)* reported that RBC folate levels strongly interacted with HPV infection; and HPV infection was not associated with risk among women with a high RBC folate concentration, it was significantly associated with a fivefold increase in risk of cervical dysplasia among women with a low RBC folate concentration. Similar associations were found in a clinical trial conducted by Butterworth et al. *(153)*. At baseline, the prevalence of HPV 16 infection was 16% among patients in the upper tertile of RBC folate, 32%

Table 5
Epidemiologic Studies of Folate and Cervical Dysplasia Risk

Study (Reference), Year	Location	Cases	Exposure	Comparison	Relative Risk (95% CI)
Prospective study					
Wideroff et al. (155), 1998	Oregon	HPV+			
		68	Dietary folate	Highest vs lowest quartile	0.7 (0.3–2.1)
		HPV⁻			
		146	Dietary folate	Highest vs lowest quartile	1.0 (0.5–1.7)
Case-control studies					
Buckley et al. (157), 1992	New Mexico	42	Dietary folate	Lowest vs highest tertile	3.31 (1.87–5.84)
Yeo et al. (158), 1998	New Mexico	CIN I			
		186	RBC folate	Lowest vs highest quartile	0.7 (0.4–1.3)
		CIN II/III			
		107	RBC folate	Lowest vs highest quartile	0.8 (0.4–1.7)
Butterworth et al. (159), 1992	Alabama	294	RBC folate	Lowest vs highest tertile	1.4 (0.8–2.4)
Liu et al. (160), 1993	Alabama	257	Dietary folate	Lowest vs highest quartile	1.4 (0.7–2.7)
VanEenwyk et al. (156), 1992	Illinois	68	RBC folate	Highest vs lowest quartile	0.1 (0.0–0.4)
		98	Serum folate		0.3 (0.1–1.1)
		100	Dietary folate		0.4 (0.1–1.1)
Kanetsky et al. (161), 1998	New York	27	RBC folate	Highest vs lowest tertile	0.76 (0.17–3.4)
		31	Serum folate		1.50 (0.37–5.8)
		32	Dietary folate		0.28 (0.05–1.7)
Goodman et al. (162), 2000	Hawaii	ASCUS*			
		184	Plasma folate	Highest vs lowest quartile	1.2 (0.6–2.2)
		LSIL†			
		92	Plasma folate	Highest vs lowest quartile	0.8 (0.3–2.3)
		HSIL‡			
		55	Plasma folate	Highest vs lowest quartile	1.5 (0.4–5.9)
Goodman et al. (163), 2001	Hawaii	150	Total folate	Highest vs lowest quartile	0.3 (0.1–0.7)

*Atypical squamous cell of undetermined significance.
†Low-grade squamous intraepithelial lesion.
‡High-grade squamous intraepithelial lesion.

in the middle tertile, and 37% in the bottom tertile; this pattern persisted after daily treatment with 10 mg folic acid for 6 mo. However, no interaction between plasma folate and HPV infection in relation to cervical dysplasia was found in a case-control study in Hawaii (162).

Epidemiologic data on the association between folate and cervical cancer risk are also inconsistent (Table 6). Three case-control studies observed no association (165,166) or a positive association (167) between folate intake and the risk of cervical cancer. The other two studies showed weak protection against

the risk of cervical cancer by dietary folate (168,169). In two case-control studies, long-term use of folate or multivitamin supplements was associated with a lower risk of cervical cancer (166,169). However, two case-control studies relating folate blood levels to the risk of cervical cancer showed no association (170) or an inverse association when blood folate levels were assayed by radiobinding but not by microbiology (171). The only published study to use prospectively collected blood related higher plasma folate levels to a nonsignificant 40% lower risk of cervical cancer; however, the study included only 39 cases (172).

Table 6
Epidemiologic Studies of Folate and Cervical Cancer Risk

Study (Reference), Year	Location	Cases	Exposure	Comparison	Relative Risk (95% CI)
Prospective study					
Alberg et al. (172), 2000	Maryland	39	Plasma folate	Highest vs lowest tertile	0.60 (0.19–1.88)
Case-control studies					
Brock et al. (167), 1988	Sydney, Australia	In situ			
		117	Dietary folate	Highest vs lowest quartile	1.3 (0.3–5.8)
Ziegler et al. (169), 1991	US	In situ			
		228	Dietary folate	Highest vs lowest quartile	0.73*
			Folate supplements	≥16 years vs nonusers	0.49*
			Multivitamins	≥16 years vs nonusers	0.42*
Ziegler et al. (166), 1990	US	218	Dietary folate	Highest vs lowest quartile	1.18*
			Folate supplements	≥15 years vs nonusers	0.74*
			Multivitamins	≥15 years vs nonusers	0.61*
Verreault et al. (168), 1989	Seattle	189	Dietary folate	Highest vs lowest quartile	0.8 (0.3–1.7)
Herrero et al. (165), 1991	Colombia, Mexico, Costa Rica, and Panama	748	Folate-rich foods	Highest vs lowest quartile	0.95 (0.7–1.3)
Potischman et al. (170), 1991	Colombia, Mexico, Costa Rica, and Panama	330	Serum folate	Highest vs lowest quartile	1.05 (0.7–1.6)
Weinstein et al. (171), 2001	US	170	Serum folate	Lowest vs highest quartile	1.27 (0.7–2.3)[†]
		169			1.63 (0.9–2.9)[‡]
		169	RBC folate	Lowest vs highest quartile	1.18 (0.6–2.2)[†]
		162			1.49 (0.8–2.7)[‡]

*95% CI was not given.
[†]Microbiologic assay.
[‡]Radiobinding assay.

4.4. Folate and Pancreatic Cancer

Limited data relate folate to pancreatic cancer risk; three (173–175) of four studies (173–176) observed an inverse association. In the ATBC Cancer Prevention Study cohort, higher dietary folate intake was associated with a significant 48% reduction in risk of pancreatic cancer comparing the highest with the lowest quintile (175). A prospective case-control study nested within this cohort found higher levels of serum folate associated with a significant 55% lower risk (174). A significant inverse association between total folate intake and the risk of pancreatic cancer was also observed in a population-based case-control study in Adelaide, South Australia (173). However, a large US population-based case-control investigation observed no association between intakes of folate or multivitamin supplements and the risk of pancreatic cancer (176).

4.5. Folate and Acute Lymphoblastic Leukemia (ALL)

A recent population-based case-control study of 83 cases of ALL in children 0–14 yr of age in western Australia from 1984–1992 showed that iron or folate supplementation during pregnancy conferred a significant 63% reduction in risk of ALL on the child (177). The protective effect is mostly the result of folate, because iron use alone was only weakly protective

(177). In a British case-control study of adult acute lymphocytic leukemia, the MTHFR 677TT genotype was associated with a significant 77% lower risk *(178)*. In this study, the authors also observed a significant 67% reduction in risk of acute lymphocytic leukemia in individuals with the MTHFR 1298AC genotype and a significant 93% reduction with the MTHFR 1298CC genotype *(178)*. As seen with the relationship between the MTHFR 677TT genotype and CRC the MTHFR 677C→T polymorphism appears to reduce risk of acute lymphocytic leukemia; both cancers are derived from rapidly proliferating tissues that have high demands for DNA synthesis.

4.6. Folate and Lung cancer

In a randomized, double-blind, placebo-controlled clinical trial among 73 male smokers, treatment with 10 mg of folate plus 500 µg of vitamin B_{12} for 4 mo significantly reduced bronchial squamous metaplasia *(179)*. In addition, lower levels of plasma folate were found among smokers with bronchial squamous metaplasia than among those without metaplasia *(180)*.

Two studies that related folate intake to the risk of lung cancer support the findings concerning premalignant lesions. In the New York State cohort, individuals in the highest tertile of folate intake had a significant 30% lower risk of lung cancer than those in the lowest tertile *(181)*. This association was limited to squamous cell carcinoma and was strong among smokers *(181)*. A nonsignificant inverse association between folate intake and the risk of lung cancer was also seen in a population-based case-control study in Hawaii *(182)*. However, three studies that related blood folate levels to the risk of lung cancer observed either no association *(183,184)* or a positive association *(185)*. In a prospective case-control study nested within the ATBC Cancer Prevention Study cohort among male smokers, higher levels of serum folate were not associated with lung cancer risk; the relative risk was 0.96 (95% CI = 0.52–1.79) comparing highest to lowest quintile *(183)*. There were no differences in serum and RBC folate levels or the MTHFR polymorphism frequencies between lung cancer cases and controls in a hospital based case-control study in Boston *(184)*. Serum folate levels were found to be higher in patients with lung cancer than in normal control subjects in a hospital-based case-control study in Turkey *(185)*. In a non-population-based case-control study, although patients with lung cancer consumed significantly less folate than controls, the MTHFR 677C→T and 1298A→C

polymorphisms were not associated with the risk of lung cancer, even among individuals with low folate intake and high alcohol consumption *(186)*.

5. FOOD FORTIFICATION POLICY IMPLICATIONS

Possible ways to improve folate status include increasing intake of vegetables and fruits, fortification of grain products, and use of folic acid or multivitamin supplements. Multivitamin supplements in the US usually contain 400 µg of folic acid per tablet. Folic acid used in fortification and supplements is in the form of monoglutamate, which bypasses deconjugation and is thus more bioavailable than dietary folate *(187)*. Cuskelly et al. *(96)* reported that RBC folate concentrations increased significantly over a period of 3 mo among women who took an additional daily 400 µg of folic acid from supplements or foods fortified with folic acid; such an increase was not seen among women taking additional daily 400 µg of dietary folate.

Mandatory fortification of grain products with folic acid by the addition of 140 µg/100 g of flour was introduced in the US in January 1998 *(188)*, a policy expected to increase average per-person intake by 100 µg/d *(189)* and to reduce the occurrence of neural tube defects *(190)*. Food fortification with folic acid was associated with a substantial improvement in folate status in the Framingham Offspring Study cohort, a middle-aged and older population *(191)*. From 1994–1998, median serum folate values in blood specimens submitted to Kaiser Permanente's southern California Endocrinology Laboratory also increased from 12.6–18.7 µg/L, and the percentage of low values decreased *(192)*. Food fortification with folic acid is a likely explanation, because these changes occurred mostly during 1997–1998 *(192)*.

Folate intake after food fortification with folic acid was estimated from two national surveys that took into consideration the food fortification and the apparently high bioavailability of synthetic folic acid *(193)*. Estimated median intakes of folate from the 1988–1994 NHANES III were 455 µg/d for women ages 20–49 yr, 441 µg/d for women ages >70 yr, 504 µg/d for men ages 45–69 yr, and 470 µg/d for men ages >70 yr *(193)*. Similar findings were also noted in another national survey, the 1994–1996 Continuing Survey of Food Intakes by Individuals (CSFII) *(193)*. With fortification, folate intake among adult populations on average meet Dietary Reference Intakes (DRIs) of 400 µg/d *(194)*, although about one-fourth of adults still consumed an amount below the DRIs *(193)*. Optimal folate intake for cancer prevention remains uncertain. Although 400 µg/d minimizes blood homocysteine levels in most people *(195)*, more may be needed to minimize cancer risk.

6. SAFETY

Folate is generally considered safe. However, folate supplementation in excess of 5 mg/d may mask the hematologic manifestations of vitamin B_{12} deficiency, allowing neurologic damage progress secondary to undiagnosed pernicious anemia *(196)*. This concern is based on numerous case reports, and some case series that suggest that the neurologic complications of vitamin B_{12} deficiency worsen when folic acid alone is supplemented and not vitamin B_{12} *(196)*.

Some medications, including methotrexate and aminopterin (anticancer, immunosuppressive, and antipsoriasis), pyrimethamine (antimalarial), trimethoprim (antibacterial), and triamterence (diuretic), directly interfere with folate metabolism by inhibiting the enzyme folate reductase *(197,198)*. Sulfasalazine, a drug used to treat rheumatic arthritis and inflammatory bowel disease, reduces folate intestinal absorption through inhibition of folate conjugase on the brush border membrane *(199–202)*. Other medications, including many anticonvulsants (phenytoin, phenobarbital, and primidone), cycloserine (antituberculosis), oral contraceptives, and colchicine (anti-acute gout), also impair folate metabolism by uncertain mechanisms *(197,198)*. Folate supplementation during drug therapy may reduce some of the side effects associated with folate deficiency *(203)*, but in some cases might interfere with the intended effects.

7. SUMMARY

Data from molecular and biological studies, animal studies, randomized trials using intermediate endpoints, and observational epidemiologic studies strongly suggest that folate may have a chemopreventive role in colon carcinogenesis. Emerging epidemiologic data also suggest that adequate folate status may reduce the risk of breast cancer, particularly among women who are at increased risk because of regular alcohol consumption. Epidemiologic data on folate and pancreatic cancer are limited but promising. The establishment of folate as a protective factor for pancreatic cancer would be important because it is difficult to treat pancreatic cancer effectively. Data on folate and acute lymphoblastic leukemia are also limited, but promising. Finally, available data do not support an important link between folate and incidence of either cervical or lung cancer.

The effectiveness of current folate fortification in the US may have an unplanned positive impact on cancer prevention. However, the impact of fortification on the incidence of cancer depends critically on the quantitative dose-response relationship between folate intake and cancer risk. Substantial evidence suggests that this dose-response relationship may vary according to alcohol consumption, the MTHFR genotypes, and other genotypes yet to be identified. Supplementation with 0.4–1.0 mg folic acid daily appears to be a safe, cheap, and effective method to improve folate status when an optimal supply of folate cannot be achieved through the diet.

REFERENCES

1. Selhub J, Rosenberg IH. Folic acid, in *Present Knowledge in Nutrition, 7th ed.* Ziegler EE, Filer LJ Jr, eds. International Life Sciences Institute Press, Washington, DC, 1996, pp. 206–219.

2. Dugdale M. Anemia. *Obstet Gynecol Clin North Am* 2001;28:363–381.

3. MRC Vitamin Study Research Group. Prevention of neural tube defects: results of the Medical Research Council Vitamin Study. *Lancet* 1991;338:131–137.

4. Czeizel AE, Dudas I. Prevention of the first occurrence of neural-tube defects by periconceptional vitamin supplementation. *N Engl J Med* 1992;327:1832–1835.

5. Kim YI. Folate and carcinogenesis: evidence, mechanisms, and implications. *J Nutr Biochem* 1999;10:66–88.

6. Halsted CH. The intestinal absorption of dietary folates in health and disease. *J Am Coll Nutr* 1989;8:650–658.

7. Said HM, Ghishan FK, Redha R. Folate transport by human intestinal brush-border membrane vesicles. *Am J Physiol* 1987;252:G229–G236.

8. Nguyen TT, Dyer DL, Dunning DD, et al. Human intestinal folate transport: cloning, expression, and distribution of complementary RNA. *Gastroenterology* 1997;112:783–791.

9. Russell RM, Dhar GJ, Dutta SK, Rosenberg IH. Influence of intraluminal pH on folate absorption: studies in control subjects and in patients with pancreatic insufficiency. *J Lab Clin Med* 1979;93:428–436.

10. Chanarin I, Perry J. Evidence for reduction and methylation of folate in the intestine during normal absorption. *Lancet* 1969;2:776–778.

11. Corrocher R, Olivieri O, Pacor ML. The folate binding proteins. *Haematologica* 1991;76:500–504.

12. Antony AC. Folate receptors. *Annu Rev Nutr* 1996;16:501–521.

13. Birn H, Selhub J, Christensen EI. Internalization and intracellular transport of folate-binding protein in rat kidney proximal tubule. *Am J Physiol* 1993;264:C302–C310.

14. Selhub J. Folate binding proteins. Mechanisms for placental and intestinal uptake. *Adv Exp Med Biol* 1994;352:141–149.

15. Hillman RS, Steinberg SE. The effects of alcohol on folate metabolism. *Annu Rev Med* 1982;33:345–354.

16. Weir DG, McGing PG, Scott JM. Folate metabolism, the enterohepatic circulation and alcohol. *Biochem Pharmacol* 1985;34:1–7.

17. Sullivan LW, Herbert V. Suppression of hematopoiesis by ethanol. *J Clin Invest* 1964;43:2048–2062.

18. Eichner ER, Pierce HI, Hillman RS. Folate balance in dietary-induced megaloblastic anemia. *N Engl J Med* 1971;284:933–938.

19. Eichner ER, Hillman RS. Effect of alcohol on serum folate level. *J Clin Invest* 1973;52:584–591.

20. Jacques PF, Sulsky S, Hartz SC, Russell RM. Moderate alcohol intake and nutritional status in nonalcoholic elderly subjects. *Am J Clin Nutr* 1989;50:875–883.

21. Shaw S, Jayatilleke E, Herbert V, Colman N. Cleavage of folates during ethanol metabolism. Role of acetaldehyde/xanthine oxidase-generated superoxide. *Biochem J* 1989;257:277–280.

22. Guynn RW, Labaume LB, Henkin J. Equilibrium constants under physiological conditions for the condensation of acetaldehyde with tetrahydrofolic acid. *Arch Biochem Biophys* 1982;217:181–190.

23. Hidiroglou N, Camilo ME, Beckenhauer HC, et al. Effect of chronic alcohol ingestion on hepatic folate distribution in the rat. *Biochem Pharmacol* 1994;47:1561–1566.

24. Barak AJ, Beckenhauer HC, Hidiroglou N, et al. The relationship of ethanol feeding to the methyl folate trap. *Alcohol* 1993;10:495–497.

25. Jokelainen K, Roine RP, Vaananen H, et al. In vitro acetaldehyde formation by human colonic bacteria. *Gut* 1994;35:1271–1274.

26. Salaspuro M. Bacteriocolonic pathway for ethanol oxidation: characteristics and implications. *Ann Med* 1996;28:195–200.

27. Salaspuro V, Nyfors S, Heine R, et al. Ethanol oxidation and acetaldehyde production in vitro by human intestinal strains of *Escherichia coli* under aerobic, microaerobic, and anaerobic conditions. *Scand J Gastroenterol* 1999;34:967–973.

28. Homann N, Tillonen J, Salaspuro M. Microbially produced acetaldehyde from ethanol may increase the risk of colon cancer via folate deficiency. *Int J Cancer* 2000;86:169–173.

29. Giovannucci E, Stampfer MJ, Colditz GA, et al. Folate, methionine, and alcohol intake and risk of colorectal adenoma. *J Natl Cancer Inst* 1993;85:875–884.

30. Baron JA, Sandler RS, Haile RW, et al. Folate intake, alcohol consumption, cigarette smoking, and risk of colorectal adenomas. *J Natl Cancer Inst* 1998;90:57–62.

31. Giovannucci E, Rimm EB, Ascherio A, et al. Alcohol, low-methionine-low-folate diets, and risk of colon cancer in men. *J Natl Cancer Inst* 1995;87:265–273.

32. Smith-Warner SA, Spiegelman D, Yaun S-S, et al. Alcohol and breast cancer in women: a pooled analysis of cohort studies. *JAMA* 1998;279:535–540.

33. Singletary KW, Gapstur SM. Alcohol and breast cancer: review of epidemiologic and experimental evidence and potential mechanisms. *JAMA* 2001;286:2143–2151.

34. Bandera EV, Freudenheim JL, Vena JE. Alcohol consumption and lung cancer: a review of the epidemiologic evidence. *Cancer Epidemiol Biomark Prev* 2001;10:813–821.

35. Wickramasinghe SN, Fida S. Bone marrow cells from vitamin B_{12}- and folate-deficient patients misincorporate uracil into DNA. *Blood* 1994;83:1656–1661.

36. Blount BC, Mack MM, Wehr CM, et al. Folate deficiency causes uracil misincorporation into human DNA and chromosome breakage: implications for cancer and neuronal damage. *Proc Natl Acad Sci USA* 1997;94:3290–3295.

37. Choi SW, Kim YI, Weitzel JN, Mason JB. Folate depletion impairs DNA excision repair in the colon of the rat. *Gut* 1998;43:93–99.

38. James SJ, Yin L, Swendseid ME. DNA strand break accumulation, thymidylate synthesis and NAD levels in lymphocytes from methyl donor-deficient rats. *J Nutr* 1989;119:661–664.

39. Pogribny IP, Basnakian AG, Miller BJ, et al. Breaks in genomic DNA and within the p53 gene are associated with hypomethylation in livers of folate/methyl-deficient rats. *Cancer* Res 1995;55:1894–1901.

40. Kim YI, Pogribny IP, Basnakian AG, et al. Folate deficiency in rats induces DNA strand breaks and hypomethylation within the p53 tumor suppressor gene. *Am J Clin Nutr* 1997;65:46–52.

41. Kim YI, Shirwadkar S, Choi SW, et al. Effects of dietary folate on DNA strand breaks within mutation-prone exons of the p53 gene in rat colon. *Gastroenterology* 2000;119:151–161.

42. Baker SJ, Fearon ER, Nigro JM, et al. Chromosome 17 deletions and p53 gene mutations in colorectal carcinomas. *Science* 1989;244:217–221.

43. Fearon ER, Vogelstein B. A genetic model for colorectal tumorigenesis. *Cell* 1990;61:759–767.

44. Fearon ER, Jones PA. Progressing toward a molecular description of colorectal cancer development. *FASEB J* 1992;6:2783–2790.

45. Soussi T. The p53 tumor suppressor gene: from molecular biology to clinical investigation. *Ann NY Acad Sci* 2000;910:137–139.

46. Vogelstein B, Lane D, Levine AJ. Surfing the p53 network. *Nature* 2000;408:307–310.

47. Kim YI, Baik HW, Fawaz K, et al. Effects of folate supplementation on two provisional molecular markers of colon cancer: a prospective, randomized trial. *Am J Gastroenterol* 2001;96:184–195.

48. Biasco G, Zannoni U, Paganelli GM, et al. Folic acid supplementation and cell kinetics of rectal mucosa in patients with ulcerative colitis. *Cancer Epidemiol Biomark Prev* 1997;6:469–471.

49. Fenech M, Aitken C, Rinaldi J. Folate, vitamin B_{12}, homocysteine status and DNA damage in young Australian adults. *Carcinogenesis* 1998;19:1163–1171.

50. Baylin SB, Herman JG. DNA hypermethylation in tumorigenesis: epigenetics joins genetics. *Trends Genet* 2000;16:168–174.

51. Wajed SA, Laird PW, DeMeester TR. DNA methylation: an alternative pathway to cancer. *Ann Surg* 2001;234:10–20.

52. Jones PA, Laird PW. Cancer epigenetics comes of age. *Nat Genet* 1999;21:163–167.

53. Robertson KD. DNA methylation, methyltransferases, and cancer. *Oncogene* 2001;20:3139–3155.

54. Herman JG, Merlo A, Mao L, et al. Inactivation of the CDKN2/p16/MTS1 gene is frequently associated with

aberrant DNA methylation in all common human cancers. *Cancer Res* 1995;55:4525–4530.

55. Herman JG, Umar A, Polyak K, et al. Incidence and functional consequences of hMLH1 promoter hypermethylation in colorectal carcinoma. *Proc Natl Acad Sci USA* 1998;95:6870–6875.

56. Veigl ML, Kasturi L, Olechnowicz J, et al. Biallelic inactivation of hMLH1 by epigenetic gene silencing, a novel mechanism causing human MSI cancers. *Proc Natl Acad Sci USA* 1998;95:8698–8702.

57. Cunningham JM, Christensen ER, Tester DJ, et al. Hypermethylation of the hMLH1 promoter in colon cancer with microsatellite instability. *Cancer Res* 1998;58:3455–3460.

58. Toyota M, Ahuja N, Ohe-Toyota M, et al. CpG island methylator phenotype in colorectal cancer. *Proc Natl Acad Sci USA* 1999;96:8681–8686.

59. Rashid A, Shen L, Morris JS, et al. CpG island methylation in colorectal adenomas. *Am J Pathol* 2001;159:1129–1135.

60. Tornaletti S, Pfeifer GP. Complete and tissue-independent methylation of CpG sites in the p53 gene: implications for mutations in human cancers. *Oncogene* 1995;10:1493–1499.

61. Frederico LA, Kunkel TA, Shaw BR. A sensitive genetic assay for the detection of cytosine deamination: determination of rate constants and the activation energy. *Biochemistry* 1990;29:2532–2537.

62. Laird PW, Jackson-Grusby L, Fazeli A, et al. Suppression of intestinal neoplasia by DNA hypomethylation. *Cell* 1995;81:197–205.

63. Feinberg AP, Vogelstein B. Hypomethylation distinguishes genes of some human cancers from their normal counterparts. *Nature* 1983;301:89–92.

64. Goelz SE, Vogelstein B, Hamilton SR, Feinberg AP. Hypomethylation of DNA from benign and malignant human colon neoplasms. *Science* 1985;228:187–190.

65. Feinberg AP, Gehrke CW, Kuo KC, Ehrlich M. Reduced genomic 5-methylcytosine content in human colonic neoplasia. *Cancer Res* 1988;48:1159–1161.

66. Cravo M, Fidalgo P, Pereira AD, et al. DNA methylation as an intermediate biomarker in colorectal cancer: modulation by folic acid supplementation. *Eur J Cancer Prev* 1994;3:473–479.

67. Glória L, Cravo M, Pinto A, et al. DNA hypomethylation and proliferative activity are increased in the rectal mucosa of patients with long-standing ulcerative colitis. *Cancer* 1996;78:2300–2306.

68. Cravo M, Pinto R, Fidalgo P, et al. Global DNA hypomethylation occurs in the early stages of intestinal type gastric carcinoma. *Gut* 1996;39:434–438.

69. Kim YI, Giuliano A, Hatch KD, et al. Global DNA hypomethylation increases progressively in cervical dysplasia and carcinoma. *Cancer* 1994;74:893–899.

70. Soares J, Pinto AE, Cunha CV, et al. Global DNA hypomethylation in breast carcinoma: correlation with prognostic factors and tumor progression. *Cancer* 1999;85:112–118.

71. Schmid M, Haaf T, Grunert D. 5-azacytidine-induced undercondensations in human chromosomes. *Hum Genet* 1984;67:257–263.

72. Feinberg AP, Vogelstein B. Hypomethylation of ras oncogenes in primary human cancers. *Biochem Biophys Res Commun* 1983;111:47–54.

73. Sharrard RM, Royds JA, Rogers S, Shorthouse AJ. Patterns of methylation of the c-*myc* gene in human colorectal cancer progression. *Br J Cancer* 1992;65:667–672.

74. Rogers AE. Methyl donors in the diet and responses to chemical carcinogens. *Am J Clin Nutr* 1995;61:659S–665S.

75. Mikol YB, Hoover KL, Creasia D, Poirier LA. Hepatocarcinogenesis in rats fed methyl-deficient, amino acid-defined diets. *Carcinogenesis* 1983;4:1619–1629.

76. Ghoshal AK, Farber E. The induction of liver cancer by dietary deficiency of choline and methionine without added carcinogens. *Carcinogenesis* 1984;5:1367–1370.

77. Wainfan E, Dizik M, Stender M, Christman JK. Rapid appearance of hypomethylated DNA in livers of rats fed cancer-promoting, methyl-deficient diets. *Cancer Res* 1989;49:4094–4097.

78. Dizik M, Christman JK, Wainfan E. Alterations in expression and methylation of specific genes in livers of rats fed a cancer promoting methyl-deficient diet. *Carcinogenesis* 1991;12:1307–1312.

79. Wainfan E, Poirier LA. Methyl groups in carcinogenesis: effects on DNA methylation and gene expression. *Cancer Res* 1992;52:2071s–2077s.

80. Christman JK, Sheikhnejad G, Dizik M, et al. Reversibility of changes in nucleic acid methylation and gene expression induced in rat liver by severe dietary methyl deficiency. *Carcinogenesis* 1993;14:551–557.

81. Cravo ML, Pinto AG, Chaves P, et al. Effect of folate supplementation on DNA methylation of rectal mucosa in patients with colonic adenomas: correlation with nutrient intake. *Clin Nutr* 1998;17:45–49.

82. Rogers AE, Nauss KM. Rodent models for carcinoma of the colon. *Dig Dis Sci* 1985;30:87S–102S.

83. Ahnen DJ. Are animal models of colon cancer relevant to human disease. *Dig Dis Sci* 1985;30:103S–106S.

84. Yander G, Halsey H, Kenna M, Augenlicht LH. Amplification and elevated expression of c-*myc* in a chemically induced mouse colon tumor. *Cancer Res* 1985;45:4433–4438.

85. Caignard A, Kitagawa Y, Sato S, Nagao M. Activated K-*ras* in tumorigenic and non-tumorigenic cell variants from a rat colon adenocarcinoma, induced by dimethylhydrazine. *Jpn J Cancer Res* 1988;79:244–249.

86. Cravo ML, Mason JB, Dayal Y, et al. Folate deficiency enhances the development of colonic neoplasia in dimethylhydrazine-treated rats. *Cancer Res* 1992;52:5002–5006.

87. Kim YI, Salomon RN, Graeme-Cook F, et al. Dietary folate protects against the development of macroscopic colonic neoplasia in a dose responsive manner in rats. *Gut* 1996;39:732–740.

88. Vogelstein B, Fearon ER, Hamilton SR, et al. Genetic alterations during colorectal-tumor development. *N Engl J Med* 1988;319:525–532.

89. Atkin WS, Morson BC, Cuzick J. Long-term risk of colorectal cancer after excision of rectosigmoid adenomas. *N Engl J Med* 1992;326:658–662.

90. Benito E, Cabeza E, Moreno V, et al. Diet and colorectal adenomas: a case-control study in Majorca. *Int J Cancer* 1993;55:213–219.

91. Bird CL, Swendseid ME, Witte JS, et al. Red cell and plasma folate, folate consumption, and the risk of colorectal adenomatous polyps. *Cancer Epidemiol Biomark Prev* 1995;4:709–714.

92. Tseng M, Murray SC, Kupper LL, Sandler RS. Micronutrients and the risk of colorectal adenomas. *Am J Epidemiol* 1996;144:1005–1014.

93. Boutron-Ruault MC, Senesse P, Faivre J, et al. Folate and alcohol intakes: related or independent roles in the adenoma-carcinoma sequence? *Nutr Cancer* 1996;26:337–346.

94. Whelan RL, Horvath KD, Gleason NR, et al. Vitamin and calcium supplement use is associated with decreased adenoma recurrence in patients with a previous history of neoplasia. *Dis Colon Rectum* 1999;42:212–217.

95. Neugut AI, Horvath K, Whelan RL, et al. The effect of calcium and vitamin supplements on the incidence and recurrence of colorectal adenomatous polyps. *Cancer* 1996;78:723–728.

96. Cuskelly GJ, McNulty H, Scott JM. Effect of increasing dietary folate on red-cell folate: implications for prevention of neural tube defects. *Lancet* 1996;347:657–659.

97. Wald DS, Bishop L, Wald NJ, et al. Randomized trial of folic acid supplementation and serum homocysteine levels. *Arch Intern Med* 2001;161:695–700.

98. Kim YI, Fawaz K, Knox T, et al. Colonic mucosal concentrations of folate correlate well with blood measurements of folate status in persons with colorectal polyps. *Am J Clin Nutr* 1998;68:866–872.

99. Kim YI, Fawaz K, Knox T, et al. Colonic mucosal concentrations of folate are accurately predicted by blood measurements of folate status among individuals ingesting physiologic quantities of folate. *Cancer Epidemiol Biomark Prev* 2001;10:715–719.

100. Paspatis GA, Kalafatis E, Oros L, et al. Folate status and adenomatous colonic polyps. A colonoscopically controlled study. *Dis Colon Rectum* 1995;38:64–67.

101. Paspatis GA, Karamanolis DG. Folate supplementation and adenomatous colonic polyps. *Dis Colon Rectum* 1994;37:1340–1341.

102. Glynn SA, Albanes D, Pietinen P, et al. Colorectal cancer and folate status: a nested case-control study among male smokers. *Cancer Epidemiol Biomark Prev* 1996;5:487–494.

103. Giovannucci E, Stampfer MJ, Colditz GA, et al. Multivitamin use, folate, and colon cancer in women in the Nurses' Health Study. *Ann Intern Med* 1998;129:517–524.

104. Kato I, Dnistrian AM, Schwartz M, et al. Serum folate, homocysteine and colorectal cancer risk in women: a nested case-control study. *Br J Cancer* 1999;79:1917–1922.

105. Su LJ, Arab L. Nutritional status of folate and colon cancer risk: evidence from NHANES I epidemiologic follow-up study. *Ann Epidemiol* 2001;11:65–72.

106. Kim DH, Smith-Warner SA, Hunter DJ. Pooled analysis of prospective cohort studies on folate and colorectal cancer. *Am J Epidemiol* 2001;153:S118.

107. Ma J, Stampfer MJ, Giovannucci E, et al. Methylenetetrahydrofolate reductase polymorphism, dietary interactions, and risk of colorectal cancer. *Cancer Res* 1997;57:1098–1102.

108. Benito E, Stiggelbout A, Bosch FX, et al. Nutritional factors in colorectal cancer risk: a case-control study in Majorca. *Int J Cancer* 1991;49:161–167.

109. Freudenheim JL, Graham S, Marshall JR, et al. Folate intake and carcinogenesis of the colon and rectum. *Int J Epidemiol* 1991;20:368–374.

110. Ferraroni M, La Vecchia C, D'Avanzo B, et al. Selected micronutrient intake and the risk of colorectal cancer. *Br J Cancer* 1994;70:1150–1155.

111. Meyer F, White E. Alcohol and nutrients in relation to colon cancer in middle-aged adults. *Am J Epidemiol* 1993;138:225–236.

112. White E, Shannon JS, Patterson RE. Relationship between vitamin and calcium supplement use and colon cancer. *Cancer Epidemiol Biomark Prev* 1997;6:769–774.

113. Slattery ML, Schaffer D, Edwards SL, et al. Are dietary factors involved in DNA methylation associated with colon cancer? *Nutr Cancer* 1997;28:52–62.

114. Ghosh S, Shand A, Ferguson A. Ulcerative colitis. *Br Med J* 2000;320:1119–1123.

115. Eaden JA, Mayberry JF. Colorectal cancer complicating ulcerative colitis: a review. *Am J Gastroenterol* 2000;95:2710–2719.

116. Eaden JA, Abrams KR, Mayberry JF. The risk of colorectal cancer in ulcerative colitis: a meta-analysis. *Gut* 2001;48:526–535.

117. Lashner BA, Heidenreich PA, Su GL, et al. Effect of folate supplementation on the incidence of dysplasia and cancer in chronic ulcerative colitis. A case-control study. *Gastroenterology* 1989;97:255–259.

118. Lashner BA. Red blood cell folate is associated with the development of dysplasia and cancer in ulcerative colitis. *J Cancer Res Clin Oncol* 1993;119:549–554.

119. Lashner BA, Provencher KS, Seidner DL, et al. The effect of folic acid supplementation on the risk for cancer or dysplasia in ulcerative colitis. *Gastroenterology* 1997;112:29–32.

120. Frosst P, Blom HJ, Milos R, et al. A candidate genetic risk factor for vascular disease: a common mutation in methylenetetrahydrofolate reductase. *Nat Genet* 1995;10:111–113.

121. Christensen B, Frosst P, Lussier-Cacan S, et al. Correlation of a common mutation in the methylenetetrahydrofolate reductase gene with plasma homocysteine in patients with premature coronary artery disease. *Arterioscler Thromb Vasc Biol* 1997;17:569–573.

122. Kang SS, Wong PW, Malinow MR. Hyperhomocyst(e)inemia as a risk factor for occlusive vascular disease. *Annu Rev Nutr* 1992;12:279–298.

123. Malinow MR, Duell PB, Hess DL, et al. Reduction of plasma homocyst(e)ine levels by breakfast cereal fortified with folic acid in patients with coronary heart disease. *N Engl J Med* 1998;338:1009–1015.

124. Botto LD, Yang Q. 5,10-Methylenetetrahydrofolate reductase gene variants and congenital anomalies: a HuGE review. *Am J Epidemiol* 2000;151:862–877.

125. Jacques PF, Bostom AG, Williams RR, et al. Relation between folate status, a common mutation in methylenetetrahydrofolate reductase, and plasma homocysteine concentrations. *Circulation* 1996;93:7–9.

126. Chen J, Giovannucci E, Kelsey K, et al. A methylenetetrahydrofolate reductase polymorphism and the risk of colorectal cancer. *Cancer Res* 1996;56:4862–4864.

127. Park KS, Mok JW, Kim JC. The 677C > T mutation in 5,10-methylenetetrahydrofolate reductase and colorectal cancer risk. *Genet Test* 1999;3:233–236.

128. Slattery ML, Potter JD, Samowitz W, et al. Methylenetetrahydrofolate reductase, diet, and risk of

colon cancer. *Cancer Epidemiol Biomark Prev* 1999;8:513–518.

129. Chen J, Giovannucci E, Hankinson SE, et al. A prospective study of methylenetetrahydrofolate reductase and methionine synthase gene polymorphisms, and risk of colorectal adenoma. *Carcinogenesis* 1998;19:2129–2132.

130. Ulrich CM, Kampman E, Bigler J, et al. Colorectal adenomas and the C677T MTHFR polymorphism: evidence for gene-environment interaction? *Cancer Epidemiol Biomark Prev* 1999;8:659–668.

131. Levine AJ, Siegmund KD, Ervin CM, et al. The methylenetetrahydrofolate reductase 677C—>T polymorphism and distal colorectal adenoma risk. *Cancer Epidemiol Biomark Prev* 2000;9:657–663.

132. Marugame T, Tsuji E, Inoue H, et al. Methylenetetrahydrofolate reductase polymorphism and risk of colorectal adenomas. *Cancer Lett* 2000;151:181–186.

133. Ulvik A, Evensen ET, Lien EA, et al. Smoking, folate and methylenetetrahydrofolate reductase status as interactive determinants of adenomatous and hyperplastic polyps of colorectum. *Am J Med Genet* 2001;101:246–254.

134. van der Put NM, Gabreels F, Stevens EM, et al. A second common mutation in the methylenetetrahydrofolate reductase gene: an additional risk factor for neural-tube defects? *Am J Hum Genet* 1998;62:1044–1051.

135. Li YN, Gulati S, Baker PJ, et al. Cloning, mapping and RNA analysis of the human methionine synthase gene. *Hum Mol Genet* 1996;5:1851–1858.

136. Leclerc D, Campeau E, Goyette P, et al. Human methionine synthase: cDNA cloning and identification of mutations in patients of the cblG complementation group of folate/cobalamin disorders. *Hum Mol Genet* 1996;5:1867–1874.

137. Chen LH, Liu ML, Hwang HY, et al. Human methionine synthase. cDNA cloning, gene localization, and expression. *J Biol Chem* 1997;272:3628–3634.

138. Ma J, Stampfer MJ, Christensen B, et al. A polymorphism of the methionine synthase gene: association with plasma folate, vitamin B12, homocyst(e)ine, and colorectal cancer risk. *Cancer Epidemiol Biomark Prev* 1999;8:825–829.

139. Zhang S, Hunter DJ, Hankinson SE, et al. A prospective study of folate intake and the risk of breast cancer. *JAMA* 1999;281:1632–1637.

140. Rohan TE, Jain MG, Howe GR, Miller AB. Dietary folate consumption and breast cancer risk. *J Natl Cancer Inst* 2000;92:266–269.

141. Sellers TA, Kushi LH, Cerhan JR, et al. Dietary folate intake, alcohol, and risk of breast cancer in a prospective study of postmenopausal women. *Epidemiology* 2001;12:420–428.

142. Negri E, La Vecchia C, Franceschi S. Re: dietary folate consumption and breast cancer risk. *J Natl Cancer Inst* 2000;92:1270–1271.

143. Ronco A, De Stefani E, Boffetta P, et al. Vegetables, fruits, and related nutrients and risk of breast cancer: a case-control study in Uruguay. *Nutr Cancer* 1999;35:111–119.

144. Freudenheim JL, Marshall JR, Vena JE, et al. Premenopausal breast cancer risk and intake of vegetables, fruits, and related nutrients. *J Natl Cancer Inst* 1996;88:340–348.

145. Graham S, Hellmann R, Marshall J, et al. Nutritional epidemiology of postmenopausal breast cancer in Western New York. *Am J Epidemiol* 1991;134:552–566.

146. Levi F, Pasche C, Lucchini F, La Vecchia C. Dietary intake of selected micronutrients and breast-cancer risk. *Int J Cancer* 2001;91:260–263.

147. Shrubsole MJ, Jin F, Dai Q, et al. Dietary folate intake and breast cancer risk: results from the Shanghai breast cancer study. *Cancer Res* 2001;61:7136–7141.

148. Wu K, Helzlsouer KJ, Comstock GW, et al. A prospective study on folate, B$_{12}$, and pyridoxal 5'-phosphate (B6) and breast cancer. *Cancer Epidemiol Biomark Prev* 1999;8:209–217.

149. Potischman N, Swanson CA, Coates RJ, et al. Intake of food groups and associated micronutrients in relation to risk of early-stage breast cancer. *Int J Cancer* 1999;82:315–321.

150. Van Niekerk WA. Cervical cytological abnormalities caused by folic acid deficiency. *Acta Cytol* 1966;10:67–73.

151. Whitehead N, Reyner F, Lindenbaum J. Megaloblastic changes in the cervical epithelium. Association with oral contraceptive therapy and reversal with folic acid. *JAMA* 1973;226:1421–1424.

152. Butterworth CE Jr, Hatch KD, Gore H, et al. Improvement in cervical dysplasia associated with folic acid therapy in users of oral contraceptives. *Am J Clin Nutr* 1982;35:73–82.

153. Butterworth CE Jr, Hatch KD, Soong SJ, et al. Oral folic acid supplementation for cervical dysplasia: a clinical intervention trial. *Am J Obstet Gynecol* 1992;166:803–809.

154. Childers JM, Chu J, Voigt LF, et al. Chemoprevention of cervical cancer with folic acid: a Phase III Southwest Oncology Group Intergroup study. *Cancer Epidemiol Biomark Prev* 1995;4:155–159.

155. Wideroff L, Potischman N, Glass AG, et al. A nested case-control study of dietary factors and the risk of incident cytological abnormalities of the cervix. *Nutr Cancer* 1998;30:130–136.

156. VanEenwyk J, Davis FG, Colman N. Folate, vitamin C, and cervical intraepithelial neoplasia. *Cancer Epidemiol Biomark Prev* 1992;1:119–124.

157. Buckley DI, McPherson RS, North CQ, Becker TM. Dietary micronutrients and cervical dysplasia in southwestern American Indian women. *Nutr Cancer* 1992;17:179–185.

158. Yeo AS, Schiff MA, Montoya G, et al. Serum micronutrients and cervical dysplasia in Southwestern American Indian women. *Nutr Cancer* 2000;38:141–150.

159. Butterworth CE Jr, Hatch KD, Macaluso M, et al. Folate deficiency and cervical dysplasia. *JAMA* 1992;267:528–533.

160. Liu T, Soong SJ, Wilson NP, et al. A case control study of nutritional factors and cervical dysplasia. *Cancer Epidemiol Biomark Prev* 1993;2:525–530.

161. Kanetsky PA, Gammon MD, Mandelblatt J, et al. Dietary intake and blood levels of lycopene: association with cervical dysplasia among non-Hispanic, black women. *Nutr Cancer* 1998;31:31–40.

162. Goodman MT, McDuffie K, Hernandez B, et al. Case-control study of plasma folate, homocysteine, vitamin B$_{12}$, and cysteine as markers of cervical dysplasia. *Cancer* 2000;89:376–382.

163. Goodman MT, McDuffie K, Hernandez B, et al. Association of methylenetetrahydrofolate reductase polymorphism C677T and dietary folate with the risk of cervical dysplasia. *Cancer Epidemiol Biomark Prev* 2001;10:1275–1280.

164. Piyathilake CJ, Macaluso M, Johanning GL, et al. Methylenetetrahydrofolate reductase (MTHFR) polymorphism increases the risk of cervical intraepithelial neoplasia. *Anticancer Res* 2000;20:1751–1757.

165. Herrero R, Potischman N, Brinton LA, et al. A case-control study of nutrient status and invasive cervical cancer. I. Dietary indicators. *Am J Epidemiol* 1991;134:1335–1346.

166. Ziegler RG, Brinton LA, Hamman RF, et al. Diet and the risk of invasive cervical cancer among white women in the United States. *Am J Epidemiol* 1990;132:432–445.

167. Brock KE, Berry G, Mock PA, et al. Nutrients in diet and plasma and risk of in situ cervical cancer. *J Natl Cancer Inst* 1988;80:580–585.

168. Verreault R, Chu J, Mandelson M, Shy K. A case-control study of diet and invasive cervical cancer. *Int J Cancer* 1989;43:1050–1054.

169. Ziegler RG, Jones CJ, Brinton LA, et al. Diet and the risk of in situ cervical cancer among white women in the United States. *Cancer Causes Control* 1991;2:17–29.

170. Potischman N, Brinton LA, Laiming VA, et al. A case-control study of serum folate levels and invasive cervical cancer. *Cancer Res* 1991;51:4785–4789.

171. Weinstein SJ, Ziegler RG, Frongillo EA Jr, et al. Low serum and red blood cell folate are moderately, but nonsignificantly associated with increased risk of invasive cervical cancer in U.S. women. *J Nutr* 2001;131:2040–2048.

172. Alberg AJ, Selhub J, Shah KV, et al. The risk of cervical cancer in relation to serum concentrations of folate, vitamin B_{12}, and homocysteine. *Cancer Epidemiol Biomark Prev* 2000;9:761–764.

173. Baghurst PA, McMichael AJ, Slavotinek AH, et al. A case-control study of diet and cancer of the pancreas. *Am J Epidemiol* 1991;134:167–179.

174. Stolzenberg-Solomon RZ, Albanes D, Nieto FJ, et al. Pancreatic cancer risk and nutrition-related methyl-group availability indicators in male smokers. *J Natl Cancer Inst* 1999;91:535–541.

175. Stolzenberg-Solomon RZ, Pietinen P, Barrett MJ, et al. Dietary and other methyl-group availability factors and pancreatic cancer risk in a cohort of male smokers. *Am J Epidemiol* 2001;153:680–687.

176. Silverman DT, Swanson CA, Gridley G, et al. Dietary and nutritional factors and pancreatic cancer: a case-control study based on direct interviews. *J Natl Cancer Inst* 1998;90:1710–1719.

177. Thompson JR, Gerald PF, Willoughby ML, Armstrong BK. Maternal folate supplementation in pregnancy and protection against acute lymphoblastic leukaemia in childhood: a case-control study. *Lancet* 2001;358:1935–1940.

178. Skibola CF, Smith MT, Kane E, et al. Polymorphisms in the methylenetetrahydrofolate reductase gene are associated with susceptibility to acute leukemia in adults. *Proc Natl Acad Sci USA* 1999;96:12810–12815.

179. Heimburger DC, Alexander CB, Birch R, et al. Improvement in bronchial squamous metaplasia in smokers treated with folate and vitamin B12. Report of a preliminary randomized, double-blind intervention trial. *JAMA* 1988;259:1525–1530.

180. Heimburger DC. Localized deficiencies of folic acid in aerodigestive tissues. *Ann NY Acad Sci* 1992;669:87–95.

181. Bandera EV, Freudenheim JL, Marshall JR, et al. Diet and alcohol consumption and lung cancer risk in the New York State Cohort (United States). *Cancer Causes Control* 1997;8:828–840.

182. Le Marchand L, Yoshizawa CN, Kolonel LN, et al. Vegetable consumption and lung cancer risk: a population-based case-control study in Hawaii. *J Natl Cancer Inst* 1989;81:1158–1164.

183. Hartman TJ, Woodson K, Stolzenberg-Solomon R, et al. Association of the B-vitamins pyridoxal 5'-phosphate (B_6), B_{12}, and folate with lung cancer risk in older men. *Am J Epidemiol* 2001;153:688–694.

184. Jatoi A, Daly BD, Kramer G, Mason JB. Folate status among patients with non-small cell lung cancer: a case-control study. *J Surg Oncol* 2001;77:247–252.

185. Gürdal-Yüksel E, Karadag M, Özyardimci N, et al. Cigarette smoking, serum lipids, folate, and vitamin B_{12} in lung cancer. *J Environ Pathol Toxicol Oncol* 1996;15:161–167.

186. Shen H, Spitz MR, Wang LE, et al. Polymorphisms of methylene-tetrahydrofolate reductase and risk of lung cancer: a case-control study. *Cancer Epidemiol Biomark Prev* 2001;10:397–401.

187. Gregory JF 3rd. Case study: folate bioavailability. *J Nutr* 2001;131:1376S–1382S.

188. Food and Drug Administration. Food standards: amendment of standards of identity for enriched grain products to require addition of folic acid. *Fed Regist* 1996;61:8781–8797.

189. Oakley GP Jr, Erickson JD, Adams MJ Jr. Urgent need to increase folic acid consumption. *JAMA* 1995;274:1717–1718.

190. Cuskelly GJ, McNulty H, Scott JM. Fortification with low amounts of folic acid makes a significant difference in folate status in young women: implications for the prevention of neural tube defects. *Am J Clin Nutr* 1999;70:234–239.

191. Jacques PF, Selhub J, Bostom AG, et al. The effect of folic acid fortification on plasma folate and total homocysteine concentrations. *N Engl J Med* 1999;340:1449–1454.

192. Lawrence JM, Petitti DB, Watkins M, Umekubo MA. Trends in serum folate after food fortification. *Lancet* 1999;354:915–916.

193. Lewis CJ, Crane NT, Wilson DB, Yetley EA. Estimated folate intakes: data updated to reflect food fortification, increased bioavailability, and dietary supplement use. *Am J Clin Nutr* 1999;70:198–207.

194. Institute of Medicine. Dietary Reference Intakes for Thiamin, Riboflavin, Niacin, Vitamin B_6, Folate, Vitamin B_{12}, Pantothenic Acid, Biotin, and Choline. A Report of the Standing Committee on the Scientific Evaluation of Dietary Reference Intakes and its Panel on Folate, Other B Vitamins, and Choline and Subcommittee on Upper Reference Levels of Nutrients, Food and Nutrition Board, Institute of Medicine, National Academy Press, Washington, DC, 2000.

195. Selhub J, Jacques PF, Wilson PW, et al. Vitamin status and intake as primary determinants of homocysteinemia in an elderly population. *JAMA* 1993;270:2693–2698.

196. Campbell RK. The unnecessary epidemic of folic acid-preventable spina bifida and anencephaly. *Pediatrics* 2001;108:1048–1050.

197. Lambie DG, Johnson RH. Drugs and folate metabolism. *Drugs* 1985;30:145–155.

198. Campbell NR. How safe are folic acid supplements? *Arch Intern Med* 1996;156:1638–1644.

199. Franklin JL, Rosenberg HH. Impaired folic acid absorption in inflammatory bowel disease: effects of salicylazosulfapyridine (Azulfidine). *Gastroenterology* 1973;64:517–525.

200. Selhub J, Dhar GJ, Rosenberg IH. Inhibition of folate enzymes by sulfasalazine. *J Clin Investig* 1978;61:221–224.

201. Reisenauer AM, Halsted CH. Human jejunal brush border folate conjugase. Characteristics and inhibition by salicylazosulfapyridine. *Biochim Biophys Acta* 1981;659:62–69.

202. Krogh Jensen M, Ekelund S, Svendsen L. Folate and homocysteine status and haemolysis in patients treated with sulphasalazine for arthritis. *Scand J Clin Lab Invest ig* 1996;56:421–429.

203. Endresen GK, Husby G. Folate supplementation during methotrexate treatment of patients with rheumatoid arthritis. An update and proposals for guidelines. *Scand J Rheumatol* 2001;30:129–134.

38 Conjugated Linoleic Acid as a Tumor Preventive Agent

David Kritchevsky, PhD and Michael W. Pariza, PhD

Contents

1. EARLY HISTORY

Carcinogens—e.g., benzo[a]pyrene (B[a]P) and 2-amino-3-methylimidazo[4,5f]-quinoline (IQ)—may be formed during flame broiling of protein-rich foods such as meat or fish (1–3). Pariza et al. (4), in the course of studying effects of controlled cooking temperature on mutagen formation in hamburger, found both mutagenic and antimutagenic activity. This activity was also found in uncooked hamburger. In further research, Pariza et al. (5) showed that the partially purified fraction (then called mutagenesis modulator) could inhibit IQ-induced mutagenicity in the Ames test (6). Before its chemical structure was established, Pariza and Hargraves (7) demonstrated that the mutagenesis modulator also inhibited 7,12-dimethylbenz[a]anthracene (DMBA)-induced epidermal neoplasia in mice (Table 1). In 1987, Ha et al. (8) established that the material they had referred to a mutagenesis modulator was a mixture of isomers of conjugated linoleic acid (CLA).

CLA was not an unknown substance. The history of CLA has been elaborated by Parodi (9). Dairy scientists had shown that cows could convert nonconjugated polyunsaturated fatty acids to their conjugated counterparts. Kepler et al. (10) showed that the principal conjugated diene formed in the rumen was 9-cis,11-trans-octadecadienoic acid, produced by the action of a common rumen bacterium, *Butyrivibrio fibrisolvens,* on linoleic acid. The enzyme that isomerized linoleic acid to CLA was isolated by Kepler and Tove (11).

2. EXPERIMENTAL CARCINOGENESIS

Until quite recently, CLA used in the studies discussed here has been obtained by base-catalyzed isomerization of oils rich in linoleic acid. The preparations most commonly used contain 40–45% each of the 9-cis,11-trans and 10-trans,12-cis isomers. The CLA isomer mixture was tested for its ability to inhibit B[a]P-induced mouse forestomach neoplasia. When CLA was compared with linoleic acid (Table 2), it was found that although CLA inhibited tumor formation by 40–50%, linoleic acid was without effect (12).

The experiments cited here (7,12) showed that CLA could affect tumorigenicity when applied directly to the tumor site. In an elegant series of experiments, Ip and his colleagues showed that dietary CLA also inhibited chemically induced mammary tumors in rats independent of type or amount of dietary fat and independent of carcinogen type. Ip et al. (13) fed female Sprague-Dawley rats a basal diet or one augmented with 0.5, 1.0, or 1.5% CLA. The dietary regimen was instituted 2 wk prior to administration of DMBA and continued to the end of the experiment (24 wk). As can be seen from Table 3, even the lowest level of CLA exerted some anti-tumorigenic effect.

From: *Cancer Chemoprevention, Volume 1: Promising Cancer Chemoprevention Agents*
Edited by: G. J. Kelloff, E. T. Hawk, and C. C. Sigman © Humana Press Inc., Totowa, NJ

Table 1
Influence of Mutagenesis Modulator on DMBA-Induced
Skin Tumors in Mice*

| Group** | Papillomas/Mouse | | |
	Control*	Test	p
A) SENCAR mice	30.2 ± 3.4	13.4 ± 2.4	0.01
B) SENCAR mice	9.6 ± 0.8	4.5 ± 0.9	0.01
C) CD-1 mice	10.0 ± 1.7	3.2 ± 1.1	0.01

*After ref. 7.
**A) 20-wk study. Modulator prepared by ion exchange.
  B) 19-wk study. Modulator prepared by extraction.
  C) 10-wk study. Modulator prepared on florisil.

Table 2
Inhibition of B[a]P-Induced Forestomach Tumors
in Female ICR Mice*

	No.	Incidence (%)	Multiplicity
Exp. 1			
Olive oil	22	90.9	3.8 ± 0.5
CLA	19	70.9**	2.0 ± 0.3**
Linoleic acid	14	78.9	4.5 ± 1.3
Exp. 2			
Olive oil	24	95.8	6.0 ± 0.07
CLA	24	95.8	3.2 ± 0.6**
Linoleic acid	22	100.0	6.3 ± 1.3
Exp. 3			
Olive oil	22	100.0	5.0 ± 0.6
CLA	24	70.8**	2.5 ± 0.3**
Linoleic acid	20	90.0	4.1 ± 0.6

*After ref. 12.
Mice given 0.1 mL CLA or linoleic acid in olive oil by
gavage. Duration: 4 wk.
**Significantly different from other groups.

To address the possibility that CLA's effect was the result of interference with the metabolic conversion of DMBA to an active form, Ip et al. (14) tested CLA effects on the carcinogenicity of N-methyl-N-nitrosourea (MNU, a direct-acting carcinogen). In a 36-wk study, they found that dietary levels of CLA as low as 0.1% significantly decreased the carcinogenicity of DMBA. They also found (Table 4) that 1% dietary CLA reduced the incidence of DMBA-induced mammary tumors by 35% and the incidence of MNU-induced mammary tumors by 32%. CLA was shown to reduce the proliferative activity of ductal and lobuloalveolar

Table 3
Effect of Different Levels of Dietary CLA
on DMBA-Induced Mammary Tumors in Sprague-Dawley
Rats (30/gp)*

| Group | CLA (%) | DMBA | Tumors | | |
			Incidence	No.	Multiplicity
1	–	+	80.0	81	2.7 ± 0.3
2	0.5	+	66.7	55**	1.8 ± 0.2**
3	1.0	+	46.7**	36**	1.2 ± 0.2**
4	1.5	+	40.0**	32**	1.1 ± 0.1**
5	1.5	0	0	0	0

*After ref. 13.
**$p < 0.05$ compared to control.

Table 4
Effect of CLA on Mammary Tumors in Sprague-Dawley
Rats Induced by DMBA OR MNU*

| Carcinogen | CLA (%) | Tumors | |
		Incidence	Number
DMBA	—	80	62
DMBA	1	52**	38**
MNU	—	88	76
MNU	1	60**	50**

*After ref. 15.
CLA fed from weaning to 1 wk post carcinogen administration (5 wk).
**$p < 0.05$ compared to control.

mammary epithelial cells by 15% and 23%, respectively. This observation suggested that CLA might affect mammary tumorigenesis through a direct effect on the target organ. CLA feeding for only a short period in the rat's life, corresponding to postweaning and puberty, was enough to reduce tumorigenesis caused by subsequent administration of MNU by about 25–30%, depending on the time of MNU treatment (15). In the same study, it was shown that feeding 1% CLA as a triglyceride or as free fatty acid had virtually the same effect on MNU-induced tumorigenesis.

The amount and type of dietary fat influence the course of experimental carcinogenesis (16). Linoleic acid enhances experimental carcinogenesis. The possibility that elevated levels of linoleic acid might swamp the CLA effect was tested in rats fed blended fat that reflecting the fatty acid composition of the American diet. The ratio of saturated to monounsaturated to polyunsaturated fatty acids in the blended fat was 1:1:1.

Inhibition of DMBA-induced mammary tumorigenesis was virtually the same in rats fed 1% CLA together with 10%, 13.3%, 16.7%, or 20% of the blended fat (17). The amount of linoleic acid in the diet (2% or 12%) did not affect the inhibition of DMBA-induced mammary cancer by CLA. There seemed to be a graded effect of CLA up to dietary concentration of 1.5%, but not beyond that level (18).

CLA's effect on experimental tumors other than mammary tumors has also received attention. Liew et al. (19) studied the effect of CLA on colon neoplasia induced by IQ in F344 rats. IQ alone yielded 100% incidence of aberrant crypt foci (ACF) (4.3 ± 2.4 ACF/rat). When CLA (0.5%) was added to the diet, ACF incidence was reduced by 40% and ACF/rat were reduced to 1.1 ± 1.3 ($p < 0.05$). When the diet contained safflower oil, ACF incidence was 100%, but ACF/rat were reduced by 26% (3.2 ± 1.7). Dietary CLA reduced IQ-DNA adducts in the liver by 27% and in the colon by 41%. Other experiments carried out in the course of the study suggest that CLA inhibited carcinogen activation.

Belury et al. (20) investigated the effects of increasing levels of dietary CLA on phorbol ester (12-O-tetradecanoyl phorbol-13-acetate) promotion on skin tumors in mice. The mice were fed diets containing 0%, 0.5%, 1.0%, or 1.5% CLA for 24 wk after tumor promotion was initiated. Over that period, all the CLA-fed mice showed reduced (by 40%) weight gain. The effects of dietary CLA on papilloma yield after 24 wk were: 0%–6.71; 0.5%–5.92; 1.0%–4.83 ($p < 0.05$); and 1.5%–4.67 ($p < 0.05$).

The severe combined immunodeficiency (SCID) mouse provides a vehicle for examining effects of human tumor cells in an experimental animal model (21). Subcutaneous injection of tumor cells into this model results in tumor growth at the site of injection as well as metastatic proliferation of the tumors. In one study, SCID mice were fed 1% CLA for 2 wk prior to subcutaneous inoculation of 1×10^7 MDA-MB468 cells (human breast adenocarcinoma). Feeding was continued for 14 wk. After 9 wk, the weight of tumors in the treated mice was 74% ($p < 0.01$) lower than in the controls and tumor area (mm^3) was reduced by 87% ($p < 0.01$). At 14 wk, tumor weight in treated mice was reduced by 30% ($p < 0.02$) and tumor weight by 62% ($p < 0.05$). There was no spread of breast cancer cells to lungs, peripheral blood, or bone marrow. In a subsequent study (23), SCID mice were fed a semipurified diet containing 1% CLA for 2 wk prior to injection

with 5×10^6 DU-145 cells (human prostatic carcinoma) and followed for 12 wk thereafter. In addition to a control group maintained on laboratory ration, a third group was fed a semipurified diet containing 1% linoleic acid. Food intake (g/d) at wk 12 was similar in the control and linoleic acid-fed groups (about 4 g) and significantly lower in the CLA group (about 3 g). However, body wt did not totally reflect food intake, which was 27 g in the linoleic acid fed group, 24.5 g in the controls, and 22 g in mice fed CLA. Tumor volume measured at 4 wk was similar in all three groups; by 8 wk, tumor volume in the linoleic acid-fed mice was slightly larger than in the controls and significantly larger ($p < 0.05$) than in the CLA-fed group. By 12 wk, tumor growth in the CLA-fed group was only slightly greater than it was at 4 wk (about 400 mm^3), whereas in the linoleic acid and control groups it had risen to 1700 mm^3 and 1500 mm^3, respectively. Tumor mass was lowest in the CLA-fed group ($p < 0.001$) against both controls and highest in the mice fed linoleic acid ($p < 0.05$) against commercial diet. CLA-fed mice exhibited a dramatically reduced number of lung metastases compared to the other two groups; they showed no metastases to any other tissue.

3. TISSUE-CULTURE STUDIES

Many in vitro studies of CLA on the growth of cells in culture have been designed to explore possible mechanisms. Visonneau et al. (24) examined the comparative effects of different concentrations of CLA or linoleic acid (1×10^{-6}, 10^{-5}, and 10^{-4} M) on a number of cell lines. Five breast carcinoma cell lines were tested: MBA-MB468, MCF7, MDA-MB 231, HS-578T, and BT-474. Except for the BT-474 line, CLA inhibited growth at every concentration. Linoleic acid at a concentration of 1×10^{-4} M stimulated cell growth. At the lower concentration, linoleic acid was generally inhibitory. With the BT-474 line, 10^{-4} M CLA inhibited growth, but lower concentrations stimulated growth. Linoleic acid inhibited growth at all concentrations. CLA inhibited growth of a prostatic carcinoma cell line (DU145) at concentrations of 1×10^{-4} or 1×10^{-5} and inhibited growth of a melanoma cell line (WM451) at all three concentrations. CLA at 10^{-4} M inhibited growth of a colon carcinoma cell line (HT-29) and a glioblastoma cell line (U87-MG). Table 5 summarizes these findings.

Shultz and colleagues (25–27) have confined their studies to three human cell lines. When CLA was

Table 5
Inhibitory or Stimulatory Activity of CLA or Linoleic Acid on Human Cancer Cells in Culture*

	CLA			Linoleic Acid		
Cell Line	10^{-4}	10^{-5}	10^{-6}	10^{-4}	10^{-5}	10^{-6}
MDA-MB468 (breast)	II	II	II	s	S	SS
MCF-7 (Breast)	II	II	I	s	S	S
MDA MB231 (Breast)	i	i	I	S	S	s
Hs578T (Breast)	II	II	II	SS	S	s
BT-474 (Breast)	I	s	s	i	i	i
DU 145 (Prostate)	I	i	s	SS	i	i
WM 451 (Melanoma)	II	i	I	SS	SS	SS
HT29 (Colon)	I	i	i	SS	SS	SS
Mesothelioma	i	I	i	s	I	i
Glioblastoma	I	I	s	s	s	S
Ovarian CA	II	II	i	SS	SS	SS

*After ref. 24.
Inhibition: i = <10%; I = 10–20%; II = >20%.
Stimulation: s = <10%; S = 10–20%; SS = >20%.

incubated with human malignant melanoma (M21-HPB), colorectal (HT-29), or breast cancer (MCF-7) cells, reduction in growth, dependent on the time and dose, was observed. All three cell lines, when incubated with CLA, incorporated less tritium-labeled leucine than did controls, suggesting cytotoxicity (25). Linoleic acid and CLA were used at concentrations of 1.78–7.14 ×10^{-5}. Linoleic acid stimulated MCF-7-cell growth initially, but became inhibitory at 8–12 d. CLA, on the other hand, was inhibitory at all concentrations; inhibition reached 100% after 12 d. The authors concluded that CLA was cytotoxic to MCF-7 cells (26). Another study (27) investigated the possibility that the CLA effect involved inhibition of eicosanoid synthesis. Their findings suggested that CLA activity was mediated through inhibition of lipoxygenase (LOX) activity. Linoleic acid, but not CLA, increased peroxide concentrations in normal human breast cells (HMEC) and MCF-7 cells. Treatment of MCF-7 cells with CLA and a cyclooxygenase (COX) inhibitor (indomethacin) stimulated cell growth, but when CLA was used together with a LOX inhibitor (nordihydroguaiaretic acid, NGDA), growth was inhibited. Durgam and Fernandes (28) attributed the inhibitory effect of CLA on growth of human breast cancer cells to interference with the hormone-regulated mitogenic pathway. They compared CLA effects on estrogen-responsive (ER) MCF-7 cells and ER-negative MDA-MB-231 cells. They found that CLA (3.5 × 10^{-5} M) decreased MCF-7

cell growth significantly, but had no effect on the growth of the MDA-MB-231 cells.

Schonberg and Krokan (29) examined the effects of 40-µM concentrations of CLA and linoleic acid on the growth of three different human lung adenocarcinoma lines (A-427, SK-LU-1, and A549) and one human glioblastoma line (A-172). Lipid peroxidation (measured as production of malondialdehyde, MDA) was 113%, 63%, and 85% higher in A427, SK-LU-1, and A549 cell lines supplemented with CLA compared to linoleic acid and 11% higher in the A-172 cells. The formation of MDA was totally abolished by the addition of 30 µM vitamin E to the medium, but cellular growth rates were not completely restored, suggesting that lipid peroxidation accounted for only part of the effect.

In contrast, Igarashi and Miyazawa (30), using a human hepatoma cell line (HepG2), attributed growth inhibition by CLA to alterations in fatty acid metabolism but not lipid peroxidation. Their indication of peroxidation was formation of thiobarbituric acid reactive substances (TBARS) rather than MDA specifically. TBARS production was 6% higher in cells incubated with linoleic acid than in those incubated with CLA. The level of TBARS production was about the same as that seen in control cells, and in every case was strongly inhibited by addition of α-tocopherol. The total fatty acid content of HepG2 cells incubated with CLA was 32% greater than controls and 53% greater than cells grown with linoleic acid. The major differences between the fatty acid composition of control cells and those grown with CLA was in the higher content of palmitic acid (+35%), palmitoleic acid (+83%), and stearic acid (+37%). As one would expect, there was a large difference in CLA content. Cellular total and free cholesterol, triglycerides, and phospholipids were all increased significantly in cells supplemented with CLA. The data suggest stimulation of *de novo* lipid synthesis.

CLA has been shown to inhibit experimental carcinogenesis and to inhibit proliferation of tumor cells in vitro. The mechanism of CLA action is moot; it can possibly exert more than one effect. Wattenberg *(31)* divided anticarcinogens into three classes: preventers of carcinogen formation, blockers of carcinogen action, or suppressors of proliferation. CLA may fit more than one of these categories.

4. MECHANISM(S) OF ACTION

Ha et al. *(12)* suggested that the anticarcinogenic effect of CLA might be partly the result of antioxidative properties. However, Ip et al. *(17)* showed that levels of hepatic malondialdehyde were not reduced in carcinogen-treated, CLA-fed rats, and van den Berg et al. *(32)* demonstrated that CLA was not a free radical scavenger or a metal chelator. Chen et al. *(33)* found that CLA, CLA methyl ester, and CLA-rich triglycerides did not affect oxidation of a heated polyunsaturated edible fat. Thus, antioxidant action would appear to be ruled out as underlying the antitumor properties of CLA. Yurawecz et al. *(34)* showed that CLA could be oxidized to yield furan derivatives; CLA furans have been reported to protect cultured fibroblasts against H_2O_2 toxicity *(35)*. This observation has not been pursued.

Schut and his colleagues (19,36–39) have studied the inhibitory effects of CLA on DNA adduct formation with IQ or 2-amino-1-methyl-6-phenylimidazo[4,5-*b*]pyridine (PhIP). In general, CLA reduces adduct formation, possibly acting as a blocking agent under certain conditions. The mechanism by which CLA blocks DNA adduct formation has not been elucidated.

One active area of research and speculation concerns the effects of CLA on eicosanoid metabolism. It has been shown by many investigators *(12,17,40,* among others) that CLA is readily incorporated into cell membrane phospholipids. CLA may thus displace arachidonic acid in phospholipids *(41)*. Liew et al. *(19)* proposed that modulation of eicosanoid metabolism

may underlie the inhibitory effect of CLA against IQ-initiated colonic ACF, and evidence has been presented indicating that the mechanism of action of the 10-*trans*,12-*cis* isomer may involve modulating LOX activity *(42)*.

In a study of effects of CLA in MCF-7 and SW480 cancer cells, Miller et al. *(43)* found that the 9-*cis*,11-*trans* isomer significantly decreased conversion of arachidonic acid to prostaglandin E_2. The underlying finding was that CLA reduced the incorporation of arachidonic acid into phosphatidyl choline (lecithin), which is the preferential substrate for phospholipase A_2, which in turn releases arachidonic acid for eicosanoid synthesis. Arachidonic acid is released from phospholipids by the action of phospholipase A_2 and converted to eicosanoids along the COX pathway (yielding prostaglandins and thromboxanes) as well as the LOX pathway (yielding leukotrienes). Eicosanoids affect cell proliferation, inflammation, and immunity, all of which may influence carcinogenesis.

CLA may induce its effects on lipid metabolism and possibly carcinogenesis via its effects on a family of peroxisome proliferator-activated receptors (PPARs), which can alter gene expression when activated. Hypolipidemic drugs of the fibrate family and some polyunsaturated fatty acids are ligands for PPARs. Belury and her colleagues have provided evidence that CLA may also be a member of the peroxisome proliferator family *(44)*. There are several PPARs (α, β/δ, γ) with different metabolic effects. CLA interaction with PPARα involves transcription of genes encoding enzymes that are involved in lipid metabolism *(45)*, and in this regard it should be noted that Peters et al. *(46)* demonstrated that CLA reduced body fat gain in PPARα-null mice. Farquharson et al. *(47)* hypothesized that the effects of CLA on gene expression may initiate events leading to reduction of free radical-induced cell damage.

Inhibition of experimental mammary carcinogenesis depends on retention of CLA within the mammary gland *(48)*. Thus, action of CLA in inhibiting one type of cancer may be related to its retention in the affected tissue, but this type of action has not been reported for CLA in other tissues.

There can be little doubt that CLA exhibits potent anticarcinogenic properties. The mechanisms by which CLA affects cancer growth are speculative. As the previous discussion shows, there are a number of possibilities regarding modes of action against specific tumors. The CLA-stimulated response may have a

Table 6

ORs and 95% CIs for Breast Cancer by Quintiles of Serum Fatty Acids in Postmenopausal Women*

	Quintile				
	1	2	3	4	5
Myristic acid (14:0)					
Mean % fatty acids	0.74	0.98	1.14	1.40	1.84
OR**	1.0	0.5 (0.2–1.3)	0.2 (0.1–0.5)	0.2 (0.1–0.4)	0.2 (0.1–0.5)
trans-vaccenic acid (18:1 t11)					
Mean % of fatty acids	0.17	0.23	0.27	0.31	0.40
OR	1.0	0.5 (0.2–1.3)	0.2 (0.1–0.6)	0.4 (0.1–0.9)	0.2 (0.1–0.6)
CLA (18:2)					
Mean % of fatty acids	0.21	0.27	0.32	0.36	0.43
OR	1.0	0.7 (0.3–1.8)	0.3 (0.1–0.7)	0.4 (0.1–1.2)	0.2 (0.1–0.6)
Arachidonic acid (20:4)					
Mean % of fatty acids	3.84	4.89	5.46	6.04	7.15
OR	1.0	1.1 (0.4–2.8)	2.0 (0.8–4.8)	2.4 (1.0–5.9)	3.1 (1.3–7.8)

*After ref. 52.

**Adjusted for age; rural or urban; age at menarche; age at first-full term pregnancy; oral contraceptive use; estrogen replacement therapy; family history of breast cancer/disease; educational level; alcohol intake; smoking; physical activity; waist/hip ratio; and BMI.

general base coupled with specific metabolic pathways evoked by specific tissues. The availability of pure specific isomers of CLA expands the field of inquiry.

5. HUMAN STUDIES

A basic concern is to relate the experimental findings to possible CLA effects on human cancers. Knekt et al. (49) reported that a high intake of milk is correlated with a reduced risk of breast cancer. Knekt and Järvinen (50) have reviewed the field exhaustively. Analysis of the epidemiological evidence relating to dairy products and the risk of breast cancer is confusing. High consumption of dairy products has been linked to both reduced and elevated risk. These studies have many modifying factors such as age, body wt, menopause, components of the specific dairy products under consideration, other components of the diet, and caloric intake. The findings are provocative, and call for more focused studies related to dairy food consumption.

Lavillonniere and Bougnoux have (51) reported preliminary data from a study of the CLA content of breast adipose tissue from women with breast cancer and controls. The CLA content of control tissue was elevated compared to that in afflicted tissue. Aro et al. (52) studied serum and dietary CLA in Finnish women with breast cancer. They examined 195 cases (35% premenopausal) and 208 controls (36% premenopausal). In postmenopausal women, dietary CLA and serum CLA, myristic acid, and trans-vaccenic acid were significantly lower in cases than in controls. Their results are summarized in Table 6.

Animal data are almost unanimous in finding CLA to inhibit experimental tumorigenesis and tumor-cell proliferation in vitro. Data in humans are sparse because they are derived reflectively rather than by targeted survey or experiment. CLA is a component of a class of dietary foods (animal products) that have taken most of the epidemiological blame for human carcinogenesis. Continuing experimental evidence from CLA research may lead to reconsideration of the dietary effects on carcinogenesis. The emphasis should be on dietary patterns, quantities of food, caloric intake, and exercise rather than on a single dietary component. The idea that we are what we eat has been voiced in many languages. This observation should relate to the total diet rather than to specific components.

ACKNOWLEDGMENT

Supported, in part, by a Research Career Award (HL-00734) from the National Institutes of Health (DK) and by gift funds administered by the University of Wisconsin-Madison Food Research Institute (MWP).

REFERENCES

1. Lijinsky W, Shubik P. Benzo(*a*)pyrene and other polynuclear hydrocarbons in charcoal broiled meat. *Science* 1974;145:53–55.

2. Dipple A. Formation, metabolism and mechanism of action of polycyclic aromatic hydrocarbons. *Cancer Res* 1983;43:2422S–2425S.

3. Wakabayashi K, Nagao M, Esumi H, Sugimura T. Food derived mutagens and carcinogens. *Cancer Res* 1992;52:2092S–2098S.

4. Pariza MW, Ashoor SH, Chu FS, Lund DB. Effects of temperature and time on mutagen formation in pan-fried hamburger. *Cancer Lett* 1979;7:63–69.

5. Pariza MW, Loretz, LJ, Storkson JM, Holland NC. Mutagens and modulator of mutagenesis in fried ground beef. *Cancer Res* 1983;43:2444S–24446S.

6. Ames BN, McCann J, Yamasaki E. Methods for detecting carcinogens and mutagens with *Salmonella*/mammalian microsomes mutagenicity tests. *Mutat Res* 1975;31:347–364.

7. Pariza MW, Hargraves WA. A beef derived mutagenesis modulator inhibits initiation of mouse epidermal tumors by 7,12-dimethylbenz(*a*) anthracene. *Carcinogenesis* 1985;6:591–593.

8. Ha YL, Grimm NK, Pariza MW. Anti-carcinogens from fried ground beef: heat altered derivatives of linoleic acid. *Carcinogenesis* 1987;8:1881–1887.

9. Parodi PW. Conjugated linoleic acid: the early years, in *Advances in Conjugated Linoleic Acid Research, vol. 1.* Yurawecz MP, Mossaba MM, Kramer JKG, et al., eds. AOCS Press, Champaign, IL, 1999, pp. 1–11.

10. Kepler CR, Hirons KP, McNeill JJ, Tove SB. Intermediates and products of the biohydrogenation of linoleic acid by *Butyrivibrio fibrisolvens. J Biol Chem* 1966;241:1350–1354.

11. Kepler CR, Tove SB. Biohydrogenation of unsaturated fatty acids. III. Purification and properties of a linoleate Δ^{12}-*cis*, Δ^{11}-*trans* from *Butyrivibrio fibrisolvens. J Biol Chem* 1967;242:5686–5692.

12. Ha YL, Storkson JM, Pariza MW. Inhibition of benzo[*a*]pyrene-induced mouse forestomach neoplasia by conjugated dienoic derivatives of linoleic acid. *Cancer Res* 1990;50:1097–1101.

13. Ip C, Chin SF, Scimeca JA, Pariza MW. Mammary cancer prevention by conjugated dienoic derivative of linoleic acid. *Cancer Res* 1991;51:6118–6124.

14. Ip C, Singh M, Thompson HJ, Scimeca JA. Conjugated linoleic acid suppresses mammary carcinogenesis and proliferative activity of the mammary gland in the rat. *Cancer Res* 1994;54:1212–1215.

15. Ip C, Scimeca JA, Thompson H. Effect of timing and duration of dietary conjugated linoleic acid on mammary cancer prevention. *Nutr Cancer* 1995;24:241–247.

16. Welsch CW. Relationship between dietary fat and experimental mammary tumorigenesis: a review and critique. *Cancer Res* 1992;52:2040S–2048S.

17. Ip C, Briggs SP, Haegele AD, et al. The efficacy of conjugated linoleic acid in mammary cancer prevention is independent of the level or type of fat in the diet. *Carcinogenesis* 1996;17:1045–1050.

18. Ip C, Scimeca JA. Conjugated linoleic acid and linoleic acid are distinctive modulators of mammary carcinogenesis. *Nutr Cancer* 1997;27:131–135.

19. Liew C, Schut HAJ, Chin SF, et al. Protection of conjugated linoleic acids against 2-amino-3-methylimidazo[4,5*f*]-quinoline-induced colon carcinogenesis in the F344 rat: a study of inhibitory mechanisms. *Carcinogenesis* 1995;16:3037–3043.

20. Belury MA, Nickel KP, Bird CE, Wu Y. Dietary conjugated linoleic acid modulation of phorbol ester skin tumor promotion. *Nutr Cancer* 1996;26:149–157.

21. Cesano A, Hoxie JA, Lange B, et al. The severe combined immunodeficient (SCID) mouse as a model for human myeloid leukemia. *Oncogene* 1992;7:827–836.

22. Visonneau S, Cesano A, Tepper SA, et al. Conjugated linoleic acid suppresses the growth of human breast adenocarcinoma cells in SCID mice. *Anticancer Res* 1997;17:969–974.

23. Cesano A, Visonneau S, Scimeca JA, et al. Opposite effects of linoleic acid and conjugated linoleic acid on human prostatic cancer in SCID mice. *Anticancer Res* 1998;18:833–838.

24. Visonneau S, Cesano A, Tepper SA, et al. Effect of different concentrations of conjugated linoleic acid (CLA) on tumor cell growth in vitro. *FASEB J* 1996;10:A182.

25. Shultz TD, Chew BP, Seaman WR, Luedecke LO. Inhibitory effect of conjugated diene derivatives of linoleic acid and β carotene on the in vitro growth of human cancer cells. *Cancer Lett* 1992;63:125–133.

26. Schultz TD, Chew BP, Seaman WR. Differential stimulatory and inhibitory responses of human MCF-7 breast cancer cells to linoleic acid and conjugated linoleic acid in culture. *Anticancer Res* 1992;12:2143–2146.

27. Cunningham DC, Harrison LY, Shultz TD. Proliferative response of normal human mammary and MCF-7 breast cancer cells to linoleic acid, conjugated linoleic acid and eicosanoid synthesis inhibitors in culture. *Anticancer Res* 1997;17:197–204.

28. Durgam VR, Fernandes G. The growth inhibitory effect of conjugated linoleic acid on MCF-7 cells is related to estrogen response system. *Cancer Lett* 1997;116:121–130.

29. Schonberg S, Krokan HE. The inhibitory effect of conjugated dienoic derivatives (CLA) of linoleic acid on the growth of human tumor cell lines is in part due to increased lipid peroxidation. *Anticancer Res* 1995;15:1241–1246.

30. Igarashi M, Miyazawa T. The growth inhibitory effect of conjugated linoleic acid on a human hepatoma cell line, HepG2 is induced by a change in fatty acid metabolism, but not the facilitation of lipid peroxidation in the cells. *Biochim Biophys Acta* 2001;1530:162–171.

31. Wattenberg L. Chemoprevention of cancer. *Cancer Res* 1985;45:1–8.

32. van den Berg JJ, Cook NE, Tribble DL. Reinvestigation of the antioxidant properties of conjugated linoleic acid. *Lipids* 1995;30:599–605.

33. Chen ZY, Chan PT, Kwan KY, Zhang A. Reassessment of the antioxidant activity of conjugated linoleic acid. J *Am Oil Chem Soc* 1997;74:719–753.

34. Yurawecz MP, Hood JK, Mossaba MM, et al. Furan fatty acids determined as oxidation products of conjugated octadecadienoic acid. *Lipids* 1995;30:595–598.

35. Wamer W, Yurawecz MP, Wei R, et al. In vitro assessment of cytotoxicity and antioxidant activity of a furan fatty acid, a novel oxidation product of conjugated linoleic acid. *FASEB J* 1996;10:A272.

36. Zu HX, Schut HAJ. Inhibition of 2-amino-3-methylimidazo[4,5*f*]quinoline-DNA adduct formation in CDF$_1$ mice by

heat altered derivatives of linoleic acid. *Food Chem Toxicol* 1992;30:9–16.

37. Schut HAJ, Cummings DA, Smale MHE, et al. DNA adducts of heterocylic amines: formation, removal and inhibition by dietary components. *Mutat Res* 1997;376:185–194.

38. Josyula S, He YH, Ruch RJ, Schut HAJ. Inhibition of DNA adduct formation of PhIP in female F344 rats by dietary conjugated linoleic acid. *Nutr Cancer* 1998;32:132–138.

39. Josyula S, Schut HAJ. Effects of dietary conjugated linoleic acid on DNA adduct formation of PhIP and IQ after bolus administration to female F344 rats. *Nutr Cancer* 1998;32:139–145.

40. Sugano M, Tsujita A, Yamasaki M, et al. Lymphatic recovery, tissue distribution, and metabolic effects of conjugated linoleic acid in rats. *J Nutr Biochem* 1997;8:38–43.

41. Cook ME, Miller CC, Park Y, Pariza M. Immune modulation by altered nutrient metabolism: nutritional control of immune-induced growth depression. *Poultry Sci* 1993;72:1301–1306.

42. Park Y, Pariza MW. Lipoxygenase inhibitors inhibit heparin-releasable lipoprotein lipase activity in 3T3-L1 adipocytes and enhance body fat reduction in mice by conjugated linoleic acid. *Biochim Biophys Acta* 2001;1534:27–33.

43. Miller A, Stanton C, Devery R. Modulation of arachidonic acid distribution by conjugated linoleic acid isomers and linoleic acid in MCF-7 and SW480 cancer cells. *Lipids* 2001;36:1161–1168.

44. Belury MA, Vanden Heuvel JP. Modulation of diabetes by conjugated linoleic acid in Yurawicz MP, Mossaba MM, Kramer JKG, et al., eds. *Advances in Conjugated Linoleic Acid Research, vol. 1.* AOCS Press, Champaign, IL,1999, pp.404–411.

45. Moody DE, Reddy JK, Lake B, et al. Peroxisomers proliferation and nongenotoxic carcinogenesis. Commentary of a symposium. *Fundam Appl Toxicol* 1991;16:233–248.

46. Peters JM, Park Y, Gonzalez FJ, Pariza MW. Influence of conjugated linoleic acid on body composition and target gene expression in peroxisome proliferator-activated receptor α-null mice. *Biochim Biophys Acta* 2001;1533:233–242.

47. Farquharson A, Wu HC, Grant I, et al. Possible mechanisms for the putative antiatherogenic and antitumorigenic effects of conjugated polyenoic fatty acids. *Lipids* 1999;34:S343.

48. Ip C, Jiang C, Thompson HJ, Scimeca JA. Retention of conjugated linoleic acid in the mammary gland is associated with tumor inhibition during the post-initiation phase of carcinogenesis. *Carcinogenesis* 1997;18:755–759.

49. Kneckt P, Järvinen R, Seppänen R, et al. Intake of dairy products and the risk of breast cancer. *Br J Cancer* 1996;73:687–691.

50. Knekt P, Järvinen R. Intake of dairy products and breast cancer risk, in Yurawecz MP, Mossaba MM, Kramer JKG, et al., eds. *Advances in Conjugated Linoleic Acid Research, vol. 1.* AOCS Press, Champaign, IL, 1999, pp.444–470.

51. Lavillonniere F, Bougnoux P. Conjugated linoleic acid (CLA) and the risk of breast cancer,. In Yurawecz MP, Mossaba MM, Kramer JKG, Pariza MW, Nelson GJ, eds. *Advances in Conjugated Linoleic Acid Research, vol. 1.* AOCS Press, Champaign, IL, 1999, pp.276–282.

52. Aro A, Männestö S, Salminen I, et al. Inverse association between dietary and serum conjugated linoleic acid and risk of breast cancer in postmenopausal women. *Nutr Cancer* 2000;38:151–157.

39 Chemopreventive Effects of Omega-3 Fatty Acids

Joanne R. Lupton, PhD and Robert S. Chapkin, PhD

CONTENTS

1. INTRODUCTION

Evidence increasingly suggests that $1\omega-3$ fatty acids, particularly eicosapentaenoic acid (20:5n–3) (EPA) and docosahexaenoic acid (22:6n–3) (DHA) are protective against cancer, and the data is strongest for breast and colon cancer. These protective effects are mediated by a variety of different mechanisms, including the incorporation of n–3 fatty acids into cell membranes, which changes membrane fluidity, may affect the association of proteins within cell membranes, and/or may initiate different signal-transduction processes. Effects of n–3 fatty acids on eicosanoid synthesis are well documented, although it is not yet determined which products of lipoxygenase (LOX) or cyclooxygenase (COX) are responsible for the observed effects and the specific role of EPA as compared to DHA on these pathways. Omega-3 fatty acids have also been shown to decrease cell proliferation and/or increase apoptosis during the tumorigenic process. Of interest is lipid peroxidation and the role it may play in initiating apoptosis. The role of n–3 fatty acids in the generation of new blood vessels is significant in both tumor growth and metastases, and these fatty acids now appear to play a role in modulating angiogenesis. With new methodology available to document changes in gene expression as a function of n–3 administration, it seems to be the right time to test hypotheses in humans that have previously been explored in vitro or in animals. It has not been determined whether the beneficial effects of n–3 fatty acids are dependent upon a specific amount of these fatty acids or on their ratio to n–6 fatty acids.

2. THE ESSENTIAL FATTY ACIDS (18:2N–6) AND (18:3N–3)

2.1. Biochemistry and Food Sources

α-Linolenic acid (18:3n–3) and linoleic acid (18:2n–6) are considered to be the two essential fatty acids, which cannot be synthesized in the body and thus must be obtained from the diet. The major polyunsaturated fatty acid (PUFA) in most diets is linoleic acid (18:2n–6), found in vegetable seeds and oils such as those from corn, soybean, safflower, and sunflower. α-Linolenic acid (18:3n–3) is the primary n–3 fatty acid and, is found in soybean and canola oils (as well as in linseed, rapeseed, walnut, and blackcurrant oils) and in dark green leafy plants (1). Deep, cold-water fatty fish such as herring, sardines, salmon, and tuna are rich sources of EPA (20:5n–3) and DHA (22:6n–3) (2), which are incorporated into the fatty acids of these fish from the plankton and algae on which they feed. The relative amounts of EPA and DHA contained in fish oils are highly variable across species (3).

Both α-linolenic acid and linoleic acid can be metabolized to longer-chain fatty acids. For example, α-linolenic acid can be elongated and desaturated to EPA (20:5n–3) and DHA (22:6n–3), and linoleic acid is the precursor of arachidonic acid (AA) (4). However, the efficiency of conversion of α-linolenic acid to the longer-chain fatty acids in the n–3 family is not optimal. A recent study addressing in vivo metabolism of n–3 fatty acids using isotope tracer methodology in healthy humans determined that only

From: Cancer Chemoprevention, Volume 1: Promising Cancer Chemoprevention Agents
Edited by: G. J. Kelloff, E. T. Hawk, and C. C. Sigman © Humana Press Inc., Totowa, NJ

about 0.2% of plasma 18:3n–3 was used for biosynthesis of 20:5n–3. In contrast, the synthesis of 22:5n–3 and 22:6n–3 from their immediate substrate precursors was highly effective. The authors concluded that dietary 18:3n–3 may be an inadequate substrate for 22:5n–3 synthesis, even under dietary conditions intended to enhance long-chain PUFA production (5). The inefficiency of the conversion of 18:3n–3 to 20 5n–3 indicates that the biosynthesis of long-chain n–3 PUFA from α-linolenic acid is limited in healthy individuals. This is significant because the primary source of 20:5n–3 and 22:6n–3 is marine fish (2), yet Americans typically do not eat high amounts of these rich sources of EPA and DHA (6). This means, as noted by Pawlosky et al., (5) that the major source of EPA and DHA for most Americans may be its production from α-linolenic acid (a highly ineffective process).

2.2. Metabolic and Functional Differences Between n–6 and n–3 Fatty Acids

An increased intake of PUFA has been promoted as being "heart healthy," as PUFA tend to lower blood cholesterol values compared to saturated fats (7), and high blood cholesterol values are considered a risk factor for coronary heart disease. However, the distinction between the major subclasses of PUFA (n–3 and n–6) is often lost in these recommendations. Clearly, with respect to their effects on cancer development (as described in Subheading 3), the two subclasses have very different effects. These two classes of PUFAs are biochemically and functionally distinct and have different physiological functions. Competition exists between the n–3 and n–6 fatty acids for the Δ 5 and Δ 6 desaturases, and the n–3 fatty acids have greater affinities for these enzymes. Thus, increasing the dietary intake of α-linolenic acid, EPA, or DHA may reduce the desaturation of linoleic acid and therefore the synthesis of AA (4,8,9). Also, n–3 fatty acids may inhibit the uptake of other fatty acids into cells. In a series of studies, Sauer et al. examined the effects of n–6 and n–3 fatty acids on the growth of a transplantable rat tumor, finding a direct relationship between the rate of linoleic acid uptake and tumor growth in vivo (10), which a later study from the same laboratory found could be inhibited by the addition of α-linolenic acid, EPA, or DHA to arterial blood during perfusion of the hepatoma, perfusion also inhibited tumor linoleic acid uptake (11).

2.2.1. METABOLIC AND FUNCTIONAL DIFFERENCES BETWEEN SUBCLASSES OF N–3 FATTY ACIDS (18:3N–3) (20:5N–3) (22:6N–3)

EPA and DHA are known to have different effects on plasma lipids (12). They also have different effects on eicosanoid production; EPA is a competitive inhibitor of both the COX and LOX pathways (13), and DHA only inhibits the COX pathway (14). Their roles in cell membranes also differ. DHA reduces membrane cholesterol content and increases membrane fluidity, an effect that is not observed with EPA (15). This may result in differential effects on tumorigenesis. For example, Kafrawy et al. (16) measured tumor cell death as a function of the incorporation of different fatty acids in different positions and in different phospholipids, and found that DHA in phosphatidylcholine is cytotoxic to T27A tumor cells, whereas EPA and α-linolenic acid did not have this effect (16).

2.3. Ratio of n–6 to n–3 Fatty Acids

Average linoleic acid intake in the United States has risen from approx 3% of energy in the 1950s to 6–7% in the 1990s (17). Simopoulos has noted that the 1950s diet contained small but approximately equal amounts of n–6 and n–3 fatty acids, in contrast to higher amounts of n–6 fatty acids that are presently consumed (3). The ratio of n–6 to n–3 fatty acids in most Western diets today is considered to be too high, with a ratio of 10–20× more n–6 than n–3 PUFAs (18,19). The rationale for lowering the ratio of n–6 to n–3 comes predominantly from studies on fatty acid intake and various cancers—e.g., which have found an increased incidence of breast cancer and colon cancer in the Japanese, which correlates with a decrease in the n–3:n–6 fatty acid ratio. However, from a meta-analysis of linoleic acid intake and cancer risk (20), the authors concluded: "It seems unlikely that a high intake of linoleic acid substantially raises the risks of breast, colorectal, or prostate cancer in humans." Others have also questioned whether or not n–6 fatty acids such as linoleic acid and AA are actually negative dietary factors (21). However, 18:2n–6 does promote colonic tumors in a rat multiorgan carcinogenesis model (22).

A compromise in recommendations for fatty acid intake centers around monounsaturated fatty acids (n–9). The Mediterranean diet (high in olive oil; 18:1n–9) is believed to be both cardioprotective and chemoprotective. In the Lyon Diet Heart Study (23), investigators compared cancer rates among patients randomized to either a Mediterranean-type diet or a control diet close to the Step 1 American Heart Association Prudent Diet. The Mediterranean diet produced a healthier profile than the American Heart Association Prudent Diet; the reduction in risk for Mediterranean diet subjects compared to those on the American Heart Association diet was 56% for total deaths ($p = 0.03$) and 61% ($p = 0.05$) for cancers. However, this does not necessarily mean that n–9 fatty acids are more protective than n–6 fatty acids, as omega-3 fatty acids were higher ($p < 0.001$) and omega-6 fatty acids were lower ($p < 0.001$) in the Mediterranean diet compared to the American Heart Association Prudent Diet.

3. CHEMOPREVENTION BY OMEGA-3 FATTY ACIDS

3.1. General

Epidemiological evidence suggests that individuals with diets rich in fish containing high levels of n–3 fatty acids have a low incidence of cancer in general, and of breast and colon cancer in particular (24–26). There are some excellent previously published reviews on the relationship of lipids to cancer (27–33).

3.2. Breast/Mammary Cancer

3.2.1. EPIDEMIOLOGICAL STUDIES

Ecological studies comparing the incidence of breast cancer and mortality rates with fish consumption have generally found an inverse association between the percentage of calories from fish and breast cancer rates (24). Sasaki et al. (34) analyzed data from 30 countries and found a significant negative correlation between fish intake and the incidence of breast cancer. In this same analysis, using the variable of dietary animal fat minus fish fat intake, a highly significant positive relationship with breast cancer mortality rates for women over 50 yr of age was detected (34). It has long been known that native Greenland Eskimos, whose diet is very high in fish and aquatic mammals and thus very rich in n–3 fatty acids (35), have a very low risk for cancer in general and breast cancer in particular (2,36), despite a high total fat intake.

Data from a number of case-control studies also suggest a protective effect of diets high in fish against the risk of breast cancer (37–40), but this is not true of all such studies (41–44). The importance of separating out n–3 fatty acids from n–6 fatty acids is illustrated by Boyd et al. (45), who evaluated the relationship between total PUFA intake and relative risk of breast

cancer in nine case-control studies published before 1993. They calculated a combined relative risk of 0.92 from the nine case-control studies; two showed a lower risk of breast cancer with higher PUFA intake, and the other seven studies showed no significant effect. As some have observed (33), the ratio of n–6 to n–3 fatty acids may be more important than the amount of n–3 fatty acids per se. In support of this hypothesis, a case-control study (46) and a cohort study (47) indicated that breast cancer patients have a lower proportion of n–6 PUFAs in their red blood cell (RBC) membranes (46) and serum phospholipids (47), but no association was found between levels of serum phospholipid n–3 PUFAs (47) and the risk of the disease. In contrast, Pala et al. (48) analyzed the association between the risk of breast cancer and fatty acid composition of erythrocyte membranes in 4,052 healthy postmenopausal women who resided in northern Italy and were enrolled in the Hormone and Diet Etiology Study of Breast Cancer (ORDET) (49). They found that DHA, inversely associated with the risk of breast cancer, was the only fatty acid associated with fish consumption. Although it has been not confirmed that the fatty acid composition of erythrocyte membranes is similar to that of breast tissue, it has been shown to be correlated in a number of animal studies (50,51).

Further confirmation for the importance of the n–6 to n–3 fatty acid ratio comes from a study in which the fatty acid content of adipose tissue in postmenopausal breast cancer cases and controls from five European countries in the European Community Multicenter Study on Antioxidants, Myocardial Infarction, and Cancer (EURAMIC) was used to test the hypothesis that n–3 fatty acids inhibit breast cancer with the degree of inhibition depending on background levels of n–6 fatty acids (52). The level of n–3 fatty acids in adipose tissue was not consistently associated with breast cancer; however, the ratio of n–3 fatty acids to total n–6 showed an inverse association with breast cancer in four of five centers in this trial (52). More recently (53), the authors examined fatty acid composition in adipose tissue from 241 patients with invasive, nonmetastatic breast carcinoma and 88 patients with benign breast disease in Tours, France. They found inverse associations between the risk of breast cancer and n–3 fatty acid levels in breast adipose tissue. Women in the highest tertile of the long-chain n–3/total n–6 ratio had an odds ratio of 0.33 compared to women in the lowest tertile ($p = 0.0002$). The authors concluded that their data suggest a protective effect of n–3 fatty acids on the risk of breast cancer and support the hypothesis that the balance between n–3 and n–6 fatty acids plays a role in breast cancer *(53)*.

3.2.2. CLINICAL STUDIES

Although the studies by Zaridze et al. *(46)*, Vatten et al. *(47)*, Pala et al. *(48)*, and Berrino et al. *(49)* tested the relationship between a biochemical parameter (fatty acid composition of erythrocyte membranes) and the incidence of breast cancer and may thus be considered epidemiological, we consider them clinical studies because of the biochemical assessment. Similarly, Simonsen et al. *(52)* and Maillard et al. *(53)* measured fatty acid composition of adipose tissue and related these data to the incidence of breast cancer. Again, these studies could be considered preclinical in nature. However, there are no clinical intervention trials in which omega-3 fatty acids are provided in the diet and measurements of the incidence of breast cancer are evaluated.

3.2.3. EXPERIMENTAL STUDIES

Although at first all PUFAs were believed to promote experimentally induced mammary cancer, n–3 fatty acids have been shown to delay their development, whereas n–6 fatty acids have the opposite effect *(54–58,* reviewed in *59,60)*. For example, Ip et al. observed a direct positive relationship between the concentration of dietary linoleate (0.5–4.4%) and breast tumor proliferation *(61)*. Karmali *(58)* was one of the first to show that n–3 fatty acids, but not n–6 fatty acids, were protective against rodent mammary tumors. Several studies after those by Karmali showed that diets high in n–6 fatty acids enhance breast and colon tumorigenesis in rodents, whereas fish oil that is high in n–3 PUFAs reduces carcinogenesis *(29)*.

With respect to individual fatty acids and mammary tumor development, both DHA and EPA have proven to be protective in a number of studies. For example, DHA was provided as a triglyceride to female nude mice, injected in their mammary fat pads with MDA-MB-231 cells *(62)*. The addition of 4% DHA to a 4% linoleic acid-containing diet reduced the tumor growth rate. Tumor weights were also reduced in the 4% DHA-fed mice compared with the 4% linoleic acid control group ($p = 0.02$) *(62)*. A separate study investigated the effects of linoleic acid, EPA, and DHA on the growth, metastasis, and cell proliferation of a murine mammary tumor transplanted into mice. Growth of the primary tumor, the number of metastatic tumors in the lung, and cell proliferation of

the tumor were significantly inhibited in EPA and DHA groups compared to control and/or linoleic acid groups *(63)*. In contrast, an in vitro study by Abdidezfuli et al. that used EPA and DHA in the medium of MCF-7 human breast cancer cells found that only EPA inhibited their proliferation.

In a number of instances, in vitro studies do not reflect the effects found in vivo. Although it did not assess the effect of DHA or EPA on mammary tumor incidence, one study *(64)* determined their effect on the recurrence and/or metastases of mammary tumors excised from female nude mice. Although there were no differences in the incidence of local recurrence between groups, EPA and DHA both inhibited the development of lung metastases.

As pioneers in the area of experimental mammary cancer and fatty acids, Rose et al. *(65)* have compared the effects of diets containing linoleic acid, EPA, and DHA on the growth and metastasis of human breast cancer cells in the nude mouse model. They have also determined how such effects relate to observed changes in the chemical content of tumor fatty acids and eicosanoid production. Results showed that growth of primary tumors was retarded in mice fed diets supplemented with EPA and DHA compared with those fed linoleic acid *(65)*. Fay et al. *(66)* conducted a meta-analysis on the incidence of mammary tumors and fat intake from 97 reports of experiments involving more than 12,800 mice and rats. Despite numerous positive effects of n–3 fatty acids against mammary cancer cited here, results of their analysis showed that n–6 PUFAs have a strong promoting effect on mammary cancer, whereas n–3 PUFAs have a small and statistically nonsignificant protective effect.

3.2.4. POTENTIAL MECHANISMS

3.2.4.1. Overview There is a growing body of literature on how n–3 fatty acids may ultimately decrease mammary carcinogenesis. These fatty acids may incorporate into cell membranes and differentially affect signaling pathways, which in turn can up- or downregulate oncogenes and tumor suppressor genes, activate cell death pathways, or inactivate events that lead to an increase in cell proliferation. In addition, these long-chain PUFAs undergo lipid peroxidation, resulting in oxidative products that may be cytotoxic to tumor cells. Omega-3 fatty acids may inhibit COX activity and depress synthesis of certain prostaglandins (PG), known stimulants to cell proliferation. Examples of each of these follow.

3.2.4.2. Alterations in Signaling Pathways Both the protein kinase C (PKC) and protein kinase A (PKA) signaling pathways have been shown to be affected by administration of n–3 fatty acids. For example, the human breast cancer cell line MDA-MB-231 exposed to physiological concentrations of EPA and DHA significantly decreased expression of the RIa regulatory subunit of PKA and PKCa isozyme *(67)*, which are capable of modulating cell cytokinetics. n–3 Fatty acids may also mediate the development of mammary cancer through their effect on the epidermal growth-factor receptor (EGFR) mitogen-activated PK signal-transduction cascade (reviewed in *68*). The effectiveness of n–3 fatty acids to inhibit growth of human breast cancer cells may depend upon expression of a mammary-derived growth inhibitor (MRG) (a DHA-selective fatty acid binding protein). In one study, MRG-transfected cells or MRG-protein treated cells were more sensitive to DHA-induced growth inhibition than MRG-negative or untreated control cells *(69)*. Another pathway that may be affected by n–3 fatty acids is production of mevalonate, an intermediate in cholesterol biosynthesis. Mevalonate production was shown to be decreased in mammary glands of fish oil-fed rats *(70)*. This may be significant because inhibitors of cholesterol synthesis (such as isoprenoids) are also inhibitors of tumor cell growth. The precise mechanism by which this inhibition of the key regulatory step in cholesterol biosynthesis (e.g., production of mevalonate) may be antitumorigenic is unknown, but could include such diverse outcomes as changes in membrane fluidity affecting signaling pathways to a downregulation of Ras farnesylation, which could result in a lower activity of the Ras protein that is often overexpressed during tumorigenesis.

Omega-3 fatty acids may also have a direct effect on gene expression *(71)*. Thoennes et al. *(71)* tested a variety of fatty acids for their effects on the transcriptional activity of peroxisome proliferator-activated receptor γ (PPARγ), in human breast cancer cell lines. Omega-3 fatty acids inhibited transactivation of PPARγ to levels below controls, and omega-6 fatty acids stimulated the activity of the transcriptional reporter *(71)*.

Although not specific to mammary tumorigenesis, Palakurthi et al. *(72)* have elucidated a relationship between EPA-induced depletion of intracellular calcium stores and the inhibition of cell proliferation and tumor growth. A series of experiments showed that EPA may release calcium from inositol-tris-1,4,5-phosphate-sensitive calcium pools and prevent the refilling of these pools. This in turn triggers PKR-mediated phosphorylation of eIF2α, with the ultimate effect of cell-cycle arrest in G_1.

3.2.4.3. Alterations in Eicosanoid Synthesis The literature on breast carcinoma and n–3 fatty acids is reviewed in Noguchi et al. *(73)*. A number of studies in both cell lines and rodents have shown a link between downregulation of eicosanoid synthesis and protection against mammary tumor growth. In one study, rats fed a menhaden oil diet and treated with 7,12-dimethyl-benz[*a*]anthracene (DMBA) had both lower mammary tumor incidence and lower levels of PGE_2, 6-keto-$PGF_{1\alpha}$, and LTB_4 than their corn oil-fed counterparts *(74)*. Which eicosanoids may be responsible for the enhanced tumorigenesis seen with corn oil-supplemented rats has not been determined, but LOX rather than COX inhibitors have proven to be effective in inhibiting human breast cancer cell growth both in vivo *(75)* and in vitro *(76,77)*. For example, in one study, inhibition of DMBA-induced rat mammary tumorigenesis was associated with both reduction of tumor LTB_4 production and inhibition of 5-LOX *(56)*. Treatment of W256 cells with LOX, but not COX, inhibitors induced apoptosis that was partially reversed by exogenous 12-hydroxyeicosatetraenoic acid (HETE) or 15-HETE *(78)*. In fact, it is hypothesized that promotive effects of linoleic acid (high in corn oil) are really the result of its conversion to 13-hydroxyoctadecadienoic acid (HODE) by LOX rather than to linoleic acid itself *(79)*. This hypothesis is supported by findings that ^{14}C linoleic acid added to arterial blood is recovered as ^{14}C13-HODE in tumor venous blood *(10)*; the addition of a LOX inhibitor to drinking water inhibited formation of 13-HODE in the tumor and caused regression of growth, but had no effect on linoleic acid uptake.

However, other studies have shown that PGE_2 concentrations are elevated in mammary tumors *(80,81)*; fish oil has been shown to decrease PGE_2 levels by 90% in human mammary tumor MX-1 in the athymic nude mouse *(82)*. Similarly, inhibitors of COX (e.g., indomethacin) decrease the growth of tumors *(83,84)*.

Also unresolved is the mechanism by which downregulation of either COX-2 or 12-LOX expression results in a lower incidence of mammary tumors. One connection appears to be through downregulation of apoptosis, when 12-LOX or COX-2 is overexpressed. For example, treatment of nude mice with MCF-7 breast cancer cells that overexpress 12-LOX resulted in increased tumor cell growth and inhibition of apoptosis *(85)*. Rose summarizes these data accordingly: "With this background, it seems reasonable to postulate that dietary n–3 fatty acids, which inhibit 12-HETE, 15-HETE, and PGE$_2$ production by human breast cancer cells growing as solid tumors in nude mice, may exert their suppressive effect on tumor-mass acquisition, at least in part, by activation of the apoptotic pathway" *(86)*.

3.2.4.4. Alterations in Cell Kinetics Both EPA and DHA inhibit growth of human breast cancer cell lines in vitro, although DHA has been more effective than EPA in suppressing growth of certain estrogen-independent breast cancer cells *(76)*. With respect to an estrogen-dependent breast cancer cell line, EPA, DHA, and a-linolenic acid all inhibited growth, although a-linolenic acid did so to a lesser degree than the other two longer-chain n–3 fatty acids *(87)*. There appears to be a fine line between the inhibition of growth by non-cytotoxic means seen at low concentrations of n–3 fatty acids, and cytotoxic effects seen at higher levels *(88)*.

The growth of human breast cancer cell lines in vitro, or mammary tumors in vivo, is dependent upon an increase in cell proliferation and/or a decrease in apoptosis. One study addressed the kinetics of cell proliferation in vivo using a double label (BrdU labeling and DNA analysis by flow cytometry) *(89)*. They found a longer S-phase duration (15.0 vs 9.1 h, p < 0.001) in cells from fish oil-fed rats than in those from safflower oil-fed rats, accounting for the difference in tumor growth rates. A study in nude mice with the MDA-MB-231 human breast cancer cell line growing as solid tumors showed reduced tumor growth, decreased cell proliferation, and increased apoptosis when 4% DHA was added to a 20% fat diet containing 4% linoleic acid *(90)*. The relationship of n–3 fatty acids to cell kinetics is reviewed in *(59,60)*.

3.2.4.5. Lipid Peroxidation and Cytostatic and/or Cytotoxic Effects Oxidation of n–3 fatty acids can produce a number of products that may have cytostatic or cytotoxic effects on tumor cells (reviewed in *91,92*). In one study, female athymic nude mice were implanted with human breast carcinoma MDA-MB-231 *(93)* and provided with diets containing various amounts of corn oil and fish oil (plus or minus antioxidants). Tumor volume and thiobarbituric acid reactive substances (TBARS) were evaluated after 6–8 wk. Tumor growth was suppressed in mice that received fish oil diets without antioxidants in a dose-dependent manner. However, the addition of antioxidants to the fish oil reversed the benefits of fish oil feeding *(93)*. The level

of increase in TBARS was directly related to the increase in dietary fish oil, suggesting that lipid peroxidation products were responsible for the depression in tumor growth. The effect of n–3 fatty acids on mammary tumorigenesis as a function of lipid peroxidation has been reviewed by Welsch *(94)*. The mechanism(s) by which these lipid peroxidation products of n–3 fatty acids may inhibit breast cancer cell growth is unclear, and could be a direct or indirect cytotoxic effect that initiates an apoptotic cascade.

3.2.4.6. Effects on Hormones Surprisingly, there is little information on the effect of n–3 fatty acids on hormones associated with breast cancer, although steroid hormones are known to play a role in breast cancer development. In one study *(95)*, women with either a predisposition to breast cancer or a carcinoma *in situ* were given fish oil, which reduced the 16α-hydroxylation of estradiol. This is significant because studies in women have shown that elevated 16α-hydroxylation of estradiol may be a biomarker for an increased risk of breast cancer *(96)*.

3.2.4.7. Effects on Angiogenesis In order for a tumor to grow and for cancers to metastasize, the formation of new blood vessels is required. Thus, inhibition of neovascularization is considered to be an important target for chemoprevention and/or cancer therapy. High angiogenic activity was seen in athymic nude mice injected with MCF-7 human breast carcinoma cells that stably overexpressed 12-LOX (and secreting high levels of 12-HETE) *(85)*. In contrast, a number of factors known to promote blood vessel growth are also known to be downregulated by n–3 fatty acids. Examples of these factors include COX and LOX products—e.g., PGs *(97)* and 12-HETE *(98)*. This suggests a role for n–3 fatty acids as antiangiogenic agents *(99)*.

3.3. Colon Cancer

3.3.1. EPIDEMIOLOGICAL STUDIES

As noted in Subheading 3.2.1., it has long been known that native Alaskan and Greenland Eskimos, whose consumption of 20:5n–3 and 22:6n–3 fatty acids is higher than that of other North Americans *(2,35,100)*, have a very low risk for cancer in general and breast and colon cancer in particular *(2,36,35)*, despite a high total fat intake. Also, fish consumption in 24 European countries was found to be inversely related to colorectal cancer (CRC) in males, although a similar trend for females was not significant *(25)*. Interestingly, when the data from these 24 countries were reanalyzed to consider both n–3 and n–6 fatty acid consumption into account, high fish intake had a protective effect relative to sources of n–6 fatty acids for both colon and breast cancer (26). This suggests, as noted in Subheading 2.3., that the ratio of n–6 to n–3 fatty acids rather than the absolute amounts of either of these classes of PUFAs may determine their protective effect.

An epidemiological study on diet and colon cancer from South Africa (101) is illuminating for a variety of reasons. This study compared 101 men and women with a low incidence of colon cancer, who fished for their livelihood on the west coast of South Africa, to 99 age- and sex-matched urban Cape Town inhabitants with a higher rate of this disease. The daily intake of n–3 fatty acids was more than 5 × higher in the fishing population than in the urban Cape Town inhabitants ($p < 0.0001$). Surprisingly, despite the lower incidence of colon cancer, a higher proportion of those who fished were smokers and had hypertension, and they consumed fewer fruits and vegetables and fiber than did the urban population. Of particular interest is the finding that none of those who fished took vitamin supplements, compared to one-third of the urban Cape Town population who took supplements. This may be significant because of the ability of peroxidation products of n–3 fatty acids to either initiate apoptotic removal of DNA damaged cells and/or to delete DNA damaged cells by cytotoxic mechanisms (91,92) as noted in Subheading 3.2.4.5. Support for the potentially negative effect of antioxidant supplementation on tumor development was from the previously discussed study in female athymic nude mice implanted with human breast carcinoma MDA-MB-231 and fed diets containing various amounts of corn oil and fish oil (plus or minus antioxidants). Adding antioxidants to the fish oil reversed the benefits of fish-oil feeding (93). This is consistent with the South African fishing community that did not consume vitamin supplements and yet had a low incidence of colon cancer, in contrast to the urban Cape Town inhabitants with a higher rate of this disease (one-third of these did consume such supplements).

Similar to the effects observed in breast cancer, a stepwise increase in EPA concentrations in plasma phospholipids and in colonic mucosal phospholipids was associated with a stepwise reduction in colon tumorigenesis assessed in patients as CRC, sporadic adenoma, or a normal colon. A stepwise increase in EPA concentrations was seen from the most advanced colon cancer to the most benign adenoma ($p = 0.009$) (102).

3.3.2. CLINICAL STUDIES

Clinical intervention trials on n–3 fatty acid consumption and intermediate markers for colon cancer are limited. Ulcerative colitis (UC) is considered to be a risk factor for colon cancer, and thus interventions that reduce the severity of this disease may be considered protective against later colon cancer development. In one such study (103), patients were randomized into two groups (either fish oil or sunflower oil supplementation) for 6 mo. At the end of 6 mo, the fish oil-supplemented group had a significant reduction in sigmoidoscopic and histological scores for UC compared to controls (103).

Individuals with sporadic adenomatous colorectal polyps are also considered at increased risk to develop colon cancer. Anti et al. found that humans with sporadic adenomatous colorectal polyps who took fish oil in capsule form for 12 wk had lower indices of cell proliferation in the upper colonic crypt compared to placebo controls (104). In later work, the same group studied patients with sporadic adenomatous colorectal polyps to establish an optimal dose of fish oil for achieving a chemopreventive effect (105). After 30 d, the n–3 fatty acid-supplemented group showed dose-related increases in rectal mucosal EPA and DHA levels. These changes in rectal mucosal n–3 fatty acids were accompanied by decreased cell proliferation, but this effect was not dose-related. This study also compared n–3 fatty acid supplementation with a placebo over a 6-mo period. As in the first study, rectal cell-proliferative indices were reduced by n–3 fatty acid supplementation in those with elevated cell proliferation prior to intervention.

Unlike breast cancer, colon cancer is affected by the constituents passing through the gastrointestinal (GI) tract. Data are unclear on which fecal bile acids (if any) promote colon cancer, and what the appropriate fecal bacterial content may be. In one study (106), 24 healthy volunteers were supplemented for 4 wk with either fish oil or corn oil. Effects of these diet interventions were investigated with respect to fecal excretion of secondary bile acids, certain neutral sterols, and bacterial enzyme activities. No significant differences were noted for fecal microbial enzyme activities measured, and fecal bile acid excretion was not affected by treatment (107).

Changes in rectal cell proliferation have been used as intermediate markers for later tumor development to evaluate whether or not a diet intervention is protective against colon cancer. Diets that decrease rectal cell proliferation are considered to be protective of colon cancer development. Two human studies were performed to determine the effect of fish oil supplementation on rectal cell proliferation and PGE$_2$ biosynthesis *(107,108)*. A decrease in rectal cell proliferation was observed when the dietary n–3:n–6 ratio was 0.4, but not with the same absolute level of fish oil intake and an n–3:n–6 fatty acid ratio of 0.25. This further supports the previously discussed concept, that the ratio of n–6 to n–3 fatty acids is more important in terms of chemoprevention than is the absolute amount of either of these PUFA categories. In a separate study, Bartoli et al. *(109)* investigated the effect of fish oil supplements in a 30-d clinical trial. They found that rectal cell proliferation was lower in the fish oil group than in the placebo group.

3.3.3. EXPERIMENTAL STUDIES

Fish oil high in n–3 fatty acids has been shown to be protective against experimentally induced colon cancer in a large number of studies *(110–117)*. This protective effect of fish oil has been shown to occur at initiation *(118)* and during promotion *(111,112)*, and with fish oil and n–3 fatty acid supplementation *(119)*. Athymic mice fed high-fat diets rich in coconut oil, olive oil, safflower oil, or fish oil were inoculated with HT29 cells to initiate colon tumor growth *(120)* and compared to mice fed a low-fat diet. There was no difference between resulting tumor sizes of mice fed fish oil compared to the low-fat diet, yet all other diets resulted in an increase in tumor size. Similarly, other investigators *(115)* found that a diet high in fish oil (23% by weight) did not enhance colon tumor development in rats injected with azoxymethane (AOM) compared with a diet low in corn oil (5%), whereas a diet high in corn oil did increase tumor incidence. We have found that fish oil-fed rats had higher levels of colonic epithelial cell differentiation and increased apoptosis, with no difference in proliferation compared to corn oil-fed rats *(121)*. Fish oil-fed rats also had a lower incidence of tumors than their corn oil-fed counterparts *(112)*.

In one of the few studies that tested the effects of various ratios of n–3 to n–6 fatty acids, Deschner et al. *(110)* looked at both early and late stages of tumor development in rats injected with AOM. Providing 16% of the total 20.4% fat as fish oil (n–3:n–6 ratio of 1.5) partially suppressed the increase in cell proliferation, which occurred as a function of the carcinogen injection at the early stages of tumorigenesis. Similarly, the occurrence of early dysplastic foci was reduced significantly in AOM-injected animals fed either 16% or 10.2%, but not 4.4%, fish oil. The highest tumor incidence occurred in rats fed 20.4% corn oil or 16% corn oil with the lowest (4.4%) level of fish oil. Diets containing 4.4% corn oil without any n–3 fatty acids, or 10.2% or 16% fish oil, resulted in a similarly low incidence of colon tumors.

The specific effect of DHA was tested in a study by Takahashi et al. *(119)*. DHA was provided as the ethyl ester by intragastric intubation in single doses 5 × weekly in rats injected with 1,2-dimethylhydrazine, and the development of aberrant crypt foci (ACF) was assessed. DHA treatment reduced the formation of ACF using this experimental paradigm. We have also provided purified n–3 fatty acid ethyl esters to rats in ratios that mimic those found in fish oil (122) in an attempt to determine whether purified fatty acids produce the same physiological effects as intact fish oil. We found that that these fatty acids incorporated similarly into mitochondrial phospholipids, and also had similar effects on mitochondrial membrane potential and caspase 3 activation (an early event in the apoptotic cascade) *(122)*. This suggests that the benefits of fish oil seen in experimental studies are indeed the result of fatty acids, rather than some contaminant of fish oil itself.

3.3.4. POTENTIAL MECHANISMS

3.3.4.1. Overview Most potential mechanisms by which n–3 fatty acids may protect against colon cancer are common to breast cancer—alterations in signaling pathways, eicosanoid synthesis, cell kinetics, lipid peroxidation, effect on hormones, and effect on angiogenesis. In addition, n–3 fatty acids may have a direct effect on lumenal constituents within the GI tract and on colonic microflora. This class of PUFA also uniquely influences the immune system *(123–125)*. As noted previously, n–3 fatty acids accumulate in biological membranes and may initiate signal-transduction processes or modify membrane structure *(123)*, which may also be linked to changes in gene expression.

3.3.4.2. Alterations in Signaling Pathways One of the most important signaling pathways that may be modified during tumorigenesis is *ras*-mediated. *Ras* genes code for 21-Kd guanine nucleotide-binding proteins that play an important role in colonic epithelial-cell growth, differentiation, and tumor formation *(126,127)*. Singh et al. *(128)* investigated the effect of various types and amounts of dietary fat on Ras-p21 expression during AOM-induced colon carcinogenesis in rats. They found higher levels of Ras-p21 expression with advancing stages of colon tumorigenesis. However, feeding fish oil inhibited Ras-p21 expression, and decreased both the incidence and multiplicity of colon tumors. Ras protein is only active in the plasma membrane, and Singh et al. also found that fish oil feeding resulted in lower levels of membrane-bound Ras. Davidson et al. *(129)*, using the rat AOM tumor model, demonstrated that colonic membrane Ras levels were decreased in fish oil- compared to corn oil-fed rats. This is important because prolonged Ras activation could result in a stimulation of cell proliferation *(130)*. Another documented effect of prolonged Ras activation is a reduced susceptibility to apoptosis *(131)* and another signaling pathway shown to be affected by fish oil feeding is PKC *(132)*. Specific PKC isoforms have different effects in colonocytes *(133)*, and altered PKC isoform signaling appears to be involved in colon cancer development *(134–136)*.

A necessary prerequisite to cell proliferation and thus to tumor growth is polyamine synthesis. Ornithine decarboxylase (ODC) is considered to be the rate-limiting enzyme for polyamine biosynthesis, and this inducible enzyme is elevated during colon carcinogenesis *(137)*. Craven and DeRubertis *(138)* reported an increase in ODC activity and PKC activation in colonic epithelial cells exposed to n–6 fatty acids. In an AOM rat colon cancer study, Reddy and Sugie *(117)* detected an inverse relationship between ODC activity and the level of menhaden oil in the diet. Investigators from the same laboratory *(139)* showed that an n–6 fatty acid-rich diet upregulated ODC activity in the colonic mucosa of rats exposed to AOM, whereas an n–3 fatty acid-rich diet resulted in relative suppression of the enzyme.

3.3.4.3. Alterations in Eicosanoid Synthesis

Although it is not known how fish oil decreases cell division and enhances apoptosis (Subheading 3.3.4.4.), one hypothesis is that n–3 fatty acids inhibit PG production, which in turn decreases colonic cell proliferation and tumor formation *(107,139)*. COX catalyzes the conversion of AA to PGs, and COX-2 expression is increased in colorectal adenomas and carcinomas compared to normal mucosa *(140)*. Elevated levels of PGs have been observed in human colon carcinomas compared to normal mucosa *(141)*, and in the colonic mucosa of rats injected with AOM during the initiation and postinitiation stages of carcinogenesis *(142)*. Similarly, elevated levels of AA (the precursor for PG synthesis) have been reported in colon tumors from rats injected with the colon carcinogen *(143)*.

We have reported that fish oil diets result in lower levels of AA in colonic mucosal phospholipids of rats

than corn oil diets *(144)*, and significantly lower levels of colonic mucosal PGE_2 with fish oil-supplemented diets compared with those supplemented with corn oil or beef tallow *(144)*. Similarly, Minoura et al. *(145)* found that partial suppression of rat colon carcinogenesis by EPA was associated with a reduction in PGE_2 content in tumors of EPA-supplemented rats. PGE_2 levels also have been shown to be lower in colonic biopsies from humans after fish oil consumption compared to corn oil consumption *(107)*. Singh et al. *(146)* showed that COX-2 expression was positively correlated with the incidence and multiplicity of colon tumors in the rat AOM model, and that enzyme expression and the incidence of tumors were enhanced by feeding a high-fat, n–6 PUFA-rich diet, but suppressed by a high-fat, 20% menhaden oil diet.

Corey et al. have reported that DHA is a strong inhibitor of PG but not leukotriene synthesis *(147)*. In an in vitro study, Hussey and Tisdale *(148)* showed that growth of two murine colon adenocarcinoma cell lines was enhanced by linoleic acid and AA but blocked by a selective LOX inhibitor. Subsequent in vivo studies using a 12-LOX inhibitor provided similar results *(149)*. The protective effect of nonsteroidal antiinflammatory drugs (NSAIDs) on CRC is believed to be mediated in part by inhibition of COX-2 *(141,150,151)*. Epidemiological studies show a protective effect of aspirin ingestion on colon cancer incidence *(152)*. Selective COX-2 inhibitors are also effective in experimental colon cancer chemoprevention *(153,154)*. In a recent study, both EPA and DHA were shown to be potent inhibitors of COX-2-catalyzed PG biosynthesis *(155)*. Rao et al. tracked the effects of diets high in n–3 and n–6 fatty acids on PG and thromboxane formation during different stages of AOM-induced colon tumorigenesis *(156)*. They found that compared to saline injection, AOM treatment increased the formation of PG and thromboxane during the tumorigenic process. In contrast, both a high-fat n–3 fatty acid-enriched diet and a low-fat corn oil diet resulted in lower amounts of PG and thromboxane B_2 than a high-fat corn oil diet *(156)*.

The connection between PG synthesis and apoptosis was explored by Tsujii and DuBois *(157)*, who overexpressed COX-2 in epithelial cells, and found that cells that overexpressed COX-2 were resistant to apoptosis induction by butyrate. In a separate study, Shiff et al. *(158)* reported that the PG synthesis inhibitor sulindac sulfide inhibits proliferation and induces apoptosis in HT-29 colon adenocarcinoma cells.

3.3.4.4. Alterations in Cell Kinetics We have shown *(121)* that fish oil has a greater effect on increasing apoptosis than on decreasing cell proliferation, and that this may be an important mechanism by which fish oil supplementation results in fewer colon tumors than corn oil *(112)*. Inhibition of apoptosis now is believed to be an integral component of the genesis of colorectal adenomas and carcinomas *(159)*. Of course, different signal transduction processes (*see* subheading 3.3.4.2.) may affect changes in both cell proliferation and apoptosis. In addition, COX-2 expression has been shown to downregulate apoptosis *(160)* (Subheading 3.3.4.3.).

In an attempt to determine changes in gene expression related to cell kinetics as a function of n–3 fatty acids *(161)*, CaCo-2 cells (a colon cancer cell line) were incubated with DHA for 48 h; gene-expression profiles were determined using DNA oligonucleotide arrays. The investigators reported elevated levels of a number of genes associated with apoptosis (e.g., cytochrome C and caspases), and also elevation of a number of growth arrest-specific proteins. Finally, consistent with studies reported in Subheading 3.3.4.3., there was an inactivation of the PG family of genes by DHA treatment.

3.3.4.5. Effect on Angiogenesis As shown previously for breast cancer, a high degree of angiogenic activity in colonic carcinomas has also been associated with a poor prognosis *(162)*. Similarly, microvessel density is higher in aggressively invasive colon cancers than in less invasive cases *(163)*. Nitric oxide (NO) is known to activate COX-2 and regulate PG biosynthesis *(164)*, which in turn affects angiogenesis. One study *(114)* reports that both inducible and constitutive endothelial nitric oxide synthases (NOS) were elevated in rat colon tumors induced by AOM. Thus, it appears that the downregulation of COX by n–3 fatty acids, in addition to upregulating apoptosis (*see* Subheading 3.3.4.3.) may also lead to antiangiogenic effects.

3.3.4.6. Effects Specific to the Colon Fish oil feeding in rats has resulted in a different mixed population of colonic microflora relative to corn oil feeding *(165)*. This in turn could result in differential bacterial metabolism in the colon. In one study, for example, a diet high in corn oil compared to one high in fish oil increased activity of the bacterial enzyme 7α-dehydroxylase, which converts primary bile acids to secondary bile acids. Lower levels of secondary bile acids were found with fish oil vs corn oil feeding *(166)*, which may be significant because secondary bile acids are considered to be colon tumor promoters *(167)*. Bartram et al. *(168)* conducted a clinical study in which healthy volunteers were supplemented with either 11 g of fish oil or corn oil, and fecal bile acid excretion was determined. After 4 wk, excretion of lithocholic acid (a secondary bile acid) was lower after n–3 fatty acid than n–6 fatty acid administration, although the difference was not statistically significant.

3.4. Other Cancers

3.4.1. PROSTATE CANCER

There is some epidemiological support for a protective effect of n–3 fatty acids on prostate cancer. Clinical trials, generally of short duration, with small numbers of participants, suggest that consumption of diets that are high in omega-3 fatty acids reduce the risk of prostate cancer. For example, in one study, 25 patients with prostate cancer *(169)* supplemented with 30 g per d of flaxseed (rich in n–3 fatty acids) who consumed 20% or less kilocalories from fat were compared to historic cases. Low fat combined with flaxseed supplementation resulted in lower levels of total testosterone, free androgen, and cell proliferation indices than historic controls. In addition, apoptotic indices were higher in this n–3 supplemented group. In an outpatient clinic-based study of 89 cases of prostate cancer and 38 controls *(170)*, fatty acids in erythrocyte membranes and adipose tissue fatty acids from subcutaneous fat samples were analyzed and used to calculate odds ratios for the association of each fatty acid with prostate cancer. Linoleic acid in erythrocyte membranes was positively associated with prostate cancer ($p < 0.04$). n–3 Fatty acids had no significant protective effect, yet their sample size was quite small.

One study that reported on the effects of diets containing different unsaturated fatty acids on human prostate cancer cell growth in nude mice *(171)* that consumed menhaden oil found a 30% reduction in tumor growth compared to mice that received corn oil or linseed oil diets ($p < 0.001$). Of the long chain n–3 fatty acids, it appears that both DHA and EPA inhibited androgen-stimulated cell growth, and prostate-specific antigen (PSA) was reduced by DHA and EPA in a dose-dependent manner *(172)*. The amount of fatty acid administered also appears to be important. For example, in one study *(173)*, EPA at lower concentrations had a promotive effect on human prostate cancer cell line growth. In contrast, EPA at higher concentrations inhibited prostate cell growth.

3.4.2. Lung Cancer

A study conducted in 36 countries found a significant inverse correlation between fish consumption and lung cancer mortality rates in nine of the 10 time periods studied, but only for men *(174)*. Interestingly, this association of fish consumption with a reduced risk of lung cancer mortality was only observed in countries with high levels of cigarette smoking. Although the reason for this finding is not clear, it is interesting to note that smoking increases reactive oxygen species (ROS), which supports a protective effect of n–3 fatty acids by raising ROS production and perhaps initiating apoptosis through this process. In a separate epidemiological study in Norway *(175)*, the relationship between the incidence of lung cancer and intake of fish and fish products was studied in 25,956 men and 25,496 women. A significantly lower risk for lung cancer was found for cod liver oil supplementation (RR = 0.5).

3.4.3. Cervical and Pancreatic Cancer

These cancers have not been addressed in a concerted way with respect to the effect of fatty acid intake on their occurrence. With cervical cancer, one study examined the effect of linoleic acid, EPA, or DHA on human precancerous cervical keratinocytes immortalized with the oncogenic human papillomavirus (HPV) *(176)*. Results showed that DHA inhibited growth of these cells in a dose-dependent manner to a greater extent than EPA; linoleic acid had no effect. Studies in human pancreatic cancer cell lines showed that EPA arrests cell growth and upregulates apoptosis *(177,178)*.

4. TREATMENT OF CANCER WITH OMEGA-3 FATTY ACIDS

4.1. Inhibition of Metastases and Tumor Growth

The growth of a tumor at the original site or at a new site depends on a number of factors, including changes in cell kinetics, angiogenesis, and adhesion properties of tumor cells. n–3 Fatty acids can affect all these factors, as described in detail in the sections on cell kinetics and angiogenesis. The growth of a transplanted Morris hepatocarcinoma was reduced by providing rats with low doses of either EPA or DHA, but these reductions were apparently achieved by different mechanisms *(179)*. EPA reduced cell proliferation of the tumor cells, and DHA upregulated apoptosis. In a separate study *(180)*, DHA-containing liposomes were injected into tumor-bearing mice, and mouse survival was charted. DHA-containing liposomes caused a statistically significant increase in the survival of tumor-bearing mice compared with those containing oleic acid. Treatment with n–3 fatty acids may also alter tumor-cell sensitivity to immune cytolysis *(181)*. An in vivo mouse study *(182)* correlated the incorporation of DHA into T27A leukemia cells grown as an ascites tumor in mice with an increased susceptibility to tumor cytolysis by T-lymphocytes.

The adhesion of colon cancer cells to endothelial cells was tested in vitro by growing cells in an n–3 fatty acid-enriched medium. Binding of colon cancer cells to endothelial cells was reduced after incubation *(183)*. Similarly, Connolly and Rose *(184)* used an in vitro invasion assay system to test the effect of linoleic acid, EPA, and DHA on the invasive capacity of MDA-MB-435 human breast cancer cells. Both n–3 fatty acids inhibited tumor cell invasion, whereas invasion was stimulated by linoleic acid. McCarty *(185)* suggests that one of the mechanisms by which n–3 fatty acids may exert their antitumor growth and antimetastatic effects is through the downregulation of PKC. According to McCarty, PKC can induce collagenase that aids angiogenesis; n–3 fatty acids reduce PKC.

With respect to metastasis, angiogenesis plays an important role (*see* Subheadings 3.2.4.7. and 3.3.4.5.). Some researchers suggest that COX-2 upregulates the expression of vascular endothelial growth factor (VEGF), which is required for angiogenesis. As described previously, n–3 fatty acids downregulate COX-2 expression. In a recent study *(186)*, COX-2, VEGF, PGE_2, and microvessel density were immunohistochemically measured in tumors and adjacent normal mucosa from 31 surgical specimens. Both COX-2 and VEGF were significantly correlated with microvessel density, and COX-2 and VEGF genes were overexpressed in tumor specimens as compared to normal mucosa. Also, PGE_2 levels were significantly higher in metastatic tumors than in nonmetastatic ones.

4.2. Immunonutrition

A number of papers have appeared in the literature on recovery from surgery (for cancer and other surgical interventions) using normal enteral feeding, standard total parenteral nutrition, and what is called "immunonutrition" with an enteral formula enriched with arginine, omega-3 fatty acids, and RNA *(187)*. In one such study *(188)*, patients who had undergone surgery for GI cancers were provided with a standard diet or the same diet supplemented with glutamine, arginine, and omega–3 fatty acids, within 38 h after surgery. The supplement had a positive effect on post-surgical immunosuppressive and inflammatory responses. Supplementation with n–3 fatty acids has also been shown to improve patient histological scores in UC (considered a risk factor for later colon cancer development) by suppressing immune reactivity *(189)*. In addition, fish oil supplementation has reduced the rate of relapse in patients with Crohn's disease *(190)*.

Diet interventions have differed in their timing and length of intervention. In most instances, immunonutrition has resulted in lower postoperative complications and less severe infectious complications *(187,191)*. However, it has not shown an effect on overall mortality. Supplements of EPA have also been used to reduce the weight loss that is often associated with cancer *(192)*. A recent review *(193)* summarized whether or not immunonutrition translates into an improvement in clinical outcomes, concluding that immunonutrition may decrease infectious complication rates, but is not associated with an overall mortality advantage. A similar conclusion was reached in a previous meta-analysis *(194)*. A small intervention study *(195)* investigated the effect of dietary n–3 PUFA on T-cell subsets and natural killer (NK) cells of patients with solid tumors. Twenty (20) patients with solid tumors received 18 g fish oil/d for 40 d. At the end of 40 d, a significant increase in T-helper/T-suppressor cell ratio was seen, because of mainly a decrease in the number of suppressor T cells. The authors concluded that n–3 fatty acids may have a beneficial effect on the already compromised immune systems of patients with solid tumors.

Also of interest is reversal of tumor cell drug resistance, as drug resistance has a profoundly negative impact on effective cancer chemotherapy. For example, in one study *(196)*, EPA and DHA were shown to kill tumor cells in vitro and also to increase anticancer drug influx and decrease efflux in tumor cells. Similarly, a separate study *(197)* found that addition of DHA to cultured lymphoma cells enhanced the toxicity of chemotherapeutic agents. Bougnoux et al. *(198)* tested the association between levels of fatty acids in breast adipose tissue and tumor response to chemotherapy in 56 patients with an initially localized breast carcinoma. Levels of n–3 PUFA in adipose tissue were higher in the group of patients with complete or partial response to chemotherapy than in patients with no response or with tumor progression ($p < 0.004$). Specifically, DHA (22:6n–3) was an independent predictor for chemosensitivity. In a double-blind, randomized study in dogs treated for lymphoblastic lymphoma with doxorubicin chemotherapy, increasing DHA blood levels were associated with a longer disease-free interval and survival time *(199)*.

5. CONCLUSION

Cogent evidence indicates that dietary n–3 PUFAs found in fish oil—e.g., EPA and DHA—confer protection against several forms of cancer, in part by activating apoptosis to enhance deletion of cells, and by suppressing the cell proliferation and gene functions associated with angiogenesis. These data support the contention that dietary n–3 PUFAs have chemoprotective value and should be adopted by health professionals who strive for cancer prevention. Therefore, it is essential to understand precisely how an important dietary constituent modulates cell phenotypes, so that recommendations regarding the health benefits derived from nutritional manipulation can be based on a firm scientific foundation.

REFERENCES

1. Hunter JE. n–3 Fatty acids from vegetable oils. *Am J Clin Nutr* 1990;51:809–814.
2. Bang HO, Deyerberg J, Hjorne N. The composition of food consumed by Greenland Eskimos. *Acta Med Scand* 1976;200:69–73.
3. Simopoulos A. Omega-3 fatty acids in health and disease and in growth and development. *Am J Clin Nutr* 1991;54:438–463.
4. de Gomez Dumm IN, Brenner RR. Oxidative desaturation of alpha-linolenic, linoleic, and stearic acids by human liver microsomes. *Lipids* 1975;10:315–317.
5. Pawlosky RJ, Hibbeln JR, Novotny JA, Salem NJ. Physiological compartmental analysis of alpha-linolenic acid metabolism in adult humans. *J Lipid Res* 2001;42:1257–1265.
6. Lands WE, Hamazaki T, Yamazaki K, et al. Changing dietary patterns. *Am J Clin Nutr* 1990;51:991–993.
7. Consensus conference. Lowering blood cholesterol to prevent heart disease. *JAMA* 1985;253:2080–2086.
8. Hague TA, Christoffersen BO. Effect of dietary fats on arachidonic acid and eicosapentaenoic acid biosynthesis and conversion of C_{22} fatty acids in isolated liver cells. *Biochim Biophys Acta* 1984;796:205–217.
9. Christiansen EN, Lund JS, Rortviet T, Rustan AC. Effect of dietary n–3 and n–6 fatty acids on fatty acid desaturation in rat liver. *Biochim Biophys Acta* 1991;1082:57–62.
10. Sauer LA, Dauchy RT, Blask DE. Dietary linoleic acid intake controls the arterial blood plasma concentration and the rates of growth and linoleic acid uptake and metabolism in hepatoma 7288CTC in Buffalo rats. *J Nutr* 1997;127:1412–1421.
11. Sauer LA, Dauchy RT, Blask DE. Mechanism for the antitumor and anticachectic effects of n–3 fatty acids. *Cancer Res* 2000;60:5289–5295.

12. Subbaiah PV, Kaufman D, Bagddade JD. Incorporation of dietary n–3 fatty acids into molecular species of phosphatidyl choline and cholesteryl esters in normal human plasma. *Am J Clin Nutr* 1993;58:360–368.

13. Karmali RA. Fatty acids: inhibition. *Am J Clin Nutr* 1987;45:225–229.

14. Corey RJ, Shih C, Cashman JR. Docosahexaenoic acid is a strong inhibitor of prostaglandin but not leukotriene synthesis. *Proc Natl Acad Sci USA* 1980;80:3581–3584.

15. Brown ER, Subbaiah PV. Differential effects of eicosapentaenoic acid and docosahexaenoic acid on human skin fibroblasts. *Lipids* 1994;29:825–829.

16. Kafrawy O, Zerouga M, Stillwell W, Jenski LJ. Docosahexaenoic acid in phosphatidylcholine mediates cytotoxicity more effectively than other omega 3 and omega 6 fatty acids. *Cancer Lett* 1998;132:23–29.

17. McDowell MA, Briefel RR, Alaimo K, et al. Energy and macronutrient intakes of person ages 2 months and over in the United States: Third National Health and Nutrition Examination Survey, Phase I, 1988–1991. *Advance Data* 1994;255:1–24.

18. Kang ZB, Ge YL, Chen ZH, et al. Adenoviral gene transfer of *Caenorhabditis elegans* n–3 fatty acid desaturase optimizes fatty acid composition in mammalian cells. *Proc Natl Acad Sci USA* 2001;98:4050–4054.

19. Spector AA. Essentiality of fatty acids. *Lipids* 1999;34:S1–S3.

20. Zock PL, Katan MB. Linoleic acid intake and cancer risk: a review and meta-analysis. *Am J Clin Nutr* 1998;68:142–153.

21. Horrobin DF. Workshop statement on the essentiality of and recommended dietary intakes for omega-6 and omega-3 fatty acids—Commentary on the workshop statement—Are we really sure that arachidonic acid and linoleic acid are bad things. *Prostaglandins Leukot Essent Fatty Acids* 2000;63:145–147.

22. Toriyama-Baba H, Iigo M, Asamoto M, et al. Organotropic chemopreventive effects of n–3 unsaturated fatty acids in a rat multi-organ carcinogenesis model. *Jpn J Cancer Res* 2001;92:1175–1183.

23. Delorgeril M, Salen P, Martin JL, et al. Mediterranean dietary pattern in a randomized trial—prolonged survival and possible reduced cancer rate. *Arch Intern Med* 1998;158:1181–1187.

24. Kaizer L, Boyd NF, Kriukov V, Tritchler DL. Fish consumption and breast cancer risk: an ecological study. *Nutr Cancer* 1989;12:61–68.

25. Caygill CPJ, Hill MJ. Fish, n–3 fatty acids and human colorectal and breast cancer. *Eur J Cancer Prev* 1995;4:329–332.

26. Caygill CPJ, Charlett A, Hill MJ. Fat, fish, fish oil and cancer. *Br J Cancer* 1996;74:159–164.

27. Bartsch H, Nair J, Owen RW. Dietary polyunsaturated fatty acids and cancers of the breast and colorectum: emerging evidence for their role as risk modifiers. *Carcinogenesis* 1999;20:2209–2218.

28. Potter JD. Risk factors for colon neoplasia: epidemiology and biology. *Eur J Cancer* 1995;31A:1033–1038.

29. Rose DP. Effects of dietary fatty acids on breast and prostate cancer: evidence from in vitro experiments and animal studies. *Am J Clin Nutr* 1997;66:1513S–1522S.

30. Rose DP. Dietary fatty acids and cancer. *Am J Clin Nutr* 1997;66:998S–1003S.

31. Wynder EL, Cohen LA, Muscat JE, et al. Breast cancer: weighing the evidence for a promoting role of dietary fat. *J Natl Cancer Inst* 1997;89:766–775.

32. Ip C. Review of the effects of trans fatty acids, oleic acid, n–3 polyunsaturated fatty acids, and conjugated linoleic acid on mammary carcinogenesis in animals. *Am J Clin Nutr* 1997;66:1523S–1529S.

33. Rose DP, Connolly JM. Omega-3 fatty acids as cancer chemopreventive agents. *Pharmacol Ther* 1999;83:217–244.

34. Sasaki S, Horacesk M, Kesteloot H. An ecological study of the relationship between dietary fat intake and breast cancer mortality. *Prev Med* 1993;22:187–202.

35. Bang HO, Dyerberg J. Lipid metabolism and ischemic heart disease in Greenland Eskimos, in *Advances in Nutritional Research*, Vol. 3. Draper HH, ed. Plenum, New York, NY, 1980,pp.1–22.

36. Kromann N, Green A. Epidemiological studies in the Upernavik District, Greenland: incidence of some chronic diseases 1960–1974. *Acta Med Scand* 1980;208:401–406.

37. Ingram DM, Nottage E, Roberts T. The role of diet in the development of breast cancer: a case-control study of patients with breast cancer, benign epithelial hyperplasia and fibrocystic disease of the breast. *Br J Cancer* 1991;64:187–191.

38. Landa MC, Frago N, Tres A. Diet and the risk of breast cancer in Spain. *Eur J Cancer Prev* 1994;3:313–320.

39. Franceschi S, Favero A, La Vecchia C, et al. Influence of food groups and food diversity on breast cancer risk in Italy. *Int J Cancer* 1995;63:785–789.

40. Braga C, La Vecchia C, Negri E, et al. Intake of selected foods and nutrients and breast cancer risk: an age- and menopause-specific analysis. *Nutr Cancer* 1997;28:258–263.

41. Willett WC. Specific fatty acids and risks of breast and prostate cancer: dietary intake. *Am J Clin Nutr* 1997;66:1557S–1563S.

42. Vatten LJ, Solvoll K, Loken EB. Frequency of meat and fish intake and risk of breast cancer in a prospective study of 14,500 Norwegian women. *Int J Cancer* 1990;46:12–15.

43. Petrek JA, Hudgins LC, Levine B, et al. Breast cancer risk and fatty acids in the breast and abdominal adipose tissues. *J Natl Cancer Inst* 1994;86:53–56.

44. London SJ, Sacks FM, Stampfer MJ, et al. Fatty acid composition of the subcutaneous adipose tissue and risk of proliferative benign breast disease and breast cancer. *J Natl Cancer Inst* 1993;85:785–793.

45. Boyd NF, Martin LJ, Noffel M, et al. A meta-analysis of studies of dietary fat and breast cancer risk. *Br J Cancer* 1993;68:627–636.

46. Zaridze DG, Chevchenko VE, Levtshuk AA, et al. Fatty acid composition of phospholipids in erythrocyte membranes and risk of breast cancer. *Int J Cancer* 1990;45:807–810.

47. Vatten LJ, Bjerve KS, Andersen A, Jellum E. Polyunsaturated fatty acids in serum phospholipids and risk of breast cancer: a case-control study from the Janus serum bank in Norway. *Eur J Cancer* 1993;29A:532–538.

48. Pala V, Krogh V, Muti P, et al. Erythrocyte membrane fatty acids and subsequent breast cancer: a prospective Italian study. *J Natl Cancer Inst* 2001;93:1088–1095.

49. Berrino F, Muti P, Micheli A, et al. Serum sex hormone levels after menopause and subsequent breast cancer. *J Natl Cancer Inst* 1996;88:291–296.

50. Lu J, Pei H, Kaeck M, Thompson HJ. Gene expression changes associated with chemically induced rat mammary carcinogenesis. *Mol Carcinog* 1997;20:204–215.

51. Khoo DE, Fermor B, Miller J, et al. Manipulation of body fat composition with sterculic acid can inhibit mammary carcinomas in vivo. *Br J Cancer* 1991;63:97–101.

52. Simonsen N, Vantveer P, Strain JJ, et al. Adipose tissue omega-3 and omega-6 fatty acid content and breast cancer in the EURAMIC study. *Am J Epidemiol* 1998;147:342–352.

53. Maillard V, Bougnoux P, Ferrari P, et al. N-3 and N-6 fatty acids in breast adipose tissue and relative risk of breast cancer in a case-control study in Tours, France. *Int J Cancer* 2002;98:78–83.

54. Jurkowski JJ, Cave WT. Dietary effects of menhaden oil on the growth and membrane lipid composition of rat mammary tumors. *J Natl Cancer Inst* 1985;74:1145–1150.

55. Braden LM, Carroll KK. Dietary polyunsaturated fat in relation to mammary carcinogenesis in rats. *Lipids* 1986;21:285–288.

56. Abou-El-Ela SH, Prasse KW, Farrell RL, et al. Effects of d,l-2-difluoromethylornithine and indomethacin on mammary tumor promotion in rats fed high n–3 and/or n–6 fat diets. *Cancer Res* 1989;49:1434–1440.

57. Cohen LA, Chen-Backlund JY, Sepkovic DV, Sugie S. Effect of varying proportions of dietary menhaden and corn oil on experimental rat mammary tumor promotion. *Lipids* 1993;28:449–456.

58. Karmali RA, Marsh J, Fuchs C. Effect of omega-3 fatty acids on growth of a rat mammary tumor. *J Natl Cancer Inst* 1984;73:457–461.

59. Cave WT. Omega 3 fatty acid diet effects on tumorigenesis in experimental animals, in *Health Effects of Omega 3 Polyunsaturated Fatty Acids in Seafoods, Vol. 66.* Simopoulos AP, Kifer RR, Martin RE, Barlow SM, eds. Basel: Karger, 1991:pp.462–476.

60. Fernandes G, Venkatraman JT. Modulation of breast cancer growth in nude mice by omega 3 lipids, in *Health Effects of Omega 3 Polyunsaturated Fatty Acids in Seafoods, Vol. 66.* Simopoulos AP, Kifer RR, Martin RE, Barlow SM, eds. Karger, Basel 1991, pp.488–503.

61. Ip C, Carter CA, Ip MM. Requirement of essential fatty acid for mammary tumorigenesis in the rat. *Cancer Res* 1985;45:1997–2001.

62. Connolly JM, Gilhooly EM, Rose DP. Effects of reduced dietary linoleic acid intake, alone or combined with an algal source of docosahexaenoic acid, on MDA-MB-231 breast cancer cell growth and apoptosis in nude mice. *Nutr Cancer* 1999;35:44–49.

63. Kinoshita K, Noguchi M, Tanaka M. Effects of linoleic acid, eicosapentaenoic acid, and docosahexaenoic acid on the growth and metastasis of MM48 mammary tumor transplants in mice. *Int J Oncol* 1996;8:575–581.

64. Rose DP, Connolly JM, Coleman M. Effect of omega-3 fatty acids on the progression of metastases after the surgical excision of human breast cancer cell solid tumors growing in nude mice. *Clin Cancer Res* 1996;2:1751–1756.

65. Rose DP, Connolly JM, Rayburn J, Coleman M. Influence of diets containing eicosapentaenoic or docosahexaenoic acid on growth and metastasis of breast cancer cells in nude mice. *J Natl Cancer Inst* 1995;87:587–592.

66. Fay MP, Freedman LS, Clifford CK, Midthune DN. Effect of different types and amounts of fat on the development of

67. mammary tumors in rodents: a review. *Cancer Res* 1997;57:3979–3988.

67. Moore NG, Wang-Johanning F, Chang PL, Johanning GL. Omega-3 fatty acids decrease protein kinase expression in human breast cancer cells. *Breast Cancer Res Treat* 2001;67:279–283.

68. Cowing BE, Saker KE. Polyunsaturated fatty acids and epidermal growth factor receptor mitogen-activated protein kinase signaling in mammary cancer. *J Nutr* 2001;131:1125–1128.

69. Wang MS, Liu YLE, Ni J, et al. Induction of mammary differentiation by mammary-derived growth inhibitor-related gene that interacts with an omega-3 fatty acid on growth inhibition of breast cancer cells. *Cancer Res* 2000;60:6482–6487.

70. El-Sohemy A, Archer MC. Regulation of mevalonate synthesis in rat mammary glands by dietary n–3 and n–6 polyunsaturated fatty acids. *Cancer Res* 1997;57:3685–3687.

71. Thoennes SR, Tate PL, Price TM, Kilgore MW. Differential transcriptional activation of peroxisome proliferator-activated receptor gamma by omega-3 and omega-6 fatty acids in MCF-7 cells. *Mol Cell Endocrinol* 2000;160:67–73.

72. Palakurthi SS, Fluckiger R, Aktas H, et al. Inhibition of translation initiation mediates the anticancer effect of the n–3 polyunsaturated fatty acid eicosapentaenoic acid. *Cancer Res.* 2000;60:2919–2925.

73. Noguchi M, Rose DP, Earashi M, Miyazaki I. The role of fatty acids and eicosanoid synthesis inhibitors in breast carcinoma. *Oncology* 1995;52:265–271.

74. Abou-El-Ela SH, Prasse KW, Carroll R, et al. Eicosanoid synthesis in 7,12-dimethyl-benz(*a*)anthracene-induced mammary carcinomas in Sprague-Dawley rats fed primrose oil, menhaden oil or corn oil. *Lipids* 1988;23:948–954.

75. Kitagawa H, Noguchi M. Comparative effects of piroxicam and esculetin on incidence, proliferation, and cell kinetics of mammary carcinomas induced by 7,12-dimethylbenz[*a*]anthracene in rats on high-and-low-fat diets. *Oncology* 1994;51:401–410.

76. Rose DP, Connolly JM. Effects of fatty acids and inhibitors of eicosanoid synthesis on the growth of a human breast cancer cell line in culture. *Cancer Res* 1990;50:7139–7144.

77. Buckman DK, Hubbard NE, Erickson KL. Eicosanoids and linoleate-enhanced growth of mouse mammary tumor cells. *Prostaglandins Leukot Essent Fatty Acids* 1991;44:177–184.

78. Tang DG, Chen YQ, Honn KV. Arachidonate lipoxygenases as essential regulators of cell survival and apoptosis. *Proc Natl Acad Sci USA* 1996;93:5241–5246.

79. Sauer LA, Dauchy RT, Blask DE. Polyunsaturated fatty acids, melatonin, and cancer prevention. *Biochem Pharmacol* 2001;61:1455–1462.

80. Karmali RA. Eicosanoids in neoplasia. *Prev Med* 1987;16:493–502.

81. Karmali RA. Eicosanoids in cancer, in *Dietary Fat and Cancer.* Ip C, Birt DF, Rogers AE, Mettlin C, eds. Alan R. Liss, Inc., New York, NY, 1986:pp.687–697.

82. Colombo DT, Tran LK, Speck JJ, Reitz RC. Comparison of hexadecylphosphocholine with fish oil as an antitumor agent. *J Lipid Mediat Cell Signal* 1997;17:47–63.

83. Carter CA, Milholland RJ, Shea W, Ip MM. Effect of the prostaglandin synthetase inhibitor indomethacin on 7,12-

dimethylbenz(*a*)anthracene-induced mammary tumorigenesis in rats fed different levels of fat. *Cancer Res* 1983;43:3559–3562.

84. Kollmorgen GM, King MM, Kosanke SD, Do C. Influence of dietary fat and indomethacin on the growth of transplantable mammary tumors in rats. *Cancer Res* 1983;43:4714–4719.

85. Connolly JM, Rose DP. Enhanced angiogenesis and growth of 12-lipoxygenase gene-transfected MCF-7 human breast cancer cells in athymic nude mice. *Cancer Lett* 1998;132:107–112.

86. Rose DP, Connolly JM. Dietary fat and breast cancer metastasis by human tumor xenografts. *Breast Cancer Res Treat* 1997; 46:225–237.

87. Grammatikos SI, Subbaiah PV, Victor TA, Miller WM. n–3 and n–6 fatty acid processing and growth effects in neoplastic and non-cancerous human mammary epithelial cell lines. *Br J Cancer* 1994;70:219–227.

88. Begin ME, Ells G, Horrobin DF. Polyunsaturated fatty acid-induced cytotoxicity against tumor cells and its relationship to lipid peroxidation. *J Natl Cancer Inst* 1988;80:188–194.

89. Istfan NW, Wan JM, Bistrian BR, Chen ZY. DNA replication time accounts for tumor growth variation induced by dietary fat in a breast carcinoma model. *Cancer Lett* 1994;86:177–186.

90. Rose DP, Connolly JM. Antiangiogenicity of docosahexaenoic acid and its role in the suppression of breast cancer cell growth in nude mice. *Int J Oncol* 1999;15:1011–1015.

91. Gonzalez MJ. Fish oil, lipid peroxidation and mammary tumor growth. *J Am Coll Nutr* 1995;14:325–335.

92. Gonzalez MJ, Schemmel RA, Gray JI, et al. Effect of dietary fat on growth of MCF-7 and MDAA-MB231 human breast carcinomas in athymic nude mice: relationship between carcinoma growth and lipid peroxidation product levels. *Carcinogenesis* 1991;12:1231–1235.

93. Gonzalez MJ, Schemmel RA, Dugan J Jr, et al. Dietary fish oil inhibits human breast carcinoma growth: a function of increased lipid peroxidation. *Lipids* 1993;28:827–832.

94. Welsch CW. Review of the effects of dietary fat on experimental mammary gland tumorigenesis: role of lipid peroxidation. *Free Radic Biol Med* 1995;18:757–773.

95. Osborne MP, Karmali RA, Herschcopf RJ, et al. Omega-3 fatty acids: modulation of estrogen metabolism and potential for breast cancer prevention. *Cancer Invest* 1988;6:629–632.

96. Telang NT, Katdare M, Bradlow HL, Osborne MP. Estradiol metabolism: an endocrine biomarker for modulation of human mammary carcinogenesis. *Environ Health Perspect* 1997;105 (Suppl 3):559–564.

97. Form DM, Auerbach R. PGE$_2$ and angiogenesis. *Proc Soc Exp Biol Med* 1983;172:214–218.

98. Tang DG, Renaud C, Stojakovic S, et al. 12-(S)-HETE is a mitogenic factor for microvascular endothelial cells: its potential role in angiogenesis. *Biochem Biophys Res Commun* 1995;211:462–468.

99. Connolly JM, Liu X-H, Rose DP. Effects of dietary menhaden oil, soy, and a cyclooxygenase inhibitor on human breast cancer cell growth and metastasis in nude mice. *Nutr Cancer* 1997;29:48–54.

100. Blot WJ, Lanier A, Fraumeni JF, Bender TR. Cancer mortality among Alaska natives, 1960–69. *J Natl Cancer Inst* 1975;55:547–554.

101. Schloss I, Kidd MSG, Tichelaar HY, et al. Dietary factors associated with a low risk of colon cancer in coloured west coast fishermen. *S Afr Med J* 1997;87:152–158.

102. Fernandez-Banares F, Esteve M, Navarro E, et al. Changes of the mucosal n–3 and n–6 fatty acid status occur early in the colorectal adenoma-carcinoma sequence. *Gut* 1996;38:254–259.

103. Almallah YZ. Distal procto-colitis, natural cytotoxicity, and essential fatty acids. *Am J Gastroenterol* 1998;93:804–809.

104. Anti M, Marra G, Armelao F, et al. Effect of n–3 fatty acids on rectal mucosal cell proliferation in subjects at risk of colon cancer. *Gastroenterology* 1992;103:883–891.

105. Anti M, Armelao F, Marra G, et al. Effects of different doses of fish oil on rectal cell proliferation in patients with sporadic colonic adenomas. *Gastroenterology* 1994;107:1709–1718.

106. Bartram HP, Gostner A, Kelber E, et al. Effects of fish oil on fecal bacterial enzymes and steroid excretion in healthy volunteers—implications for colon cancer prevention. *Nutr Cancer* 1996;25:71–78.

107. Bartram HP, Gostner A, Scheppach W, et al. Effects of fish oil on rectal cell proliferation, mucosal fatty acids, and prostaglandin E$_2$ release in healthy subjects. *Gastroenterology* 1993;105:1317–1322.

108. Bartram HP, Gostner A, Reddy BS, et al. Missing antiproliferative effect of fish oil on rectal epithelium in healthy volunteers consuming a high-fat diet: potential role of the n–3:n–6 fatty acid ratio. *Eur J Cancer Prev* 1995; 4:231–237.

109. Bartoli GM, Palozza P, Marra G, et al. n–3 PUFA and α-tocopherol control of tumor cell proliferation. *Mol Aspects Med* 1993;14:247–252.

110. Deschner EE, Lytle JS, Wong G, et al. The effect of dietary omega-3 fatty acids (fish oil) on azoxymethanol-induced focal areas of dysplasia and colon tumor incidence. *Cancer* 1990;66:2350–2356.

111. Reddy BS, Burill C, Rigotty J. Effect of diets high in ω-3 and ω-6 fatty acids on initiation and postinitiation stages of colon carcinogenesis. *Cancer Res* 1991;51:487–491.

112. Chang W-CL, Chapkin RS, Lupton JR. Fish oil blocks azoxymethane-induced rat colon tumorigenesis by increasing cell differentiation and apoptosis rather than decreasing cell proliferation. *J Nutr* 1998;128:491–497.

113. Reddy BS. Chemoprevention of colon cancer by dietary fatty acids. *Cancer Metastasis Rev* 1994;13:285–302.

114. Takahashi M, Fukutake M, Isoi T, et al. Suppression of azoxymethane-induced rat colon carcinoma development by a fish oil component, docosahexaenoic acid (DHA). *Carcinogenesis* 1997;18:1337–1342.

115. Reddy BS, Maruyama H. Effect of dietary fish oil on azoxymethane-induced colon carcinogenesis in male F344 rats. *Cancer Res* 1986;55:3785–3789.

116. Nelson RL, Tanure JC, Andrianopoulos G, et al. A comparison of dietary fish oil and corn oil in experimental colorectal carcinogenesis. *Nutr Cancer* 1988;11:215–220.

117. Reddy BS, Sugie S. Effect of different levels of ω-3 and ω-6 fatty acids on azoxymethane-induced colon carcinogenesis in F344 rats. *Cancer Res* 1988;48:6642–6647.

118. Hong MY, Lupton JR, Morris JS, et al. Dietary fish oil reduces O^6-methylguanine DNA adduct levels in rat colon in part by increasing apoptosis during tumor initiation. *Cancer Epidemiol Biomark Prev* 2000;9:819–826.

119. Takahashi M, Minamoto T, Yamashita N, et al. Reduction in the formation and growth of 1,2-dimethylhydrazine-induced

aberrant crypt foci in rat colon by docosahexaenoic acid. *Cancer Res* 1993;53:2786–2789.

120. Calder PC, Davis J, Yaqoob P, et al. Dietary fish oil suppresses human colon tumour growth in athymic mice. *Clin Sci* 1998;94:303–311.

121. Chang W-CL, Chapkin RS, Lupton JR. Predictive value of proliferation, differentiation and apoptosis as intermediate markers for colon tumorigenesis. *Carcinogenesis* 1997;18:721–730.

122. Chapkin RS, Hong MY, Fan Y-Y, et al. Dietary n–3 PUFA alter colonocyte mitochondrial membrane composition and function. *Lipids* 2002;37:193–199.

123. Jenski LJ. Omega-3 fatty acids and the expression of membrane proteins: emphasis on molecules of immunologic importance. *Curr Org Chem* 2000;4:1185–1200.

124. Chapkin RS, McMurray DN, Jolly CA. Dietary n–3 polyunsaturated fatty acids modulate T-lymphocyte activation: clinical relevance in treating diseases of chronic inflammation, in *Nutrition and Immunology: Principles and Practice*. Gershwin ME, German B, Keen C, eds. Plenum Publishing, New York, NY, 1999:pp.121–134.

125. McMurray DN, Jolly CA, Chapkin RS. Effect of dietary n–3 fatty acids on T cell activation and T cell receptor mediated signalling in a murine model. *J Infect Dis* 2000;182(Suppl 1):S103–S107.

126. Lowy DR, Willumsen BM. Function and regulation of *ras*. *Annu Rev Biochem* 1993;62:851–891.

127. White MA, Nicollete C, Minden A, et al. Multiple ras functions can contribute to mammalian cell transformation. *Cell* 1995;80:553–541.

128. Singh J, Hamid R, Reddy BS. Dietary fat and colon cancer—modulating effect of types and amount of dietary fat on ras-p21 function during promotion and progression stages of colon cancer. *Cancer Res* 1997;57:253–258.

129. Davidson LA, Lupton JR, Jiang Y-H, Chapkin RS. Carcinogen and dietary lipid regulate ras expression and localization in rat colon without affecting farnesylation kinetics. *Carcinogenesis* 1999;20:785–791.

130. Maher J, Colonna F, Baker D, et al. Retroviral-mediated gene transfer of a mutant H-ras gene into normal human bone marrow alters myeloid cell proliferation and differentiation. *Exp Hematol* 1994;22:8–12.

131. Chen CY, Faller DV. Direction of p21ras-generated signals towards cell growth or apoptosis is determined by protein kinase C and Bcl-2. *Oncogene* 1995;11:1487–1498.

132. Chapkin RS, Gao J, Lee DYK, Lupton JR. Dietary fibers and fats alter rat colon protein kinase C activity: correlation to cell proliferation. *J Nutr* 1993;123:649–655.

133. Davidson LA, Jiang Y-H, Derr JN, et al. Protein kinase C isoforms in human and rat colonic mucosa. *Arch Biochem Biophys* 1994;312:547–553.

134. Jiang Y-H, Lupton JR, Chapkin RS. Dietary fish oil blocks carcinogen-induced down-regulation of colonic protein kinase C isoenzymes. *Carcinogenesis* 1997;18:351–357.

135. Murray NR, Davidson LA, Chapkin RS, et al. Protein kinase C βII and TGFαRII in ω-3 fatty acid-mediated inhibition of colon carcinogenesis. *J Cell Biol* 2002;157:915–920.

136. Murray NR, Davidson LA, Chapkin RS, et al. Overexpression of protein kinase C bII in the colonic epithelium causes hyperproliferation and increased sensitivity to colon carcinogenesis. *J Cell Biol* 1999;145:699–711.

137. Hixson LJ, Garewal HS, McGee DL, et al. Ornithine decarboxylase and polyamines in colorectal neoplasia mucosa. *Cancer Epidemiol Biomark Prev* 1993;2:369–374.

138. Craven PA, DeRubertis FR. Role of activation of protein kinase C in the stimulation of colonic epithelial proliferation by unsaturated fatty acids. *Gastroenterology* 1988;95:676–685.

139. Rao CV, Reddy BS. Modulating effect of amount and types of dietary fat on ornithine decarboxylase, tyrosine protein kinase and prostaglandins production during colon carcinogenesis in male F344 rats. *Carcinogenesis* 1993;14:1327–1333.

140. Eberhart CE, Coffey RJ, Radhika A, et al. Up-regulation of cyclooxygenase 2 gene expression in human colorectal adenomas and adenocarcinomas. *Gastroenterology* 1994;107:1183–1188.

141. Rigas B, Goldman IS, Levine L. Altered eicosanoid levels in human colon cancer. *J Lab Clin Med* 1993;122:518–523.

142. Kulkarni N, Zang E, Kelloff G, Reddy BS. Effect of chemopreventive agents piroxicam and D,L-α-difluoromethylornithine on intermediate biomarkers of colon carcinogenesis. *Carcinogenesis* 1992;13:995–1000.

143. Sakaguchi M, Hiramatsu Y, Takada H, et al. Effect of dietary unsaturated and saturated fats on azoxymethane-induced colon carcinogenesis in rats. *Cancer Res* 1984;44:1472–1477.

144. Lee DY, Lupton JR, Aukema HM, Chapkin RS. Dietary fat and fiber alter rat colonic mucosal lipid mediators and cell proliferation. *J Nutr* 1993;123:1808–1817.

145. Minoura T, Takata T, Sakaguchi M, et al. Effect of dietary eicosapentaenoic acid on azoxymethane-induced colon carcinogenesis in rats. *Cancer Res* 1988;48:4790–4794.

146. Singh J, Hamid R, Reddy BS. Dietary fat and colon cancer: modulation of cyclooxygenase-2 by types and amount of dietary fat during the postinitiation stage of colon carcinogenesis. *Cancer Res* 1997;57:3465–3470.

147. Corey EJ, Chuan S, Cashman JR. Docosahexaenoic acid is a strong inhibitor of prostaglandin but not leukotriene biosynthesis. *Proc Natl Acad Sci USA* 1983;80:3581–3584.

148. Hussey HJ, Tisdale MJ. Effect of polyunsaturated fatty acids on the growth of murine colon adenocarcinomas in vitro and in vivo. *Br J Cancer* 1994;74:6–10.

149. Hussey HJ, Tisdale MJ. Inhibition of tumour growth by lipoxygenase inhibitors. *Br J Cancer* 1996;74:683–687.

150. Giardiello FM, Offerhaus GJA, DuBois RN. The role of nonsteroidal anti-inflammatory drugs in colorectal cancer prevention. *Eur J Cancer* 1995;31A:1071–1076.

151. Potter JD, Slattery ML, Bostick RM, Gapstur SM. Colon cancer: a review of the epidemiology. *Epidemiol Rev* 1993;15:499–545

152. Schreinemachers DM, Everson RB. Aspirin use and lung, colon, and breast cancer incidence in a prospective study. *Epidemiology* 1994;5:138–146.

153. Reddy BS, Rao CV, Seibert K. Evaluation of cyclooxygenase-2 inhibitor for potential chemopreventive properties in colon carcinogenesis. *Cancer Res* 1996;56:4566–4569.

154. Yoshimi N, Kawabata K, Hara A, et al. Inhibitory effect of NS-398, a selective cyclooxygenase-2 inhibitor, on azoxymethane-induced aberrant crypt foci in colon carcinogenesis of F344 rats. *Jpn J Cancer Res* 1997;88:1044–1051.

155. Ringbom T, Huss U, Stenholm A, et al. COX-2 inhibitory effects of naturally occurring and modified fatty acids. *J Nat Prod* 2001;64:745–749.

156. Rao CV, Simi B, Wynn TT, et al. Modulating effect of amount and types of dietary fat on colonic mucosal phospholipase, phosphatidylinositol-specific phospholipase C activities, and cyclooxygenase metabolite formation during different stages of colon tumor promotion in male F344 rats. *Cancer Res* 1996;56:532–537.

157. Tsujii M, DuBois RN. Alterations in cellular adhesions and apoptosis in epithelial cells overexpressing prostaglandin endoperoxide synthase 2. *Cell* 1995;83:493–501.

158. Shiff SJ, Qiao L, Tsai L-L, Rigas B. Sulindac sulfide, an aspirin-like compound, inhibits proliferation, causes cell cycle quiescence, and induces apoptosis in HT-29 colon adenocarcinoma cells. *J Clin Investig* 1995;96:491–503.

159. Bedi A, Pasricha PJ, Akhtar AJ, et al. Inhibition of apoptosis during development of colorectal cancer. *Cancer Res* 1995;55:1811–1816.

160. Sheng H, Shao J, Morrow JD, et al. Modulation of apoptosis and Bcl-2 expression by prostaglandin E_2 in human colon cancer cells. *Cancer Res* 1998;58:362–366.

161. Narayanan BA, Narayanan NK, Reddy BS. Docosahexaenoic acid regulated genes and transcription factors inducing apoptosis in human colon cancer cells. *Int J Oncol* 2001;19:1255–1262.

162. Takebayashi Y, Aklyama S, Yamada K, et al. Angiogenesis is an unfavorable prognostic factor in human colorectal carcinoma. *Cancer* 1996;78:226–231.

163. Saeki T, Tanada M, Takashima S, et al. Correlation between expression of platelet-derived endothelial cell growth factor (thymidine phosphorylase) and microvessel density in early-stage human colon carcinomas. *Jpn J Clin Oncol* 1997;27:227–230.

164. Salvemini D, Misko TP, Masferrer JL, et al. Nitric oxide activates cyclooxygenase enzymes. *Proc Natl Acad Sci USA* 1993;90:7240–7244.

165. Maciorowski KG, Turner ND, Lupton JR, et al. Diet and carcinogen alter the fecal microbial populations of rats. *J Nutr* 1997;127:449–457.

166. Reddy BS, Simi B, Patel N, et al. Effect of amount and types of dietary fat on intestinal bacterial 7 α-dehydroxylase and phosphatidylinositol-specific phospholipase C and colonic mucosal diacylglycerol kinase and PKC activities during different stages of colon tumor promotion. *Cancer Res* 1996;56:2314–2320.

167. Reddy BS, Watanabe K, Weisburger JH, Wynder EL. Promoting effect of bile acids in colon carcinogenesis in germ-free and conventional F344 rats. *Cancer Res* 1977;37:3238–3242.

168. Bartram HP, Gostner A, Scheppach W, et al. Modification of fecal bile acid excretion by fish oil in healthy probands. *Z Ernahrungswiss* 1995;34:231–235.

169. Demark-Wahnefried W, Price DT, Polascik TJ, et al. Pilot study of dietary fat restriction and flaxseed supplementation in men with prostate cancer before surgery: exploring the effects on hormonal levels, prostate-specific antigen, and histopathologic features. *Urology* 2001;58:47–52.

170. Godley PA, Campbell MK, Gallagher P, et al. Biomarkers of essential fatty acid consumption and risk of prostatic carcinoma. *Cancer Epidemiol Biomark Prev* 1996;5:889–895.

171. Connolly JM, Coleman M, Rose DP. Effects of dietary fatty acids on DU145 human prostate cancer cell growth in athymic nude mice. *Nutr Cancer* 1997;29:114–119.

172. Chung BH, Mitchell SH, Zhang JS, Young CYF. Effects of docosahexaenoic acid and eicosapentaenoic acid on androgen-mediated cell growth and gene expression in LNCaP prostate cancer cells. *Carcinogenesis* 2001;22:1201–1206.

173. Pandalai PK, Pilat MJ, Yamazaki K, et al. The effects of omega-3 and omega-6 fatty acids on in vitro prostate cancer growth. *Anticancer Res* 1996;16:815–820.

174. Zhang JJ, Temme EHM, Kesteloot H. Fish consumption is inversely associated with male lung cancer mortality in countries with high levels of cigarette smoking or animal fat consumption. *Int J Epidemiol* 2000;29:615–621.

175. Veierod MB, Laake P, Thelle DS. Dietary fat intake and risk of lung cancer—a prospective study of 51,452 Norwegian men and women. *Eur J Cancer Prev* 1997;6:540–549.

176. Chen DZ, Auborn K. Fish oil constituent docosahexaenoic acid selectively inhibits growth of human papillomavirus immortalized keratinocytes. *Carcinogenesis* 1999;20:249–254.

177. Falconer JS, Ross JA, Fearon KC, et al. Effect of eicosapentaenoic acid and other fatty acids on the growth in vitro of human pancreatic cancer cell lines. *Br J Cancer* 1994;69:826–832.

178. Lai PB, Ross JA, Fearon KC, et al. Cell cycle arrest and induction of apoptosis in pancreatic cancer cells exposed to eicosapentaenoic acid in vitro. *Br J Cancer* 1996;74:1375–1383.

179. Calviello G, Palozza P, Piccioni E, et al. Dietary supplementation with eicosapentaenoic and docosahexaenoic acid inhibits growth of morris hepatocarcinoma 3924A in rats—effects on proliferation and apoptosis. *Int J Cancer* 1998;75:699–705.

180. Jenski LJ, Zerouga M, Stillwell W. Omega-3 fatty acid-containing liposomes in cancer therapy. *Proc Soc Exp Biol Med* 1995;210:227–233.

181. Pascale AW, Ehringer WD, Stillwell W, et al. Omega-3 fatty acid modification of membrane structure and function. II. Alteration by docosahexaenoic acid of tumor cell sensitivity to immune cytolysis. *Nutr Cancer* 1993;19:147–157.

182. Jenski LJ, Sturdevant LK, Ehringer WD, Stillwell W. Omega-3 fatty acid modification of membrane structure and function. I. Dietary manipulation of tumor cell susceptibility to cell- and complement-mediated lysis. *Nutr Cancer* 1993;19:135–146.

183. Kontogiannea M, Gupta A, Ntanios F, et al. Omega-3 fatty acids decrease endothelial adhesion of human colorectal carcinoma cells. *J Surg Res* 2000;92:201–205.

184. Connolly JM, Rose DP. Effects of fatty acids on invasion through reconstituted basement membrane (matrigel) by a human breast cancer cell line. *Cancer Lett* 1993;75:137–142.

185. McCarty MF. Fish oil may impede tumour angiogenesis and invasiveness by down-regulating protein kinase C and modulating eicosanoid production. *Med Hypotheses* 1996;46:107–115.

186. Cianchi F, Cortesini C, Bechi P, et al. Up-regulation of cyclooxygnase 2 gene expression correlates with tumor angiogenesis in human colorectal cancer. *Gastroenterology* 2001;121:1339–1347.

187. Di Carlo V, Gianotti L, Balzano G, et al. Complications of pancreatic surgery and the role of perioperative nutrition. *Dig Surg* 1999; 16:320–326.

188. Wu GH, Zhang YW, Wu ZH. Modulation of postoperative immune and inflammatory response by immune-enhancing enteral diet in gastrointestinal cancer patients. *World J Gastroenterol* 2001;7:357–362.

189. Almallah YZ, Ewen SW, El-Tahir A, et al. Distal proctocolitis and n–3 polyunsaturated fatty acids (n–3 PUFAs): the mucosal effect in situ. *J Clin Immun* 2000;20:68–76.

190. Belluzzi A, Brignola C, Campieri M, et al. Effect of an enteric-coated fish oil preparation on relapses in Crohn's disease. *N Engl J Med* 1996;334:1557–1560.

191. Braga M, Gianotti L, Radaelli G, et al. Perioperative immunonutrition in patients undergoing cancer surgery—Results of a randomized double-blind phase 3 trial. *Arch Surg* 1999;134:428–433.

192. Wigmore SJ, Barber MD, Ross JA, et al. Effect of oral eicosapentaenoic acid on weight loss in patients with pancreatic cancer. *Nutr Cancer* 2000;36:177–184.

193. Heyland DK, Novak F, Drover JW, et al. Should immunonutrition become routine in critically ill patients. A systematic review of the evidence. *JAMA* 2001;286:944–953.

194. Heys SD, Walker LG, Smith I, Eremin O. Enteral nutritional supplementation with key nutrients in patients with critical illness and cancer—A meta-analysis of randomized controlled clinical trials. *Ann Surg* 1999; 229:467–477.

195. Gogos CA, Ginopoulos P, Zoumbos NC, et al. The effect of dietary omega-3 polyunsaturated fatty acids on T-lymphocyte subsets of patients with solid tumors. *Cancer Detect Prev* 1995;19:415–417.

196. Das UN, Madhavi N, Sravan Kumar G, et al. Can tumour cell drug resistance be reversed by essential fatty acids and their metabolites? *Prostaglandins Leukot Essent Fatty Acids* 1998;58:39–54.

197. Kinsella JE, Black JM. Effects of polyunsaturated fatty acids on the efficacy of antineoplastic agents toward L5178Y lymphoma cells. *Biochem Pharmacol* 1993;45:1881–1887.

198. Bougnoux P, Germain E, Chajes V, et al. Cytotoxic drugs efficacy correlates with adipose tissue docosahexaenoic acid level in locally advanced breast carcinoma. *Br J Cancer* 1999;79:1765–1769.

199. Ogilvie GK, Fettman MJ, Mallinckrodt CH, et al. Effect of fish oil, arginine, and doxorubicin chemotherapy on remission and survival time for dogs with lymphoma. *Cancer* 2000;88:1916–1928.

VI AGENTS TARGETING BIOLOGICAL PROCESSES IMPORTANT IN CANCER

40 Tumor Angiogenesis as a Target for Early Intervention and Cancer Prevention

William W. Li, MD

CONTENTS

1. INTRODUCTION

Cancer now affects as many as 22 million people worldwide, and results in six million deaths each year *(1)*. Men have a 43% chance, and women a 38% chance, of being diagnosed with any type of cancer during their lifetime *(2,3)*. Despite advances in the early detection of cancer, most malignancies are still diagnosed and treated at advanced stages, with a limited range of therapeutic options and poor overall survival. Cancer prevention and early intervention are thus important long-range strategies for managing the cancer pandemic.

Major advances in understanding the biology of tumor growth have led to the development of targeted therapies for cancer. Key insights into the molecular pathways of tumorigenesis enable targeted intervention at early stages of disease. Early interventions should ideally employ agents with high target specificity and low systemic toxicity, inhibiting tumor growth with minimal adverse effects on healthy tissues *(4)*. Prevention strategies might use similar agents or even bioactive dietary factors to suppress the development of incipient cancers in high-risk patients.

It is now well-established that solid tumor growth is dependent upon angiogenesis, the growth of new blood vessels *(5–10)*. During the early stages of tumorigenesis, induction of angiogenesis by cancer cells is a critical event separating the preinvasive from the invasive phase of malignant growth. The degree of vascularity within a tumor correlates positively with disease stage, likelihood of metastases, and cancer recurrence *(11,12)*. Angiogenesis also plays a role in hematogenous malignancies, such as leukemia, lymphoma, and multiple myeloma, as well as in premalignant myelodysplastic syndromes *(13–17)*. In these pathologies, vascular endothelial cells sustain and promote malignant cell growth by secreting paracrine survival factors *(18,19)*.

The inhibition of angiogenesis suppresses primary tumor growth and metastases and improves survival in experimental laboratory models *(5)*. Phase II clinical trials of angiogenesis inhibitors in cancer patients have increasingly shown clinical benefit *(20–23)*. Preclinical and clinical data suggest that angiogenesis inhibition may also be useful for cancer prevention *(24)*.

This chapter reviews the role of angiogenesis in early cancer development, and discusses the scientific and clinical evidence supporting antiangiogenesis as a rational strategy for the early intervention and prevention of cancer.

2. GROWTH CONTROL OF NORMAL AND NEOPLASTIC TISSUE BY THE VASCULATURE

All normal cells in the body are no more than 100–200 µm—the diffusion limit of oxygen—from the nearest capillary *(25)*. Capillary blood vessels serve two major functions: they bathe tissues in oxygen and

From: Cancer Chemoprevention, Volume 1: Promising Cancer Chemoprevention Agents
Edited by: G. J. Kelloff, E. T. Hawk, and C. C. Sigman © Humana Press Inc., Totowa, NJ

Table 1
Angiogenic Growth Factors

Angiogenin

Adrenomedullin

Fibroblast growth factor-1 (acidic FGF, FGF1)

Fibroblast growth factor-2 (basic FGF, FGF2)

Follistatin

Granulocyte-colony-stimulating factor (G-CSF)

Hepatocyte growth factor/scatter factor (HGF/SF)

Interleukin-3 (IL-3)

Interleukin-8 (IL-8)

Keratinocyte growth factor (FGF-7)

Midkine

Neuregulin

Osteogenic protein-1

Placental growth factor (PlGF)

Platelet-derived endothelial-cell growth factor (PD-ECGF)

Platelet-derived growth factor (PDGF)

Pleiotrophin

Proliferin

Transforming growth factor-α (TGFα)

Transforming growth factor-β (TGFβ)

Tumor necrosis factor-α (TNFα)

Vascular endothelial growth factor/vascular permeability factor (VEGF/VPF)

micronutrients, and their endothelial cells produce and secrete paracrine growth and survival signals *(18)*. Under physiological conditions, the rate of cell proliferation in tissues is balanced with the rate of cell death (apoptosis), so there is no net tissue growth. Expansion of tissue mass requires angiogenesis to support increased metabolic demand *(9)*. In normal healthy adults, angiogenesis occurs only during the female reproductive cycle (endometrial regeneration, corpus luteum formation), pregnancy (placentation), and wound healing (granulation) *(26–29)*.

2.1. Molecular Regulators of Angiogenesis

2.1.1. Angiogenic Growth Factors

More than 20 endogenous molecules have been identified as angiogenic growth factors (Table 1). These share the ability to stimulate neovascularization in vivo, and induce endothelial proliferation, migration, or capillary tube formation in vitro. Basic fibroblast growth factor (bFGF or FGF2), an 18-kDa polypeptide, was the first angiogenic factor to be identified from a

tumor extract *(30)*. Vascular endothelial growth factor (VEGF), also called vascular permeability factor (VPF), is a potent hypoxia-mediated endothelial mitogen. It increases vascular hyperpermeability with a potency 50,000 × that of histamine, and also induces Bcl-2, promoting vascular survival *(31–33)*. VEGF is expressed by all human tumors studied and its receptor, Flk-1/KDR, is expressed selectively on angiogenic endothelial cells *(34)*. Placental growth factor (PlGF) plays a specific role in pathological neovascularization by recruiting bone marrow-derived vascular stem cells to disease sites *(35,36)*. Other factors include platelet-derived growth factor (PDGF), platelet-derived endothelial cell growth factor (PD-ECGF), interleukin-3 (IL-3), interleukin-8 (IL-8), transforming growth factor-β (TGFβ), and tumor necrosis factor-alpha (TNFα) *(37,38)*. Other angiogenic factors are neuregulin, a ligand for the ErbB receptor, and keratinocyte growth factor (KGF or FGF-7) *(39,40)*. Studies in normal, healthy subjects show that most angiogenic factors are present at low levels or are undetectable in the circulation. By contrast, markedly elevated levels of factors such as bFGF, VEGF, and PD-ECGF are present in the serum, urine, and cerebrospinal fluid of cancer patients *(41)*.

2.1.2. Endogenous Inhibitors of Angiogenesis

A diverse array of endogenous angiogenesis inhibitors exists throughout the body (Table 2). Angiogenesis inhibitory activity was first identified in 1975 through studies of cartilage, a naturally avascular tissue *(42)*. Subsequently, numerous distinct antiangiogenic molecules have been characterized within cartilage, including troponin-1, tissue inhibitors of matrix metalloproteinases (TIMPs), chondromodulin I, connective tissue-growth factor (CTGF), decorin, and metastatin *(43–48)*. In the eye, pigment epithelium-derived factor (PEDF), another avascular tissue, suppresses vascular growth and preserves optical clarity *(49–52)*. Within vascularized tissues, growth factor effects are counterbalanced by angiogenesis inhibitors, such as thrombospondin-1 and -2, interferons, tetrahydrocortisol-S, platelet factor-4, and protamine *(53–58)*. Other inhibitors, such as canstatin, tumstatin, and arresten, are present in the basement membrane surrounding established blood vessels *(59–61)*.

A unique group of inhibitors are comprised of proteolytic fragments of larger molecules. Angiostatin is an internal fragment of plasminogen and specifically inhibits endothelial cell proliferation *(62)*. Enzymes such as macrophage-derived elastase and serine proteases

Table 2
Endogenous Inhibitors of Angiogenesis

Angiopoietin-2 (in the absence of VEGF)

Angiostatin

Antithrombin III fragment

Arresten

Canstatin

Chondromodulin I

Connective tissue growth factor (CTGF)

Decorin

Endostatin

Fibronectin 20-kDa fragment

Interferons-α, β, and γ

Interleukin-4 (IL-4)

Interleukin-10 (IL-10)

Interleukin-12 (IL-12)

Interferon-inducible protein-10 (IP-10)

Kringle 5

Metastatin

METH-1

METH-2

2-Methoxyestradiol

Osteopontin cleavage product

Pigment epithelium-derived factor (PEDF)

Plasminogen activator inhibitor (PAI)

Platelet factor-4

Prolactin 16-KDa fragment

Proliferin-related protein

Maspin

Restin

SPARC cleavage product

Tetrahydrocortisol-S

Tissue inhibitors of matrix metalloproteinases (TIMPs)

Thrombospondin-1 and -2

Transforming growth factor-β (TGF-β) (*activated form*)

Troponin-1

Tumstatin

Vascular endothelial growth inhibitor (VEGI)

Vasostatin

generate angiostatin or angiostatin-like fragments *(63,64)*. Endostatin, a 20-kDa fragment of collagen XVIII, is a specific angiogenesis inhibitor that induces endothelial apoptosis *(65,66)*. Both angiostatin and endostatin were initially discovered in the serum of tumor-bearing experimental mice, suggesting that tumor-associated protease activity generates these inhibitors. Removal of the primary tumor led to a marked decline in serum angiostatin and endostatin, followed by rapid angiogenic growth of metastatic lesions *(9,67)*. Endostatin is present at a low circulating level in normal healthy subjects *(68)*. Thus, some endogenous angiogenesis inhibitors are believed to play a role in maintaining tumor dormancy in cancer patients.

2.1.3. THE BALANCE CONCEPT OF ANGIOGENESIS REGULATION

Vascular growth is physiologically governed by a homeostatic balance between positive and negative angiogenesis regulators, so that neovascularization is normally suppressed *(69)*. Vascular proliferation occurs when angiogenic growth factor production is upregulated, when expression of endogenous inhibitors is downregulated, or when both events occur simultaneously *(70–72)*.

The genetic regulators of angiogenesis are closely related to tumor growth promotion and suppression (Table 3). Gene knockout studies in mice have shown that Id1 and Id3, peptides that control cell differentiation by interfering with DNA binding of transcription factors, are required for normal vascular formation and induction of angiogenesis in tumor-bearing animals *(73)*. The activated forms of the oncogenes H-*ras*, v-*raf*, c-*myc*, c-*src*, Her-2/neu, and p73 are associated with cellular production of VEGF as well as tumorigenesis *(74–81)*. Several tumor-suppressor genes regulate angiogenesis inhibition, including p53, Rb, vHL, phosphatase and tensin homolog (PTEN), and *trk* B *(82)*. Wild-type p53 controls expression of the angiogenesis inhibitor thrombospondin and decreases tumor neovascularization; mutant p53 leads to the opposite effect *(71)*. The retinoblastoma (Rb) gene and the von Hippel-Lindau (vHL) gene both downregulate VEGF expression; their mutation leads to VEGF production, angiogenesis, and tumor growth *(83,84)*.

2.2. The Avascular Phase of Cancer

Solid tumors arise as clusters of abnormal cells, dividing above the basement membrane of organs. To acquire sustenance, incipient tumors (60–80 cells) may migrate toward existing host vessels, a process known as vessel cooption, but their growth remains limited *(85–87)*. Tumors are capable of growth to approx 2.0 mm in diameter (500,000–1,000,000 cells) before reaching a steady state of growth. Beyond this size,

Table 3
Genetic Control of Angiogenesis

Positive Regulation	Negative Regulation
Id1	p53
Id3	Rb
HIF-1a	VHL
K-*ras*	PTEN
N-*myc*	*trk* B
c-*myc*	p16INK4a
c-*fos*	
c-*src*	
c-*myb*	
c-*jun*	
HER2/*neu*	
EGFT	
Raf	
Mek	
p73	
Del-1	
FzD	
Bcl2	
MDNM2	
PML-RAR	
ElF-4E	

their metabolic demands exceed the supply of oxygen and nutrients obtained by passive diffusion from nearby blood vessels. This state corresponds to carcinoma *in situ*, and the rate of tumor cell proliferation is balanced by apoptosis *(88)*. Such dormant cancers may exist for years without clinical detection.

2.3. The "Switch" to the Angiogenic Phenotype During Multistep Tumorigenesis

To expand beyond the limits of the preexisting vascular supply, tumors recruit new blood vessels from surrounding vessels, an event known as the "switch" to the angiogenic phenotype *(89)* (Fig. 1). Three classic studies employing transgenic mice have delineated this switch as normal cells undergo the transition from normalcy to hyperplasia to dysplasia, and finally to frank carcinoma.

In a model of spontaneous β-islet cell tumor formation, Rip1-Tag2 transgenic mice selectively express the SV40 T-antigen oncogene in their insulin-producing β cells and undergo a predictable sequence of multi-step tumorigenesis *(69, 90,91)*. The transformed β-cells are localized to approx 400 islets in the pancreas, of which 100% express the oncogene. Over time, 50–70% of these islets become hyperplastic nodules. A distinct angiogenic stage occurs at 6–7 wk of age between the hyperplastic stage and the time at which subset islets become invasive carcinomas at 12–16 wk. The angiogenic capacity of these lesions is observed as visible intense tumor vascularization, accompanied by induction of capillary sprouting, endothelial proliferation, and a starburst-like convergence of capillaries when islets are harvested in vivo and co-cultured with endothelial cells in vitro (Fig. 2). Importantly, non-angiogenic islets are unable to grow beyond 0.6–0.8 mm³ in size, whereas the small subset of angiogenic islets can expand into a lethal tumor burden *(92)*.

A second study utilized the bovine papillomavirus oncogene in a transgenic mouse model of dermal fibrosarcoma *(93,94)*. Distinct stages of tumorigenesis are observed, from normal cells to a proliferative hyperplastic stage (mild and aggressive fibromas) to neoplasia (fibrosarcoma). The preneoplastic fibromas grow horizontally within the dermis as thin avascular lesions, and the fibrosarcomas are expansile and densely vascularized. Angiogenesis is first observed during the late preneoplastic stage (aggressive fibroma) and sustained until death of the animals by fibrosarcoma. Aggressive fibromas and fibrosarcomas secrete bFGF. By contrast, bFGF is not secreted by normal cells or mild fibromas.

A third study involved K14-HPV16 transgenic mice in which the human papillomavirus (HPV) type 16 oncogene is targeted to expression in basal cells of the epidermis by regulatory elements of the human keratin-14 promoter *(95)*. These basal keratinocytes undergo sequential changes from normal cells (no vascularization) to hyperplasia (mild vascularization from the underlying dermis) to dysplasia (abundant vessels under the basement membrane in close apposition to aberrant keratinocytes) to squamous cell carcinoma (intense angiogenesis breaching the basement membrane into the tumor). In hyperplasia, dysplasia, and at the invading cancer front, angiogenesis is associated with mast cell infiltration and degranulation *(96)*. Mast cells contain numerous angiogenic stimulators in their secretory granules, such as the serine protease MCP-4, VEGF, bFGF, TGFβ, TNFα, and IL-8 *(97,98)*. In dysplasia and carcinoma, tissue expression of VEGF was increased, correlating to increased tumor vessel density *(99)*.

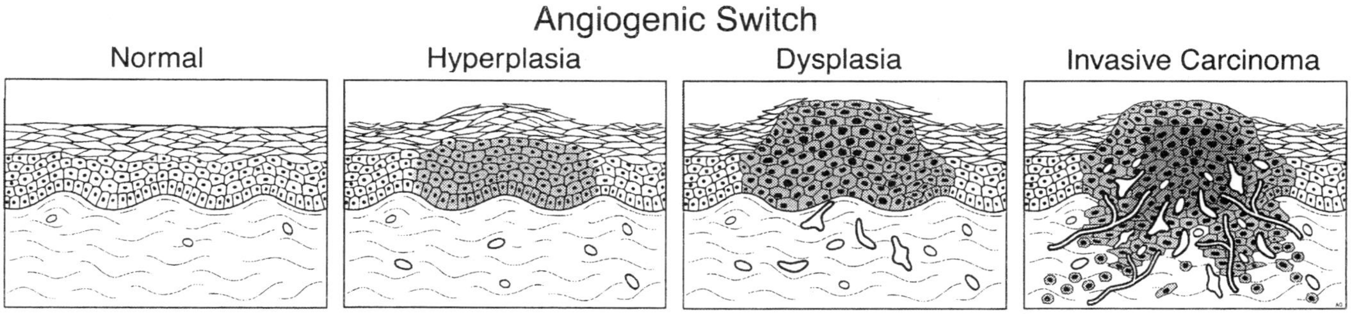

Angiogenic Switch

Fig. 1. The switch to the angiogenic phenotype occurs during multi-stage tumorigenesis. As malignancy develops, cells progress from a prevascular stage (normal to early hyperplasia) to a vascular stage (late hyperplasia to dysplasia to invasive carcinoma). Angiogenesis becomes clearly evident during dysplasia, and is permissive for further growth. When the rates of tumor cell proliferation exceed that of apoptosis, tumor expansion and local invasion occur. Intense neovascularization is observed in invasive carcinomas. (Reprinted by permission from the Angiogenesis Foundation. Copyright © 2004. The Angiogenesis Foundation. All rights reserved).

Together, these data demonstrate that angiogenesis is a discrete, genetically regulated and rate-limiting step during multi-step tumorigenesis; that the transition from prevascular to vascular phase is accompanied by the production and release of one or more angiogenic growth factors; and that host inflammatory cells may amplify the angiogenic switch by contributing additional stimuli.

2.4. The Vascular Phase of Cancer

The onset of angiogenesis precedes an exponential phase of tumor growth accompanied by local organ invasion. The velocity of angiogenic capillary growth ranges from 0.223–0.8 mm/day *(100–102)*. Studies of avascular tumor explants placed in the anterior chamber of the eye show that once new vessels reach the explant, tumors can expand 16,000 × in size in 2 wk *(103)*. During this expansion, cancer cells grow as a cuff around each new microvessel with a thickness of 50–200 µm. In this configuration, one endothelial cell supports the metabolic needs of 5–100 cancer cells *(104–105)*. Eventually, invading blood vessels occupy 1.5% of the tumor volume *(106)*. Tumor angiogenesis also facilitates cancer metastases by allowing cells to exit through the neovascular network into the systemic circulation *(107)*. Elegant studies of mammary carcinomas in mice have shown that a 1 cm tumor sheds 2×10^6 malignant cells into the circulation every 24 h *(108)*.

3. TARGETING TUMOR ANGIOGENESIS

The concept of antiangiogenesis was first proposed in 1971 by Judah Folkman, who hypothesized that inhibition of neovascularization could prevent tumor growth and metastases *(7)*. A vast literature establishes that angiogenesis inhibition is an effective antitumor strategy in animal models bearing a wide variety of cancers *(8,109)*. To date, more than 300 angiogenesis-inhibitory molecules have been identified as potential drug candidates, including many natural and synthetic chemical entities (reviewed in *53*). Selective targeting of angiogenic blood vessels is possible as a result of differential proliferation rates between normal and tumor-associated endothelium. The normal vasculature is highly quiescent, with only one in every 10,000 endothelial cells dividing at any given time, and a physiological doubling time ranging from 47–20,000 d *(110–112)*. In contrast, the doubling rate for tumor endothelium is 2–13 d. Thus, antiangiogenic agents selectively inhibit proliferating tumor vasculature, but do not affect normal blood vessels.

3.1. Angiogenesis Mechanisms and Targets

Specific molecular and cellular targets have been identified for tumor angiogenesis (Fig. 3). The function of these targets is best understood in the context of the orderly events characterizing new blood vessel growth *(113)*, as described here.

3.1.1. ANGIOGENIC GROWTH FACTOR PRODUCTION AND RELEASE

Cancer cells produce and release angiogenic growth factors that diffuse to and activate endothelial cells within existing venular blood vessels (parent vessels). Hypoxia in the tumor microenvironment is a potent

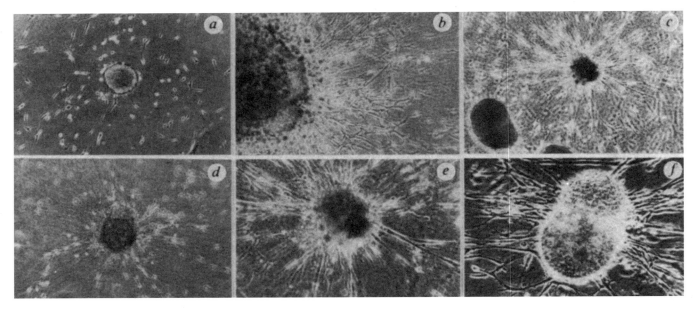

Fig. 2. In vitro studies of transgenic β-islet tumor cells co-cultured with capillary endothelial cells illustrate the switch to the angiogenic phenotype and different stages of angiogenic activity during β-cell tumorigenesis. A normal islet (**a**) is surrounded by randomly distributed endothelial cells. By contrast, a tumor (**b**) has induced extensive capillary ingrowth. Before this stage is reached, the angiogenic switch occurs, in which hyperplastic islets (**c**) induce a radial pattern of endothelial cell alignment and the formation of convergent vascular tubes in a starburst-like configuration (center islet). The progressive formation of angiogenic capillary networks by a hyperplastic islet is seen in (**d-f**). Magnification, **a-d**, X47; **e,f**, X93. (Reprinted by permission from *Nature*, Vol 339 (6219):58–61, copyright © 1989, Macmillan Publishers Ltd.)

stimulus for production of the growth factors VEGF, bFGF, TGFβ, TNFα, and IL-8 *(114)*. Peritumoral inflammation also contributes to neovascularization because monocytes and activated macrophages release growth factors and angiogenic chemokines *(115,116)*. Inducible enzymes are expressed in tumors. Cyclooxygenase-2 (COX-2) is one such enzyme, leading to prostaglandin E2-mediated generation of VEGF and other growth factors *(117,118)*. The inhibition of growth factor production and their neutralization in malignant tissues is an important antiangiogenic strategy.

3.1.2. ENDOTHELIAL RECEPTOR BINDING AND CELLULAR ACTIVATION

Growth factors bind to cognate receptors on endothelial cells, activating signal transduction pathways and inducing downstream nuclear events. Tyrosine kinase signaling is induced by VEGF through its receptor flk-KDR *(34)*. VEGF signaling also upregulates expression of Bcl-2, a survival signal *(119)*. The blockade of growth factor receptor binding and steps in the intracellular signaling pathway are major antiangiogenic strategies.

3.1.3. DEGRADATION OF VASCULAR BASEMENT MEMBRANE

Endothelial cells secrete proteases, such as plasminogen activator, collagenases, and heparanases, that focally degrade the vascular basement membrane surrounding parent vessels *(53,113,120)*. This enables endothelial cells to sprout from the parent vessel. Protease inhibition suppresses angiogenesis by impeding this process.

3.1.4. VASCULAR PROLIFERATION, MIGRATION AND SURVIVAL

Once activated, endothelial cells proliferate and migrate towards the tumor. Cell surface adhesion molecules known as vascular integrins ($\alpha_v\beta_3, \alpha_v\beta_5, \alpha_5\beta_1$) are specifically expressed on angiogenic vessels, and these mediate vascular outgrowth. Inhibition of endothelial proliferation suppresses angiogenesis. The inhibition of vascular integrins prevents endothelial cell-extracellular matrix interaction and interferes with vessel migration. Because ligation of integrins by matrix components also promotes endothelial survival signaling, integrin targeting induces vascular apopto-

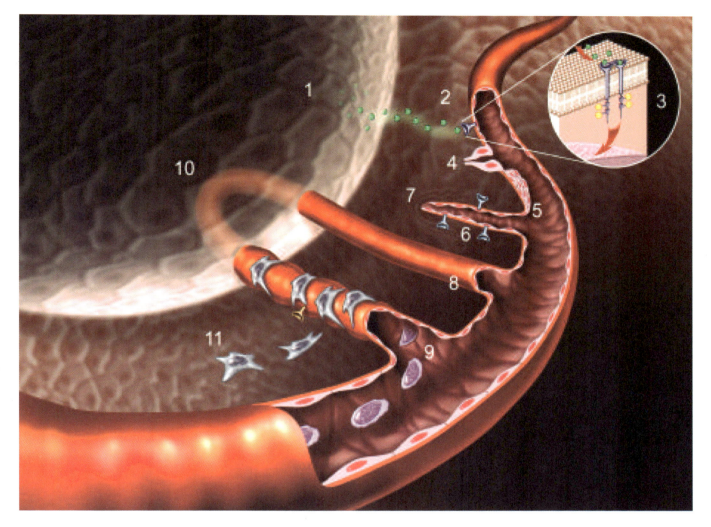

Fig. 3. The angiogenesis cascade of events. Tumors induce angiogenesis through a discrete series of molecular and cellular events: 1) production and release of angiogenic growth factors; 2) growth factor-receptor binding on venular endothelial cells; 3) endothelial intracellular signal transduction; 4) local protease secretion and vascular basement membrane degradation; 5) endothelial cell proliferation; 6) vascular sprouting and migration via integrins; 7) secretion of matrix metalloproteinases at growing vessel tips; 8) tubular morphogenesis; 9) incorporation of endothelial progenitor cells; 10) vascular loop formation (arterial-venous patterning); 11) recruitment of smooth-muscle cells and pericytes for vascular maturation. (Reprinted by permission from the Angiogenesis Foundation. Copyright © 2004. The Angiogenesis Foundation. All rights reserved.)

sis *(121)*. Pro-apoptotic designer agents also induce death of the angiogenic endothelium *(122,123)*.

3.1.5. Vascular Invasion

Matrix metalloproteinases (MMPs) are secreted at the growing tips of sprouting vessels. These proteases dissolve extracellular matrix at the advancing vascular front and facilitate tissue invasion *(124)*. Four specific MMPs (MMP-2, MMP-9, MMP-12, and MMP-21) are associated with angiogenesis *(125,126)*. Because MMP activity is also required for tumor cell invasion,

inhibitors of MMP activity can suppress both angiogenesis and tumor invasion.

3.1.6. Tubular Morphogenesis

Angiogenic blood vessels form tube-like structures through complex interactions between cell surface molecules and the extracellular matrix. Mediators of capillary tubular morphogenesis include hybrid oligosaccharides, galectin-3, PECAM-1, and VE-cadherin *(127–131)*. Targeting these moieties impairs the formation of functional vascular tubular networks.

3.1.7. ARTERIAL-VENOUS PATTERNING

Vascular loops are formed by anastomoses of individual vessel sprouts. These loops undergo a patterning process, mediated by ephrin-B2 and its receptor Eph-B4, to define the afferent (arterial) and efferent (venous) limbs *(132–135)*. Inhibition of vascular patterning alters blood vessel functionality and tumor blood flow.

3.1.8. VASCULAR MATURATION

Vascular maturation of newly formed vessels occurs by recruitment of perivascular mural cells (smooth muscle cells, pericytes) to the ablumenal vessel wall. These cells provide architectural stability as well as paracrine signals. The recruitment process occurs when angiopoietin-1 (Ang-1) binds to the endothelial Tie-2 receptor, leading to expression of PDGF and other chemokines that stimulate migration of smooth muscle cells and pericytes to the vessel *(136)*. Disruption of these events leads to immature, dilated, and dysfunctional vessels that are prone to apoptosis *(137–139)*.

3.1.9. CONTRIBUTION OF ENDOTHELIAL STEM CELLS

Bone marrow-derived endothelial progenitor cells (EPC) contribute to post-natal pathological neovascularization *(140–141)*. EPCs are mobilized from bone marrow into the circulation by PlGF and other chemokines expressed by tumor and activated endothelial cells, and they are home to sites of angiogenesis *(36)*. Attenuation of EPCs or their signals is another antiangiogenic strategy *(142)*. Alternatively, EPCs might be harvested, bioengineered, and injected to deliver antiangiogenic gene therapies directed at tumor blood vessels *(143)*.

3.2. Clinical Principles of Antiangiogenic Therapy

The clinical development of antiangiogenic therapy began in the late 1980s. The first successful treatment of a vascular tumor (pulmonary hemangiomatosis) occurred in 1989 using interferon α2a as an anti-endothelial agent *(144)*. The first drug to enter formal clinical trials as an angiogenesis inhibitor was TNP-470 in 1992 *(145)*. During the past decade, more than sixty different antiangiogenic agents have entered clinical trials, primarily in the setting of advanced disease and in heavily pretreated patient populations (Table 4).

Table 4
Major Antiangiogenic Agents That Have Reached Clinical Development

Drugs	Sponsor
Anti-Growth Factor Agents	
Actimid	Celgene Corporation
Angiozyme	Ribozyme Pharmaceuticals
Aplidine	Biomira
Avastin	Genentech
Celecoxib	Pharmacia/Pfizer
CEP-701	Cephalon
Neovastat	Aeterna Laboratories
Penicillamine	U.S. National Cancer Institute
PTK787	Novartis
Revimid	Celgene Corporation
SU11248	Pharmacia/Pfizer
TAS-102	Taiho Pharmaceuticals
Tetrathiomolybdate	University of Michigan
Thalidomide	Celgene Corporation
VEGF Trap	Regeneron Pharmaceuticals
ZD6474	AstraZeneca
Anti-Endothelial-Cell Agents	
ABT-510	Abbott Laboratories
Angiostatin	Entremed
Cilengitide	EMD Pharmaceuticals
CGP-41251	Novartis
CP-564,959	OSI Pharmaceuticals
CT-2584	Cell Therapeutics
Endostatin	Entremed
GBC-590	Glycogenesis
IMC-1C11	ImClone Systems
2-Methoxyestradiol	Entremed
Neovastat	Aeterna Laboratories
NM-3	ILEX Oncology
Rosiglitazone	GlaxoSmithKline
Squalamine	Genaera
TNP-470	TAP Pharmaceuticals
Vitaxin (Medi-522)	MedImmune
YH-16	Collgard Pharmaceuticals
Matrix Metalloproteinase Inhibition	
BMS 275291	Bristol-Myers Squibb
Col-3	CollaGenex
Neovastat	Aeterna Laboratories
Vascular Targeting Agents	
AVE8062	Aventis
Combretastatin A4 Prodrug	OXiGENE

Source: Angiotracker, The Angiogenesis Foundation (www.angio.org).

From scientific data and clinical trial experience, several important guiding principles have emerged concerning the application of antiangiogenic agents as an antitumor strategy.

3.2.1. LONG-TERM ADMINISTRATION OF ANTIANGIOGENIC THERAPY IS REQUIRED FOR EFFICACY

Because angiogenesis inhibition is a cytostatic treatment affecting proliferating blood vessels, the antitumor effect is indirect. Current experience suggests that long-term drug exposure (months) is required for pharmacological actions to translate into clinical effect *(146–148)*. Premature withdrawal of treatment may lead to both vascular and tumor regrowth *(144,149)*.

3.2.2. ANTIANGIOGENIC STRATEGIES OFFER A LOW-TOXICITY APPROACH TO CANCER TREATMENT

To date, most agents that are specific or selective for angiogenesis are well tolerated in humans, with fewer serious (Grade 3 and 4) toxicities observed in their clinical trials when compared to cytotoxic chemotherapy drugs *(150–152)*. Because only proliferating endothelium is targeted, the traditional side effects of chemotherapy, such as leukopenia, alopecia, and mucositis, are rarely observed. With some antiangiogenic agents, a maximum tolerated dose (MTD) cannot be determined *(68)*. This has led some clinical investigations to incorporate pharmacodynamic techniques for determining the optimal biological dose (OBD) of agents in early stage trials.

3.2.3. ANTIANGIOGENIC DRUGS ARE COMPATIBLE WITH AND MAY ENHANCE STANDARD CHEMOTHERAPY AND RADIOTHERAPY REGIMENS

Animal and human studies have shown that antiangiogenic agents may be safely combined with standard chemotherapy and radiation regimens, and may potentiate their efficacy *(153–156)*. Paradoxically, the inhibition of angiogenesis actually improves intratumoral delivery of chemotherapy drugs. This phenomenon occurs because the reduction of hyperpermeable microvessels leads to decreased tumor interstitial pressure, and the unpacking of compressed perfusing vessels can then more efficiently transport chemotherapy drugs into the tumor *(157–158)*.

3.2.4. MULTI-TARGETING STRATEGIES ARE ADVANTAGEOUS FOR ANTIANGIOGENESIS

Although many antiangiogenic drugs are designed to strike a single target (e.g., VEGF, its receptor, or the VEGF signaling pathway), tumors are known to possess redundant angiogenic pathways *(159–160)*. For example, an immunohistochemical profiling of human primary breast cancers from 64 patients showed that all the tumors were capable of expressing six of seven studied angiogenic factors (VEGF, aFGF, bFGF, TGFβ1, PD-ECGF, PlGF, pleiotrophin) *(161)*. Different growth factors also function via distinct cytokine-dependent angiogenic pathways. The $\alpha_v\beta_3$ integrin mediates neovascularization induced by bFGF or TNFα, whereas the $\alpha_v\beta_5$ integrin facilitates VEGF and TGFα signaling *(162)*. Inhibition of a single target or pathway is thus unlikely to completely block tumor angiogenesis. Combinatorial strategies that attack multiple points in the angiogenesis cascade offer a conceptual advantage over mono-targeting agents.

3.2.5. THE CLINICAL RESPONSE TO ANTIANGIOGENIC THERAPY DIFFERS FROM CLASSICAL CHEMOTHERAPY RESPONSE

Antiangiogenic agents alter tumor growth kinetics via a different mechanism than cytotoxic chemotherapies. Human and animal studies have shown that the antiangiogenic treatment of tumors leads to a variety of beneficial outcomes that are presently difficult to predict: slowed or delayed tumor growth; reduction of tumor size; or less frequently, complete remissions *(163–170)*. The biological basis for remission is believed to be related to induction of tumor apoptosis through deprivation of endothelial-derived survival factors *(88)*. Because tumor shrinkage is not a reliable response to angiogenesis inhibition, the use of classical tumor response (RECIST) criteria to monitor treatment underestimates the full range of efficacy of antiangiogenic agents *(89,171)*. For clinical trial design, time-dependent outcomes, such as time-to-disease progression or overall survival, are important to consider as clinically relevant endpoints. Aggregate endpoints that incorporate multiple parameters, including patient-reported outcomes (quality of life) may be another useful measure. The determination of valid surrogate biomarkers reflecting the clinical response to antiangiogenic therapy is a major research goal. Functional imaging techniques are in development to assess drug-induced changes in tumor blood flow, tumor blood volume, or vascular permeability *(89,172–173)*.

3.2.6. ANTIANGIOGENIC STRATEGIES MAY BE MORE EFFICACIOUS FOR EARLY-STAGE DISEASE COMPARED TO ADVANCED DISEASE

Overall disease burden in a patient is important to consider in the evaluation of the clinical benefit of any antiangiogenic agent. Advanced cancers contain well-established, extensive vascular networks that may respond minimally to angiogenesis inhibitors. Vascular destructive agents, also known as vascular targeting agents, may be required to achieve a clinically significant effect on tumor perfusion *(174–176)*. Indeed, most pre-clinical studies of angiogenesis inhibitors demonstrate drug efficacy in the setting of incipient disease (prevention) or small tumors (early intervention). Clinical trials of the same agents, however, have often enrolled patients with advanced, metastastic, and heavily pretreated disease, perhaps explaining differences between mice studies and the results of human trials *(177)*. Antiangiogenic therapy in the adjuvant setting to suppress minimal residual disease, or as an intervention for early-stage disease or cancer prevention, has been proposed as the scenario of the greatest clinical benefit using angiogenesis inhibitors *(178)*.

The remainder of this chapter is devoted to discussing the rationale for applying angiogenesis inhibitors for early intervention and prevention of cancer.

4. EARLY INTERVENTION AND CANCER PREVENTION

4.1. Early Intervention

Angiogenesis inhibition offers an opportunity to interrupt an early, rate-limiting step in tumorigenesis *(179–180)*. Suppression of pathological blood-vessel growth prevents early tumors from progressing to the malignant phenotype. Clinical correlates to preinvasive angiogenic lesions are commonly encountered in breast (ductal carcinoma *in situ*—DCIS), cervix (cervical intraepithelial neoplasia—CIN), skin (actinic keratosis), oropharynx (late Barrett's esophagus), lung (squamous metaplasia with dysplasia in bronchial mucosa), colon (premalignant adenoma), and prostate (high-grade prostate intraepithelial neoplasia, HGPIN) *(181–186)*. Microscopic metastases are also present in many cancer patients who are undergoing tumor resection with curative intent. For example, 25% of

colon cancer patients eventually develop hepatic metastases after primary tumor resection emerging from pre-angiogenic lesions that were present at the time of surgery *(148,187–188)*. By suppressing tumor neovascularization at subclinical stages, tumor progression and metastatic growth may be halted.

4.1.1. SUPERIORITY OF EARLY AND PROLONGED THERAPY

Animal studies have demonstrated that early administration of angiogenesis inhibitors is highly efficacious. The drug TNP-470 (*O*-[chloroacetyl-carbonyl] fumagillol) is a potent antiangiogenic analog of the antibiotic fumagillin *(177,189)*. A rat model of liver metastasis using K12/TRb rat colon adenocarcinoma cells was employed to study the differential efficacy of early, early prolonged, or delayed administration of TNP-470 (15 mg/kg) on metastatic burden and survival *(148)*. Treatment initiated at d 1 after tumor inoculation (early intervention) and maintained for 28 d (prolonged therapy) led to a 46% reduction in liver metastases and improved survival time compared to controls ($p = 0.011$). Another study showed a superior reduction in metastases with early (d 0–6) compared to delayed (d 7–13) TNP-470 treatment in rabbits bearing VX2 carcinoma *(190)*.

The effect of TNP-470 on subclinical disease has also been elegantly studied by Shusterman and colleagues *(191)*. In the first study, xenografts of human neuroblastoma-derived CHP-134 were implanted into athymic (*nu/nu*) mice, with initiation of antiangiogenic treatment 12 h following grafting (early primary tumor model). Treated tumors were reduced by 90%, compared to control animals. The second study involved administration of TNP-470 12 h following tail vein injection of CHP-134 cells into SCID/Beige mice (metastatic model). Autopsy of saline-treated control mice showed neuroblastoma deposits in the kidney, liver, adrenal gland, and ovaries in 75% of subjects, whereas TNP-470-treated mice showed no evidence of metastases. A third study evaluated TNP-470 effects in mice whose tumors were initially 0.35 mm^3, but then became difficult to palpate following 10 d of cyclophosphamide treatment (minimal residual disease model). TNP-470 was then administered subcutaneously. Tumor growth was suppressed in the TNP-470-treated group by 82%, compared to saline-treated controls. Histopathological analyses showed increased apoptosis by TdT-mediated nick-end labeling (TUNEL) assay in treated animals, but no difference in tumor cell proliferation by Ki-67 assessment

(88,191). These data demonstrate the importance of timing in antiangiogenic therapy and its efficacy in subclinical disease.

4.1.2. DIFFERENTIAL EFFECTS BETWEEN AGENTS AND TIMING OF THEIR ADMINISTRATION

The increasing number of angiogenesis inhibitors available for research study has enabled comparative efficacy testing of different agents at various disease stages. Bergers and colleagues studied four angiogenesis inhibitors (AGM-1470/TNP-470, BB-94, Fc-angiostatin, and Fc-endostatin) in the Rip1-Tag2 transgenic mouse model, with treatment beginning at the stage of small, vascularized tumors *(192)*. When administered during a short treatment period (3.5 wk), all the inhibitors reduced tumor size compared to controls, but to different degrees: 82%, 83%, 88%, and ~60% for AGM-1470/TNP-470, BB-94, Fc-endostatin, and Fc-angiostatin, respectively. When these same agents were given to mice with more advanced, invasive disease (12 wk of age) their efficacy profile changed significantly. Reductions in tumor size of 72%, 1%, 8%, and 4% were achieved for AGM-1470/TNP-470, BB-94, Fc-endostatin, and Fc-angiostatin, respectively. The basis for loss of efficacy in three of four agents between early and late intervention is unclear. Early intervention appears to have superior efficacy across all agents.

4.2. Cancer Prevention

Cancer chemoprevention is defined as the use of pharmacological, natural, or dietary agents to inhibit the development of invasive cancer by blocking DNA damage caused by carcinogens or by arresting the progression of premalignant cells after damage has already occurred *(4)*. Angiogenesis inhibition blocks carcinogenesis by preventing progression to the invasive phenotype *(109,193)*.

A number of well-known chemopreventive agents have antiangiogenic properties in vivo and in vitro (Table 5). These include retinoids, tamoxifen, oltipraz, curcumin, linoleic acid, ellagic acid, selenium, α-difluoromethylornithine (DFMO), N-acetyl-l-cysteine (NAC), catechins, and celecoxib *(194–201)*. Classical angiogenesis assay systems, such as the chorioallantoic membrane assay (CAM), the corneal micropocket assay, and modified rat aortic ring assay, have been used to screen for biological activity of established chemopreventive agents *(202,203)*. Known angiogenesis inhibitors such as endostatin have also been shown to suppress carcinogen-induced tumor devel-

Table 5
Chemopreventive Agents That Possess Antiangiogenic Properties

Alpha-difluoromethylornithine (DFMO)
Aspirin
Brassinin
Celecoxib
Curcumin
1 α,25-dihydroxyvitamin D$_3$
Ellagic acid
Epigallocatechin 3-gallate
Finisteride
Genistein
N-acetylcysteine (NAC)
Naringenin
Oltipraz
Resveratrol
Retinoids
Selenium
Silymarin
Statins
Sulindac
Tamoxifen

opment in rodent models *(204)*. The antiangiogenic properties of select chemopreventive molecules shall be discussed.

4.2.1. ANTIANGIOGENIC PREVENTION AGENTS

4.2.1.1. Retinoids Retinoids, a class of more than 2,000 chemical entities including active metabolites of vitamin A (retinol) and synthetic derivatives, are well-known chemopreventive agents that are clinically validated for cancers of the skin, head and neck, and oropharynx *(205–207)*. Low levels of 13-*cis*-retinoic acid, 9-*cis*-retinoic acid, and all-*trans*-retinoic acid are present endogenously *(207)*. These molecules act through binding to ligand-dependent, DNA-binding, transcriptional transactivator nuclear retinoid receptors, the retinoic acid receptor (RAR), and retinoid X receptor (RXR) *(208,209)*.

Retinol and its relatives etretin, etretinate, and isotretinoin are potent inhibitors of angiogenesis, affecting cell shape and suppressing endothelial proliferation *(210–212)*. Exposure to retinoids creates avascular zones in the chick CAM assay and suppresses corneal neovascularization *(196,213)*. Systemic administration of retinoid acid has been shown to suppress tumor growth and vascularization (214–215). Another antiangiogenic mechanism of action is retinoid-induced destruction of lysosomes that leads to hydrolysis and neutralization of endocytosed intracellular bFGF (216). In clinical practice, the most common retinoids in use are natural vitamin A, Vesanoid, Accutane, and 9-cis-retinoic acid.

4.2.1.2. COX-2 Inhibitors Inhibitors of the inducible enzyme COX-2 possess chemopreventive and antiangiogenic activity. Many studies have implicated COX-2 in a wide spectrum of cancers, including meningioma, breast, non-small-cell lung, pancreatic, prostate, esophageal, gastric, colorectal, and other tumor types (217–221). The enzyme is also expressed in preneoplastic lesions, such as DCIS, CIN, PIN, Barrett's esophagus, and actinic keratosis, but not in normal tissues (222–223). COX-2 promotes carcinogenesis through prostaglandin and non-prostaglandin-related mechanisms, including: conversion of xenobiotics into carcinogens (benzo[a]pyrene from tobacco); upregulation of Bcl-2 survival signaling; induction of MMP-2, and -9 facilitating tumor and vascular invasion; suppression of immune surveillance by IL-10 and -12; production of growth factors VEGF, bFGF, and PDGF; potentiation of epidermal growth factor receptor (EGFR) tyrosine kinase phosphorylation and MAP kinase signaling; and enhancing $\alpha_v\beta_3$-mediated angiogenesis (224–227). COX-2 inhibition interferes with these events, and suppresses neovascularization and tumor growth via multiple mechanisms (117,201). The COX-2 inhibitor celecoxib potently inhibits angiogenesis in the rat aortic ring assay, and inhibits corneal neovascularization.

Celecoxib has been clinically validated as a prevention agent for familial adenomatous polyposis (FAP), an autosomal dominant genetic disorder characterized by formation of hundreds of colon adenomas linked to a mutation in the APC gene. Colon adenomas represent a vascular premalignant stage in multistage carcinogenesis, and FAP patients have a 100% chance of developing colorectal cancer by age 50. Genetic studies in which COX-2 knockout mice were mated with APC $^{\Delta716}$ Min mice, a colon polyposis model, showed a dramatic polyp reduction in COX-2 null (– / –) compared to COX-2 (+ / +) or (+ / –) progeny (228). A landmark prevention trial enrolling 77 FAP patients with known polyps, randomized to receive celecoxib (100 mg or 400 mg bid) or placebo, showed a 28% significant reduction in polyp numbers

Table 6
Prevention and Intervention Trials of the COX-2 Inhibitor, Celecoxib

Intervention
Breast cancer, metastatic or recurrent
Cervical cancer, advanced
Colorectal cancer
Glioblastoma multiforme, newly diagnosed
Non-small-cell lung cancer, advanced
Malignant glioma, refractory
Prostate cancer

Prevention Studies
Actinic keratosis
Barrett's esophagus
Basal-cell nevus syndrome
Cutaneous carcinogenesis in Fitzpatrick Type I-IV skin
Familial adenomatous polyposis
Non-small-cell lung cancer, in high-risk smokers
Premalignant rectal polyps
Prior sporadic colorectal neoplasia
Superficial transitional-cell bladder carcinoma, recurrence

Sources: The Angiogenesis Foundation Clinical Trials Database, 2002; www.clinicaltrials.gov (Accessed October 15, 2002); www.cancer.gov (Accessed October 15, 2002).

after 6 mo of high-dose treatment, compared to baseline colonoscopy evaluations (229). On the basis of laboratory and clinical data, more than 100 cancer intervention and prevention trials using celecoxib are underway (Table 6).

4.2.1.3. Tamoxifen Tamoxifen, an estrogen analog used for hormonal treatment of breast cancer, is the first chemopreventive agent to be approved by the FDA for women with a previous history of breast cancer or those at high risk. The Breast Cancer Prevention Trial (BCPT), studied 13,388 women at high risk for breast cancer, who took tamoxifen (20 mg daily) vs placebo for 5 yr, and found an overall 49% reduction in the risk of breast cancer among those taking tamoxifen (230–231). A similar reduction was seen in the appearance of DCIS. In women with atypical ductal hyperplasia, the risk of breast cancer was reduced by 80%. Tamoxifen's mechanism is primarily attributed to blockade of estrogen-induced growth stimulation in patients with estrogen receptor (ER)-positive breast cancer. However, antitumor effects are seen with tamoxifen treatment in estrogen receptor-negative (ER-negative) breast cancer *(232)*.

The antiangiogenic effects of tamoxifen are well established *(233)*. Tamoxifen inhibits vascular sprouting in the rat aortic ring assay, decreases corneal neovascularization in rats, and creates avascular zones in the CAM assay independent of the presence of 17β-estradiol (E2) *(234–235)*. In animal models, tamoxifen treatment decreases tumor microvessel density by as much as 57%, even in ER-negative systems *(234,236)*. Oral tamoxifen (290 mg/d) inhibits endothelial proliferation and migration in subcutaneous Matrigel implants in rats *(233)*. These results correlate with clinical findings. A study was conducted in 57 patients with operable primary breast cancer who were treated with tamoxifen (20 mg/d) in the neoadjuvant setting, 3–6 mo prior to surgery. Patients whose tumors responded (> 25% reduction in tumor volume) to tamoxifen had significantly decreased intratumoral microvessel density, as evaluated by comparing pretreatment wedge biopsies with tissue obtained at surgical resection *(194)*. By comparison, microvessel density increased in nonresponding tumors.

The antiangiogenic mechanisms of tamoxifen include interference with E2-mediated VEGF transcription in tumor cells; inhibition of VEGF and bFGF-stimulated endothelial proliferation; and suppression of nitric oxide (NO) production *(237–241)*. Notably, exposure to tamoxifen increases uterine expression of VEGF, and increased production of three growth factors (aFGF, bFGF, and adrenomedullin) as well as vascular density in endometrium *(242,243)*. This may explain the increased risk of uterine hyperplasia and cancer in some patients who take tamoxifen on a long-term basis *(244–247)*.

4.2.2. Dietary Prevention

4.2.2.1. Green Tea Polyphenols After water, tea is the second most popular liquid in the world, and its consumption is linked with a decreased risk of colon, prostate, lung, esophageal, and other cancers *(248–250)*. Laboratory studies have demonstrated that green tea and its components prevent mutagenesis, tumorigenesis, cancer invasion and metastases, and angiogenesis *(251–255)*. Polyphenols in tea, predominantly flavones, possess chemopreventive and antiangiogenic activity. Epigallocatechin-3-gallate (EGCG) is a potent tea flavonoid that specifically inhibits endothelial cell proliferation stimulated by

bFGF; induces avascular zones in the chick CAM assay; inhibits VEGF-stimulated corneal neovascularization by as much as 70% in mice that consume 1.25% green tea (human equivalent of drinking 2–3 cups of tea/d); and reduces tumor cell invasion by 50% at levels equivalent to that in plasma of moderate green tea drinkers *(255)*.

The molecular mechanism of EGCG is the result of its inhibition of urokinase and two gelatinases (MMP-2 and -9) involved in vascular as well as tumor invasion *(256,257)*. The MMP inhibitory activity is independent of zinc or calcium binding by EGCG. High doses of EGCG induce apoptosis when topically applied to SKH-1 hairless mice bearing UVB-induced squamous cell carcinomas *(258)*. Clinical trials are underway in Western and Asian nations to study the chemopreventive potential of green tea for oral, prostate, skin, and other cancers.

4.2.2.2. Genistein Genistein (4',5,7-trihydroxy-isoflavone), an isoflavonoid found in soybeans, has both chemopreventive and antiangiogenic activity. It suppresses carcinogenesis in a variety of animal models of mammary and prostate carcinoma following oral and parenteral administration *(259–261)*. Multiple antitumor mechanisms of action have been identified, including induction of apoptosis, G_2 cell-cycle arrest, inhibition of c-*fos* expression and NF-κB activation, angiogenesis inhibition, and modulation of sex steroid receptors and growth factor signaling pathways *(262–264)*.

The antiangiogenic activity of genistein was initially detected in a study of healthy Japanese individuals who consumed a traditional soy-rich Japanese diet *(265,266)*. Urine from these subjects was collected, fractionated, and examined for activity to inhibit bFGF-stimulated endothelial cell proliferation. Of two fractions with anti-endothelial activity, one contained genistein, daidzein, and *O*-desmethylangolensin. The impact of dietary soy intake was significant. In men who consumed a Japanese vs Western diet, urinary genistein was 7052 nmol/d compared to 184.4 nmol/d, respectively *(267)*. Soy intake is known to be inversely associated with cancer risk. Japanese women who live in Hawaii and consume a traditional soy-based diet have a low incidence of breast cancer *(266,268)*. Similarly, Japanese men in Hawaii who consume a high soy diet have low mortality from prostate cancer, although the incidence at autopsy of *in situ* prostate neoplasia is similar to men in Western societies *(269)*.

The decreased cancer risk is attributed to dietary soy elements.

Genistein inhibits angiogenesis by inhibition of bFGF- and VEGF-driven endothelial cell proliferation, migration, and tube formation; inhibition of extracellular matrix degradation by suppression of bFGF-induced endothelial production of plasminogen activator (PA) and plasminogen activator inhibitor (PAI); and suppression of receptor tyrosine kinase activity for VEGF, EGF and PDGF (266,270–273). Based on laboratory findings and epidemiological data, genistein and a manufactured derivative known as genistein concentrated polysaccharide (GCP), are being evaluated in prevention trials for prostate cancer (274).

4.2.2.3. Curcumin

Curcumin (diferuloylmethane) is a flavonoid derived from the plant *Curcuma longa*, and is present in the spice tumeric. It has potent chemopreventive and antiangiogenic activity, and inhibits carcinogenesis in skin, stomach, intestines, and liver. Dietary ingestion of curcumin has been shown to prevent the formation of colon polyps, suppress proliferation of colon cancer and prostate cancer cells, and decrease intratumoral microvessel density (275–277). Studies of endothelial cells exposed in vitro to curcumin show induction of apoptosis; downregulation of gene transcripts for VEGF, bFGF, and MMP-2; COX-2 inhibition; upregulation of TIMP; disruption of vascular tube formation; and inhibition of endothelial cell motility by interfering with the Ras-mediated c-Jun N-terminal kinase (JNK) pathway (278–282). A Phase I prevention trial of curcumin (500–800 mg/d) showed histological improvement of lesions in patients with various malignant and premalignant lesions, including recently resected bladder cancer, oral leukoplakia, intestinal metaplasia, CIN, and Bowen's disease (283).

4.2.2.4. Resveratrol

Resveratrol (3,4',5-trihydroxystilbene) is a natural phytoalexin and polyphenol found in more than 72 plant species, such as mulberries, peanuts, grapes, and grape products, including red, white, and rose wine. Fresh grape skins contain 50–100 µg resveratrol per g, and yield a concentration in Italian red wine of 1.5–3 mg/L (284). Resveratrol inhibits chemically induced mammary carcinogenesis, skin cancer tumorigenesis, and tumor growth and metastasis in mice bearing Lewis lung carcinoma (284–285).

Resveratrol inhibits angiogenesis in the chick CAM assay, suppresses VEGF- and bFGF-induced corneal neovascularization (at ~3–4 mg, equivalent to 3–4 glasses red wine/d), and inhibits tumor vascularization in T241 fibrosarcoma growing in mice (285–286). In mice with full thickness skin wounds, resveratrol delays wound healing angiogenesis and the time required for complete wound closure (286). A number of antiangiogenic mechanisms have been identified, including suppression of capillary tube formation; inhibition of endothelial cell DNA synthesis and binding of VEGF to human endothelial cells; reduction of vascular cell adhesion molecule-1 (VCAM-1); interference with phosphorylation of endothelial mitogen-activated kinases; suppression of COX-2 enzyme; and inhibition of MMP-9 expression (285,287–289).

4.2.2.5. Linoleic Acid

Linoleic acid is a chemopreventive agent that inhibits mammary carcinogenesis by inhibiting epithelial proliferation and inducing apoptosis. The bioactive form of this agent is present as dietary-conjugated linoleic acid (CLA). Dietary ingestion of CLA (1–2%) inhibits angiogenesis and normal microvascular morphology in Matrigel pellets implanted in mice (290). The same regimen decreases expression of VEGF and its flk-1 receptor in mammary glands. At least four isomers of CLA exhibit dose-dependent antiangiogenic effects.

4.2.2.6. Other Novel Dietary Inhibitors

We have identified antiangiogenic activity in a number of other dietary-derived chemopreventive molecules. These include brassinin, a phytoalexin found in Chinese cabbage; the citrus-derived bioflavonoids hesperidin and naringenin; ellagic acid from berries, pomegranate, and grapes; silymarin from milk thistle and artichoke; and the organosulfur allyl disulfide derived from garlic (291–296). Further studies are underway to define their molecular targets in angiogenesis, their optimal biological doses, and efficacy in inhibiting tumor vascularity. The diverse natural sources of these and other antiangiogenic chemopreventive molecules raise the possibility of designing scientific diets for patients at high risk for cancer, or for those with known disease to chronically suppress angiogenesis and tumorigenesis.

5. CONCLUSION AND FUTURE DIRECTIONS

Angiogenesis is a critical, rate-limiting step in the development of all known cancers, and its inhibition suppresses tumor growth, progression, and metastases. Antiangiogenic therapy represents a new approach to the early intervention and prevention of malignant disease. During the next 50 yr, the total yearly number of newly diagnosed cases of cancer is projected to rise from 10 million new cases per year in 2000 to 24 million in 2050, and the number of annual deaths is projected to increase 2.7-fold to 16 million. The implementation of effective chemoprevention strategies based on angiogenesis inhibition may decrease these numbers significantly.

Importantly, most antiangiogenic agents appear to be safe and well tolerated in humans. Their application as preventive agents represent a paradigm shift in oncology, away from reliance on high doses of cytoxic drugs toward chronic suppressive treatment. The success of tamoxifen as an effective prevention agent for breast cancer paves the way for future studies and approval of other agents in other tumor types. Because cancer prevention trials are challenging to design and conduct for new molecular entities in large healthy populations, an opportunity exists to mine the existing pharmacopoeia for drugs with angiogenesis-inhibitory activity. COX-2 inhibitors (celecoxib, rofecoxib), peroxisome proliferator-activated receptor (PPAR)-γ ligands (rosiglitazone), and statins (cerivastatin) are examples of widely used oral drugs that inhibit tumor neovascularization *(117,297–298)*. As new antiangiogenic agents become approved for the treatment of advanced cancer, these should be studied in trials focused on cancer prevention and early stages of disease. A novel concept in preclinical development is an antiangiogenic DNA vaccine directed against VEGF receptor-2. In animals, this vaccine confers long-term resistance to tumor vascularization and protection against cancer *(299)*.

In summary, tumor angiogenesis is an important target for early cancer intervention and prevention. Antiangiogenic agents are in development, and represent a variety of compound types. The desirable attributes of an antiangiogenic preventive agent are established efficacy in preventing cancer; knowledge about its mechanism of action; evidence for efficacy in humans from epidemiological and clinical observations; documented efficacy in experimental animal models; lack of toxicity or undesirable side effects; status as an FDA-approved agent or an agent likely to be readily approved based on existing dosing and toxicity studies; or the natural occurrence of the agent in foods or beverages. Dietary antiangiogenic strategies are already in development in Asia. The molecular control of blood vessel growth promises to shape the future approach to cancer as a disease that can be prevented or effectively suppressed throughout an individual's lifetime.

ACKNOWLEDGMENTS

The author would like to thank Drs. Gary Kelloff, Lee Rosen, Richard Beliveau, Lee Ellis, Jaime Masferrer, Yihai Cao, Raymond DuBois, Vincent Li, and Gerald Gehr for their helpful discussions and insights, Andrew Grivas for scientific illustrations, and Kathy Trull for assistance with the manuscript. The original experimental work described is supported by grants from the Angiogenesis Foundation and the American Academy of Feline Practitioners.

REFERENCES

1. Schwartsmann G, Ratain MJ, Cragg GM, et al. Anticancer drug discovery and development throughout the world. *J Clin Oncol* 2002;20:47S–59S.
2. Ries LAG, Eisner MP, Kosary CL, et al. SEER Cancer Statistics Review, 1973–1998, National Cancer Institute, Bethesda, MD. http://seer.cancer.gov/Publications/CSR 1973–1998, 2001.
3. Lifetime risk of being diagnosed with cancer. *J Natl Cancer Inst* 2001;93:742.
4. Chemoprevention Working Group. Prevention of cancer in the next millennium: report of the Chemoprevention Working Group to the American Association for Cancer Research. *Cancer Res* 1999;59:4743–4758.
5. Folkman J. What is the evidence that tumors are angiogenesis dependent? *J Natl Cancer Inst* 1990;82:4–6.
6. Folkman J, Merler E, Abernathy C, et al. Isolation of a tumor fraction responsible for angiogenesis. *J Exp Med* 1971;133:275–288.
7. Folkman J. Tumor angiogenesis: therapeutic implications. *N Engl J Med* 1971;285:1182–1186.
8. Ribatti D, Vacca A, Dammacco F. The role of the vascular phase in solid tumor growth: a historical review. *Neoplasia* 1999;1(4):293–302.
9. Folkman J. Angiogenesis in cancer, vascular, rheumatoid and other disease. *Nat Med* 1995;1:27–31.
10. Kerbel RS. Tumor angiogenesis: past, present, and the near future. *Carcinogenesis* 2000;21:505–515.
11. Weidner N. Angiogenesis as a predictor of clinical outcome in cancer patients. *Hum Pathol* 2000;31(4):403–405.
12. Folkman J. Tumor angiogenesis, in *Harrison's Textbook of Internal Medicine*, 15th ed. Braunwald E, Fauci AS, Kasper DL, et al., eds. McGraw-Hill, New York, NY, 2000 pp.132–152.
13. Mangi MH, Newland AC. Angiogenesis and angiogenic markers in haematological malignancies. *Br J Haematol* 2000;111:43–51.
14. Brandvold KA, Neiman P, Rudell A. Angiogenesis is an early event in the generation of myc-induced lymphomas. *Oncogene* 2000;19:2780–2785.
15. Padro T, Ruiz S, Bieker R, et al. Increased angiogenesis in the bone marrow of patients with acute myeloid leukemia. *Blood* 2000;95:2637–2644.
16. Rajkumar SV, Greipp PR. Angiogenesis in multiple myeloma. *Br J Haematol* 2001;113:565.
17. Pruneri G, Bertolini F, Soligo D, et al. Angiogenesis in myelodysplastic syndromes. *Br J Cancer* 1999;81:1398–1401.

18. Rak J, Filmus J, Kerbel RS. Reciprocal paracrine interactions between tumour cells and endothelial cells: the 'angiogenesis progression' hypothesis. *Eur J Cancer* 1996;32A:2438–2450.

19. Folkman J. Angiogenesis-dependent diseases. *Semin Oncol* 2001;28:536–542.

20. Singhal S, Mehta J, Desikan R et al. Antitumor activity of thalidomide in refractory multiple myeloma. *N Engl J Med* 1999;341:1565–1571.

21. DeVore RF, Fehrenbacher L, Herbst RS, et al. A randomized phase II trial comparing rhuMab VEGF (recombinant humanized monoclonal antibody to vascular endothelial cell growth factor) plus carboplatin/paclitaxel (CP) to CP alone in patients with stage IIIB/IV NSCL. *Proc Am Soc Clin Oncol* 2000;19:485a, abst. no. 1896.

22. Batist G, Patenaude F, Champagne P, et al. (AE-941) in refractory renal cell carcinoma patients: report of a phase II trial with two dose levels. *Ann Oncol* 2002;13:1259–1263.

23. Kerbel R, Folkman J. Clinical translation of angiogenesis inhibitors. *Nature Rev Cancer* 2002;2:727–739.

24. Tosetti F, Ferrari N, De Flora S, et al. Angioprevention: angiogenesis is a common and key target for cancer chemopreventive agents. *FASEB J* 2002;16:2–14.

25. Helmlinger G, Yuan F, Dellian M, et al. Interstitial pH and pO2 gradients in solid tumors in vivo: high-resolution measurements reveal a lack of correlation. *Nat Med* 1997;3:177–182.

26. Gargett CE, Rogers PA. Human endometrial angiogenesis. *Reproduction* 2001;121:181–186.

27. Hazzard TM, Stouffer RL. Angiogenesis in ovarian follicular and luteal development. *Baillieres Clin Obstet Gynaecol* 2000;14:883–900.

28. Reynolds LP, Redmer DA. Angiogenesis in the placenta. *Biol Reprod* 2001;64:1033–1040.

29. Tonnesen MG, Feng X, Clark RA. Angiogenesis in wound healing. *J Investig Dermatol Symp Proc* 2000;5:40–46.

30. Shing Y, Folkman J, Sullivan R, et al. Heparin affinity: purification of a tumor-derived capillary endothelial growth factor. *Science* 1984;223:1296–1298.

31. Senger DR, Galli SJ, Dvorak AM, et al. Tumor cells secrete a vascular permeability factor that promotes accumulation of ascites fluid. *Science* 1983;219:983–985.

32. Leung DW, Cachianes G, Kuang WJ, et al. Vascular endothelial growth factor is a secreted angiogenic mitogen. *Science* 1989;246:1306–1309.

33. Nor JE, Christensen J, Mooney DJ, et al. Vascular endothelial growth factor (VEGF)-mediated angiogenesis is associated with enhanced endothelial cell survival and induction of Bcl-2 expression. *Am J Pathol* 1999;154:375–384.

34. Risau W. Mechanisms of angiogenesis. *Nature* 1997;386:671–674.

35. Adini A, Kornaga T, Firoozbakht F, et al. Placental growth factor is a survival factor for tumor endothelial cells and macrophages. *Cancer Res* 2002;62:2749–2752.

36. Hattori K, Heissig B, Wu Y, et al. Placental growth factor reconstitutes hematopoiesis by recruiting VEGFR1(+) stem cells from bone-marrow microenvironment. *Nat Med* 2002;8:841–849.

37. Folkman J, Klagsbrun M. Angiogenic factors. *Science* 1987;235:442–447.

38. Thommen R, Humar R, Misevic G, et al. PDGF-BB increases endothelial migration on cord movements during angiogenesis in vitro. *J Cell Biochem* 1997;64:403–413.

39. Russell KS, Stern DF, Polverini PJ, et al. Neuregulin activation of ErbB receptors in vascular endothelium leads to angiogenesis. *Am J Physiol* 1999;277:H2205–H2211.

40. Gillis P, Savla U, Volpert OV, et al. Keratinocyte growth factor induces angiogenesis and protects endothelial barrier function. *J Cell Sci* 1999;112:2049–2057.

41. Nguyen M. Angiogenic factors as tumor markers. *Investig New Drugs* 1997;15:29–37.

42. Brem H, Folkman J. Inhibition of tumor angiogenesis mediated by cartilage. *J Exp Med* 1975;141:427–439.

43. Moses MA, Wiederschain D, Wu I, et al. Troponin I is present in human cartilage and inhibits angiogenesis. *Proc Natl Acad Sci USA* 1999;96:2645–2650.

44. Feldman L, Rouleau C. Troponin I inhibits capillary endothelial cell proliferation by interaction with the cell's bFGF receptor. *Microvasc Res* 2002;63:41–49.

45. Inoki I, Shiomi T, Hashimoto G, et al. Connective tissue growth factor binds vascular endothelial growth factor (VEGF) and inhibits VEGF-induced angiogenesis. *FASEB J* 2002;16:219–221.

46. Kusafuka K, Hiraki Y, Shukunami C, et al. Cartilage-specific matrix protein, chondromodulin-I (ChM-I), is a strong angio-inhibitor in endochondral ossification of human neonatal vertebral tissues in vivo: relationship with angiogenic factors in cartilage. *Acta Histochem* 2002;104:167–175.

47. Davies C, de L, Melder RJ, Munn LL, et al. Decorin inhibits endothelial migration and tube-like structure formation: role of thrombospondin-1. *Microvasc Res* 2001;62(1):26–42.

48. Liu N, Lapcevich RK, Underhill CB, et al. Metastatin: a hyaluronan-binding complex from cartilage that inhibits tumor growth. *Cancer Res* 2001;61:1022–1028.

49. Dawson DW, Volpert OV, Gillis P, et al. Pigment epithelium-derived factor: a potent inhibitor of angiogenesis. *Science* 1999;285:245–248.

50. Lutty GA, Thompson DC, Gallup JY, et al. Vitreous: an inhibitor of retinal extract-induced neovascularization. *Invest Ophthalmol Vis Sci* 1983;24:52.

51. Williams GA, Eisenstein R, Schumacher B, et al. Inhibitor of vascular endothelial cell growth in the lens. *Am J Ophthalmol* 1984;97:366–371.

52. Mun EC, Doctrow SR, Carter R, et al. An angiogenesis inhibitor from the cornea. *Investig Ophthalmol Vis Sci* 1989;30(Suppl):151.

53. Auerbach W, Auerbach R. Angiogenesis inhibition: a review. *Pharmacol Ther* 1994;63:265–311.

54. Dameron KM, Volpert OV, Tainsky MA, et al. Control of angiogenesis in fibroblasts by p53 regulation of thrombospondin-1. *Science* 1994;265:1582–1584.

55. Nor JE, Mitra RS, Sutorik MM, et al. Thrombospondin-1 induces endothelial cell apoptosis and inhibits angiogenesis by activating the caspase death pathway. *J Vasc Res* 2000;37:209–218.

56. Streit M, Riccardi L, Velasco P, et al. Thrombospondin-2: a potent endogenous inhibitor of tumor growth and angiogenesis. *Proc Natl Acad Sci USA* 1999;96:14,888–14,893.

57. Singh RK, Gutman M, Bucana CD, et al. Interferons alpha and beta down-regulate the expression of basic fibroblast growth factor in human carcinomas. *Proc Natl Acad Sci USA* 1995;92:4562–4566.

58. Friesel R, Komoriya A, Maciag T. Inhibition of endothelial cell proliferation by gamma-interferon. *J Cell Biol* 1987;104:689–696.

59. Kamphaus GD, Colorado PC, Panka DJ, et al. Canstatin, a novel matrix-derived inhibitor of angiogenesis and tumor growth. *J Biol Chem* 2000;275:1209–1215.

60. Maeshima Y, Manfredi M, Reimer C, et al. Identification of the anti-angiogenic site within vascular basement membrane-derived tumstatin. *J Biol Chem* 2001;276:15,240–15,248.

61. Colorado PC, Torre A, Kamphaus G, et al. Anti-angiogenic cues from vascular basement membrane collagen. *Cancer Res* 2000;60:2520–2526.

62. O'Reilly MS, Holmgren L, Shing Y, et al. Angiostatin: a novel angiogenesis inhibitor that mediates the suppression of metastases by a Lewis lung carcinoma. *Cell* 1994;79:315–328.

63. Heidtmann HH, Nettelbeck DM, Mingels et al. Generation of angiostatin-like fragments from plasminogen by prostate-specific antigen. *Br J Cancer* 1999;81:1269–1272.

64. Gately S, Twardowski P, Stack MS, et al. The mechanism of cancer-mediated conversion of plasminogen to the angiogenesis inhibitor angiostatin. *Proc Natl Acad Sci USA* 1997;94:10,868–10,872.

65. O'Reilly MS, Boehm T, Shing Y, et al. Endostatin: an endogenous inhibitor of angiogenesis and tumor growth. *Cell* 1997;88:277–285.

66. Dixelius J, Larsson H, Sasaki T, et al. Endostatin-induced tyrosine kinase signaling through the Shb adaptor protein regulates endothelial cell apoptosis. *Blood* 2000;95:3403–3411.

67. O'Reilly MS, Holmgren L, Shing Y, et al. Angiostatin: a circulating endothelial cell inhibitor that suppresses angiogenesis and tumor growth. *Cold Spring Harb Symp Quant Biol* 1994;59:471–482.

68. Herbst RS, Hess KR, Tran HT, et al. Phase I study of recombinant human endostatin in patients with advanced solid tumors. *J Clin Oncol* 2002;20:3792–3803.

69. Hanahan D, Folkman J. Patterns and emerging mechanisms of the angiogenic switch during tumorigenesis. *Cell* 1996;86:353–364.

70. Plate KH, Breier G, Millauer B, et al. Up-regulation of vascular endothelial growth factor and its cognate receptors in a rat glioma model of tumor angiogenesis. *Cancer Res* 1993;53:5822–5827.

71. Rastinejad F, Polverini PJ, Bouck NP. Regulation of the activity of a new inhibitor of angiogenesis by a cancer suppressor gene. *Cell* 1989;56:345–355.

72. Ohno-Matsui K, Morita I, Tombran-Tink J, et al. Novel mechanism for age-related macular degeneration: an equilibrium shift between the angiogenesis factors VEGF and PEDF. *J Cell Physiol* 2001;189:323–333.

73. Lyden D, Young AZ, Zagzag D, et al. Id1 and Id3 are required for neurogenesis, angiogenesis and vascularization of tumor xenografts. *Nature* 1999;401:670–677.

74. Baudino TA, McKay C, Pendeville-Samain H, et al. c-Myc is essential for vasculogenesis and angiogenesis during development and tumor progression. *Genes Dev* 2002;16:2530–2543.

75. Vikhanskaya F, Bani MR, Borsotti P, et al. p73 Overexpression increases VEGF and reduces thrombospondin-1 production: implications for tumor angiogenesis. *Oncogene* 2001;20:7293–7300.

76. Lu L, Holmqvist K, Cross M, et al. Role of the src homology 2 domain-containing protein Shb in murine brain endothelial cell proliferation and differentiation. *Cell Growth Differ* 2002;13:141–148.

77. Rak J, Mitsuhashi Y, Bayko L, Mutant ras oncogenes upregulate VEGF/VPF expression: implications for induction and inhibition of tumour angiogenesis. *Cancer Res* 1995;55:4575–4580.

78. Grugel D, Finkenzeller G, Weindel K, et al. Both v-Ha-ras and v-raf stimulate expression of the vascular endothelial growth factor in NIH 3T3 cells. *J Biol Chem* 1995;270:25,915–25,919.

79. Arbiser JL, Moses MA, Fernandez CA, et al. Oncogenic H-ras stimulates tumour angiogenesis by two distinct pathways. *Proc Natl Acad Sci USA* 1997;94:861–866.

80. Schlessinger J. New roles for Src kinases in control of cell survival and angiogenesis. *Cell* 2000; 100: 293–296.

81. Kumar R, Yarmand-Bagheri R. The role of HER2 in angiogenesis. *Semin Oncol* 2001;28(Suppl 16):27–32.

82. Giri D, Ittmann M. Inactivation of the PTEN tumor suppressor gene is associated with increased angiogenesis in clinically localized prostate carcinoma. *Hum Pathol* 1999;30:419–424.

83. Claudio PP, Stiegler P, Howard CM, et al. RB2/p130 gene-enhanced expression down-regulates vascular endothelial growth factor expression and inhibits angiogenesis in vivo. *Cancer Res* 2001;6:462–468.

84. Blancher C, Moore JW, Robertson N et al. Effects of ras and von Hippel-Lindau (VHL) gene mutations on hypoxia-inducible factor (HIF)-1alpha, HIF-2alpha, and vascular endothelial growth factor expression and their regulation by the phosphatidylinositol 3'-kinase/Akt signaling pathway. *Cancer Res* 2001;61:7349–7355.

85. Li CY, Shan S, Huang O, et al. Initial stages of tumor cell-induced angiogenesis: evaluation via skin window chambers in rodent models. *J Natl Cancer Inst* 2000;92:143–147.

86. Holash J, Maisonpierre PC, Compton D, et al. Vessel cooption, regression, and growth in tumors mediated by angiopoietins and VEGF. *Science* 1999;284:1994–1998.

87. Folkman J. Incipient angiogenesis. *J Natl Cancer Inst* 2000;92:94–95.

88. Holmgren L, O'Reilly MS, Folkman J. Dormancy of micrometastases: balanced proliferation and apoptosis in the presence of angiogenesis suppression. *Nat Med* 1995;1:149–153.

89. Li W. Tumor angiogenesis: molecular pathology, therapeutic targeting and imaging. *Acad Radiol* 2000;7:800–811.

90. Hanahan D. Heritable formation of pancreatic beta-cell tumours in transgenic mice expressing recombinant insulin/simian virus 40 oncogenes. *Nature* 1985;315:115–122.

91. Folkman J, Hanahan D. Expression of the angiogenic phenotype during development of murine and human cancer, in *Origins of Human Cancer: A Comprehensive Review*. Brugge J, Curran T, Harlow E, et al, eds. Cold Spring Harbor Laboratory Press, Cold Spring Harbor, NY, 1991:pp.803–814.

92. Folkman J, Watson K, Ingber D, et al. Induction of angiogenesis during the transition from hyperplasia to neoplasia. *Nature* 1989;339:58–61.

93. Lacey M, Alpert S, Hanahan D. Bovine papillomavirus genome elicits skin tumours in transgenic mice. *Nature* 1986;322:609–612.

94. Kandel J, Bossy-Wetzel E, Radvanyi F, et al. Neovascularization is associated with a switch to the export of bFGF in the multistep development of fibrosarcoma. *Cell* 1991;66:1095–1104.

95. Bergers G, Hanahan D, Coussens LM. Angiogenesis and apoptosis are cellular parameters of neoplastic progression

in transgenic mouse models of tumorigenesis. *Int J Dev Biol* 1998;42(7 Spec No):995–1002.

96. Coussens LM, Raymond WW, Bergers G, et al. Inflammatory mast cells up-regulate angiogenesis during squamous epithelial carcinogenesis. *Genes Dev* 1999;13:1382–1397.

97. Norrby K. Mast cells and angiogenesis. *APMIS* 2002;110:355–371.

98. Ribatti D, Crivellato E, Candussio L, et al. Mast cells and their secretory granules are angiogenic in the chick embryo chorioallantoic membrane. *Clin Exp Allergy* 2001;31:602–608.

99. Smith-McCune K, Zhu YH, Hanahan D, et al. Cross-species comparison of angiogenesis during the premalignant stages of squamous carcinogenesis in the human cervix and K14-HPV16 transgenic mice. *Cancer Res* 1997;57:1294–1300.

100. Folkman J. Tumor angiogenesis, in *Cancer Biology, Vol 3: Biology of Tumors*. FF Becker, ed. Plenum Press, New York, NY; 1975, pp.355–388.

101. Wurschmidt F, Beck-Bornholdt HP, Vogler H. Radiobiology of the rhabdomyosarcoma R1H of the rat: influence of the size of irradiation field on tumor response, tumor bed effect, and neovascularization kinetics. *Int J Radiat Oncol Biol Phys* 1990;18:879–882.

102. Yamaura H, Yamada K, Matsuzawa T. Radiation effect on the proliferating capillaries in rat transparent chamber. *Int J Radiat Biol* 1976;30:179.

103. Gimbrone MA Jr, Cotran R, Leapman S, et al. Tumor dormancy in vivo by prevention of neovascularization. *J Exp Med* 1972;136:261–276.

104. Folkman J. Tumor angiogenesis and tissue factor. *Nat Med* 1996;2:167–168.

105. Modzelewski RA, Davies P, Watkins SC, et al. Isolation and purification of fresh tumor-derived endothelial cells from a murine RIF-1 fibrosarcoma. *Cancer Res* 1994;54:336–339.

106. Thompson WD, Shiach KJ, Fraser RA, et al. Tumours acquire their vasculature by vessel incorporation, not vessel ingrowth. *J Pathol* 1987;151:323–332.

107. Fidler IJ, Ellis LM. The implications of angiogenesis for the biology and therapy of cancer metastasis. *Cell* 1994;79:185–188.

108. Butler TP, Gullino PM. Quantitation of cell shedding into efferent blood of mammary adenocarcinoma. *Cancer Res* 1975;35:512–516.

109. Folkman J. Antiangiogenesis Agents, in *Cancer: Principles & Practice of Oncology, 6th ed.* DeVita VT, Hellman S, Rosenberg SA, eds. Lippincott Williams & Wilkins, Philadelphia, PA, 2001, pp.509–519.

110. Engerman RL, Pfaffenbach D, Davis MD. Cell turnover in capillaries. *Lab Investig* 1967;17:738–743.

111. Hobson B, Denekamp J. Endothelial proliferation in tumours and normal tissues: continuous labelling studies. *Br J Cancer* 1984;49:405–413.

112. Tannock IF. Population kinetics of carcinoma cells, capillary endothelial cells, and fibroblasts in a transplanted mouse mammary tumor. *Cancer Res* 1970;30:2470–2476.

113. Ausprunk D, Folkman J. Migration and proliferation of endothelial cells in preformed and newly formed blood vessels during tumor angiogenesis. *Microvasc Res* 1977;14:53–65.

114. Carmeliet P, Dor Y, Herbert JM, et al. Role of HIF-1 in hypoxia-mediated apoptosis, cell proliferation and tumor angiogenesis. *Nature* 1998;394:485–490.

115. Polverini PJ, Leibovich SJ. Induction of neovascularization in vivo and endothelial proliferation in vitro by tumor-associated macrophages. *Lab Investig* 1984;51:635–642.

116. Dias S, Choy M, Rafii S. The role of CXC chemokines in the regulation of tumor angiogenesis. *Cancer Investig* 2001;19:732–738.

117. Masferrer JL, Leahy KM, Koki AT, et al. Antiangiogenic and antitumor activities of cyclooxygenase-2 inhibitors. *Cancer Res* 2000; 60:1306–1311.

118. Leahy KM, Koki AT, Masferrer JL. Role of cyclooxygenases in angiogenesis. *Curr Med Chem* 2000;7:1163–1170.

119. Nor JE, Christensen J, Liu J, et al. Up-regulation of Bcl-2 in microvascular endothelial cells enhances intratumoral angiogenesis and accelerates tumor growth. *Cancer Res* 2001;61:2183–2188.

120. Mignatti P, Tsuboi R, Robbins E, et al. In vitro angiogenesis on the human amniotic membrane: requirement for basic fibroblast growth factor-induced proteinases. *J Cell Biol* 1989;108:671–682.

121. Brooks PC, Montgomery AM, Rosenfeld M, et al. Integrin $\alpha_v\beta_3$ antagonists promote tumor regression by inducing apoptosis of angiogenic blood vessels. *Cell* 1994;79(7):1157–1164.

122. Van Der Schaft DW, Dings RP, De Lussanet QG, et al. The designer anti-angiogenic peptide anginex targets tumor endothelial cells and inhibits tumor growth in animal models. *FASEB J* 2002;16:1991–1993.

123. Huang S, Pettaway CA, Uehara H, et al. Blockade of NF-kappaB activity in human prostate cancer cells is associated with suppression of angiogenesis, invasion, and metastasis. *Oncogene* 2001;20:4188–4197.

124. Nelson AR, Fingleton B, Rothenberg ML, et al. Matrix metalloproteinases: biologic activity and clinical implications. *J Clin Oncol* 2000;18:1135–1149.

125. Sang QXA. Complex role of matrix metalloproteinases in angiogenesis. *Cell Res* 1998;8:171–177.

126. Koolwijk P, Sidenius N, Peters E, et al. Proteolysis of the urokinase-type plasminogen activator receptor by metalloproteinase-12: implication for angiogenesis in fibrin matrices. *Blood* 2001;97:3123–3131.

127. Nguyen M, Folkman J, Bischoff J. 1-Deoxymannojirimycin inhibits capillary tube formation in vitro. Analysis of N-linked oligosaccharides in bovine capillary endothelial cells. *J Biol Chem* 1992;267:26,157–26,165.

128. Nguyen M, Strubel NA, Bischoff J. A role for sialyl Lewis-X/A glycoconjugates in capillary morphogenesis. *Nature* 1993;365:267–269.

129. Nangia-Makker P, Honjo Y, Sarvis R, et al. Galectin-3 induces endothelial cell morphogenesis and angiogenesis. *Am J Pathol* 2000;156:899–909.

130. DeLisser HM, Christofidou-Solomidou M, Strieter RM, et al. Involvement of endothelial PECAM-1/CD31 in angiogenesis. *Am J Pathol* 1997;151:671–677.

131. Bach TL, Barsigian C, Chalupowicz DG, et al. VE-Cadherin mediates endothelial cell capillary tube formation in fibrin and collagen gels. *Exp Cell Res* 1998;238:324-334.

132. Wang HU, Chen ZF, Anderson DJ. Molecular distinction and angiogenic interactions between embryonic arteries and veins revealed by ephrin-B2 and its receptor Eph-B4. *Cell* 1998;93:741–753.

133. Yancopoulos GD, Klagsbrun M, Folkman J. Vasculogenesis, angiogenesis and growth factors: ephrins enter the fray at the border. *Cell* 1998;93:661–664.

134. Adams RH, Wilkinson GA, Weiss C, et al. Roles of ephrinB ligands and EphB receptors in cardiovascular development: demarcation of arterial/venous domains, vascular morphogenesis, and sprouting angiogenesis. *Genes Dev* 1999;13:295–306.

135. Shin D, Garcia-Cardena G, Hayashi S, et al. Expression of ephrinB2 identifies a stable genetic difference between arterial and venous vascular smooth muscle as well as endothelial cells, and marks subsets of microvessels as sites of adult neovascularization. *Dev Biol* 2001;230:139–150.

136. Folkman J, D'Amore PA. Blood vessel formation: what is its molecular basis? *Cell* 1996;87:1153–1155.

137. Hayes AJ, Huang WQ, Mallah J, et al. Angiopoietin-1 and its receptor Tie-2 participate in the regulation of capillary-like tubule formation and survival of endothelial cells. *Microvasc Res* 1999;58:224–237.

138. Benjamin LE, Golijanin D, Itin A, et al. Selective ablation of immature blood vessels in established human tumors follows vascular endothelial growth factor withdrawal. *J Clin Investig* 1999;103:159–165.

139. Lindahl P, Johansson BR, Leveen P, et al. Pericyte loss and microaneurysm formation in PDGF-B-deficient mice. *Science* 1997;277:242–245.

140. Asahara T, Murohara T, Sullivan A, et al. Isolation of putative progenitor endothelial cells for angiogenesis. *Science* 1997;275:964–967.

141. Asahara T, Masuda H, Takahashi T, et al. Bone marrow origin of endothelial progenitor cells responsible for postnatal vasculogenesis in physiological and pathological neovascularization. *Circ Res* 1999;85:221–228.

142. Lyden D, Hattori K, Dias S, et al. Impaired recruitment of bone-marrow-derived endothelial and hematopoietic precursor cells blocks tumor angiogenesis and growth. *Nat Med* 2001:1194–1201.

143. Iwaguro H, Yamaguchi J-I, Kalka C, et al. Endothelial progenitor cell vascular endothelial growth factor transfer for vascular regeneration. *Circulation* 2002;105:732–738.

144. White CW, Sondheimer HM, Crouch EC, et al. Treatment of pulmonary hemangiomatosis with recombinant interferon alpha-2a. *N Engl J Med* 1989;320:1197–1200.

145. Kruger EA, Figg WD. TNP-470: an angiogenesis inhibitor in clinical development for cancer. *Expert Opin Invest Drugs* 2000;9:1383–1396.

146. Ezekowitz RBA, Mulliken JB, Folkman J. Interferon alpha-2a therapy for life-threatening hemangiomas of infancy. *N Engl J Med* 1992;326:1456–1463.

147. Li WW, Li VW, Tsakayannis D. Angiogenesis therapies: concepts, clinical trials, and considerations for new drug development, in *The New Angiotherapy*. Fan T-PD, Kohn EC, eds. Humana Press, Totowa, NJ, 2002, pp. 547–571.

148. Watson JC, Sutanto-Ward E, Osaku M, et al. Importance of timing and length of administration of angiogenesis inhibitor TNP-470 in the treatment of K12/TRb colorectal hepatic metastases in BD-IX rats. *Surgery* 1999;126:358–363.

149. Boehm T, Folkman J, Browder T, et al. Antiangiogenic therapy of experimental cancer does not induce acquired drug resistance. *Nature* 1997;390:404–407.

150. Pluda JM. Tumor-associated angiogenesis: mechanisms, clinical implications, and therapeutic strategies. *Semin Oncol* 1997;24:203–218.

151. Folkman J, Hahnfeldt P, Hlatky L. The logic of anti-angiogenic gene therapy, in *The Development of Human Gene Therapy*. Friedman T, ed. Cold Spring Harbor Laboratory Press, Cold Spring Harbor, NY, 1998, pp. 527–543.

152. Herbst RS, Lee AT, Tran HT, Abbruzzese JL. Clinical studies of angiogenesis inhibitors: the University of Texas MD Anderson Center Trial of Human Endostatin. *Curr Oncol Rep* 2001;3:131–140.

153. Teicher BA, Sotomayor EA, Huang ZD. Antiangiogenic agents potentiate cytotoxic cancer therapies against primary and metastatic disease. *Cancer Res* 1992;52:6702–6704.

154. Mauceri HJ, Hanna NN, Beckett MA, et al. Combined effects of angiostatin and ionizing radiation in antitumour therapy. *Nature* 1998;394:287–291.

155. Bergsland E, Hurwitz H, Fehrenbacher L, et al. A randomized phase II trial comparing rhuMAb VEGF (recombinant humanized monoclonal antibody to vascular endothelial cell growth factor) plus 5-fluorouracil/leucovorin (FU/LV) to FU/LV alone in patients with metastatic colorectal cancer. *Proc Am Soc Clin Oncol* 2000;19:939a, abst. no 939.

156. Burke PA, DeNardo SJ, Miers LA, et al. Cilengitide targeting of alpha(v)beta(3) integrin receptor synergizes with radioimmunotherapy to increase efficacy and apoptosis in breast cancer xenografts. *Cancer Res* 2002;62:4263–4272.

157. Boucher Y, Leunig M, Jain RK. Tumor angiogenesis and interstitial hypertension. *Cancer Res* 1996;56:4264–4266.

158. Jain RK. Normalizing tumor vasculature with anti-angiogenic therapy: a new paradigm for combination therapy. *Nat Med* 2001;7:987–989.

159. Kumar R, Kuniyasu H, Bucana CP, et al. Spatial and temporal expression of angiogenic molecules during tumor growth and progression. *Oncol Res* 1998;10:301–311.

160. Kumar R, Yoneda J, Bucana CP, et al. Regulation of distinct steps of angiogenssis by different angiogenic molecules. *Int J Oncol* 1998;12:749–757.

161. Relf M, LeJeune S, Scott PA, et al. Expression of the angiogenic factors vascular endothelial cell growth factor, acidic and basic fibroblast growth factor, tumor growth factor b-1, platelet-derived endothelial cell growth factor, placenta growth factor, and pleiotrophin in human primary breast cancer and its relation to angiogenesis. *Cancer Res* 1997;57:963–969.

162. Friedlander M, Brooks PC, Shaffer RW, et al. Definition of two angiogenic pathways by distinct alpha v integrins. *Science* 1995;270:1500–1502.

163. Kaban LB, Mulliken JB, Ezekowitz RA, et al. Antiangiogenic therapy of a recurrent giant cell tumor of the mandible with interferon alfa-2a. *Pediatrics* 1999;103:1145–1149.

164. Fine HA, Figg WD, Jaeckle K, et al. Phase II trial of the antiangiogenic agent thalidomide in patients with recurrent high-grade gliomas. *J Clin Oncol* 2000;18:708–715.

165. Tulpule A, Scadden DT, Espina BM, et al. Results of a randomized study of IM862 nasal solution in the treatment of AIDS-related Kaposi's sarcoma. *J Clin Oncol* 2000;18:716–723.

166. Kudelka AP, Verschraegen CF, Loyer E. Complete remission of metastatic cervical cancer with the angiogenesis inhibitor TNP-470. *N Engl J Med* 1998;338:991–992.

167. Marler JJ, Rubin JB, Trede NS, et al. Successful antiangiogenic therapy of giant cell angioblastoma with interferon alfa 2b: report of 2 cases. *Pediatrics* 2002;109:E37.

168. Patt YZ, Hassan MM, Lozano RD, et al. Durable clinical response of refractory hepatocellular carcinoma to orally administered thalidomide. *Am J Clin Oncol* (CCT) 2000;23:319–321.

169. Mesters RM, Padro T, Bieker R, et al. Stable remission after administration of the receptor tyrosine kinase inhibitor SU5416 in a patient with refractory acute myeloid leukemia. *Blood* 2001;98:241–243.

170. Barlogie B, Desikan R, Eddlemon P, et al. Extended survival in advanced and refractory multiple myeloma after single-agent thalidomide: identification of prognostic factors in a phase 2 study of 169 patients. *Blood* 2001;98:492–494.

171. Tatum JL, Hoffman JM. Role of imaging in clinical trials of antiangiogenesis therapy in oncology. *Acad Radiol* 2000;7:798–799.

172. Sipkins DA, Cheresh DA, Kazemi MR, et al. Detection of tumor angiogenesis in vivo by alpha-Vbeta3-targeted magnetic resonance imaging. *Nat Med* 1998;4:623–626.

173. Jayson GC, Zweit J, Jackson A, et al. Molecular imaging and biological evaluation of HuMV833 anti-VEGF antibody: implications for trial design for antiangiogenic antibodies. *J Natl Cancer Inst* 2002;94:1484–1493.

174. Hill SA, Toze GM, Petit GR, et al. Preclinical evaluation of the antitumor activity of the novel vascular targeting agent Oxi 4503. *Anticancer Res* 2002;22:1453–1458.

175. Goto H, Yano S, Zhang H, et al. Activity of a new vascular targeting agent, ZD6126, in pulmonary metastases by human lung adenocarcinoma in nude mice. *Cancer Res* 2002;62:3711–3715.

176. Siemann DW, Mercer E, Lepler S, et al. Vascular targeting agents enhance chemotherapeutic agent activities in solid tumor therapy. *Int J Cancer* 2002;99:1–6.

177. Brem H, Folkman J. Analysis of experimental antiangiogenic therapy. *J Pediatr Surg* 1993;28:445–451.

178. Li, WW, Li VW, Casey R, et al. Clinical trials of angiogenesis-based therapies: overview and new guiding principles, in *Angiogenesis: Models, Modulators and Clinical Application.* Maragoudakis M, ed. Plenum Press, New York, NY, 1998, pp.475–492.

179. Teo NB, Shoker BS, Martin L, et al. Angiogenesis in pre-invasive cancers. *Anticancer Res* 2002;22:2061–2072.

180. Vajkoczy P, Farhadi M, Gaumann A, et al. Microtumor growth initiates angiogenic sprouting with simultaneous expression of VEGF, VEGF receptor-2, and angiopoietin-2. *J Clin Investig* 2002;109:777–785.

181. Lee AH, Happerfield LC, Bobrow LG, et al. Angiogenesis and inflammation in ductal carcinoma in situ of the breast. *J Pathol* 1997;181:200–206.

182. Fisseler-Eclchoff A, Rothstein D, Muller KM. Neovascularization in hyperplastic, metaplastic and potentially preneoplastic lesions of the bronchial mucosa. *Virchows Arch* 1996;429:95–100.

183. Wong MP, Cheung N, Yuen ST, et al. Vascular endothelial growth factor is up-regulated in the early pre-malignant stage of colorectal tumour progression. *Int J Cancer* 1999;81(6):845–850.

184. Dellas A, Moch H, Schultheiss E. Angiogenesis in cervical neoplasia: microvessel quantification in precancerous lesions and invasive carcinomas with clinicopathological correlations. *Gynecol Oncol* 1997;67:27–33.

185. Smith-McCune KK, Weidner N. Demonstration and characterization of the angiogenic properties of cervical dysplasia. *Cancer Res* 1994;54:800–804.

186. Chodak GW, Haudenschild C, Gittes RF, et al. Angiogenic activity as a marker of neoplastic and preneoplastic lesions of the human bladder. *Ann Surg* 1980;192(6):762–771.

187. Fong Y, Blumgart L, Cohen A. Surgical treatment of colorectal metastases to liver. *CA Cancer J Clin* 1995;45:50–62.

188. Paku S, Lapis K. Morphological aspects of angiogenesis in experimental liver metastases. *Am J Pathol* 1993;143:926–936.

189. Ingber D, Fujita T, Kishimoto S, et al. Synthetic analogs of fumagillin that inhibit angiogenesis and suppress tumour growth. *Nature* 1990;348:555–557.

190. Suganuma Y, Takahashi T, Taniguchi H, et al. Inhibitory effect of anti-angiogenic agent TNP-470 (AGM-1470) on liver metastasis of VX2 carcinoma in rabbits. *Reg Cancer Treat* 1994;7:160–162.

191. Shusterman S, Grupp SA, Barr R, et al. The angiogenesis inhibitor TNP-470 effectively inhibits human neuroblastoma xenograft growth, especially in the setting of subclinical disease. *Clin Cancer Res* 2001;7:977–984.

192. Bergers G, Javaherian K, Lo K-M, et al. Effects of angiogenesis inhibitors on multistage carcinogenesis in mice. *Science* 1999;284:808–812.

193. Joseph IB, Vukanovic J, Isaacs JT. Antiangiogenic treatment with linomide as chemoprevention for prostate, seminal vesicle, and breast carcinogenesis in rodents. *Cancer Res* 1996;56:3404–3408.

194. Marson LP, Kurian KM, Millere WR, et al. The effect of tamoxifen on breast tumour vascularity. *Breast Cancer Res Treat* 2001;66:9–15.

195. Ruggeri BA, Robinson C, Angeles T, et al. The chemopreventive agent oltipraz possesses potent antiangiogenic activity in vitro, ex vivo, and in vivo and inhibits tumor xenograft growth. *Clin Cancer Res* 2002;8:267–274.

196. Lingen MW, Polverini PJ, Bouck NP. Inhibition of squamous cell carcinoma angiogenesis by direct interaction of retinoic acid with endothelial cells. *Lab Investig* 1996;74:476–483.

197. Takahashi Y, Mai M, Nishioka K. Alpha-difluoromethylornithine induces apoptosis as well as antiangiogenesis in the inhibition of tumor growth and metastasis in a human gastric cancer model. *Int J Cancer* 2000;85:243–247.

198. Jiang C, Jiang W, Ip C, et al. Selenium-induced inhibition of angiogenesis in mammary cancer at chemopreventive levels of intake. *Mol Carcinog* 1999;26:213–225.

199. Cai T, Fassina G, Morini M, et al. *N*-acetylcysteine inhibits endothelial cell invasion and angiogenesis. *Lab Investig* 1999;79:1151–1159.

200. Ebeler SE, Brenneman CA, Kim GS, et al. Dietary catechin delays tumor onset in a transgenic model. *Am J Clin Nutr* 2002;76:865–872.

201. Wang Z, Fuentes CF, Shapshay SM. Antiangiogenic and chemopreventive activities of celecoxib in oral carcinoma cell. *Laryngoscope* 2002;112:839–842.

202. Sharma S, Ghoddoussi M, Gao P, et al. A quantitative angiogenesis model for efficacy testing of chemopreventive agents. *Anticancer Res* 2001;21:3829–3837.

203. Kruger EA, Duray PH, Price DK, et al. Approaches to pre-clinical screening of antiangiogenic agents. *Semin Oncol* 2001;28:570–576.

204. Perletti G, Concari P, Giardini R, et al. Antitumor activity of endostatin against carcinogen-induced rat primary mammary tumors. *Cancer Res* 2000;60:1793–1796.

205. Hong WK, Lippman SM, Itri LM, et al. Prevention of second primary tumors with isotretinoin in squamous-cell carcinoma of the head and neck. *N Engl J Med* 1995;332:1405–1410.

206. Hong WK, Endicott J, Itri LM. 13-*cis*-Retinoic acid in the treatment of oral leukoplakia. *N Engl J Med* 1986;315:1501–1505.

207. Singh DK, Lippman SM. Cancer chemoprevention, part 1: retinoids and carotenoids and other classic antioxidants. *Oncology* 1998;12:1643–1660.

208. Petkovich M, Brand NJ, Krust A, et al. A human retinoic acid receptor which belongs to the family of nuclear receptors. *Nature* 1987; 330:444–450.

209. Lotan R. Retinoids in cancer chemoprevention. *FASEB J* 1996;10:1031–1039.

210. Braunhut SJ, Palomares M. Modulation of endothelial cell shape and growth by retinoids. *Microvasc Res* 1991;41:47–62.

211. Ingber DE. Extracellular matrix and cell shape: potential control points for inhibition of angiogenesis. *J Cell Biochem* 1991;87:3579–3583.

212. Imcke E, Ruszczak Z, Mayer-Da Silva A, et al. Cultivation of human dermal microvascular endothelial cells *in vitro*: immunocytochemical and ultrastructural characterization and effect of treatment with three synthetic retinoids. *Arch Dermato Res* 1991;283:149–157.

213. Arensman RM and Stolar CJH. Vitamin A effect on tumor angiogenesis. *J Ped Surg* 1979;14:809–812.

214. Liaudet-Coopman EDE, Berchem GJ, Wellstein A. In vivo inhibition of angiogenesis and induction of apoptosis by retinoid acid in squamous cell carcinoma. *Clin Cancer Res* 1997;3:179–84.

215. Majewski S, Szmurlo A, Marczak M, et al. Inhibition of tumor cell-induced angiogenesis by retinoids, 1,25-dihydroxyvitamin D_3 and their combination. *Cancer Lett* 1993;75:35–39.

216. Yasuda Y, Nishi N, Takahashi JA, et al. Induction of avascular yolk sac due to reduction of basic fibroblast growth factor by retinoic acid in mice. *Dev Biol* 1992;150:397–413.

217. Kirkpatrick K, Ogunkolade W, Elkak A, et al. The mRNA expression of cyclo-oxygenase-2 (COX-2) and vascular endothelial growth factor (VEGF) in human breast cancer. *Curr Med Res Opin* 2002;18:237–241.

218. Changching DL, Kenyon L, Hyslop T, et al. Cyclooxygenase-2 (COX-2) expression in human meningioma: correlation with malignant progression and potential target. *Proc Am Soc Clin Oncol* 2002: Abstract #296.

219. Soslow RA, Dannenberg AJ, Rush D, et al. COX-2 is expressed in human pulmonary, colonic, and mammary tumors. *Cancer* 2000;89:2637–2645.

220. Krishnan K, Arnett D, Youngberg G. Expression of Bcl-2, CD95, VEGF, Ki-67 and COX-2 in Barrett's esophagus and esophageal carcinoma: markers for esophageal cancer chemoprevention trials. *Proc Am Soc Clin Oncol* 2002: Abstract #2276.

221. Kang J, Kim E, Shin H, et al. The overexpression of cyclooxygenase-2 (COX-2) and antitumor effect of selective COX-2 inhibitor (SC-236) in gastric cancer. *Proc Am Soc Clin Oncol* 2000; Abstract #1279.

222. Half E, Tang XM, Gwyn K, et al. Cyclooxygenase-2 expression in human breast cancers and adjacent ductal carcinoma in situ. *Cancer Res* 2002;62:1676–1681.

223. Dannenberg AJ, Altorki NK, Boyle JO, et al. Cyclo-oxygenase 2: a pharmacological target for the prevention of cancer. *Lancet Oncol* 2001;2:544–551.

224. Amano H, Hayashi I, Yoshida S, et al. Cyclooxygenase-2 and adenylate cyclase/protein kinase A signaling pathway enhances angiogenesis through induction of vascular endothelial growth factor in rat sponge implants. *Hum Cell* 2002;15:13–24.

225. Leahy KM, Ornberg RL, Wang Y, et al. Cyclooxygenase-2 inhibition by celecoxib reduces proliferation and induces apoptosis in angiogenic endothelial cells in vivo. *Cancer Res* 2002;62:625–631.

226. Fosslien E. Review: molecular pathology of cyclooxygenase-2 in cancer-induced angiogenesis. *Ann Clin Lab Sci* 2001;31:325–348.

227. Dormand O, Bezzi M, Mariotti A, et al. Prostaglandin E2 promotes integrin avb3-dependent endothelial cell adhesion, Rac activation and spreading through cAMP/PKA-dependent signaling. *J Biol Chem* 2002;277:4S838–4S846.

228. Oshima M, Dinchuk JE, Kargman SL, et al. Suppression of intestinal polyposis in Apc 716 knockout mice by inhibition of cyclooxygenase-2 (COX-2). *Cell* 1996;87:803–809.

229. Steinbach G, Lynch PM, Phillips RK, et al. The effect of celecoxib, a cyclooxygenase-2 inhibitor, in familial adenomatous polyposis. *N Engl J Med* 2000;342:1946–1952.

230. Fisher B, Costantino JP, Wickerham DL, et al. Tamoxifen for prevention of breast cancer: Report of the National Surgical Adjuvant Breast and Bowel Project P-1 study. *J Natl Cancer Inst* 1998;90:1371–1388.

231. Hershman D, Sundararajan V, Jacobson JS, et al. Outcomes of tamoxifen chemoprevention for breast cancer in very high-risk women: a cost effectiveness analysis. *J Clin Oncol* 2002;20:9–16.

232. Gelmann EP. Tamoxifen induction of apoptosis in estrogen receptor-negative cancers: new tricks for an old dog? *J Natl Cancer Inst* 1996;88:224–226.

233. McNamara DA, Harmey J, Wang JH, et al. Tamoxifen inhibits endothelial cell proliferation and attenuates VEGF-mediated angiogenesis and migration in vivo. *Eur J Surg Oncol* 2001;27:714–718.

234. Blackwell KL, Haroon ZA, Shan S, et al. Tamoxifen inhibits angiogenesis in estrogen receptor-negative animal models. *Clin Cancer Res* 2000;6(11):4359–4364.

235. Gagliardi A, Collins DC. Inhibition of angiogenesis by antiestrogens. *Cancer Res* 1993;53(3):533–535.

236. Haran EF, Maretzek AF, Goldberg I, et al. Tamoxifen enhances cell death in implanted MCF7 breast cancer by inhibiting endothelium growth. *Cancer Res* 1994;54:5511–5514.

237. Gagliardi AR, Hennig B, Collins DC. Antiestrogens inhibit endothelial cell growth stimulated by angiogenic growth factors. *Anticancer Res* 1996;16:1101–1106.

238. Buteau-Lozano H, Ancelin M, Lardeux B, et al. Transcriptional regulation of vascular endothelial growth factor by estradiol and tamoxifen in breast cancer cells: a

complex interplay between estrogen receptors alpha and beta. *Cancer Res* 2002;62:4977–4984.

239. Thamrongwittawatpong L, Sirivatanauksorn Y, Batten JJ, et al. The effect of N(G)-monomethyl-L-arginine and tamoxifen on nitric oxide production in breast cancer cells stimulated by estrogen and progesterone. *Eur J Surg* 2001;167:484–489.

240. Gallo O, Masini E, Morbidelli L, et al. Role of nitric oxide in angiogenesis and tumor progression in head and neck cancer. *J Natl Cancer Inst* 1998;90(8):587–596.

241. Garcia-Cardena G, Folkman J. Is there a role for nitric oxide in tumor angiogenesis? *J Natl Cancer Inst* 1998;90:560–561.

242. Hyder SM, Stancel GM, Chiappetta C, et al. Uterine expression of vascular endothelial growth factor is increased by estradiol and tamoxifen. *Cancer Res* 1996;56:3954–3960.

243. Hague S, Manek S, Oehler MK, et al. Tamoxifen induction of angiogenic factor expression in endometrium. *Br J Cancer* 2002;86:761–767.

244. Neis KJ, Brandner P, Schlenker M. Tamoxifen-induced hyperplasia of the endometrium. *Contrib Gynecol Obstet* 2000;20:60–68.

245. Maugeri G, Nardo LG, Campione C, et al. Endometrial lesions after tamoxifen therapy in breast cancer women. *Breast J* 2001;7:240–244.

246. Deligdisch L, Kalir T, Cohen CJ, et al. Endometrial histopathology in 700 patients treated with tamoxifen for breast cancer. *Gynecol Oncol* 2000;78:181–186.

247. Gail MH, Costantino JP, Bryant J, et al. Weighing the risks and benefits of tamoxifen treatment for preventing breast cancer. *J Natl Cancer Inst* 1999;91:1829–1846.

248. Yang CS, Wang Z-Y. Tea and cancer. *J Natl Cancer Inst* 1993;85:1038–1049.

249. Wang ZY, Wang LD, Lee MJ, et al. Inhibition of *N*-nitrosomethylbenzylamine-induced esophageal tumorigenesis in rats by green and black tea. *Carcinogenesis* 1995;16:2143–2148.

250. Yang G, Wang ZY, Kim S, et al. Characterization of early pulmonary hyperproliferation and tumor progression and their inhibition by black tea in a 4-(methylnitrosamino)-1-(3-pyridyl)-1-butanone-induced lung tumorigenesis model with A/J mice. *Cancer Res* 1997;57:1889–1894.

251. Wang ZY, Cheng SI, Zhou ZC, et al. Antimutagenic activity of green tea polyphenols. *Mutat Res* 1989;223:273–285.

252. Wang ZY, Hong JY, Huang MT, et al. Inhibition of *N*-nitrosodiethylamine- and 4-(methylnitrosoamino)-1-(3-pyridyl)-1-butanone-induced tumorigenesis in A/J mice by green tea and black tea. *Cancer Res* 1992;52:1943–1947.

253. Sazuka M, Murakami S, Isemura M, et al. Inhibitory effects of green tea infusion on in vitro invasion and in vivo metastasis of mouse lung carcinoma cells. *Cancer Lett* 1995;98:27–31.

254. Taniguchi S, Fujiki H, Kobayashi K, et al. Effect of (-)-epigallocatechin gallate, the main constituent of green tea, on lung metastasis with mouse B16 melanoma cell lines. *Cancer Lett* 1992;65:51–54.

255. Cao Y, Cao R. Angiogenesis inhibited by drinking green tea. *Nature* 1999;398:381.

256. Garbisa S, Biggin S, Cavallarin N, et al. Tumor invasion: molecular shears blunted by green tea. *Nat Med* 1999;5:1216.

257. Garbisa S, Sartor L, Biggin S, et al. Tumor gelatinases and invasion inhibited by the green tea flavanol epigallocatechin-3-gallate. *Cancer* 2001;91:822–832.

258. Lu YP, Lou YR, Xie JG, et al. Topical applications of caffeine or (-)-epigallocatechin gallate (EGCG) inhibit carcinogenesis and selectively increase apoptosis in UVB-induced skin tmors in mice. *Proc Natl Acad Sci USA* 2002;99:12,455–12,460.

259. Lamartiniere CA, Cotroneo MS, Fritz WA, et al. Genistein chemoprevention: timing and mechanisms of action in murine mammary and prostate. *J Nutr* 2002;132:552S–558S.

260. Cotroneo MS, Wang J, Fritz WA, et al. Genistein action in the prepubertal mammary gland in a chemoprevention model. *Carcinogenesis* 2002;23:1467–1474.

261. Constantinou AI, Lantvit D, Hawthorne M, et al. Chemopreventive effects of soy protein and purified soy isoflavones on DMBA-induced mammary tumors in female Sprague-Dawley rats. *Nutr Cancer* 2001;41:75–81.

262. Brown A, Jolly P, Wei H. Genistein modulates neuroblastoma cell proliferation and differentiation through induction of apoptosis and regulation of tyrosine kinase activity and N-myc expression. *Carcinogenesis* 1998;19:991–997.

263. Davis JN, Kucuk O, Sarkar FH. Genistein inhibits NF-kappa B activation in prostate cancer cells. *Nutr Cancer* 1999;35:167–174.

264. Dixon RA, Ferreira D. Genistein. *Phytochemistry* 2002;60:205–211.

265. Adlercreutz H, Honjo H, Higashi A, et al. Urinary excretion of lignans and isoflavanoid phytoestrogens in Japanese men and women consuming traditional Japanese diet. *Am J Clin Nutr* 1991;54:1093–1100.

266. Fotsis T, Pepper M, Adlercreutz H, et al. Genistein, a dietary-derived inhibitor of in vitro angiogenesis. *Proc Natl Acad Sci USA* 1993;90:2690–2694.

267. Fotsis T, Pepper M, Adlercreutz H, et al. Genistein, a dietary ingested isoflavanoid, inhibits cell proliferation and in vitro angiogenesis. *J Nutr* 1995;125:790S–797S.

268. Muir C, Waterhouse J, Mack T, et al. Cancer Incidence in Five Continents, Vol. 5. Lyon France: International Agency for Research on Cancer, 1987.

269. Severson RK, Nomura AMY, Grove JS, et al. A prospective study of demographics and prostate cancer among men of Japanese ancestry in Hawaii. *Cancer Res* 1989;49:1857–1860.

270. Akiyama T, Ishida J, Nakagawa S, et al. Genistein, a specific inhibitor of tyrosine-specific protein kinases. *J Biol Chem* 1987;262:5592–5595.

271. Guo D, Jia Q, Song HY, et al. Vascular endothelial growth factor promotes tyrosine phosphorylation of mediators of signal transduction that contain SH2 domains. Association with endothelial cell proliferation. *J Biol Chem* 1995;270:6729–6733.

272. Levy AP, Levy NS, Goldberg MA. Post-transcriptional regulation of vascular endothelial growth factor by hypoxia. *J Biol Chem* 1996;271:113–131.

273. Xia P, Aiello LP, Ishii H, et al. Characterization of vascular endothelial growth factor's effect on the activation of protein kinase C, its isoforms, and endothelial cell growth. *J Clin Investig* 1996;988:2018–2026.

274. Angiogenesis Foundation Clinical Trials Database, 2003. http:// www.clinicaltrials.gov

275. Perkins S, Verschoyle RD, Hill K, et al. Chemopreventive efficacy and pharmacokinetics of curcumin in the min/+ mouse, a model of familial adenomatous polyposis. *Cancer Epidemiol Biomark Prev* 2002;11:535–540.

276. Goel A, Boland CR, Chauhan DP. Specific inhibition of cyclooxygenase-2 (COX-2) expression by dietary curcumin in HT-29 human colon cancer cells. *Cancer Lett* 2001;172:111–118.

277. Dorai T, Cao YC, Dorai B, et al. Therapeutic potential of curcumin in human prostate cancer. III. Curcumin inhibits proliferation, induces apoptosis, and inhibits angiogenesis of LNCaP prostate cancer cells in vivo. *Prostate* 2001;47:293–303.

278. Gururaj A, Belakavadi M, Venkatesh D, et al. Molecular mechanisms of anti-angiogenic effect of curcumin. *Biochem Biophys Res Commun* 2002;297:934–942.

279. Shao ZM, Shen ZZ, Liu CH, et al. Curcumin exerts multiple suppressive effects on human breast carcinoma cells. *Int J Cancer* 2002;98:234–240.

280. Mohan R, Sivak J, Ashton P, et al. Curcuminoids inhibit the angiogenic response stimulated by fibroblast growth factor-2, including expression of matrix metalloproteinase gelatinase B. *J Biol Chem* 2000;275:10,405–10,412.

281. Shin EY, Kim SY, Kim EG. c-Jun N-terminal kinase is involved in motility of endothelial cells. *Exp Mol Med* 2001;33:276–283.

282. Thaloor D, Singh AK, Sidhu GS, et al. Inhibition of angiogenic differentiation of human umbilical vein endothelial cells by curcumin. *Cell Growth Differ* 1998;9:305–312.

283. Cheng AL, Hsu CH, Lin JK, et al. Phase I clinical trial of curcumin, a chemopreventive agent, in patients with high-risk or pre-malignant lesions. *Anticancer Res* 2001;21:2895–2900.

284. Jang M, Cai L, Udeani GO, et al. Cancer chemopreventive activity of resveratrol, a natural product derived from grapes. *Science* 1997;275:218–220.

285. Kimura Y, Okuda H. Resveratrol isolated from *Polygonum cuspidatum* root prevents tumor growth and metastasis to lung and tumor-induced neovascularization in Lewis lung carcinoma-bearing mice. *J Nutr* 2001;13:1844–1849.

286. Brakenhielm E, Cao R, Cao Y. Suppression of angiogenesis, tumor growth, and wound healing by resveratrol, a natural compound in red wine and grapes. *FASEB J* 2001;10:1798–1800.

287. Bertelli AA, Baccalini R, Battaglia E, et al. Resveratrol inhibits TNF alpha-induced endothelial cell activation. *Therapie* 2001;56:613–616.

288. Igura K, Ohta T, Kuroda Y, et al. Resveratrol and quercetin inhibit angiogenesis in vitro. *Cancer Lett* 2001;171:11–16.

289. Banerjee S, Bueso-Ramos C, Aggarwal BB. Suppression of 7,12-dimethylbez(a)anthracene-induced mammary carcinogenesis in rats by resveratrol: role of nuclear factor-kappaB, cyclooxygenase 2, and matrix metalloprotease 9. *Cancer Res* 2002;62:4945–4954.

290. Masso-Welch PA, Zangani D, Ip C, et al. Inhibition of angiogenesis by the chemopreventive agents conjugated linoleic acid. *Cancer Res* 2002;62:4383–4389.

291. Mehta RG, Liu J, Constantinou A, et al. Cancer chemopreventive activity of brassinin, a phytoalexin from cabbage. *Carcinogenesis* 1995;16:399–404.

292. Garg A, Garg S, Zaneveld LJ, et al. Chemistry and pharmacology of the citrus bioflavanoid herperidin. *Phytother Res* 2001;15:655–669.

293. So FV, Guthrie N, Chambers AF, et al. Inhibition of human breast cancer cell proliferation and delay of mammary tumorigenesis by flavanoids and citrus juices. *Nutr Cancer* 1996;26:167–181.

294. Akagi K, Hirose M, Hoshiya T, et al. Modulating effects of ellagic acid, vanillin and quercetin in a rat medium term multi-organ carcinogenesis model. *Cancer Lett* 1995;94:113–121.

295. Kohno H, Tanaka T, Kawabata K, et al. Silymarin, a naturally occurring polyphenolic antioxidant flavanoid, inhibits azoxymethane-induced colon carcinogenesis in male F344 rats. *Int J Cancer* 2002;101:461–468.

296. Kwon KB, Yoo SJ, Ryu DG, et al. Induction of apoptosis by allul disulfide through activation of caspase-3 in human leukemia HL-60 cells. *Biochem Pharmacol* 2002;63:41–47.

297. Panigrahy D, Singer S, Shen LQ, et al. PPARγ ligands inhibit primary tumor growth and metastasis by inhibiting angiogenesis. *J Clin Investig* 2002;110:923–932.

298. Weis M, Heeschen C, Glassford AJ, et al. Statins have biphasic effects on angiogenesis. *Circulation* 2002;105:739–745.

299. Niethammer AG, Xiang R, Becker JC, et al. A DNA vaccine against VEGF receptor 2 prevents effective angiogenesis and inhibits tumor growth. *Nat Med* 2002;8(12):1369–1375.

41 Proteasome Inhibitors in Cancer Therapy

Julian Adams, PhD

Contents

1. INTRODUCTION

The proteasome is a multicatalytic enzyme complex responsible for the majority of protein degradation in cells. Traditionally believed to be a mere recycler of damaged or misfolded proteins, the proteasome's importance in modulating cell cycle and survival pathways is now recognized. By degrading regulatory proteins, the proteasome helps to remove signals that promote transcription, cell growth, angiogenesis, and cell adhesion. Preclinical studies have found that agents that inhibit the proteasome's activity will promote cell cycle arrest and induce apoptosis in tumor cells, thus establishing the proteasome as a promising potential target for anticancer therapy *(1)*. This evidence has led to the examination of these compounds for the treatment of human cancer, and one such proteasome inhibitor, bortezomib (VELCADE™, formerly PS-341, LDP-341, MLN341), has entered human clinical trials.

2. THE PROTEASOME

The proteasome is present in the cytoplasm and nucleus of all eukaryotic cells. This key regulatory enzyme is responsible for up to 80% of protein degradation that occurs in the cell. The proteasome comprises a 20S core catalytic complex and one or two 19S regulatory subunits (*see* Fig.1), which cap either end of the 20S subunit and recognize ubiquitinated proteins.

In order for a protein to be recognized by the proteasome a small peptide known as ubiquitin must first be attached to the target protein. This process is carried out by a family of enzymes (E1, E2, and E3) that activate free ubiquitin and carry it to the target protein. E1 activates and transfers ubiquitin to the carrier protein E2, which presents ubiquitin to E3. E3 binds to the target protein and interacts with E2 to covalently attach ubiquitin to the target protein. This sequence is repeated several times, resulting in a polyubiquitin chain that flags the protein for destruction by the proteasome *(2,3)*.

To date, only one E1 enzyme has been identified, but about 20 known E2 enzymes exist in yeast and humans, and hundreds of E3 ligases have been identified *(3)*. This hierarchical structure, with a small number of E2s and a larger number of substrate-specific E3s, allows the cell to regulate coordinated protein degradation with the high degree of precision necessary to ensure that the proteins are degraded at the appropriate time. This pathway by which proteins are ubiquitinated and degraded by the proteasome is known as the ubiquitin-proteasome pathway, and is critical to the cell cycle as well as to inflammatory response and antigen presentation. The ubiquitin-proteasome pathway is only beginning to be elucidated, and may provide additional targets for drug development, particularly upstream of the proteasome.

Once recognized by the 19S cap, the targeted protein is fed into the barrel-shaped catalytic core. The 20S core is composed of two β rings sandwiched between two α

From: Cancer Chemoprevention, Volume 1: Promising Cancer Chemoprevention Agents
Edited by: G. J. Kelloff, E. T. Hawk, and C. C. Sigman © Humana Press Inc., Totowa, NJ

20S Proteasome   **26S Proteasome**

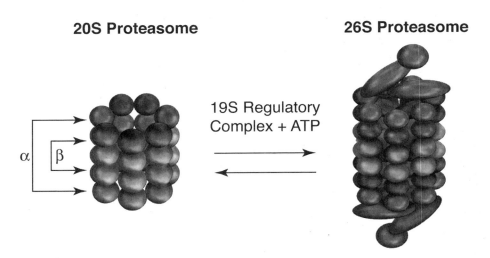

19S Regulatory
Complex + ATP

Fig. 1. The 26S proteasome. **(A)** The 26S proteasome is a multisubunit complex comprised of a proteolytically active core unit sandwiched between two regulatory units.

rings and has a total of six active sites, three per β ring. Inside the catalytic core, proteins are exposed to the proteolytic activities of the proteasome and are cleaved to generate peptides 3–22 residues in length *(4,5)*. The proteasome is unique among proteases because it has three distinct proteolytic activities, which can break bonds on the carboxyl side of basic, hydrophobic, and acidic amino acid residues (named trypsin-like, chymotrypsin-like, and post-acidic or peptidyl-glutamyl peptide hydrolyzing (PGPH), respectively) *(6,7)*. The 20S subunit is a member of the group of *N*-terminal hydrolases that use the side chains of *N*-terminal serines, threonines, or cysteines to break peptide bonds *(8)*. Unlike the other members of this class, the proteasome has threonines at each of its active sites.

A wide array of proteins are targets of the proteasome (*see* Table 1; *7*), including tumor suppressors such as p53 *(9)*, cell-cycle regulators such as p27 and p21 *(10)*, transcription factors *(11)*, or their inhibitors such as IκB *(12)* and Id *(13)*, and anti-apoptosis proteins such as Bcl-2 *(14)*. Because of its far-reaching impact, the proteasome is fundamental to the cell's metabolic processes, and interference with its function results in death of cells and organisms.

3. PROTEASOME INHIBITORS

A number of compounds, both natural and synthetic, inhibit proteasomal function. Among the earliest proteasome inhibitors were the peptide aldehydes (e.g., ALLN, MG-132, PSI), which are structurally similar to a number of proteasome substrates and reversibly bind to the proteasome, inhibiting its chymotrypsin-like

activity. They have slow on-off binding rates and poor metabolic stability. They are also nonspecific, and inhibit cysteine proteases such as cathepsin B and the calpains. This class of proteasome inhibitors is typically used only for basic research, and has not been evaluated for clinical therapeutic use.

Lactacystin—a fungal product—and the β-lactone that results from its hydrolysis, along with other derivative molecules, constitute another class of proteasome inhibitors. Lactacystin and its β-lactone inhibit all three proteolytic activities of the proteasome in an irreversible fashion *(15)*. Like the peptide aldehydes, these compounds are nonspecific and unstable; however, other β-lactone-related molecules have been engineered (e.g., PS-519), and have been shown to be more potent in inhibiting chymotrypsin-like activity of the proteasome in preclinical disease models *(16,17)*. Peptide epoxyketones, which include epoxomicin and eponemycin among others, make up another class of inhibitors discovered from products of fungal organisms *(18,19)*. These agents are extremely selective and potent inhibitors of the proteasome *(18,20)*. More in vitro and in vivo research is needed to evaluate their activity and potential toxicities. Peptide boronate proteasome inhibitors, which are similar in structure to peptide aldehydes with a boronic acid substituted for the terminal aldehyde moiety, block chymotrypsin-like activity of the proteasome in a reversible manner, but dissociate more slowly than their aldehyde analogs *(7)*; they are both more potent and more selective for the proteasome than are peptide aldehydes *(21)*.

Table 1
Proteasome Substrates

Protein Name	Protein Function	Reference
Cell Division		
Topoisomerase II	DNA "unwinding"	*42*
Topoisomerase I	DNA "unwinding"	*43*
Pro- and Anti-Apoptosis Factors		
XIAP	Inhibitor of apoptosis	*44*
Bax	Pro-apoptosis factor	*14*
Bcl-2	Inhibitor of apoptosis	*45*
Survivin	Inhibitor of apoptosis	*38*
Securin	Anaphase-promoting factor	*46*
Cell-Cycle Progression		
Cyclin E	Kinase activator	*10*
p27 KIP1	Cyclin-dependent kinase inhibitor	*47*
p21 CIP1/WAF1	Cyclin-dependent kinase inhibitor	*48*
Transcriptional Regulation		
Androgen receptor	Nuclear steroid receptor transcription factor	*49*
Fos/Jun	Transcription factor; early immediate gene	*11*
Id	Transcription-factor inhibitor	*13*
IκB-α	Inhibitor of NF-κB	*12*
Tumor Suppression		
p53	Multiple functions	*9*
Rb	Multiple functions	*50*

The most widely studied of the peptide boronate class is bortezomib, a dipeptidyl boronic acid that is a selective, water-soluble, and potent competitive inhibitor of the proteasome's chymotrypsin-like active site (*see* Fig.2). A number of qualities make bortezomib especially suitable for clinical use. It binds to its target site with high affinity ($K_i = 0.6$ nM), and is a reversible inhibitor of proteasome inhibition *(21)*. Its compact size and low molecular wt allow for ease of synthesis *(21)*. Furthermore, when the National Cancer Institute (NCI) performed an in vitro cytotoxicity assay in 60 cell lines derived from human tumors *(1)*, bortezomib was found to have potent anticancer activity, achieving 50% inhibition of cancer cell growth at 7 nM.

4. PRECLINICAL RATIONALE FOR PROTEASOME INHIBITION IN CANCER THERAPY

The first in vivo study involving a proteasome inhibitor (Z-LLF-CHO) in a xenograft model was reported in 1998 by Orlowski and colleagues *(22)*. Severe combined immunodeficiency (SCID) mice were implanted with human Burkitt's lymphoma tumors and then given single doses of Z-LLF-CHO (a peptide aldehyde) or Z-LLF-OH (the equivalent peptide alcohol, which does not inhibit the proteasome or induce apoptosis). Mice treated with the aldehyde experienced a delay in tumor growth of 42% compared with mice treated with the alcohol. This study established that proteasome inhibition had potential in vivo antitumor activity.

As stated here, Bortezomib's potential was first suggested by the results of NCI's cancer cell line screen showing that bortezomib had potent anticancer activity in vitro *(1)* and that it penetrated cancer cells, reduced the degree of protein proteolysis, and inhibited cell growth. Importantly, a comparison of the cytotoxic profile of bortezomib with historical results of 60,000 other compounds found it to be unique, with little similarity to standard chemotherapeutic drugs or other investigational agents *(1)*.

The in vitro and in vivo activity of bortezomib has been evaluated by numerous investigators. As a single agent, bortezomib clearly resulted in apoptosis in myeloma cells *(23)* as well as pancreatic *(24,25)*, prostate *(1,26)*, ovarian *(26)*, and head and neck *(27)* cancer cells. The precise mechanisms by which proteasome inhibitors induce cell death have not yet been established. Although stabilization of p21, p27, and p53 are common responses to proteasome inhibition *(25,28,29)*, involvement of these regulatory proteins in apoptosis varies between cell types. Initiation of programmed cell death (PCD) is not necessarily mediated by any one protein, but rather by the ratio of anti-apoptotic to pro-apoptotic signals within a cell. Proteasome inhibition may therefore induce apoptosis, or increase sensitivity to apoptosis, by disturbing this balance.

In preclinical studies of solid tumors, bortezomib has shown additive activity when combined with other chemotherapeutic agents. When bortezomib was administered with irinotecan to mice bearing colon cancer (LoVo) xenografts, Cusack and colleagues showed that tumor growth inhibition was greater than

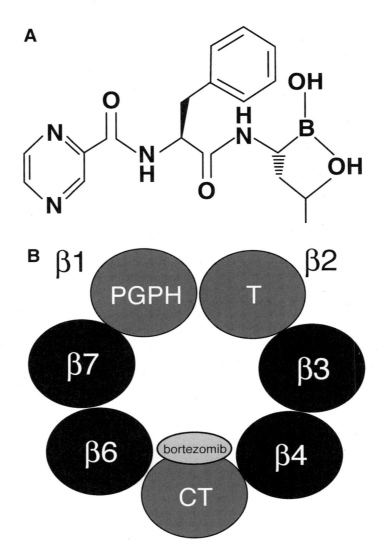

Fig. 2. Bortezomib: structure and binding. **(A)** The structure of the dipeptidyl boronic acid proteasome inhibitor bortezomib. **(B)** A cross-section of the core shows the orientation of the three active sites within a single β ring. Abbreviations: CT = chymotrypsin-like; PGPH = peptidyl-glutamyl peptide hydrolyzing; T = trypsin-like. Copyright Millennium Pharmaceuticals Inc., Cambridge, Massachusetts.

that of either agent administered alone *(30)*. The reason for this additive activity is not known, but an explanation may lie in the role of NFκB, a transcription factor that initiates prosurvival pathways. Irinotecan, like many other chemotherapeutic agents and radiation, induces an NFκB stress response in cancer cells. Cusack and colleagues also noted that NFκB levels were dramatically reduced in LoVo cancer cells when bortezomib was given with SN38, the active metabolite of irinotecan in vivo. Although bortezomib induces apoptosis as a single agent, its effect on NFκB may provide an additional antitumor effect in tumors that constitutively express NFκB or have high-induced

expression of NFκB in response to chemotherapy, thus providing a rationale for the use of bortezomib in combination with other chemotherapeutic drugs. Other investigators have shown similar antitumor activity when bortezomib was combined with gemcitabine *(24)* or irinotecan *(25)* in pancreatic cancer models or given alone *(27)* in squamous cell carcinoma (head and neck cancer) models. In all three tumor types, investigators noted NFκB downregulation with bortezomib. In myeloma—a highly NFκB-dependent malignancy—single-agent activity of bortezomib against myeloma xenografts has been reported by LeBlanc and colleagues *(31)* and Steiner and colleagues *(32)*. In a preliminary

Table 2
Early Phase I Bortezomib Trials[a]

Testing Center	Schedule	Cycle Length	DLT	MTD
M.D. Anderson Cancer Center	1x /wk × 4	35 d	2.0 mg/m^2	1.8 mg/m^2
Memorial Sloan-Kettering Cancer Center	2x /wk × 2	21 d	1.56 mg/m^2	1.3 mg/m^2
University of North Carolina/MSKCC	2x /wk × 4	42 d	1.38 mg/m^2	1.04 mg/m^2

[a]Sponsored by Millennium Pharmaceuticals, Inc.

report from Steiner and colleagues, in vivo activity was noted even against xenografts derived from myeloma cell lines that were first cultured in vitro to be resistant to bortezomib. Other investigators have shown that bortezomib was active in vitro against doxorubicin-, melphalan-, and dexamethasone-resistant myeloma cells *(33)*, and was able to bypass Bcl-2-mediated resistance *(34)*.

5. DIFFERENTIAL SENSITIVITY OF TUMOR CELLS AND NORMAL CELLS TO BORTEZOMIB

Preclinical studies have shown that proteasome inhibitors in general and bortezomib in particular may be more active against cancer cells than normal cells. Differential sensitivity has been observed in models using various proteasome inhibitors (bortezomib, lactacystin, LLnV, PSI, Z-LLF-CHO) and tumor types such as myeloma *(23,31,35)*, leukemia *(35–37)* lymphoma *(22)*, and squamous cell carcinoma *(38)*. Recently, LeBlanc and colleagues quantitated the degree of proteasome inhibition with bortezomib in myeloma xenografts vs that in blood, liver, and spleen samples. Despite significant antitumor activity with minimal toxicity to animals, proteasome inhibition was higher in normal tissue than in tumor tissue, suggesting that normal cells have an intrinsic resistance to proteasome inhibition and cancer cells do not *(39)*.

6. CLINICAL STUDIES OF BORTEZOMIB

6.1. Phase I Study in Advanced Hematologic Malignancies

Patients with histologically confirmed refractory hematologic malignancies received intravenous bortezomib on an intensive dosing schedule of twice weekly for 4 wk, followed by 1 wk of rest, in a Phase I multicenter trial. A total of 27 patients were enrolled in this study; they received 293 doses of bortezomib and 24 complete cycles of therapy *(40)*. The maximum

tolerated dose (MTD) in this trial was determined to be 1.04 mg/m^2, and dose-limiting toxicities (DLTs) were thrombocytopenia, hyponatremia, hypokalemia, fatigue, and malaise. Serious adverse events (AE), observed in three of 10 patients during Cycle 2, included postural hypotension, hypersensitivity reaction, and grade 4 transaminitis. Among the common AEs (occurring in at least 10% of patients) were the cytopenias thrombocytopenia (74%), anemia and leukopenia (48%), and neutropenia (37%). Fatigue and nausea were also frequently reported (59% and 52% of patients, respectively).

At least one cycle of therapy was completed by nine patients with heavily pretreated plasma cell dyscrasias. One patient had a complete response to treatment (tumor response [RECIST] criteria); the other eight patients had a reduction in paraprotein levels and/or marrow plasmacytosis. In addition, one patient with mantle cell lymphoma and another with follicular lymphoma had shrinkage of nodal disease.

6.2. Phase I Study in Advanced Solid Tumors

In a Phase I trial in patients with advanced solid tumors *(41)*, intravenous doses of bortezomib were administered twice weekly for 2 wk, followed by 1 wk of rest. A total of 43 heavily pretreated patients received 89 treatment cycles, with doses ranging from 0.13–1.56 mg/m^2.

The MTD with this dosing regimen was found to be 1.3–1.56 mg/m^2, with DLTs of grade 3 diarrhea and grade 3 sensory neuropathy. Diarrhea occurred in two of 12 patients at the 1.56 mg/m^2 dose level, and was treatable with loperamide. Sensory neuropathy also occurred in two of 12 patients at the 1.56 mg/m^2 dose level; however, both patients had pre-existing neuropathy from prior therapies that included taxanes. No hematologic DLTs were reported, although higher dose levels were correlated with the occurrence of thrombocytopenia and neutropenia. All seven episodes of thrombocytopenia occurred in patients who received 1.56 mg/m^2 bortezomib: grade 1 thrombocytopenia occurred in three patients, grade 2 occurred in two patients, and grade 3 occurred in two patients; no patient required transfusion or experienced bleeding. There were three episodes of neutropenia overall: one patient with metastatic prostate cancer receiving 0.9 mg/m^2 bortezomib experienced grade 3 neutropenia, one patient receiving 1.08 mg/m^2 bortezomib experienced grade 2 febrile neutropenia (which resolved in 24 h), and one patient receiving 1.56 mg/m^2 bortezomib experienced grade 3 neutropenia.

Thus, bortezomib is seen to have predictable toxicities on a schedule of twice-weekly doses for 2 wk, and a pharmacodynamic assay revealed a dose-related inhibition of 20S proteasome activity at levels associated with preclinical antitumor activity. Furthermore, one patient with non-small-cell lung cancer experienced a partial response.

6.3. Efficacy Trials of Bortezomib in Multiple Myeloma

The hematologic and solid tumor Phase I studies described here, and an unpublished Phase I study primarily in patients with advanced hormone-refractory prostate cancer, assessed different dose intensities: twice-weekly for 2 wk, twice weekly for 4 wk, and once-weekly for 4 wk. Based on an analysis of these studies, a twice-weekly schedule with 1 wk of rest seemed to strike the best balance between potential antitumor efficacy and safety. A twice-weekly schedule at 1.3 mg/m^2 was thus used in a Phase II trial of multiple myeloma in 202 patients with heavily pretreated relapsed and refractory disease. Preliminary data from this trial showed antitumor activity and manageable toxicities (8). An international Phase III trial (APEX) in patients with relapsed or refractory myeloma who have received 1–3 prior therapies is now enrolling patients.

7. FUTURE DIRECTIONS

Proteasome inhibitors have been used for basic research with increased frequency in the last few years, and topics of study have included cell biology and the mechanisms of cell growth and death in the treatment of solid and hematologic cancers and stroke. However, because they have become available only recently, reports are limited on the mechanisms by which proteasome inhibitors induce apoptosis and on their potential therapeutic activities. Bortezomib, PS-519, and the epoxyketones such as YU-101, epoxomicin, and TMC-95 are the most clinically promising proteasome inhibitors currently in commercial development. Despite their differing structural characteristics and origins, these agents share a number of qualities: nanomolar active-site binding capabilities, low mol wts, and favorable solubility characteristics with sufficient hydrophobicity to allow access into cells.

Currently, NCI is sponsoring more than 20 trials of bortezomib as monotherapy and in combination with standard chemotherapies in solid and hematologic tumors, and development of other agents for human therapy continues. The results of these ongoing studies will help to clarify the potential role of bortezomib in the management of cancer. The role of proteasome inhibition in the prevention and treatment of early disease has not yet been defined. The mechanism of proteasome inhibition holds promise for maintaining normal cellular regulating functions, because cancer (abnormal) cells have increased sensitivity to proteasome inhibition compared with normal cells. However, the drugs developed to date, particulary bortezomib, are not ideal for administration to subjects without disease (e.g., patients with monoclonal gammopathies of undetermined significance, the precursor to multiple myeloma), since they require intravenvous injection and have toxicities that could threaten quality of life. Therefore, further developmental efforts are needed.

REFERENCES

1. Adams J, Palombella VJ, Sausville EA, et al. Proteasome inhibitors: a novel class of potent and effective antitumor agents. *Cancer Res* 1999;59:2615–2622.
2. Wilkinson KD. Ubiquitin-dependent signaling: the role of ubiquitination in the response of cells to their environment. *J Nutr* 1999;129:1933–1936.
3. Pickart CM. Mechanisms underlying ubiquitination. *Annu Rev Biochem* 2001;70:503–533.
4. Wilkinson KD. Ubiquitination and deubiquitination: targeting of proteins for degradation by the proteasome. *Semin Cell Dev Biol* 2000;11:141–148.
5. Larsen CN, Price JS, Wilkinson KD. Substrate binding and catalysis by ubiquitin C-terminal hydrolases: identification of two active site residues. *Biochemistry* 1996;35:6735–6744.
6. Lupas A, Koster AJ, Baumeister W. Structural features of 26S and 20S proteasomes. *Enzyme Protein* 1993;47:252–273.
7. Kisselev AF, Goldberg AL. Proteasome inhibitors: from research tools to drug candidates. *Chem Biol* 2001;8:739–758.
8. Richardson PG, Barlogie B, Berenson J, et al. Phase II study of the proteasome inhibitor PS-341 in multiple myeloma patients (pts) with relapsed/refractory disease: results from cohort 1 analysis. *Proc Annu Meet Am Soc Clin Oncol* 2002;21:11a.

9. Maki CG, Huibregtse JM, Howley PM. In vivo ubiquitination and proteasome-mediated degradation of p53(1). *Cancer Res* 1996;56:2649–2654.

10. Clurman BE, Sheaff RJ, Thress K, et al. Turnover of cyclin E by the ubiquitin-proteasome pathway is regulated by cdk2 binding and cyclin phosphorylation. *Genes Dev* 1996;10:1979–1990.

11. Nesbit CE, Tersak JM, Prochownik EV. MYC oncogenes and human neoplastic disease. *Oncogene* 1999;18:3004–3016.

12. Palombella VJ, Rando OJ, Goldberg AL, Maniatis T. The ubiquitin-proteasome pathway is required for processing the NF-kappa B1 precursor protein and the activation of NF-kappa B. *Cell* 1994;78:773–785.

13. Bounpheng MA, Dimas JJ, Dodds SG, Christy BA. Degradation of Id proteins by the ubiquitin-proteasome pathway. *FASEB J* 1999;13:2257–2264.

14. Li B, Dou QP. Bax degradation by the ubiquitin/proteasome-dependent pathway: involvement in tumor survival and progression. *Proc Natl Acad Sci USA* 2000;97:3850–3855.

15. Dick LR, Cruikshank AA, Grenier L, et al. Mechanistic studies on the inactivation of the proteasome by lactacystin: a central role for clasto-lactacystin beta-lactone. *J Biol Chem* 1996;271:7273–7276.

16. Elliott PJ, Pien CS, McCormack TA, et al. Proteasome inhibition: a novel mechanism to combat asthma. *J Allergy Clin Immunol* 1999;104:294–300.

17. Campbell B, Adams J, Shin YK, Lefer AM. Cardioprotective effects of a novel proteasome inhibitor following ischemia and reperfusion in the isolated perfused rat heart. *J Mol Cell Cardiol* 1999;31:467–476.

18. Meng L, Mohan R, Kwok BH, et al. Epoxomicin, a potent and selective proteasome inhibitor, exhibits in vivo antiinflammatory activity. *Proc Natl Acad Sci USA* 1999;96:10,403–10,408.

19. Meng L, Kwok BH, Sin N, Crews CM. Eponemycin exerts its antitumor effect through the inhibition of proteasome function. *Cancer Res* 1999;59:2798–2801.

20. Myung J, Kim KB, Crews CM. The ubiquitin-proteasome pathway and proteasome inhibitors. *Med Res Rev* 2001;21:245–273.

21. Adams J, Behnke M, Chen S, et al. Potent and selective inhibitors of the proteasome: dipeptidyl boronic acids. *Bioorg Med Chem Lett* 1998;8:333–338.

22. Orlowski RZ, Eswara JR, Lafond-Walker A, et al. Tumor growth inhibition induced in a murine model of human Burkitt's lymphoma by a proteasome inhibitor. *Cancer Res* 1998;58:4342–4348.

23. Hideshima T, Richardson P, Chauhan D, et al. The proteasome inhibitor PS-341 inhibits growth, induces apoptosis, and overcomes drug resistance in human multiple myeloma cells. *Cancer Res* 2001;61:3071–3076.

24. Bold RJ, Virudachalam S, McConkey DJ. Chemosensitization of pancreatic cancer by inhibition of the 26S proteasome. *J Surg Res* 2001;100:11–17.

25. Shah SA, Potter MW, McDade TP, et al. 26S proteasome inhibition induces apoptosis and limits growth of human pancreatic cancer. *J Cell Biochem* 2001;82:110–122.

26. Frankel A, Man S, Elliott P, et al. Lack of multicellular drug resistance observed in human ovarian and prostate carcinoma treated with the proteasome inhibitor PS-341. *Clin Cancer Res* 2000;6:3719–3728.

27. Sunwoo JB, Chen Z, Dong G, et al. Novel proteasome inhibitor PS-341 inhibits activation of nuclear factor-kappaB, cell survival, tumor growth, and angiogenesis in squamous cell carcinoma. *Clin Cancer Res* 2001;7:1419–1428.

28. Kurland JF, Meyn RE. Protease inhibitors restore radiation-induced apoptosis to Bcl-2-expressing lymphoma cells. *Int J Cancer* 2001;96:327–333.

29. Fan XM, Wong BC, Wang WP, et al. Inhibition of proteasome function induced apoptosis in gastric cancer. *Int J Cancer* 2001;93:481–488.

30. Cusack JC Jr, Liu R, Houston M, et al. Enhanced chemosensitivity to CPT-11 with proteasome inhibitor PS-341: implications for systemic nuclear factor-κB inhibition. *Cancer Res* 2001;61:3535–3540.

31. LeBlanc R, Catley LP, Hideshima T, et al. Proteasome inhibitor PS-341 inhibits human myeloma cell growth in vivo and prolongs survival in a murine model. *Cancer Res* 2002;62:4996–5000.

32. Steiner P, Neumeier H, Lightcap ES, et al. Generation of PS-341-adapted human multiple myeloma cells as experimental tools for analysis of proteasome function in cancer. *Blood* 2001;98:310a.

33. Hideshima T, Chauhan D, Podar K, et al. Novel therapies targeting the myeloma cell and its bone marrow microenvironment. *Semin Oncol* 2001;28:607–612.

34. Feinman R, Aris VM, Vergano S, et al. Transcriptional gene expression profiles in drug-sensitive and Bcl-2-resistant myeloma cells in response to dexamethasone, arsenic trioxide, and PS-341. *Blood* 2001;98:368a.

35. Soligo D, Servida F, Delia D, et al. The apoptogenic response of human myeloid leukaemia cell lines and of normal and malignant haematopoietic progenitor cells to the proteasome inhibitor PSI. *Br J Haematol* 2001;113:126–135.

36. Masdehors P, Merle-Beral H, Magdelenat H, Delic J. Ubiquitin-proteasome system and increased sensitivity of B-CLL lymphocytes to apoptotic death activation. *Leuk Lymphoma* 2000;38:499–504.

37. Delic J, Masdehors P, Omura S, et al. The proteasome inhibitor lactacystin induces apoptosis and sensitizes chemo- and radioresistant human chronic lymphocytic leukaemia lymphocytes to TNF-alpha-initiated apoptosis. *Br J Cancer* 1998;77:1103–1107.

38. Kudo Y, Takata T, Ogawa I, et al. p27Kip1 accumulation by inhibition of proteasome function induces apoptosis in oral squamous cell carcinoma cells. *Clin Cancer Res* 2000;6:916–923.

39. Kumatori A, Tanaka K, Inamura N, et al. Abnormally high expression of proteasomes in human leukemic cells. *Proc Natl Acad Sci USA* 1990;87:7071–7075.

40. Orlowski RZ, Stinchcombe TE, Mitchell BS, et al. Phase I trial of the proteasome inhibitor PS-341 in patients with refractory hematologic malignancies. *J Clin Oncol* 2002;20:4420–4427.

41. Aghajanian C, Soignet S, Dizon DS, et al. A phase I trial of the novel proteasome inhibitor PS341 in advanced solid tumor malignancies. *Clin Cancer Res* 2002;8:2505–2511.

42. Mao Y, Desai SD, Ting CY, et al. 26 S proteasome-mediated degradation of topoisomerase II cleavable complexes. *J Biol Chem* 2001;276:40,652–40,658.

43. Desai SD, Liu LF, Vazquez-Abad D, D'Arpa P. Ubiquitin-dependent destruction of topoisomerase I is stimulated by the antitumor drug camptothecin. *J Biol Chem* 1997;272:24,159–24,164.

44. Yang Y, Fang S, Jensen JP, et al. Ubiquitin protein ligase activity of IAPs and their degradation in proteasomes in response to apoptotic stimuli. *Science* 2000;288:874–877.

45. Chadebech P, Brichese L, Baldin V, et al. Phosphorylation and proteasome-dependent degradation of Bcl-2 in mitotic-arrested cells after microtubule damage. *Biochem Biophys Res Commun* 1999;262:823–827.

46. Tatebe H, Yanagida M. Cut8, essential for anaphase, controls localization of 26S proteasome, facilitating destruction of cyclin and Cut2. *Curr Biol* 2000;10:1329–1338.

47. Pagano M, Tam SW, Theodoras AM, et al. Role of the ubiquitin-proteasome pathway in regulating abundance of the cyclin-dependent kinase inhibitor p27. *Science* 1995;269:682–685.

48. Cayrol C, Ducommun B. Interaction with cyclin-dependent kinases and PCNA modulates proteasome-dependent degradation of p21. *Oncogene* 1998;17:2437–2444.

49. Segnitz B, Gehring U. The function of steroid hormone receptors is inhibited by the hsp90-specific compound geldanamycin. *J Biol Chem* 1997;272:18,694–18,701.

50. Boyer SN, Wazer DE, Band V. E7 protein of human papilloma virus-16 induces degradation of retinoblastoma protein through the ubiquitin-proteasome pathway. *Cancer Res* 1996;56:4620–4624.

42 Modulation of DNA Methylation for the Treatment and Prevention of Cancer

David S. Schrump, MD

CONTENTS

INTRODUCTION
DNA METHYLATION
DNA METHYLATION AND CANCER
DNMTs
DNMT INHIBITORS IN CANCER THERAPY
CONCLUSIONS AND FUTURE DIRECTIONS
REFERENCES

1. INTRODUCTION

Alterations in chromatin structure represent early and critical events that perturb gene expression during multistep carcinogenesis *(1)*. The nucleosome—the basic structure of chromatin—is composed of 146 basepairs of DNA coiled around an octamer of core histones (H2A, H2B, H3, and H4); nucleosomes are separated by variable lengths of linker DNA bound to histone H1. In association with additional proteins, nucleosomes are assembled into higher order chromatin *(2)*. The modulation of histone proteins by acetylation, phosphorylation, or methylation influences the nature and specificity of DNA-histone interactions, thus influencing gene activity *(2–4)*. For example, deacetylation of core histone proteins by histone deacetylases (HDACs) increases DNA-histone interactions, resulting in chromatin compaction and repression of transcription, whereas acetylation of histones by histone acetyl transferases (HATs) diminishes DNA-histone binding, resulting in chromatin relaxation and enhanced gene expression *(5,6)*.

DNA methylation is a major epigenetic mechanism that regulates gene expression and chromatin structure in normal as well as malignant cells *(1,7,8)*. Recent studies have established that DNA methylation is mechanistically linked to histone acetylation *(5,9)*. In general, transcriptionally active regions of chromatin contain hypomethylated DNA sequences associated with acety-lated core histones, whereas transcriptionally silent regions contain hypermethylated DNA associated with deacetylated histone proteins *(10–12)*. DNA methylation promotes HDAC-mediated histone deacetylation and inactivation of chromatin *(1,13,14)*; conversely, acetylation of core histones within active chromatin facilitates DNA demethylation via DNA demethylases *(9)*. These highly dynamic processes are modulated by proto-oncogenes as well as tumor suppressor genes during normal cell cycle progression. For instance, Ras, Fos, and the promyelocytic leukemia-retinoic acid receptor (PML-RAR) fusion protein modulate DNA methyltransferase (DNMT) activity *(15–17)*. Ras also mediates the activation and localization of several HDACs *(18)*. Furthermore, Rb and its related pocket proteins p107 and p130 associate with DNA methyltransferase, and recruit HDAC 1 to repress E2F-mediated transcription of cyclin E *(19,20)*.

The emerging relationships between epigenetics, cell cycle regulation, and cancer *(21)* have prompted considerable research efforts directed toward evaluating agents that modulate chromatin structure for cancer therapy. This chapter focuses on the rationale for using DNA demethylating agents to treat and prevent cancer.

2. DNA METHYLATION

DNA methylation regulates gene expression during embryogenesis and differentiation, and is a principal

From: Cancer Chemoprevention, Volume 1: Promising Cancer Chemoprevention Agents
Edited by: G. J. Kelloff, E. T. Hawk, and C. C. Sigman © Humana Press Inc., Totowa, NJ

mechanism in mediating X chromosome inactivation and silencing of imprinted alleles (22,23). In mammalian cells, methylation of DNA occurs exclusively at the 5' position of cytosine (24). Approximately 4% of cytosines are methylated in the human genome (25,26). Cytosine methylation normally occurs in the context of CpG dinucleotides, many of which are clustered in CpG islands that constitute approx 1–2% of the genome (12,27). CpG islands are characterized by high G+C content (65%) and CG:GC ratios of one compared to bulk DNA that contains a G+C content of approx 40% and CG:GC ratios of approx 0.2 (28). The low CG:GC ratios in bulk DNA reflect a tendency for methylcytosine to be deaminated to thymine, which is repaired by thymine-DNA glycosylase much less effectively than the corresponding deamination of unmethylated cytosine to uracil, which is repaired by uracil-DNA glycosylase (29).

Nearly 50% of all genes contain CpG islands (30). Although most CpG islands occur in promoter and proximal coding regions, some are located solely within transcribed gene sequences. For instance, the human tumor-suppressor gene p16 contains a CpG island lying within the promoter that extends into the first exon; in contrast, the human APOE gene has a CpG island located only in the transcribed region (31). Many housekeeping genes contain CpG islands, but rarely are these islands downstream from transcriptional start sites (31). On the other hand, nearly 50% of genes with more limited expression contain downstream CpG islands (30). In general, genes with limited expression contain CpG islands that are shorter than those within housekeeping genes (32).

Methylation of CpG islands within promoter regions represses transcription; however, methylation of downstream CpG islands appears to have no inhibitory effect on normal gene expression in mammalian cells (7,31,33–35). Methylation of downstream CpG islands as well as CpG dinucleotides outside of CpG islands serves to inhibit the expression of parasitic DNA, including endogenous retroviruses, ALU sequences, L1 elements, and juxtacentromeric satellite sequences, thereby maintaining genomic stability (36–38).

DNA methylation represses gene expression through several different mechanisms. First, DNA methylation may directly inhibit binding of transcription factors to promoter regions (7,39). Methylated cytosines protrude into the major groove of DNA, directly inhibiting binding of AP2, ATS/CREB, c-myc, and SP1 to their respective regulatory elements

(40–42). DNA methylation may also alter gene expression via indirect inhibition of transcription-factor binding; methylated DNA facilitates recruitment of methylcytosine-binding proteins that associate with multi-protein complexes containing corepressors as well as histone deacetylases to render chromatin inactive (5,43). For instance, MeCP2, which can bind DNA sequences with a single methylated CpG site, recruits the sin3a complex containing seven proteins (including sin3a, MBD2, HDAC1, and HDAC2) to methylated DNA, rendering promoter sequences inaccessible to transcription factors (6,7,44). MeCP2 may also directly compete with transcription-factor binding to DNA via its repressor domain (45). Additional complexes including MeCP1, and MI-2 (NURD) are recruited to methylated DNA (7), establishing a direct mechanistic link between DNA methylation and histone acetylation. Recent observations that HDAC inhibitors can potentiate the induction of tumor-suppressor genes mediated by DNA demethylating agents (46) attest to the cooperation of DNA methylation and histone acetylation in regulating gene expression in cancer cells.

3. DNA METHYLATION AND CANCER

Aberrant DNA methylation patterns have been observed in numerous cancers as well as a variety of premalignant lesions, indicating that alterations in chromatin structure occur early during multistep carcinogenesis (1,47). In general, cancer cells exhibit global DNA demethylation with site-specific hypermethylation (31,48,49). Global DNA demethylation occurs passively during DNA replication; however, methylation patterns in normal cells are rapidly restored by specific DNA methyltransferases (47). Regional DNA demethylation occurring in the context of chromatin remodeling may be attributable to specific DNA demethylases such as 5-methylcytosine-DNA glycosylase (5-MCDG), which catalyze excision repair of methylated cytosines in the absence of DNA replication (50).

Although the mechanisms have not been fully defined, the effects of genome-wide demethylation have profound consequences during malignant transformation. Global demethylation enhances genomic instability, in part by enabling expression of parasitic DNA sequences (51). Furthermore, genome-wide demethylation facilitates expression of a variety of genes, including melanoma antigen-encoding gene (MAGE) and NY-ESO-1 tumor antigens, which are encoded on the X chromosome, and normally silenced

Table 1
Genes Hypermethylated in Cancer

Gene	Function	Gene	Function
APC	Signal transduction	MDR-1	Drug transport
Androgen receptor	Signal transduction	O-6MGMT	DNA repair
c-Abl	Signal transduction	p14/ARF	Cell cycle regulation
BRCA-1	DNA repair	p15INK4b	Cell cycle regulation
DAP-kinase	Apoptosis	p16INK4a	Cell cycle regulation
E-cadherin	Adhesion/metastasis	p73	Cell cycle regulation
Endothelin receptor	Signal transduction	Progesterone receptor	Signal transduction
Estrogen receptor	Signal transduction	RAR-β	Signal transduction
GST-π	Detoxification	RASSF1A	Apoptosis
HIC-1	Chromatin remodeling	THBS-1	Angiogenesis
hMLH-1	DNA mismatch repair	TIMP-3	Metastasis

in somatic tissues, yet aberrantly expressed in a variety of cancers (52–54). Recently, Jang et al. (55) observed promoter hypomethylation of MAGE-A1, -A3, and -B2 in 75%, 80%, and 80% of resected lung cancers, and 35%, 50%, and 55% of histologically normal tissues adjacent to these cancers, indicating that genomic demethylation occurs as an early event during multistep pulmonary carcinogenesis.

In addition to genome-wide demethylation, cancer cells exhibit site-specific DNA methylation that results in the inactivation of numerous genes regulating cell progression, stress response, and apoptosis (1,48); (Table 1); many of these genes are inactivated in aging normal tissues and premalignant lesions. For instance, the estrogen receptor (ER) gene is silenced by promoter hypermethylation in a significant percentage of colon cancers as well as a subpopulation of normal colonic epithelial cells in an age-specific manner (56). Methylation of p16 has been observed in 25–40% of non-small-cell lung carcinomas, 20–25% of respiratory epithelial tissues adjacent to primary lung cancers, and 20–40% of histologically normal bronchial biopsies from current or former smokers (57–60); in addition, methylation of p16 is frequently observed in esophageal adenocarcinomas (61) as well as 20–60% of biopsies from Barrett's esophagus (62,63). Inactivation of RASSF1A by promoter methylation mechanisms occurs in 50% of SV40 T antigen-positive malignant pleural mesotheliomas (64), and aberrant methylation of this tumor-suppressor gene has been observed in SV40-transformed mesothelial cells in vitro (65). Whereas a "methylator phenotype" has been

observed in leukemia and colon cancers (66,67), specific methylation profiles for other common malignancies have not yet been defined.

Increasing evidence indicates that aberrant DNMT activity directly contributes to site-specific DNA methylation during malignant transformation. Several investigators (68,69) have detected overexpression of DNMTs in cancer specimens; others (70,71) have observed no correlation between DNMT levels and gene silencing in cancer cells, indicating that DNMT overexpression alone may be insufficient to account for aberrant promoter hypermethylation during malignant transformation. Nevertheless, observations that DNMT overexpression induces DNA methylation and malignant transformation of NIH-3T3 cells (72), and that abrogation of DNMT expression by antisense techniques inhibits the malignant phenotype of cancer cells (15,73), have clearly established the significance of DNMTs in the pathogenesis of cancer. Laird et al. (74) observed that APC MIN/+ mice heterozygous for expression of DNMT 1 (approx 50% reduction in DNMT levels) exhibited a 60% reduction in intestinal adenomas relative to APC MIN/+ mice that expressed normal levels of DNMT; adenoma development in APC MIN/+ DNMT+/– mice could be further reduced by treatment with the DNA demethylating agent 5-deoxyazacytidine (DAC). Collectively, these data indicate that DNMT1 contributes to intestinal adenoma development in mice.

Belinsky et al. (75) examined the relationship between DNMT activity and lung cancer using the well-established A/J mouse model (76). Briefly, DNMT activity in type II pneumocytes (target cells) and Clara cells (nontarget cells) from A/J mice exposed to the tobacco carcinogen 4-(methylnitrosamino)-1-(3-pyridyl)-1-butanone (NNK), were compared to those from C3H mice, which are resistant to NNK-induced pulmonary carcinogenesis. Increased DNMT activity and enhanced DNA methylation were observed in type II pneumocytes, but not Clara cells, within 7 d following NNK administration in A/J mice. Increasing DNMT activity in type II pneumocytes, which was not attributable to the proliferation status of these cells, coincided with progression to malignancy in A/J mice. Although endogenous DNMT levels in type II pneumocytes and Clara cells from A/J and C3H mice were comparable, no significant increase in DNMT levels was detected in type II pneumocytes from NNK-treated C3H mice; however, enhanced DNMT activity was observed in the rare tumors that developed in these animals. Although not directly demonstrated in this series of experiments, enhanced DNMT activity in preneoplastic lesions coincided temporally with K-*ras* mutations that are known to be early events in NNK- as well as urethane-induced pulmonary carcinogenesis in A/J mice (76,77).

Lantry et al. (78) examined the chemopreventive effects of DAC in (C3H/HeJ × A/J) F1 hybrid mice. Following NNK exposure, animals were treated 3× weekly for 24 wk with 1 mg DAC/kg administered intraperitoneally. The incidence and multiplicity of lung tumors were reduced by 23% and 42%, respectively, in DAC-treated mice. Hammond et al. (79) examined the effects of DNA demethylating agent 5-azacytidine (5-AC) on tumor formation in a hamster model of bronchogenic carcinoma. Early administration of 5-AC (3–5 d following carcinogen exposure) resulted in smaller tumors than when treatment was administered later during cancer development. Collectively, these data suggest that aberrant DNMT activity contributes to pulmonary carcinogenesis, and that abrogation of DNMT expression may be efficacious in treating and preventing lung cancer.

4. DNMTS

In mammalian cells, DNA methylation is mediated by the opposing actions of DNMTs and DNA demethylases. To date, four DNMTs have been identified, and three of these (DNMT1, 3a, and 3b) mediate transfer of the methyl group from *S*-adenosylmethionine (SAM) to the 5'-position of cytosine; although homologous to the other DNMTs, DNMT2 exhibits minimal methyltransferase activity (7,47).

DNMT1 is composed of approx 1,620 amino acids with a C-terminal domain containing a catalytic site and an *N*-terminal domain containing a nuclear localization signal, a zinc-finger region, and a DNA-binding domain, as well as a domain that targets DNMT1 to the replication fork. Alternative splicing results in several isoforms of DNMT1 that are differentially expressed in somatic tissues. DNMT1 exhibits preferential binding to hemimethylated DNA, and predominantly mediates methyltransferase activity during the S phase. Although DNMT1 plays a major role in maintenance of DNA methylation during DNA replication, and contributes to X chromosome inactivation and imprinting (7,80,81), this methyltransferase may also mediate *de novo* methylation of DNA. Overexpression of DNMT1 increases DNA methylation in myocytes as well as fibroblasts (82,83), and upregulation of DNMT1 in lymphocytes following HIV infection results in methylation of the interferon gamma receptor (84). Targeted disruption of DNMT1 results in embryonic lethality in mice (85). Embryonic stem (ES) cells with DNMT1 mutations grow normally in vitro, but undergo apoptosis when induced to differentiate. These cells maintain low-level DNA methylation and retain cytosine methyltransferase activity (86); as such, DNMT1-deficient ES cells retain the ability to methylate endogenous viral sequences, as well as newly integrated retroviral DNA. DNMT1 associates with several cell cycle related proteins, including proliferating cell nuclear antigen (PCNA), E2F, and Rb, as well as HDAC1 and HDAC2 (19,87).

DNMT3a and 3b contribute to methylation of unmethylated as well as hemimethylated DNA in vitro, and are required for *de novo* methylation in vivo (88). Although they exhibit overlapping activities, DNMT3a and 3b have different patterns of expression in the embryo, suggesting that these isoforms have unique functions during development (69). DNMT3a knockout mice are normal at birth but die shortly thereafter; DNMT3b knockouts die *in utero* from multiple developmental defects (88). Methylation of endogenous retroviral DNA is maintained in DNMT3a knockout mice, and slightly decreased in DNMT3b knockouts. Markedly hypomethylated satellite repeat DNA sequences have been observed in ES cells derived from DNMT3b knockout mice. ES cells that are deficient for DNMT3a and 3b exhibit aberrant methylation of some CpG sites within the imprinted insulin growth factor-2 (IGF-2) gene. Although the role of *de novo* methylation in nonembryonic tissues is unclear, DNMT3a and 3b have been observed in normal tissues.

Robertson et al. *(69)* utilized Northern blot and RT-PCR techniques to examine levels of expression of DNMT 1, 3a, and 3b in a variety of normal and malignant human tissues. Northern blot analysis demonstrated coordinate expression of DNMT1, 3a, and 3b in normal tissues, and DNMT1 was the predominant methyltransferase, which was expressed in all adult tissues except the small intestine. Although DNMT3a and 3b were also expressed in all normal tissues examined, the levels of these enzymes were considerably lower than DNMT1. Various isoforms of DNMT3b that resulted from alternative splicing were differentially expressed in normal cells. Relative to corresponding normal tissues, 6 of 10, 5 of 10, and 8 of 10 tumors exhibited overexpression of DNMT1, DNMT3a, and DNMT3b, respectively; several tumors overexpressed all three methyltransferases. Average levels of DNMT1, 3a, and 3b were 4-, 3.1-, and sevenfold higher in tumors than normal cells. The magnitude of DNMT overexpression in cancer cells was not attributable to proliferation status.

In a subsequent study, Robertson et al. *(89)* examined the pattern of DNMT expression during G_0/G_1 to S-phase progression in normal and malignant cells. DNMT1 and 3b levels were significantly reduced during G_0/G_1; DNMT3a levels did not vary significantly during cell cycle progression. Whereas overall DNMT activity was diminished during G_0/G_1 arrest, tumor cells exhibited a higher methylation capacity relative to normal cells.

A series of elegant experiments was performed to determine the role of specific DNMTs in cancer cells. Rhee et al. *(90)* examined HCT116 colon cancer cells in which DNMT1 had been silenced by homologous recombination. DNMT1 cancer cells grew slightly more slowly than parental HCT116 cells, and exhibited normal morphology during more than 75 passages in cell culture (300 cell generations). Compared to parental HCT116 cells, DNMT activity was diminished by 66% and 96% in DNMT1+/− and DNMT1−/− cells, respectively. However, despite the marked decrease in DNA methyltransferase activity, total 5-methylcytosine content was diminished by only 20% in DNMT1 −/− cells. Methylation of satellite 2 and 3 DNA sequences at juxtacentromeric regions of chromosomes 1, 9, 15, and 16 was decreased in DNMT1-/- cells relative to parental HCT116 cells. In contrast, no demethylation of ALU repeats or alphoid satellite sequences at centromeric regions of chromosomes 3, 4, 7, 10, 12, 17, 18, 22, and X was observed in DNMT1

−/− cells; these sequences were readily demethylated following deoxyazacytidine treatment. In addition, *p16* and tissue inhibitor of matrix metalloproteinases (TIMP)-3 genes remained methylated in DNMT1−/− cells. Furthermore, methylation of endogenous retroviral DNA sequences remained intact in DNMT −/− cells. No difference in DAC-mediated cytotoxicity was observed in DNMT1-deficient cells compared to parental HCT116 cells.

In a subsequent study, Rhee et al. *(91)* disrupted DNMT1 as well as DNMT3b in HCT116 cells. Relative to parental HCT116 cells, DNMT activity was decreased by 93% in DNMT1−/− cells, and nearly 100% in the double knockouts. Although there was no significant change from parental cells regarding methylcytosine content in DNMT1−/− or the DNMT3b −/− cells, a 95% reduction in 5-methylcytosine content was observed in double knockout cells. The loss of DNA methylation in the double knockout cells was associated with abnormal methylation of multiple genes. For instance, although hypermethylated in DNMT1−/− or DNMT3b−/− cells, the *p16* promoter was 98% demethylated in double knockouts, resulting in re-expression of this tumor-suppressor gene. Furthermore, in double knockout cells, TIMP-3 was demethylated to a level comparable to that observed following DAC treatment of parental HCT116 cells. In addition, the normally silenced allele of the imprinted gene IGF-2 was activated in the double knockouts, indicating a complete loss of imprinting in these cells. Interestingly, double knockout cells retained the ability to silence retroviral elements (presumably because of DNMT3a), and remained sensitive to DAC. Collectively, these experiments clearly demonstrate cooperation between DNMT1 and DNMT3b with regard to repression of gene expression under normal as well as pathologic conditions.

McLeod and Szyf *(15)* observed that murine adrenocortical cells transfected with a 600-BP sequence of DNMT1 in antisense orientation exhibited decreased DNA methylation, reduced proliferation in vitro, and diminished tumorigenicity relative to untransfected control cells. In subsequent experiments, Ramchandani et al. *(92)* observed that a phosphorothioate-modified antisense oligonucleotide directed against the 5' end of DNMT1 mRNA inhibited DNMT1 expression, induced adrenocortical-specific C21 expression, and diminished the tumorigenicity of murine Y1 adrenocortical carcinoma cells.

More recently, Beaulieu et al. *(73)* developed specific and potent antisense constructs that recognized DNMT3a and DNMT3b. The antisense oligos targeted 3'-UTR sequences of DNMT3a and 3b that were common to all of the splice variants, resulting in depletion of all DNMT3a and 3b transcripts. Although the antisense DNMT3a oligo had no antiproliferative effects, antisense to DNMT3b mediated dose-dependent growth inhibition and apoptosis in lung and breast cancer cells. Whereas DNMT3b depletion did not result in dramatic global demethylation, and did not induce demethylation of classic satellite 2 region juxtacentromeric DNA, abrogation of DNMT3b expression coincided with induction of p21 and PCNA, as well as caspases 7 and 10, in cultured cancer cells. In addition, the antisense DNMT3b oligo mediated demethylation of the RASSF1A promoter, resulting in reexpression of this tumor suppressor gene, which may have contributed to the pro-apoptotic effects of the DNMT3b antisense oligo.

Data from experiments by Beaulieu et al. *(73)* indicate that abrogation of DNMT3b expression can diminish proliferation of cultured cancer cells. In contrast, Rhee et al. *(92)* observed no significant decrease in proliferation of DNMT3b-deficient colon cancer cells. This discrepancy may be the result of differences in cell lines, as well as the methods used to silence DNMT3b in the two studies (antisense oligos in the experiments by Beaulieu et al. *[73]* , vs site-directed mutagenesis with selection in the experiments performed by Rhee and colleagues *[91]*). Nevertheless, available data suggest that DNMT1 as well as DNMT3b are required for *de novo* methylation and repression of genes that regulate cell cycle progression and apoptosis in cancer cells.

Inhibition of DNMT expression may directly inhibit cancer cell growth via demethylation of tumor suppressor genes, yet the antiproliferative effects of DNMT depletion may be mediated by indirect mechanisms as well. Multinovic et al. *(93)*, as well as Fournel et al. *(94)*, examined mechanisms of p16 and p21 induction in A549 lung cancer and T24 bladder cancer cells following exposure to antisense DNMT oligos. Restoration of p16 expression was directly related to promoter demethylation; in contrast, induction of p21 expression following DNMT depletion was independent of methylation changes within the p21 promoter. Recent studies indicate that p21 exists in a complex with PCNA, cyclin D, and *cdk4*; this quaternary complex is stable in normal cells but not transformed cells *(95)*. When complexed with PCNA, p21 inhibits DNA synthesis.

DNMT1 competes with p21 for binding to PCNA *(96)*. As such, DNMT1 may exert its oncogenic effects in part by destabilizing this quaternary complex, thereby enabling promiscuous G_1/S transit and aberrant DNA methylation during S phase. Increased p21 levels observed in cancer cells following DNMT1 depletion may reflect enhanced stability of the quarternary complex. These observations highlight the intricacies of the emerging interrelationships between chromatin structure and cell cycle regulation in normal and transformed cells, and the complexities of the mechanisms by which DNA demethylating agents mediate growth arrest and apoptosis in cancer cells.

5. DNMT INHIBITORS IN CANCER THERAPY

In light of the fact that many cancers exhibit hypermethylation of multiple genes that regulate cell cycle progression and apoptosis, inhibition of aberrant DNMT activity represents an attractive strategy for cancer treatment and prevention. To date, several DNA demethylating agents have been studied extensively in clinical settings. The cytidine derivatives 5-AC, DAC, and dihydroazacytidine (DHAC) compete with cytidine triphosphate for incorporation into DNA, and covalently trap DNMT onto DNA, thereby effectively diminishing free DNMT levels, resulting in DNA hypomethylation *(97,98)*. As such, DNA replication is required for DNA demethylation mediated by these agents. In addition, 5-AC is incorporated into RNA, resulting in the inhibition of protein synthesis via several mechanisms *(99–101)*. Because 5-AC is incorporated into RNA more efficiently than DNA, this cytidine analog is a less potent DNA demethylating agent than DAC *(97)*. All three derivatives are inactivated by cytidine deaminase. Although more resistant to deamination, DHAC is not efficiently phosphorylated and incorporated into DNA; as such, this cytidine analog is a considerably less potent DNA demethylating agent than DAC or 5-AC *(97,102)*.

Numerous studies have demonstrated induction of tumor suppressor genes such as VHL, p16, p14/ARF, RASSF1A, TIMP-3, and hMLH-1 in cancer cells in vitro or tumor xenografts following 5-AC or DAC exposure *(35,64,103–106)*. Additional studies have indicated that doses of DAC that induce tumor-suppressor gene expression can mediate *de novo* induction of cancer-testis antigens in tumor cells. Weiser et al. *(53,54)* reported that low-dose DAC (0.1 µg/mL ×

72 h) mediated induction of MAGE-3 and NY-ESO-1 in cultured cell lines derived from a variety of epithelial malignancies; following DAC exposure, cancer cells were recognized by HLA-restricted cytolytic T lymphocytes specific for NY-ESO-1. No induction of MAGE-3 or NY-ESO-1 was observed in cultured normal human bronchial epithelial (NHBE) cells following DAC exposure. DAC mediated growth arrest and apoptosis regardless of of Rb, p53, p16, p14/ARF, and RAS expression in cancer cells, but not NHBE cells; these observations and those reported by Bender et al. *(104)* suggest that DNA demethylating agents may mediate cytotoxicity preferentially in cancer cells.

Whereas the induction of tumor suppressor gene expression may contribute to growth inhibition in cancer cells mediated by DNA demethylating agents, the cytotoxic effects of 5-AC, DAC, and DHAC appear to be related primarily to covalent trapping of DNMT on the DNA *(98)*. Thus, the cytotoxic effects of these agents may not be caused by demethylation per se; indeed, cancer cells deficient for DNMT1, 3b, or both do not appear more susceptible to DAC than parental cancer cells *(90,91)*. In addition, some of the changes in chromatin structure mediated by DNA demethylating agents may not be attributable solely to genomic hypomethylation. For instance, DAC can induce alterations of murine heterochromatin by mechanisms that are independent of DNA methylation *(107)*.

A number of clinical trials have been performed to determine the effects of DNA demethylating agents in cancer patients; representative trials involving patients with hematologic malignancies and solid tumors are summarized in Tables 2 and 3, respectively. In five published studies, including 430 individuals receiving 5-d continuous intravenous infusion of 5-AC at doses ranging from 150–750 mg/m² as salvage therapy for acute myelogenous leukemia (AML), approx 33% of patients exhibited response to treatment *(108–112)*; in one large series, complete (CR) and partial response (PR) rates were 20% and 16%, respectively *(109)*. Administration of conventional chemotherapy agents has not enhanced the efficacy of 5-AC in this setting *(113,114)*. Rivard et al. *(115)* observed responses in three of nine AML patients treated with 36–80 mg/kg DAC via 36–44 h continuous intravenous infusion; Momparler et al. *(116)* reported responses in five of six AML patients who received 45–100 mg/kg DAC via 40–90 h continuous infusion. Response rates ranging from 40–70% have been observed in three trials eval-

uating DAC (250–1000 mg/m² via 6 d continuous intravenous infusion) in conjunction with amsacrine or idarubicin as salvage therapy for AML *(117–119)*. Petti et al. *(120)* observed a response rate of 33% when DAC was administered alone as induction therapy for AML. Schwartsmann et al. *(121)* observed complete remission in six of eight individuals who received DAC (90 mg/m² via 5 d continuous intravenous infusion) in conjunction with daunorubicin as first-line therapy for AML.

Several studies have been undertaken to evaluate 5-AC and DAC in chronic myelogenous leukemia (CML). In two studies totaling nearly 70 patients, Schiffer et al. *(122)* and Dutcher et al. *(123)* observed response rates of 58% and 23% respectively, in CML patients in blastic phase treated with 5-AC (150 mg/m²) in conjunction with etoposide or mitoxantrone; six patients had complete responses, whereas 17 individuals exhibited partial remissions. Kantarjian et al. *(124)* observed overall response rates of 10% and 25%, respectively, in 20 patients with CML in blastic phase; reversion to chronic phase was observed in six of 17 patients with accelerated-phase CML.

5-AC and DAC appear to have significant activity in myelodysplastic syndrome (MDS). Silverman et al. *(125)* treated 43 patients with 5-AC (75 mg/m² via 7-d infusion) and observed responses in 21 patients, five of whom experienced complete remission. In a subsequent study *(126)*, Silverman treated 36 patients with 5-AC administered at a dose of 75 mg/m² subcutaneously qd × 7. Trilineage responses were observed in approx 40% of patients; four individuals experienced complete responses, and eight individuals exhibited partial remissions. Later, Silverman et al. *(127)* randomized 191 patients to receive 5-AC (75 mg/m² subcutaneously q 4h qd × 3) or observation alone. Sixty-three percent of patients who received 5-AC exhibited a response to treatment (6% CR, 10% PR, 47% hematologic improvement); only 7% of patients in the observation arm responded. Median time to leukemia formation, as well as survival times, were improved in patients who received 5-AC.

Additional trials have been performed to examine the effects of DAC in patients with MDS. In three trials, Wijerman et al. treated approx 125 patients with varying regimens of DAC (total dose, 120–150 mg/m² per course) *(128–130)*. Responses were observed in 59 of 121 evaluable patients (49%); 24 patients (20%) exhibited complete remission, and 12 individuals (10%) had partial remissions. Twenty-three (23) patients (19%)

Table 2
Representative Clinical Trials Evaluating DNA Demethylating Agents in Hematologic Malignancies

Authors	Disease	Number of Patients	Agent	Total Dose	Response (%)
McCredie et al. (108)	AML	28	5-AC	400 mg/m^2 over 5d	28
Von Hoff et al. (109)	AML	200	5-AC	150–400 mg/m^2 over 5 d	36
Karan et al. (110)	AML	37	5-AC	150–300 mg/m^2 over 5 d	36
Saiki et al. (111)	AML	120	5-AC	300–750 mg/m^2 over 5 d	9
Vogler et al. (112)	AML	45	5-AC	100–300 mg/m^2 over 5 d	33
Goldberg et al. (113)	AML	53	5-AC with mitoxantrone	200 mg/m^2 over 3 d	15
Winton et al. (114)	AML	128	5-AC with amsacrine	112–200 mg/m^2 over 2 d	16
Rivard et al. (115)	AML	9	DAC	36–80 mg/kg over 36-44 h	33
Momparler et al. (116)	AML	6	DAC	45–100 mg/kg over 40-90 h	89
Willemze et al. (117)	AML	22	DAC with amsacrine or idarubicin	250 mg/m^2 over 6 d	68
Willemze et al. (118)	AML	63	DAC with amsacrine or idarubicin	250 mg/m^2 over 6 d	39
Richel et al. (119)	AML	16	DAC $^+$/–amsacrine	250–1000 mg/m^2 over 6 d	62
Petti et al. (120)	AML	12	DAC	90–120 mg/m^2 over 3 d	33
Schwartsmann et al. (121)	AML	8	DAC + daunorubicin	90 mg/m^2 over 5 d	75
Shiffer et al. (122)	CML	27	5-AC with etoposide	150 mg/m^2 over 5 d	58
Dutcher et al. (123)	CML	40	5-AC with mitoxantrone	150 mg/m^2 over 5 d	23
Kantarjean et al. (124)	CML	47	5-AC	100–200 mg/m^2 over 5 h	25 (blastic phase) Accelerated phase: 53
Silverman et al. (125)	MDS	43	5-AC	75–150 mg/m^2 over 7 d	49
Silverman et al. (126)	MDS	36	5-AC	75 mg/m^2 SQ over 7 d	40
Silverman et al. (127)	MDS	99	5-AC	75 mg/m^2 SQ over 7 d	63
Wijermans et al. (128)	MDS	29	DAC	40–55 mg/m^2 over 3 d	54
Wijermans et al. (129)	MDS	66	DAC	45 mg/m^2 over 3 d	48

experienced hematologic improvement. Median duration of response was 9 mo, and median survival was 15 mo.

Lubbert et al. (131) characterized cytogenetic responses in patients with MDS treated with DAC. Of 115 karyotyped patients, 61% exhibited clonal chromosomal abnormalities. Major cytogenetic responses were observed in 19 individuals, including three of five International Prognostic Screening System (IPSS) "low-risk" patients, six of 30 "interme-diate-risk" patients, and 10 of 26 "high-risk" patients. The median duration of cytogenetic response was 7.5 mo. Median survivals in low-, intermediate-, and high-risk patients were 30, 8, and 13 mo, respectively.

Daskalakis et al. (132) evaluated the methylation status of $p15^{ink4b}$ in bone marrow cells from high-risk MDS patients who received DAC treatment. Using methylation-sensitive primary extension assays (MSnuPE), denaturing gradient gel electrophoresis, and bisulfite sequencing techniques, these investigators

Table 3
Representative Clinical Trials Evaluating DNA Demethylating Agents in Solid Tumors

Authors	Disease	Number of Patients	Agent	Total Dose	Response (%)
Cunningham et al. (133)	Breast cancer	27	5-AC	600 mg/m² over 10 d	2 PR (7%)
Weiss et al. (134)	Breast cancer	11	5-AC	5–24 mg/m² over 8 d	7 PR (63%)
Weiss et al. (135)	Breast cancer	29	5-AC	160 mg/kg over 10 d	6 PR (20%)
Sessa et al. (137)	Ovarian cancer	24	DAC	225 mg/m² over 10 d	1 PR (8%)
Pohlmann et al. (138)	Cervical cancer	21	DAC	150 mg/m² over 3 d	8 PR (38%)
			CDDP	90–120 mg/m² over 3 d	5 stable disease
Moertel et al. (140)	Colon cancer	27	5-AC	500–750 mg/m² over 10 d	0 (0%)
Abele et al. (141)	Colon cancer	42	DAC	225 mg/m² over 10 d	0 (0%) 3 stable disease
Thibault et al. (139)	Prostate cancer	12	DAC	225 mg/m² over 24 h	2 stable disease
Weiss et al. (134)	Melanoma	5	5-AC	160 mg/m² over 10 d	2 PR (40%)
Abele et al. (141)	Melanoma	18	DAC	225 mg/m² over 10 d	0 (0%) 4 stable disease
Creagan et al. (142)	Melanoma	40	DHAC	5 g/m² over 24 h	8 PR (20%)
Vogelzang et al. (143)	Mesothelioma	41	DHAC	7.5 g/m² over 5 d	1 CR, 2 PR (7%) (+4 regression of evaluable disease)
Samuels et al. (144)	Mesothelioma	41	DHAC/ CDDP	7.5 g/m² over 5 d/ 75 mg/m² over 5 d	2 PR (8%) (+3 regression of evaluable disease) 13 stable disease
Momparler et al. (145)	Lung	15	DAC 8-h infusion	200–660 mg/m² via	3 stable disease
Schrump et al. (148)	Lung/esophagus mesothelioma	22	DAC	60–75 mg/m² over 3 d	7 stable disease

observed hypermethylation of p15 in 12 of 19 patients with high-risk MDS. Hypomethylation of p15 was observed in nine of these patients following DAC treatment. Immunohistochemistry analysis revealed that four of eight patients exhibiting p15 hypermethylation had low or undetectable p15 protein expression in bone marrow cells; in these patients, *p15* protein expression was restored following DAC treatment. Complete remissions were observed in three of nine patients in whom p15 hypermethylation was reversed by DAC treatment. The fact that hematologic responses (including one PR) were seen in four of seven patients without p15 hypermethylation indicates that demethylation of p15 alone is insufficient to account for the effects of DAC in myelodysplastic syndrome.

A number of trials have been performed to determine the effects of DNA demethylating agents in solid tumors. In an early clinical trial, Cunningham et al. (133) randomized 58 breast cancer patients to receive 5-AC or *N*-(2-chloroethyl)-*N*'-cyclohexyl-*N*-nitrosourea (CCNU) therapy. Thirty-one (31) individuals received 5-AC at a dose of 60 mg/m² intravenously q d × 10 d and twice weekly thereafter. Most patients who received 5-azacytidine therapy experienced severe nausea and vomiting; this gastrointestinal toxicity precluded administration of full doses of 5-AC in four patients. Two of 27 patients (7%) who received full-dose 5-AC exhibited PRs; four patients experienced stabilization of disease of variable duration. In contrast, of 27 patients who received CCNU therapy, three exhibited PR and six experienced stabilization of disease.

Weiss et al. (134) treated 30 patients with a variety of solid tumors with 5-AC (0.5–2.4 mg/kg/d × 10–15 d). Major toxicities included leukopenia and thrombocytopenia; nausea, mild diarrhea, and hepato-toxicity were also observed. No CRs were seen; however, PRs were observed in seven of 11 breast cancer patients, two of five melanoma patients, and two of six colon cancer patients. In a subsequent study, Weiss et al. *(135)* treated 177 patients with 5-AC (1.6 mg/kg/d × 10 d) followed by a maintenance regimen. A total of 148 individuals received the drug by rapid intravenous infusion, whereas 29 received the drug via 18–24 h infusion. Nearly 20% of evaluable patients with breast cancer, and 21% of lymphoma patients exhibited partial responses of limited durations. Response rates of 8% and 25% have been observed in two trials totaling 28 ovarian cancer patients treated with 5-AC (275–800 mg/m^2 total dose administered subcutaneously over the course of 10 d), or DAC (225 mg/m^2 total dose administered intravenously over the course of 10 d) *(136,137)*. In a more recent Phase II trial involving patients with cervical carcinomas receiving sequential DAC (50 mg/m^2 qd × 3) and cisplatin (30–60 mg/m^2 qd × 3), Pohlmann et al. *(138)* observed PRs in eight of 21 evaluable patients (38%); stabilization of disease was noted in five additional patients.

In a recent study, Thibault et al. *(139)* observed stabilization of disease in two of 12 patients with hormone-independent prostate cancer following DAC therapy (75 mg/m^2 administered every 1 h q 8h × 3 doses). Moertel et al. *(140)* and Abele and colleagues *(141)* observed no objective responses in nearly 70 colon cancer patients treated with 5-AC (*n* = 27; total dose = 500–750 mg/m2 administered over a period of 5–10 d) or DAC (*n* = 42; total dose = 225 mg/m^2 administered by three 1-h infusions over a period of 24 h). Whereas Weiss et al. *(134)* reported PRs in two of five melanoma patients receiving 5-AC, Abele et al. *(141)* observed no objective responses in 18 melanoma patients who received DAC (225 mg/m^2 total dose); Creagan et al. *(142)* observed a 20% response rate in 40 melanoma patients who received DHAC (5 g/m^2 administered by 24-h continuous infusion). Vogelzang et al. *(143)* observed an overall response rate of 17% (including one CR and two PRs) in 41 patients with malignant mesothelioma treated with DAC (1500 mg/m^2/d × 5 d). In a subsequent trial, Samuels et al. *(144)* observed two PRs in 26 evaluable mesothelioma patients following DHAC (1500 mg/m^2/d × 5 d) administered in conjunction with cisplatin.

In a recent Phase I/II study, Momparler et al. *(145)* treated 15 lung cancer patients with DAC (200–660 mg/m^2) administered via 1–8-h infusion. Stabilization of disease was observed in three patients, one of whom experienced prolonged survival (>60 mo). Dose-limiting toxicities (DLTs) included myelosuppression; non-hematologic toxicities included transient nausea and vomiting, asthenia, and myalgias. The mean DAC plasma concentration following 8-h infusion of 660 mg/m^2 DAC was 0.94 µg per mL (approx 4 µm).

In light of the fact that DAC's half-life in plasma is relatively short (t$_{1/2\alpha}$ = 7 min, t$_{1/2\beta}$ = 35 min) *(146)*, the efficacy of this agent in clinical settings may be contingent on total dose as well as the duration of infusion. Indeed, studies involving leukemia patients suggest that duration of DAC exposure may be more important than total dose *(147)*. This issue may be particularly relevant for treating solid tumors with a low fraction of cycling cells.

Recently, Schrump et al. *(148)* conducted a Phase I study of tumor antigen and tumor-suppressor gene induction mediated by 72-h DAC infusion in patients with inoperable thoracic malignancies. Quantitative reverse transcriptase-polymerase chain reaction (RT-PCR), methylation-specific PCR (MSP), immunohistochemistry, and enzyme-linked immuno sorbent assay (ELISA) techniques were used to evaluate NY-ESO-1 and *p16* expression in tumor biopsies, and to examine immune response to NY-ESO-1. Twenty-three (23) patients received DAC infusions, of whom 22 were evaluable. The maximum tolerated dose (MTD) was 75 mg/m^2 for individuals with two or less prior treatments, and 60 mg/m^2 for patients with three or more prior therapies. Plasma DAC concentrations approximated 10 to 20 ng/mL (25–50 n*M*). No major responses were observed; however, stabilization of disease was noted in seven patients. Two lung cancer patients experienced prolonged stabilization of disease (>6 mo and 12 mo). Grade III leukopenia, thrombocytopenia, or anemia were observed in 9/22, 2/22, and 3/22 patients, respectively. Grade IV neutropenia was observed in eight patients, and was dose limiting in four individuals. Grade III nonhematologic toxicities occurred in three patients. One individual developed an infected malignant pleural effusion. Quantitative RT-PCR analysis revealed induction of NY-ESO-1 and p16 in one of nine, and none of nine patients, respectively. This analysis, as well as MSP, proved unreliable using DNA extracted from biopsies, because of the extent of inflammatory cells and necrosis in these specimens. Immunohistochemistry analysis revealed induction of NY-ESO-1 and p16 in nine of 15 and eight of 17 patients, respectively. Post-treatment antibodies to NY-ESO-1 were observed in two of 13 patients, and both of these had NY-ESO -1 expression in post-treatment biopsy specimens. Collectively, these data indicate that plasma concentrations of DAC sufficient to mediate target-gene induction are achievable in thoracic oncology patients, and support further evaluation of gene-induction strategies for treating thoracic malignancies.

Because HDAC inhibitors can potentiate gene expression and apoptosis mediated by DNA demethylating agents *(46,54,149)*, Schrump and colleagues have commenced a Phase I study of sequential DAC/depsipeptide FK228 infusion in patients with cancers involving lungs or pleura. The overall goals of this study include definition of the MTD of DAC and depsipeptide administered by sequential infusion, as well as analysis of NY-ESO-1, p16, and p21 expression, and apoptosis in tissue specimens before and after treatment. Laser capture microdissection techniques have been refined to allow more precise assessment of molecular endpoints in this trial.

On the basis of impressive preclinical data utilizing antisense oligos targeting DNMT1 *(15,92)*, several trials have been initiated to evaluate MG-98, an antisense oligo that targets the 3'-untranslated region (UTR) of DNMT1 mRNA in cancer patients*(151)*. Two Phase I dose escalation studies have been performed thus far in patients with solid tumors. One trial employed a continuous 21-d infusion every 4 wk and the second study used a 2-h infusion twice weekly for 3 of every 4 wk. In the first trial, 14 patients with solid tumors received a total number of 25 cycles of therapy; the highest number of cycles received by any one patient was three. The MTD of continuous 21-d administration of MG-98 was 80 mg/m^2/d. Grade III hepatotoxicity was observed at 160 mg/m^2/d, and grade IV fatigue with grade III thrombocytopenia was observed in patients who received 200 mg/m^2/d. Most individuals experienced delayed thrombocytopenia. No evidence of clinical activity was observed in this trial *(150,151)*. In the second study, 19 patients received a total of 74 cycles of therapy; the maximum number of cycles in any one patient was 18. The MTD of MG-98 observed in this trial was 360 mg/m$^{2\cdot}$ The DLTs included fevers, chills, diaphoresis, and fatigue; hematologic toxicities were minimal. Two patients developed hypersensitivity reactions. Pharmacokinetics of MG-98 appeared to be independent of the dose administered; significant decreases in DNMT1 levels in peripheral-blood mononuclear cells (PBMC) were observed in approximately 40% of patients. One PR was seen in a renal

cell carcinoma patient, commencing approximately eight cycles into therapy, and lasting more than 6 mo. These data suggest that prolonged infusion of MG-98 may be necessary in order to mediate antitumor effects *(150,152)*. On the basis of these Phase I data, a Phase II trial has been initiated to further evaluate MG-98 administered by intermittent dose regimen in patients with oropharyngeal and renal cell carcinomas. In addition, a dose-refining trial has been initiated in patients with late-stage MDS or AML *(150)·*

6. CONCLUSIONS AND FUTURE DIRECTIONS

Recent insights regarding the mechanisms that regulate chromatin structure in normal and malignant cells provide new opportunities for development of potent and specific therapies based on targeting aberrant DNMT activity in cancer cells. Available data indicate that as single agents, 5-AC and DAC have significant activity in established hematologic malignancies as well as myelodysplastic syndrome. In contrast, 5-AC, DAC, and DHAC appear to have little activity in advanced solid tumors; furthermore, preliminary data indicate that antisense oligos targeting DNMT1 also have limited efficacy in treating solid neoplasms. Nevertheless the finding that 5-AC and DAC, as well as antisense oligos that target DNMTs—modulate expression of tumor suppressor genes known to be silenced by hypermethylation mechanisms early in the course of multistep carcinogenesis suggests that DNA demethylating agents administered via regional techniques may be efficacious for chemoprevention of a variety of common malignancies, including lung, esophageal, and oropharyngeal carcinomas *(153–155)*.

Because hMLH1 and mdr-1 expression can be restored in cancer cells following DNA demethylation, DAC, 5-AC, or related compounds may prove useful for enhancing the efficacy of conventional chemotherapeutic agents in cancer patients. Indeed, recent studies indicate that DAC treatment sensitizes ovarian and colorectal carcinoma xenografts to a variety of standard chemotherapeutic agents, including cisplatin, carboplatin, temozolamide, and epirubicin, but not paclitaxel *(106)*. Well-designed clinical trials are necessary to determine whether DNA demethylating agents can be administered with acceptable toxicities at doses that will modulate mdr-1 or hMLH-1 expression in solid tumors, and to determine whether DNA demethylating agents can enhance the efficacy of conventional cytotoxic agents in cancer patients. All clinical trials utilizing DNA demethylating agents should include analysis of appropriate target genes in pre- and post-treatment biopsies in order to validate mechanisms pertaining to treatment effects, and to generate hypotheses for future research efforts. Without question, we are witnessing a new era regarding cancer epigenetics; it remains to be seen whether potent and specific inhibitors of DNMTs will prove efficacious for the treatment and prevention of cancer.

REFERENCES

1. Jones PA, Baylin SB. The fundamental role of epigenetic events in cancer. *Nat Rev Genet* 2002;3:415–428.
2. Annunziato AT, Hansen JC. Role of histone acetylation in the assembly and modulation of chromatin structures. *Gene Expr* 2000;9:37–61.
3. Rice JC, Allis CD. Histone methylation *versus* histone acetylation: new insights into epigenetic regulation. *Curr Opin Cell Biol* 2001;13:263–273.
4. Nakayama T, Takami Y. Participation of histones and histone-modifying enzymes in cell functions through alterations in chromatin structure. *J Biochem (Tokyo)* 2001;129:491–499.
5. Nguyen CT, Gonzales FA, Jones PA. Altered chromatin structure associated with methylation-induced gene silencing in cancer cells: correlation of accessibility, methylation, MeCP2 binding and acetylation. *Nucleic Acids Res* 2001;29:4598–4606.
6. Nan X, Ng HH, Johnson CA, et al. Transcriptional repression by the methyl-CpG-binding protein MeCP2 involves a histone deacetylase complex. *Nature* 1998;393:386–389.
7. Attwood JT, Yung RL, Richardson BC. DNA methylation and the regulation of gene transcription. *Cell Mol Life Sci* 2002;59:241–257.
8. Clark SJ, Melki J. DNA methylation and gene silencing in cancer: which is the guilty party? *Oncogene* 2002;21:5380–5387.
9. Cervoni N, Szyf M. Demethylase activity is directed by histone acetylation. *J Biol Chem* 2001;276:40,778–40,787.
10. Eden S, Hashimshony T, Keshet I, et al. DNA methylation models histone acetylation. *Nature* 1998;394:842.
11. Jones PA, Laird PW. Cancer epigenetics comes of age. *Nat Genet* 1999;21:163–167.
12. Razin A, Cedar H. Distribution of 5-methylcytosine in chromatin. *Proc Natl Acad Sci USA* 1977;74:2725–2728.
13. Novik KL, Nimmrich I, Genc B, et al. Epigenomics: genome-wide study of methylation phenomena. *Curr Issues Mol Biol* 2002;4:111–128.
14. Urnov FD, Wolffe AP. Chromatin remodeling and transcriptional activation: the cast (in order of appearance). *Oncogene* 2001;20:2991–3006.
15. MacLeod AR, Szyf M. Expression of antisense to DNA methyltransferase mRNA induces DNA demethylation and inhibits tumorigenesis. *J Biol Chem* 1995;270:8037–8043.
16. Bakin AV, Curran T. Role of DNA 5-methylcytosine transferase in cell transformation by fos. *Science* 1999;283:387–390.
17. Di Croce L, Raker VA, Corsaro M, et al. Methyltransferase recruitment and DNA hypermethylation of target promoters

18. Zhou X, Richon VM, Wang AH, et al. Histone deacetylase 4 associates with extracellular signal-regulated kinases 1 and 2, and its cellular localization is regulated by oncogenic Ras. *Proc Natl Acad Sci USA* 2000;97:14,329–14,333.
19. Robertson KD, Ait-Si-Ali S, Yokochi T, et al. DNMT1 forms a complex with Rb, E2F1 and HDAC1 and represses transcription from E2F-responsive promoters. *Nat Genet* 2000;25:338–342.
20. Brehm A, Miska EA, McCance DJ, et al. Retinoblastoma protein recruits histone deacetylase to repress transcription. *Nature* 1998;391:597–601.
21. Wade PA. Transcriptional control at regulatory checkpoints by histone deacetylases: molecular connections between cancer and chromatin. *Hum Mol Genet* 2001;10:693–698.
22. Jones PA, Takai D. The role of DNA methylation in mammalian epigenetics. *Science* 2001;293:1068–1070.
23. Robertson KD, Wolffe AP. DNA methylation in health and disease. *Nat Rev Genet* 2000;1:11–19.
24. Bird A. DNA methylation patterns and epigenetic memory. *Genes Dev* 2002;16:6–21.
25. Razin A, Riggs AD. DNA methylation and gene function. *Science* 1980;210:604–610.
26. Ehrlich M, Wang RY. 5-Methylcytosine in eukaryotic DNA. *Science* 1981;212:1350–1357.
27. McClelland M, Ivarie R. Asymmetrical distribution of CpG in an 'average' mammalian gene. *Nucleic Acids Res* 1982;10:7865–7877.
28. Cooper DN, Taggart MH, Bird AP. Unmethylated domains in vertebrate DNA. *Nucleic Acids Res* 1983;11:647–658.
29. Lindahl T. DNA repair enzymes. *Annu Rev Biochem* 1982;51:61–87.
30. Larsen F, Gundersen G, Prydz H. Choice of enzymes for mapping based on CpG islands in the human genome. *Genet Anal Tech Appl* 1992;9:80–85.
31. Jones PA. The DNA methylation paradox. *Trends Genet* 1999;15:34–37.
32. Larsen F, Gundersen G, Lopez R, Prydz H. CpG islands as gene markers in the human genome. *Genomics* 1992;13:1095–1107.
33. Gonzalgo ML, Hayashida T, Bender CM, et al. The role of DNA methylation in expression of the p19/p16 locus in human bladder cancer cell lines. *Cancer Res* 1998;58:1245–1252.
34. Larsen F, Solheim J, Prydz H. A methylated CpG island 3' in the apolipoprotein-E gene does not repress its transcription. *Hum Mol Genet* 1993;2:775–780.
35. Robertson KD, Jones PA. The human ARF cell cycle regulatory gene promoter is a CpG island which can be silenced by DNA methylation and down-regulated by wild-type p53. *Mol Cell Biol* 1998;18:6457–6473.
36. Yoder JA, Walsh CP, Bestor TH. Cytosine methylation and the ecology of intragenomic parasites. *Trends Genet* 1997;13:335–340.
37. Matzke MA, Mette MF, Aufsatz W, et al. Host defenses to parasitic sequences and the evolution of epigenetic control mechanisms. *Genetica* 1999;107:271–287.
38. Liang G, Chan MF, Tomigahara Y, et al. Cooperativity between DNA methyltransferases in the maintenance methylation of repetitive elements. *Mol Cell Biol* 2002;22:480–491.

by an oncogenic transcription factor. *Science* 2002;295:1079–1082.

39. Siegfried Z, Eden S, Mendelsohn M, et al. DNA methylation represses transcription in vivo. *Nat Genet* 1999;22:203–206.

40. Comb M, Goodman HM. CpG methylation inhibits proenkephalin gene expression and binding of the transcription factor AP-2. *Nucleic Acids Res* 1990;18:3975–3982.

41. Iguchi-Ariga SM, Schaffner W. CpG methylation of the cAMP-responsive enhancer/promoter sequence TGACGTCA abolishes specific factor binding as well as transcriptional activation. *Genes Dev* 1989;3:612–619.

42. Prendergast GC, Ziff EB. Methylation-sensitive sequence-specific DNA binding by the c-Myc basic region. *Science* 1991;251:186–189.

43. Lewis JD, Meehan RR, Henzel WJ, et al. Purification, sequence, and cellular localization of a novel chromosomal protein that binds to methylated DNA. *Cell* 1992;69:905–914.

44. Jones PL, Veenstra GJ, Wade PA, et al. Methylated DNA and MeCP2 recruit histone deacetylase to repress transcription. *Nat Genet* 1998;19:187–191.

45. Yu F, Thiesen J, Stratling WH. Histone deacetylase-independent transcriptional repression by methyl-CpG-binding protein 2. *Nucleic Acids Res* 2000;28:2201–2206.

46. Cameron EE, Bachman KE, Myohanen S, et al. Synergy of demethylation and histone deacetylase inhibition in the re-expression of genes silenced in cancer. *Nat Genet* 1999;21:103–107.

47. Robertson KD. DNA methylation, methyltransferases, and cancer. *Oncogene* 2001;20:3139–3155.

48. Baylin SB, Herman JG, Graff JR, et al. Alterations in DNA methylation: a fundamental aspect of neoplasia. *Adv Cancer Res* 1998;72:141–196.

49. Ehrlich M. DNA methylation in cancer: too much, but also too little. *Oncogene* 2002;21:5400–5413.

50. Jost JP, Siegmann M, Sun L, Leung R. Mechanisms of DNA demethylation in chicken embryos. Purification and properties of a 5-methylcytosine-DNA glycosylase. *J Biol Chem* 1995;270:9734–9739.

51. Costello JF, Plass C. Methylation matters. *J Med Genet* 2001;38:285–303.

52. De Smet C, De Backer O, Faraoni I, et al. The activation of human gene MAGE-1 in tumor cells is correlated with genome-wide demethylation. *Proc Natl Acad Sci USA* 1996;93:7149–7153.

53. Weiser TS, Ohnmacht GA, Guo ZS, et al. Induction of MAGE-3 expression in lung and esophageal cancer cells. *Ann Thorac Surg* 2001;71:295–301.

54. Weiser TS, Guo ZS, Ohnmacht GA, et al. Sequential 5-Aza-2 deoxycytidine-depsipeptide FR901228 treatment induces apoptosis preferentially in cancer cells and facilitates their recognition by cytolytic T lymphocytes specific for NY-ESO-1. *J Immunother* 2001;24:151–161.

55. Jang SJ, Soria JC, Wang L, et al. Activation of melanoma antigen tumor antigens occurs early in lung carcinogenesis. *Cancer Res* 2001;61:7959–7963.

56. Issa JP, Ottaviano YL, Celano P, et al. Methylation of the oestrogen receptor CpG island links ageing and neoplasia in human colon. *Nat Genet* 1994;7:536–540.

57. Zochbauer-Muller S, Fong KM, Virmani AK, et al. D. Aberrant promoter methylation of multiple genes in non-small cell lung cancers. *Cancer Res* 2001;61:249–255.

58. Soria JC, Rodriguez M, Liu DD, et al. Aberrant promoter methylation of multiple genes in bronchial brush samples from former cigarette smokers. *Cancer Res* 2002;62:351–355.

59. Lamy A, Sesboue R, Bourguignon J, et al. Aberrant methylation of the CDKN2a/p16INK4a gene promoter region in preinvasive bronchial lesions: a prospective study in high-risk patients without invasive cancer. *Int J Cancer* 2002;100:189–193.

60. Belinsky SA, Palmisano WA, Gilliland FD, et al. Aberrant promoter methylation in bronchial epithelium and sputum from current and former smokers. *Cancer Res* 2002;62:2370–2377.

61. Schrump DS, Altorki NK, Forastiere AA, Minsky BD. Esophageal Cancer, in: *Cancer: Principles and Practice of Oncology, 6th ed.* DeVita VT, Hellman S, Rosenberg SA, eds. Lippincott, Williams & Wilkins Philadelphia, PA, 2001 pp.1051–1091.

62. Wong DJ, Paulson TG, Prevo LJ, et al. p16(INK4a) lesions are common, early abnormalities that undergo clonal expansion in Barrett's metaplastic epithelium. *Cancer Res* 2001;61:8284–8289.

63. Bian YS, Osterheld MC, Fontolliet C, et al. p16 inactivation by methylation of the CDKN2A promoter occurs early during neoplastic progression in Barrett's esophagus. *Gastroenterology* 2002;122:1113–1121.

64. Toyooka S, Pass HI, Shivapurkar N, et al. Aberrant methylation and simian virus 40 tag sequences in malignant mesothelioma. *Cancer Res* 2001;61:5727–5730.

65. Toyooka S, Carbone M, Toyooka KO, et al. Progressive aberrant methylation of the RASSF1A gene in simian virus 40 infected human mesothelial cells. *Oncogene* 2002;21:4340–4344.

66. Toyota M, Kopecky KJ, Toyota MO, et al. Methylation profiling in acute myeloid leukemia. *Blood* 2001;97:2823–2829.

67. Toyota M, Ahuja N, Ohe-Toyota M, et al. CpG island methylator phenotype in colorectal cancer. *Proc Natl Acad Sci USA* 1999;96:8681–8686.

68. Issa JP, Vertino PM, Wu J, et al. Increased cytosine DNA-methyltransferase activity during colon cancer progression. *J Natl Cancer Inst* 1993;85:1235–1240.

69. Robertson KD, Uzvolgyi E, Liang G, et al. The human DNA methyltransferases (DNMTs) 1, 3a and 3b: coordinate mRNA expression in normal tissues and overexpression in tumors. *Nucleic Acids Res* 1999;27:2291–2298.

70. Lee PJ, Washer LL, Law DJ, et al. Limited up-regulation of DNA methyltransferase in human colon cancer reflecting increased cell proliferation. *Proc Natl Acad Sci USA* 1996;93:10,366–10,370.

71. Sato M, Horio Y, Sekido Y, et al. The expression of DNA methyltransferases and methyl-CpG-binding proteins is not associated with the methylation status of p14(ARF), p16(INK4a) and RASSF1A in human lung cancer cell lines. *Oncogene* 2002;21:4822–4829.

72. Wu J, Issa JP, Herman J, et al. Expression of an exogenous eukaryotic DNA methyltransferase gene induces transformation of NIH 3T3 cells. *Proc Natl Acad Sci USA* 1993;90:8891–8895.

73. Beaulieu N, Morin S, Chute I, et al. An essential role for DNA methyltransferase DNMT3b in cancer cell survival. *J Biol Chem* 2002;277:28,176–28,181.

74. Laird PW, Jackson-Grusby L, Fazeli A, et al. Suppression of intestinal neoplasia by DNA hypomethylation. *Cell* 1995;81:197–205.

75. Belinsky SA, Nikula KJ, Baylin SB, Issa JP. Increased cytosine DNA-methyltransferase activity is target-cell-specific and an early event in lung cancer. *Proc Natl Acad Sci USA* 1996;93:4045–4050.

76. Malkinson AM. Primary lung tumors in mice: an experimentally manipulable model of human adenocarcinoma. *Cancer Res* 1992;52:2670s–2676s.

77. Horio Y, Chen A, Rice P, et al. K-*ras* and *p53* mutations are early and late events respectively in urethane-induced pulmonary carcinogenesis in A/J mice. *Mol Carcinog* 1996;17:217–223.

78. Lantry LE, Zhang Z, Crist KA, et al. 5-Aza-2'-deoxycytidine is chemopreventive in a 4-(methyl-nitrosamino)-1-(3-pyridyl)-1-butanone-induced primary mouse lung tumor model. *Carcinogenesis* 1999;20:343–346.

79. Hammond WG, Yellin A, Gabriel A, et al. Effects of 5-azacytidine in Syrian golden hamsters: toxicity, tumorigenicity, and differential modulation of bronchial carcinogenesis. *Exp Mol Pathol* 1990;53:34–51.

80. Yoder JA, Soman NS, Verdine GL, Bestor TH. DNA (cytosine-5)-methyltransferases in mouse cells and tissues. Studies with a mechanism-based probe. *J Mol Biol* 1997;270:385–395.

81. Howell CY, Bestor TH, Ding F, et al. Genomic imprinting disrupted by a maternal effect mutation in the Dnmt1 gene. *Cell* 2001;104:829–838.

82. Takagi H, Tajima S, Asano A. Overexpression of DNA methyltransferase in myoblast cells accelerates myotube formation. *Eur J Biochem* 1995;231:282–291.

83. Vertino PM, Yen RW, Gao J, Baylin SB. De novo methylation of CpG island sequences in human fibroblasts overexpressing DNA (cytosine-5-)-methyltransferase. *Mol Cell Biol* 1996;16:4555–4565.

84. Mikovits JA, Young HA, Vertino P, et al. Infection with human immunodeficiency virus type 1 upregulates DNA methyltransferase, resulting in de novo methylation of the gamma interferon (IFN-gamma) promoter and subsequent downregulation of IFN-gamma production. *Mol Cell Biol* 1998;18:5166–5177.

85. Li E, Bestor TH, Jaenisch R. Targeted mutation of the DNA methyltransferase gene results in embryonic lethality. *Cell* 1992;69:915–926.

86. Lei H, Oh SP, Okano M, et al. De novo DNA cytosine methyltransferase activities in mouse embryonic stem cells. *Development* 1996;22:3195–3205.

87. Chuang LS, Ian HI, Koh TW, et al. Human DNA-(cytosine-5) methyltransferase-PCNA complex as a target for p21WAF1. *Science* 1997;277:1996–2000.

88. Okano M, Bell DW, Haber DA, Li E. DNA methyltransferases Dnmt3a and Dnmt3b are essential for de novo methylation and mammalian development. *Cell* 1999;99:247–257.

89. Robertson KD, Keyomarsi K, Gonzales FA, et al. Differential mRNA expression of the human DNA methyltransferases (DNMTs) 1, 3a and 3b during the G(0)/G(1) to S phase transition in normal and tumor cells. *Nucleic Acids Res* 2000;28:2108–2113.

90. Rhee I, Jair KW, Yen RW, et al. CpG methylation is maintained in human cancer cells lacking DNMT1. *Nature* 2000;404:1003–1007.

91. Rhee I, Bachman KE, Park BH, et al. DNMT1 and DNMT3b cooperate to silence genes in human cancer cells. *Nature* 2002;416:552–556.

92. Ramchandani S, MacLeod AR, Pinard M, et al. Inhibition of tumorigenesis by a cytosine-DNA, methyltransferase, antisense oligodeoxynucleotide. *Proc Natl Acad Sci USA* 1997;94:684–689.

93. Milutinovic S, Knox JD, Szyf M. DNA methyltransferase inhibition induces the transcription of the tumor suppressor p21(WAF1/CIP1/sdi1). *J Biol Chem* 2000;275:6353-6359.

94. Fournel M, Sapieha P, Beaulieu N, et al. Down-regulation of human DNA-(cytosine-5) methyltransferase induces cell cycle regulators p16(ink4A) and p21(WAF/Cip1) by distinct mechanisms. *J Biol Chem* 1999;274:24,250–24,256.

95. Baylin SB. DNA Methylation: tying it all together: epigenetics, genetics, cell cycle, and cancer. *Science* 1997;277:1948–1949.

96. Chuang LS, Ian HI, Koh TW, et al. Human DNA-(cytosine-5) methyltransferase-PCNA complex as a target for p21 WAF1. *Science* 1997;277:1996–2000.

97. Jones PA, Taylor SM. Cellular differentiation, cytidine analogs and DNA methylation. *Cell* 1980;20:85–93.

98. Juttermann R, Li E, Jaenisch R. Toxicity of 5-aza-2'-deoxycytidine to mammalian cells is mediated primarily by covalent trapping of DNA methyltransferase rather than DNA demethylation. *Proc Natl Acad Sci USA* 1994;91:11,797–11,801.

99. Lee TT, Karon MR. Inhibition of protein synthesis in 5-azacytidine-treated HeLa cells. *Biochem Pharmacol* 1976;25:1737–1742.

100. Glazer RI, Peale AL, Beisler JA, Abbasi MM. The effect of 5-azacytidine and dihydro-5-azacytidine on nuclear ribosomal RNA and poly(A) RNA synthesis in L1210 cells in vitro. *Mol Pharmacol* 1980;17:111–117.

101. Cihak A, Vesely J. Prolongation of the lag period preceding the enhancement of thymidine and thymidylate kinase activity in regenerating rat liver by 5-azacytidine. *Biochem Pharmacol* 1972;21:3257–3265.

102. McGregor DB, Brown AG, Cattanach P, et al. TFT and 6TG resistance of mouse lymphoma cells to analogs of azacytidine. *Carcinogenesis* 1989;10:2003–2008.

103. Herman JG, Latif F, Weng Y, et al. Silencing of the VHL tumor-suppressor gene by DNA methylation in renal cell carcinoma. *Proc Natl Acad Sci USA* 1994;91:9700–9704.

104. Bender CM, Pao MM, Jones PA. Inhibition of DNA methylation by 5-aza-2'-deoxycytidine suppresses the growth of human tumor cell lines. *Cancer Res* 1998;58:95–101.

105. Bachman KE, Herman JG, Corn PG, et al. Methylation-associated silencing of the tissue inhibitor of metalloproteinase-3 gene suggest a suppressor role in kidney, brain, and other human cancers. *Cancer Res* 1999;59:798–802.

106. Plumb JA, Strathdee G, Sludden J, Kaye SB, Brown R. Reversal of drug resistance in human tumor xenografts by 2'-deoxy-5-azacytidine-induced demethylation of the hMLH1 gene promoter. *Cancer Res* 2000;60:6039–6044.

107. Takebayashi S, Nakao M, Fujita N, et al. 5-Aza-2'-deoxycytidine induces histone hyperacetylation of mouse centromeric heterochromatin by a mechanism independent of DNA demethylation. *Biochem Biophys Res Commun* 2001;288:921–926.

108. McCredie KB, Bodey GP, Burgess MA, et al. Treatment of acute leukemia with 5-azacytidine (NSC-102816). *Cancer Chemother Rep* 1973;57:319–323.

109. Von Hoff DD, Slavik M, Muggia FM. 5-Azacytidine. A new anticancer drug with effectiveness in acute myelogenous leukemia. *Ann Intern Med* 1976;85:237–245.

110. Karon M, Sieger L, Leimbrock S, et al. 5-Azacytidine: a new active agent for the treatment of acute leukemia. *Blood* 1973;42:359–365.

111. Saiki JH, Bodey GP, Hewlett JS, et al. Effect of schedule on activity and toxicity of 5-azacytidine in acute leukemia: a Southwest Oncology Group Study. *Cancer* 1981;47:1739–1742.

112. Vogler WR, Miller DS, Keller JW. 5-Azacytidine (NSC 102816): a new drug for the treatment of myeloblastic leukemia. *Blood* 1976;48:331–337.

113. Goldberg J, Gryn J, Raza A, et al. Mitoxantrone and 5-aza-cytidine for refractory/relapsed ANLL or CML in blast crisis: a leukemia intergroup study. *Am J Hematol* 1993;43:286–290.

114. Winton EF, Hearn EB, Martelo O, et al. Sequentially administered 5-azacitidine and amsacrine in refractory adult acute leukemia: a phase I-II trial of the Southeastern Cancer Study Group. *Cancer Treat Rep* 1985;69:807–811.

115. Rivard GE, Momparler RL, Demers J, et al. Phase I study on 5-aza-2'-deoxycytidine in children with acute leukemia. *Leuk Res* 1981;5:453–462.

116. Momparler RL, Rivard GE, Gyger M. Clinical trial on 5-aza-2'-deoxycytidine in patients with acute leukemia. *Pharmacol Ther* 1985;30:277–286.

117. Willemze R, Archimbaud E, Muus P. Preliminary results with 5-aza-2'-deoxycytidine (DAC)-containing chemotherapy in patients with relapsed or refractory acute leukemia. The EORTC Leukemia Cooperative Group. *Leukemia* 1993;7(Suppl 1):49–50.

118. Willemze R, Suciu S, Archimbaud E, et al. A randomized Phase II study on the effects of 5-Aza-2'-deoxycytidine combined with either amsacrine or idarubicin in patients with relapsed acute leukemia: an EORTC Leukemia Cooperative Group Phase II study (06893). *Leukemia* 1997;11:S24–S27.

119. Richel DJ, Colly LP, Kluin-Nelemans JC, Willemze R. The antileukaemic activity of 5-Aza-2 deoxycytidine (Aza-dC) in patients with relapsed and resistant leukaemia. *Br J Cancer* 1991;64:144–148.

120. Petti MC, Mandelli F, Zagonel V, et al. Pilot study of 5-aza-2'-deoxycytidine (Decitabine) in the treatment of poor prognosis acute myelogenous leukemia patients: preliminary results. *Leukemia* 1993;7(Suppl 1):36–41.

121. Schwartsmann G, Fernandes MS, Schaan MD, et al. Decitabine (5-Aza-2'-deoxycytidine; DAC) plus daunorubicin as a first line treatment in patients with acute myeloid leukemia: preliminary observations. *Leukemia* 1997;11:S28–S31.

122. Schiffer CA, DeBellis R, Kasdorf H, Wiernik PH. Treatment of the blast crisis of chronic myelogenous leukemia with 5-azacitidine and VP-16-213. *Cancer Treat Rep* 1982;66:267–271.

123. Dutcher JP, Eudey L, Wiernik PH, et al. Phase II study of mitoxantrone and 5-azacytidine for accelerated and blast crisis of chronic myelogenous leukemia: a study of the Eastern Cooperative Oncology Group. *Leukemia* 1992;6:770–775.

124. Kantarjian HM, O'Brien SM, Keating M, et al. Results of decitabine therapy in the accelerated and blastic phases of chronic myelogenous leukemia. *Leukemia* 1997;11:1617–1620.

125. Silverman LR, Holland JF, Weinberg RS, et al. Effects of treatment with 5-azacytidine on the in vivo and in vitro hematopoiesis in patients with myelodysplastic syndromes. *Leukemia* 1993;7(Suppl 1):21–29.

126. Silverman L, Holland J, Demakos E, et al. 5-azacytidine in myelodysplastic syndromes (MDS): the experience at Mount Sinai Hospital, New York. *Leuk Res* 1994;18:21.

127. Silverman LR, Demakos EP, Peterson B, et al. A randomized controlled trial of subcutaneous azacitidine (AZA C) in patients with myelodysplastic syndromes (MDS): a study of the cancer and leukemia group B. *Proc Amer Soc Clin Oncol* 1998;17:14a..

128. Wijermans PW, Krulder JW, Huijgens PC, Neve P. Continuous infusion of low-dose 5-Aza-2'-deoxycytidine in elderly patients with high-risk myelodysplastic syndrome. *Leukemia* 1997;11:S19–S23.

129. Wijermans P, Lubbert M, Verhoef G, et al. Low-dose 5-aza-2'-deoxycytidine, a DNA hypomethylating agent, for the treatment of high-risk myelodysplastic syndrome: a multicenter Phase II study in elderly patients. *J Clin Oncol* 2000;18:956–962.

130. Wijermans P, Lubbert M, Verhoef G, et al. DNA demethylating therapy in MDS—the experience with 5-aza-2'-deoxycytidine (decitabine). *Blood* 1999;94:306a.

131. Lubbert M, Wijermans P, Kunzmann R, et al. Cytogenetic responses in high-risk myelodysplastic syndrome following low-dose treatment with the DNA methylation inhibitor 5-aza-2'-deoxycytidine. *Br J Haematol* 2001;114:349–357.

132. Daskalakis M, Nguyen TT, Nguyen C, et al. Demethylation of a hypermethylated P15/INK4B gene in patients with myelodysplastic syndrome by 5-Aza-2'-deoxycytidine (decitabine) treatment. *Blood* 2002;100:2957–2964.

133. Cunningham TJ, Nemoto T, Rosner D, et al. Comparison of 5-azacytidine (NSC-102816) with CCNU (NSC-79037) in the treatment of patients with breast cancer and evaluation of the subsequent use of cyclophosphamide (NSC-26271). *Cancer Chemother Rep* 1974;58:677–681.

134. Weiss A, Stambaugh J, Mastrangelo M, et al. Phase I study of 5-azacytidine (NSC-102816). *Cancer Chemother Rep* 1972;56:413–419.

135. Weiss AJ, Metter GE, Nealon TF, et al. Phase II study of 5-azacytidine in solid tumors. *Cancer Treat Rep* 1977;61:55–58.

136. Bellet RE, Mastrangelo MJ, Engstrom PF, et al. Clinical trial with subcutaneously administered 5-azacytidine (NSC-102816). *Cancer Chemother Rep* 1974;58:217–222.

137. Sessa C, ten Bokkel HW, Stoter G, et al. Phase II study of 5-aza-2'-deoxycytidine in advanced ovarian carcinoma. The EORTC Early Clinical Trials Group. *Eur J Cancer* 1990;26:137–138.

138. Pohlmann P, DiLeone LP, Cancella AI, et al. Phase II trial of cisplatin plus decitabine, a new DNA hypomethylating agent, in patients with advanced squamous cell carcinoma of the cervix. *Am J Clin Oncol* 2002;25:496–501.

139. Thibault A, Figg WD, Bergan RC, et al. A Phase II study of 5-aza-2'deoxycytidine (decitabine) in hormone independent metastatic (D2) prostate cancer. *Tumori* 1998;84:87–89.

140. Moertel CG, Schutt AJ, Reitemeier RJ, Hahn RG. Phase II study of 5-azacytidine (NSC-102816) in the treatment of advanced gastrointestinal cancer. *Cancer Chemother Rep* 1972;56:649–652.

141. Abele R, Clavel M, Dodion P, et al. The EORTC Early Clinical Trials Cooperative Group experience with 5-aza-2'-

deoxycytidine (NSC 127716) in patients with colo-rectal, head and neck, renal carcinomas and malignant melanomas. *Eur J Cancer Clin Oncol* 1987;23:1921–1924.

142. Creagan ET, Schaid DJ, Hartmann LC, Loprinzi CL. A Phase II study of 5,6-dihydro-5-azacytidine hydrochloride in disseminated malignant melanoma. *Am J Clin Oncol* 1993;6:243–244.

143. Vogelzang NJ, Herndon JEI, Cirrincione C, et al. Dihydro-5-azacytidine in malignant mesothelioma: a phase II trial demonstrating activity accompanied by cardiac toxicity. *Cancer* 1997;9:237–242.

144. Samuels BL, Herndon JE, Harmon DC, et al. Dihydro-5-azacytidine and cisplatin in the treatment of malignant mesothelioma: a Phase II study by the Cancer and Leukemia Group B. *Cancer* 1998;82:1578–1584.

145. Momparler RL, Bouffard DY, Dionne J, et al. Pilot Phase I-II study on 5-aza-2'-deoxycytidine (Decitabine) in patients with metastatic lung cancer. *Anticancer Drugs* 1997;8:358–368.

146. van Groeningen CJ, Leyva A, O'Brien AMP, et al. Phase I and pharmacokinetic study of 5-Aza-2'-deoxycytidine (NSC 127716) in cancer patients. *Cancer Res* 1986;46:4831–4836.

147. Santini V, Kantarjian HM, Issa JP. Changes in DNA methylation in neoplasia: pathophysiology and therapeutic implications. *Ann Intern Med* 2001;134:573–586.

148. Schrump D, Fischette MR, Nguyen D, et al. Decitabine-mediated induction of tumor antigen and tumor suppressor gene expression in patients with inoperable thoracic malignancies. *Lung Cancer* 2002;38:S31.

149. Zhu WG, Lakshmanan RR, Beal MD, Otterson GA. DNA methyltransferase inhibition enhances apoptosis induced by histone deacetylase inhibitors. *Cancer Res* 2001;61:1327–1333.

150. Reid GK, Besterman JM, MacLeod AR. Selective inhibition of DNA methyltransferase enzymes as a novel strategy for cancer treatment. *Curr Opin Mol Ther* 2002;4:130–137.

151. Davis A, Moore MJ, Gelmon K, et al. Phase I and pharmacodynamic study of human DNA methyltransferase (MeTase) antisense oligodeoxynucleotide (ODN), MG98, administered as 21-day infusion q4 weekly. *Clin Cancer Res* 2000;6:P257.

152. Stewart D, Donehower RC, Eisenhauer E., et al. A Phase I pharmacokinetic and pharmacodynamic study of the DNA methyltransferase 1 inhibitor MG98 administered twice weekly. *Ann Oncol* 2003;14:755–774.

153. Schrump DS, Nguyen DM. Targets for molecular intervention in multistep pulmonary carcinogenesis. *World J Surg* 2001;25:174–183.

154. Schrump DS, Nguyen DM. Strategies for molecular intervention in esophageal cancers and their precursor lesions. *Dis Esophagus* 1999;12:181–185.

155. McGregor F, Muntoni A, Fleming J, et al. Molecular changes associated with oral dysplasia progression and acquisition of immortality: potential for its reversal by 5-azacytidine. *Cancer Res* 2002;62:4757–4766.

43 Targeting Histone Deacetylase as a Strategy for Cancer Prevention

Ho Jung Oh, PhD, Eun Joo Chung, PhD, Sunmin Lee, MS Andrea Loaiza-Perez, PhD, Edward A. Sausville, MD, PhD, and Jane B. Trepel, MD

CONTENTS

1. INTRODUCTION

Histone proteins were identified in 1884 *(1)*. For many years, the material that encoded genetic diversity was believed to consist of histones *(2)*. Posttranslational modification of histones by acetylation, and detection of histone deacetylase (HDAC) activity (enzymatic removal of acetyl moieties from internal lysines in the *N*-terminal tails of core histones), was described more than 40 years ago (reviewed in *3*), and more than 30 years ago, acetylation of histone tails was shown to be associated with transcriptionally active chromatin *(4)*. However, in the past 10 years, interest in HDAC has increased dramatically, both as a key component of the transcription-regulatory apparatus and as a target for anticancer drug development. The *Tetrahymena* Gcn5 protein, which is highly homologous to the well-characterized yeast transcriptional activator Gcn5, was discovered to be a histone acetyltransferase (HAT), thus providing a mechanism for linking histone acetylation with transcriptional activation *(5)*. Use of the HDAC inhibitor trapoxin in an affinity matrix to isolate and subsequently clone HDAC1 *(6)* revealed the relationship between HDAC1 and the yeast transcriptional repressor RPD3, providing a link between histone deacetylation and transcriptional repression. Contemporaneously, molecular genetic studies of acute promyelocytic leukemia (APL) demonstrated that the gene-encoding retinoic acid receptor alpha (RARα) is involved in a reciprocal chromosomal translocation, producing oncogenic fusion proteins that aberrantly repress retinoic acid-responsive promoters and obstruct normal myeloid differentiation via inappropriate recruitment of HDAC to RARα-responsive promoters, thus associating deregulated HDAC activity and cancer *(7)*.

It is now clear that HDACs and HATs are critical regulators of gene expression, that these enzymatic functions are frequently subverted in cancer, and that small-molecule drugs are available that have HDAC-inhibitory activity and promising activity in preclinical and early clinical trials. In light of their ability to selectively regulate gene expression, HDAC-directed agents have the potential to occupy an important niche in anticancer therapy, either as single agents or in combination. This review summarizes aspects of the

From: Cancer Chemoprevention, Volume 1: Promising Cancer Chemoprevention Agents
Edited by: G. J. Kelloff, E. T. Hawk, and C. C. Sigman © Humana Press Inc., Totowa, NJ

HDAC literature to facilitate evaluation of HDAC inhibitors as potential chemopreventive agents.

2. HISTONE ACETYLATION, CHROMATIN, AND GENE EXPRESSION

The mammalian genome is compacted in the nucleus by approx 100,000-fold, creating steric challenges for chromatin-templated functions, including transcription. DNA is organized around histone proteins in the nucleosome *(2)*, a dynamic structure that is essential in regulated transcription. The nucleosome core particle contains 146 basepairs of DNA wrapped around the histone octamer, composed of two copies each of core histones H2A, H2B, H3, and H4 arranged as an H3-H4 tetramer flanked by H2A-H2B dimers *(8)*. On either side of the core particle is approx 20 bp of linker DNA associated with linker histone H1. Among the most positively charged proteins in the cell, histones bind tightly to the negatively charged DNA-phosphate backbone. Core histones have a globular domain and a long, lysine-rich, positively charged amino-terminal tail, which contains sites for an array of posttranslational modifications, including acetylation, methylation, phosphorylation, ubiquitination, and ADP-ribosylation *(9)*. The combinatorial pattern of posttranslational modifications of the core histone tail acts as a flag for recruitment of chromatin-regulatory proteins, and thus affects most chromatin-templated processes. It has been speculated that this pattern of histone modifications forms a histone code, which dictates specific biological responses *(10)*. Signaling pathways that converge on gene-regulatory regions affect histone tail modifications. For example, mitogen-activated protein (MAP) kinase activation, an important signal-transduction response to extracellular cues, ultimately impacts transcription-factor activation as well as the state of histone modification of chromatin of promoters of MAP kinase-regulated genes *(11)*. There is also cross-communication between DNA methylation and the histone code status. Methylation of lysine 9 of histone H3 has been shown to be required for function of DNA methyltransferase (DNMT); thus, histone methyltransferase controls methylation-dependent gene silencing *(12)*. The layer of information encoded in posttranslational modifications of DNA and histones is referred to as the epigenome. Interestingly, science has moved from viewing histones as the actual genetic material, to regarding them as passive structural components, to an appreciation of the complexity and importance of modified histones in the regulation of gene expression.

Among histone tail modifications, acetylation has been the most intensively studied. Acetylation neutralizes positively charged lysines and reduces the affinity of histone amino-terminal tail domains for DNA. In general, histone acetylation is associated with an open chromatin configuration and active transcription, and histone deacetylation is associated with chromatin condensation and transcriptional repression. Acetylation of histone tails can remodel nucleosome structure locally, making DNA more accessible to the transcription apparatus. Interactions among nucleosomes further compact chromatin. Extended tails of core histones can reach to adjacent nucleosomes *(8)*, facilitating organization of chromatin into progressively higher-order states and resulting, for example, in the highly condensed metaphase chromosome. Thus, histone tail acetylation can weaken internucleosomal interactions and regulate higher-order states of chromatin condensation.

2.1. Histone Acetyltransferases

Two classes of enzymes, HATs and HDACs, reciprocally regulate the acetylation of histones. HATs have been divided into two categories based on subcellular localization *(13)*, although some HATs may function in multiple compartments *(14)*. A-type HATs are nuclear and acetylate chromatin-associated histones. B-type HATs are cytoplasmic and acetylate newly synthesized histones prior to their transport to the nucleus, where they are deacetylated and incorporated into chromatin *(15)*. Most human HATs are transcriptional coactivators that are recruited to chromatin by sequence-specific transcription factors and function as part of large, multi-protein activator complexes *(14)*. HATs have other substrates in addition to histones, including many transcription factors, as discussed in Subheading 2.3.

HAT proteins have been organized into families on the basis of conserved structural features. The GNAT (Gcn5-related *N*-acetyltransferase) superfamily includes GCN5 and the highly homologous p300/ CREB-binding protein (CBP)-associated factor (PCAF). The first identified A-type, transcription-related HAT was Gcn5 of *Tetrahymena* and yeast. The human homolog GCN5 *(16)* has HAT activity and is a transcriptional coactivator that occurs in multiple alternatively spliced versions. As indicated by its name, PCAF can be found in association with p300 and CBP *(17)*. The viral oncoprotein E1A competes with PCAF for binding to two other histone acetyltransferases, p300 and CBP. E1A inhibits PCAF-regulated gene expression, and exogenous expression of PCAF opposes the positive effect of E1A on cell-cycle progression, suggesting that targeting PCAF and p300/CBP may be a mechanism of viral oncogenesis *(17)*.

HATs often have substrate preferences. For example, PCAF acetylates both histone H3 and H4, but among the many available lysines, it preferentially acetylates lysine 14 of histone H3 and, less robustly, lysine 8 of histone H4 *(18)*. In addition to associating with p300 and CBP, PCAF can be found in the nucleus as part of the macromolecular PCAF complex, which consists of more than 20 polypeptides *(19)*. Linker histones inhibit the acetylation of mono- and oligonucleosomes, but this linker histone-mediated repression is overcome by the PCAF macromolecular complex *(20)*. PCAF functions in a HAT-dependent manner to regulate gene expression associated with myogenesis, nuclear hormone, and growth-factor signaling *(14)*.

The discovery that yeast transcriptional coactivator Gcn5 has HAT activity resulted in a search for HAT activity associated with other previously characterized coactivators. CBP and p300, closely related coactivators, were discovered to possess inherent HAT activity *(21,22)*. These proteins acetylate all core histones in free form or within nucleosomes. Ubiquitously expressed, they are potent acetyltransferases that act as global coactivators and regulate a variety of cellular events, including cell cycle, differentiation, and apoptosis *(23)*. CBP and p300 are recruited to DNA by an array of transcriptional activators, including c-Jun, c-Fos, CREB, and nuclear-hormone receptors. When tethered to DNA, these coactivators can hyperacetylate nucleosomal histones, facilitating chromatin remodeling and transcriptional activation. As described in Subheading 3, mutations and translocations involving CBP and p300 have been detected in human cancers, and in some cases these events appear to be critical to oncogenesis.

The MYST family is named for its principal members, monocyte leukemia zinc finger protein (MOZ), YBF2/SAS3, SAS2, and TAT-interactive protein-60 (Tip60). Tip60, the first identified human MYST protein, was found in a yeast two-hybrid screen for proteins that interact with HIV-1 transactivator protein Tat *(24)*. The Tip60 activated gene, superoxide dismutase (SOD), is repressed by Tat, and Tat-mediated repression is dependent on Tat inhibition of Tip60 HAT activity. Thus HIV-1 Tat appears to subvert the gene-expression program coactivated by Tip60 by inhibiting Tip60 HAT activity *(25)*. MOZ is a HAT involved in the 8;16 translocation of acute myeloid leukemia (AML), and in a leukemia-associated translocation with the co-activator TIF2, as described in Subheading 3.

The nuclear receptor coactivator family includes HATs, SRC-1, and ACTR *(14)*. SRC-1 interacts with a wide variety of nuclear receptors, including estrogen receptor (ER), retinoic acid X receptor (RXR), and glucocorticoid receptor, and stimulates ligand-dependent nuclear receptor transcriptional activation *(26)*. SRC-1 also interacts with other HATs, including p300/CBP and PCAF, and is itself a substrate for p300/CBP, suggesting that multiple HATs cooperate to regulate hormone signaling. Similarly, ACTR associates with multiple nuclear receptors, stimulates transactivation, and is a substrate for acetylation by CBP (*see* Subheading 2.3.).

TAF$_{II}$250 *(27)* and TFIIIC *(28)*, general transcription factors that possess HAT activity, further connect HAT activity with transcriptional regulation. TAF$_{II}$250 is a component of the TATA box-associated basal transcription factor TFIID, required for assembly of RNA polymerase II preinitiation complex and activation of mRNA synthesis. TFIIIC is a general transcription factor for transcription of tRNA precursors by RNA polymerase III; multiple TFIIIC subunits have been shown to have HAT activity. Nucleosomes are repressive to transcription, and acetylation of core histones within promoter-associated nucleosomes serves to destabilize nucleosome structure. Thus, the data suggest that for both pol II- and pol III-dependent transcription, HAT recruitment is part of the first step of transcription complex binding to DNA, and during this time, HAT activity serves to destabilize promoter-associated nucleosomes and relieve nucleosome-mediated transcriptional repression *(14)*.

2.2. Histone Deacetylases

Two families of eukaryotic deacetylases have been identified; the HDACs and the Sir2-like deacetylases or sirtuins, and these have been subdivided into three classes *(29,30;* Table 1). The first class of human HDAC to be isolated (Class I) has high homology to yeast Rpd3 protein and includes HDAC1, 2, 3, and 8, with molecular sizes ranging from 42–55 kDa *(6)*. Class I HDACs are nuclear proteins, and are expressed ubiquitously.

Class II HDACs (HDAC4, 5, 6, 7, 9, 10) are larger proteins (100–130 kDa) related to the yeast Hda1 protein, which can shuttle between the nucleus and cytoplasm *(31,32)*. Novel HDAC11 has properties of both Class I and Class II enzymes *(33)*. HDAC4, 5, and 7 harbor a highly conserved C-terminal catalytic domain and constitute a subfamily, whereas HDAC6 is distinct in containing a duplicated catalytic domain. The nuclear export of Class II HDACs has been associated with highly conserved serine residues among this class, and their association with 14-3-3 proteins *(34,35)*. The expression patterns of HDAC4, 5, and 7

Table 1
Histone Deacetylases

HDAC	Catalytic Domains	Chromosome	Protein Length (Amino Acids)	Subcellular Localization	Expression[6]
HDAC1	1	1p34.1	482	nuclear	ubiquitous
HDAC2	1	6q21	488	nuclear	ubiquitous
HDAC3[1]	1	5q31.1–5q31.3	428	nucleocytoplasmic shuttling	ubiquitous
HDAC8	1	Xq13	377	nuclear	ubiquitous
HDAC11[3]	1	3p25.1	347	nuclear/cytoplasmic	ND
HDAC4	1	2q37.2	1084	nucleocytoplasmic shuttling	tissue-specific
HDAC5	1	17q21	1122	nucleocytoplasmic shuttling	tissue-specific
HDAC6[4]	2	Xp11.23	1215	nucleocytoplasmic shuttling	tissue-specific
HDAC7[1]	1	12q13.1	952	nucleocytoplasmic shuttling	tissue-specific
HDAC9[1]	1	7p21–p15	1011	nucleocytoplasmic shuttling[5]	tissue-specific
HDAC10	1	22q13.31	669	nuclear/cytoplasmic[2]	ubiquitous
SIRT1	1	10q22.2	747	ND	ubiquitous
SIRT2	1	19q13	373	ND	ubiquitous
SIRT3	1	11p15.5	399	ND	ubiquitous
SIRT4	1	12q	314	ND	ubiquitous
SIRT5	1	6p22.3	310	ND	ubiquitous
SIRT6	1	19p13.3	355	ND	ND
SIRT7	1	17q25	400	ND	ND

[1] Isoforms reported.

[2] Nucleocytoplasmic shuttling has not been proven for HDAC10 but is likely to occur.

[3] Since HDAC11 shows conserved residues compared to both Class I and Class II HDACs, this classification was made based on amino acid length similarities.

[4] HDAC6 is primarily cytoplasmic.

[5] Alternative splicing of HDAC9 removes the nuclear localization signal from some of its isoforms.

[6] All tissue expression characterizations were made through the use of northern blots of human tissues except of HDAC7 in which mouse tissues were used.

are tissue specific, and heart, lung, and skeletal muscle show the greatest abundance of mRNA (36–40). Class II HDACs have been shown to regulate the activity of myocyte enhancer factor 2, a protein family involved in muscle differentiation and heart development (31, 41–43). Both Class I and II HDACs function, in part, through direct or indirect association with transcriptional corepressors, such as silencing mediator for retinoid and thyroid hormone receptor (SMRT), NCoR, and mSin3A (38,44). When recruited to chromatin, HDACs deacetylate histone tails and induce chromatin condensation and transcriptional repression. Few studies have demonstrated specificity of HDAC isozymes for gene-specific regulation. However, in yeast, cDNA microarray studies of cells with specific isozyme knockouts demonstrated distinct functions for Rpd3, Sir2 and Hda1 in cell-cycle progression, amino acid biosynthesis, and carbohydrate transport (45).

Sirtuins, the second family of deacetylases, can be divided into five classes based on their primary structure (46). They have a conserved 275 amino acid catalytic domain that is unrelated to the HDAC family, and a distinct catalytic mechanism. To catalyze deacetylation, HDACs activate a water molecule with a divalent zinc cation coupled to a histidine-aspartate charge-relay system (47). In contrast, sirtuins require hydrolysis of the adenosine 5' diphosphate (ADP)-ribose/nicotinamide glycosidic bond of one molecule of nicotinamide adenine dinucleotide

Table 2
FAT Substrates

Transcriptional Activators	Nonhistone Chromatin Proteins
p53 (165–167)	HMG1 (168)
b-Myb (169)	HMG2 (168)
c-Myb (170)	HMG14 (171)
GATA-1 (172,173)	HMG17 (52,171)
EKLF (174)	HMGI(Y) (55)
MyoD (59)	
E2F (57)	Coactivators
DTCF (175)	ACTR (176)
HIV Tat (177)	SRC-1 (176)
c-Jun (178)	TIF2 (176)
p50 (179)	PCAF (180)
YY1 (181)	p300
STAT6 (182,183)	PC4 (184)
IRF-2 (185)	β-catenin (186)
GATA-3 (187)	
Sp3 (188)	General Transcription Factors
NF-E2 (189)	TFIIE (190)
RelA (191)	TFIIF (190)
CIITA (192)	
Androgen receptor (193)	Others
	PRB (194)
	HNF-4 (195)
	Importin-α7, Rch1 (196)
	UBF (197)
	α tubulin (198)
	TAF(I)68 (199)
	RIP140 (200)
	Tal1 (201)
	Fen-1 (202)

(NAD) for each molecule of acetyl lysine that is deacetylated. Interestingly, because NAD is used as a substrate rather than as a component of the catalytic machinery, levels of NAD are related in a 1:1 manner to the level of Sir2-catalyzed deacetylation. This allows Sir2 to sense the intracellular level of NAD and to regulate transcription adaptively, consistent with the proposed link between Sir2 deacetylase and metabolic activity (48,49).

2.3. Factor Acetylation

HATs and HDACs can also acetylate and deacetylate non-histone substrates (14). This activity has been called factor acetyltransferase or FAT (50). Thus far, the majority of these substrates have been transcription-regulatory proteins. The impact of acetylation on protein function is not yet clear for every substrate. FAT protein substrates are listed in Table 2, and several are discussed here to give an idea of the range of impact of acetylation on protein function.

The first described non-histone nuclear substrates were the high-mobility group (HMG) class of architectural proteins that bind DNA and induce conformational changes in chromatin (51). HMG14 and 17 bind to nucleosomes through interactions with histone N-terminal tails and regulate higher-order chromatin structure. Acetylation of HMG17 has been shown to reduce its interaction with nucleosomes (52). The interferon-β enhanceosome, a macromolecular complex of activators and coactivators that control activated transcription, contains HMGI(Y) (53,54), a substrate for acetylation by PCAF and p300/CBP. Acetylation by p300/CBP but not by PCAF decreases the association of HMGI(Y) with transcription factors and with DNA. However HMGI(Y) acetylation by p300/CBP is required for full activation and termination of interferon-β gene expression, and PCAF is required for full activation but not termination (55).

Transcription factor E2F1, a critical regulator of cell cycle and apoptosis (56), is acetylated by PCAF; this acetylation increases the affinity of E2F1 for DNA, increases E2F1 half-life, and correspondingly enhances E2F1-activated transcription (57).

The activator myoD is required for transcription of muscle-specific genes (58). MyoD is acetylated by PCAF (59), requiring both p300/CBP and PCAF for its transcriptional activity (60,61). However, though PCAF HAT activity is required, p300 HAT activity is dispensable. Mutation of myoD lysines that are acetylated by PCAF to nonacetylatable arginines results in loss of transcription activity and failure of myogenesis (61).

Acetylation of the nuclear receptor coactivator HAT ACTR by p300 inhibits ACTR binding to nuclear receptors and induces loss of ACTR coactivation function. Thus, one HAT, p300, regulates activity of a second HAT, ACTR, through its FAT activity (14).

Tubulin, a cytoplasmic protein, is a substrate for deacetylation by the Class II enzyme HDAC6 (62). Associated with decreased cell motility and thus presumably decreased metastatic potential, acetylated microtubules are less dynamic *(63)*. Overexpression of HDAC6 promoted chemotactic cell motility. These data demonstrate that FAT activity can regulate non-transcriptional functions that are associated with features of the malignant phenotype.

3. HAT AND HDAC DEREGULATION IN CANCER

HAT inactivation through mutations, translocations, or expression of viral oncoproteins has been associated with various cancers *(64)*. Missense mutations or truncations of one p300 allele, frequently in association with inactivation of the other allele, have been detected in colorectal and gastric cancers *(65,66)*. Rubinstein-Taybi syndrome, a condition that predisposes to cancer, is characterized by functional inactivation of one CBP allele *(67)*. Viral oncoproteins such as SV40 T antigen and adenovirus E1A can bind to and antagonize the activity of PCAF, p300 and CBP, thus antagonizing coactivators that are critical in the action of tumor suppressors such as p53 and the growth-inhibitory TGFβ signaling pathway *(68)*. The majority of glioblastomas exhibit loss of heterozygosity of p300; loss of heterozygosity (LOH) around the CBP locus has been observed in hepatocellular carcinomas *(69)*.

A variety of chromosomal translocations involving p300 or CBP occur in leukemia *(69,70)*. The 8;16 translocation of AML fuses the HAT MOZ with the C-terminal 90% of CBP *(71)*. MOZ fusion with transcriptional intermediary factor-2 (TIF2) has also been observed in AML *(72,73)*, as have fusion of mixed-lineage leukemia (MLL) and CBP *(74)*, MLL and p300 *(75)*, and monocytic leukemia zinc finger protein-related factor (MORF) and CBP *(76)*. Translocations of CBP and p300 have been detected in treatment-related leukemia and myelodysplastic syndrome (MDS) *(77)*. These translocations are believed to affect transcription via inhibition of the HAT partner, or through fusion of the HAT to a DNA-binding protein such as MLL, resulting in aberrant activation of genes whose suppression is important for the non-transformed phenotype.

APL is a particularly compelling example of HDAC's role in malignant transformation. All patients with APL have a translocation involving RARα *(7)*. The t(15;17) translocation of APL produces a fusion protein of RARα and promyelocytic leukemia (PML) protein, and the APL t(11;17) translocation produces a fusion of RARα and PML zinc finger (PLZF). These fusion proteins bind to retinoic acid response elements in the promoters of genes that are believed to be critically important in myeloid differentiation. They are non-responsive to retinoic acid, the physiologic activator of RAR, but bind with high affinity to HDAC, inducing constitutive repression of RAR target genes and a block in myeloid maturation. HDAC inhibitors have been shown to restore the sensitivity of APL cells to retinoic acid ex vivo, and produced a prolonged response in one APL patient who was resistant to retinoic acid alone. The molecular and clinical studies in APL demonstrate the role of dysregulated histone deacetylation in leukemogenesis and the potential for its reversal with HDAC-targeted agents.

Further examples of HDAC deregulation in acute leukemia include the AML1-ETO and TEL-AML1 fusion proteins of AML and acute lymphocytic leukemia (ALL) respectively, in which the transcription factor AML1 is converted from an activator to a repressor through aberrant recruitment of HDAC by ETO and TEL *(78,79)*. In non-Hodgkin's lymphoma and diffuse large-cell lymphoma, chromosomal rearrangements within the LAZ3/B-cell lymphoma 6 (BCL6) promoter induce overexpression of BCL6, a potent transcriptional repressor that recruits HDAC through binding of corepressor proteins *(80)*.

Several signaling pathways further demonstrate the importance of HDAC in tumorigenesis. The proto-oncogene c-*myc* is overexpressed in many cancers as a result of translocations, gene amplifications, or activating point mutations. Myc activates the transcription of growth-promoting genes with its heterodimer partner Max. Myc/Max transcription is repressed by the heterodimer Mad/Max, which recruits HDAC to Myc-regulated promoters. The cellular protein c-Ski is a component of the mSin3/nuclear receptor corepressor (NCoR)/HDAC complex required for transcriptional repression by Mad. The oncogenic form of c-Ski, v-Ski, lacks the mSin3A-binding domain and acts in a dominant-negative manner to abrogate transcriptional repression by Mad *(81)*.

Two of the most important tumor suppressors, p53 and Rb, utilize HDAC to regulate gene expression. Transcriptional repression by p53 utilizes HDAC recruited by the corepressor Sin3A *(82)*. In turn, p53 is a substrate for acetylation; in response to stress, p53 is inactivated through deacetylation by the sirtuin Sir2, a mechanism for promoting cell survival *(83)*. The tumor suppressor Rb binds to the E2F family of cell-cycle transcription factors that regulate progression of cells into and through S-phase *(84)*. The Rb-E2F complex actively represses transcription at least in part through recruitment of HDAC *(85–87)*. This active repression by Rb-E2F is important for growth suppression by Rb *(88)*. Rb can form repressor complexes with BRG1 and hBRM, members of the SWI/SNF family of ATP-dependent chromatin remodeling factors that use adenosine 5' triphosphate (ATP) hydrolysis to reposition nucleosomes on promoters. Rb also forms a repressor complex with hSWI/SNF and HDAC, and another complex with only hSWI/SNF. The specific composition of these complexes serves to regulate the order of expression of cyclins and cyclin-dependent kinases (CDKs) during the cell cycle, and thus regulates cell-cycle progression *(89)*.

4. HDAC INHIBITORS

HDAC inhibitors can be classified into six structurally diverse classes (Table 3; *90*). They include: short-chain fatty acids, e.g., butyrate *(91)*; valproic acid *(92)*; hydroxamic acids e.g., trichostatin A (TSA) *(93,94)*; oxamflatin *(95)*; suberoylanilide hydroxamic acid (SAHA) *(96)*; cyclic tetrapeptides containing a 2-amino-8-oxo-9,10-epoxy-decanoyl (AOE) moiety e.g., trapoxin (TPX) *(97)*; cyclic peptides that do not contain an AOE moiety e.g., depsipeptide *(98)*; apicidin *(99)*; benzamides, e.g., MS-275 *(100,101)*; CI-994 *(102)*; and epoxides, e.g., depudecin *(103–105)*.

Butyrate, which has HDAC inhibitory activity, is generated by the fermentation of dietary fibers in the lumen of the large intestine. The aromatic fatty acids phenylbutyrate and phenylacetate, which have been used to treat patients with disorders of urea metabolism, have been evaluated in anticancer trials, as described in Subheading 6. Valproic acid, which was identified as an anticonvulsant, has been shown to have HDAC inhibitory activity at relatively high concentrations *(92,106)*. Short-chain fatty acids have a short plasma half-life and are the least potent of HDAC inhibitors, requiring millimolar plasma concentrations.

Essential characteristics of hydroxamic acid-based inhibitors are the polar hydroxamic group—a six-carbon hydrophobic methylene spacer, a second polar site, and a terminal hydrophobic group. Crystallographic studies of the hydroxamic-acid containing the HDAC inhibitors TSA and SAHA indicate that they inhibit HDAC by interacting with the catalytic site and blocking substrate access *(47)*. TSA, which was developed as an antifungal agent *(93)*, inhibits HDAC at nanomolar concentrations. It has relatively high reactivity and

instability, making it a poor drug candidate, but has been a useful probe of HDAC activity in vitro *(94)*. Oxamflatin inhibits HDAC activity at micromolar concentrations *(95)*. Cyclic hydroxamic acid containing peptide (CHAP) compounds, rationally designed hybrid derivatives of TSA and cyclic tetrapeptides, inhibit HDAC at nanomolar concentrations *(107)*. This is the first example of a synthetic HDAC inhibitor more potent than TSA. Extensive structure-activity studies performed to optimize hydroxamates such as SAHA, suberic bishydroxamic acid (SBHA), m-carboxy cinnamic acid bishydroxamic acid (CBHA), and pyroxamide have yielded some compounds with subnanomolar activity *(69)*.

Cyclic tetrapeptides containing an AOE moiety, which may mimic an acetylated lysine substrate, can also inhibit HDAC at nanomolar concentrations *(107)*. Trapoxin irreversibly inhibits HDAC activity at nanomolar concentrations by covalently binding to the enzyme catalytic site *(97)*. Cyclic peptides such as depsipeptide (also known as FK-228 or FR901228) isolated from *Chromobacterium violaceum (108)* and apicidin, which exhibits antiprotozoal activity, inhibit HDAC activity at nanomolar concentrations *(109)*.

A newly synthesized benzamide derivative with HDAC inhibitory activity, MS-275 (originally designated as MS-27-275) is believed to enter the catalytic site and bind the active zinc, inhibits HDAC at micromolar concentrations *(100,101)*. CI-994 (*N*-acetyl dinaline), originally synthesized as an anticonvulsant, does not seem to directly inhibit HDAC, but causes accumulation of acetylated histones by an unknown mechanism *(110)*. The naturally occurring epoxide depudecin irreversibly binds to HDAC *(105)* and inhibits its activity at micromolar concentrations.

4.1. Genes Regulated by HDAC Inhibitors

The anticancer effect of HDAC inhibitors is believed to derive largely from their ability to selectively regulate gene expression. First analysis of global transcriptional response to an HDAC inhibitor, which was performed by differential display of a limited number of genes, suggested that the response was limited to 2% of the genome *(111)*. A subsequent study performed by DNA microarray suggests that in a different setting the number of regulated genes may encompass 10% of the genome *(70)*. Analysis of genes regulated by HDAC inhibitors provides a clue to their mechanism of action and offers potential surrogate markers for monitoring drug effects in clinical trials. The genes associated with

Table 3
Histone Deacetylase Inhibitors

Classes	Name	Structure	Source	Inhibitory Conc	Activity** In vitro	Activity** In vivo	Activity** Clinical trials
Short-chain fatty acids	Butyrate Phenylbutyrate Valproic acid		Synthetic	mM mM mM	O O O	O O O	O O O
Hydroxamic acids	Trichostatin A (TSA)		Streptomyces hygroscopicus	nM	O	O	ND***
	Oxamflatin		Synthetic	μM	O	O	ND
	Cyclic hydroxamic acid-containing peptide (CHAP) compounds		Synthetic	nM	O	O	ND***
	Scriptaid		Synthetic	μM	O	O	ND***
	Suberoylanilide hydroxamic acid (SAHA)		Synthetic	μM	O	O	O

Class	Compound	Source				
	Suberic bishydroxamic acid (SBHA)	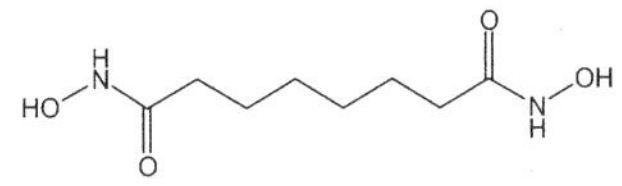 Synthetic	μM	O	ND	ND***
	m-Carboxy cinnamic acid bishydroxamic acid (CBHA)	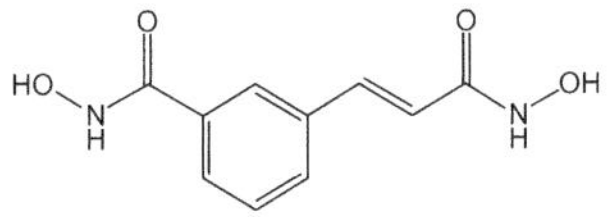 Synthetic	μM	O	O	ND***
	Pyroxamide	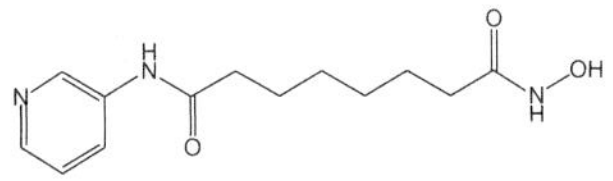 Synthetic	μM	O	O	O
Cyclic tetrapeptides containing an AOE*	Trapoxin (TPX)	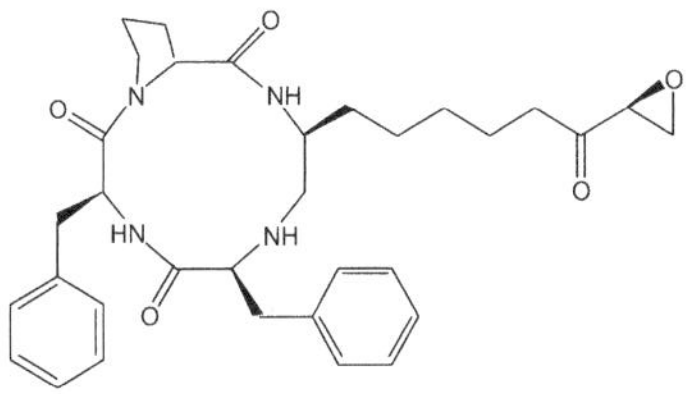 Helioma ambiens	nM	O	ND	ND***
Cyclic peptides not containing an AOE	Depsipeptide (FK-228, FR901228	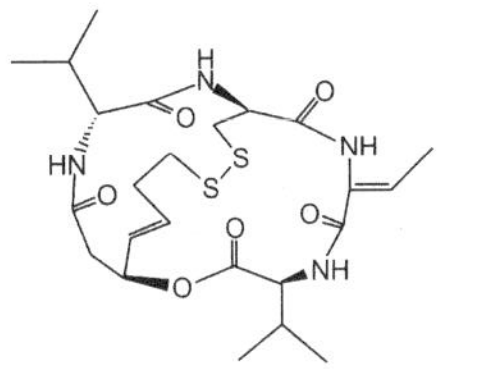 Chromobacterium violaceum	nM	O	O	O
	Apicidin	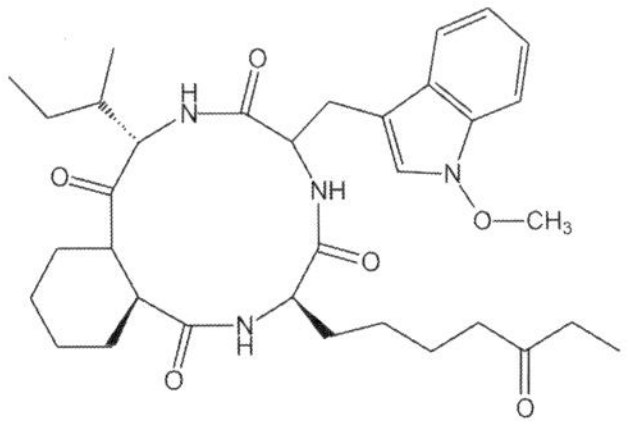 Fusarium species	nM	O	O	ND***
Benzamides	MS-275	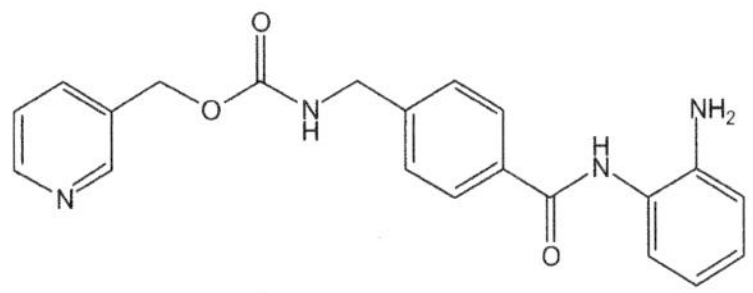 Synthetic	μM	O	O	O

667

(continued)

Table 3 (*continued*)

Classes	Name	Structure	Source	Inhibitory Conc	Activity**		
					In vitro	*In vivo*	*Clinical trials*
	CI-994 (*N*-acetyl-dinaline)		Synthetic	µM	O	O	O
Epoxides	Depudecin		Alternaria brassicicola	µM	O	O	ND***

* AOE: 2-amino-8-oxo-9, 10-epoxy-decanoyl moiety.
** Activity: shown to inhibit the growth of transformed cells in culture or in vivo timor growth in animal studies, phase I or II clinical trials
*** ND: no data reported.

differentiation, apoptosis, or growth arrest in tumor cells are common targets for regulation by HDAC inhibitors, as the inhibitors typically induce these processes. Numerous studies have reported the induction of differentiation markers in response to HDAC treatment, such as induction by SAHA of hemoglobin in MEL erythroleukemia cells, and milk proteins in MCF-7 breast carcinoma cells *(112)*. HDAC inhibitors have been reported to induce genes associated with the death-receptor pathway, such as *fas* and *fas ligand (113,114)*. In addition, HDAC inhibitors have been shown to upregulate the proapoptotic bcl2 gene, and downregulate the anti-apoptotic genes of the BCL2 family of the intrinsic apoptotic pathway *(115–117)*.

Perhaps the most universal target for transcriptional regulation by HDAC inhibitors is the cyclin-dependent kinase CDK inhibitor p21, which is markedly upregulated by HDAC inhibitors in association with p21 promoter histone hyperacetylation *(118)*. The induction of p21, along with downregulation of cyclin A and D expression, are probably central to the commonly observed loss of S-phase cells and growth arrest in response to HDAC inhibitor treatment *(119,120)*. Some tumor cells do not arrest in G_1 after HDAC inhibitors; they undergo apoptosis after progressing through S-phase, potentially after failing to trigger a G_2 checkpoint that is intact in normal cells and protects them from HDAC inhibitor-induced cell death *(70)*.

The HDAC inhibitor MS-275 upregulates signaling of the TGF-β pathway via transcriptional activation of the TGF-β type II receptor (TβRII) *(121)*, as a result of PCAF recruitment to the NF-Y complex on the type II receptor promoter and selective hyperacetylation of histones associated with the TβRII promoter *(122)*. TGFβ signaling is a potent negative growth regulator of epithelial cells. The loss of TGFβ signaling, typically through inactivation of the TβRII, is a hallmark of epithelially derived tumors. Although this gene is often inactivated by mutation, it is more often transcriptionally repressed in many forms of cancer, such as prostate cancer, and is therefore a potential candidate for reactivation by HDAC inhibitor treatment *(123,124)*.

HDAC inhibitors have also been shown to have the potential to boost tumor-cell immunogenicity through transcriptional activation of MHC Class I and II genes, costimulatory molecules (CD40, CD80, CD86), intercellular adhesion molecule ICAM1, and type I and II interferons *(70)*. HDAC inhibitors also modulate angiogenesis in a potentially therapeutic manner. HDAC1 downregulates expression of *p53* and the von Hippel-Lindau tumor-suppressor gene and stimulates angiogenesis of human endothelial cells. TSA upregulates p53 and von Hippel-Lindau expression, downregulates hypoxia-inducible factor-1α (HIF-1α) and vascular endothelial growth factor (VEGF), and blocks angiogenesis in vitro and in vivo *(125)*.

In addition to elucidating the genes regulated by HDAC inhibitors, several important issues are raised by expression profiling studies. Considering that most of the genome appears to be unaffected, what determines whether an individual gene will respond to an HDAC inhibitor? Are the histones associated with promoters of non-induced genes that are differentially non-acetylated in response to HDAC inhibitors, or are other factors such as other posttranslational modifications of histone or factor acetylation of greater regulatory significance? What is the molecular basis of gene downregulation by HDAC inhibition? Through the technique of chromatin immunoprecipitation *(126)*, polymerase chain reaction (PCR) amplification can now be used to approach these questions on a promoter-specific basis.

5. DIET AND MODULATION OF HDAC

In 1971, Dennis Burkitt first reported an epidemiologically based observation associating a high-fiber diet with a lower incidence of colorectal cancer (CRC) *(127)*. Evidence indicates that a diet high in fresh fruits and vegetables decreases risk of certain cancers, including CRC; these protective effects have been suggested to be the result of fiber, folate, and vitamins with antioxidant activity. Meta-analyses of observational epidemiologic and case-control studies have reported that dietary fiber provided a protective effect against colon cancer *(128,129)*. However, prospective data have not generally supported the hypothesis that either dietary or supplemental fiber is protective against development of colorectal adenomas or colorectal carcinomas *(130)*. Nevertheless, there is ample evidence that fermentation of dietary fiber in the lumen of the colon produces the short-chain fatty acid n-butyrate, which has anticarcinogenic activity on a variety of cellular functions, including differentiation, motility, invasion, adhesion, proliferation, and apoptosis. Experimentally induced, high fecal butyrate levels decrease tumor incidence and tumor growth *(131–133)*. Butyrate arrests the growth of neoplastic colonocytes and inhibits the preneoplastic hyperproliferation induced by some tumor promoters *(134)*. Butyrate induces differentiation of colon cancer-cell lines and regulates expression of several proto-oncogenes that are relevant to colorectal carcinogenesis in vitro *(135)*. Although the molecular mechanism by which butyrate mediates its effects are not fully understood, it is known to modulate activities in addition to HDAC, including DNA methylation *(136,137)*. Butyrate induces expression of the CDK inhibitor p21 through a process involving histone hyperacetylation and recruitment of Sp3 to the proximal p21 promoter *(138)*, and p21 is required for butyrate-mediated growth arrest in colon carcinoma cells *(139)*. Although p21 is a critical p53 target gene, p21 induction by butyrate and other HDAC inhibitors is p53-independent *(140)*. Thus HDAC inhibitors can induce p21-associated growth arrest in the absence of wild-type p53 function.

6. CLINICAL STUDIES WITH HDAC INHIBITORS

Despite intense biological interest in the cellular effects of HDAC inhibitors described in the previous section, advancing suitable candidates to the clinic is in the early stages. A number of studies have appeared with butyrates, phenylbutyrate, or tributyrin (as a prodrug for butyrates), and an initial Phase I evaluation of depsipeptide has recently appeared. However, initial studies with SAHA, pyroxamide, MS-275, and others are still in progress.

6.1. Butyrates and Derivatives

Initial enthusiasm for exploration of butyric acid as a differentiating agent in the clinic was fueled by Novogrodsky and colleagues, who reported a favorable yet limited response in a pediatric patient whose leukemia was treated with sodium butyrate *(141)*. This was followed up by more detailed studies *(142)* in Europe using the same regimen in adults with leukemia. This study documented that though concentrations of approximately 50 μ*M* could be achieved, this was unfortunately less than 10% of the butyrate concentrations needed to elicit differentiation in even the most sensitive preclinical models; moreover, the compound's half-life (~6 min) required continuous intravenous administration. Investigators in this country employed arginine butyrate infusions and defined administration schedules that achieved analogous concentrations of butyrate, but did demonstrate favorable modulation of Hgb F expression in patients with hemoglobinopathies *(143)*.

In an effort to define a potential oral-acting prodrug of butyrate, tributyrin, a triglyceride with three butyrate moieties per molecule, was shown to have potent differentiating effects and to be orally bioavailable. A Phase I trial of orally administered tributyrin once every 3 wk demonstrated that grade 3 toxicities of nausea, vomiting, and myalgia occurred at 400 mg/kg/d. Although a dose-limiting toxicity (DLT)-producing dose was not formally defined in this trial *(144)*, peak plasma butyrate concentrations were reached between 0.25 and 3 h, and ranged from 0–0.45 m*M*. As the latter concentration approached those necessary for recapitulation of in vitro differentiation effects, doses of 250–400 mg/kg/dose were considered suitable for devising more frequent administration schedules, although the capsule size and number of capsules required for the higher dose ranges (at 500 mg/capsule) were considered potentially problematic for widespread routine use.

Phenylbutyrate is a compound with the potential to act as a differentiating agent after hydrolysis of butyrate, although a clear delineation of its capacity to only affect HDACs as opposed to affecting pathways metabolizing amino acids is a matter of current research. A Phase I evaluation *(145)* of orally administered phenylbutyrate in patients with solid tumors revealed that a recommended Phase II dose of 27 g/d could be defined, and the most common toxicities were nausea or dyspepsia and fatigue; DLTs of nausea/vomiting and hypocalcemia were seen at 36 g/d. Interestingly, the ~0.5 m*M* concentration of phenylbutyrate achieved in this trial was quite close to the concentration that elicited cytotoxic and differentiating effects in vitro. When administered on a 120-h infusion schedule *(146)*, the dose was escalated from 150–515 mg/kg/d, and the DLT was defined as neuro-cortical effects, including somnolence and confusion, with the noteworthy occurrence of hypocalcemia, hyponatremia, and hyperuricemia. The maximum tolerated dose (MTD) was 410 mg/kg/d over a period of 5 d, at which the drug remained above the targeted 0.5 m*M* threshold for activity. This dose was used to construct a feasibility study *(147)* for more protracted administration schedules in patients with MDS and AML. Prolonged infusions of 14 or 21 d were well tolerated, with maintenance of the 0.5 m*M* target and only one of 23 patients experiencing dose-limiting neuro-cortical toxicity. Two patients on the 21-of-28 d schedule demonstrated some evidence of hematological improvement.

In summary, although certain butyrate derivatives and prodrugs do appear to achieve concentrations associated with differentiating activity characteristic of HDAC inhibition, the butyrates are generally cumbersome to use clinically, and therefore clinical interest in other chemotypes with HDAC inhibitor activity remains quite keen.

6.2. Depsipeptide

Clinical evaluation of depsipeptide (FR901228; NSC630176) is underway. In an initial Phase I study *(148)*, 37 patients received the drug as two 4-h infusions on days one and five, with each cycle intended to be repeated every 21 d. DLT was exceeded by 24.9 mg/m^2, and included fatigue, nausea and vomiting, thrombocytopenia, and atrial fibrillation. Non-dose-limiting ST-T wave flattening or inversions occurred at or below 17.8 mg/m^2, as well as non-dose-limiting neutropenia of relatively brief and clinically insignificant duration. Other toxicities included hypocalcemia and hypophosphatemia. The drug was cleared with a $t_{1/2}$ of ~8 h. Encouragingly, at 17.8 mg/m^2 there was clear evidence of induction of histone acetylation in either ex vivo treated reporter cells using patient plasma, or in patient's own peripheral-blood mononuclear cells (PBMC). Encouragingly, one patient with renal carcinoma attained a documented partial response. Noteworthy instances of activity in cutaneous T-cell lymphoma have also been achieved with variants of this schedule *(149)*.

6.3. Summary of Clinical Directions

Clearly, the full range of tools needed to explore the family of HDAC inhibitors is still being defined. Key issues in early clinical trials will be understanding which toxicities reflect an HDAC-related effect, and which reflect adventitious effects of the newer agents. Nonetheless, a real opportunity to bring a full range of biologic correlative tests to real-time use in the clinic presents itself with this class of agents, as well as their evaluation, should usefully incorporate as many of these biological correlates as possible at early phases of their clinical evaluation.

7. CONSIDERATIONS IN DEVELOPMENT OF HDAC INHIBITORS AS CHEMOPREVENTIVE AGENTS

Genetic changes are central to carcinogenesis. Therefore, a wide range of populations may benefit from HDAC-targeted intervention. MDS—clonal hematologic disorders characterized by ineffective hematopoiesis—have a natural history ranging from a chronic course that spans years to a rapid course of leukemic progression *(150)*. An estimated 15,000–20,000 new cases are diagnosed annually, which is probably an underestimate because patients with low-grade disease have few symptoms and subtle bone marrow changes *(151)*. At present, there is no Food and Drug Administration (FDA)-approved agent with an indication for this disease *(152)*. Bone marrow in MDS is hypercellular, with aberrant differentiation and concomitant bone marrow failure *(147)*. This observation, coupled with the ability of HDAC inhibitors to induce hematopoietic cell differentiation *(7,69,70,153)*, supports the investigation of HDAC inhibitors in MDS. In a completed Phase I study of MDS, prolonged infusion of sodium phenylbutyrate was well tolerated *(147)*.

Butyrate and butyrate analogs have been shown to decrease proliferation and induce differentiation in normal mammary epithelial cells and in breast cancer cells in vitro. These events are associated with down-regulation of cyclin D1 and ER expression *(154)*. Phenylbutyrate has been shown to inhibit proliferation of normal cells in the murine mammary gland in vivo *(155)*. When given in the diet continuously during carcinogenesis, SAHA has been shown to inhibit the development of *N*-methylnitrosourea (MNU)-induced rat mammary tumors *(156)*. The effect of SAHA was subsequently studied during initiation and progression phases, and its effects unexpectedly occurred at phases of tumor development subsequent to initiation. SAHA administered in the diet also inhibited growth of established tumors *(157)*. Their ability to arrest growth and induce differentiation in normal mammary epithelial cells and ER-positive and ER-negative breast cancer cells suggests that HDAC inhibitors may be useful as chemoprevention agents in women who are at high risk of developing breast cancer *(154)*. SAHA has also been reported to inhibit the development of lung tumors in mice induced by the tobacco smoke carcinogen 4-(methylnitrosamino)-1-(3-pyridyl)-1-butanone *(158)*.

Butyrate is a physiological regulator of colonic epithelial cell proliferation, differentiation, and survival. High-throughput microarray analysis of the impact of HDACs butyrate and TSA vs non-HDAC agents curcumin and sulindac in SW620 colon carcinoma cells has been used to identify agents for colon cancer chemoprevention. Expression profiling has the potential to predict mechanisms of action, potential toxicities, and potential synergies in prevention trials *(159)*.

An important issue in HDAC inhibitor development is identification of appropriate biomarkers to monitor response. Most studies currently monitor hyperacetylation of histones in PBMC chromatin. Although HDAC inhibitor activity can be monitored in this manner, several caveats should be considered. First, histone acetylation may be too sensitive, and thus may not be indicative of a therapeutic response (160). Second, chromatin of non-neoplastic, resting-state PBMC is likely to differ markedly from normal epithelial-cell chromatin, dysplastic epithelial cell chromatin, or epithelial tumor-cell chromatin. Gene-expression changes may be useful to monitor efficacy, but again, the transcriptional response of PBMC is potentially not a good indicator of epithelial cell response. Newer techniques for obtaining cells for study, such as ductal lavage or periareolar random fine-needle aspiration in breast cancer chemoprevention studies (161), may provide appropriate cells. It is also possible that histones are not the only or the most relevant protein substrate for determining a biologically effective dose; perhaps other substrates such as transcription factors, or even cytoplasmic proteins such as tubulin, should be evaluated. Proteomic analysis of the effect of different HDAC inhibitors on protein expression profiles and on protein acetylation will be helpful in identifying critical substrates.

Several of the large number of HDAC isozymes (48) have alternatively spliced isoforms. For example, the gene that encodes HDAC9 can generate six different proteins by alternative splicing, and transcript levels of the isoforms differs in different tissues (162). Splice variants of HDAC9 differ in function, and one variant, HDRP, is a transcriptional repressor without HDAC activity. Alternative splicing of HDAC9 could control intracellular localization and function, depending on whether the nuclear localization signal is spliced out (162). Considerably more research is needed to determine the distribution of HDAC isozymes in normal tissue and tumor cells. Studies are just beginning to identify the isozyme specificity of known HDAC inhibitors and design new inhibitors with isozyme specificity (48,107,109). Also be of interest is to search for polymorphisms that predict response to HDAC inhibitors. Discoveries in this field will be accelerated by development of tools for genome-wide genetic analysis of gene-based single nucleotide polymorphisms (SNPs) (163,164).

Inappropriate recruitment of HDAC to promoters of critical proliferation—or differentiation—regulatory genes is a continually recurring motif in neoplasia, suggesting that HDAC inhibitors have the potential to intervene in a wide variety of cancers. HDAC inhibitors are both important probes of the molecular mechanisms of carcinogenesis, and promising agents for intervention in carcinogenesis.

REFERENCES

1. Kossel A. Ueber einen peptoartigen bestandheil des zellkerns. *Z Physiol Chem* 1884;8:511–515.
2. Kornberg RD, Lorch Y. Twenty-five years of the nucleosome, fundamental particle of the eukaryote chromosome. *Cell* 1999;98:285–294.
3. Allfrey VA. Functional and metabolic aspects of DNA-associated proteins, in *Histones and Nucleohistones.* Phillips DMP, ed. Plenum Publishing Co., London, 1971, pp. 241–294.
4. Pogo BG, Pogo AO, Allfrey VG, et al. Changing patterns of histone acetylation and RNA synthesis in regeneration of the liver. *Proc Natl Acad Sci USA* 1968;59:1337–1344.
5. Brownell JE, Zhou J, Ranalli T, et al. *Tetrahymena* histone acetyltransferase A: a homolog to yeast Gcn5p linking histone acetylation to gene activation. *Cell* 1996;84:843–851.
6. Taunton J, Hassig CA, Schreiber, SL. A mammalian histone deacetylase related to the yeast transcriptional regulator Rpd3p. *Science* 1996;272:408–411.
7. Minucci S, Nervi C, Lo Coco F, et al. Histone deacetylases: a common molecular target for differentiation treatment of acute myeloid leukemias? *Oncogene* 2001;20:3110–3115.
8. Luger K, Mader AW, Richmond RK, et al. Crystal structure of the nucleosome core particle at 2.8 A resolution. *Nature* 1997;389:251–260.
9. Henry KW, Berger SL. Trans-tail histone modifications: wedge or bridge? *Nat Struct Biol* 2002;9:565–566.
10. Strahl BD, Allis CD. The language of covalent histone modifications. *Nature* 2000;403:41–45.
11. Hazzalin CA, Mahadevan LC. MAPK-regulated transcription: a continuously variable gene switch? *Nat Rev Mol Cell Biol* 2002;3:30–40.
12. Tamaru H, Selker EU. A histone H3 methyltransferase controls DNA methylation in *Neurospora crassa. Nature* 2001;414:277–283.
13. Brownell JE, Allis CD. Special HATs for special occasions: linking histone acetylation to chromatin assembly and gene activation. *Curr Opin Genet Dev* 1996;6:176–184.
14. Sterner DE, Berger SL. Acetylation of histones and transcription-related factors. *Microbiol Mol Biol Rev* 2000;64:435–459.
15. Chang L, Loranger SS, Mizzen C, et al. Histones in transit: cytosolic histone complexes and diacetylation of H4 during nucleosome assembly in human cells. *Biochemistry* 1997;36:469–480.
16. Candau R, Moore PA, Wang L, et al. Identification of human proteins functionally conserved with the yeast putative adaptors ADA2 and GCN5. *Mol Cell Biol* 1996;16:593–602.
17. Yang XJ, Ogryzko VV, Nishikawa J, et al. A p300/CBP-associated factor that competes with the adenoviral oncoprotein E1A. *Nature* 1996;382:319–324.

18. Schiltz RL, Mizzen CA, Vassilev A, et al. Overlapping but distinct patterns of histone acetylation by the human coactivators p300 and PCAF within nucleosomal substrates. *J Biol Chem* 1999;274:1189–1192.

19. Vassilev A, Yamauchi J, Kotani T, et al. The 400 kDa subunit of the PCAF histone acetylase complex belongs to the ATM superfamily. *Mol Cell* 1998;2:869–875.

20. Herrera JE, West KL, Schiltz RL, et al. Histone H1 is a specific repressor of core histone acetylation in chromatin. *Mol Cell Biol* 2000;20:523–529.

21. Bannister AJ, Kouzarides T. The CBP co-activator is a histone acetyltransferase. *Nature* 1996;384:641–643.

22. Ogryzko VV, Schiltz RL, Russanova V, et al. The transcriptional coactivators p300 and CBP are histone acetyltransferases. *Cell* 1996;87:953–959.

23. Chan HM, La Thangue NB. p300/CBP proteins: HATs for transcriptional bridges and scaffolds. *J Cell Sci* 2001;114:2363–2373.

24. Kamine J, Elangovan B, SubramanianT, et al. Identification of a cellular protein that specifically interacts with the essential cysteine region of the HIV-1 Tat transactivator. *Virology* 1996;216:357–366.

25. Westendorp MO, Shatrov VA, Schulze-Osthoff K, et al. HIV-1 Tat potentiates TNF-induced NF-kappa B activation and cytotoxicity by altering the cellular redox state. *EMBO J* 1995;14:546–554.

26. Onate SA, Tsai ST, Tsai MJ, O'Malley BW. Sequence and characterization of a coactivator for the steroid hormone receptor superfamily. *Science* 1995;270:1354–1357.

27. Mizzen CA, Yang XJ, Kokubo T, et al. The TAF(II)250 subunit of TFIID has histone acetyltransferase activity. *Cell* 1996;87:1261–1270.

28. Kundu TK, Wang Z, Roeder RG. Human TFIIIC relieves chromatin-mediated repression of RNA polymerase III transcription and contains an intrinsic histone acetyltransferase activity. *Mol Cell Biol* 1999;19:1605–1615.

29. Cress WD, Seto E. Histone deacetylases, transcriptional control, and cancer. *J Cell Physiol* 2000;184:1–16.

30. Gray SG, Ekstrom TJ. The human histone deacetylase family. *Exp Cell Res* 2001;262:75–83.

31. Wang AH, Bertos NR, Vezmar M, et al. HDAC4, a human histone deacetylase related to yeast HDA1, is a transcriptional corepressor. *Mol Cell Biol* 1999;19:7816–7827.

32. McKinsey TA, Zhang CL, Lu J, Olson EN. Signal-dependent nuclear export of a histone deacetylase regulates muscle differentiation. *Nature* 2000;408:106–111.

33. Gao L, Cueto MA, Asselbergs F, Atadja P. Cloning and functional characterization of HDAC11, a novel member of the human histone deacetylase family. *J Biol Chem* 2002;277:25,748–25,755.

34. Grozinger CM, Schreiber SL. Regulation of histone deacetylase 4 and 5 and transcriptional activity by 14-3-3-dependent cellular localization. *Proc Natl Acad Sci USA* 2000;97:7835–7840.

35. Zhao X, Ito A, Kane CD, et al. The modular nature of histone deacetylase HDAC4 confers phosphorylation-dependent intracellular trafficking. *J Biol Chem* 2001;276:35,042–35,048.

36. Grozinger CM, Hassig CA, Schreiber SL. Three proteins define a class of human histone deacetylases related to yeast Hda1p. *Proc Natl Acad Sci USA* 1999;96:4868–4873.

37. Verdel A, Khochbin S. Identification of a new family of higher eukaryotic histone deacetylases. Coordinate expression of differentiation-dependent chromatin modifiers. *J Biol Chem* 1999;274:2440–2445.

38. Kao HY, Downes M, Ordentlich P, Evans RM. Isolation of a novel histone deacetylase reveals that class I and class II deacetylases promote SMRT-mediated repression. *Genes Dev* 2000;14:55–66.

39. Fischle W, Emiliani S, Hendzel MJ, et al. A new family of human histone deacetylases related to *Saccharomyces cerevisiae* HDA1p. *J Biol Chem* 1999;274:11,713–11,720.

40. Fischle W, Dequiedt F, Fillion M, et al. Human HDAC7 histone deacetylase activity is associated with HDAC3 in vivo. *J Biol Chem* 2001;276:35,826–35,835.

41. Lu J, McKinsey TA, Zhang CL, Olson EN. Regulation of skeletal myogenesis by association of the MEF2 transcription factor with class II histone deacetylases. *Mol Cell* 2000;6:233–244.

42. Lemercier C, Verdel A, Galloo B, et al. mHDA1/HDAC5 histone deacetylase interacts with and represses MEF2A transcriptional activity. *J Biol Chem* 200;.275:15,594–15,599.

43. Bodmer R, Venkatesh TV. Heart development in *Drosophila* and vertebrates: conservation of molecular mechanisms. *Dev Genet* 1998;22:181–186.

44. Alland L, Muhle R, Hou H Jr, et al. Role for N-CoR and histone deacetylase in Sin3-mediated transcriptional repression. *Nature* 1997;387:49–55.

45. Robyr D, Suka Y, Xenarios I, et al. Microarray deacetylation maps determine genome-wide functions for yeast histone deacetylases. *Cell* 2002;109:437–446.

46. Frye RA. Phylogenetic classification of prokaryotic and eukaryotic Sir2-like proteins. *Biochem Biophys Res Commun* 2000;273:793–798.

47. Finnin MS, Donigian JR, Cohen A, et al. Structures of a histone deacetylase homologue bound to the TSA and SAHA inhibitors. *Nature* 1999;401:188–193.

48. Grozinger CM, Schreiber SL. Deacetylase enzymes: biological functions and the use of small-molecule inhibitors. *Chem Biol* 2002;9:3–16.

49. Imai S, Armstrong CM, Kaeberlein M, Guarente L. Transcriptional silencing and longevity protein Sir2 is an NAD-dependent histone deacetylase. *Nature* 2000;403:795–800.

50. Roth SY, Denu JM, Allis CD. Histone acetyltransferases. *Annu Rev Biochem* 2001;70:81–120.

51. Bustin M, Reeves R. High-mobility-group chromosomal proteins: architectural components that facilitate chromatin function. *Prog Nucleic Acid Res Mol Biol* 1996;54:35–100.

52. Herrera JE, Sakaguchi K, Bergel M, et al. Specific acetylation of chromosomal protein HMG-17 by PCAF alters its interaction with nucleosomes. *Mol Cell Biol* 1999;19:3466–3473.

53. Falvo JV, Thanos D, Maniatis T. Reversal of intrinsic DNA bends in the IFN beta gene enhancer by transcription factors and the architectural protein HMG I(Y). *Cell* 1995;83:1101–1111.

54. Thanos D, Maniatis T. Virus induction of human IFN beta gene expression requires the assembly of an enhanceosome. *Cell* 1995;83:1091–1100.

55. Munshi N, Merika M, Yie J, et al. Acetylation of HMG I(Y) by CBP turns off IFN beta expression by disrupting the enhanceosome. *Mol Cell* 1998;2:457–467.

56. Trimarchi JM, Lees JA. Sibling rivalry in the E2F family. *Nat Rev Mol Cell Biol* 2002;3:11–20.

57. Martinez-Balbas MA, Bauer UM, Nielsen SJ, et al. Regulation of E2F1 activity by acetylation. *EMBO J* 2000;19:662–671.

58. Puri PL, Sartorelli V. Regulation of muscle regulatory factors by DNA-binding, interacting proteins, and post-transcriptional modifications. *J Cell Physiol* 2000;185:155–173.

59. Sartorelli V, Puri PL, Hamamori Y, et al. Acetylation of MyoD directed by PCAF is necessary for the execution of the muscle program. *Mol Cell* 1999;4:725–734.

60. Puri PL, Avantaggiati ML, Balsano C, et al. p300 is required for MyoD-dependent cell cycle arrest and muscle-specific gene transcription. *EMBO J* 1997;16:369–383.

61. Puri PL, Sartorelli V, Yang XJ, et al. Differential roles of p300 and PCAF acetyltransferases in muscle differentiation. *Mol Cell* 1997;1:35–45.

62. Hubbert C, Guardiola A, Shao R, et al. HDAC6 is a microtubule-associated deacetylase. *Nature* 2002;417:455–458.

63. Piperno G, LeDizet M, Chang XJ. Microtubules containing acetylated alpha-tubulin in mammalian cells in culture. *J Cell Biol* 1987;104:289–302.

64. Kouzarides T. Histone acetylases and deacetylases in cell proliferation. *Curr Opin Genet Dev* 1999;9:40–48.

65. Giles RH, Peters DJ, Breuning MH. Conjunction dysfunction: CBP/p300 in human disease. *Trends Genet* 1998;14:178–183.

66. Gayther SA, Batley SJ, Linger L, et al. Mutations truncating the EP300 acetylase in human cancers. *Nat Genet* 2000;24:300–303.

67. Petrij F, Giles RH, Dauwerse HG, et al. Rubinstein-Taybi syndrome caused by mutations in the transcriptional co-activator CBP. *Nature* 1995;376:348–351.

68. Chakravarti D, Ogryzko V, Kao HY, et al. A viral mechanism for inhibition of p300 and PCAF acetyltransferase activity. *Cell* 1999;96:393–403.

69. Marks P, Rifkind RA, Richon VM, et al. Histone deacetylases and cancer: causes and therapies. *Nature Rev Cancer* 2001;1:194–202.

70. Johnstone RW. Histone-deacetylase inhibitors: novel drugs for the treatment of cancer. *Nat Rev Drug Discov* 2002;1:287–299.

71. Borrow J, Stanton VP Jr, Andresen JM, et al. The translocation t(8;16)(p11;p13) of acute myeloid leukaemia fuses a putative acetyltransferase to the CREB-binding protein. *Nat Genet* 1996;14:33–41.

72. Carapeti M, Aguiar RC, Goldman JM, Cross NC. A novel fusion between MOZ and the nuclear receptor coactivator TIF2 in acute myeloid leukemia. *Blood* 1998;91:3127–3133.

73. Liang J, Prouty L, Williams BJ, et al. Acute mixed lineage leukemia with an inv(8)(p11q13) resulting in fusion of the genes for MOZ and TIF2. *Blood* 1998;92:2118–2122.

74. Taki T, Sako M, Tsuchida M, Hayashi Y. The t(11;16)(q23;p13) translocation in myelodysplastic syndrome fuses the MLL gene to the CBP gene. *Blood* 1997;89:3945–3950.

75. Ida K, Kitabayashi I, Taki T, et al. Adenoviral E1A-associated protein p300 is involved in acute myeloid leukemia with t(11;22)(q23;q13). *Blood* 1997;90:4699–4704.

76. Panagopoulos I, Fioretos T, Isaksson M, et al. Fusion of the MORF and CBP genes in acute myeloid leukemia with the t(10;16)(q22;p13). *Hum Mol Genet* 2001;10:395–404.

77. Rowley JD, Reshmi S, Sobulo O, et al. All patients with the T(11;16)(q23;p13.3) that involves MLL and CBP have treatment-related hematologic disorders. *Blood* 1997;90:535–541.

78. Heibert SW, Lutterbach B, Durst K, et al. Mechanisms of transcriptional repression by the t(8;21)-, t(12;21)-, and inv(16)-encoded fusion proteins. *Cancer Chemother Pharmacol* 2001;48 Suppl 1:S31–S34.

79. Licht JD. AML1 and the AML1-ETO fusion protein in the pathogenesis of t(8;21) AML. *Oncogene* 2001;20:5660–5679.

80. Dhordain P, Albagli O, Lin RJ, et al. Corepressor SMRT binds the BTB/POZ repressing domain of the LAZ3/BCL6 oncoprotein. *Proc Natl Acad Sci USA* 1997;94:10,762–10,767.

81. Nomura T, Khan MM, Kaul SC, et al. Ski is a component of the histone deacetylase complex required for transcriptional repression by Mad and thyroid hormone receptor. *Genes Dev* 1999;13:412–423.

82. Murphy M, Ahn J, Walker KK, et al. Transcriptional repression by wild-type p53 utilizes histone deacetylases, mediated by interaction with mSin3a. *Genes Dev* 1999;13:2490–2501.

83. Luo J, Nikolaev AY, Imai S, et al. Negative control of p53 by Sir2alpha promotes cell survival under stress. *Cell* 2001;107:137–148.

84. Nevins JR. E2F: a link between the Rb tumor suppressor protein and viral oncoproteins. *Science* 1992;258:424–429.

85. Brehm A, Miska EA, McCance DJ, et al. Retinoblastoma protein recruits histone deacetylase to repress transcription. *Nature* 1998;391:597–601.

86. Luo RX, Postigo AA, Dean DC. Rb interacts with histone deacetylase to repress transcription. *Cell* 1998;92:463–473.

87. Magnaghi-Jaulin L, Groisman R, Naguibneva I, et al. Retinoblastoma protein represses transcription by recruiting a histone deacetylase. *Nature* 1998;391:601–605.

88. Zhang HS, Postigo AA, Dean DC. Active transcriptional repression by the Rb-E2F complex mediates G_1 arrest triggered by p16INK4a, TGFbeta, and contact inhibition. *Cell* 1999;97:53–61.

89. Zhang HS, Gavin M, Dahiya A, et al. Exit from G_1 and S phase of the cell cycle is regulated by repressor complexes containing HDAC-Rb-hSWI/SNF and Rb-hSWI/SNF. *Cell* 2000;101:79–89.

90. Vigushin DM, Coombes RC. Histone deacetylase inhibitors in cancer treatment. *Anticancer Drugs* 2002;13:1–13.

91. Warrell RP Jr, He LZ, Richon V, et al. Therapeutic targeting of transcription in acute promyelocytic leukemia by use of an inhibitor of histone deacetylase. *J Natl Cancer Inst* 1998;90:1621–1625.

92. Gottlicher M, Minuci S, Zhu P, et al. Valproic acid defines a novel class of HDAC inhibitors inducing differentiation of transformed cells. *EMBO J* 2001;20:6969–6978.

93. Tsuji N, Kobayashi M, Nagashima K, et al. A new antifungal antibiotic, trichostatin. *J Antibiot (Tokyo)* 1976;29:1–6.

94. Yoshida M, Kijima M, Akita M, Beppu T. Potent and specific inhibition of mammalian histone deacetylase both in vivo and in vitro by trichostatin A. *J Biol Chem* 1990;265:17,174–17,179.

95. Kim YB, Lee KH, Sugita K, et al. Oxamflatin is a novel antitumor compound that inhibits mammalian histone deacetylase. *Oncogene* 1999;18:2461–2470.

96. Richon VM, Emiliani S, Verdin E, et al. A class of hybrid polar inducers of transformed cell differentiation inhibits

histone deacetylases. *Proc Natl Acad Sci USA* 1998;95:3003–3007.

97. Kijima M, Yoshida M, Sugita K, et al. Trapoxin, an antitumor cyclic tetrapeptide, is an irreversible inhibitor of mammalian histone deacetylase. *J Biol Chem* 1993;268:22,429–22,435.

98. Nakajima H, Kim YB, Terano H, et al. FR901228, a potent antitumor antibiotic, is a novel histone deacetylase inhibitor. *Exp Cell Res* 1998;241:126–133.

99. Darkin-Rattray SJ, Gurnett AM, Myers RW, et al. Apicidin: a novel antiprotozoal agent that inhibits parasite histone deacetylase. *Proc Natl Acad Sci USA* 1996;93:13,143–13,147.

100. Suzuki T, Ando T, Tsuchiya K, et al. Synthesis and histone deacetylase inhibitory activity of new benzamide derivatives. *J Med Chem* 1999;42:3001–3003.

101. Saito A, Yamashita T, Mariko Y, et al. A synthetic inhibitor of histone deacetylase, MS-27-275, with marked in vivo antitumor activity against human tumors. *Proc Natl Acad Sci USA* 1999;96:4592–4597.

102. el-Beltagi HM, Martens AC, Lelieveld P, et al. Acetyldinaline: a new oral cytostatic drug with impressive differential activity against leukemic cells and normal stem cells—preclinical studies in a relevant rat model for human acute myelocytic leukemia. *Cancer Res* 1993;53:3008–3014.

103. Oikawa T, Onozawa C, Inose M, Sasaki M. Depudecin, a microbial metabolite containing two epoxide groups, exhibits anti-angiogenic activity in vivo. *Biol Pharm Bull* 1995;18:1305–1307.

104. Shimada J, Kwon HJ, Sawamura M, Schreiber SL. Synthesis and cellular characterization of the detransformation agent, (–)-depudecin. *Chem Biol* 1995;2:517–525.

105. Kwon HJ, Owa T, Hassig CA, et al. Depudecin induces morphological reversion of transformed fibroblasts via the inhibition of histone deacetylase. *Proc Natl Acad Sci USA* 1998;95:3356–3361.

106. Phiel CJ, Zhang F, Huang EY, et al. Histone deacetylase is a direct target of valproic acid, a potent anticonvulsant, mood stabilizer, and teratogen. *J Biol Chem* 2001;276: 36,734–36,741.

107. Furumai R, Komatsu Y, Nishino N, et al. Potent histone deacetylase inhibitors built from trichostatin A and cyclic tetrapeptide antibiotics including trapoxin. *Proc Natl Acad Sci USA* 2001;98:87–92.

108. Ueda H, Manda T, Matsumoto S, et al. FR901228, a novel antitumor bicyclic depsipeptide produced by *Chromobacterium violaceum* No. 968. III. Antitumor activities on experimental tumors in mice. *J Antibiot (Tokyo)* 1994;47:315–323.

109. Furumai R, Matsuyama A, Kobashi N, et al. FK228 (depsipeptide) as a natural prodrug that inhibits class I histone deacetylases. *Cancer Res* 2002;62:4916–4921.

110. Prakash S, Foster BJ, Meyer M, et al. Chronic oral administration of CI-994: a phase 1 study. *Investig New Drugs* 2001;19:1–11.

111. Van Lint C, Emiliani S, Verdin E. The expression of a small fraction of cellular genes is changed in response to histone hyperacetylation. *Gene Expr* 1996;5:245–253.

112. Marks PA, Richon VM, Rifkind RA. Histone deacetylase inhibitors: inducers of differentiation or apoptosis of transformed cells. *J Natl Cancer Inst* 2000;92:1210–1216.

113. Kwon SH, Ahn SH, Kim YK, et al. Apicidin, a histone deacetylase inhibitor, induces apoptosis and Fas/Fas ligand expression in human acute promyelocytic leukemia cells. *J Biol Chem* 2002;277:2073–2080.

114. Glick RD, Swendeman SL, Coffey DC, et al. Hybrid polar histone deacetylase inhibitor induces apoptosis and CD95/CD95 ligand expression in human neuroblastoma. *Cancer Res* 1999;59:4392–4399.

115. Ruefli AA, Ausserlechner MJ, Bernhard D, et al. The histone deacetylase inhibitor and chemotherapeutic agent suberoylanilide hydroxamic acid (SAHA) induces a cell-death pathway characterized by cleavage of Bid and production of reactive oxygen species. *Proc Natl Acad Sci USA* 2001;98:10,833–10,838.

116. Suzuki T, Yokozaki H, Kuniyasu H, et al. Effect of trichostatin A on cell growth and expression of cell cycle- and apoptosis-related molecules in human gastric and oral carcinoma cell lines. *Int J Cancer* 2000;88:992–997.

117. Cao XX, Mohuiddin I, Ece F, et al. Histone deacetylase inhibitor downregulation of bcl-xl gene expression leads to apoptotic cell death in mesothelioma. *Am J Respir Cell Mol Biol* 2001;25:562–568.

118. Richon VM, Sandhoff TW, Rifkind RA, Marks PA. Histone deacetylase inhibitor selectively induces p21WAF1 expression and gene-associated histone acetylation. *Proc Natl Acad Sci USA* 2000;97:10,014–10,019.

119. Sandor V, Senderowicz A, Mertins S, et al. P21-dependent g(1)arrest with downregulation of cyclin D1 and upregulation of cyclin E by the histone deacetylase inhibitor FR901228. *Br J Cancer* 2000;83:817–825.

120. Rosato RR, Wang Z, Gopalkrishnan RV, et al. Evidence of a functional role for the cyclin-dependent kinase-inhibitor p21WAF1/CIP1/MDA6 in promoting differentiation and preventing mitochondrial dysfunction and apoptosis induced by sodium butyrate in human myelomonocytic leukemia cells (U937). *Int J Oncol* 2001;19:181–191.

121. Lee BI, Park SH, Kim JW, et al. MS-275, a histone deacetylase inhibitor, selectively induces transforming growth factor beta type II receptor expression in human breast cancer cells. *Cancer Res* 2001;61:931–934.

122. Park SH, Lee SR, Kim BC, et al. Transcriptional regulation of the transforming growth factor beta type II receptor gene by histone acetyltransferase and deacetylase is mediated by NF-Y in human breast cancer cells. *J Biol Chem* 2002;277:5168–5174.

123. Park K, Kim SJ, Bang YJ, et al. Genetic changes in the transforming growth factor beta (TGF-beta) type II receptor gene in human gastric cancer cells: correlation with sensitivity to growth inhibition by TGF-beta. *Proc Natl Acad Sci USA* 1994;91:8772–8776.

124. Markowitz S, Wang J, Myeroff L, et al. Inactivation of the type II TGF-beta receptor in colon cancer cells with microsatellite instability. *Science* 1995;268:1336–1338.

125. Kim MS, Kwon JH, Lee YM, et al. Histone deacetylases induce angiogenesis by negative regulation of tumor suppressor genes. *Nat Med* 2001;7:437–443.

126. Kuo MH, Allis CD. In vivo cross-linking and immunoprecipitation for studying dynamic protein:DNA associations in a chromatin environment. *Methods* 1999;19:425–433.

127. Lewin MR. Is there a fibre-depleted aetiology for colorectal cancer? Experimental evidence. *Rev Environ Health* 1991;9:17–30.

128. Trock B, Lanza E, Greenwald P. Dietary fiber, vegetables, and colon cancer: critical review and meta-analyses of the

epidemiologic evidence. *J Natl Cancer Inst* 1990;82:650–661.

129. Howe GR, Benito E, Castelleto R, et al. Dietary intake of fiber and decreased risk of cancers of the colon and rectum: evidence from the combined analysis of 13 case-control studies. *J Natl Cancer Inst* 1992;84:1887–1896.

130. Janne PA, Mayer RJ. Chemoprevention of colorectal cancer. *N Engl J Med* 2000;342:1960–1968.

131. McIntyre A, Gibson PR, Young GP. Butyrate production from dietary fibre and protection against large bowel cancer in a rat model. *Gut* 1993;34:386–391.

132. Cassidy A, Bingham SA, Cummings JH. Starch intake and colorectal cancer risk: an international comparison. *Br J Cancer* 1994;69:937–942.

133. Hylla S, Gostner A, Dusel G, et al. Effects of resistant starch on the colon in healthy volunteers: possible implications for cancer prevention. *Am J Clin Nutr* 1998;67:136–142.

134. Bartram HP, Englert S, Scheppach W, et al. Antagonistic effects of deoxycholic acid and butyrate on epithelial cell proliferation in the proximal and distal human colon. *Z Gastroenterol* 1994;32:389–392.

135. Young GP, Gibson PR. Butyrate and colorectal cancer cell, in *Short-Chain Fatty Acids, Vol. 6.* Binder JH, Cummings JH, Soergel KH, eds. Kluwer, Boston, MA, 1994, pp. 148–160.

136. Riggs MG, Whitaker RG, Neumann JR, Ingram VM. n-Butyrate causes histone modification in HeLa and Friend erythroleukaemia cells. *Nature* 1977;268:462–464.

137. de Haan JB, Gevers W, Parker MI. Effects of sodium butyrate on the synthesis and methylation of DNA in normal cells and their transformed counterparts. *Cancer Res* 1986;46:713–716.

138. Sowa Y, Orita T, Minamikawa-Hiranabe S, et al. Sp3, but not Sp1, mediates the transcriptional activation of the p21/WAF1/Cip1 gene promoter by histone deacetylase inhibitor. *Cancer Res* 1999;59:4266–4270.

139. Archer SY, Meng S, Shei A, Hodin RA. p21(WAF1) is required for butyrate-mediated growth inhibition of human colon cancer cells. *Proc Natl Acad Sci USA* 1998;95:6791–6796.

140. Xiao H, Hasegawa T, Miyaishi O, et al. Sodium butyrate induces NIH3T3 cells to senescence-like state and enhances promoter activity of p21WAF/CIP1 in p53-independent manner. *Biochem Biophys Res Commun* 1997;237:457–460.

141. Novogrodsky A, Dvir A, Ravid A, et al. Effect of polar organic compounds on leukemic cells. Butyrate-induced partial remission of acute myelogenous leukemia in a child. *Cancer* 1983;51:9–14.

142. Miller AA, Kurschel E, Osieka R, Schmidt CG. Clinical pharmacology of sodium butyrate in patients with acute leukemia. *Eur J Cancer Clin Oncol* 1987;23:1283–1287.

143. Perrine SP, Ginder GD, Faller DV, et al. A short-term trial of butyrate to stimulate fetal-globin-gene expression in the beta-globin disorders. *N Engl J Med* 1993;328:81–86.

144. Conley BA, Egorin MJ, Tait N, et al. Phase I study of the orally administered butyrate prodrug, tributyrin, in patients with solid tumors. *Clin Cancer Res* 1998;4:629–634.

145. Gilbert J, Baker SD, Bowling MK, et al. A phase I dose escalation and bioavailability study of oral sodium phenylbutyrate in patients with refractory solid tumor malignancies. *Clin Cancer Res* 2001;7:2292–2300.

146. Carducci MA, Gilbert J, Bowling MK, et al. A Phase I clinical and pharmacological evaluation of sodium phenylbutyrate on an 120-h infusion schedule. *Clin Cancer Res* 2001;7:3047–3055.

147. Gore SD, Weng LJ, Figg WD, et al. Impact of prolonged infusions of the putative differentiating agent sodium phenylbutyrate on myelodysplastic syndromes and acute myeloid leukemia. *Clin Cancer Res* 2002;8:963–970.

148. Sandor V, Bakke S, Robey RW, et al. Phase I trial of the histone deacetylase inhibitor, depsipeptide (FR901228, NSC 630176), in patients with refractory neoplasms. *Clin Cancer Res* 2002;8:718–728.

149. Piekarz RL, Robey R, Sandor V, et al. Inhibitor of histone deacetylation, depsipeptide (FR901228), in the treatment of peripheral and cutaneous T-cell lymphoma: a case report. *Blood* 2001;98:2865–2868.

150. Heaney ML, Golde DW. Myelodysplasia. *N Engl J Med* 1999;340:1649–1660.

151. Aul C, Germing U, Gattermann N, Minning H. Increasing incidence of myelodysplastic syndromes: real or fictitious? *Leuk Res* 1998;22:93–100.

152. List AF. New approaches to the treatment of myelodysplasia. *Oncologist* 2002;7 Suppl 1:39–49.

153. Melnick A, Licht JD. Histone deacetylases as therapeutic targets in hematologic malignancies. *Curr Opin Hematol* 2002;9:322–332.

154. Davis T, Kennedy C, Chiew YE, et al. Histone deacetylase inhibitors decrease proliferation and modulate cell cycle gene expression in normal mammary epithelial cells. *Clin Cancer Res* 2000;6:4334–4342.

155. Longacre TA, Bartow SA. A correlative morphologic study of human breast and endometrium in the menstrual cycle. *Am J Surg Pathol* 1986,10 382–393.

156. Cohen LA, Amin S, Marks PA, et al. Chemoprevention of carcinogen-induced mammary tumorigenesis by the hybrid polar cytodifferentiation agent, suberanilohydroxamic acid (SAHA). *Anticancer Res* 1999;19:4999–5005.

157. Cohen LA, Marks PA, Rifkind RA, et al. Suberoylanilide hydroxamic acid (SAHA), a histone deacetylase inhibitor, suppresses the growth of carcinogen-induced mammary tumors. *Anticancer Res* 2002;22:1497–1504.

158. Desai D, El-Bayoumy K, Amin S. Chemopreventive efficacy of suberanilohydroxamic acid (SAHA), a cytodifferentiating agent, against tobacco-specific nitrosamine 4-(methylnitrosamino)-1-(3-pyridyl)-1-butanone (NNK)-induced lung tumorigenesis in female A/J mice. *Proc Am Assoc Cancer Res* 1999;40:A2396.

159. Mariadason JM, Corner GA, Augenlicht LH. Genetic reprogramming in pathways of colonic cell maturation induced by short chain fatty acids: comparison with trichostatin A, sulindac, and curcumin and implications for chemoprevention of colon cancer. *Cancer Res* 2000;60:4561–4572.

160. Jing Y, Xia L, Waxman S. Targeted removal of PML-RARalpha protein is required prior to inhibition of histone deacetylase for overcoming all-trans retinoic acid differentiation resistance in acute promyelocytic leukemia. *Blood* 2002;100:1008–1013.

161. Fabian CJ, Kimler BF. Beyond tamoxifen new endpoints for breast cancer chemoprevention, new drugs for breast cancer prevention. *Ann NY Acad Sci* 2001;952:44–59.

162. Zhou, X, Marks PA, Rifkind RA, Richon VM. Cloning and characterization of a histone deacetylase, HDAC9. *Proc Natl Acad Sci USA* 2001;98:10,572–10,577.

163. Buetow KH, Edmonson M, MacDonald R, et al. High-throughput development and characterization of a genomewide collection of gene-based single nucleotide polymorphism markers by chip-based matrix-assisted laser desorption/ionization time-of-flight mass spectrometry. *Proc Natl Acad Sci USA* 2001;98:581–584.

164. Kwok PY. Methods for genotyping single nucleotide polymorphisms. *Annu Rev Genomics Hum Genet* 2001;2:235–258.

165. Gu W, Roeder RG. Activation of p53 sequence-specific DNA binding by acetylation of the p53 C-terminal domain. *Cell* 1997;90:595–606.

166. Sakaguchi K, Herrera JE, Saito S, et al. DNA damage activates p53 through a phosphorylation-acetylation cascade. *Genes Dev* 1998;12:2831–2841.

167. Liu L, Scolnick DM, Trievel RC, et al. p53 sites acetylated in vitro by PCAF and p300 are acetylated in vivo in response to DNA damage. *Mol Cell Biol* 1999;19:1202–1209.

168. Sterner R, Vidali G, Allfrey VG. Studies of acetylation and deacetylation in high mobility group proteins. Identification of the sites of acetylation in HMG-1. *J Biol Chem* 1979;254:11,577–11,583.

169. Johnson LR, Johnson TK, Desler M, et al. Effects of B-Myb on gene transcription: phosphorylation-dependent activity and acetylation by p300. *J Biol Chem* 2002;277:4088–4097.

170. Tomita A, Towatari M, Tsuzuki S, et al. c-Myb acetylation at the carboxyl-terminal conserved domain by transcriptional co-activator p300. *Oncogene* 2000;19:444–451.

171. Sterner R, Vidali G, Allfrey VG. Studies of acetylation and deacetylation in high mobility group proteins. Identification of the sites of acetylation in high mobility group proteins 14 and 17. *J Biol Chem* 1981;256:8892–8895.

172. Boyes J, Byfield P, Nakatani Y, Ogryzko V. Regulation of activity of the transcription factor GATA-1 by acetylation. *Nature* 1998;396:594–598.

173. Hung HL, Lau J, Kim AY, et al. CREB-binding protein acetylates hematopoietic transcription factor GATA-1 at functionally important sites. *Mol Cell Biol* 1999;19: 3496–3505.

174. Zhang W, Bieker JJ. Acetylation and modulation of erythroid Kruppel-like factor (EKLF) activity by interaction with histone acetyltransferases. *Proc Natl Acad Sci USA* 1998;95:9855–9860.

175. Waltzer L, Bienz M. Drosophila CBP represses the transcription factor TCF to antagonize Wingless signalling. *Nature* 1998;395:521–525.

176. Chen H, Lin RJ, Xie W, et al. Regulation of hormone-induced histone hyperacetylation and gene activation via acetylation of an acetylase. *Cell* 1999;98:675–686.

177. Kiernan RE, Vanhulle C, Schiltz L, et al. HIV-1 tat transcriptional activity is regulated by acetylation. *EMBO J* 1999;18:6106–6118.

178. Vries RG, Prudenziati M, Zwartjes C, et al. A specific lysine in c-Jun is required for transcriptional repression by E1A and is acetylated by p300. *EMBO J* 2001;20:6095–6103.

179. Furia B, Deng L, Wu K, et al. Enhancement of nuclear factor-kappa B acetylation by coactivator p300 and HIV-1 Tat proteins. *J Biol Chem* 2002;277:4973–4980.

180. Herrera JE, Bergel M, Yang XJ, et al. The histone acetyltransferase activity of human GCN5 and PCAF is stabilized by coenzymes. *J Biol Chem* 1997;272:27,253–27,258.

181. Yao YL, Yang WM, Seto E. Regulation of transcription factor YY1 by acetylation and deacetylation. *Mol Cell Biol* 2001;21:5979–5991.

182. McDonald C, Reich NC. Cooperation of the transcriptional coactivators CBP and p300 with Stat6. J Interferon *Cytokine Res* 1999;19:711–722.

183. Shankaranarayanan P, Chaitidis P, Kuhn H, Nigam S. Acetylation by histone acetyltransferase CREB-binding protein/p300 of STAT6 is required for transcriptional activation of the 15-lipoxygenase-1 gene. *J Biol Chem* 2001;276: 42,753–42,760.

184. Kumar BR, Swaminathan V, Banerjee S, Kundu TK. p300-mediated acetylation of human transcriptional coactivator PC4 is inhibited by phosphorylation. *J Biol Chem* 2001;276:16,804–16,809.

185. Masumi A, Ozato K. Coactivator p300 acetylates the interferon regulatory factor-2 in U937 cells following phorbol ester treatment. *J Biol Chem* 2001;276:20,973–20,980.

186. Wolf D, Rodova M, Miska EA, et al. Acetylation of beta-catenin by CREB-binding protein (CBP). *J Biol Chem* 2002;277:25,562–25,567.

187. Yamagata T, Mitani K, Oda H, et al. Acetylation of GATA-3 affects T-cell survival and homing to secondary lymphoid organs. *EMBO J* 2000;19:4676–4687.

188. Braun H, Koop R, Ertmer A, et al. Transcription factor Sp3 is regulated by acetylation. *Nucleic Acids Res* 2001;29:4994–5000.

189. Hung HL, Kim AY, Hong W, et al. Stimulation of NF-E2 DNA binding by CREB-binding protein (CBP)-mediated acetylation. *J Biol Chem* 2001;276:10,715–10,721.

190. Imhof A, Yang XJ, Ogryzko VV, et al. Acetylation of general transcription factors by histone acetyltransferases. *Curr Biol* 1997;7:689–692.

191. Chen L, Fischle W, Verdin E, Greene WC. Duration of nuclear NF-kappaB action regulated by reversible acetylation. *Science* 2001;293:1653–1657.

192. Spilianakis C, Papamatheakis J, Kretsovali A. Acetylation by PCAF enhances CIITA nuclear accumulation and transactivation of major histocompatibility complex class II genes. *Mol Cell Biol* 2000;20:8489–8498.

193. Fu M, Wang C, Reutens AT, et al. p300 and p300/cAMP-response element-binding protein-associated factor acetylate the androgen receptor at sites governing hormone-dependent transactivation. *J Biol Chem* 2000;275:20, 853–20,860.

194. Chan HM, Krstic-Demonacos M, Smith L, et al. Acetylation control of the retinoblastoma tumour-suppressor protein. *Nat Cell Biol* 2001;3:667–674.

195. Soutoglou E, Katrakili N, Talianidis I. Acetylation regulates transcription factor activity at multiple levels. *Mol Cell* 2000;5:745–751.

196. Bannister AJ, Miska EA, Gorlich D, Kouzarides T. Acetylation of importin-alpha nuclear import factors by CBP/p300. *Curr Biol* 2000;10:467–470.

197. Pelletier G, Stefanovsky VY, Faubladier M, et al. Competitive recruitment of CBP and Rb-HDAC regulates UBF acetylation and ribosomal transcription. *Mol Cell* 2000;6:1059–1066.

198. L'Hernault SW, Rosenbaum JL. Chlamydomonas alpha-tubulin is posttranslationally modified by acetylation on the epsilon-amino group of a lysine. *Biochemistry* 1985;24:473–478.

199. Muth V, Nadaud S, Grummt I, Voit R. Acetylation of TAF(I)68, a subunit of TIF-IB/SL1, activates RNA polymerase I transcription. *EMBO J* 2001;20:1353–1362.

200. Vo N, Fjeld C, Goodman RH. Acetylation of nuclear hormone receptor-interacting protein RIP140 regulates binding of the transcriptional corepressor CtBP. *Mol Cell Biol* 2001;21:6181–6188.

201. Huang S, Qiu Y, Shi Y, et al. P/CAF-mediated acetylation regulates the function of the basic helix-loop-helix transcription factor TAL1/SCL. *EMBO J* 2000;19:6792–6803.

202. Hasan S, Stucki M, Hassa PO, et al. Regulation of human flap endonuclease-1 activity by acetylation through the transcriptional coactivator p300. *Mol Cell* 2001;7:1221–1231.

Index